Recommended Dietary Allowances (RDAs) and Adequate Intakes (AIs) for Vitamins

Life-Stage Group	Thiamin (mg/day) RDA	Riboflavin (mg/day) RDA	Niacin (mg/day)a RDA	Biotin (µg/day) AI	Pantothenic acid (mg/day) AI	Vitamin B6 (mg/day) RDA	Folate (µg/day)b RDA	Vitamin B12 (µg/day) RDA	Choline (mg/day) AI	Vitamin C (mg/day) RDA	Vitamin A (µg/day)c RDA	Vitamin D (µg/day)d RDA	Vitamin E (mg/day)e RDA	Vitamin K (µg/day) AI
Infants														
0–6 mo	0.2	0.3	2	5	1.7	0.1	65	0.4	125	40	400	10	4	2.0
7–12 mo	0.3	0.4	4	6	1.8	0.3	80	0.5	150	50	500	10	5	2.5
Children														
1–3 y	0.5	0.5	6	8	2	0.5	150	0.9	200	15	300	15	6	30
4–8 y	0.6	0.6	8	12	3	0.6	200	1.2	250	25	400	15	7	55
Males														
9–13 y	0.9	0.9	12	20	4	1.0	300	1.8	375	45	600	15	11	60
14–18 y	1.2	1.3	16	25	5	1.3	400	2.4	550	75	900	15	15	75
19–30 y	1.2	1.3	16	30	5	1.3	400	2.4	550	90	900	15	15	120
31–50 y	1.2	1.3	16	30	5	1.3	400	2.4	550	90	900	15	15	120
51–70 y	1.2	1.3	16	30	5	1.7	400	2.4	550	90	900	15	15	120
> 70 y	1.2	1.3	16	30	5	1.7	400	2.4	550	90	900	20	15	120
Females														
9–13 y	0.9	0.9	12	20	4	1.0	300	1.8	375	45	600	15	11	60
14–18 y	1.0	1.0	14	25	5	1.2	400	2.4	400	65	700	15	15	75
19–30 y	1.1	1.1	14	30	5	1.3	400	2.4	425	75	700	15	15	90
31–50 y	1.1	1.1	14	30	5	1.3	400	2.4	425	75	700	15	15	90
51–70 y	1.1	1.1	14	30	5	1.5	400	2.4	425	75	700	15	15	90
> 70 y	1.1	1.1	14	30	5	1.5	400	2.4	425	75	700	20	15	90
Pregnancy														
14–18 y	1.4	1.4	18	30	6	1.9	600	2.6	450	80	750	15	15	75
19–30 y	1.4	1.4	18	30	6	1.9	600	2.6	450	85	770	15	15	90
31–50 y	1.4	1.4	18	30	6	1.9	600	2.6	450	85	770	15	15	90
Lactation														
14–18 y	1.4	1.6	17	35	7	2.0	500	2.8	550	115	1200	15	19	75
19–30 y	1.4	1.6	17	35	7	2.0	500	2.8	550	120	1300	15	19	90
31–50 y	1.4	1.6	17	35	7	2.0	500	2.8	550	120	1300	15	19	90

Note: For all nutrients, values for infants are AIs.
a Niacin recommendations are expressed as niacin equivalents (NE), except for recommendations for infants younger than six months, which are expressed as preformed niacin.
b Folate recommendations are expressed as dietary folate equivalents (DFE).
c Vitamin A recommendations are expressed as retinol activity equivalents (RAE).
d Vitamin D recommendations are expressed as cholecalciferol.
e Vitamin E recommendations are expressed as α-tocopherol.

Recommended Dietary Allowances (RDAs) and Adequate Intakes (AIs) for Minerals

Life-Stage Group	Sodium (mg/day) AI	Chloride (mg/day) AI	Potassium (mg/day) AI	Calcium (mg/day) RDA	Phosphorus (mg/day) RDA	Magnesium (mg/day) RDA	Iron (mg/day) RDA	Zinc (mg/day) RDA	Iodine (µg/day) RDA	Selenium (µg/day) RDA	Copper (µg/day) RDA	Manganese (mg/day) AI	Fluoride (mg/day) AI	Chromium (µg/day) AI	Molybdenum (µg/day) RDA
Infants															
0–6 mo	120	180	400	200	100	30	0.27	2	110	15	200	0.003	0.01	0.2	2
7–12 mo	370	570	700	260	275	75	11	3	130	20	220	0.6	0.5	5.5	3
Children															
1–3 y	1000	1500	3000	700	460	80	7	3	90	20	340	1.2	0.7	11	17
4–8 y	1200	1900	3800	1000	500	130	10	5	90	30	440	1.5	1	15	22
Males															
9–13 y	1500	2300	4500	1300	1250	240	8	8	120	40	700	1.9	2	25	34
14–18 y	1500	2300	4700	1300	1250	410	11	11	150	55	890	2.2	3	35	43
19–30 y	1500	2300	4700	1000	700	400	8	11	150	55	900	2.3	4	35	45
31–50 y	1500	2300	4700	1000	700	420	8	11	150	55	900	2.3	4	35	45
51–70 y	1300	2000	4700	1000	700	420	8	11	150	55	900	2.3	4	30	45
> 70 y	1200	1800	4700	1200	700	420	8	11	150	55	900	2.3	4	30	45
Females															
9–13 y	1500	2300	4500	1300	1250	240	8	8	120	40	700	1.6	2	21	34
14–18 y	1500	2300	4700	1300	1250	360	15	9	150	55	890	1.6	3	24	43
19–30 y	1500	2300	4700	1000	700	310	18	8	150	55	900	1.8	3	25	45
31–50 y	1500	2300	4700	1000	700	320	18	8	150	55	900	1.8	3	25	45
51–70 y	1300	2000	4700	1200	700	320	8	8	150	55	900	1.8	3	20	45
> 70 y	1200	1800	4700	1200	700	320	8	8	150	55	900	1.8	3	20	45
Pregnancy															
14–18 y	1500	2300	4700	1300	1250	400	27	12	220	60	1000	2.0	3	29	50
19–30 y	1500	2300	4700	1000	700	350	27	11	220	60	1000	2.0	3	30	50
31–50 y	1500	2300	4700	1000	700	360	27	11	220	60	1000	2.0	3	30	50
Lactation															
14–18 y	1500	2300	5100	1300	1250	360	10	13	290	70	1300	2.6	3	44	50
19–30 y	1500	2300	5100	1000	700	310	9	12	290	70	1300	2.6	3	45	50
31–50 y	1500	2300	5100	1000	700	320	9	12	290	70	1300	2.6	3	45	50

Tolerable Upper Intake Levels (ULs) for Vitamins

Life-Stage Group	Niacin (mg/day)[a]	Vitamin B6 (mg/day)	Folate (µg/day)[a]	Choline (mg/day)	Vitamin C (mg/day)	Vitamin A (µg/day)[b]	Vitamin D (µg/day)	Vitamin E (mg/day)[c]
Infants								
0–6 mo	—	—	—	—	—	600	25	—
7–12 mo	—	—	—	—	—	600	38	—
Children								
1–3 y	10	30	300	1000	400	600	63	200
4–8 y	15	40	400	1000	650	900	75	300
Adolescents								
9–13 y	20	60	600	2000	1200	1700	100	600
14–18 y	30	80	800	3000	1800	2800	100	800
Adults								
19–70 y	35	100	1000	3500	2000	3000	100	1000
>70 y	35	100	1000	3500	2000	3000	100	1000
Pregnancy								
14–18 y	30	80	800	3000	1800	2800	100	800
19–50 y	35	100	1000	3500	2000	3000	100	1000
Lactation								
14–18 y	30	80	800	3000	1800	2800	100	800
19–50 y	35	100	1000	3500	2000	3000	100	1000

[a] The ULs for niacin and folate apply to synthetic forms obtained from supplements, fortified foods, or a combination of the two.

[b] The UL for vitamin A applies to the preformed vitamin only.
[c] The UL for vitamin E applies to any form of supplemental α-tocopherol, fortified foods, or a combination of the two.

Tolerable Upper Intake Levels (ULs) for Minerals

Life-Stage Group	Sodium (mg/day)	Chloride (mg/day)	Calcium (mg/day)	Phosphorus (mg/day)	Magnesium (mg/day)[d]	Iron (mg/day)	Zinc (mg/day)	Iodine (µg/day)	Selenium (µg/day)	Copper (µg/day)	Manganese (mg/day)	Fluoride (mg/day)	Molybdenum (µg/day)	Boron (mg/day)	Nickel (mg/day)
Infants															
0–6 mo	—[e]	—[e]	1000	—	—	40	4	—	45	—	—	0.7	—	—	—
7–12 mo	—[e]	—[e]	1500	—	—	40	5	—	60	—	—	0.9	—	—	—
Children															
1–3 y	1500	2300	2500	3000	65	40	7	200	90	1000	2	1.3	300	3	0.2
4–8 y	1900	2900	2500	3000	110	40	12	300	150	3000	3	2.2	600	6	0.3
Adolescents															
9–13 y	2200	3400	3000	4000	350	40	23	600	280	5000	6	10	1100	11	0.6
14–18 y	2300	3600	3000	4000	350	45	34	900	400	8000	9	10	1700	17	1.0
Adults															
19–70 y	2300	3600	2500[f]	4000	350	45	40	1100	400	10,000	11	10	2000	20	1.0
>70 y	2300	3600	2000	3000	350	45	40	1100	400	10,000	11	10	2000	20	1.0
Pregnancy															
14–18 y	2300	3600	3000	3500	350	45	34	900	400	8000	9	10	1700	17	1.0
19–50 y	2300	3600	2500	3500	350	45	40	1100	400	10,000	11	10	2000	20	1.0
Lactation															
14–18 y	2300	3600	3000	4000	350	45	34	900	400	8000	9	10	1700	17	1.0
19–50 y	2300	3600	2500	4000	350	45	40	1100	400	10,000	11	10	2000	20	1.0

[d] The UL for magnesium applies to synthetic forms obtained from supplements or drugs only.
[e] Source of intake should be from human milk (or formula) and food only.
[f] The UL for calcium for 19–50 y is 2500 mg/day; the UL for calcium is reduced to 2000 mg/day for 51–70 y.

Source: Adapted with permission from the *Dietary Reference Intakes* series, National Academies Press. Copyright 1997, 1998, 2000, 2001, 2011, by the National Academy of Sciences. Courtesy of the National Academies Press, Washington, D.C.

Note: An upper limit was not established for vitamins and minerals not listed and for those age groups listed with a dash (—) because of a lack of data, not because these nutrients are safe to consume at any level of intake. All nutrients can have adverse effects when intakes are excessive.

SEVENTH **edition**

Community Nutrition in Action

AN ENTREPRENEURIAL APPROACH

Marie A. Boyle, PhD, RD
College of Saint Elizabeth

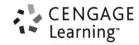

CENGAGE
Learning™

Australia • Brazil • Mexico • Singapore • United Kingdom • United States

CENGAGE
Learning™

Community Nutrition in Action, Seventh Edition
Marie A. Boyle

Product Manager: Krista Mastroianni

Content Developer: Suzannah Alexander

Marketing Manager: Tom Ziolkowski

Content Project Manager: Carol Samet

Art Director: Michael Cook

Manufacturing Planner: Karen Hunt

Production Service: Amy Saucier, SPi-Global

Photo Researcher: Lumina Datamatics

Text Researcher: Lumina Datamatics

Text Designer: Riezebos Holzbaur/Andrei Pasternak; Ellen Pettengell Design

Cover Designer: Michael Cook

Compositor: SPi-Global

Cover Image: Istock/FangXiaoNuo (main), Istock/SolStock (top), Istock/gpointstudio (middle), Istock/monkeybusinessimages (bottom

Library of Congress Control Number: 2016936074

ISBN: 978-1-305-63799-3

Loose-leaf Edition:

ISBN: 978-1-305-88235-5

Cengage Learning
20 Channel Center Street
Boston MA 02210
USA

Cengage Learning is a leading provider of customized learning solutions with employees residing in nearly 40 different countries and sales in more than 125 countries around the world. Find your local representative at **www.cengage.com.**

Cengage Learning products are represented in Canada by Nelson Education, Ltd.

To learn more about Cengage Learning Solutions, visit **www.cengage.com.** Purchase any of our products at your local college store or at our preferred online store **www.cengagebrain.com.**

Printed in the United States of America
Print Number: 03   Print Year: 2017

Dedication

In memory of Jesse, Dylan, Kate, and McCauley—my twinkling stars in the night sky. And to Maggie, Rex, Elvis, and Tess—may there always be time for footprints in the sand.

—Marie A. Boyle

About the Author

MARIE A. BOYLE, PhD, RD, received her BA in psychology from the University of Southern Maine and her MS and PhD in nutrition from Florida State University. She is author of the basic nutrition textbook *Personal Nutrition*. Dr. Boyle serves as Chair of the Foods and Nutrition Program and Director of the Graduate Program in Nutrition at the College of Saint Elizabeth in Morristown, New Jersey. Her other professional activities include serving as an author and reviewer for the Academy of Nutrition and Dietetics and the Society for Nutrition Education and Behavior. Dr. Boyle coauthored the current position paper of the Academy of Nutrition and Dietetics, titled *Nutrition Security in Developing Nations: Sustainable Food, Water and Health*, and serves as editor-in-chief of the *Journal of Hunger and Environmental Nutrition* by Taylor & Francis. She is a member of the Academy of Nutrition and Dietetics, the American Public Health Association, and the Society for Nutrition Education and Behavior.

Contents in Brief

Contents

Preface   xi

Section *Two*

Community Nutritionists in Action: Delivering Programs   367

Section *Three*

Community Nutritionists in Action: Planning Nutrition Interventions 595

Preface

To succeed in community nutrition today, you must be committed to lifelong learning: every day brings new research findings, new legislation, new ideas about health promotion, and new technologies, all of which affect the ways in which community nutritionists gather information, solve problems, and reach vulnerable populations. You will probably be an entrepreneur—one who uses innovation and creativity to guide individuals and communities to optimal nutrition and good health. You will work well as a member of teams to lobby policymakers, gather information about your community, and design nutrition programs and services. You will be skilled in assessing the activities of "the competition"—the myriad messages about foods, dietary supplements, and research findings that appear in the media.

We spoke, in the first edition of this book, about a sea change—a shift toward globalization of the workforce and communications, reflected in the growth of the Internet—a virtual tsunami in communications, and a shift from clinical dietetics to community-based practice. In the last two decades, the public health arena in the United States has documented the possibilities of health care reform, the rise of complementary and alternative medicine, and the sequencing of all of the human genes—together known as the human genome.

Food insecurity has not significantly changed in the last 20 years, while obesity, diabetes, and other chronic diseases, including heart disease, are increasingly prevalent in both developed and developing countries. Our society acknowledges that current modes of food production have contributed to some of the adverse environmental changes that we see. The concept of sustainable food systems is gaining mainstream attention—with numerous groups encouraging consumers to increase their awareness of sustainability issues and how these apply to food systems and the health of communities. The growing connectedness of the human race—through increasing use of mobile devices and social media—promises to create new opportunities for community nutritionists to enhance the nutrition and health of all peoples.

Since the last edition was published, our society has developed wellness policies for its schools; proposed new policies and legislation to prevent obesity and overweight in school, workplace, and community environments; rallied behind the various *Let's Move!* initiatives to address the epidemic of childhood obesity; embraced social marketing and evidence-based guidelines for practice; and gathered evidence and data to improve public health practice and policies—in an effort to achieve the nation's health objectives by the year 2020.

This new seventh edition includes new features and some reorganization:

- The epidemiology chapter (Chapter 2) has been moved up to follow the introductory community nutrition discussion so that the incidence, distribution, and control of disease in a population may be examined before trying to understand and achieve behavior change (Chapter 3). The chapter also precedes the program planning chapter (Chapter 5) to showcase the role of research in developing an evidence base on which to build policy and programming.
- Chapter 3 "Understanding and Achieving Behavior Change" describes several evidence-based theories and strategies to consider when designing a nutrition intervention program targeting lifestyle change related to eating patterns and physical activity and includes practical applications of motivational interviewing, the transtheoretical model (stages of change), health belief model, theory of planned behavior, social-cognitive theory, and cognitive-behavioral theory. The chapter is now positioned before the program planning chapter to provide students with a theoretical base for planning program activities.
- The material on community needs assessment is now presented in one chapter (Chapter 4) so that this important topic is as clear and concise as possible. A new case study "Planning a Needs Assessment Focused on School Children" helps guide students through a sample needs assessment scenario. A new Appendix D provides a sample community needs assessment assignment, as well as an example of a completed assignment.
- The text's program planning chapter (Chapter 5) follows the chapter on community needs assessment in order to facilitate students' projects in program planning earlier in the semester. The program planning chapter includes more examples to help students write objectives for the program planning process, and new tools used in program

evaluation. In the case study following Chapter 5, students practice their program planning skills for designing and implementing a worksite wellness program.

- The text further illustrates the importance of demonstrating meaningful outcomes for nutrition services by including a Professional Focus following Chapter 5 that introduces the nutrition care process (NCP) to enable community nutrition professionals to compete successfully in a rapidly changing environment. Examples of applying the nutrition care process for heart disease in different community practice settings are given. Two case studies also incorporate the NCP to give students practice in writing a nutrition diagnosis as a problem, etiology, signs, and symptoms (PES) statement.

New and expanded topics include:

- Coverage of the nation's new guidelines for healthy meals and snacks in schools.
- Expanded inclusion of medical nutrition therapy as a benefit to certain Medicare recipients; new legislative priorities and the current strategic plan of the Academy of Nutrition and Dietetics.
- Complete coverage of the *2015–2020 Dietary Guidelines for Americans*, which emphasize healthy eating patterns and other recommendations to improve the nutrition and health status of Americans.
- A detailed discussion of the *Healthy People 2020* initiative and its emphasis on health disparities and the social and physical determinants of health.
- The social–ecological model, which illustrates how diverse factors converge to influence food and physical activity choices. The Centers for Disease Control and Prevention's "Social Ecological Model: A Framework for Prevention" is introduced in Chapter 1, connected to the *2015–2020 Dietary Guidelines for Americans* in Chapter 7, and applied to child obesity in Chapter 8.
- Expanded coverage of cultural competence and health disparities with specific examples of health disparities.
- Coverage of health and media literacy and informatics; a Programs in Action feature "The Food Literacy Partners Program" focuses on food and nutrition information to help individuals make appropriate eating decisions.
- The most recent recommendations for obesity prevention as found in the IOM report, *Accelerating Progress in Obesity Prevention: Solving the Weight of the Nation*; new coverage of proposed policies and legislation to prevent obesity and overweight in the school, workplace, and community environments; a Programs in Action feature "The Farm to Work Initiative: An Innovative Approach to Obesity Prevention" describes a worksite wellness program that was created to change the worksite environment in order to make opting for fruits and vegetables an easy choice for employees.

- The Programs in Action feature "Whole School, Whole Community, Whole Child Programs" describes a model that views the school in a multidimensional and systems-level fashion, in which all components at the school level work together to maintain consistent, healthful messages, including the surrounding community and environment.
- Nutrition-related environmental concerns and sustainability issues such as how our food and agricultural system impacts our food choices, nutrition, and environment.
- Program planning tools including community nutrition mapping tools and the Logic Model; the Logic Model is included to provide a framework for planning, implementing, managing, and evaluating community nutrition programs.
- Breastfeeding promotion efforts by WIC, including efforts to improve exclusive breastfeeding rates; UNICEF's Programming for Infant and Young Child Feeding, including interventions for improved breastfeeding and complementary feeding.
- Since connecting program objectives with appropriate activities is an important program planning skill, new tips for linking objectives with program activities for achieving the objectives are included; several chapters place new emphasis on the three levels of intervention—building awareness, changing lifestyles, or creating a supportive environment—when linking objectives and activities. In a new case study: "Developing a Nutrition Education Plan for Older Adults at Congregate Feeding Sites," students use literature and formative evaluation data to develop topics and objectives for nutrition lessons, and include strategies that address each of the three levels of intervention.
- In the case study following Chapter 17, students incorporate social media and social marketing tools in developing a marketing plan for a weight-loss program.
- Appendix A now includes both the WHO Child Growth Standards to monitor growth for infants and children from birth to two years of age in the U.S. and the CDC growth charts for use with children age two years and older in the U.S.

Several terms surface repeatedly in this text: *change, innovation, creativity, evidence-based, community, policymaking, networking,* and *entrepreneurship.* These watchwords herald the unprecedented challenges that lie ahead of us in this decade. Community nutritionists who succeed in this challenging environment are flexible, innovative, and versatile. They are *focused* on recognizing opportunities for improving people's nutrition status and health and on helping society meet its obligation to alleviate food insecurity and malnutrition. It is an exciting time for community nutritionists. It is a time for learning new skills and moving into new areas of practice. It is a time of great opportunity and incredible need.

The Seventh Edition

In this seventh edition, we continue to discuss the important issues in community nutrition practice and to present the core information needed by students who are interested in solving nutrition and health problems. The book is organized into three sections. Section One shows the community nutritionist in action within the community. Chapter 1 describes the activities and responsibilities of the community nutritionist and introduces the principles of entrepreneurship and the three arenas of community nutrition practice: people, policy, and programs. Chapter 2 reviews the basic principles of epidemiology. Chapter 3 introduces several behavior change theories and discusses what research tells us about how to influence behavior. Chapter 4 gives a step-by-step analysis of the community needs assessment process and describes the types and sources of data collected about the community, as well as the questions you'll ask in obtaining information about your target population, including diet assessment methods. Chapter 5 describes the program planning process, covering everything from the factors that trigger program planning, to tools such as the Logic Model to guide the planning process, to the types of evaluations undertaken to improve program design and delivery. Chapter 6 makes it perfectly clear that if you're a community nutritionist, you're involved in policy-making. Chapter 7 focuses on the nuts and bolts of national nutrition policy, including national nutrition monitoring and dietary recommendations. Chapter 8 discusses the epidemic of obesity, examining some societal and environmental determinants of the epidemic, current public health policies, and proposed policies and legislation to prevent obesity and overweight. Chapter 9 discusses today's health care system, health care reform, and the challenge of eliminating health disparities and providing quality health care to all citizens, and the necessity of outcomes assessment in nutrition services.

Section Two describes current federal and non-governmental programs designed to meet the food and nutritional needs of vulnerable populations. Chapter 10 examines some of the issues surrounding poverty and food insecurity in the domestic arena, considers how these contribute to nutritional risk and malnutrition, and outlines the major domestic food and nutrition assistance programs designed to help with achieving food security. Chapter 11 focuses on programs for pregnant and lactating women and for infants. Chapter 12 describes programs for children and adolescents. Chapter 13 covers a host of programs for adults, including older adults. Chapter 14 examines the issue of global food insecurity.

Section Three focuses on the tools used by community nutritionists to address nutritional and health problems in their communities. Chapter 15 addresses the need for cultural competence and explains strategies for providing culturally

competent nutrition services. Chapter 16 gets to the heart of any program: the nutrition messages used in community interventions. Chapter 17 introduces the principles of marketing, including social marketing, an important endeavor in community nutrition practice. You are more likely to get good results if your program is marketed successfully! Chapter 18 addresses such important management issues as how to control costs and manage people. Finally, Chapter 19 closes the text with a discussion of grantsmanship—everything you need to know about finding and managing funding for community programs and interventions.

Many of the unique features of the previous editions have been retained:

- **Professional Focus.** This feature is designed to help you develop personal and professional skills and attitudes that will boost your effectiveness and confidence in community settings. The topics range from utilizing the Academy of Nutrition and Dietetic's nutrition care process in community settings, goal setting, and time management to public speaking, working with the media, using social media, and leadership.

- **Programs in Action.** This feature—found in most chapters—highlights award-winning, innovative, grassroots nutrition programs. It offers a unique perspective on the practice of community nutrition. Our hope is that the insights you gain from these initiatives will inspire you to get involved in learning about your community and its health and nutritional problems and to design similar programs to address the needs you uncover. The feature highlights such programs as Eat Healthy: Your Kids Are Watching, a program designed to remind parents that they serve as role models for their children; the Farm to Work Initiative, an innovative approach to obesity prevention; the Food Literacy Partners Program, a "learn-and-serve" program that provides nutrition education to volunteers in exchange for community nutrition education service; and Food on the Run, a program to empower teens to make healthful decisions about their nutrition and physical activity patterns. This feature discusses each program's goals, objectives, and rationale; the practical aspects of its implementation; and its effectiveness in serving the needs of its intended audience.

- **Case Studies.** The book's case studies make use of a transdisciplinary, developmental problem-solving model as a learning framework to enhance students' critical thinking skills.* They are designed to help students develop competence in applying their knowledge and skills to contemporary nutrition issues with real-life uncertainties—such issues as might

---

* See C. L. Lynch, S. K. Wolcott, and G. E. Huber, *Steps for Better Thinking: A Developmental Problem Solving Process*, May 31, 2002; available at *www.WolcottLynch.com*.

be found in the workplace. Each case emphasizes the need to evaluate the information presented, identify and describe uncertainties in the case, locate and distinguish between relevant and irrelevant information, identify assumptions, prioritize alternatives, make decisions, and communicate and evaluate conclusions. Many of the case questions are open-ended.

- **Entrepreneur in Action.** This feature—found in every chapter—focuses on professionals actively engaged in community nutrition. Each story is highlighted in brief in the text with instructions on how students can access the full articles online at *www.cengagebrain.com*.
- **Chapter Summaries.** Each chapter presents the major points in a concise, section-by-section bulleted list. The design enables students to easily identify content that requires further review and locate where the information is located in the chapter.
- **Internet Resources.** Each chapter ends with a list of relevant Internet addresses. You'll use these websites to obtain data about your community and to scout for ideas and educational materials. Moreover, you can link with the Internet addresses presented in this book through the publisher's website at *www.cengagebrain.com*.

In the seventh edition, the following feature has been added:

- **NEW! Think Like a Community Nutritionist.** This feature—found in most chapters—provides questions and activities to help you think analytically and critically about the chapter topics, giving you the opportunity to step into the role of a community nutritionist to further explore scenarios that you may encounter in the field.

Finally, we hope that the people, policies, and programs presented in this text inspire you to consider a rewarding career path in community nutrition. We want you to think of yourself as a planner, manager, change agent, thinker, and leader—in short, a nutrition entrepreneur—who has the energy and creativity to open up new vistas for improving the public's health through good nutrition.

Instructor and Student Resources

Please consult your local Cengage Learning sales representative for more information on the key resources that accompany this text, or visit the book's website at *www.cengagebrain.com*.

- **Instructor Companion Site.** Everything you need for your course in one place! This collection of book-specific lecture and class tools is available online via *www.cengage.com/login*. Access and download PowerPoint® presentations, images, the instructor's manual, videos, and more.

- **Cengage Learning Testing Powered by Cognero.** This flexible online system allows the instructor to author, edit, and manage test bank content from multiple Cengage Learning solutions; create multiple test versions in an instant; and deliver tests from an LMS, a classroom, or wherever the instructor wants.
- **Diet & Wellness Plus.** Diet & Wellness Plus helps you understand how nutrition relates to your personal health goals. Track your diet and activity, generate reports, and analyze the nutritional value of the food you eat. Diet & Wellness Plus includes over 75,000 foods as well as custom food and recipe features. The new Behavior Change Planner helps you identify risks in your life and guides you through the key steps to make positive changes.
- **MindTap.** A new approach to highly personalized online learning. Beyond an eBook, homework solution, digital supplement, or premium website, MindTap is a digital learning platform that works alongside your campus LMS to deliver course curriculum across the range of electronic devices in your life. MindTap is built on an "app" model, allowing enhanced digital collaboration and delivery of engaging content across a spectrum of Cengage and non-Cengage resources.
- **Global Nutrition Watch.** Bring currency to the classroom with Global Nutrition Watch from Cengage Learning! This student-friendly website provides convenient access to thousands of trusted sources, including academic journals, newspapers, videos, and podcasts, for students to use for research projects or classroom discussion. Global Nutrition Watch is updated daily to offer the most current news about topics related to nutrition. Available standalone, or as activities within MindTap.
- **Community Needs Assessment Workbook.** This workbook, available online via MindTap, helps nutrition and allied health students to apply text concepts by guiding them step-by-step through the process of organizing and conducting a community nutrition needs assessment. The workbook provides exercises for each stage of the assessment outlined in the text, reference information, and three fully developed sample assessments.

Acknowledgments

This book was a community effort. Family and friends provided encouragement and support. Colleagues shared their insights, program materials, and experiences about the practice of community nutrition and the value of focusing on entrepreneurship.

We are grateful to our entrepreneurs who are highlighted in the Entrepreneur in Action feature found in every chapter and in the book's online materials:

Bonnie Taub-Dix, MA, RDN, CDN
Erin Palinski-Wade, RD, CDE, LDN, CPT
Mary Kay Hunt, MPH
David Strefling, MPH, RD
Frances Galasyn Miller, MPH, RD
Christine Carroll, MPH, RD
Nicole Geurin, MPH, RD
Tracy Fox, MPH, RD
Dawn Crayco, MPH
Carolyn O'Neil, MS, RD
Susan Mitchell, PhD, RDN, LDN, FAND
Dan Jaris, MPH, ACSM-HFS, ACE-LWMC, AFPA-NWC
Nancy Munoz, DCN, MHA, RD, LDN
Janelle L'Heureux, MS, RD
Shailja Mathur, MS, MEd, RD
Teri Underwood, MS, RD, CD
Celestine Onyango, RDN, LD
Laura Sprauer, MPH, RD, IBCLC, LCCE
Hallie Halsey, RD, SNS
Kristine Smith, MS, RD
Alberta Scruggs, RDN, LDN, DTR
Stacia Nordin, RD
Tracy Gregg, MPH, RD, LD, CLC
Jaime Schwartz Cohen, MS, RD
Amanda Archibald, RD
Natalia Hancock, RD
Lucille Beseler, MS, RD, LD/N, CDE
Constance Brown-Riggs, MSEd, RD, CDE, CDN
Becky Dorner, RD, LD
Helen E. Costello, MS, RD, LD

We also are grateful to this text's contributing authors:

- Kathleen Bauer, PhD, RD, Professor, Montclair State University, Montclair, New Jersey, for Chapter 15, "Gaining Cultural Competence in Community Nutrition."
- Carol Byrd-Bredbenner, PhD, RD, FAND, Professor and Extension Specialist in Nutrition, Rutgers—The State University of New Jersey, New Brunswick, New Jersey, for Chapter 19, "Building Grantsmanship Skills."
- Virginia Gray, PhD, RD, Assistant Professor, Nutrition and Dietetics, Graduate Coordinator, Department of Family and Consumer Sciences, California State University, Long Beach, for the new Think Like a Community Nutritionist activities and for the new Appendix D, "Community Needs Assessment Assignment"; as well as for her revision of both Chapter 4, "Community Needs Assessment" and Chapter 16, "Principles of Nutrition Education".
- Deanna M. Hoelscher, PhD, RD, LD, John P. McGovern Professor in Health Promotion and Director, Michael and Susan Dell Center for Healthy Living, University of Texas School of Public Health, Austin Regional Campus, Austin, Texas; and Christine McCullum-Gómez, PhD, RD, LD, food and nutrition consultant, Houston, Texas, for Chapter 8, "Addressing the Obesity Epidemic: An Issue for Public Health Policy."
- Kathy Roberts, MS, RD, former Clinical Coordinator, Dietetic Internship Program, College of Saint Elizabeth, Morristown, New Jersey, for her revisions to Chapter 3, "Understanding and Achieving Behavior Change" as well as Chapter 12, "Children and Adolescents: Nutrition Issues, Services, and Programs."
- Joanne Spahn, MS, RD, Director, Evidence Analysis Library, United States Department of Agriculture, Alexandria, Virginia, for her contributions to Chapter 3, "Understanding and Achieving Behavior Change," as well as her work in creating the Professional Focus feature that follows Chapter 5, "The Nutrition Care Process: A Road Map to Quality Care."
- Nicole Geurin, MPH, RD, nutrition consultant, Sacramento, California, and Jessica Anderson for their work in creating the Professional Focus feature that follows Chapter 17, "Social Media for Nutrition Professionals."
- Alice Fornari, EdD, RD, Director of Faculty Development and Associate Dean of Medical Education, Hofstra North Shore–LIJ School of Medicine, Hempstead, New York; Alessandra Sarcona, EdD, RD, director, Dietetic Internship, Long Island University Post, Brookville, New York; and Alison Barkman, MS, RD, adjunct faculty at Long Island University Post, Brookville, New York, for their development of the case studies that accompany many of this text's chapters.

The text is richer for the contributions made by these authors. Finally, we are grateful for the work that Diane Morris, PhD, RD, and David Holben, PhD, RD, LD, contributed to the previous editions of this text; their expertise and insights are still reflected in this new edition. We thank the many people who have prepared the ancillaries for this book, especially Melanie Burns, Jamie Benedict, and Chimborazo Publishing, Inc., for their expertise in preparing the Online Instructor's Manual and Test Bank that accompany this text, and Patricia Beffa-Negrini, Nicole Geurin, Denine Stracker, and Amanda Sylvie for preparing the Community Needs Assessment Workbook, now available in MindTap.

Special thanks go to our Cengage Learning team—Krista Mastroianni, product manager; Carol Samet, content project manager; Victor Luu, product assistant; Tom Ziolkowski, marketing manager; Michael Cook, art director; and Karen Hunt, manufacturing planner—for their support and assistance. We are grateful to Suzannah Alexander, Alexandria Brady, and Kellie Petruzzelli for their coordination of this book's revision and ancillaries. We appreciate Christine Myaskovsky and Betsy

Hathaway's help in finalizing the text and photo permissions and the work of Lumina Datamatics in researching photos. We also offer our thanks to Amy Saucier and everyone at SPi Global for skillfully producing a text to be proud of. Last, but not least, we owe much to our colleagues who provided articles and course outlines, their favorite Internet addresses, and expert reviews of the manuscript. Their ideas and suggestions are woven into every chapter. We appreciate their time, energy, and enthusiasm, and we hope they take as much pride in this book as all of us with Cengage Learning do. Thanks to all of you:

Debra Barone Sheats, MPH, RD, LD, St. Catherine University

Jamie A. Benedict, PhD, RD, University of Nevada, Reno

Virginia Bennett, PhD, RD, Central Washington University

Laura Calderon, DrPH, RD, California State University, Los Angeles

Cinda J. Catchings, MS, MPH, CHES, RD, LD, Alcorn State University

Jenell Ciak, PhD, RD, LD, Northwest Missouri State University

Alana D. Cline, University of Northern Colorado

Nancy Cohen, PhD, RD, LDN, University of Massachusetts

Nancy Cotugna, DrPH, RD, University of Delaware

Lynn Duerr, PhD, RD, CD, Indiana State University

Jerald Foote, PhD, RD, University of Arkansas

Virginia Gray, PhD, RD, California State University, Long Beach

Melissa Gutschall, Radford University

Lauren Haldeman, The University of North Carolina at Greensboro

Nancy Harris, East Carolina University

Terryl J. Hartman, The Pennsylvania State University

M. Jane Heinig, University of California, Davis

Tanya M. Horacek, PhD, RD, Syracuse University

Tay Kennedy, Oklahoma State University

Deborah Marino, University of Akron

Diana McGuire, MS, RD, CD, CNSD, Brigham Young University

Pamela S. McMahon, University of Florida

Teresa Motlas, South Dakota State University

Valentina M. Remig, Kansas State University

Padmini Shankar, PhD, RD, LD, Georgia Southern University

Suzanne Stluka, South Dakota State University

Kim S. Stote, PhD, MPH, RD, State University of New York, College at Oneonta

Tamara S. Vitale, Utah State University

Sandia Waller, PhD, RD, Texas Southern University

Marie Boyle

Community Nutritionists in Action:
Working in the Community

On Saturday morning, Irene H. opens her kitchen cabinet and takes down six small bottles. She lines them up on the countertop and works their caps off. The process takes a few minutes because her fingers are stiff from arthritis. Let's see, there's cod liver oil, chondroitin sulfate, and glucosamine for arthritis; ginkgo biloba and St. John's wort to relieve anxiety and depression; and DHEA to restore youthful vigor. Irene knows her doctor would be surprised—maybe shocked—to learn that she takes these supplements regularly. She knows, too, that her doctor would not approve of her consultations with a naturopath whose office is just a couple of miles from her home.

At 48, Irene figures she is doing all she can to manage the pain from her arthritis and the depression that has afflicted her since her divorce. The supplements and naturopathic counseling are expensive, but she stretches the income from her job as a checkout clerk at a paint supply store to pay for them. After washing down the pills with orange juice, she pops two frozen waffles in the toaster and pours another cup of coffee. She figures she shouldn't eat the waffles—she was diagnosed with type 2 diabetes just three months ago—but she wants them. After breakfast, she'll enjoy a cigarette with her coffee and then call her oldest daughter. Maybe they can drive out to the mall.

Irene is a typical consumer in many respects. She has chronic health problems for which she has sought traditional medical advice and treatment. Like one in three U.S. adults, she has also sought help from an alternative practitioner. She smokes cigarettes, she is overweight, and about the only exercise she gets is browsing the sale stalls out at the mall. She could do more to improve her health, but she isn't motivated to change her diet or quit smoking. She's looking for the quick fix.

Irene and the thousands of other consumers like her are a challenge for the community nutritionist. To help Irene make changes in her lifestyle—changes that will reduce her demands on the health care system and improve her physical well-being—the community nutritionist must be familiar with a broad spectrum of clinical and epidemiologic research, understand the health care system, and draw on the principles of public health and health promotion. The community nutritionist must know where Irene and people like her live and work, what they eat, and what their attitudes and values are. The community nutritionist must know about the community itself and how it delivers health services to people like Irene. And the community nutritionist must know how to influence policymakers. Perhaps now is the time to call for tighter regulation of dietary supplements and greater government support for health promotion and disease prevention programs.

This section describes the work that community nutritionists do in their communities. It outlines the principles of public health, health promotion, and policymaking and reviews the current health care environment. You will learn strategies to influence—and eventually change—the behavior of a target population. The incorporation of behavior change theories in program planning is critical to the nutrition care process because the theories suggest the questions that community nutritionists should ask to understand why consumers do what they do. This section also outlines some of the tools you might use to assess the nutrition status of a target population and describes how to conduct a needs assessment in your community. You'll learn how to lay out a plan for designing a program or intervention and how to write program goals and objectives.

This section describes how to use the results of a community needs assessment by reviewing several important questions: *Who* has a nutritional problem that is not being met? *How* did this problem develop? *What* programs and services exist to alleviate this problem? *Why* do existing services fail to help the people who experience this problem? The answers to these and other questions help community nutritionists understand the many factors that influence the health and nutrition status of a particular group.

The section also focuses on entrepreneurship—the discipline founded on creativity and innovation—and how entrepreneurial principles can be used to reach Irene and other people in the community with health and nutritional problems. The material in this section sets the stage and lays the groundwork for understanding what community nutritionists do: focus on people, policies, and programs.

CHAPTER 1

Opportunities in Community Nutrition

LEARNING **OBJECTIVES**

After you have read and studied this chapter, you will be able to:

- Describe the three arenas of community nutrition practice.
- Explain how community nutrition practice fits into the larger realm of public health.
- Describe the three types of prevention efforts and identify an example of each.

- List three major health objectives for the nation and explain why each is important.
- Outline the educational requirements, practice settings, and roles and responsibilities of community and public health nutritionists.
- Discuss the role of entrepreneurship in the practice of community nutrition.

CHAPTER **OUTLINE**

*Something
to think
about. . .*

"Education and health are the two great keys. We must use all public sector institutions, flawed though they may be, to close the gap between rich and poor. We must work with the political sector to convincingly paint the breadth and depth of the problem and the size of the opportunity as well. . . . Above all, we must not abandon the hope of progress."

—*SIR GUSTAV NOSSAL,*
writing on health and the biotechnology revolution in Public Health Reports, *March/April 1998*

For a complete list of references, please access the MindTap Reader within your MindTap course.

Introduction

Community nutritionists face many challenges in the practice of their science and art. There is the challenge of improving the nutrition status of different kinds of people with different education and income levels and different health and nutritional needs: teenagers with anorexia nervosa, pregnant women living in public housing, the homeless, new immigrants from Southeast Asia, older adult women alone at home, middle-class adults with high blood cholesterol, professional athletes, and children with disabilities. There is the challenge of forming partnerships with colleagues, business leaders, and the public to advocate for change. There is the challenge of influencing lawmakers and other key citizens to enact laws, regulations, and policies that protect and improve the public's health. There is the challenge of studying the scientific literature for new angles on how to help people make good food choices for good health. And there is the challenge of mastering new technologies to help meet the needs of clients and communities.

In addition to these challenges, certain social and economic trends also present challenges for community nutritionists. Immigrants from Mexico, Asia, Africa, and the Caribbean, many of whom have poor English skills, have streamed into North America in recent years, searching for jobs and improved living conditions.[1] The North American population is aging rapidly as "baby boomers" mature and life expectancy increases.[2] Financial pressures and increased global competition have forced governments, businesses, and organizations to be creative in the face of scarce resources. Indeed, according to one survey of employers undertaken by the Academy of Nutrition and Dietetics, the single greatest challenge for the food and nutrition practitioner today is "the need to do more and better with less."[3] Community nutritionists in all practice settings face rising costs, changing consumer expectations about health care services, increased competition in the market, and greater cultural diversity among their clients. They are pressured by downsizing, mergers, cross-training, and managed health care.

Community nutritionists who succeed in this changing environment are flexible, innovative, and versatile. They are *focused* on recognizing opportunities for improving people's nutrition status and health and on helping society meet its obligation to alleviate hunger and malnutrition. It is an exciting time for community nutritionists. It is a time for learning new skills and moving into new areas of practice. It is a time of great opportunity and incredible need.

The Concept of Community

"There is no complete agreement as to the nature of community," wrote G. A. Hillery, Jr.[4] Such diverse locales as isolated rural hamlets, mountain villages, prairie towns, state capitals, industrial cities, suburbs or ring cities, resort towns, and major metropolitan areas can all be lumped into a single category called "community."[5] The concept of community is not always circumscribed by a city limits sign or zoning laws. Sometimes the term describes people who share certain interests, beliefs, or values, even though they live in diverse geographical locations; examples include the academic community, the gay community, and the immigrant community. For our purposes in this book, a **community** is a grouping of people who reside in a specific locality and who interact and connect through a definite social structure to fulfill a wide range of daily needs. By this definition, a community has four components: people, a location in space (which can include the realm of cyberspace), social interaction, and shared values.

Community A group of people who are located in a particular space (including cyberspace), have shared values, and interact within a social system.

Communities can be viewed on different scales: global, national, regional, and local. Each of these can be further segmented into specialized communities or groups, such as those individuals who speak Spanish, those who own smartphones, and those who observe Hanukkah. In the health arena, communities tend to be segmented around particular wellness, disease, or risk factors—for example, adults who exercise regularly, children infected with HIV, black men with high blood pressure, and people with a peanut allergy.

Opportunities in Community Nutrition

Founded on the sciences of epidemiology, food, nutrition, and human behavior, **community nutrition** is a discipline that strives to improve the health, nutrition, and well-being of individuals and groups within communities. Its practitioners develop policies and programs that help people improve their eating patterns and health. Indeed, these three arenas—people, policy, and programs—are the focus of community nutrition. As an example, low-income pregnant women benefit from nutritious foods, nutrition counseling, and breastfeeding support provided by the Special Supplemental Nutrition Program for Women, Infants, and Children (WIC), which is supported by federal policy that authorizes a specific amount of funds each year for the program.

Community nutrition
A discipline that strives to prevent disease and to improve the health, nutrition, and well-being of individuals and groups within communities.

People Individuals who benefit from community nutrition programs and services range from young single mothers on public assistance to senior business executives, from immigrants with poor English skills to college graduates, from pregnant teenagers with iron-deficiency anemia to grandfathers with Alzheimer's disease. They are found in worksites, schools, community centers, health clinics, churches, apartment buildings—virtually any community setting. Through community nutrition programs and services, these individuals and their families have access to food in times of need or learn skills that improve their eating patterns. It is the community nutritionist who identifies a group of people with an unmet nutritional need; gathers information about the group's socioeconomic background, ethnicity, religion, geographical location, and cultural food patterns; and then develops a program or service tailored to the needs of this group.

Policy Policy is a key component of community nutrition practice. **Policy** is a course of action chosen by public authorities to address a given problem.[6] Policy is what governments and organizations intend to accomplish through their laws, regulations, and programs.

Policy A course of action chosen by public authorities to address a given problem.

How does policy apply to the practice of community nutrition? Consider a situation in which a group of community nutritionists address food waste in their community. The impetus for their action came from learning the results of a U.S. Department of Agriculture study that found that one-fourth of all food produced in the United States is wasted[7] and from reading about a successful food assistance program called *gleaning*. Gleaning began as a project to deliver an abundance of apples from communities with apple orchards to food banks in neighboring states where apples were scarce.[8] The community nutritionists wanted to try gleaning on a small scale, using farmers' markets in their community. Unfortunately, there was no city bylaw that allowed surplus foods from farmers' markets to be made available to local food banks and soup kitchens. After gaining the support of the farmers' markets, food banks, and soup kitchens, the community nutritionists lobbied the city council to enact a bylaw to allow such transactions. The city council members voted to pass a bylaw to support gleaning projects. In other words, the city council altered its *policy* about recovering and recycling surplus foods.

Community nutritionists are involved in policy when they write letters to their state legislators, lobby Congress to secure expanded Medicare coverage for medical nutrition therapy, advise their municipal governments about food banks and soup kitchens, and use the results of research to influence policymakers. Many aspects of the community nutritionist's job involve policy issues.

Programs Programs are the instruments used by community nutritionists to seek behavior changes that improve nutrition status and health. They are wide-ranging and varied. They may target small groups of people—children with developmental disabilities in Nevada schools or teenagers living in a Brooklyn residential home—or they may target large groups, such as all adults with high blood cholesterol concentrations. Programs may be as widespread as the U.S. federal Supplemental Nutrition Assistance Program (SNAP; formerly called the Food Stamp Program), or as local as a diabetes prevention program for Mohawk people living in the Akwesasne community in northern New York State. They may be tailored to address the specific health and nutritional needs of people with obesity or osteoporosis, or they may be aimed at the general population. Two examples of population-based programs are "ParticipACTION," a Canadian program designed to get people moving and fit for health; and "Fruits & Veggies—More Matters," a program of the Centers for Disease Control and Prevention and its partners aimed at making people more aware of how eating fruits and vegetables can improve their health and may reduce their cancer risk. Regardless of the setting or target audience, community nutrition programs have one desired outcome: behavior change.

Public Health and Community Interventions

Community nutritionists promote good nutrition as one avenue for achieving good health. They develop programs to help people improve their eating habits, and they seek environmental changes (in the form of policy) to support good health habits. But community nutritionists do not work in a vacuum. They work closely with other practitioners, particularly those in public health, to help consumers achieve and maintain behavior change.

Public health Focuses on protecting and promoting people's health through the actions of society.

Public health can be defined as an effort organized by society to protect, promote, and restore the people's health through the application of science, practical skills, and collective actions. "Public health is what we, as a society, do collectively to assure the conditions in which people can be healthy," wrote the authors of a report for the Institute of Medicine.[9] In the nineteenth century, the scope of public health was generally restricted to matters of general sanitation, including building municipal sewer systems, purifying the water supply, and controlling food adulteration. Major public health efforts focused on controlling infectious diseases such as tuberculosis, smallpox, yellow fever, cholera, and typhoid. In 1900, the leading causes of death and disability in the United States were pneumonia, tuberculosis, and diarrhea/enteritis. The morbidity and mortality linked with these disease outbreaks shaped public health practice for many years. Such runaway epidemics, which sometimes killed thousands of people in a single outbreak, are uncommon today because of large-scale public efforts to improve water quality, control the spread of communicable diseases, and enhance personal hygiene and the sanitation of the environment.

The leading causes of morbidity and mortality in the United States today are chronic diseases such as heart disease, cancer, and chronic lung disease (**Figure 1-1**). Cardiovascular disease (mainly heart disease and stroke) causes about 29% of all deaths, killing 740,000 U.S. adults and 17.5 million people worldwide every year.[10] Cancer kills almost 585,000 people each year in the United States and about 8.2 million people worldwide.[11] Other serious chronic diseases that reduce the quality of life, disable, or kill include arthritis, diabetes mellitus, osteoporosis, and Alzheimer's disease.[12]

Infectious diseases remain a problem, however. An estimated 35 million people are living with HIV/AIDS worldwide, with approximately 1.1 million cases in the United States and about 35,000 new HIV infections occurring in the United States every year.[13] HIV/AIDS is among the top ten causes of death for people ages 25–44.[14]

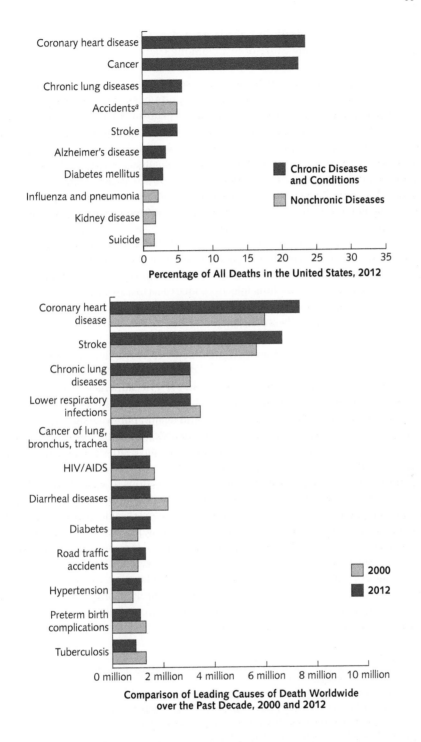

FIGURE 1-1 Leading Causes of Death, United States and Worldwide

Many of the major chronic disease killers—such as heart disease, some types of cancer, stroke, and diabetes—are influenced by a number of factors, including a person's genetic makeup, eating habits, and physical activity, and other lifestyle habits.

[a] The leading cause of death for persons ages 15–24 is motor vehicle and other accidents, followed by homicide, suicide, cancer, and heart disease. About half of all accident fatalities are alcohol-related.

Sources: Centers for Disease Control and Prevention, *National Vital Statistics Report, 2012*; available at *www.cdc.gov/nchs*; World Health Organization, *The Top Ten Causes of Death*, Fact Sheet No. 310 (Geneva, Switzerland: World Health Organization, May 2014).

Another infectious disease is tuberculosis, whose incidence has been declining in the general U.S. population since the resurgence of TB cases peaked in 1992. An estimated 13 million people are infected with TB bacteria, with the potential to develop active TB disease in the future. About 10% of these infected individuals will develop TB at some point in their lives.[15] The AIDS epidemic is partly responsible for the reemerging outbreaks of tuberculosis, although there are other causes, such as increases in homelessness and immigration from other countries where tuberculosis is widespread.[16]

The leading causes of death in Canada mirror those of the U.S. population in many respects.[17] The top-ranking cause of death among Canadian men and women is cancer followed by cardiovascular disease.

Many of the major killers—such as heart disease, some types of cancer, chronic lung disease, stroke, and diabetes—are influenced by a number of factors, including a person's genetic makeup, eating and physical activity habits, exposure to tobacco, and other lifestyle practices. Five of the 15 leading causes of death in the United States—heart disease, cancer, stroke, diabetes, and hypertension—have been linked to diet. Another three are associated with excessive alcohol consumption: accidents, suicide, and liver disease.[18] Because obesity and a sedentary lifestyle are linked with chronic diseases, such as diabetes, heart disease, and certain cancers, it can be projected that increased rates of obesity will lead to increased deaths each year, not to mention hospitalizations, disability, time lost from jobs, and poor quality of life for many Americans.[19]

In contrast to high-income countries, where more than two-thirds of the population live beyond the age of 70 and predominantly die of chronic diseases, less than a quarter of all people in low-income countries reach the age of 70. People in low-income countries predominantly die of infectious diseases: lung infections, diarrheal diseases, HIV/AIDS, tuberculosis, and malaria—and over a third of all deaths are among children under the age of 14.[20] Chronic diseases cause increasing numbers of deaths worldwide as well. Chronic diseases were responsible for 68% (38 million) of all deaths globally in 2012, up from 60% (31 million) in 2000.[21] The four main types of chronic diseases worldwide are cardiovascular diseases (heart attacks and stroke), cancers, chronic lung diseases, and diabetes (see Figure 1-1).[22]

These changes in disease patterns over the last few decades have spawned changes in public health actions. Because the goals of public health reflect the values and beliefs of society and existing knowledge about disease and health, public health initiatives change as society's perception of health needs changes. In order to ensure the health of the public in the twenty-first century, public health initiatives have shifted from financing basic population-based measures, such as immunization, to efforts focused on achieving universal health services, responding rapidly to new infectious diseases such as Ebola, and responding to new threats from antibiotic-resistant germs or **bioterrorism**.

Recognizing the need for increased emphasis on preventive health measures, new efforts are underway to foster better collaboration between public health agencies and other organizations involved in protecting and promoting the public's health.[23] Under the leadership of the World Health Organization (WHO), more than 190 countries have agreed upon global mechanisms to reduce the avoidable chronic disease burden.[24] This plan aims to reduce the number of premature deaths from chronic diseases by 25% by 2025 through nine voluntary global targets (**Table 1-1**). The nine targets address factors such as tobacco and alcohol use, unhealthy diet, and physical inactivity that increase people's risk of developing chronic diseases.[25]

Bioterrorism The intentional release of disease-causing toxins, microorganisms, or other substances.

TABLE 1-1 Nine Voluntary Global Targets for Prevention and Control of Chronic Diseases to be Attained by 2025

1. A 25% relative reduction in the overall mortality from cardiovascular diseases, cancer, diabetes, or chronic respiratory diseases
2. At least 10% relative reduction in the harmful use of alcohol
3. A 10% relative reduction in prevalence of insufficient physical activity
4. A 30% relative reduction in mean population intake of salt/sodium
5. A 30% relative reduction in prevalence of current tobacco use
6. A 25% relative reduction in the prevalence of high blood pressure
7. Halt the rise in diabetes and obesity
8. At least 50% of eligible people receive drug therapy and counseling to prevent heart attacks and strokes
9. An 80% availability of the affordable basic technologies and essential medicines, including generics, required to treat major chronic diseases in both public and private facilities

Source: Adapted from WHO, Global Status Report on Noncommunicable Diseases, 2014.

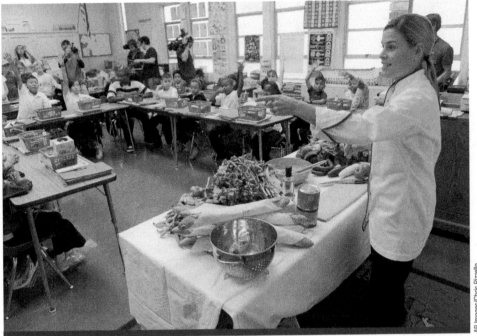

A cooking demonstration is an intervention that promotes awareness of the importance of healthful eating and teaches heart-healthy cooking skills. In this example, a chef gives a cooking demonstration to students during an event for The Teaching Garden—a program that uses gardens to teach children about healthy eating.

The Concept of Health

Most of us equate health with "feeling good," a concept we understand intuitively but cannot define exactly. The term *health* is a derivative of the old English word for "hale," which means whole, hearty, sound of mind and body.[26] Health can be viewed as the absence of disease and pain, or it can be pictured as a continuum along which the total living experience can be placed, with the presence of disease, impairment, or disability at one end of the spectrum and freedom from disease or injury at the other. These extremes in the health continuum are shown in **Figure 1-2**.[27]

Health is properly defined from an ecological viewpoint—that is, one that focuses on **ecology**, or the interaction of humans among themselves and with their environment. In this sense, **health** is a state characterized by "anatomic integrity; ability to perform

Ecology The interrelations between individuals and their environments.

Health According to the World Health Organization, a state of complete physical, mental, and social well-being, not merely the absence of disease.

Population by stages of disease continuum →			
Well population	**At risk**	**Established disease**	**Controlled chronic disease**
Primary Prevention	**Secondary Prevention/ Early Detection**	**Disease Management and Tertiary Prevention**	
• Promote healthy behaviors and environments across the lifespan • Create supportive environments	• Screening • Periodic health examinations • Early intervention • Control risk factors–lifestyle and medication	• Treatment and acute care • Complications management • Self-management	• Continuing care • Maintenance • Rehabilitation • Self-management
Health Promotion	**Health Promotion**	**Health Promotion**	**Health Promotion**

↑ Prevent disease incidence   ↑ Prevent progression to established disease   ↑ Reduce complications or disability

FIGURE 1-2 The Health Continuum and Types of Prevention to Promote Health and Prevent Disease

Source: Adapted from National Public Health Partnership, *Preventing Chronic Disease: A Strategic Framework Background Paper* (National Public Health Partnership: Melbourne, Australia), 2001, 6.

▶ **THINK LIKE A COMMUNITY** NUTRITIONIST

Community nutritionists use tailored strategies to affect each of the levels of prevention. For instance, consider the following examples related to prevention of heart disease.

• Primary prevention: A school-based program that promotes fruit and vegetable consumption among children aims to help establish heart healthy eating habits in early life.
• Secondary prevention: A workplace-based wellness fair provides free cholesterol screenings.
• Tertiary prevention: A clinic-based nutrition education program for patients with established cardiovascular disease aims to reduce the risk of cardiac events.

Now it's your turn. List a primary, secondary, and tertiary prevention strategy related to cancer risk.

personally valued family, work, and community roles; ability to deal with physical, biological, and social stress; a feeling of well-being; and freedom from the risk of disease and untimely death."[28] A healthy individual, then, has the physical, mental, and spiritual capacity to live, work, and interact joyfully with other human beings.

But how is good health achieved? Why does one child in a family become addicted to cocaine, whereas another never touches illicit drugs? Why do people start smoking? Why do some people overeat? Why do some teenagers consume adequate amounts of iron and calcium, whereas others do not? Why is one 90-year-old healthy and vigorous and another 70-year-old infirm? The answers to these questions still elude epidemiologists and other scientists. We know that a constellation of factors, shown in **Table 1-2**, influence health. Certain individual factors such as age, sex, and race are fixed, inherited traits that influence an individual's health potential. Other factors—such as lifestyle, housing, working conditions, social networks, community services, and even national health policies—represent layers of influence that can theoretically be changed to improve the health of individuals. In truth, however, less is known about the specific determinants of health than about the factors that contribute to disease, injury, and disability. And understanding the causes of disease and ill health does not necessarily lead to an understanding of the causes of good health.

TABLE 1-2 Determinants of Health

BIOLOGY AND GENETICS	LIFESTYLE	LIVING, WORKING, AND SOCIAL CONDITIONS	COMMUNITY CONDITIONS	BACKGROUND CONDITIONS
Sex	Physical activity	Housing	Climate and geography	National food and nutrition policy
Race	Diet	Education	Water supply	State and local food and nutrition policy
Age	Hobbies	Occupation	Type and condition of housing	National minimum wage
Other hereditary factors	Leisure-time activities	Income	Community design	Cultural beliefs
	Use of drugs:	Employment status	Number and type of hospitals and clinics	Cultural values
	• Cigarettes, cigars, chewing tobacco	Social networks such as family, friends, coworkers	Health and medical services	Cultural attitudes
	• Alcohol	Socioeconomic status/ class	Social services	Advertising
	• Prescription medications	Economic inequality	Leading industries	Media messages
	• Illicit drugs such as cocaine, marijuana, etc.	Racial and ethnic health disparities	Political/government structure	Food distribution system
	Religion	Access to nutritious foods	Community health groups and organizations	
	Safety practices such as handwashing, wearing seat belts, and wearing wrist guards and knee pads	Access to health services	Number, type, and location of grocery stores, etc.	
	Medical self-care	Public safety	Recreational settings	
	Stress management		Transportation systems	
			Built environment (buildings, sidewalks, bike lanes, and roads)	

Source: Adapted from G. Pickett and J. J. Hanlon, *Public Health: Administration and Practice* (St. Louis, MO: Times Mirror/Mosby College Publishing, 1990), 50; M. P. O'Donnell, "Definition of Health Promotion," *American Journal of Health Promotion* 1 (1986): 4–5; Institute of Medicine, *The Future of Public Health in the 21st Century* (Washington, D.C.: National Academy Press, 2003).

Health Promotion

Some people do things that are not good for their health. They overeat, smoke, refuse to wear a helmet when riding a bicycle, never wear seat belts when driving, fail to take their blood pressure medication—the list is endless. These behaviors reflect personal choices, habits, and customs that are influenced and modified by social forces. Such "lifestyle behaviors" can be changed if the individual is so motivated. Educating people about healthful and unhealthful behaviors is one way to help them adopt positive health behaviors.

Health promotion focuses on changing human behavior by encouraging people to eat healthful diets, be active, get regular rest, develop leisure-time hobbies for relaxation, strengthen social networks with family and friends, and achieve a balance among family, work, and play.[29] It is "the science and art of helping people change their lifestyle to move toward a state of optimal health."[30] Behavior change is the desired outcome of a health promotion activity—what we call an **intervention**—aimed at a target audience. Interventions focus on promoting health and preventing disease and are designed to change a preexisting condition related to the target audience's behavior.[31]

There are three types of prevention efforts, as shown in Figure 1-2. Primary prevention is aimed at preventing disease by controlling **risk factors** that are related to injury and disease. Heart-healthy cooking classes, for example, help people change their eating and cooking patterns to reduce their risk of cardiovascular disease. Secondary prevention focuses on detecting disease early through screening and other forms of risk appraisal. Public screenings for hypertension at a health fair identify people whose blood pressure is high; these individuals are then referred to a physician or other health professional for follow-up and treatment. Tertiary prevention aims to treat and rehabilitate people who have experienced an illness or injury. Education programs for people recently diagnosed with diabetes help prevent further disability and health problems, such as blindness and end-stage renal disease, from arising from the condition and improve overall health.[32] Prevention has become increasingly important as the medical community moves away from conventional medicine, which focuses on diagnosing and treating diseases, to a holistic approach that encompasses all aspects of the health spectrum.

Many questions about why people make the choices they make remain unanswered, but the ways to promote good health are widely recognized. Born of decades, if not centuries, of scientific observation and testing, the strategies for promoting good health are outlined in **Table 1-3**. Although these strategies seem relatively straightforward, putting them into practice is a major challenge for most communities and nations.

Health Objectives

The challenge of improving nutrition, health, and quality of life for humans is complex. As outlined by the nations of the world in a 1978 conference on primary health care convened by the WHO and the United Nations Children's Fund (UNICEF), the goal of the world community is to "protect and promote the health of all people of the world."[33] The commitment to the WHO goal of "health for all" through global improvements in health, especially for the most disadvantaged populations, was

Health promotion The process of enabling people to achieve their maximum potential for good health.

Intervention A health promotion activity aimed at changing the behavior of a target audience.

Risk factors Factors associated with an increased probability of acquiring a disease.

• Safe environment	Control physical, chemical, and biological hazards.
• Enhance immunity	Immunize to protect individuals and communities.
• Sensible behavior	Encourage healthful habits and discourage harmful habits.
• Good nutrition	Eat a well-balanced diet, containing neither too much nor too little.
• Well-born children	Every child should be a wanted child, and every mother fit and healthy.
• Prudent health care	Cautious skepticism is better than uncritical enthusiasm.

TABLE 1-3 Ways to Promote Good Health

Source: Adapted from J. M. Last, *Public Health and Human Ecology*, 2nd ed. (Stamford, CT: Appleton & Lange, 1998), 10.

renewed by nations in 1998.[34] At the World Summit on Sustainable Development, health was recognized as both a resource for and an outcome of sustainable development: "The goals of sustainable development cannot be achieved when there is a high prevalence of debilitating illness and poverty, and the health of a population cannot be maintained without a responsive health system and a healthy environment."[35]

When translating the global goal of "health for all" into action at the local level, one challenge is to understand the many physical, biological, social, and behavioral factors that influence the health of individuals and communities. Another challenge is to change human behavior.

Nations differ in how they formulate health objectives in an effort to help their people achieve behavior change, although there are common themes. Working groups in the European Region of the WHO, for example, outlined the following prerequisites for health:[36]

- Freedom from the fear of war—"the most serious of all threats to health"
- Equal opportunity for all peoples
- The satisfaction of basic needs for food, clean water and sanitation, decent housing, and education
- The right to find meaningful work and perform a useful role in society

Achieving these necessities requires both political will and public support, according to the working groups, which translated these prerequisites into specific targets for health. One such target, for example, called for enhancing life expectancy by reducing infant and maternal mortality. Other targets focused on enhancing social networks, promoting healthful behaviors, controlling water and air pollution, and improving the primary health care system.

In Canada, a new vision for promoting health and preventing disease among Canadians was expressed in documents released by Health Canada that aim to promote a balance between individual and societal responsibilities for health. These documents, *Achieving Health for All: A Framework for Health Promotion* and *Toward a Healthy Future*, cite goals to be met in achieving health for all: reducing inequities in access to and use of the health care system, increasing prevention efforts to change unhealthful behaviors, and enhancing the individual's ability to cope with chronic illnesses and disabilities. A key focus of the proposed implementation strategies is the strengthening of community-based health services, including worksite programs.[37] This vision for health in Canada is a window of opportunity for community nutritionists to promote food and nutrition policies in all Canadian communities.

Social–Ecological Models of Health Behavior

Although traditionally, much emphasis was placed on strategies to change nutrition and health-related behaviors by focusing on individual-level factors such as knowledge and skills, more recent interventions focus on the contribution of environmental factors to the development of obesity and other chronic diseases. Increasingly, ecological approaches to improving health have directed intervention strategies to target factors at several levels of influence, such as improving the health-promoting features of communities and reducing the abundance of high-calorie, nutrient-poor food choices. The combination of environmental, policy, social, and individual intervention strategies is credited with the major reductions in tobacco use in the United States since the 1960s, and this success has led to the application of similar approaches to many chronic health conditions today.[38] One way to frame this current thinking is the **social–ecological model (SEM)**, as shown in **Figure 1-3**, in which various levels of influence are arranged by relative proximity to the individual.[39] Thus, interpersonal relationships such as family factors are more proximal to the individual, while structures, policies, and systems, such as changes in food labeling or food costs, are more distant.

Social–ecological models (SEMs) Focus on the nature of people's interactions with their surrounding physical and sociocultural environments.

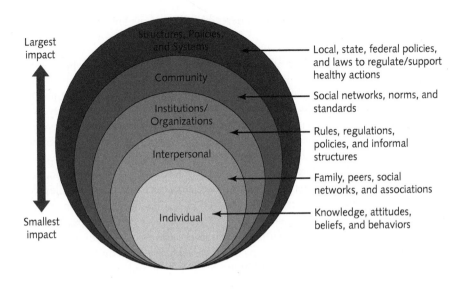

Largest impact

Smallest impact

- Local, state, federal policies, and laws to regulate/support healthy actions
- Social networks, norms, and standards
- Rules, regulations, policies, and informal structures
- Family, peers, social networks, and associations
- Knowledge, attitudes, beliefs, and behaviors

FIGURE 1-3 The Social–Ecological Model Health promotion activities that focus on policy-, system-, and environmental-level settings (community and institutions/organizations) are more likely to have a greater impact on health behaviors and health disparities than individual-level interventions.

Source: Adapted from the Centers for Disease Control and Prevention (CDC), The Social Ecological Model: A Framework for Prevention.

The SEM emphasizes multiple levels of influence (such as individual, interpersonal, organizational, community, and public policy) and the idea that all elements of society combine to shape an individual's food and physical activity choices or other health behaviors, and ultimately one's chronic disease risk. **Table 1-4** provides a brief description of each

TABLE 1-4 A Description of Social–Ecological Model (SEM) Levels of Influence

	DESCRIPTION	EXAMPLES OF INTERVENTIONS TO DECREASE OBESITY AT EACH SEM LEVEL OF INFLUENCE
Individual	Characteristics of an individual that influence behavior change, such as knowledge, attitudes, behavior, beliefs, lifestyle, self-efficacy, gender, age, genetics, religion, race/ethnicity, sexual orientation, economic status, financial resources, values, goals, priorities, literacy, body image, and other personal factors.	• A social media campaign to educate adolescents and young adults about the benefits of regular moderate physical activity. • A health educator seeks to increase the target population's knowledge and subsequently help form positive attitudes toward physical activity. • Public health nutritionist endeavors to increase knowledge about healthy food choices and skills in food shopping and meal preparation.
Interpersonal	Social networks and social support systems that can influence individual behaviors, including family, friends, peers, coworkers, health professionals, religious and/or social networks, customs or traditions.	• Programs utilize relationships between individuals to influence change. For example, peer support groups, recipe swaps, and walking groups encourage members to keep each other accountable to nutrition and physical activity goals.
Institutional/ Organizational Settings	Organizations or social institutions with policies and regulations that affect how, or how well, resources, services, or other items are provided to an individual or group (e.g., policy for school vending machines).	• A private business park replaces fast-food and soft-drink options in the cafeteria with water, fresh sandwiches, and salad bars to encourage employees to replace unhealthy options with more healthy ones.
Community Settings	Relationships among organizations, institutions, and informational networks within defined boundaries, including the built environment (e.g., parks), community leaders, businesses, and transportation.	• In a town with disproportionately low access to fresh fruits and vegetables, a working group of local school officials, community leaders, and business owners help establish a food cooperative as well as a biweekly farmers' market.
Structures, Policies, and Systems	Local, state, national and global laws and policies, including policies regarding the allocation of resources (e.g., eligibility requirements for food assistance programs).	• Structural changes are made for the development of safe parks, recreational areas, and sidewalks statewide to help facilitate physical activity.

Source: Adapted from CDC's Ecological Framework for Addressing Disparities in Obesity, 2013.

of the SEM levels. The following section describes the various levels of influence found within the model.[40]

Cognitions The knowledge and awareness that people have of their environment and the judgments they make related to it.

Attitudes An individual's positive or negative evaluation of performing a behavior or engaging in an activity.

- **Individual level.** The primary circle of the SEM is the individual—ultimately affected by all other levels of influence. Factors such as age, gender, income, race and ethnicity, genetics, and the presence of a disability can all influence an individual's food intake and physical activity patterns. Food intake is influenced by a constellation of biological, psychosocial, cultural, and lifestyle factors listed in Table 1-2, as well as by our personal food preferences, **cognitions, attitudes,** and health beliefs and practices. In order to change one's knowledge, attitudes, beliefs, and behaviors, these individual factors should be addressed.

- **Interpersonal level.** The next level in the SEM represents individuals' interactions with one another, or relationships shared within social networks such as families, friends, peer groups, and health professionals. Food choices are strongly influenced by social groups. Primary social groups such as families, friends, and work groups also influence health and nutrition status. The family is a paramount source of values for its members, and its values, attitudes, and traditions can have lasting effects on the members' food choices and health. This is especially true for children and teenagers. The calcium intakes of teenagers, for example, are higher in families in which teenagers perceive their parents' attention, care, support, and understanding than in families with low family connectedness.[41] Likewise, children whose parents did not regularly drink soft drinks were much less likely to consume soft drinks than children whose parents drank soft drinks on a regular basis.[42]

- **Institutional–organizational-level settings.** People regularly make decisions about food, physical activity, and health in a variety of settings, such as schools, worksites, faith-based organizations, and health care organizations. Health promotion activities implemented at this level facilitate individual behavior change by influencing organizational systems and policies. Health care systems, worksites, insurance plans, local health clinics, and professional organizations represent potential sources of organizational messages and supportive environments.[43] Examples of interventions appropriate for this level include: encouraging the expansion of insurance benefits for medical nutrition therapy or adopting worksite policies that support healthy behaviors.

- **Community-level settings.** Communities are composed of individuals as they participate in interpersonal relationships within various groups of institutions and organizations.[44] Healthy eating and lifestyle patterns can be influenced by availability and access to recreational facilities, restaurants, fast-food outlets, supermarkets, convenience stores, and other food retail establishments. Social and cultural norms and values are guidelines that govern our thoughts, beliefs, and behaviors. These shared assumptions of appropriate behavior are based on the values of a society and are reflected in everything from laws to personal expectations. Making healthy choices can be more difficult if those healthy choices are not strongly valued within a society. As mentioned earlier, communities may be viewed on different scales: global, national, regional, local, cultural, or by other shared characteristics.

- **Structures, policies, and systems.** The outermost tier of the SEM represents the local, state, and federal structures and systems that affect the built environment surrounding communities and individuals.[45] Communities are influenced by many factors, such as government and its programs and policies, public health and health care systems, agriculture and its food and agricultural policies, industry, and media. Many of these sectors determine the degree to which individuals have access to healthy food and opportunities to be physically active in their own communities.

The social–ecological model helps explain the roles that various segments of society can play in making healthy choices more widely accessible and desirable. Such a framework encourages a paradigm shift to a society oriented around health promotion and chronic disease prevention. To this end, the 2010 *Dietary Guidelines* included the following call to action:[46]

" *Ultimately, Americans make their own food and physical activity choices at the individual (and family) level. In order for Americans to make healthy choices, however, they need to have opportunities to purchase and consume healthy foods and engage in physical activity. Although individual behavior change is critical, a truly effective and sustainable improvement in the nation's health will require a multi-sector approach that applies the social–ecological model to improve the food and physical activity environment. This type of approach emphasizes the development of coordinated partnerships, programs, and policies to support healthy eating and active living. Interventions should extend well beyond providing traditional education to individuals and families about healthy choices, and should help build skills, reshape the environment, and re-establish social norms to facilitate individuals' healthy choices.* "

The social–ecological model provides guidance for developing successful programs. The most effective approach to health promotion and disease prevention uses a combination of interventions at all levels of the model. Creating a social environment conducive to change is important to making it easier for individuals to adopt healthy behaviors.

Healthy People: A Report Card for the Nation's Health

The health objectives for the peoples of the United States differ slightly from those of the European and Canadian communities, reflecting the health needs of the U.S. population. A national strategy for improving the health of the United States—known as **Healthy People**—is released by the U.S. Department of Health and Human Services each decade. For the past three decades, *Healthy People* has provided a framework for promoting health and avoiding preventable disease. Chronic diseases, such as heart disease, cancer, and diabetes, are responsible for 7 out of every 10 deaths among people in the United States each year and account for 75% of the nation's health spending. Many of the risk factors that contribute to the development of these diseases are preventable.[47] The *Healthy People* initiative is grounded in the principle that setting national objectives and monitoring progress can motivate action.

Healthy People A set of goals and objectives with 10-year targets designed to guide national health promotion and disease prevention efforts to improve the health of all people in the United States.

How did the nation do in terms of meeting the *Healthy People 2010* goals? When *Healthy People 2010* was released in 2000, life expectancy was 76 years. Today, the average life expectancy at birth is 78 years and death rates for heart disease, stroke, and certain types of cancer have declined.[48] However, health disparities remain evident among individuals, with significant differences between whites and minorities in mortality, morbidity, health insurance coverage, and the use of health services.[49]

Almost no progress was made toward the *Healthy People 2010* targets for objectives in the nutrition and overweight focus area.[50] Only one objective (calcium intake) showed positive movement. In addition, statistically significant health disparities were observed among racial and ethnic populations, as well as by sex, income, and disability status.

Since the 1980s, the prevalence of overweight has soared (see Chapter 8). In fact, overweight increased among all ethnic and age subgroups of the population. One contributing factor is that people seem to be taking fewer steps to control their weight by adopting sound dietary patterns and being physically active. Little or no improvements are noted for dietary fat intake and consumption of fruits, vegetables, and whole grains. Additional health promotion efforts are also needed to reduce the prevalence of iron deficiency and anemia and to increase the number of women who breastfeed their infants early in the postpartum period.[51] Progress toward meeting the *Healthy People* objectives is also discussed in Chapters 8, 11, 12, and 13. Chapter 7 provides the final status of the *Healthy People 2010* objectives for nutrition.

Looking Ahead: *Healthy People 2020*

Healthy People 2020 is the national health agenda for the current decade. It was developed by a consortium of national health organizations, state health departments, the Institute of Medicine, and the U.S. Public Health Service. The initiative identifies health improvement goals and objectives to be reached by the year 2020. It builds on the accomplishments and challenges in meeting the *Healthy People 2010* health objectives and communicates a strategy for achieving health equity.[52] *Healthy People 2020* assists federal and state agencies in setting priorities and in providing funding and support to organizations and institutions that are able to help achieve the *Healthy People 2020* objectives. A recent report has demonstrated that for the United States to become a healthier nation, *prevention* must become a driving force in our health care strategy.[53] To this end, *Healthy People 2020* aims to redirect our attention from health care to the **determinants of health** in our social and physical environments.[54]

Goals of *Healthy People 2020*

The goals for *Healthy People 2020* continue the tradition of earlier *Healthy People* initiatives and advocate for improvements in the health of all people (**Figure 1-4**).[55] The goals address the environmental factors that contribute to health and disease by placing particular emphasis on the determinants of health. As was shown in Table 1-2, health determinants are the range of personal, social, economic, and environmental factors that determine the health status of individuals or populations. Social determinants include family, community, income, education, geographic location, and access to health care, among others. Determinants in the physical environment include our natural and built environments.

Determinants of health The range of personal, social, economic, and environmental factors that influence health status. It is the interrelationships among these factors that determine individual and population health.

FIGURE 1-4 The *Healthy People 2020* Framework: Vision and Overarching Goals This figure depicts the ecological and determinants approach that *Healthy People 2020* takes in framing the national health objectives. It illustrates the fundamental degree of overlap among the determinants of health and shows their collective impact and influence on health outcomes.
Source: *Healthy People* Framework, November 2010; *www.healthypeople.gov*.

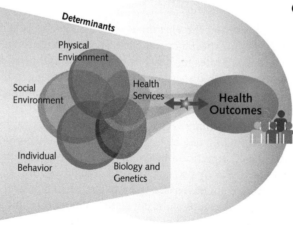

Healthy People 2020

A society in which all people live long, healthy lives

Overarching Goals:

- Attain high quality, longer lives free of preventable disease, disability, injury, and premature death.

- Achieve health equity, eliminate disparities, and improve the health of all groups.

- Create social and physical environments that promote good health for all.

- Promote quality of life, healthy development, and healthy behaviors across all life stages.

The overarching goals of *Healthy People 2020* include:[56]

- **Goal 1:** *Attain high-quality, longer lives free of preventable disease, disability, injury, and premature death.* This goal emphasizes the importance of prevention and health promotion for all people. Even people with diseases that cannot be prevented or cured can benefit from health promotion efforts that slow functional declines or improve the ability to live independently and participate in community life.

  This goal also considers problems such as violence or lack of preparedness for natural and manmade disasters. Since the 2000 launch of *Healthy People 2010*, the attacks of September 11, 2001; the subsequent anthrax attacks; the devastating effects of natural disasters such as Hurricanes Katrina and Ike; and concerns about an influenza pandemic have added urgency to the importance of *preparedness* as a public health issue. Being prepared for any emergency is a high priority for public health in the current decade.

- **Goal 2:** *Achieve health equity, eliminate disparities, and improve the health of all groups.* This goal reflects the increasing diversity of the population and recognizes that gender, race, and ethnicity; income and education; rural or urban location; disability; and sexual orientation are major factors that affect access to health care services and contribute to health disparities.

  To eliminate health disparities and promote health equity, it is necessary to address all determinants of health disparities that can be influenced by institutional policies and practices. These include disparities in health care as well as other health determinants, such as the conditions of daily life and the circumstances in which people are born, grow, work, and age.[57]

- **Goal 3:** *Create social and physical environments that promote good health for all.* This goal takes an ecological approach to health promotion. Health and health behaviors are determined by influences at multiple levels, including personal, organizational/institutional, environmental, and policy levels. Because dynamic interrelationships exist among these different levels of health determinants, interventions are most likely to be effective when they address determinants at all levels. Policies that can increase the income of low-income persons and communities (e.g., through education, job opportunities, and improvement in public infrastructure) may improve population health. Reducing inequalities in the physical environment (e.g., access to healthful foods, safe recreational areas, and transportation) can also improve key health behaviors and other determinants, thereby helping to meet numerous health objectives.

- **Goal 4:** *Promote quality of life, healthy development, and healthy behaviors across every stage of life.* This goal emphasizes promotion of health throughout the life cycle and highlights the importance of tailoring strategies to fit a particular age group, since the determinants of health change as a person develops. New topic areas include maternal, infant, and child health; early and middle childhood; adolescent health; and older adults.

Healthy People in Healthy Communities

The *Healthy People 2020* goals represent the nation's hope for the improved health of its citizens, and they can serve as the foundation for all work toward health promotion and disease prevention. As stated, however, they are too broad to implement. The working groups therefore also laid out objectives with specific, measurable targets to be achieved by the year 2020. These objectives are grouped into 42 broad topic areas, such as access to health services, cancer, diabetes, food safety, heart disease and stroke, nutrition and weight status, and physical activity, as shown in **Table 1-5.** *Healthy People 2020* balances the comprehensive set of health objectives with a smaller list of public health priorities for the decade, known as *leading health indicators.*

TABLE 1-5 *Healthy People 2020* Topic Areas
The 42 topic areas identify and group objectives of related content, highlighting specific issues and populations. Each topic area is assigned to one or more lead agencies within the federal government that is responsible for developing, tracking, monitoring, and periodically reporting on objectives.

1. Access to health services
2. Adolescent health
3. Arthritis, osteoporosis, and chronic back conditions
4. Blood disorders and blood safety
5. Cancer
6. Chronic kidney disease
7. Dementias, including Alzheimer's disease
8. Diabetes
9. Disability and health
10. Early and middle childhood
11. Educational and community-based programs
12. Environmental health
13. Family planning
14. Food safety
15. Genomics
16. Global health
17. Health care–associated infections
18. Health communication and health information technology
19. Health-related quality of life and well-being
20. Hearing and other sensory or communication disorders
21. Heart disease and stroke
22. HIV
23. Immunization and infectious diseases
24. Injury and violence prevention
25. Lesbian, gay, bisexual, and transgender health
26. Maternal, infant, and child health
27. Medical product safety
28. Mental health and mental disorders
29. Nutrition and weight status
30. Occupational safety and health
31. Older adults
32. Oral health
33. Physical activity
34. Preparedness
35. Public health infrastructure
36. Respiratory diseases
37. Sexually transmitted diseases
38. Sleep health
39. Social determinants of health
40. Substance abuse
41. Tobacco use
42. Vision

Source: U.S. Department of Health and Human Services, *Healthy People 2020*.

For each of the leading health indicators, specific objectives from *Healthy People 2020* are used to track the progress made in improving the nation's health and to provide periodic "snapshots" of the nation and its communities during the decade (**Table 1-6**).[58]

Many nutrition-related activities are considered essential to the overall *Healthy People 2020* initiative because four of the leading causes of death in the United States are related to dietary imbalance and excess (coronary heart disease, some types of cancer, stroke, and

TABLE 1-6 Leading Health Indicator Topic Areas and Objectives Used to Track Progress on *Healthy People 2020*
Healthy People 2020 includes a small set of high-priority health issues called *leading health indicators (LHIs)* that can result in significant public health problems if not addressed. However, addressing these critical health issues—such as tobacco use, health disparities, and obesity—will help reduce some of the leading causes of preventable deaths and major illnesses. Selected from the *Healthy People 2020* objectives, the 26 leading health indicators are organized under 12 topic areas. Access and track *Healthy People 2020* data online at *www.healthypeople.gov*. You can search the Health Indicators Warehouse for data related to *Healthy People 2020* objectives at *http://healthindicators.gov*.

PROGRESS TOWARD TARGET	LEADING HEALTH TOPIC AND INDICATOR	BASELINE (YEAR)	MOST RECENT (YEAR)	TARGET
	Access to Health Services			
○	**AHS-1.1** Persons with medical insurance (percent, < 65 years)	83.2% (2008)	83.1% (2012)	100.0%
○	**AHS-3** Persons with a usual primary care provider (percent)	76.3% (2007)	77.3% (2011)	83.9%
	Clinical Preventive Services			
+	**C-16** Adults receiving colorectal cancer screening based on most recent guidelines (age adjusted, percent, 50–75 years)	52.1% (2008)	59.2% (2010)	70.5%
+	**HDS-12** Adults with hypertension whose blood pressure is under control (age adjusted, percent, 18+ years)	43.7% (2005–08)	48.9% (2009–12)	61.2%
○	**D-5.1** Persons with diagnosed diabetes whose A1c value is > 9 percent (age adjusted, percent, 18+ years)	17.9% (2005–08)	21.0% (2009–12)	16.1%
+	**IID-8** Children receiving the recommended doses of DTaP, polio, MMR, Hib, hepatitis B, varicella, and PCV vaccines (percent, aged 19–35 months)	44.3% (2009)	68.5% (2011)	80.0%

PROGRESS TOWARD TARGET	LEADING HEALTH TOPIC AND INDICATOR	BASELINE (YEAR)	MOST RECENT (YEAR)	TARGET
	Environmental Quality			
✓	**EH-1** Air Quality Index (AQI) exceeding 100 (number of billion person days, weighted by population and Air Quality Index value)	2.237 (2006–08)	1.252 (2009–11)	1.980
✓	**TU-11.1** Children exposed to secondhand smoke (percent; nonsmokers, 3–11 years)	52.2% (2005–08)	41.3% (2009–12)	47.0%
	Injury and Violence			
+	**IVP-1.1** Injury deaths (age adjusted, per 100,000 population)	59.7 (2007)	57.1 (2010)	53.7
✓	**IVP-29** Homicides (age adjusted, per 100,000 population)	6.1 (2007)	5.3 (2010)	5.5
	Maternal, Infant, and Child Health			
+	**MICH-1.3** Infant deaths (per 1,000 live births, < 1 year)	6.7 (2006)	6.1 (2010)	6.0
+	**MICH-9.1** Total preterm live births (percent, < 37 weeks gestation)	12.7% (2007)	11.5% (2012)	11.4%
	Mental Health			
−	**MHMD-1** Suicide (age adjusted, per 100,000 population)	11.3 (2007)	12.1 (2010)	10.2
−	**MHMD-4.1** Adolescents with major depressive episodes (percent, 12–17 years)	8.3% (2008)	9.1% (2012)	7.5%
	Nutrition, Physical Activity, and Obesity			
✓	**PA-2.4** Adults meeting aerobic physical activity and muscle-strengthening Federal guidelines (age adjusted, percent, 18+ years)	18.2% (2008)	20.6% (2012)	20.1%
○	**NWS-9** Obesity among adults (age adjusted, percent, 20+ years)	33.9% (2005–08)	35.3% (2009–12)	30.5%
○	**NWS-10.4** Obesity among children and adolescents (percent, 2–19 years)	16.1% (2005–08)	16.9% (2009–12)	14.5%
○	**NWS-15.1** Mean daily intake of total vegetables (age adjusted, cup equivalents per 1,000 calories, 2+ years)	0.8 (2001–04)	0.8 (2007–10)	1.1
	Oral Health			
−	**OH-7** Persons who visited the dentist in the past year (age adjusted, percent, 2+ years)	44.5% (2007)	41.8% (2011)	49.0%
	Reproductive and Sexual Health			
Baseline data only	**FP-7.1** Sexually experienced females receiving reproductive health services in the past 12 months (percent, 15–44 years)	78.6% (2006–10)	Not available	86.5%
+	**HIV-13** Knowledge of serostatus among HIV-positive persons (percent, 13+ years)	80.9% (2006)	84.2% (2010)	90.0%
	Social Determinants			
+	**AH-5.1** Students awarded a high school diploma four years after starting 9th grade (percent)	74.9% (2007–08)	78.2% (2009–10)	82.4%
	Substance Abuse			
+	**SA-13.1** Adolescents using alcohol or illicit drugs in past 30 days (percent, 12–17 years)	18.4% (2008)	17.4% (2012)	16.6%
○	**SA-14.3** Binge drinking in past 30 days—adults (percent, 18+ years)	27.1% (2008)	27.1% (2012)	24.4%
	Tobacco			
+	**TU-1.1** Adult cigarette smoking (age adjusted, percent, 18+ years)	20.6% (2008)	18.2% (2012)	12.0%
○	**TU-2.2** Adolescent cigarette smoking in past 30 days (percent, grades 9–12)	19.5% (2009)	18.1% (2011)	16.0%

✓ Target met
+ Improving
○ Little or no detectable change
− Getting worse
* Each of the 26 indicators listed for the 12 topics will be tracked, measured, and reported on regularly throughout the decade.

Source: U.S. Department of Health and Human Services, *Healthy People 2020*.

diabetes mellitus). Diet also contributes to the development of other conditions, such as hypertension, osteoporosis, obesity, dental caries, and diseases of the gastrointestinal tract.[59]

Some of the *Healthy People 2020* nutrition-related objectives focus on improving health status. For example, one objective calls for increasing the proportion of adults who are at a healthy weight. Several objectives focus on health risk reduction and specify targets for the intake of nutrients such as sodium, saturated fat, and calcium and of foods such as fruits, vegetables, and whole grains. Other nutrition-related objectives set targets for the prevalence of iron deficiency and anemia and the proportion of worksites that offer nutrition or weight management counseling.[60] Some objectives address the special needs of various age groups, such as adolescents or older adults, whereas others focus on special population groups, such as women who are pregnant.

Surveillance An approach to collecting data on a population's health and nutrition status in which data collection occurs regularly and repeatedly.

Each *Healthy People 2020* objective has a target for specific improvements to be achieved by the year 2020. The **surveillance** and data-tracking systems of *Healthy People 2020* systematically collect and analyze health data to understand the nation's health status and plan prevention programs.[61]

The ultimate objective of public health is to lower the risk of disease and disability and to discourage risky behaviors in the first place.[62] Thus, many of the nutrition and educational programs and services developed by public health practitioners to meet the objectives of *Healthy People* focus on people in groups, whether they be families, schools, workplaces, cities, or nations. Such strategies target people of all ages and segments within the community. Refer to the Internet Resources at the end of this chapter for sites related to *Healthy People* initiatives and other sites of interest to community nutritionists.

Community Nutrition Practice

Earlier in the chapter, we defined community nutrition as a discipline that strives to improve the nutrition and health of individuals and groups within communities. How do community nutritionists do this? What skills are needed to accomplish this goal? What job responsibilities do community nutritionists have? This book answers these questions and introduces you to the challenges of working in communities today. Imagine for a moment that you are a community nutritionist in each of the following situations:

- An article in the *New York Times* describes the high rates of substance abuse, teen pregnancy, HIV infection, sexually transmitted diseases, smoking, and eating disorders among U.S. adolescents. Long concerned about this issue, your public health department plans an assessment of the health and nutrition status of teenagers in your county. Your job is to coordinate and lead the community assessment. Where do you start? What is the purpose of your assessment? What types of data do you collect? What information already exists about this population? Should your department work with other agencies to collect data? How will the results of your assessment be used to improve the health of teenagers in your community?
- As the director of health promotion for a large nonprofit health organization, you are responsible for developing and implementing programs to reduce the risk of cardiovascular diseases among people living in your state. Your organization's board of directors has called for an assessment of the effectiveness of all programs in your area. How do you evaluate program effectiveness? What types of data should be collected to show that each program reaches an appropriate number of people at a reasonable cost and helps them make behavioral changes to reduce their risk of heart attack and stroke? How will you present your findings to the board?

- You are attracted to the challenge of building a business and believe that your training in nutrition and exercise physiology can help people in your community get fit and improve their lifestyles. What is an attractive name for your business? Where should it be located? What services will you offer and to whom? Who are your competitors? How will you market your services? Can you use the Internet to enhance your business?
- You are employed by the Special Supplemental Nutrition Program for Women, Infants, and Children (WIC) in your state, and you have noticed that Spanish is the first language for an increasing number of your clients. You and your colleagues want to offer these clients more materials and services in Spanish. Should you adapt existing English-language materials for these clients or develop new materials from scratch? Are the existing English-language materials culturally appropriate for your Hispanic clients? What are other state WIC programs doing to address this issue?

Common themes are apparent in these situations. All refer to gathering information about the community itself or about people who use or implement community-based programs and services. Although it may not be clear to you now, all involve issues of policy, program management, and cost. All entail making decisions about how to use scarce resources. All are concerned with determining whether nutrition programs and services are reaching the right audience with the right messages and having the desired effect. All describe challenges of a trained professional—the community nutritionist—who identifies a nutritional need in the community and then puts into place a program or service designed to meet that need.

Community versus Public Health Nutrition

"Community nutrition" and "public health nutrition" are sometimes considered synonymous terms. In this book, *community nutrition* is the broader of the two and encompasses any nutrition program whose target is the community, whether the program is funded by the federal government, as are the WIC program and the National School Lunch program, or sponsored by a private group, such as a worksite weight management program. *Public health nutrition* refers to those community-based programs conducted by a government agency (federal, state, provincial, territorial, county, or municipal) whose official mandate is the delivery of health services to individuals living in a particular area.

The confusion over these terms stems partly from the traditional practice settings of **community dietitians** and **public health nutritionists**, as shown in **Figure 1-5**. Community dietitians, who are always registered dietitians (RDs) or licensed dietitians (LDs), tend to be situated in hospitals, clinics, health maintenance organizations, voluntary health organizations, worksites, and other nongovernment settings. Some community dietitians work in federal, state, and municipal health agencies. Public health nutritionists, only some of whom are RDs or LDs, more often provide nutrition services through government agencies, and often have a master's degree in public health nutrition.

In today's practice environment, these two designations overlap considerably, and practitioners in both areas share many goals, responsibilities, target groups, and practice settings. The community dietitian plans, coordinates, directs, manages, and evaluates the nutrition component of his or her organization's programs and services. The public health nutritionist carries out similar activities in a government agency.[63] For our purposes, all nutritionists whose major orientation is community-based programming will be called community nutritionists, whether their official title is community dietitian, public health nutritionist, nutrition education specialist, or some other designation.

Essential Practices of the Community Nutritionist

- Manage nutrition care for diverse population groups across the lifespan.
- Participate in nutrition surveillance and monitoring of communities.
- Develop and implement community-based food and nutrition programs.
- Conduct outcome assessment and evaluation of community-based food and nutrition programs.
- Collaborate in community-based research.
- Participate in food and nutrition policy development and evaluation based on community needs and resources.
- Consult with organizations regarding food access for target populations.
- Develop and implement a health promotion/disease prevention intervention project.
- Participate in screening activities such as measuring hematocrit and cholesterol levels.

Community dietitians/ public health nutritionists Nutrition professionals who plan and evaluate food and nutrition programs; develop food and nutrition policies; plan, implement, and evaluate health promotion and disease prevention programs; and provide nutrition services to all age groups in a community setting.

FIGURE 1-5 Practice Settings of Community Dietitians and Public Health Nutritionists

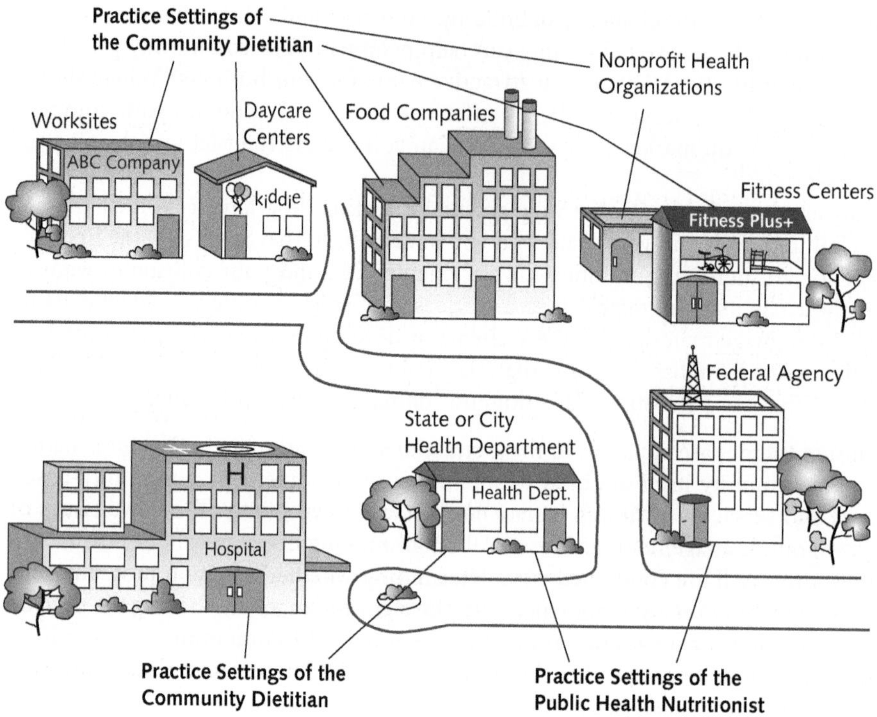

Practice Settings of the Community Dietitian

Nonprofit Health Organizations

Worksites

Daycare Centers

Food Companies

Fitness Centers

Fitness Plus+

ABC Company

kiddie

Federal Agency

State or City Health Department

Health Dept.

Hospital

Practice Settings of the Community Dietitian

Practice Settings of the Public Health Nutritionist

► **THINK LIKE A COMMUNITY** NUTRITIONIST

Particular skills and competencies are important for success in the field of community nutrition. Use the box on pages 23–24 to review the skill set of a community nutritionist. Then list knowledge and competencies you believe you already have, ones that you are working on developing, and ones that are not yet developed. Lastly, circle the knowledge and competency items you would like to further develop during this course. You can reevaluate your progress at the end of the course.

Educational Requirements Community nutritionists have a solid background in the nutrition sciences. They have competencies in such areas as nutritional biochemistry, nutrition requirements, nutritional assessment, medical nutrition therapy, nutrition throughout the life cycle, food composition, food safety, and food habits and customs. They are knowledgeable about the theories and principles of health education, epidemiology, community organization, management, and marketing. Marketing skills are especially important because it is no longer sufficient merely to know *which* nutrition messages to deliver. It is also necessary to know *how* to deliver them effectively in a variety of media formats to a variety of audiences.

The minimum educational requirements for a community nutritionist include a bachelor's degree in community nutrition, foods and nutrition, or dietetics from an accredited college or university. Most community nutrition positions require registration as a dietitian by the Academy of Nutrition and Dietetics. Some positions also require graduate-level training to obtain additional competencies in areas such as quality assurance, biostatistics, research methodology, health program planning and management, survey design and analysis, and the behavioral sciences. Community nutritionists who are registered dietitians are expected to have the core competencies listed on page 23.

Although dietetic technicians, registered (DTRs), are most often employed in the food-service sector and clinical settings, some do work in the community arena. Community-based DTRs assist the community nutritionist in determining the community's nutritional needs and in delivering community nutrition programs and services. DTRs must have at least an associate's degree and must pass the registration examination developed by the Commission on Dietetic Registration (CDR).

Basic Competencies of the Community Dietitian

▶ *Scientific and Evidence Base of Practice: Integration of scientific information and research into practice*
  - Select indicators of program quality and/or customer service and measure achievement of objectives (*Tip:* Outcomes may include clinical, programmatic, quality, productivity, economic, or other outcomes in wellness, management, sports, clinical settings, etc.)
  - Apply evidence-based guidelines, systematic reviews, and scientific literature in the nutrition care process and model and other areas of dietetics practice
  - Justify programs, products, services, and care using appropriate evidence or data
  - Evaluate emerging research for application in dietetics practice
  - Conduct projects using appropriate research methods, ethical procedures, and data analysis

▶ *Professional Practice Expectations: Beliefs, values, attitudes, and behaviors for the professional dietitian level of practice*
  - Practice in compliance with current federal regulations and state statutes and rules, as applicable and in accordance with accreditation standards and the Scope of Dietetics Practice and Code of Ethics for the Profession of Dietetics
  - Demonstrate professional writing skills in preparing professional communications (*Tip:* Examples include research manuscripts, project proposals, education materials, policies, and procedures.)
  - Design, implement, and evaluate presentations to a target audience (*Tip:* A quality presentation considers life experiences, cultural diversity, and educational background of the target audience.)
  - Use effective education and counseling skills to facilitate behavior change
  - Demonstrate active participation, teamwork, and contributions in group settings
  - Assign patient care activities to DTRs and/or support personnel as appropriate
  - Refer clients and patients to other professionals and services when needs are beyond individual scope of practice
  - Apply leadership skills to achieve desired outcomes
  - Participate in professional and community organizations
  - Establish collaborative relationships with other health professionals and support personnel to deliver effective nutrition services
  - Demonstrate professional attributes within various organizational cultures (*Tip:* Professional attributes include showing initiative and proactively developing solutions, advocacy, customer focus, risk taking, critical thinking, flexibility, time management, work prioritization, and work ethic.)
  - Perform self-assessment, develop goals and objectives, and prepare a draft portfolio for professional development as defined by the Commission on Dietetics Registration
  - Demonstrate negotiation skills (*Tip:* Demonstrating negotiation skills includes showing assertiveness when needed while respecting the life experiences, cultural diversity, and educational background of the other parties.)

▶ *Clinical and Customer Services: Development and delivery of information, products, and services to individuals, groups, and populations*
  - Perform the Nutrition Care Process (steps a through e below) and use standardized nutrition language for individuals, groups, and populations of differing ages and

continued

health status, in a variety of settings (See the Professional Focus feature in Chapter 5 for more about the Nutrition Care Process.)

a. Assess the nutrition status of individuals, groups, and populations in a variety of settings where nutrition care is or can be delivered

b. Diagnose nutrition problems and create problem, etiology, and signs and symptoms (PES) statements

c. Plan and implement nutrition interventions to include prioritizing the nutrition diagnosis, formulating a nutrition prescription, establishing goals, and selecting and managing the intervention

d. Monitor and evaluate problems, etiologies, signs, symptoms, and the impact of interventions on the nutrition diagnosis

e. Complete documentation that follows professional guidelines, guidelines required by health care systems, and guidelines required by the practice setting

- Demonstrate effective communications skills for clinical and customer services in a variety of formats (*Tip:* Formats include oral, print, visual, electronic, and mass media methods for maximizing client education, employee training, and marketing.)
- Develop and deliver products, programs, or services that promote consumer health, wellness, and lifestyle management (*Tip:* Consider health messages and interventions that integrate the consumer's desire for taste, convenience, and economy with the need for nutrition and food safety.)
- Deliver respectful, science-based answers to consumer questions concerning emerging trends
- Coordinate procurement, production, distribution, and service of goods and services (*Tip:* Demonstrate and promote responsible use of resources including employees, money, time, water, energy, food, and disposable goods.)
- Develop and evaluate recipes, formulas, and menus for acceptability and affordability that accommodate the cultural diversity and health needs of various populations, groups, and individuals

▶ *Practice Management and Use of Resources: Strategic application of principles of management and systems in the provision of services to individuals and organizations*
- Participate in management of human resources
- Perform management functions related to safety, security, and sanitation that affect employees, customers, patients, facilities, and food
- Participate in public policy activities, including both legislative and regulatory initiatives
- Conduct clinical and customer service quality management activities
- Use current informatics technology to develop, store, retrieve, and disseminate information and data
- Analyze quality, financial, or productivity data and develop a plan for intervention
- Propose and use procedures as appropriate to the practice setting to reduce waste and protect the environment
- Conduct feasibility studies for products, programs, or services with consideration of costs and benefits
- Analyze financial data to assess utilization of resources
- Develop a plan to provide or develop a product, program, or service that includes a budget, staffing needs, equipment, and supplies
- Code and bill for dietetic/nutrition services to obtain reimbursement from public or private insurers

Source: Core Knowledge & Competencies for the RD, ACEND accrediting agency of the Academy of Nutrition and Dietetics (formerly the American Dietetic Association). Reproduced with permission.

Licensure of Nutrition Practitioners Licensure of physicians has been the principal social mechanism for quality control in health care. In the past three decades, increasing numbers of licensed, nonphysician health care providers—such as nurse practitioners, physician assistants, midwives, physical therapists, dietitians, and dental hygienists—have appeared. They provide at a lower cost many services formerly performed only by doctors.[64]

In medicine, the educational standards for the medical degree (MD) are governed by law. Unfortunately, in some states the term "nutritionist" is not legally defined, and as a result, the public can be the hapless prey of anyone who wishes to use this title. Some nutritionists obtain their diplomas and titles without the rigorous training required for a legitimate nutrition degree. Because of lax state laws, it is even possible for an irresponsible "correspondence school"—a diploma mill—to pass out degrees to anyone who pays a fee.

Licensure of qualified nutritionists protects consumers from unqualified practitioners, particularly those who have no training in nutrition but nevertheless refer to themselves as "nutritionists." Licensure is designed to protect the public, control malpractice, and ensure minimum standards of practice. Its aim is legal recognition of health care professionals with the training and experience to deliver nutrition services.

Today, better consumer protection with respect to nutrition services is evident in many states. As of 2015, 44 states, the District of Columbia, and Puerto Rico had enacted legislation regulating the practice of dietetics. Several states have passed legislation restricting the fraudulent use of the title "dietitian." Several other states have passed legislation to prohibit people from calling themselves nutritionists without a license that requires a background in dietetics.

The advantages of licensure are clear. People are accustomed to identifying licensed health professionals. States that regulate nutrition services by means of licensure or **certification** assure consumers, health professionals, and insurance companies that the people providing those services meet the specific professional standards established by the state's Department of Professional Regulation.

Practice Settings The practice settings of community nutritionists include schools, worksites, cooperative extension agencies, universities, colleges, medical schools, voluntary and nonprofit health organizations, public health departments, home health care agencies, daycare centers, residential facilities, fitness centers, sports clinics, hospital outpatient facilities, food companies, wellness programs, and homes (their own or those of their clients). Some community nutritionists work as consultants, providing nutrition expertise to government agencies, food companies, foodservice companies, or other groups who are planning community-based services or programs with a nutrition component.

Community nutritionists are also employed by world and regional health organizations. WHO's Division of Family Health, located at WHO headquarters in Geneva, Switzerland, includes an office of nutrition. Likewise, the North American regional WHO office in Washington, D.C., which is known officially as the Pan American Sanitary Bureau and coexists with the Pan American Health Organization (PAHO), has a strong nutrition mandate. The PAHO directs its efforts toward solving nutritional problems in Latin America and the Caribbean. Another prominent organization in global community nutrition is the Food and Agriculture Organization (FAO) of the United Nations. The programs of the Food Policy and Nutrition Division of FAO are directed toward improving the nutrition status of at-risk populations and ensuring access to adequate supplies of safe, good-quality foods.[65] For more about global nutrition issues, see Chapter 14.

Roles and Responsibilities Community nutritionists play many roles: educator, counselor, advocate, coordinator, generator of ideas, facilitator, and supervisor. They interpret and incorporate new scientific information into their practice and provide nutrition

Licensure Dietetics practitioners are licensed to ensure that only qualified, trained professionals provide nutrition services or advice to individuals requiring or seeking nutrition counseling or information; nonlicensed practitioners may be subject to prosecution for practicing without a license.

Certification Limits the use of particular titles (e.g., dietitian or nutritionist) to persons meeting predetermined requirements, but persons not certified can still practice the occupation or profession. For a list of states with laws that regulate dietitians or nutritionists through licensure or certification, go to *www.cdrnet.org/certifications/licensure/index.htm*.

Bonnie Taub-Dix

ENTREPRENEUR
IN ACTION

Bonnie Taub-Dix, MA, RDN, CDN is the award-winning author of *Read It Before You Eat It* and owner of BTD Nutrition Consultants, LLC. She is a media personality, spokesperson, motivational speaker, journalist, and corporate consultant whose messages are laced with her culinary passion as a foodie, her credible guidance as an advisor, and her wit and wisdom as a mom. Bonnie is a health and wellness blogger and contributor for *TODAY.com*, *US News & World Report*, *Everyday Health*, and *Sonima.com*. Her stories, quotes, and interviews have appeared in all forms of media comprised of television and radio shows and print and online platforms. She is an advisor to global corporations, food companies, and media outlets, writing stories, creating media/social media campaigns, devising wellness programs, and conducting workshops for health professionals and consumers. On a personal note, Bonnie is grateful to be able to do what she loves every day. She is married and has three sons . . . all foodies! Visit her website at *www.BetterThanDieting.com* and find out more about her social media presence at *www.cengagebrain.com*.

information to individuals, specialized groups, and the general population. Their focus is normal nutrition, although they sometimes cover the principles of medical nutrition therapy and nutritional care in disease for certain groups (e.g., HIV-positive children or people with diabetes).[66] In addition to serving the general public, community nutritionists refer clients to other health professionals when necessary and participate in professional activities.

Community nutritionists are responsible for planning, evaluating, managing, and marketing nutrition services, programs, and interventions. Nutrition services range from individual counseling for weight management, blood cholesterol reduction, and eating disorders to consulting services provided for food companies and institutions such as residential centers and nursing homes. Nutrition programs may be national in focus, such as the WIC program, or local, such as Healthy Start for Mom and Me, a Winnipeg prenatal nutrition program for low-income, high-risk pregnant women.[67] Community nutritionists who develop programs identify nutrition problems within the community, obtain screening data on target groups, locate information on community resources, develop education materials, disseminate nutrition information through the media, evaluate the effectiveness of programs and services, negotiate contracts for nutrition programs, train staff and community workers, and document program services.[68] Examples of essential practices of the community nutritionist are listed on page 21.[69]

The job responsibilities of community nutritionists are similar across practice settings. The community nutritionists whose responsibilities are shown in **Table 1-7** are all involved in assessing the nutrition status of individuals or identifying a nutritional problem within a community. They all have opportunities for teaching their clients about foods, diet, nutrition, and health and for addressing emerging issues in community nutrition. Some are involved in the budget process and in developing marketing strategies; others are not. The community nutritionist in private practice does it all!

In today's market, community nutritionists are increasingly expected to manage projects, resources, and people. One survey of 350 community dietitians found that more than two-thirds had mid- to upper-level management responsibilities. Community dietitians in management positions reported spending more time planning, coordinating, and evaluating programs and less time interacting with clients than did those in lower-level positions.[70] A role delineation study conducted by the Academy of Nutrition and Dietetics found that RDs working in community settings also had advising and policy-setting roles.[71] The time allocated to these activities varied somewhat by practice level. Community dietitians reported having major responsibility for teaching students, other dietitians, and health professionals. Their roles overlapped significantly with those of RDs in clinical dietetics.

Community nutritionists are also expected to be multiskilled or cross-trained (**Table 1-8**). Multiskilled practitioners perform more than one function, often in more than one discipline.[72] The multiskilled community nutritionist knows not only how to conduct a needs assessment and provide dietary guidance but also how to design and conduct a survey, use an Internet website for marketing health messages, and obtain funding to support a

Position: Child Nutrition Specialist, State Department of Education

Responsibilities

1. Interprets USDA's regulations, policies, and procedures related to the National School Lunch Program for users of the program
2. Trains program users in such areas as how to count meals and keep records accurately, how to determine that menus meet current nutrition requirements, and which foods can be ordered through the commodities program
3. Revises training manuals
4. Audits program user compliance with USDA's regulations and procedures, including assessing whether student eligibility for participation in the program was determined correctly, ensuring that proper accounting procedures have been followed, and creating an action plan when the program user has not complied with the USDA regulations and procedures

Position: Nutritionist, Special Supplemental Nutrition Program for Women, Infants, and Children (WIC)

Responsibilities

1. Determines client's eligibility for program, using WIC program criteria (e.g., presence of anemia, underweight/overweight, prior pregnancies, inadequate diet)
2. Assesses the nutrition status of clients
3. Determines the adequacy of the client's diet
4. Provides one-on-one diet counseling
5. Conducts group sessions for clients on basic nutrition topics such as food sources of iron and calcium
6. Helps clients understand how to use the WIC-approved foods in their daily diets
7. Assists in developing educational materials as required
8. Assists in reviewing client records and monitoring health data posted to records as required

Position: Director of Health Promotion, First-Rate Spa and Health Resort

Responsibilities

1. Develops, implements, and evaluates programs in the areas of nutrition, fitness, weight management, and risk reduction (e.g., blood cholesterol reduction, stress management, smoking cessation)
2. Assists the director in developing marketing strategies for programs
3. Prepares program budgets
4. Tracks program expenses
5. Teaches nutrition/fitness to groups of clients
6. Supervises dietitians and other staff involved in counseling clients and fitness assessments

Position: President/Owner, Cornerstone Nutrition Services

Responsibilities

1. Sets business goals and objectives
2. Manages all aspects of company's programs and services, including developing programs and services, developing educational materials and teaching tools, and evaluating the success of programs and services
3. Develops and evaluates a marketing plan
4. Identifies new business opportunities
5. Tracks income (including billings) and expenses for tax purposes
6. Maintains client records
7. Networks with colleagues in business and the community

TABLE 1-7

Responsibilities of Community Nutritionists in Diverse Practice Settings

program's promotional plan. Survey design and analysis, marketing, Internet technology, and grant writing are important disciplines for community nutritionists. And in today's culturally diverse environment, bilingual community nutritionists are in demand. Being fluent in a language other than English helps the nutritionist gather information from at-risk or hard-to-reach populations and develop programs that meet their needs.

- Basic understanding of the epidemiology and surveillance of health conditions such as diabetes, including the origin and availability of data sets
- Knowledge of how to influence policy development
- Ability to do an evaluation that will drive program changes
- Knowledge of how to effect change by developing broad-based community partnerships
- Knowledge of how to write grant applications
- Familiarity with budget development, justification, and management skills
- Knowledge of how to work with different cultures and adapt approaches based on the specific needs of each culture
- Knowledge of how to promote health through social marketing
- Knowledge of how to facilitate health system change

TABLE 1-8

Multiskilling in Community Dietetics

Source: Public Health and Community Nutrition Practice Group, *www.eatright.org*.

Entrepreneurship in Community Nutrition

Entrepreneurship is important in community nutrition. What is entrepreneurship? Who is an entrepreneur? How is entrepreneurship related to community nutrition? In the business world, entrepreneurship is defined as the act of starting a business or the process of creating new "values," be they goods, services, methods of production, technologies, or markets.[73] The essence of entrepreneurship is innovation. Consider the late Ray Kroc of McDonald's. He did not invent the hamburger, but he did develop an entirely new way of marketing and delivering it to his customers. In the process, he revolutionized the foodservice industry.

Entrepreneurship Creating something of value through the creation of organization.

Entrepreneurship, then, is the creation of something of value, be it a product or a service, through the creation of organization. In this context, *organization* means orchestration of the materials, people, and capital required to deliver a product or service. This definition encompasses the myriad actions of individuals—the entrepreneurs—who invent or develop some new product or service that is valued by the community or marketplace.[74]

Entrepreneurs and Intrapreneurs

Entrepreneur One who undertakes the risk of a business or enterprise.

An **entrepreneur** is an innovator, initiator, promoter, and coordinator. Entrepreneurs are change agents who seek, recognize, and act on opportunities. They ask, "What if?" and "Why not?" and translate their ideas into action. They tend to be creative, are able to see an old problem in a new light, and are willing to break new ground in delivering a product or service. When they spot an opportunity to fill a niche in the marketplace, they work to bring together the expertise, materials, labor, and capital necessary to meet the perceived need or want. Two entrepreneurs in community nutrition are Oklahoma dietitians Kellie Bryant, MS, RD, LD, and Mary S. Callison, MS, RD, LD, who developed a nutrition newsletter for Head Start programs. They observed that Head Start programs, particularly on Indian reservations and in rural areas, lacked practical information pieces on child health and on how to shop for, cook, store, and serve healthful foods. Their *Primarily Nutrition* newsletter is marketed to Head Start programs, which distribute it to clients and their families.[75] Janet Helm, MS, RD, and Lori Fromm, MS, RD, the two registered dietitians who launched the Nutrition Blog Network—a collection of blogs written by registered dietitians—are also entrepreneurs.[76] They spotted a new social media trend and learned how to harness it for educating consumers with trusted advice from nutrition experts on topics ranging from pregnancy to senior nutrition, gluten-free to "green," and diabetes to diet myths. The blog directory helps dietitians network and become more visible online.

Entrepreneurs share some common personality traits. They are achievers, setting high goals for themselves. They work hard, are good organizers, enjoy managing a project to completion, and accept responsibility for their ventures. They strive for excellence and are optimistic, believing that now is the best of times and anything is possible. Finally, entrepreneurs are reward oriented, seeking recognition and respect for their ventures and ideas. Recognition and respect are often more important than money to entrepreneurs.[77]

Intrapreneur A risk taker whose job is located within a corporation, company, or other organization.

These qualities are typically applied to the self-starting, independent entrepreneur in business, but they also describe the **intrapreneur**, the corporate employee who is creative and innovative. Intrapreneurs are seldom solely responsible for the financial risk associated with a new venture, but they share the same entrepreneurial spirit as their more independent counterparts. Like entrepreneurs, intrapreneurs use innovation to exploit change as an opportunity for creating something of value. In other words, intrapreneurs seek to better the existing state of affairs within their organizations through creative problem solving.[78] A good example of intrapreneurship is the action of Dr. Cheryl Sonnenberg at the

Economic Opportunity Board of Clark County in Las Vegas, Nevada. Dr. Sonnenberg had been struggling to find ways of delivering WIC services to clients in remote areas of Clark County. She had read of a Texas experiment in which a renovated Cadillac had been used to deliver WIC services in rural areas, but when she discovered that the renovation costs far exceeded her budget, she began exploring other innovative delivery systems. Eventually, she arranged to buy a used Winnebago, which was renovated with the help of engineers in the transportation division. Her solution became known as WIC on Wheels. Her intrapreneurial initiative helped solve a problem and improve rural service delivery to 450 WIC clients.[79]

What do entrepreneurs do? (In this book, innovators in both the private [corporate] and public [government] sectors who embody the spirit and principles of entrepreneurship will be considered entrepreneurs.) One study of entrepreneurs identified at least 57 separate activities associated with launching a new venture—a clear indication of how complex entrepreneurial behavior can be. Entrepreneurs have wide-ranging competencies in areas such as planning, marketing, networking, budgeting, and team building. They turn their creative vision into deliberate decision-making and problem-solving actions to accomplish their goals. They are not just managers, although they typically "manage" themselves well. Their high self-esteem stems from a strong belief in their own personal worth, which strengthens their capacity for self-management. Successfully managing oneself means being in control (i.e., having willpower), knowing one's personal strengths and weaknesses, and being willing to change one's behavior and graciously make use of feedback and criticism.

Community nutritionists who are RDs and entrepreneurs are expected to have competencies in addition to the core competencies expected of all dietitians. These business competencies include the following:[80]

- Perform organizational and strategic planning
- Develop and implement a business or operating plan
- Supervise procurement of resources
- Manage the integration of financial, human, physical, and material resources
- Supervise coordination of services
- Supervise marketing functions

What relevance does entrepreneurship have to community nutrition? The answer to this question will become increasingly clear as you read the remaining chapters of this book. Suffice it to say at this point that creativity and innovation—the essence of entrepreneurship—are as important to the discipline of community nutrition as to any other field. Consider the entrepreneurial activities listed in the margin above. Nearly all are relevant for the community nutritionist: recognizing an opportunity to deliver nutrition and health messages, developing an action plan for a target audience, building the team for delivering a nutrition program or service, developing a marketing plan, and evaluating the effectiveness of the nutrition program or service.[81]

Photo courtesy, Erin Palinski. © Digital Edge Photography

ENTREPRENEUR IN ACTION

Erin Palinski-Wade, RD, CDE, LDN, felt the entrepreneurial spirit early on, opening her private nutrition counseling practice less than one year after graduating from her dietetic internship. Since then, her practice has grown to include a team of dietitians counseling thousands of individuals in the areas of weight management, diabetes, cardiovascular disease, pediatric obesity, and sports nutrition. Erin says, "To be successful in private practice, you need to find your niche, excel in it, and develop a counseling style or program that works for the clients in your niche. To find your niche, you have to find what area of nutrition you are passionate about. You also need to be constantly evolving, learning, and fine-tuning your techniques and your business approach. In order to best serve your community, it is important not only to stay abreast of the latest nutrition information, but also to learn how to best relay that message to your target population. Perhaps in the past newspaper articles and mailings were best, whereas now perhaps a social media campaign to relay new information would be most effective." Find out what she has to say about entrepreneurship online at *www.cengagebrain.com*.

Activities of Entrepreneurs and Intrapreneurs

- Identify an opportunity
- Create a solution
- Conduct market research
- Establish business objectives
- Set up an organizational structure
- Determine personnel requirements
- Prepare a financial plan
- Locate financial resources
- Prepare a production plan
- Prepare a management plan
- Prepare a marketing plan
- Produce and test-market the product
- Build an organization

Community nutritionists who want to change people's eating habits must be able to see new ways of reaching desired target groups. The strategy that works well with Hmong adolescents in California will probably not be successful with institutionalized older adult women living in Ohio. Community nutritionists must draw on theories and skills from the disciplines of sociology, educational psychology, medicine, communications, health education, technology, and business to develop programs for improving people's eating patterns. The twin stanchions of entrepreneurship—creativity and innovation—assist the community nutritionist in achieving the broad goal of improved health for all.

Social and Economic Trends for Community Nutrition

Recent social and economic trends have important consequences for community nutrition. For example, the demographic profile of many communities is changing rapidly, along with the client mix served by community nutritionists.

Leading Indicators of Change

A worldwide increase in the educational level of the workforce is anticipated. In 2000, 25% of the U.S. population were college graduates. By 2020, more than 55% are expected to have completed some college study.[82] Women have entered the global workforce in unprecedented numbers, a trend that has led to changes in traditional family norms and structures and thus may affect the format and delivery of nutrition programs and services. Consequently, a variety of alternative educational strategies will be needed to reach consumers whose education, training, income, language skills, time pressures, and economic potential will be highly diverse.[83] See also the discussion in Chapter 6 of emerging policy issues, including sustainable food systems, complementary nutrition and health therapies, functional foods, genetics, and biotechnology.

An Aging Population In North America, the aging of the population, coupled with a more ethnically diverse society, will challenge community nutritionists to develop new products and services. Forty percent of our population—some 117 million people—have a chronic disease or condition.[84] In the United States, for example, the fastest-growing segment of the nation's population consists of people over 65 years of age. Indeed, the most rapidly growing segment is the 80-plus age group, which, compared with younger groups, tends to have more chronic health problems and to use more hospital health services such as inpatient and outpatient care.[85] See Chapter 13 for more about nutrition issues and programs for older adults.

Generational Diversity Many of the so-called baby boomers—those people born between 1946 and 1964—have reached their peak earning years and are expected to be a leading market force in redefining how to live as older adults.[86] At the same time, the younger generations are emerging with new values and attitudes about health, lifestyles, and society. The generations can differ in workplace values, lifestyle and social values, motivation, learning and communication styles, and technical competence (**Table 1-9**).[87] Community dietitians will need to understand the characteristics of these distinct generations in order to develop skills, tools, and resources for communicating nutrition and health information most effectively to individuals throughout these groups.

By the Year 2020 . . .

- Another 50 to 80 million people will probably have been added to the U.S. population, which was 319 million in 2014.
- The population and labor force will continue to diversify as immigration continues to account for a sizable part of the population growth. Certain states and cities, especially those on the East and West Coasts, can be expected to receive a disproportionately large number of immigrants.
- The growing diversity of food choices is likely to echo the increasing diversity of the population. Between 1980 and 2020, the Hispanic population will have grown from 6.5 to 18% of the population; blacks will have grown from 11.6 to 12.9%; and Asian or Pacific Islanders will have grown from 1.5 to 5%. For the same time period, whites will have declined from 79.9 to 62.5% of the population.
- The world's population will have grown by about 2.2 billion people. How to feed these additional people adequately will be one of the main challenges facing the global system of agricultural production and trade.
- The number of people over 65 years of age will have grown from 35 million in 2000 to 55 million because of aging baby boomers and longer life expectancies.
- People ages 65–74 will have increased from 6 to 10% of the population, and those ages 75 and older will have increased from 6 to 7%.
- Total national spending on long-term health care will have risen to $207 billion—up from $115 billion in 1997; spending on home care will account for about one-third of spending on long-term care.

Sources: U.S. Department of Health and Human Services, Public Health Service, *Healthy People 2010: Understanding and Improving Health* (Washington, D.C.: U.S. Government Printing Office, 2000); U.S. Bureau of the Census, *Population Projections of the United States by Age, Sex, Race, and Hispanic Origin: 1995 to 2050*, Current Population Reports, P25–1130.

TABLE 1-9

Characteristics and Insights Regarding Current U.S. Generations

GENERATION AND BIRTH YEARS	CHARACTERISTICS AND INSIGHTS
Matures/Traditionalists, Pre-1946	Respect authority; avoid challenging the system; place duty before pleasure; value honor, integrity, personal ties and relationships; give information on a "need-to-know" basis; not completely comfortable with technology-based delivery of information and services.
Baby Boomers, 1946–1964	Live to work; committed to climbing the ladder of success; optimistic; strive for convenience and personal fulfillment; first wave of dual-income, dual-career families; interested in interpersonal communication; gently question status quo; team- and process-oriented; want to see big picture of an organization; will crusade for a cause; desire to preserve their youth and be nostalgic about it; enjoy unprecedented influence on government, corporate, and organizational policies and consumer products because of their numbers; comfortable with technology.
Generation X (the Baby Bust), 1965–1980	Work to live, not live to work; first generation of latchkey kids; independent, resourceful, entrepreneurial, and focused on personal growth; desire versatility, challenging work, and substantial financial rewards; aggressively question status quo and authority, interested in removing outdated work models; believe in clear, consistent expectations.

continued

TABLE 1-9

Characteristics and Insights Regarding Current U.S. Generations —*continued*

GENERATION AND BIRTH YEARS	CHARACTERISTICS AND INSIGHTS
Generation Y (the Baby Boom Echo), 1981–1995	Live in the moment; earn to spend; rely on immediacy of technology; grew up with the Internet; comfortable in getting, using, and sharing information that is visual, fast-paced, and conceptual; prefer to be tech-savvy and multitasking; enjoy collaborative efforts; more culturally diverse than other generations; social-minded and altruistic; demand respect and often question everything; need clear and consistent expectations to ensure productivity.
Generation Z (i-Generation, digital natives), 1996–2014	First generation to be born into a digital world and the most electronically connected generation in history; from an early age, have used the Internet, laptops, cell phones, text messaging, multimedia players, wireless, video games, YouTube, and weblogs; communicate and collaborate in real-time regardless of physical location; access information easily.

Sources: Adapted from J. Jarratt and J. B. Mahaffie, "Key trends affecting the dietetics profession and the American Dietetic Association," *Journal of the American Dietetic Association* 102 (2002): 1825; C. Alexander, "Understanding generational differences helps you manage a multi-age workforce," *The Digital Edge*, July 2001; D. Brown, "Ways dietitians of different generations can work together," *Journal of the American Dietetic Association* 103 (2003): 1461.

Increasing Demands for Nutrition and Health Care Services As they move into their retirement years over the next two decades, baby boomers are expected to seek out information and opportunities to live healthier and longer lives. This represents a growing opportunity for community nutritionists to deliver sound nutrition and health promotion information to this emerging group of seniors. The aging population will probably place many demands on health care services, home care services, and food assistance programs.[88] See Chapter 9 for more about health care reform and related nutrition issues.

Increasing Ethnic Diversity Analysts predict that the global workforce will become even more ethnically diverse in the next few years, the result of massive relocations of people—including immigrants, refugees, retirees, temporary workers, and visitors—across national borders. As society becomes more ethnically diverse, more knowledge of health beliefs, cultural foods, and values is needed. An interesting consequence of the influx of immigrants into Canada and the United States is an anticipated change in consumer marketing strategies as a consequence of the family-oriented shopping behaviors of Asian and Hispanic consumers. The cultural values and lifestyles of these ethnic groups tend to reinforce family decision making and collective buying behavior. Marketers will have to change their strategies to appeal to the decision style of the extended family. They will need to market their products and services to groups rather than individuals.[89] See Chapter 15 for more about gaining cultural competence in community nutrition practice.

Increasing Emphasis on Addressing Health Disparities Not all cultural groups have the same health status. There are substantial **health disparities** in segments of the population—disparities based on gender, age, race or **ethnicity**, education, income, religion, disability, geographic location, sexual orientation, or other characteristics historically linked to discrimination or exclusion. Disparities can exist in regard to access to health care; delivery of quality, competent health care services; and health outcomes. The incidence of chronic disease, disability, and death is higher

Health disparities Health disparities exist when a segment of the population bears a disproportionate incidence of a health condition or illness.

Ethnicity A property of a group that consists of its sharing cultural traditions, having a common linguistic heritage, and originating from the same land.

among American Indian or Alaska Native, Asian American, black or African American, Hispanic or Latino, and Native Hawaiian or Other Pacific Islander.[90] See Table 15-2 in Chapter 15 for specific examples of health disparities among these groups. The Patient Protection and Affordable Care Act of 2010 has a number of provisions to improve the health of underserved populations, including insurance reform, improved access to health care, quality improvement, cost containment, and public health initiatives.[91] The Act also specifies support for the development and implementation of programs that aim to reduce health disparities, improve prevention techniques, and focus on health care for disabled individuals.[92]

Challenges of the Twenty-First-Century Lifestyle
The WHO describes obesity as "an escalating epidemic" and one of the greatest neglected public health problems of our time. Many factors, including genetics, influence body weight, but excess calorie intake and physical inactivity are the leading causes of overweight and obesity and represent the best opportunities for prevention and treatment. Consider how the following lifestyle trends have either increased opportunities for poor nutrition (particularly excess calories) or decreased opportunities for physical activity:[93]

- Food portion sizes and obesity rates have grown in parallel. In the 1960s, an average fast-food meal of a hamburger, fries, and a 12-ounce cola provided 590 calories; today, many super-sized, "extra-value" fast-food meals deliver 1,500 calories or more.
- Vending machines selling soft drinks, high-fat snacks, and sweet snacks are common on college campuses and in workplaces. Milk, juices, water, and healthful snacks are far less accessible than their unhealthful counterparts.
- Both adults and children spend more time in sedentary activities, such as watching television, sitting at the computer, or commuting to and from work and school, and schools offer fewer physical education classes for children.
- Increasing numbers of families live in communities designed for car use that are unsuitable (lack of green space for recreation) and often unsafe (lack of sidewalks, inadequate street lighting) for activities such as walking, biking, and running.

No doubt the causes of obesity are complex and many causes may contribute to the problem in a single person. Given this complexity, it is obvious that there is no panacea for successful weight management. The top priority should be prevention, but where prevention has failed, the treatment of obesity represents a "crisis opportunity" for community dietitians to gain the public's attention by delivering effective health promotion and intervention programs.[94] See Chapter 8 for a detailed discussion of the obesity epidemic and descriptions of current public health policies, as well as proposed policies and legislation to prevent obesity and overweight.

Increasing Awareness of Environmental Nutrition Issues
Eat fresh. Eat local. It's Saturday morning in Anytown, USA, and in the center of the old "downtown" a large gathering of community members bustle around, chat, and enjoy their morning out.[95] These people are buying locally grown produce and goods from farmers in their community. Farmers' markets have existed in different forms for many years and have enjoyed excellent growth over the past decade. Through these markets, farmers are able to build a local clientele and reap profits without a middleman. Farmers' markets encourage healthier food choices by promoting fresh-picked seasonal fruit and vegetables. Additionally, less packaging is used. This creates less waste, which is good for the environment. Moreover, energy resources used to transport foods produced in more distant areas can be saved, thus helping to diminish the size of the region's ecological footprint.

Take the *Ecological Footprint Quiz* at *www.myfootprint.org* to estimate how much productive land and water you need to support what you use and what you discard. Communities as a whole benefit from farmers' markets because of the small investment and potential boost to their economies. Through farm-to-cafeteria programs in schools, colleges, hospitals, and corporations, and chef–farmer relationships in restaurants, a growing number of additional opportunities exist to buy and eat food that is locally produced as well.[96] For more information, see the Professional Focus feature in Chapter 10: Moving Toward Community Food Security.

Global Environmental Challenges for Public Health Many global environmental indicators affecting public health are now deteriorating.[97] These include climate change, depletion and degradation of topsoil, accelerated loss of species and of fresh water and sources of energy, and increased use of and persistence of many chemical pollutants. Recent and current modes of food production have made major contributions to these adverse environmental changes.[98] A diverse group of international scholars and food and nutrition experts have come together to work on a project titled New Nutrition Science; they argue that the field of nutrition—and particularly public health nutrition practice because of its work in developing food and nutrition policies—is necessarily involved with these environmental challenges facing the world.[99] Additional challenges exist as well. Global food insecurity has not significantly changed in the last 20 years. New epidemics of obesity, diabetes, and other chronic diseases including heart disease, osteoporosis, and certain types of cancer are now prevalent in both developed and developing countries and among high-, middle-, and low-income populations and communities. These diseases, all of which are related to nutrition, impose an enormous burden on today's health care systems.[100] The nutrition field can successfully address these challenges, but it can do so only by means of an integrated biological, social, and environmental approach (see the box that follows).

"How food is grown, processed, distributed, sold, prepared, cooked, and consumed is crucial to its quality and to its effect on well-being and health, society, and the environment."[101] The concepts of **sustainability** and **sustainable food systems** are gaining mainstream attention—with numerous groups encouraging consumers to increase their awareness of sustainability issues and how these apply to food systems and the health of communities—both locally and around the world. As a result, more and more people are embracing the personal, environmental, and public health benefits that come with sustainable food choices, and demand for more sustainably produced products (e.g., local and organic foods) is increasing.

Sustainability The capacity of being maintained over the long term in order to meet the needs of the present without jeopardizing the ability of future generations to meet their needs.[85]

Sustainable food systems A sustainable food system exists when production, processing, distribution, and consumption are integrated and related practices that regenerate rather than degrade natural resources, are socially just and accessible, and support the development of local communities and economies.[86]

Principles, Dimensions, and Purpose of the New Nutrition Science

The Giessen Declaration specifies the principles, dimensions, and purpose of a new nutrition science as follows:

- The overall principles that should guide nutrition science are ethical in nature. All principles should also be guided by the philosophies of co-responsibility and sustainability . . .
- The biological dimension should . . . be one of the three dimensions of nutrition science. The other two dimensions are social and environmental.
- Nutrition science is defined as the study of food systems, foods and drinks, and their nutrients and other constituents; and of their interactions within and between all relevant biological, social, and environmental systems.

- The purpose of nutrition science is to contribute to a world in which present and future generations fulfill their human potential, live in the best of health, and develop, sustain, and enjoy an increasingly diverse human, living, and physical environment.
- Nutrition science should be the basis for food and nutrition policies. These should be designed to identify, create, conserve, and protect rational, sustainable, and equitable communal, national, and global food systems to sustain the health, well-being, and integrity of humankind and of the living and physical worlds.

Source: "The Giessen Declaration," *Public Health Nutrition* 8 (2005): 783–86.

"It is the position of the Academy of Nutrition and Dietetics to encourage environmentally responsible practices that conserve natural resources, minimize the quantity of waste generated and support the ecological sustainability of the food system—the process of food production, transformation, distribution, access and consumption. . . . Conserving and protecting resources will contribute to the sustainability of the global food system now and in the future."[102] The Academy of Nutrition and Dietetics has published a primer for food and nutrition practitioners, stating that educating ourselves about the food system and sustainability is critical if we are to guide consumers toward making sustainable food choices.[103]

Watchwords for the Future

Several terms have surfaced repeatedly in this chapter: *change, innovation, creativity, community, entrepreneurship*. These watchwords herald the early decades of a century marked by unprecedented global social change. The world is growing smaller, and its peoples seem to be moving toward the birth of a single, global nation. "Citizen of the world," a phrase popular during the mid-twentieth century, takes on added meaning as we move forward in the twenty-first century. Where once a community was circumscribed by a distant ridge or the next valley, today the "information highway" links us via satellite and optic fibers to seen and unseen faces on the other side of the earth. The growing connectedness of the human race promises to create new challenges for community nutritionists in their efforts to enhance the nutrition and health of all peoples.

case study

Ethics and You

by Alice Fornari, EdD, RD, Alessandra Sarcona, MS, RD, CSSD, and Alison Barkman, MS, RD, CDN

Scenario

A dietetics student is placed in an urban community rotation as part of a field practicum that focuses on the nutritional needs of HIV clients. This city agency provides supportive services to the clients and also meals for clients who do not have assistance at home. This community practicum is a new exposure for the student in terms of the role of a nutritionist in an urban community setting. The many hats the nutritionist must wear in one day overwhelm her. The student attended a suburban private high school and a small, rural college. She always thought of community nutrition as cooperative extension agencies reaching out to the local community. This type of community-based service to a specific at-risk population is certainly eye-opening. Of course she has studied HIV in her clinical nutrition courses and understands the disease process and nutrition implications. However, the diversity of the staff and clients is a new experience. In addition, she is taken aback by the professional peer group at the agency: many are gay.

As part of her practicum, there are biweekly reports to the faculty coordinator and presentations to the other students. During the first presentation, the student makes disparaging remarks about the staff and clients, regarding sexual preference, past use of IV drugs by some clients, economic disadvantage, and the communal nature of HIV illness. Another student in the practicum class comments that her view seems provincial. The faculty coordinator encourages the student to be more open and to value the diversity of the placement and the professional challenges it entails.

The final evaluation completed by the site preceptor clearly indicates that the preceptor perceives a prejudice on the part of this student regarding HIV and the population affected. The student's self-evaluation indicates that she does not see her role as a nutritionist within this specialized practice setting.

Learning Outcomes

- Identify the three arenas of community nutrition practice.
- Recognize that a code of ethics developed by the Academy of Nutrition and Dietetics exists and is specific for the dietetics profession.
- Identify how a practice situation can violate or be supported by the Academy's Code of Ethics.

Foundation: Acquisition of Knowledge and Skills

1. Outline the three arenas of community nutrition practice presented in this case. Include a description of each arena specific to the type of community agency presented.
2. Identify the determinants of health (as defined here in Chapter 1) that may contribute to HIV in the agency population presented in this case.

3. Access the Code of Ethics by using the search function at *www.eatright.org/codeofethics* and the supporting narrative from the *Journal of the Academy of Nutrition and Dietetics*, 2009. The new version of the Code of Ethics also appears in Chapter 9's Professional Focus feature.

Step 1: *Identify Relevant Information and Uncertainties*

1. Why does the Code of Ethics of the Academy of Nutrition and Dietetics apply to the scenario? (All students enrolled in the practicum course are student members of the Academy.)
2. Under what circumstances would the Code of Ethics not apply?
3. Which characteristics of the student make her vulnerable to bias and violation of the Code?
4. Specifically, which principle(s) in the Code of Ethics applies (or apply) to the issue raised?

Step 2: *Interpret Information*

1. How can the preceptor and faculty coordinator help the student recognize that she is violating the Code?
2. Brainstorm characteristics of individuals that can contribute to personal biases and affect decision making and actions.

Step 3: *Draw and Implement Conclusions*

1. To ensure that this is a learning experience for the student, she is asked to communicate her understanding of the ethical issue to her peers. Indicate one way she could do this as part of the practicum class.

Step 4: *Engage in Continuous Improvement*

1. From a student perspective, suggest one or two strategies that will help the student and her peers in the practicum class to reflect on the values and ethical principles supported by the Code of Ethics.
2. Reflect on how working with a variety of populations can help dietitians become more competent as professionals. Develop a list of essential qualities dietitians need when working with diverse clients.

PROFESSIONAL **FOCUS**

Community-Based Dietetics Professionals

There are many steps that dietetics professionals who are interested in working in a community setting can take to achieve and maintain a successful career. And for professionals already established in a nonclinical setting, there are key points to focus on when working to keep a high caliber of community dietitians.

Karen Ensle

Longtime community dietitian Karen Ensle, EdD, RD, is a family and consumer sciences educator and department head for Rutgers Cooperative Extension of Union County in New Jersey. She has been an educator at the secondary and collegiate levels for 30 years, and her chosen career path has led her to develop and teach programs in nutrition and family resource management. She is a project investigator for her county's Supplemental Nutrition Assistance Program's Nutrition Education Program (SNAP-Ed), where she supervises several community dietetics professionals and other staff members. The program reaches over 4,000 youth and adults every year. Ensle is also in charge of the Union County Senior Meals Program.

Ensle says that one key to success in community dietetics is to follow the old adage, "Know thyself." (For more on this topic, see the Professional Focus feature "Getting Where You Want to Go" in Chapter 4.) Professionals interested in working outside the clinical setting need to be flexible self-starters who are comfortable creating their own schedules and cooperating with many different types of people. On any given day, Ensle's job may take her from putting on a PowerPoint presentation for a local group of senior citizens to working with children in an inner-city school. "You have to be a very independent person with good people skills," says Ensle. "You've got to piece together ideas and look at the big picture—not micromanage."

Strong advocacy skills are also important. Ensle's SNAP-Ed program is funded by a $539,000 grant. Community dietetics professionals must be comfortable seeking and lobbying for funding on both the federal and state levels. Ensle says the public policy workshop offered annually by the Academy of Nutrition and Dietetics is so beneficial in this area that it should be required.

Christine McCullum

But for community nutrition practitioners to make an impact, their numbers have to be strong. Echoing Ensle's concerns is Christine McCullum-Gómez, PhD, RD, a food and nutrition consultant in Houston, Texas. In the past, she worked on a strategic plan for the prevention and treatment of overweight children in Houston and Harris County, Texas, which was carried out under the auspices of St. Luke's Episcopal Health Charities.

"I think it's important to have the people who are overseeing the future of dietetics understand the importance of marketing the profession," says McCullum-Gómez. "There's a tendency to market dietetics as a primarily clinically based occupation. In the future, we're going to have to do a better job of marketing a broader range of job opportunities, including those that are community based."

Like many food and nutrition practitioners, when she began her training Christine says she assumed she would enter the clinical arena. But after earning her master's degree in nutrition, she says she was drawn to the idea of policy work and prevention. Helping create the strategic plan for the prevention and treatment of overweight children was particularly enjoyable because it enabled her to connect her academic research to a community-building process. "It gives me a lot of energy," she says. "It keeps you in tune with the needs of people who live in underserved communities."

McCullum-Gómez says that current community nutrition practitioners can help recruit future colleagues by taking on an active role as a mentor in the dietetics community as well as the broader community. That may include everything from attending a high school career day to encouraging promising young food and nutrition practitioners to consider doing an internship or taking a full-time position with a community-based organization.

She also adds that future practitioners who may be interested in working with the community should take sociology and political science courses or classes that teach communication and negotiation skills while they are still in school, along with their required biomedical and health science courses. They might also consider participating in a community service project. These experiences can benefit them later on, especially when working with a diverse group of people.

Because the country is becoming so ethnically diverse, being able to work with all kinds of populations is going to be key, says Karen Ensle, who adds that recruiting minorities to the profession is very important. Ensle recently worked with one intern of Sioux descent who created a food wheel that took into consideration the diet of her native people. The wheel was later presented at a U.S. Department of Agriculture (USDA) conference.

Tracy Fox

Although it is important to recruit new dietitians into the community setting, many practitioners who started out in a clinical setting have successfully navigated the transition into a nonclinical one. One such professional is Tracy Fox, MPH, RD. Fox began her career in the United States Navy, doing outpatient work in naval hospitals for five years. As much as she enjoyed her clinical experience, she says her transition into the policy work that followed felt like a "natural progression." She simply found it compelling, so after her clinical experience she took an entirely different path, taking a job doing policy and analysis work for the Food and Nutrition Service (FNS) of the USDA, where she helped develop and implement major school lunch regulations and served in other positions at FNS.

From there, she went to work for the Government Relations office of the Academy of Nutrition and Dietetics in Washington, D.C., where she was responsible for regulatory affairs and helped define the association's position on a range of topics, including child nutrition, dietary supplements and functional foods, food safety, and food labeling.

Her experience led her to believe that undergraduates preparing to enter the field need to learn more about policy work. Agreeing with Ensle, Fox says it would be a terrific idea if all food and nutrition practitioners, especially those just starting out, understood more about lobbying and whom they need to reach to influence change.

Fox says her diverse employment history helped prepare her to start her own consulting company that focuses on nutrition policy. Like many who choose a nonclinical setting, she found the flexible nature of the job appealing, along with the work itself. But that first year, Fox had a lot to learn about setting up her own business. She took a course specifically geared toward women starting their own companies and learned the nuts and bolts of certain important issues, such as how to market herself and how to bill clients.

During her first year of self-employment, Fox cast her potential client net far and wide by getting involved in her local community. She did everything from volunteering for her county's school health council to joining task forces of the Academy of Nutrition and Dietetics. Her past employment history also generated work. "My initial clients came from other jobs," says Fox. "Don't burn any bridges. You are marketing yourself any time you talk to someone."

Currently, as president of Food, Nutrition & Policy Consultants, Fox utilizes her extensive experience in federal nutrition policy and the legislative and regulatory process. Her clients include federal, state, and local agencies, such as the U.S. Department of Agriculture and the Centers for Disease Control and Prevention; nonprofit organizations, such as the Produce for Better Health Foundation and the Action for Healthy Kids Foundation; and public relations firms, where she provides advice and expertise on policy and nutrition initiatives. Most recently, she has been selected to serve on the Institute of Medicine's Committee on Childhood Obesity Prevention Actions for Local Governments.

Nancy Clark

Nancy Clark, MS, RD, an internationally known sports nutritionist and nutrition author, specializes in nutrition for exercise, health, and the nutritional management of eating disorders. Clark has a successful private practice in which she counsels casual exercisers and competitive athletes.

Along with acquiring marketing skills, she recommends getting a strong clinical background (i.e., working for two years in a clinical setting); the experience will be invaluable for an aspiring community and/or sports nutritionist who will be dealing with heart disease, cancer, pregnancy, diabetes, hypertension, and a myriad of health conditions. Although she had little interest in hospital dietetics, Clark saw the importance of developing a strong clinical background, so she worked for two years in a hospital environment. She then worked with the New England Dairy and Food Council as a nutrition education consultant. Concurrent with her personal interests in hiking, biking, and other outdoor sports activities, she recognized a professional interest in counseling people active in sports. She next completed a master's degree in nutrition, with a special focus on exercise physiology.

In addition to individually counseling fitness exercisers and competitive athletes, Clark gives talks to local high school and college teams and sports clubs, presents workshops for health professionals, and writes sports nutrition articles. She also has created several teaching tools for food and nutrition practitioners throughout the country and has written two popular books with information for the serious athlete or the active person who wants to eat optimally for health and energy.

For Ensle, McCullum-Gómez, Fox, Clark, and others like them, working outside the traditional model of a clinically based practitioner has been rewarding both personally and professionally. They hope that their career paths inspire others in the field to consider community dietetics. "The whole training process and mindset needs to shift," says Ensle. "We need to stimulate interest in this in young people. It's critical for the profession."

Sources: Adapted from Jennifer Mathieu, "Community-Based Dietetics Professionals," *Journal of the American Dietetic Association* 103 (2003): 1126–27; and personal communication with Chris McCullum, Tracy Fox, and Nancy Clark, *www.nancyclarkrd.com*.

CHAPTER SUMMARY

The Concept of Community

▶ A community is a group of people who are located in a particular space, have shared values, and interact within a social system. A community has four components: people, a location in space (which can include the realm of cyberspace), social interaction, and shared values.

▶ Community nutrition is a discipline that strives to prevent disease and to improve the health, nutrition, and well-being of individuals and groups within communities. Its practitioners develop policies and programs that help people improve their eating patterns and health. Three arenas—people, policy, and programs—are the focus of community nutrition.

▶ The World Health Organization defines health as a state of complete physical, mental, and social well-being, not merely the absence of disease.

▶ Health promotion is the process of enabling people to achieve their maximum potential for good health. An intervention is a health promotion activity aimed at changing the behavior of a target audience.

▶ There are three types of prevention efforts:

- Primary prevention is aimed at preventing disease by controlling risk factors that are related to disease.
- Secondary prevention focuses on detecting disease early through screening and other forms of risk appraisal.
- Tertiary prevention aims to treat and rehabilitate people who have experienced an illness or injury.

▶ Although traditionally, much emphasis was placed on strategies to change nutrition and health-related behaviors by focusing on individual-level factors such as knowledge and skills, more recent interventions focus on the contribution of environmental factors to the development of chronic diseases. The social–ecological model (SEM) emphasizes multiple levels of influence (such as individual, interpersonal, organizational, community, and public policy) and the idea that all elements of society combine to shape an individual's food and physical activity choices or other health behaviors, and ultimately one's chronic disease risk.

▶ *Healthy People* is a set of goals and objectives with 10-year targets designed to guide national health promotion and disease prevention efforts. *Healthy People 2020* redirects our attention from health care to prevention and the determinants of health in our social and physical environments.

Community Nutrition Practice

▶ Public health and community nutritionists plan and evaluate food and nutrition programs; develop food and nutrition policies; plan, implement, and evaluate health promotion and disease prevention programs; and provide nutrition services to all age groups in a community setting. They work in a variety of practice settings at the local, state, national, and international levels.

▶ In most states, dietetics practitioners are licensed to ensure that only qualified, trained professionals provide nutrition services or advice to individuals requiring or seeking nutrition counseling or information. Licensure is designed to protect the public, control malpractice, and ensure minimum standards of practice.

Entrepreneurship in Community Nutrition

▶ Community nutritionists who want to change people's eating habits must be able to see new ways of reaching desired target groups. The twin stanchions of entrepreneurship—creativity and innovation—assist the community nutritionist in achieving the broad goal of improved health for all.

▶ Entrepreneurs are change agents who seek, recognize, and act on opportunities. Intrapreneurs seek to better the existing state of affairs within their organizations through creative problem solving.

Social and Economic Trends for Community Nutrition

▶ Recent social and economic trends have important consequences for community nutrition. The demographic profile of many communities is changing rapidly, along with the client mix served by community nutritionists.

▶ Leading indicators of change include a worldwide increase in the educational level of the workforce; an aging population; generational diversity; increasing demands for nutrition and health care services; increasing ethnic diversity and health disparities; challenges associated with the increasing prevalence of obesity and diabetes among children and adults; and an increasing awareness of environmental nutrition issues and how these apply to the health of communities—both locally and around the world.

SUMMARY **QUESTIONS**

1. Describe the three arenas of community nutrition practice.
2. Define "health" based on the World Health Organization definition.
3. Describe and give an example of the three types of prevention to promote health and prevent disease.
4. Review the determinants of health listed in Table 1-2. For each category (e.g., Biology and Genetics, Lifestyle, and so on), list one factor that could have a positive impact on health and one factor that could have a negative impact on health.
5. Choose a health behavior or chronic health condition of your choice, and describe the multiple levels of influence that may contribute to the behavior or condition based on the social–ecological model described in this chapter.
6. List the overarching goals for the *Healthy People 2020* initiative.
7. Outline the educational requirements, practice settings, and roles and responsibilities of community nutritionists.
8. Describe the personality characteristics of the entrepreneur/intrapreneur.
9. Consider the social and economic trends presented at the end of this chapter. What types of skills do community nutritionists need for working well in the current context?

INTERNET **RESOURCES**

Check out these Internet addresses for resources relevant to community nutrition and public health.

Professional Organizations

Academy of Nutrition and Dietetics
www.eatright.org

American Public Health Association
www.apha.org

Society for Nutrition Education and Behavior
www.sneb.org

Canadian Public Health Association
www.cpha.ca

Dietitians of Canada
www.dietitians.ca

Health Organizations

Food and Agriculture Organization of the United Nations
www.fao.org

Pan American Health Organization
www.paho.org

World Health Organization
www.who.int

Canadian Government Agencies

Canadian Food Inspection Agency
www.inspection.gc.ca

Health Canada
www.hc-sc.gc.ca

U.S. Government Agencies and Other Sites

Centers for Disease Control and Prevention
www.cdc.gov

Department of Health and Human Services
www.hhs.gov

Food and Drug Administration
www.fda.gov

Food and Nutrition Information Center
http://fnic.nal.usda.gov

Healthy People 2020
www.healthypeople.gov

National Center for Chronic Disease Prevention
www.cdc.gov/chronicdisease/index.htm

National Institutes of Health
www.nih.gov

National Library of Medicine Databases
www.nlm.nih.gov/databases/index.html

Office of Minority Health
www.minorityhealth.hhs.gov

Consumer Health Sites

Healthfinder
http://healthfinder.gov

Kids Health
http://kidshealth.org

Medline Plus
www.nlm.nih.gov/medlineplus

National Health Information Center
http://health.gov/nhic

Consumer Health Information
www.nih.gov/health-information

Gateway to Nutrition Information from U.S. Government
www.nutrition.gov

CHAPTER 2

Principles of Epidemiology

LEARNING **OBJECTIVES**

After you have read and studied this chapter, you will be able to:

- Define epidemiology.
- Describe various vital statistics used by epidemiologists to monitor a population's health status.
- Explain prevalence rates and how they differ from incidence rates.
- Describe the strengths and weaknesses of various types of epidemiologic studies.
- Explain why the day-to-day variation in an individual's nutrient intake can have important

implications for nutritional epidemiologic studies.

- List the advantages and disadvantages of various dietary assessment methods.

This chapter addresses such issues as research methodologies, the scientific method, interpreting current research, collecting pertinent information for nutrition assessments, and current information technologies that have been designated by the Accreditation Council for Education in Nutrition and Dietetics (ACEND) as Foundation Knowledge and Learning Outcomes for dietetics education.

CHAPTER **OUTLINE**

Something to think about...

"The argument that we should wait for certainty [in making public health recommendations] is an argument for never taking action—we shall never be certain."

—*M. G. MARMOT*

For a complete list of references, please access the MindTap Reader within your MindTap course.

Introduction

In 1855, Dr. John Snow of London wrote an account of his discovery of the link between contaminated water and a local outbreak of cholera, one of the greatest scourges of modern times. Snow observed that people who had drunk water from a pump on Broad Street in central London were attacked by the disease. He formulated a hypothesis about the mode of cholera transmission, suggesting that the intestinal discharges of people sick with cholera were seeping into the Thames River—the source of Broad Street drinking water—and were turning it into a cesspool. To test his hypothesis, he tracked down cholera cases and interviewed family members about their source of drinking water. He identified common events that linked cholera patients and established the ways in which they differed from healthy individuals in the same neighborhood. Snow observed that the rate of cholera was significantly lower in communities consuming water drawn from the Thames River upstream, which he therefore presumed was uncontaminated. His recommendation for stopping the cholera epidemic was simple: Remove the handle from the Broad Street pump so that it could not be used. Medical publishers were so skeptical of Snow's theory that he was forced to publish the particulars of his discovery at his own expense.[1]

Snow described the mode of transmission of this dreaded infection nearly 30 years before the cholera bacterium, *Vibrio cholerae*, was discovered. Thanks in part to Snow's careful observations, London took a major step toward controlling cholera epidemics

John Snow (1813–1858) is considered one of the founders of epidemiology for his work identifying the source of a London cholera outbreak in 1854. At the time, it was assumed that cholera was airborne. However, Snow argued that the mode of transmission was through the mouth. After careful investigation, including plotting cases of cholera on the dot map of the area shown here, Snow was able to identify a water pump in Broad Street as the source of the disease. Note that nearly all the clusters of deaths had taken place within a short distance of the Broad Street pump. Although there were a few deaths in houses situated decidedly nearer to another street-pump, Snow's investigation revealed that these individuals preferred the water from the Broad Street pump to that of the pump nearer to their homes.

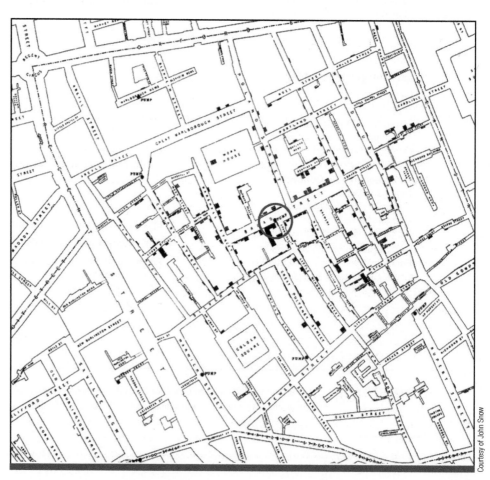

Courtesy of John Snow

and improving the public's health by installing new water supply systems. This story is an example of how the classic epidemiologic method was applied to determining the cause and course of a disease outbreak. In fact, the word **epidemiology** is derived from *epidemic*, which, translated from the Greek, means "upon the people." As this derivation indicates, the epidemiologic method was initially used to investigate, control, and prevent epidemics of infectious diseases such as cholera, plague, smallpox, typhoid, tuberculosis, and poliomyelitis. Although investigating infectious disease outbreaks is still part of epidemiology, today it is also applied to the study of injuries, especially those occurring in the home and at work; chronic diseases such as cancer, coronary heart disease, and arthritis; and social problems such as teenage pregnancies, homicide, alcoholism, and cocaine abuse. The primary reason for investigating and analyzing these health problems is to work toward controlling and preventing them, typically through the formulation of specific health policies.

> **Epidemiology** From the Greek word meaning "upon the people"; the study of epidemics; the basic science of public health; "the study of the distribution and determinants of health-related states in specified populations, and the application of this study to control health problems."

The Practice of Epidemiology

The discipline of epidemiology has expanded from its origin as the study of epidemics to include the control and prevention of all types of health problems. It is similar to clinical medicine and laboratory science in its concern with understanding the processes of health and disease in humans, but it differs from these disciplines in its focus on the health problems of populations rather than of individual patients. A panel of international experts offers the following definition of epidemiology:[2]

> Epidemiology is the study of the distribution and determinants of health-related states and events in specified populations and the application of this study to the control of health problems.

This definition requires some explanation. The term *distribution* refers to the relationship between the health problem or disease and the population in which it exists. The distribution includes the persons affected and the place and time of the occurrence. It also encompasses such population parameters as age, sex, race, occupation, income and educational levels, exposure to certain agents, and other social and environmental features. Distribution is concerned with population trends or patterns of disease or exposure to a specific agent among groups of people.

The term *determinants* refers to the causes and factors that affect the risk of disease. Infectious diseases have a single, necessary cause. Shigellosis, for example, is an infection of the bowel caused by *Shigella* organisms. Rubella, or German measles, is a highly contagious disease caused by a virus spread by airborne droplets or close contact. Many conditions, however, have multiple determinants, as in the contribution of gender, race, dietary intake, and hormonal status to osteoporosis. Determinants of disease are typically divided into two groups: (1) host factors, such as age, sex, race, genetic makeup, nutrition status, and physiologic state, which determine an individual's susceptibility to disease; and (2) environmental factors, such as living conditions, occupation, geographical location, and lifestyle, which determine the host's exposure to a specific agent.

Investigating Causes of Diseases

Whereas the clinician is concerned with an individual patient and with the host and environmental factors that affect that patient's health status, the epidemiologist is concerned with groups of individuals or populations. The epidemiologist measures or counts those elements that are common to individuals, so that the magnitude and

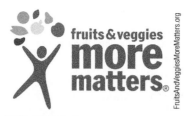

FruitsAndVeggiesMoreMatters.org

FIGURE 2-1

The Fruits & Veggies—More Matters® initiative is focused on helping Americans increase fruit and vegetable consumption for better health. This public health initiative is spearheaded by the Produce for Better Health Foundation, which partners with the CDC to help communicate the health benefits of adding more fruits and vegetables to the diet.

Fetal alcohol spectrum disorder (FASD) A broad range of birth defects and developmental disabilities caused by prenatal alcohol exposure. The following are the disorders under the FASD category:
• Fetal alcohol syndrome (FAS)—This diagnosis requires a characteristic pattern of facial abnormalities, growth deficits, and central nervous system abnormalities.
• Partial FAS—includes some signs and symptoms of FAS but not all three of the characteristics noted above.
• Alcohol-related birth defects (ARBD)—includes alcohol-related physical abnormalities.
• Alcohol-related neurodevelopmental disorder (ARND)—includes central nervous system abnormalities, as well as cognitive and behavioral problems.

effects of individual variation within a population can be accounted for in studying a disease process. Differences in rates of disease in populations are then used to formulate hypotheses about the cause of a health problem or to assess exposure to a specific agent. Working closely with clinicians, laboratory scientists, biostatisticians, and other health professionals, the epidemiologist works to identify the causes of disease and to propose strategies for controlling or preventing health problems.

For example, in the 1990s, epidemiologic studies established that women could reduce their risk of bearing a child with a neural tube birth defect such as spina bifida by increasing their intake of folic acid.[3] Consequently, the Food and Drug Administration now mandates that grain products be fortified with folic acid to improve intakes in the United States. Epidemiologic studies have also associated low intakes of fruits and vegetables with increased risks of some types of cancer. Although the mechanisms by which these foods may protect against cancer are not completely known, the epidemiologic evidence provides a reasonable basis for action. As a result, both the National Cancer Institute's National Fruit and Vegetable program and the Fruits & Veggies—More Matters® initiative urge consumers to eat five to nine servings (or more) of fruits and vegetables rich in fiber, vitamins, minerals, antioxidants, and phytochemicals every day to help protect against cancer (**Figure 2-1**).

Examining a Community's Health Status In addition to enhancing our understanding of health and disease and searching for the causes of disease, epidemiology has several other uses. The epidemiologic method can be used to describe a community's particular health problems and to determine whether a community's overall health is improving or getting worse. Diagnosing a community's health problems is important to health agencies. The public health department, for example, may need to know whether the number of low-birthweight infants born within the community decreased, increased, or remained the same compared with the previous year. The agency may want to compare the community's current rate of births of underweight infants with the rate from the previous decade or with the state or national average. This information can be used to evaluate the agency's current programs and services and thereby determine whether they are meeting the health needs of pregnant women in the community. Potential health problems may also be spotted through this ongoing examination of a community's health status. For example, in the early 1980s an unusual illness was observed mostly among gay men living in San Francisco, Los Angeles, and New York. The finding of an unusually high number of cases of Kaposi's sarcoma, a rare cancer affecting primarily middle-aged men of Jewish or Italian ancestry, led to the discovery of the acquired immunodeficiency syndrome (AIDS). Chapter 4 provides a detailed discussion on the assessment of a community's health status.

Surveillance and Related Activities Alcohol consumption among pregnant women is a public health concern, as prenatal alcohol exposure is a leading preventable cause of birth defects and developmental disabilities in the United States.[4] Over the past decade, epidemiologic data have been used to develop surveillance methods for identifying women at high risk for giving birth to a child with **fetal alcohol spectrum disorder (FASD)** and to design and implement prevention activities.[5] In order to characterize trends in alcohol use among women of childbearing age, the Centers for Disease Control and Prevention (CDC) analyzed representative survey data from the Behavioral Risk

Factor Surveillance System (BRFSS) from 1991 to 2010. The rate of any alcohol use (e.g., at least one drink) during pregnancy has declined since 1995. However, rates of binge drinking (e.g., four or more drinks on any one occasion) during pregnancy have not declined and remain higher than the *Healthy People 2020* objective.[6] Additionally, the frequency and intensity of binge drinking (e.g., approximately three times per month and six drinks on an occasion) have not declined among nonpregnant women of childbearing age who may become pregnant. **Figure 2-2** illustrates findings from the BRFSS examining alcohol use and binge drinking among pregnant and nonpregnant women of childbearing age (18–44 years) in the United States. Prevalence estimates for any alcohol use in the past 30 days during 2006–2010 were 7.6% among pregnant women and 51.5% among nonpregnant women. The prevalence estimates for binge drinking in the past 30 days were 1.4% among pregnant women and 15.0% among nonpregnant women. Greater binge-drinking prevalence was observed among younger women, non-Hispanic whites, and unmarried women.[7] As a result of these findings, and to ensure more uniform dissemination of prenatal alcohol prevention messages, the CDC is conducting targeted media campaigns to increase public awareness of the adverse effects of alcohol use during pregnancy among diverse geographical, racial, and ethnic populations and among younger women (**Figure 2-3**). Public health interventions, such as alcohol screening and brief interventions and community-level policy interventions (e.g., increasing alcohol excise taxes) may also help reduce alcohol misuse by pregnant and nonpregnant women of childbearing age.[8]

Based on the **vital statistics** (such as age at death and cause of death) recorded on death certificates, the epidemiologic method can also be used to calculate an individual's risk of dying before a certain age. **Table 2-1** provides indices commonly used in determining key types of vital statistics. This type of risk assessment is the foundation of the actuarial

Vital statistics Figures pertaining to life events, such as births, deaths, and marriages.

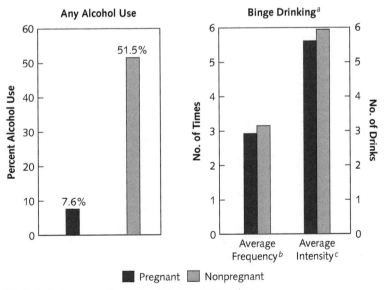

Any Alcohol Use

Binge Drinking[a]

a Defined as having consumed four or more drinks on an occasion at least one time in the past 30 days.
b Number of times respondent reported consuming four or more drinks on an occasion in the past 30 days.
c Largest number of drinks consumed on an occasion in the past 30 days.

FIGURE 2-2

Percentage of Women, Aged 18 to 44 Years, Who Reported Alcohol Use, United States, 2006–2010
Prenatal exposure to alcohol is one of the leading preventable causes of mental retardation in the United States. One of the *Healthy People 2020* national health objectives is to increase from 89% (2007–2008) to 98% the percentage of pregnant women abstaining from alcohol use.
Source: CDC

FIGURE 2-3 Tools to Help Spread the Word: Pregnancy and Alcohol Don't Mix.

Targeted ads can be used in a health organization's newsletter or magazine to help raise awareness about alcohol use during pregnancy and fetal alcohol spectrum disorders (FASDs). FASDs are completely preventable if a woman does not drink alcohol during pregnancy. All women of childbearing age should be informed of the adverse effects of alcohol use in order to avert early prenatal exposure before women become aware of pregnancy. Additional information about CDC's activities to prevent alcohol-exposed pregnancies is available at *www.cdc.gov/fasd*.
Source: CDC

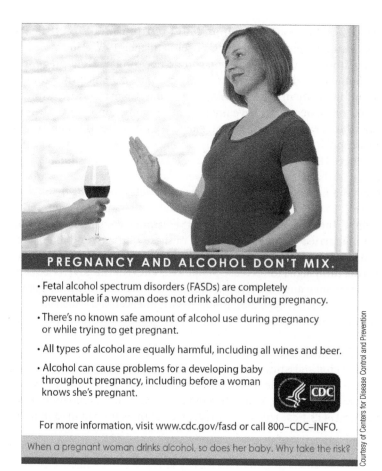

TABLE 2-1 Vital Statistics: Equations for Commonly Used Population Data

1. Crude birth rate[a] $= \dfrac{\text{Number of live births during year}}{\text{Average (midyear) population}} \times 1{,}000$

2. Crude death rate[a] $= \dfrac{\text{Number of deaths during year}}{\text{Average (midyear) population}} \times 1{,}000$

3. Age-specific death rate $= \dfrac{\text{Number of deaths to people in a particular age group}}{\text{Average (midyear) population in specified age group}} \times 1{,}000$

4. Cause-specific death rate $= \dfrac{\text{Number of deaths due to a particular cause during year}}{\text{Average (midyear) population}} \times 1{,}000$

5. Infant mortality rate $= \dfrac{\text{Number of deaths to infants} < 1 \text{ year during year}}{\text{Number of live births in same year}} \times 1{,}000$

6. Neonatal mortality rate $= \dfrac{\text{Number of deaths to infants} < 28 \text{ days during year}}{\text{Number of live births in same year}} \times 1{,}000$

7. Fetal death rate $= \dfrac{\text{Number of fetal deaths} (> 20 \text{ weeks gestation}) \text{ during year}}{\text{Number of live births and fetal deaths in same year}} \times 1{,}000$

8. Maternal mortality rate $= \dfrac{\text{Number of pregnancy-related deaths during year}}{\text{Number of live births in same year}} \times 100{,}000$

[a] In general, *crude rates* apply to an entire population and are not useful for comparisons because population characteristics may differ greatly, particularly with respect to age.

Source: Adapted from CDC; available at *www.cdc.gov/nchs/nvss.htm*.

tables developed by life insurance companies. A related use occurs in clinical decision making when, for example, a particular drug or surgical intervention is evaluated for its effectiveness in treating a certain condition and for its association with side effects or other health risks. Sometimes the epidemiologic method is used to identify the characteristics of a disease and determine whether some syndromes are related to one another or represent distinct conditions. A good example of this use was the development of a working case definition that outlined the clinical, behavioral, and physiological manifestations of chronic fatigue syndrome.[9]

Basic Epidemiologic Concepts

To put it simply, "the basic operation of the epidemiologist is to count cases and measure the population in which they arise" in order to calculate rates of occurrence of a health problem and compare the rates in different groups of people.[10] This section presents key epidemiologic concepts that illustrate how data about disease processes are obtained and analyzed.

Rates and Risks

A middle-aged woman is admitted to the emergency room, complaining of chest pain, nausea, and dizziness. The attending physician orders a diagnostic workup, which confirms that the woman has had a heart attack. For the emergency room physician, this woman is a patient requiring immediate critical care. For the epidemiologist studying the factors that contribute to coronary heart disease, this woman is a **case**—a single individual with a confirmed diagnosis of myocardial infarction. The physician and the epidemiologist share a common concern about this woman: her risk status. Does she possess certain characteristics that placed her at high risk for heart attacks? If so, can these characteristics be modified to reduce her chance of having another? If the woman does not appear to belong in a high-risk group, why did she have a heart attack at this particular time?

In epidemiology, **risk** refers to the likelihood that people who are without a disease, but are exposed to certain **risk factors**, will acquire the disease at some point in their lives.[11] These risk factors may be inherited. Others are found in the physical environment in the form of infectious agents, toxins, or drugs. Some risk factors are derived from the social environment—that is, the family, community, or culture. Others are behavioral, such as not wearing seat belts, smoking, or gaining excess weight.

The *relative risk (RR)* is a comparison of the risk of some health-related event, such as disease or death, in two groups. The two groups might be differentiated by gender, age, or exposure to a suspected risk factor (e.g., tobacco or high dietary intake of saturated fat). The risk for disease or death will be greater in the exposed group if an exposure is harmful (as in the case of a diet high in saturated fat) or will be smaller if an exposure is protective (as in the case of a diet high in soluble fiber).

If the relative risk is greater than 1, people exposed to the factor have an increased risk of the outcome under investigation.[12] If the relative risk is less than 1, people exposed to the factor have a decreased risk of the outcome. For example, in a Spanish study of bladder cancer, subjects with high intake of saturated fat had a relative risk of 2.25, meaning they had more than double the risk of developing bladder cancer than those with low intake of saturated fat had. In an Italian study of colorectal cancer, subjects with high intakes of beta-carotene had a relative risk of 0.38, which means that they had about one-third the risk of developing colorectal cancer compared to those

Case A particular instance of a disease or outcome of interest.

Risk The probability or likelihood of an event occurring—in this case, the probability that people will acquire a disease.

Risk factors Clinically important signs associated with an increased likelihood of acquiring a disease.

A general formula for relative risk is as follows:

$$\text{Relative risk}^* = \frac{\text{Risk of disease or death for exposed persons}}{\text{Risk of disease or death for unexposed persons}}$$

* If RR = 1.0, there is no association; the risk in the exposed group and that in the unexposed group are the same.

If RR > 1.0, the exposed group is at greater risk of dying than the unexposed group. If RR > 1, it has a direct relationship with the disease and poses a risk for the subject. The farther away from 1 the RR, the stronger the association.

If RR < 1.0, the exposed group has smaller risk than the unexposed group—possibly because of a protective effect from the "exposure." A RR of 0.82 means an inverse relationship between disease and exposure. In other words, it is protective.

with low beta-carotene intakes. Relative risks can be used to compare the strengths of different associations. The relative risk of lung cancer in people with low fruit and vegetable intake compared to those with high intake is about 2.0. The relative risk of lung cancer in smokers compared to nonsmokers is at least 10.0. Clearly, the association of cancer with smoking is stronger than its association with low intake of fruits and vegetables.

Some of us are exposed to certain risk factors more than other individuals are.[13] For example, workers in photographic laboratories, dry-cleaning establishments, and some industrial processing plants are exposed daily to chloroform, a highly volatile liquid that has been shown to cause tumors in mice and rats. Workers in office buildings and schools are typically not exposed to chloroform. These different rates of exposure to a risk factor (in this case, chloroform) allow for basic comparisons of disease rates among individuals. One expression of how frequently a disease occurs in a population is **incidence**, the fraction or proportion of a group initially free of a disease or condition that develops the disease or condition over a period of time. Incidence is measured by a two-step process:

> **Incidence** The number of *new* cases of a disease during a specific time period in a defined population.

1. Identify a group of susceptible people who are initially free of the disease or condition.

2. Examine them periodically over a period of time to discover and count the new cases of the disease that develop during that interval.

> **Prevalence** The number of *existing* cases of a disease or other condition in a given population. *Point prevalence* is the amount of a particular disease present in a population at a particular point in time—usually the time a survey was done. *Period prevalence* is the amount of a particular disease in a population over a period of time. The *prevalence rate* is the proportion (usually the percentage) of persons in a population who have a particular disease or attribute at a particular point in time.

Another common measure of frequency of occurrence of an event is **prevalence**, or the fraction or proportion of a group possessing a disease or condition at a specific time. The prevalence rate is measured by a single examination or survey of a group. The characteristics of these two measures are summarized in **Table 2-2**. Incidence and prevalence rates describe the frequency with which particular events occur. By calculating and comparing rates, epidemiologists can determine the strength of the association between risk factors and the health problem being studied.

The Epidemiologic Method

In its study of disease processes, epidemiology uses a variety of tools: clinical, microbiological, pathological, demographic, sociological, and statistical. None of these is exclusive to epidemiology, but the manner in which they are used uniquely defines the epidemiologic

TABLE 2-2

Characteristics of Incidence Rates and Prevalence Rates

RATE	NUMERATOR	DENOMINATOR	TIME	HOW MEASURED
Incidence	New cases occurring during the follow-up period in a group initially free of the disease	All susceptible individuals present at the beginning of the follow-up period (often called the population at risk)	Duration of the follow-up period	Cohort study
Prevalence	All cases counted in a single survey or examination of a group	All individuals examined, including cases and noncases	Single point in time	Prevalence or cross-sectional study

Source: R. H. Fletcher, S. W. Fletcher, and G. S. Fletcher, *Clinical Epidemiology—The Essentials*, 5th ed.

method. The following example uses the investigation of the "diet–heart" hypothesis to illustrate the rigorous, scientific approach of the epidemiologist:

1. **Observing.** Many years of investigation had shown that atherosclerosis could be induced in laboratory animals, particularly rabbits and monkeys, by feeding them a diet rich in fats and cholesterol. Physicians working in India, Africa, and Latin America also observed that coronary heart disease (CHD) was fairly rare in human populations whose diet tended to be high in vegetables and grains.[14]

2. **Counting cases or events.** Vital statistics obtained from the World Health Organization showed marked differences in deaths from CHD among countries, with Finland having one of the highest and Greece and Japan among the lowest CHD death rates, as shown graphically in **Figure 2-4**. The habitual diets of the peoples in these countries differed as well.

3. **Relating cases or events to the population at risk.** Public health officials in the United States became increasingly concerned about the number of deaths attributable to CHD, which was (and remains) the leading cause of death in the U.S. population. Identifying the risk factors for CHD became a public health priority.

4. **Making comparisons.** One of the first large population studies to examine the relationship between blood cholesterol levels and risk of CHD was the Seven Countries Study.[15] This project was undertaken in the late 1950s to examine the effects of differences in lifestyle, culture, diet, and general health habits on risk factors such as serum cholesterol levels, morbidity, and mortality from CHD. Sixteen population groups, involving about 11,000 men aged 40 to 59 years, were studied in seven countries that had reliable census data and well-organized medical systems: Greece, the Netherlands, Yugoslavia, Italy, Japan, the United States, and Finland. The **cohort** of adult men was followed for 10 years. One of the main study findings, shown in **Figure 2-5**, was that the population risk of CHD death, after adjusting for age, rose in a stepwise manner with increasing total blood cholesterol level. In addition, an analysis of dietary intakes of the

Cohort A well-defined group of people who are studied over a period of time to determine their incidence of disease, injury, or death.

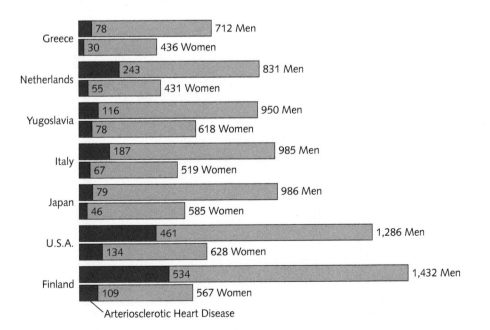

FIGURE 2-4 Deaths per 100,000 in 1965 from CHD and from All Causes for Ages 35 to 64 Years (age-standardized)
Source: A. Keys, "Coronary Heart Disease in Seven Countries," *Circulation* 41 and 42 (Supplement 1): 1–4. Copyright © 1970 by Lippincott, Williams, & Wilkins. Reprinted by permission.

FIGURE 2-5 Total Blood Cholesterol and CHD Deaths in Men (*Note:* A recent analysis of 30-year follow-up data revealed that longevity in men aged 50 years or more was not related to serum cholesterol in any of the cohorts, indicating the importance of factors other than those related to cholesterol. —Ancel Keys, personal communication)

Source: Reprinted by permission of the publishers from *Seven Countries: A Multivariate Analysis of Death and Coronary Heart Disease* by Ancel Keys. Cambridge, MA: Harvard University Press. Copyright © 1980 by the President and Fellows of Harvard College.

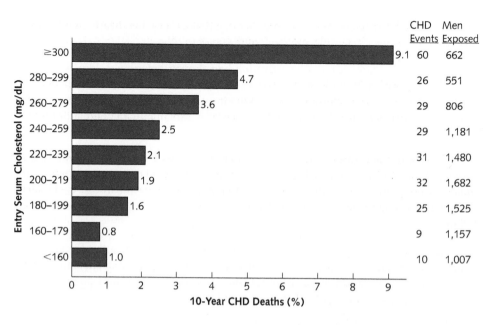

study population showed that the serum cholesterol level increased progressively as the level of saturated fat in the diet rose.

Figure 2-6 shows that Finland, with the highest reported intake of saturated fat (expressed as a percentage of total calories), had the highest mean population serum cholesterol level (about 260 mg/dL). (*Note:* The *r* value in the upper left-hand corner is the correlation coefficient. The correlation coefficient is a number between −1 and +1 that is used to quantify the strength of an association between two variables—in this case, dietary saturated fat and serum cholesterol level. The stronger the relationship of the two variables, the closer *r* is to 1; the weaker the relationship, the closer *r* is to 0. An *r* value of 0.89 means that although dietary saturated fat intake is strongly correlated with serum

FIGURE 2-6 Median Serum Cholesterol Values of the Seven Countries Cohort Plotted versus the Percentage of Total Calories from Saturated Fat

Source: A. Keys, "Coronary Heart Disease in Seven Countries," *Circulation* 41 and 42 (Supplement 1): 1–4. Copyright © 1970 by Lippincott, Williams, & Wilkins.

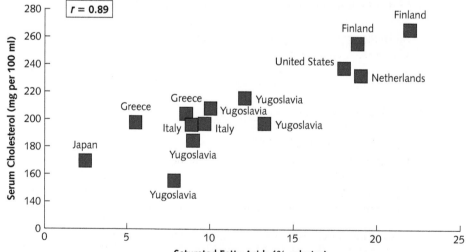

The seven countries cohort was drawn from the following seven regions and cities: Finland = east, west; Greece = Crete, Corfu; Italy = Crevalcone, Montegiorgio; Japan = Tanushimaru; Netherlands = Zutphe; U.S.A. = U.S. railroad; Yugoslavia = Belgrade, Dalmatia, Slavonia, Velika Krsna, Zrenjanin.

cholesterol level, the relationship between the two variables isn't perfect because of measurement errors [e.g., in calculating the dietary intake of saturated fat or determining the serum cholesterol level] or other factors [e.g., genetic determinants].[16])

5. **Developing the hypothesis.** The results of animal studies and large-scale population studies such as the Seven Countries Study were used to formulate the hypothesis that a diet high in saturated fat increases blood cholesterol levels and contributes to the development of CHD.

6. **Testing the hypothesis.** Many studies were undertaken to test this hypothesis. In one migration study, groups of Japanese living in Japan were compared with groups of Japanese who were originally from the same regions in Japan but had emigrated to Hawaii or California.[17] The study design used standardized protocols for measuring blood cholesterol and the number of existing and new cases of CHD. It showed that the intake of saturated fat as a percentage of total calories in the three populations varied widely, with Japanese living in Japan having a saturated fat intake of 7% of total calories and Japanese living in Hawaii and California having an intake of 23 and 26%, respectively. Japanese living in Japan had the lowest blood cholesterol level, followed by those living in Hawaii; Japanese living in California had the highest blood cholesterol level. These differences in blood cholesterol paralleled the rates of CHD, suggesting that changes in diet after migration were partly responsible for the differences in blood cholesterol levels and the incidence of CHD.

Other population studies—such as the Western Electric Study,[18] the Framingham Heart Study,[19] the Bogalusa Heart Study,[20] and the Puerto Rico Heart Health Program[21]—helped confirm the relationship of diet to blood cholesterol levels and CHD risk.

7. **Drawing scientific inferences.** The results of these and other large-scale population studies provided convincing evidence that the rates of CHD differ among populations and that these differences are due partly to environmental (diet) factors. However, the data have not been entirely consistent. The famous Ireland–Boston brothers study provided only weak support for the diet–heart hypothesis. This study did not find significant differences in CHD mortality between Irish brothers who were born and remained in Ireland and those who, although born in Ireland, had lived in Boston for at least 10 years. It did, however, underscore the increased risk of death from CHD among study subjects consuming a diet high in saturated fat. Furthermore, it found that the consumption of a high-fiber, vegetable-rich diet decreased the risk of CHD death.[22]

It is unrealistic to expect total agreement among the results of epidemiologic or clinical studies. Many genetic, environmental, social, and experimental factors affect a study's outcome. On balance, however, many studies conducted over the last five decades have strengthened the evidence for the link among diet, blood cholesterol, and CHD.[23]

8. **Conducting experimental studies.** Studies with rabbits, pigs, and nonhuman primates showed that these species are susceptible to diet-induced hypercholesterolemia. In addition, the blood cholesterol levels of some laboratory animals were affected by the types of fatty acids in the diet. In primates, for example, blood cholesterol levels rose when a diet rich in cholesterol and saturated fatty acids was consumed; a diet rich in polyunsaturated fatty acids lowered them.[24] Animal studies provided compelling support for a role of saturated fat and cholesterol in the atherogenic process.

9. **Intervening and evaluating.** One of the most ambitious interventions undertaken to modify CHD risk factors was the Multiple Risk Factor Intervention Trial (MRFIT), commonly called Mister Fit. This six-year clinical trial was directed toward the primary prevention of CHD among middle-aged men determined to be at high risk for CHD

because they had hypertension or high blood cholesterol or smoked cigarettes. The 12,866 eligible men were randomly assigned to a special-intervention group or a usual-care group. Men in the special-intervention group received extensive nutrition counseling to help them make dietary changes to reduce their saturated fat and cholesterol intake. Participants in the special-intervention group who smoked received counseling to help them stop smoking.[25] Although the mean reduction in blood cholesterol in the intervention group was less than the predicted response, MRFIT showed that serum cholesterol reductions and dietary changes could be sustained over a period of several years.[26]

The mounting experimental (animal) and epidemiologic evidence supporting the diet–heart hypothesis led to the formulation of dietary advice designed to reduce CHD risk in the general population. Voluntary and nonprofit health agencies, such as the American Heart Association[27] and the American Medical Association,[28] published statements for health professionals describing the known risk factors for CHD and strategies for reducing CHD risk (**Table 2-3**). These were followed by the report of the National

TABLE 2-3 Leading Risk Factors for Heart Disease

RISK FACTOR	HOW TO MINIMIZE THE RISK
High LDL cholesterol	Consume a diet emphasizing vegetables, fruits, and whole grains; include low-fat dairy products, poultry, fish, legumes, nontropical vegetable oils, and nuts; limit intake of sweets, sugar-sweetened beverages, and red meats; avoid *trans* fats.
Low HDL cholesterol	Avoid *trans* fat; lose weight if necessary; do not smoke; and maintain a physically active lifestyle.
High blood pressure	Control high blood pressure with medication and a heart-healthy diet. Maintain a healthy weight. Losing just 5 to 10 pounds may lower your blood pressure. Compare sodium in soups, frozen meals, and other foods—and choose the foods with less sodium.
Cigarette smoking	Stop smoking. Nicotine constricts blood vessels and forces your heart to work harder. Carbon monoxide reduces oxygen in blood and damages the lining of blood vessels.
Diabetes	Maintain proper weight. Losing excess weight helps control blood sugar level. Eat high-fiber foods. Limit solid fats and added sugars. Get regular physical activity.
Physical inactivity	Increase physical activity by seeking ways to be more physically active every day. Aim for the equivalent of 150 minutes (2 hours and 30 minutes) of moderate-intensity aerobic activity (such as brisk walking) each week.
Obesity	Maintain a healthy weight and be physically active. Being only 10% overweight increases heart disease risk.
"Atherogenic" diet	To lower LDL cholesterol, keep saturated fat to less than 5% to 6% of daily calories. Substitute olive and canola oils for saturated fat. Avoid *trans* fat. Limit consumption of foods with solid fats and added sugars. Increase soluble fiber intake by eating whole grains, legumes, fruits, and vegetables. Eat a variety of fruits and vegetables each day to receive the beneficial antioxidants, vitamins, minerals, and phytochemicals they contain.
Stress	Get regular physical activity. Avoid excessive caffeine and alcohol. Practice relaxation techniques. Maintain good social relationships.
RISK FACTORS YOU CAN'T CHANGE	
Age	Men over age 45 and women over age 55 are at increased risk.
Gender	Men are at higher risk. Estrogen may protect women before menopause.
Genetics	Increased risk if you have a father or brother under age 55 or a mother or sister under age 65 who had heart disease.

Source: M. Boyle, *Personal Nutrition*, 9th ed. (Belmont, CA: Wadsworth/Cengage Learning, 2016), 148.

Cholesterol Education Program on the detection, evaluation, and treatment of high blood cholesterol in adults.[29] The science supporting the diet–heart link was eventually incorporated into the *Dietary Guidelines for Americans*, which advised the public to consume fewer calories from saturated fatty acids and to keep *trans* fatty acid consumption as low as possible by limiting foods that contain synthetic sources of *trans* fats, such as partially hydrogenated oils, as a means of reducing the risk of chronic disease and improving health.[30]

In November 2013, in response to increasing pressure to eliminate the use of artificial *trans* fat, the U.S. Food and Drug Administration (FDA) took the first step toward banning the use of *trans* fats in foods. The FDA published a preliminary ruling in the *Federal Register* stating: "Partially hydrogenated oils, which are the primary dietary source of industrially produced *trans* fatty acids, are not *generally recognized as safe* (GRAS)* for any use in food based on current scientific evidence establishing the health risks associated with the consumption of *trans*-fat, and therefore . . . partially hydrogenated oils are food additives."[31] When the FDA finalizes this ruling, food manufacturers will no longer be permitted to use partially hydrogenated oils in food products without prior FDA approval.

Hypothesis Testing

Another precept of the epidemiologic method is hypothesis testing. Its importance to the experimental process cannot be overstated. In planning an experimental trial, the investigator identifies a cause–effect comparison to be tested as the research hypothesis. For example, a study might be designed to determine whether a vaccine for hepatitis A is effective among children or whether a protein in cow's milk is responsible for triggering type 1 diabetes mellitus. In a community-based nutrition study, one hypothesis might be stated thus: "There will be a significant decrease in the calories from saturated fat and an increase in the grams of fiber consumed by employees in the eight intervention worksites receiving nutrition programming compared with employees in the eight control worksites."[32]

Once the specific research question (hypothesis) has been formulated, the investigators design a study to obtain information that will enable them to make inferences about the original hypothesis, as illustrated in **Figure 2-7**. In some epidemiologic studies, however, not all hypotheses are specified at the beginning. Rather, one or more hypotheses are generated retrospectively, after the research data have been collected and analyzed. The temptation to do this is compelling. A typical epidemiologic study produces reams of data about individuals (age, sex, race, educational level, occupation), specific agents (diet, vitamins, tobacco, alcohol, drugs, pesticides), and outcomes (death, heart attack, colon cancer, impairment of renal function). When the data are downloaded into a computer for statistical analysis, the investigator may consider rummaging around in the data, searching for statistical associations among various groups that may suggest a cause–effect relationship. This activity, sometimes called "data dredging," is worth avoiding. The statement of a clear, precise hypothesis (or hypotheses) at the beginning of the study ensures that the appropriate data are collected to answer the research question(s) and helps avoid the pitfall of drawing spurious conclusions from the data set.[33]

---

* A substance is GRAS if it is generally recognized "among qualified experts as having been adequately shown through scientific procedures to be safe under the conditions of its intended use." GRAS items are not food additives and can be lawfully used without FDA review and approval.

FIGURE 2-7 The Scientific Method: Hypothesis Testing

Note that most research generates new questions, not final answers. Thus, the sequence begins anew, and research continues in a somewhat cyclical way.

Source: E. Whitney and S. Rolfes, *Understanding Nutrition*, 14th ed. (Belmont, CA: Wadsworth/Cengage Learning, 2013), 13.

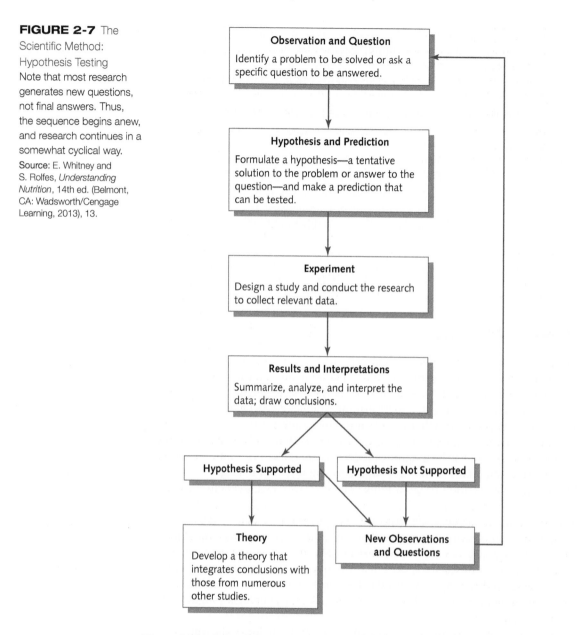

Explaining Research Observations

An important aspect of the epidemiologic method—and, indeed, of the scientific method in general—is determining whether the data are valid. That is, do the data represent the true state of affairs or are they distorted in some fashion? Research data can have three possible explanations, as shown in **Table 2-4**. Consider the following research project:

> A study was designed to determine whether a worksite-sponsored physical activity program resulted in a lower percentage of body fat and lower blood lipids among overweight adults. Employees in two companies were invited to enroll in the three-month program. Those who agreed to participate underwent several clinical measurements at the beginning and end of the study: height, weight, skin folds, and total blood cholesterol. The 156 employees who participated in the physical activity program showed a reduction in percentage of body fat and total blood cholesterol, compared with 210 adults who did not participate.

Bias	The observation is incorrect because a systematic error was introduced by: 1. Selection bias—the method by which patients or study subjects were selected for observation 2. Measurement bias—the method by which the observation or measurement was made 3. Confounding bias—the presence of another variable that accounts for the observation
Chance	The observation is incorrect because of error arising from random variation.
Truth	The observation is correct. This explanation should be accepted only after the others have been excluded.

TABLE 2-4 Possible Explanations for Research Observations

Source: R. H. Fletcher, S. W. Fletcher, and G. S. Fletcher, *Clinical Epidemiology—The Essentials*, 5th ed.

One possible explanation for these results is that the data are incorrect because they are biased; in other words, a systematic error was made in measuring one or more outcome variables, or there were systematic differences in the populations studied. Although there are probably dozens of possible biases, most fall into one of the three categories listed in Table 2-4. More than one bias may operate at one time. In the study just described, *selection bias* may have occurred because the study participants were self-selected. In other words, employees who were interested in improving their fitness level or losing weight were more inclined to join the program than those who were less interested in improvements in fitness or weight loss. *Measurement bias* may have occurred if the technician responsible for obtaining skin-fold measurements was an enthusiastic supporter of vigorous exercise and took more pains to make careful measurements in the exercising adults than in the sedentary adults. Finally, *confounding bias* may have existed because the study focused on physical activity as the sole determinant of changes in total blood cholesterol and body fat. It is possible that employees entering the physical activity program made significant, but unconscious, alterations in their eating patterns that contributed to the changes in blood lipids and body composition. Thus, the presence of (unmeasured or unidentified) **confounding factors** may have influenced the study outcome.

Another possible explanation for the study results is that they are due simply to chance and do not represent the true state of affairs; that is, that the observations made on these employees arose from random variation within the sample. Many factors could have contributed to the differences between the groups, including the manner in which the clinical or laboratory measurements were made and differences in the makeup of the workforce (e.g., a manufacturing plant versus a company that develops computer software programs). Random variation cannot be totally eliminated and usually occurs in tandem with some form of bias. The influence of these two sources of error can be reduced by careful study design and statistical analysis.

The final possible explanation for the study results is that they represent the truth: Participating in a physical activity program resulted in reductions in body fat and total blood cholesterol among employees in these two companies. To say that the data are valid, then, means that they are neither biased nor incorrect due to chance and that they represent the true state of affairs regarding the physiologic effects of physical activity.

Confounding factors (confounder) A "hidden" factor or characteristic that is distributed differently in the study and control groups and may cause an association that the researchers attribute to other factors. Common confounding factors—such as age, gender, race, ethnicity, and dietary or lifestyle factors—can make it difficult to distinguish between a response to treatment and the effect of some other factor. Confounders may be due to bias or to chance.

Types of Epidemiologic Studies

When a nutritional problem is suspected, an investigation is undertaken "to find out something." The hypothesis to be tested is defined, the population to be studied is selected, measurements are taken or cases are counted, and the data are analyzed to determine whether the established facts support the hypothesis. The type of investigation undertaken depends to a large extent on the research question being asked and the type of data needed to answer the question. The major types of nutritional epidemiological studies are described next.[34]

> ## Miniglossary of Research Design Categories

Epidemiological studies, as a research category, are analytical studies of the determinants of health and illness in specific populations. Studies are designed to determine the relationship among exposure factors (which can be risk factors or protective factors) and outcomes. The most common epidemiological study designs are case–control, cohort, and cross-sectional studies.

Observational Study	Examines causes, preventions, and treatments for diseases; investigator passively observes as nature takes its course.
Case–Control Study	A type of observational analytic study; involves identifying patients who have the outcome of interest (cases) and matching them with individuals who have similar characteristics, but do not have the outcome of interest (controls). Characteristics, such as previous exposure to a factor (i.e., the hypothesized causal or contributing factors), are then compared between cases and controls.
Cohort Study	A type of observational analytic study that can be retrospective or prospective in nature. Enrollment in the study is based on exposure characteristics (e.g., past exposure to risk factors) or on membership in a group. Disease, death, and/or other health-related outcomes are then determined and compared. Comparison groups can be defined at the beginning or created later using data from the study (e.g., age group, smokers/nonsmokers, amount of a specific food group consumed). **Prospective cohort** studies (i.e., Nurses Health Study) enroll individuals and then collect data at many intervals. **Retrospective cohort** studies use an existing longitudinal data set to look back for a temporal relationship between exposure factors and outcome development.
Cross-Sectional Study	A study where exposure factors (e.g., individual or environmental risk factor, nutrition education) and outcomes (e.g., disease occurrence, eating behavior) are observed or measured at one point in time in a sample from the population of interest, usually by survey or interview. In this design, a researcher examines the association among factors and outcomes using a statistical test for association, but cannot infer cause and effect. An example is the BRFSS.
Trend Study	A study in which the same or similar data about exposures and outcomes are collected from the same population many times, but each time a different sample is used. A trend study is like a series of cross-sectional studies. An example is NHANES.
Ecological/Correlational Study	An ecological study focuses on groups of people (rather than individuals) and examines the relationship between exposure and disease with population-level rather than individual-level data. Can be used as the first step in exploring the relationship between an exposure and a disease. An example is the Coronary Heart Disease in Seven Countries Study.
Experimental Study	Examines preventions and treatments for diseases; investigator actively manipulates which groups receive the agent under study.
Randomized Controlled Trial (RCT)	Individuals meeting eligibility requirements are randomly assigned into an experimental group or a control group. The experimental intervention (protocol, method, or treatment) and its alternative(s) are clearly defined and their implementation is closely managed by the researcher. An example is the Dietary Approaches to Stop Hypertension (DASH) Study. An experimental study in which intact communities (worksites, schools, villages) are the units of randomization is known as a *community trial/community intervention study*; used to evaluate interventions that are more naturally administered at the community level.
Nonrandomized Controlled Trial	A study where subjects are assigned to intervention (protocol, method, or treatment) alternatives by a method that is not random. The researcher does define and manage the alternatives, which could be treatment and control or two or more different interventions.

Other Systematic Review   A summary of the scientific literature on a specific topic or question that uses explicit methods to conduct a comprehensive literature search and identify relevant studies, critically appraise the quality of each study, and summarize the body of literature or evidence to answer the question. A *meta-analysis* is a systematic, quantitative method that combines the results of all relevant studies to produce an overall estimate. A meta-analysis can be part of a systematic review, but not all systematic reviews include meta-analysis.

Sources: Adapted from Academy of Nutrition and Dietetics, *Evidence Analysis Manual: Steps in the Academy Evidence Analysis Process* (Chicago, IL: Academy of Nutrition and Dietetics, 2012): 85–87; and A. Aschengrau and G. R. Seage III, *Essentials of Epidemiology in Public Health* (Sudbury, MA: Jones and Bartlett, 2008).

Ecological or Correlational Studies

Ecological or **correlational studies** compare the frequency of events (or disease rates) in different populations with the per capita consumption of certain dietary factors (e.g., saturated fat, total fat, and beta-carotene). The dietary data collected in this type of study are usually *disappearance data*—that is, the national figures for food produced for human consumption minus the food that is exported, fed to animals, wasted, or otherwise not available for human consumption.

An example of an ecological study is an investigation of the correlation between fish consumption and breast cancer incidence and mortality rates in humans.[35] In this study, incidence and mortality rates were derived from the cancer registries of various countries. Food consumption for each country was estimated from food availability data averaged over three years. Although there were some exceptions, as **Figure 2-8** shows, the risk for breast cancer tended to be high in countries where the relative proportion of calories derived from fish was low and the consumption of animal fat was high, such as the United States, Canada, and Switzerland. In countries where fish was consumed frequently and the animal fat intake was low, such as Japan, the breast cancer death rate was low.

Do these results mean that diets high in animal fat *cause* breast cancer, whereas diets high in fish protect against cancer? No, the data from an ecological study cannot be used to draw conclusions about the role of foods or nutrients in the development of cancer

Ecological or **correlational studies** Compare the frequency of events (or disease rates) in different populations with the per capita consumption of certain dietary factors.

FIGURE 2-8 Breast Cancer Death Rate (per 100,000) Plotted versus Fish Consumption (percentage of caloric intake)

Points include Australia (AS), Austria (AU), Belgium (BE), Bulgaria (BU), Canada (CA), Chile (CH), Czechoslovakia (CZ), Denmark (DE), Federal Republic of Germany (FG), Finland (FI), France (FR), German Democratic Republic (GE), Greece (GR), Hong Kong (HK), Hungary (HU), Iceland (IC), Ireland (IR), Israel (IS), Italy (IT), Japan (JA), Netherlands (NE), Norway (NO), New Zealand (NZ), Philippines (PH), Poland (PL), Portugal (PO), Romania (R), Sweden (SW), Switzerland (SZ), United Kingdom (UK), United States (US), and Yugoslavia (YU).

Source: From "Fish Consumption and Breast Cancer Risk: An Ecological Study," by L. Kaizer, N. F. Boyd, V. Kruikov, and D. Tritchler, 1989, *Nutrition and Cancer* 12, p. 53.

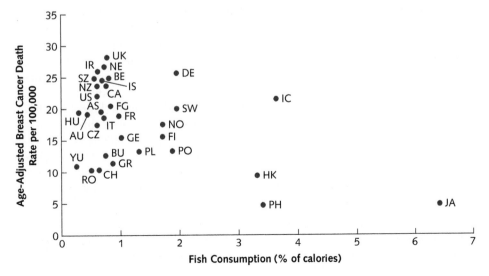

(or other diseases). Why not? One reason is that the dietary data obtained in such a study are based on population food disappearance data and are therefore not particularly specific. Ecological studies can be used, however, to generate hypotheses about the relationship of dietary components to the disease process, and these hypotheses can then be tested with a more rigorous study design.

Cross-Sectional or Prevalence Studies

Cross-sectional studies
Examine the relationships among dietary intake, diseases, and other variables as they exist in a population at a particular time.

Cross-sectional studies or prevalence studies examine the relationships among dietary intake, diseases, and other variables as they exist in a population at a particular time. This type of study is much like a camera snapshot. It gives a picture of what is happening within a particular population at a specific time.

One example of a cross-sectional study is the investigation of nutrient intakes and growth of predominantly breastfed infants living in Capulhuac, Mexico, a farming community of about 5,500 Otomi Indians. A representative sample of four- to six-month-old infants, together with their mothers, was enrolled in the study. The infants' weight, length, and intake of human breast milk were measured, and information about their health and morbidity (e.g., diarrhea or respiratory illness) was recorded. The study found that despite these infants having milk intakes similar to or greater than those of infants from more economically privileged populations (e.g., infants living in Houston, Texas), the nutrient intake from breast milk among the Otomi infants was not sufficient for normal growth. Growth faltering was evident by six months of age in this population.[36]

Cohort Studies

Cohort studies Identify and examine a group of people free of the disease or condition of interest.

Whereas cross-sectional studies are like a snapshot, **cohort studies** are like moving pictures of events occurring within populations. In these studies, a group of people free of the disease or condition of interest is identified and examined. This group is called the *cohort*. The members of the cohort are followed for months or even years, during which time they are examined periodically to determine which individuals develop the characteristics of interest and which do not. Cohort studies may look back in time to reconstruct exposures and health outcomes; such studies are called *retrospective cohort studies*. Those that follow a group into the future are called *prospective cohort studies*. Consult **Table 2-5** for a list of the advantages and disadvantages of this type of study.

An example of a cohort study (in this case, a prospective study) is the Framingham Heart Study, which was begun in 1949 in Framingham, Massachusetts. The study was undertaken to identify the factors associated with increased risk of coronary heart disease. A representative sample of 5,209 men and women, 30 to 59 years of age, was selected from the 10,000 or so residents of that age group living in the Framingham community. Of these, 5,127 were free of CHD when they were first examined. The cohort underwent complete physical examinations every two years for more than 30 years. The study has shown that the risk of developing CHD is associated with cigarette smoking, serum cholesterol, glucose intolerance, and blood pressure.[37] An analysis of the cohort's high-density lipoprotein cholesterol (HDL-C) levels taken over a period of 12 years revealed that HDL-C is a consistent predictor of CHD risk in both men and women. Individuals with a high HDL-C level (> 60 mg/dL) had a low risk of CHD, regardless of their total cholesterol level.[38] Individuals with a low total blood cholesterol level (< 200 mg/dL) had a high risk of CHD if their HDL-C levels were also low (< 40 mg/dL). The risk of CHD increases with higher total cholesterol levels, but even more strongly with low HDL levels. The ratio of total cholesterol to HDL cholesterol (total cholesterol divided by HDL cholesterol) provided the strongest prediction of relative risk. Thus, in the words of the investigators, "a low total cholesterol level per se does not necessarily indicate a low risk of developing CHD."

COHORT STUDIES	CASE–CONTROL STUDIES
Advantages	**Advantages**
May provide complete data on cases, stages	Excellent way to study rare diseases and diseases
Allow study of more than one effect of exposure	with long latency periods
Can calculate and compare rates in exposed and	Relatively quick
unexposed	Relatively inexpensive
Choice of factors available for study	Require relatively few study subjects
Quality control of data	Can often use existing records
In prospective studies, exposure is assessed prior	Can study many possible causes of disease
to diagnosis of disease	
Disadvantages	**Disadvantages**
Need to study large numbers	Rely on recall or existing records about past
May take many years	exposures
Circumstances may change during study	Difficult or impossible to validate data
Expensive	Control of extraneous factors incomplete
Control of extraneous factors may be incomplete	Difficult to select suitable comparison group
Rarely possible to study mechanism of disease	Cannot calculate rates
May provide incomplete data from subject	Cannot study mechanisms of disease
nonresponse and loss to follow-up	Disease may affect the exposure being studied

TABLE 2-5

Advantages and Disadvantages of Cohort and Case–Control Studies

Source: Adapted from R. B. Wallace, "Epidemiology and Public Health," *Maxcy-Rosenau-Last Public Health and Preventive Medicine*, 15th ed., ed. R. B. Wallace (Columbus, OH: McGraw-Hill, 2008).

A Sampling of Diet-Related Studies from the National Institutes of Health*

Name/Type of Study/Support/Year Begun	Purpose/Objectives
The Bogalusa Heart Study: Long-term, cross-sectional study of cardiovascular risk factors in children, adolescents, and young adults (1972–2002). More than 16,000 individuals, many with multiple exams, participated in the study. Subjects ranged in age from birth to 38 years (NHLBI) (*https://biolincc.nhlbi.nih.gov/studies/bhs*).	Investigate the early natural history of cardiovascular disease (CVD) in a cohort of children and young adults in a semirural community (Bogalusa, LA). The examination included standardized questionnaires to determine education, occupation, smoking habits, family medical history, and physical activity. Examination components included blood pressure, anthropometry, lipid profile, and other blood lab values. Study established lifelong adverse effects of lifestyle factors on CVD risks.
Diabetes Prevention Program: Randomized clinical trial conducted at 25 centers nationwide involving 4,000 people at risk of type 2 diabetes (NIDDK), 1997 (*www.niddk.nih.gov/about-niddk/research-areas/diabetes/diabetes-prevention-program-dpp/Pages/default.aspx*).	Prevent or delay the development of type 2 diabetes in people who are at high risk of the disease because of impaired glucose tolerance, by means of intensive lifestyle changes and drug interventions; follow subjects for three to six years to observe the potential development of diabetes.
Nurses' Health Study I (1976): Cohort study of 121,700 married female registered nurses aged 30 to 55 years; *Nurses' Health Study II* (1989): Cohort study of 116,686 female registered nurses aged 25 to 42 years (NHLBI, NCI) (*http://www.channing.harvard.edu/nhs/*).	Investigate diet and lifestyle risk factors for major chronic diseases in women; investigate the potential long-term consequences of the use of oral contraceptives.
Health Professionals Follow-Up Study: Cohort study of 51,529 male health professionals aged 40 to 75 years (NHLBI, NCI), 1986 (*www.hsph.harvard.edu/hpfs/*).	Evaluate a series of hypotheses about men's health, relating nutritional factors to the incidence of serious illnesses, such as cancer, heart disease, and other vascular diseases. This all-male study is designed to complement the all-female Nurses' Health Study, which examines similar hypotheses.

continued

A Sampling of Diet-Related Studies from the National Institutes of Health*—*continued*

Name/Type of Study/Support/Year Begun	Purpose/Objectives
Child and Adolescent Trial for Cardiovascular Health (CATCH): Randomized school-based clinical trial involving 5,106 third-grade boys and girls enrolled in 96 ethnically and racially diverse elementary schools in four locations (California, Louisiana, Minnesota, and Texas) (NHLBI), 1994–1996 (*www.ncbi.nlm.nih.gov/pubmed/9408786*).	School-based study to determine whether multicomponent health promotion efforts targeting both children's behaviors and the school environment—including classroom curricula, school food service modifications, physical education changes, and family reinforcement—would reduce cardiovascular disease risk factors later in life.
Pathways Project: Randomized school-based clinical trial involving third-, fourth-, and fifth-grade students (21 schools in intervention group and 20 schools in control group) (NHLBI), 1997 (*www.cscc.unc.edu/path*).	School-based study for prevention of obesity in Native American children using four intervention components: physical activity, family involvement, food service, and classroom curriculum.
Honolulu Heart Program: Cohort study of 8,006 American men of Japanese ancestry born between 1900 and 1919 and living in Hawaii—having either migrated from Japan or been born in Hawaii (NHLBI), 1965–1996 (*https://biolincc.nhlbi.nih.gov/studies/hhp*).	A 30-year prospective study to investigate relationships among disease frequencies, pathological findings, and disease predictors in cohort and compare to other populations (e.g., men living in Japan); assess dietary factors (e.g., intake of fish, milk and calcium, coffee and caffeine, cholesterol, alcohol, and antioxidants) and incidence of CHD.
Women's Health Initiative (WHI): Clinical trial involving 93,726 postmenopausal women aged 50 to 79 years; included randomized control trial of HRT,[†] dietary modification (DM), and calcium/vitamin D supplementation (CaD); observational study (OS); and a study of community approaches to developing healthful behaviors (Community Prevention Study [CPS]). (NHLBI, NIAMS, NCI, NIA), 1991 (*www.nhlbi.nih.gov/whi*).	A 15-year study to examine the extent to which diet, hormone replacement therapy (HRT), and calcium and vitamin D might prevent heart disease, breast and colorectal cancer, and osteoporosis in postmenopausal women; identify new risk factors for these conditions; compare risk factors and presence of disease at start of study with new occurrences of disease over extended period of follow-up.
Antioxidants, Zinc, and the Age-Related Eye Disease Study (AREDS): Clinical trial involving 4,757 participants aged 55 to 80 years (NEI), 1997 (*https://nei.nih.gov/amd*).	Assess clinical course, prognosis, and risk factors for age-related macular degeneration (AMD) and cataracts; subjects receive high-dose antioxidants or zinc with follow-up for seven years.
Beat Osteoporosis: Nourish and Exercise Skeletons (BONES) Project: Randomized after-school intervention trial involving 1,500 elementary school children aged 6 to 9 years from 84 after-school programs in 33 diverse communities (NICHD), 1999 (*www.clinicaltrials.gov/ct/show/NCT00065247*).	Implement and evaluate an after-school program with exercise, education, and diet components designed to improve bone quality and muscle strength in children. Subjects were randomized to after-school programs in the BONES Project, the BONES Project plus a parent/caregiver component, or a no-intervention control group.

* NIDDK, National Institute for Diabetes and Digestive and Kidney Diseases; NHLBI, National Heart, Lung, and Blood Institute; NIA, National Institute on Aging; NEI, National Eye Institute; NIAMS, National Institute of Arthritis, Musculoskeletal and Skin Diseases; NCI, National Cancer Institute; NICHD, National Institute of Child Health and Human Development.

† The estrogen-plus-progestin (HRT) trial was stopped early in July 2002 after an average follow-up of 5.2 years on the recommendation of the Data and Safety Monitoring Board.

Sources: Adapted from J. Pennington and coauthors, "Update: Diet-Related Trials and Observational Studies Supported by the National Institutes of Health," *Nutrition Today* 35 (2000): 158–160; and information from *http://clinicaltrials.gov*.

Case–control study
Compares a group of persons or cases with the disease or condition of interest with a group of persons without the disease or condition.

Case–Control Studies

In a **case–control study**, a group of persons or cases with the disease or condition of interest are compared with a group of persons without the disease or condition. For example, in a study investigating the effects of high blood levels of homocysteine on risk of CHD, researchers found higher blood levels of homocysteine in people with CHD (cases) than in healthy individuals (controls).[39] Case–control studies are also useful when a rare condition is being studied (see Table 2-5).

One of the most thorough case–control studies of diet and cancer was a Canadian study published in 1978.[40] In this study, the diets of 400 Canadian women with breast cancer were compared with 400 women from similar neighborhoods who did not have breast cancer (the latter were called "neighborhood controls"). The investigators used three types of diet assessment techniques: the 24-hour recall, a 4-day dietary record, and a diet history questionnaire. The investigators found that only the intake of total calories differed between cases and controls when the diet was analyzed by the 24-hour recall method. There were no differences in the intakes of total fat and saturated fat between cases and controls as a function of type of diet assessment method. This study did not support the hypothesis that fat composition of the diet is associated with the incidence of breast cancer. The investigators concluded that all three diet assessment methods may have been imperfect measures of dietary intake of fat.

ENTREPRENEUR IN ACTION

Mary Kay Hunt

In mid-career Mary Kay Hunt, MPH, changed direction. Building on her experience as a clinical dietitian, she returned to graduate school in public health nutrition and entered the field of community health research with a University of Minnesota team that was one of the three National Heart, Lung, and Blood Institute (NHLBI) community heart health studies. In this capacity, she was involved in the design, implementation, and measurement of individual and organizational change focusing not only on nutrition, but also on smoking, physical activity, and occupational health. At the conclusion of these studies, she continued her work in chronic disease prevention research at the Dana-Farber Cancer Institute/Harvard School of Public Health in Boston. Currently, she is semi-retired and has formed her own company, Community Health Research Consulting. She explains that "entrepreneurship used in the context of community nutrition incorporates concepts of change, innovation, and risk taking. The exploration of research questions requires similar approaches and, thus, provides a natural setting for those with an entrepreneurial spirit. The *community* in community nutrition means that entrepreneurs need to be skilled in collaborating with representatives from diverse sectors of the community such as media, private industry, and educational institutions. Interdisciplinary collaboration requires that all disciplines learn the vocabulary, language and 'culture' of each other." Find out more about Mary Kay online at *www.cengagebrain.com*.

Controlled Trials

The **randomized controlled trial** or clinical trial conducted as a double-blind experiment is the most rigorous evaluation of a dietary hypothesis. The primary drawback of the controlled trial is its expense. The MRFIT study cited earlier is an example of a randomized controlled trial.

Randomized controlled trial (RCT) Considered the gold standard of study designs in which subjects are randomly assigned to either an experimental/treatment group or control group; used to determine causality between an exposure factor (i.e., fruit and vegetable intake) and an outcome (i.e., hypertension).

Nutritional Epidemiology

The epidemiologic method lends itself to the study of the relationship of diet to health and disease. Historically, one of the first applications of epidemiology to nutrition science was James Lind's controlled trial investigating the curative effects of citrus fruits among sailors with scurvy.[41] Like Snow's proposed intervention to control cholera epidemics, Lind's suggestion that sea vessels carry a supply of limes, oranges, and other citrus fruits to prevent scurvy came 150 years before researchers proved in the laboratory that scurvy results from a dietary deficiency.[42] Similar investigations into the health effects of vitamin C and the other 40-odd essential nutrients are being conducted today.

Epidemiology has other applications in the nutrition arena. It can be used to monitor and describe the food consumption, nutrient intake, and nutrition status of populations or specific subgroups of a population. The information obtained from large population surveys is then used to develop specific programs and services for groups whose nutrition status appears to be compromised. Furthermore, the epidemiologic method can be used to evaluate nutrition interventions. This usually involves monitoring the nutrition and health status of a high-risk group of individuals for a period of several months or even years.

Nutritional epidemiology is a fairly new area of study. Whereas its focus was once the deficiency diseases such as scurvy, beriberi, and rickets, today it is primarily concerned with the major chronic diseases of the so-called Western world. Chronic diseases, including cardiovascular diseases, diabetes, obesity, cancer, and respiratory diseases, are now the leading cause of death and disability worldwide—accounting for 60% of deaths annually worldwide.[43] Unlike nutritional deficiency states, chronic diseases tend to have many, sometimes interrelated, causes, as illustrated in **Figure 2-9**.

Relatively few risk factors—high cholesterol, high blood pressure, obesity, physical inactivity, insufficient consumption of fruits and vegetables, smoking, and alcohol use—play a key role in the development of chronic diseases.[44] Epidemiologic evidence suggests that a change in dietary habits and physical activity can substantially influence several of these risk factors.[45]

The CDC's state-based BRFSS can be a source of information on behaviors that increase the risk for chronic diseases, such as CHD.[46] As described in Chapter 7, this system gathers information from adults in all 50 states on knowledge, attitudes, and behaviors related to key health issues, such as tobacco use, dietary patterns, levels of leisure-time physical activity, and use of preventive services. Similarly, CDC's Youth Risk Behavior Surveillance System (YRBSS) provides key data, nationally and by state, about the prevalence of health risk behaviors among young people—including tobacco use, lack of physical activity, and poor nutrition. Using BRFSS and YRBSS data, states can monitor changes in health risk behaviors over time and can better target health promotion efforts to populations most at risk. Chapter 7 provides details of many of the surveys currently in use nationally and at the state level to monitor the nutrition status of Americans.

FIGURE 2-9 Risk Factors and Chronic Diseases

Source: Adapted from E. Whitney and S. Rolfes, *Understanding Nutrition*, 12th ed. (Belmont, CA: Wadsworth/Cengage Learning, 2011), 609.

The Nature of Dietary Variation

One challenge to the study of the relationship of diet to disease is the complexity of our diets. The foods we consume each day are complex mixtures of chemicals, some of which are known to be important to human health and some of which have not even been identified or measured. The chemicals found in or on foods include essential nutrients,

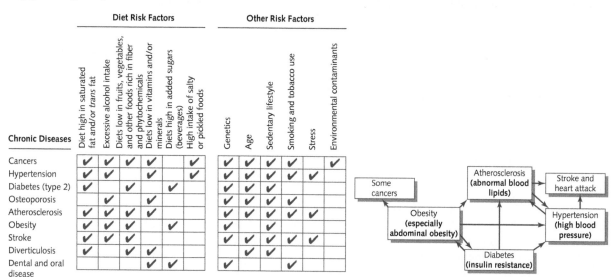

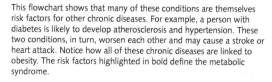

| | **Diet Risk Factors** | | | | | | **Other Risk Factors** | | | | | |
Chronic Diseases	Diet high in saturated fat and/or *trans* fat	Excessive alcohol intake	Diets low in fruits, vegetables, and other foods rich in fiber and phytochemicals	Diets low in vitamins and/or minerals	Diets high in added sugars (beverages)	High intake of salty or pickled foods	Genetics	Age	Sedentary lifestyle	Smoking and tobacco use	Stress	Environmental contaminants
Cancers	✔	✔	✔	✔		✔	✔	✔	✔	✔		✔
Hypertension	✔	✔		✔		✔	✔	✔	✔	✔	✔	
Diabetes (type 2)	✔		✔		✔		✔	✔	✔			
Osteoporosis		✔		✔			✔	✔	✔	✔		
Atherosclerosis	✔	✔	✔	✔			✔	✔	✔	✔		✔
Obesity	✔	✔	✔		✔		✔		✔			
Stroke	✔	✔	✔				✔	✔	✔	✔	✔	
Diverticulosis	✔		✔	✔				✔	✔			
Dental and oral disease					✔	✔	✔			✔		

This chart shows that the same risk factor can affect many chronic diseases. Notice, for example, how many diseases have been linked to a sedentary lifestyle. The chart also shows that a particular disease, such as atherosclerosis, may have several risk factors.

This flowchart shows that many of these conditions are themselves risk factors for other chronic diseases. For example, a person with diabetes is likely to develop atherosclerosis and hypertension. These two conditions, in turn, worsen each other and may cause a stroke or heart attack. Notice how all of these chronic diseases are linked to obesity. The risk factors highlighted in bold define the metabolic syndrome.

structural compounds (e.g., cellulose), additives, microbes, pesticides, inorganic compounds such as heavy metals, natural toxins (e.g., nicotine), and other natural compounds such as phytochemicals. The sheer diversity of the chemicals found in foodstuffs creates problems for investigators studying the relationship of diet to disease processes. When assessing the relationship of vitamin A intake to the development of lung cancer, for example, an investigator must calculate the population's intake of compounds with vitamin A activity—that is, preformed vitamin A (retinol), retinal, retinoic acid, and the carotenoids. And not only must the intake of these compounds from foods be considered, but also the intake from vitamin supplements and other sources, if they exist. In addition, for most epidemiologic investigations, it is the long-term dietary intake of foodstuffs that is important. In the case of a disease such as lung cancer, which may take 10 to 20 years to develop, the lifelong intake of vitamin A must be estimated.

Another difficulty is that people don't eat the same foods every day. Work and school schedules, illnesses, holidays, the seasons of the year, weekends, personal preferences, availability of foods, social and cultural norms, and numerous other factors influence our daily food choices. As a result, our nutrient intake varies from day to day. The magnitude of the variation differs with the nutrient.[47] Scientists with the Human Nutrition Information Services of the U.S. Department of Agriculture conducted a study to determine the number of days of food intake records needed to estimate the "true" average nutrient intake of a small number of adults.[48] The 29 men and women participating in the study completed detailed food records for 365 consecutive days. The range of days, and the average number of days, of food records required to estimate the "true" average intake for individuals are shown, for several nutrients, in **Table 2-6**. Note the gender differences in the average values. For example, more food records were needed to estimate the true average intake of calories by women than by men. Note, too, that there were differences between nutrients. Compare the average values for calories with those for vitamins A and C, sodium, and fat. Finally, note the wide ranges in food records necessary to estimate true intakes. For a reliable estimate of vitamin A intake, 115 days of food records were required for some men, whereas 1,724 days (nearly five years) were required for others! As these data demonstrate, a relatively large number of days of food intake records are needed to achieve a certain level of statistical

	RANGE AND AVERAGE NUMBER OF DAYS REQUIRED					
	Males (*n* = 13)			Females (*n* = 16)		
COMPONENT	Minimum	Average	Maximum	Minimum	Average	Maximum
Food energy	14	27	84	14	35	60
Protein	23	36	72	23	48	70
Fat	34	57	131	32	71	114
Carbohydrate	10	37	177	16	41	77
Iron	18	68	130	28	66	142
Calcium	30	74	140	35	88	168
Sodium	27	58	140	36	73	116
Vitamin A	115	390	1,724	152	474	1,372
Vitamin C	90	249	900	83	222	328
Niacin	27	53	89	48	78	126

TABLE 2-6 Range and Average Number of Days Required to Estimate the True Average Intake[a] for an Individual

[a] The "true" average intake was defined as the 365-day average for individuals.

Source: P. P. Basiotis and coauthors, "Number of Days of Food Intake Records Required to Estimate Individual and Group Nutrient Intakes with Defined Confidence," *Journal of Nutrition* 117: 1640. Copyright © 1987 American Institute of Nutrition.

significance for an individual. If the individual data are combined into groups, however, fewer days of food intake records are required, as shown in **Table 2-7**.

The day-to-day variation in an individual's nutrient intake (called within-person variation) has important implications for nutritional epidemiologic studies. If only one day's intake is determined, then the true long-term nutrient intake may be misrepresented, and, for example, an individual whose vitamin C intake over a period of several days is in fact adequate may be classified as having a low vitamin C intake. The effects of within-person variation on dietary intake must be considered when designing and evaluating studies of the relationship of diet to disease.

Food Consumption at the National Level

The primary method of assessing the available food supply at the national level is based on food balance sheets. **Food balance sheets** do not measure the food actually ingested by a population. Rather, they measure the food *available* for consumption from imports and domestic food production, less the food "lost" through exports, waste, or spoilage, on a per capita basis. The per capita figures are obtained from the population estimate for the country.

Food balance sheets tend to be affected by errors that arise in calculating production, waste, and consumption. Hence, they are not used to describe the nutritional inadequacies of countries. They can be used to formulate agricultural policies concerned with food production and consumption.[49]

Food Consumption at the Household Level

Methods of assessing **household food consumption** consider the per capita food consumption of the household, taking into account the age and sex of persons in the household (or institution), the number of meals eaten at home or away from home, income, shopping practices, and other factors. In most cases, no record is made of food obtained outside the household food supply or of food wasted, spoiled, or fed to pets.

Food Consumption by Individuals

A variety of methods are available for estimating dietary intake: diet history, 24-hour dietary recall, food record or diary, and food frequency questionnaire. None of the methods is perfect.[50] All have strong points, weak points, advantages, and disadvantages, as shown in Table 4-8 on page 126.

Food balance sheets National accounts of the annual production of food, changes in stocks, imports and exports, and distribution of food over various uses within the country.

Household food consumption The total amount of food available for consumption in the household, generally excluding food eaten away from home unless taken from home.

TABLE 2-7 Number of Days Required to Estimate the True Average Intake[a] for Groups of Individuals

| | ESTIMATED NUMBER OF DAYS REQUIRED FOR EACH GROUP | |
COMPONENT	Males (*n* = 13)	Females (*n* = 16)
Food energy	3	3
Protein	4	4
Fat	6	6
Carbohydrate	5	4
Iron	7	6
Calcium	10	7
Sodium	6	6
Vitamin A	39	44
Vitamin C	33	19
Niacin	5	6

[a] The "true" average intake was defined as the 365-day average for groups of individuals.

Source: P. P. Basiotis and coauthors, "Number of Days of Food Intake Records Required to Estimate Individual and Group Nutrient Intakes with Defined Confidence," *Journal of Nutrition* 117: 1641. Copyright © 1987 American Institute of Nutrition.

Dietary recalls are appropriate for assessing the intakes of groups of people, but a single 24-hour recall may not give an adequate picture of a specific individual's usual intake.[51] Food records are often considered the best method of assessing dietary intake, but they are time-consuming, and the results may not be accurate if subjects modify their eating habits during the time of the study. Diet histories can provide detailed information, but they require subjects to make judgments about their usual food habits. Food frequency questionnaires provide less detailed information, but they are well suited for use with large groups. These questionnaires should include all important population-specific food sources of the nutrients under investigation.

Epidemiology and the Community Nutritionist

The science of epidemiology may seem far removed from the job responsibilities of the community nutritionist, but in fact it is absolutely essential to the delivery of effective nutrition programs and services. Recall from Chapter 1 that the key roles of the community nutritionist include *identifying* nutritional problems within the community and *interpreting* the scientific literature—especially experimental, clinical, and epidemiologic nutrition research findings—for the public and other health professionals. The community nutritionist must be able to critically evaluate the scientific literature before formulating new nutrition policies or offering advice about eating patterns.

How is this accomplished, considering the number of research findings published and the complexity of the diet–disease relationship? As the criteria in **Table 2-8** indicate, it helps to consider certain elements in judging the strength of epidemiologic associations. Interpreting epidemiologic data basically involves two steps: (1) evaluate the criterion for

TABLE 2-8 Criteria for Evaluating the Strength of the Association between Variables or Outcomes

Chronological Relationship	Exposure to the causative factor must occur before the onset of the disease.
Strength of Association	The association is strong if all those with a health problem have been exposed to the agent believed to be associated with this problem and only a few in the comparison group have been so exposed.
Intensity or Duration of Exposure	The association is likely to be causal if those with the most intense, or longest, exposure to the agent have the greatest frequency or severity of illness, while those with less exposure are not as ill. This is also referred to as a dose–response relationship.
Specificity of Association	Does the removal of the agent or risk factor lead to a reduction in risk of the disease? The likelihood of a causal association is increased if an agent, or risk factor, can be isolated from others and shown to produce changes in the frequency of occurrence or severity of the disease.
Consistency of Findings	Have similar results been shown in other studies? An association is consistent if it is confirmed by different investigators, in different populations, or using different methods of study.
Plausibility	Is the association consistent with other knowledge? Evidence from experimental studies and evidence from other forms of observation are among the kinds of evidence to be considered.

Source: Adapted from R. B. Wallace, "Epidemiology and Public Health," *Maxcy-Rosenau-Last Public Health and Preventive Medicine*, 15th ed., ed. R. B. Wallace (Columbus, OH: McGraw-Hill, 2008).

► **THINK LIKE A COMMUNITY** NUTRITIONIST

Even if you are not involved as a community nutritionist in collecting or analyzing research data, interpretation and application of research findings are key responsibilities of any Registered Dietitian Nutritionist (RDN). Imagine you are tasked with writing a policy brief on dietary fat consumption for your local department of health. What types of data would you need to make this recommendation? Where would you go to find the data?

a causal association carefully and (2) assess the causal association critically for the presence of bias and the contribution of chance. Competence in this area is achieved to some degree by experience and dogged determination. This chapter's Professional Focus feature describes some of the journals and online resources that will be important to you as a community nutritionist and explains how you can critically analyze a study's results.

case study

Epidemiology of Obesity
by Alice Fornari, EdD, RD, Alessandra Sarcona, MS, RD, CSSD, and Alison Barkman, MS, RD, CDN

Scenario

You have been hired as a nutritionist by a county public health agency in southern California. This agency has never had a nutritionist. Health professionals at the agency would like to have the nutritionist implement new programs. The population served by this agency is 10% Caucasian, 15% African American, and 75% Mexican American. Your first task is to review the health programs already in place at the agency. Second, you research nutrition education programs instituted at other local community agencies. Your next step is prioritizing the nutritional needs of your target population. In your review of health records at the agency, you note a high incidence of overweight and obesity, especially among the Mexican American population. You also note that the incidence is very high in preschool-age children. You calculate that 30% of these children have a BMI that exceeds the 85th percentile of U.S. standards for body mass index (BMI). Another critical issue is the occurrence of baby bottle tooth decay (BBTD) among this age group. There are no records of any nutrition education programs conducted at this agency. The majority of your population are low income (100%); most live in apartment complexes with multiple families, and the children do not have a safe place to play and spend many hours each week on screen time (television, computer, and video games). Most speak limited English, with Spanish being their primary/native language (80%).

Learning Outcomes

- Utilize data from epidemiologic research to identify nutrient needs and concerns of a target population.
- Identify and prioritize the needs of a target population.
- Construct a nutrition diagnosis and an intervention plan for a target population.
- Demonstrate the process of program development and monitoring and evaluation that achieve desired outcomes.

Foundation: Acquisition of Knowledge and Skills

1. Define epidemiology.
2. What are the U.S. standards for defining overweight and obesity in the pediatric population? Review the American Academy of Pediatrics (AAP) definition of *overweight* and *obesity* in the pediatric population (see the Section on Obesity at *https://ihcw.aap.org*) and the definition of childhood obesity given by the Institute of Medicine (IOM). Go to *www.iom.edu/~/media/Files/Report%20Files/2004/Preventing-Childhood-Obesity-Health-in-the-Balance/GlossaryFINALBitticks.pdf* to find the IOM definition of childhood obesity.

Step 1: *Identify Relevant Information and Uncertainties*

Go to *www.cdc.gov* and click on CDC A–Z Index and search under "O" for obesity and overweight. Review obesity trends. Next, search for childhood overweight and obesity, and obesity prevalence. Review overweight trends among children and adolescents.

1. Search for the following NCHS reports:
   a. Review "Prevalence of Overweight Among Children and Obesity and Adolescents: United States, 1963–1965 through 2011–2012"; see Table 3 "Prevalence of obesity among children and adolescents aged 2–19 years, by sex and race and ethnicity" (*www.cdc.gov/nchs/data/ hestat/obesity_child_11_12/obesity_child_11_12.pdf*).
   b. Review the trend of overweight among preschool-age children and among Mexican Americans in "Prevalence of Obesity Among Children and Adolescents: United States, Trends 1963–1965 through 2009–2010"; Table 1 shows the increase in obesity that has occurred since 1976–1980 among preschool children aged 2–5 years. Also see Figure 2 "Prevalence of obesity among boys aged 12–19 years, by race and ethnicity: United States, 1988–1994 and 2009–2010," and Figure 3 "Prevalence of obesity among girls aged 12–19 years, by race and ethnicity: United States, 1988–1994 and 2009–2010" for racial and ethnic disparities (*www.cdc.gov/nchs/data/hestat/obesity_ child_09_10/obesity_child_09_10.htm*).

What are some of the determinants of obesity in the Hispanic population that may be relevant to your target population? Use the websites above and other resources relevant to your target population.

2. What are some of the uncertainties not presented in the data or the case?

Step 2: *Interpret Information*

In a memo to your agency supervisor, communicate that you wish to begin a program on overweight prevention for preschool-age Mexican American children. To support your program, include a brief review of recent epidemiologic studies that reveal the national epidemic of overweight children and the health risks that may afflict these children, with a special emphasis on data for your target population.

Step 3: *Draw and Implement Conclusions*

As part of the nutrition care process, identify the most critical nutritional needs of your target population as a general nutrition diagnosis; write two PES (Problem, Etiology, Signs and Symptoms) statements based on the data reviewed and information presented in the case. (See the Professional Focus in Chapter 5 for more about the nutrition care process.)

Step 4: *Engage in Continuous Improvement*

As part of the nutrition care process:

1. Outline your intervention plan: Set three major goals based on your desired outcomes for your target population. Include intervention strategies that coincide with these goals. Consider your nutrition diagnosis when setting up your intervention plan. What may be some limitations in carrying out your intervention strategies?
2. What areas will you monitor and evaluate to assess whether you are meeting your desired outcomes?

PROFESSIONAL **FOCUS**

The Well-Read Community Nutritionist

Here is a sobering statistic: More than 20,000 biomedical journals are published each month. If each journal published just 20 research articles, the conscientious community nutritionist would need to browse through 400,000 articles per month, or more than 13,000 articles per day, to stay abreast of current scientific findings! And this figure doesn't include editorials, review articles, and letters to the editor—all valuable reading. How can you, as a busy community nutritionist, handle this volume of information, keep yourself informed, and maintain your sanity? We don't have all the answers, but we offer the following suggestions to help you cope with the onslaught of medical, health, and nutrition information. Let's begin with a few good reasons for reading the literature.

Ten Good Arguments for Reading Journals

Consider the following 10 good reasons for reading journals regularly:[1]

1. To impress others
2. To keep abreast of professional news
3. To understand pathophysiology

4. To find out how a seasoned health practitioner handles a particular problem
5. To find out whether to use a new or an existing diagnostic test, survey instrument, or educational tool with your patients or clients
6. To learn the clinical features and course of a disorder
7. To determine etiology or causation
8. To distinguish useful from useless or even harmful therapy
9. To sort out claims concerning the need for and the use, quality, and cost-effectiveness of clinical and other health care
10. To be titillated by the letters to the editor

Regular reading of the literature, especially in your area of specialization, is a must. There is no other way to learn about the latest scientific findings, the merits of a particular intervention or assessment instrument, or current legislation and its potential impact on your programs and clients. In short, to be an effective community nutritionist, you must constantly increase and update your knowledge base through regular perusal of journals, which brings us to our next question.

Which Journals Should You Read?

There is no hard and fast rule about the "best" journals to read because so much depends on the type of work you are doing and the needs of your clients. Some journals will appear on your "must read regularly" list; others can be spot-checked every month or two. Although nutrition journals will take priority, other specialty journals—particularly in the disciplines of epidemiology, health education, and medicine—are important. Presented here is a list of journals, newsletters, and other publications that will help you stay abreast of current developments that may be useful to you in delivering community programs. Many items listed in the Internet Resource lists throughout this text allow you to sign up for regular e-mail updates, too.

Nutrition Journals
American Journal of Clinical Nutrition
Canadian Journal of Dietetic Practice and Research
Human Nutrition: Applied Nutrition
Journal of the Academy of Nutrition and Dietetics
Journal of the American College of Nutrition
Journal of Hunger and Environmental Nutrition
Journal of Nutrition
Journal of Nutrition Education and Behavior
Journal of Nutrition for the Elderly
Journal of Obesity Research
Nutrition Research
Nutrition Reviews

Public Health Nutrition
Topics in Clinical Nutrition

Nutrition Newsletters
Harvard Health Letter
Nutrition Action Health Letter
Tufts University Health & Nutrition Letter
University of California at Berkeley Wellness Letter

Specialty Journals
American Journal of Epidemiology
American Journal of Health Promotion
American Journal of Preventive Medicine
American Journal of Public Health
Annals of Internal Medicine
Bioscience
British Medical Journal
Circulation
Diabetes
Diabetes Care
Environmental Health Perspectives
Health Education Research
Health Education & Behavior
International Journal of Behavioral Nutrition and Physical Activity
International Journal of Obesity
International Journal of Pediatric Obesity
Food, Nutrition, and Agriculture
Journal of the American Medical Association
Journal of Community Practice
Journal of Human Lactation
Journal of Medicine and Science in Sports and Exercise
Journal of the National Cancer Institute
Journal of Pediatric Endocrinology & Metabolism
Journal of School Health
Lancet
New England Journal of Medicine
Pediatrics
Preventing Chronic Disease
Preventive Medicine
Public Health Reports
Science

E-Resources
Academy of Nutrition and Dietetics Evidence Analysis Library:
www.andeal.org
Academy of Nutrition and Dietetics E-Newsletters: Daily News;
Eat Right Weekly: www.eatright.org
Bulletin of the World Health Organization:
www.who.int/bulletin/en

Cochrane Library (Cochrane Database of Systematic Reviews):
www.cochrane.org
Farm-to-School Routes Newsletter:
www.farmtoschool.org
Food Research and Action Center (FRAC) E-News:
http://frac.org
Morbidity and Mortality Weekly Report (MMWR):
www.cdc.gov/mmwr
USDA Economic Research Service (ERS) Reports:
www.ers.usda.gov/Publications

How to Get the Most Out of a Journal

There is no best way to "read" a journal. Although you will want to develop your own reading style, consider the following points. A glance at the table of contents will direct you to pertinent research articles and briefs for in-depth reading. In journals that you subscribe to personally, highlight special-interest articles in the table of contents with a colored marking pen. (This simple act may make it easier for you to remember, for example, where you spotted that intriguing article on school gardens.)

After scanning the table of contents, check the professional updates and news features to keep informed about key players, committees, conferences, and events in your discipline. Consult review articles for extensive coverage of current issues. The journal's editorials will expose you to the controversies surrounding a study's findings or the implications of the findings for practitioners. Regular reading of the letters to the editor will help you appreciate the flaws that plague some study designs and will expose you to the questions raised by scientists and practitioners in interpreting study results.

In choosing articles for in-depth reading, be selective and discriminating. You only have so much time. Select those articles that appear to be directly relevant to your needs, but allow time for other articles of interest. Refrain from agonizing that you don't have time to read as much as you think you should. Be organized and disciplined in your reading, but accept the fact that no one can read everything.

How to Tease Apart an Article

Most research articles have the same basic format with the following specific sections to help you assimilate the material:[2,3]

1. **Abstract or summary.** Provides an overview of the study, highlights the results, and indicates the study's significance. It should contain a precise statement of the study's goal or purpose.

2. **Introduction.** Presents background information such as the history of the problem or relevant clinical features. It reviews the work of other scientists in the area and describes the rationale for the study.

3. **Methods.** Describes the study design, selection of subjects, methods of measurement (e.g., the diet assessment instrument used), specific hypotheses to be tested, and analytical techniques (e.g., the method used to measure blood cholesterol or the method of statistical analysis).

4. **Results.** Details the study's outcomes. The results are typically presented in tables, graphs, charts, and figures that help summarize the study's findings.

5. **Discussion.** Provides an analysis of the meaning of the findings and compares the study's findings with those of other researchers. The discussion includes a critique of the work: What were the limitations of the study design? What problems occurred that may have affected the study outcome? What were the study's strengths?

6. **Conclusions/implications.** Some, but not all, articles include a short section that summarizes the findings or considers how the study results can be applied to practice. This section may also comment on directions for future research.

7. **References/bibliography.** Cites the relevant work of other scientists that the present investigators considered in conducting their study or interpreting the results.

Reading an article involves more than simply scanning the abstract and flipping or scrolling to the last paragraph of the discussion section for the author's summary statements. If you have decided that the article is important to you, take time to read the methods section carefully, for the substance of the work is outlined there. Any new information presented in the article is only as good as the method by which it was obtained. Was the hypothesis clearly stated? Was the study design clearly described? Were the methods used appropriate for testing the hypothesis? How were the data collected and analyzed? Once you learn to review the methods section critically, you will find that in some cases you do not need to read further. Some studies are so poorly designed or seriously flawed that the results lack validity.

One other important precept remains: Learn to form your own opinions about the study findings presented in the articles you read. Do not automatically assume that the findings are valid merely because the study was published by a leading researcher or research team. Reading the letters to the editors and talking about the study results with your colleagues are good ways to help you assess the validity of a study.

What Else Should You Read?

What else should you read to be an informed, effective community nutritionist? Everything! Well, everything you can: newsletters, books, consumer magazines, food labels, newspapers, advertising, menus, junk mail, websites, and journals in other disciplines.

Are we serious? Absolutely. We said at the outset (in Chapter 1) that one of your roles as a community nutritionist is to improve the nutrition and health of individuals living in communities. To do this well, you must be able to draw on many diverse elements within your community and culture to shape a program that meets a nutritional or health need. Let's say that you have been asked to design, implement, and evaluate a program to reduce the prevalence of obesity among school children in your community. To develop a nutrition and fitness program that appeals to children, you must be able to speak their language and get inside *their* culture. You will need to think about developing programs that can be implemented during the school year and during summer vacation (e.g., at YMCA summer camps), when school is not in session. Which reading material will help you find the right approach, the right action figures, the right tone? Everything from the *Journal of the Academy of Nutrition and Dietetics*[4,5,6,7] to children's books, advertising inserts in your local newspaper, the newspaper comics, scripts of popular TV programs, fast-food menus, T-shirt logos, a *Time* magazine article on inner-city farms and food gardens, a government publication on quick snack ideas—the list is endless. You never know when something you read in a totally unrelated area will be just the thing you need to help convey a nutrition message to your clients.

CHAPTER **SUMMARY**

The Practice of Epidemiology

▶ Epidemiology is the basic science of public health, "the study of the distribution and determinants of health-related states in specified populations, and the application of this study to control health problems."

▶ Determinants of disease are divided into two groups: (1) host factors (such as age, sex, race, nutrition status) that determine an individual's susceptibility to disease; and (2) environmental factors (such as living conditions, occupation) that determine the host's exposure to a specific agent.

Investigating Causes of Diseases

▶ Differences in rates of disease in populations are used to formulate hypotheses about the cause of a health problem or to assess exposure to a specific agent and to propose strategies for controlling or preventing health problems.

▶ The epidemiologic method can be used to describe a community's particular health problems and to determine whether a community's overall health is improving or getting worse by using surveillance activities and vital statistics.

Basic Epidemiologic Concepts

▶ *Risk* refers to the likelihood that people who are without a disease, but are exposed to certain *risk factors*, will acquire the disease at some point in their lives.

▶ The *relative risk (RR)* is a comparison of the risk of some health-related event, such as disease, in two groups. If the relative risk is greater than 1, people exposed to the factor have an increased risk of the outcome under investigation.

▶ *Incidence* is the proportion of a group initially free of a disease or condition that develops the disease or condition over a period of time.

▶ Prevalence is the number of existing cases of a disease or other condition in a given population. The *prevalence rate* is the proportion of persons in a population who have a particular disease or attribute at a particular point in time.

The Epidemiologic Method

▶ The epidemiologic method involves a series of steps: observing; counting cases or events; relating cases or events to the population at risk; making comparisons; developing a hypothesis; testing the hypothesis; drawing scientific inferences; conducting experimental studies; and intervening and evaluating.

▶ An important aspect of the epidemiologic method is determining whether the data are valid. Research data can have three possible explanations: (1) the data are incorrect because they are biased due to *selection bias, measurement bias,* or *confounding bias*; (2) the study results are due simply to chance and the observations made arose from random variation within the sample; or (3) the results represent the truth.

Types of Epidemiologic Studies

▶ The type of investigation undertaken depends to a large extent on the research question being asked and the type of data needed to answer the question.

▶ Ecological or correlational studies compare the frequency of events (or disease rates) in different populations with the per capita consumption of certain dietary factors.

▶ Cross-sectional or prevalence studies examine the relationships among dietary intake, diseases, and other variables as they exist in a population at a particular time.

▶ In cohort studies, a group of people free of the disease or condition of interest is identified and examined. The members of the cohort are followed for months or even years, during which time they are examined periodically to determine which individuals develop the characteristics of interest and which do not. Cohort studies can be retrospective or prospective cohort studies.

▶ In a case–control study, a group of persons or cases with the condition of interest are compared with a group of persons without the condition.

▶ The randomized controlled trial or clinical trial conducted as a double-blind experiment is the most rigorous evaluation of a dietary hypothesis.

Nutritional Epidemiology

▶ Epidemiology can be used to monitor and describe the food consumption, nutrient intake, and nutrition status of populations. The information obtained from large population surveys is then used to develop specific programs and services for groups whose nutrition status appears to be compromised.

▶ The primary method of assessing the available food supply at the national level is based on food balance sheets.

▶ Methods of assessing household food consumption consider the per capita food consumption of the household, taking into account the age and sex of persons in the household (or institution), the number of meals eaten at home or away from home, income, shopping practices, and other factors.

▶ Food consumption by individuals is estimated by a variety of methods: diet history, 24-hour dietary recall, food record or diary, and food frequency questionnaire.

▶ The effects of within-person variation on dietary intake must be considered when designing and evaluating studies of the relationship of diet to disease.

Epidemiology and the Community Nutritionist

▶ The science of epidemiology is essential to the delivery of effective nutrition programs and services. A key role of the community nutritionist is in *identifying* nutritional problems within the community; *interpreting* and critically evaluating the scientific literature; and formulating new nutrition policies or offering advice about eating patterns.

SUMMARY **QUESTIONS**

1. Define epidemiology and its relationship to community nutrition. What is meant by the terms *distribution* and *determinants*?
2. Consider the agent, host factors, and environment as contributors to heart disease. Provide an example of a factor to represent each of these, and list an intervention strategy to mitigate risk associated with the factor.
3. Explain hypothesis testing and how data about disease processes are obtained using the epidemiological method.
4. Explain how the complexity of our diets creates challenges in studying the relationship of diet to disease.
5. Explain why the day-to-day variation in an individual's nutrient intake can have important implications for nutritional epidemiologic studies.
6. Differentiate among the different types of nutritional epidemiological studies.

INTERNET **RESOURCES** . . . .

Eating Smart: A Nutrition Resource List for Consumers
http://pubs.nal.usda.gov/eating-smart-nutrition
-resource-list-consumers
A directory of food and nutrition resources for consumers.

Centers for Disease Control and Prevention
www.cdc.gov/mmwr
Morbidity and Mortality Weekly Report.

**The Food and Nutrition Information Center Nutrition
Resources**
http://fnic.nal.usda.gov
Resources from the Food and Nutrition Information Center.

National Agricultural Library
www.nal.usda.gov/food-and-human-nutrition
*Includes online publications, nutrient databases, software,
and information centers.*

National Institutes of Health
www.nih.gov
Links to the various institutes and centers of the NIH.

Nutrition Organizations
www.nutrition.org/news/useful-links/
A list compiled by the American Society for Nutrition.

Hirsh Health Sciences Library, Nutrition
http://researchguides.library.tufts.edu/nutrition_guide
*Nutrition links include guides, databases, electronic
journals, government resources, and more.*

CHAPTER 3

Understanding and Achieving Behavior Change

LEARNING **OBJECTIVES**

After you have read and studied this chapter, you will be able to:

- Compare and contrast various behavior change theories and strategies.

- Describe the stages of the transtheoretical model and identify appropriate intervention strategies for each stage.

- Identify factors that influence an individual's intention to change a health behavior, based on the health belief model, the theory of planned behavior, and social-cognitive theory.

- Describe motivational interviewing as a style of counseling.

- Discuss the role of self-efficacy in making and maintaining health behavior changes.

- Identify counseling strategies used in cognitive-behavioral therapy.

- Define the stages involved in the innovation decision process.

This chapter addresses such issues as health promotion theories and counseling skills to facilitate behavior change, public speaking, oral communications in presenting an educational session for a group, and current information technologies, which have been designated by the Accreditation Council for Education in Nutrition and Dietetics (ACEND) as Foundation Knowledge and Learning Outcomes for dietetics education.

CHAPTER **OUTLINE**

Something to think about...

We need to have visions, visions of healthy and safe lives in healthy and safe communities—even visions that seem impossible. Robert Kennedy used to say often, "Some people see things as they are and ask, 'Why?' I dream things that never were and ask, 'Why not?'" We need to dream things that never were and ask, "Why not?"

—*BARRY S. LEVY*,
American Journal of Public Health, *February 1998*

For a complete list of references, please access the MindTap Reader within your MindTap course.

Introduction

In 1937 an inventor introduced a new product to the grocery store: the shopping cart. Until that time, people had shopped for their groceries using a small bag or basket. The inventor perceived the convenience and ease of using a cart on wheels for this activity and advertised his product with the question, "Can you imagine winding your way through a spacious food market without having to carry a cumbersome shopping basket on your arm?"[1] Unfortunately, most people answered, no, they could not imagine doing this! They refused to accept the innovation. When queried about their behavior, customers claimed that the shopping cart looked like a baby carriage and that it made them feel weak and dependent. To get around this perception, the inventor hired women and men of various ages to come into his supermarkets and use the shopping carts to buy their groceries. This simple approach had the desired effect. Other customers saw the carts being used and elected to use them, too.[2]

This story illustrates two aspects of designing interventions. First, you must have information about your target population and why they do what they do. Understanding the behavior of your target population is an important step in developing strategies to influence—and eventually change—their **behavior**. Second, you must have a variety of tools or strategies to influence behavior. Your toolbox might include a nutrition blog site, podcast or video, a community-based program, or, as in the case of the shopping cart inventor, you might choose people from the target population to "model" the desirable behavior. This inventor effectively used the strategy of "modeling" or "observational learning" to change consumer behavior.

Recall from Chapter 1 that an intervention is a health promotion activity aimed at changing the behavior of a target population. A nutrition intervention is targeted at a nutrition-related problem. This chapter describes evidence-based theories and strategies to consider when designing a nutrition intervention program that targets lifestyle change related to eating patterns and physical activity. Study each of these topics before reading how community nutritionists working on Case Study 1, on page 92, put all of the elements together.

Behavior The response of an individual to his or her environment.

Draw from Current Research on Consumer Behavior

Simply knowing the factors that affect consumers' food choices does not tell us how consumers make their decisions. Numerous *theories* and *models* have been developed and tested that attempt to explain why and how people make behavior changes. **Behavior change theories** and **models** provide **evidence-based methods** or *strategies* empirically tested and shown to be effective in facilitating health-related behavior change. Some strategies target changes in attitudes and beliefs (i.e., motivational interviewing), while others more directly target behavior change (i.e., goal setting and problem solving). Improved outcomes can be achieved if community nutrition experts understand the target population and are able to skillfully select relevant theory-based strategies to facilitate diet-related behavior change.[3] The incorporation of behavior change theories into program planning is critical to the nutrition care process because the theories provide the evidence base to guide nutrition assessment, intervention design, and program evaluation. They move the food and nutrition practitioner from experience-based to evidence-based practice by providing a systematic and scientific foundation to their work. Improved understanding of why and how intervention strategies work will facilitate better and more consistent client outcomes.

Food and nutrition practitioners are frequently challenged to persuade, instruct, and coach groups and individuals to modify their eating patterns. This may be done through

Behavior change theories A systematic explanation of why and/or how people do what they do. A set of constructs, principles, and variables is used to explain or predict behavior. Theories must explain behavior in a broad range of situations.

Models A model uses elements of multiple theories to explain behavior.

Evidence-based methods An approach based on scientific proof.

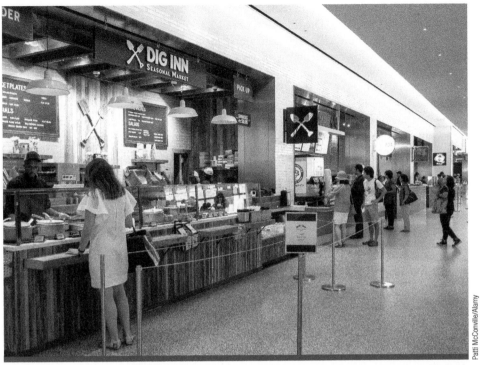

Patti McConville/Alamy

Simply knowing which food choices consumers make does not tell us *how* they make their decisions.

nutrition education, social marketing, or nutrition counseling interventions. **Nutrition education** is a formal process to instruct or train individuals in a skill or to impart knowledge to facilitate voluntary adoption of eating and other nutrition-related behaviors to improve or maintain health. Effective nutrition education generates the motivation that precedes behavior change.[4] **Social marketing** is an approach to promote healthy behaviors and improve personal and societal health and well-being that incorporates commercial marketing techniques to influence voluntary behavior.[5] The New York City Department of Health and Mental Hygiene's television ad campaign, "Are You Pouring on the Pounds?" highlights the health risks of consuming too many sugary drinks and is an example of a social marketing campaign. **Nutrition counseling** is typically conducted one-on-one, and is a collaborative activity during which a counselor and client jointly set priorities, establish goals, and create an action plan. The counselor provides coaching to foster responsibility for self-care to promote health or treat a health condition.[6]

A clear understanding of a client's or population's beliefs, attitudes, and cultural and social context permits *targeting* of educational materials to the target population (e.g., middle-aged African American women may have different needs and learning styles than men 19 to 25 years of age) and *tailoring* of nutrition information to meet the needs of a specific individual. A thorough nutrition assessment includes concepts from relevant behavior change theories (e.g., readiness to change, **self-efficacy**, perceived benefits, and barriers to change). Theories and models provide strategies that others (from diverse fields) have found effective in modifying attitudes and behavior and suggest methods for measuring the effectiveness of an intervention. A strong knowledge of behavior change theories expands a practitioner's arsenal of strategies to apply to diverse situations in order to maximize results.

It is not possible to describe every health behavior theory in this chapter, however, six deserve mention. The transtheoretical model (stages of change), the health belief model, and the theory of planned behavior each focus on individual characteristics that influence behavior, such as attitudes and beliefs. Social-cognitive theory and cognitive-behavioral

Nutrition education Any set of learning experiences designed to facilitate the voluntary adoption of food choices and other nutrition-related behaviors conducive to health and well-being.

Social marketing A method for changing consumer behavior; the design, implementation, and management of programs that seek to increase the acceptability of a social idea or practice among a target group.

Nutrition counseling A collaborative activity during which a counselor and client jointly set priorities, establish goals, and create an action plan; the counselor provides coaching to foster responsibility for self-care to promote health or treat a health condition.

Self-efficacy The belief that one can make a behavior change.

theory expand the perspective to include environmental factors, such as family, friends, and physical environment. The diffusion of innovations theory addresses the process by which people adopt new ideas and behaviors, such as seeking nutrition information on food labels or following the recommendations of the MyPlate food guidance system. Food and nutrition professionals often rely on integrating concepts and strategies related to several theories in an intervention. For example, in providing nutrition counseling for an individual, the practitioner may assess that the client is feeling ambivalent about committing to a behavior change (contemplation stage of change). The counselor may then use the motivational interviewing strategy of evocative open-ended questions to explore the client's perception of his or her susceptibility to the risks of the current behavior and the benefits of changing the behavior (health belief model) to help move the client toward committing to change. In the following sections, each theory is described briefly, and an example is given of how it can be applied to real-life situations. A summary of key concepts for several health behavior theories is provided in **Table 3-1.**

TABLE 3-1 Summary of Key Concepts of Selected Models of Behavior Change

BEHAVIOR CHANGE MODEL/ APPROACH	FOCUS	KEY CONCEPTS
Transtheoretical Model (Stages of Change Model)	Behavior change is explained as a readiness to change.	• Behavior change is described as a series of changes. • Specific behavior change strategies are identified for each stage.
Health Belief Model	Perception of the health problem and appraisal of proposed behavioral changes are central to a decision to change.	• Perceived susceptibility • Perceived impact • Perceived advantages of change • Appraisal of barriers • Self-efficacy
Theory of Planned Behavior or Theory of Reasoned Action	Behaviors are determined by a person's intentions to behave in certain ways.	• Intentions • Attitudes • Subjective norms • Perceived power and behavioral control
Social-Cognitive Theory or Social Learning Theory	People and their environment interact continuously, each influencing the other.	• Learning occurs through taking action, observations of others taking action, and evaluation of the results of those actions.
Cognitive-Behavioral Theory	Behavior is learned, so it can be unlearned; focus is on changing the environment.	• Challenge pattern of thinking. • Self-monitoring • Stress management • Identify and remove cues. • Emphasize consequences.
Diffusion of Innovation	A process by which an innovation, idea, or behavior spreads and involves an ever-increasing number of individuals in a population.	• Innovators • Early adopters • Early majority • Late majority • Laggards
Self-Efficacy	A component of numerous behavior change models; belief in ability to make a behavior change.	• Self-efficacy increases the probability of making a behavior change.
Motivational Interviewing	Client-centered approach to education and behavior change. Interviewer elicits client's intrinsic motivation to change, reinforces desire to change, seeks to diminish resistance to change, and respects client's autonomy; interviewer–client relationship is a collaborative partnership.	• Motivation is fundamental to change. • Express empathy (acceptance facilitates change). • Articulate, explore, and resolve ambivalence about change. • Self-defined behavior change goals. • Support self-efficacy.

Source: Adapted from K. Bauer, D. Liou, and C. Sokolik, *Nutrition Counseling and Education Skill Development*, 2nd ed. (Belmont, CA: Wadsworth/Cengage Learning, 2012).

The Transtheoretical Model (Stages of Change)

The Theory The transtheoretical model was developed by Prochaska and DiClemente and describes an individual's motivation and readiness to change a problem behavior. The model is founded on three assumptions: (1) behavior change involves a series of different steps or stages, (2) there are common stages and processes of change across a variety of health behaviors, and (3) tailoring an intervention to the stage of change people are in at the moment is more effective than not considering the stage people are in. The core construct of the theory is called "stages of change" and reflects a sequence of cognitive and behavioral stages through which people progress over time to change a behavior. Specific cognitive and behavioral strategies may accelerate an individual's movement along the continuum of change.[7] The transtheoretical model describes the five stages through which people move, although they don't always pass through these stages in a linear fashion and relapses are common (**Figure 3-1**).[8]

- **Precontemplation**—The individual is either unaware of or not interested in making a change.
- **Contemplation**—The individual is thinking about making a change, usually within the next six months. The individual may be weighing the risks and benefits of changing a behavior.
- **Preparation**—The individual actively decides to change and plans a change, usually within one month. The individual may have already tried changing in the recent past.
- **Action**—The individual is trying to make the desired change and has been working at making the change for less than six months. The individual has started making changes in his or her environment to support the changed behavior.
- **Maintenance**—The individual has sustained the change for six months or longer; the changed behavior has become a part of his or her daily routine.

Much work has been done to validate instruments used to assess community, group, and individual readiness to change related to specific dietary components, such as decreasing

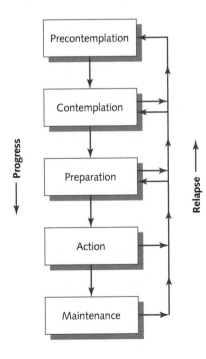

FIGURE 3-1 The Transtheoretical Stages of Change Model

Source: Adapted from S. Rollnick, P. Mason, and C. Butler, *Health Behavior Change: A Guide for Practitioners* (New York: Churchill Livingstone, 2000), 19.

fat intake, increasing fruit and vegetable intake, or maintaining a healthy weight.[9] An individual's readiness to change can quickly be assessed by asking the person to rate on a scale of 1 to 12 how interested he or she is in making a specific dietary change. A response of 1–4 can indicate unreadiness to change (precontemplation/relapse), 5–8 can indicate uncertainty regarding change (contemplation), and 9–12 may indicate readiness to change (preparation/action/maintenance). This is the type of strategy used with the nutrition algorithm outlined in Figure 15-4 (resolving phase). Asking the person why he or she gave such a score can provide insight.[10]

The model resembles a spiral in some respects, with people moving around the spiral until they eventually achieve maintenance and termination. People in the contemplation stage are typically seeking information about a behavior change, whereas people in the maintenance stage are less likely to be looking for information and more likely to be searching for methods of strengthening the behavior to avoid slipping back into old habits. The key here is to develop an intervention strategy that will meet people's needs in a manner appropriate to the stage they are in. Individuals, organizations, and communities can be assessed for their state of readiness to change.[11] **Table 3-2** outlines intervention strategies recommended for each stage of change.[12] Note that strategies targeted to the early stages of change target motivation and those used in the later stages are more consistent with strategies used in behavioral therapy.

The Application—Individual

A group of Canadian researchers sought to determine whether a new intervention program (Pathways to Change) based on the transtheoretical model would result in greater readiness to change, greater increases in self-care, and improved diabetes control as compared to standard care. Researchers recruited a total of 1,029 individuals with type 1 or type 2 diabetes who were in the precontemplation, contemplation, or preparation stages of change for self-monitoring of blood glucose, healthy eating, or smoking cessation. Clients were randomized to either usual care or the Pathways to Change program for the 12-month intervention. The Pathways to Change intervention consisted of stage-matched personalized assessment reports, self-help manuals, newsletters, and monthly individual phone counseling designed to improve readiness for self-monitoring of blood glucose, healthy eating,

TABLE 3-2 Stages of Change and Stage-Appropriate Intervention Strategies

STAGE OF CHANGE	INTERVENTION STRATEGIES
Precontemplation	• Build self-awareness and discuss risks and benefits. • Acknowledge and explore ambivalence about change. • Assess knowledge, attitudes, values, and beliefs. • Acknowledge emotions related to condition.
Contemplation	• Seek to resolve ambivalence. • Explore pros and cons of change. • Assess knowledge, attitudes, values, and beliefs. • Decrease barriers to change. • Increase confidence; reinforce past accomplishments. • Encourage a support network.
Preparation	• Resolve ambivalence about change. • Facilitate setting of small, specific, realistic goals. • Reinforce small accomplishments. • Facilitate development of an action plan.
Action	• Provide tailored self-help materials. • Refer to a behavioral program or self-management program.
Maintenance	• Coach on preparation for high-risk situations. • Link with online or community support groups. • Encourage continued self-monitoring and goal setting.

or smoking cessation. The Pathways to Change intervention targeting healthy eating proved superior over standard care in producing a significant improvement in stage of change (movement to the action or maintenance stage), decreasing intake of calories from saturated fat, and increasing daily intake of both vegetables and fruit. Clients in the action stage showed significant improvement in blood glucose measures. Use of the transtheoretical model was effective and gave practitioners insight into the mechanism of action.[13]

Fitness centers are interested in developing and implementing programs that promote fitness and health. A community nutritionist working at a local fitness club read about a study that found an association between the presence of chronic diseases such as hypertension, diabetes, heart disease, and dyslipidemia and readiness to change behavior in the areas of physical activity, fat intake, fruit and vegetable intake, and smoking. Study subjects were HMO members over the age of 40 years, a population much like the community nutritionist's own club members. The study found that members who were at highest risk of adverse health outcomes had the greatest readiness to change. A surprising finding was that members with heart disease were more ready to change their behavior to reduce disease risk than were members with diabetes.[14] Another study found that individuals in the precontemplation, contemplation, and preparation stages consumed fewer fruits and vegetables than people in the action or maintenance stages.[15]

The community nutritionist used these research findings and the stages of change model to alter certain aspects of her health promotion programming. To increase awareness among clients in the precontemplation stage, she added special lectures on heart disease and hypertension to the roster of special events and developed brochures describing the risk factors for hypertension, diabetes, and heart disease. For clients in the contemplation and preparation stages, she offered four cooking demonstrations featuring heart-healthy recipes prepared with local fresh fruits and vegetables; the cooking demos were given in the fitness center's food center on Friday nights, when club attendance was high. These activities were designed to show clients who were mainly thinking about making changes that cooking the heart-healthy way is fun and easy. For clients in the action stage—that is, those who had participated in one of the special events or attended a cooking demonstration—she offered a 20-minute individual counseling session to answer questions about reading food labels, identifying food sources of fat, and calculating saturated fat and *trans* fat intake. These actions were all designed to facilitate and support change among club members.

The Application—Communities   A university-sponsored study found that the prevalence of eating disorders among high school students in the city of Scottsville was nearly double the state average. A group of university researchers, community nutritionists, the city's chief medical officer, and a school nurse met to discuss what could be done to address the problem. The group determined that the city was in the precontemplation stage of readiness to change: No discussion of the problem among stakeholders (e.g., parents, teachers, students, administrators, health authorities) had taken place, no plan for addressing the problem had been developed, and no activities had been undertaken to reduce the prevalence of eating disorders. The group believed that the problem was urgent and that some action should be taken. As a first step in moving the community to the contemplation stage, the group decided to hold a citywide meeting of stakeholders and key community leaders to assess their perception of the problem, enhance awareness of the problem, identify pros and cons of action, identify resources for addressing the problem, and discuss desirable actions.

> **▶ THINK LIKE A COMMUNITY** NUTRITIONIST

Imagine you are a community nutritionist asked to develop a nutrition education class on the topic of fruit and vegetable consumption for parents of preschoolers attending a Head Start program in your community. You have decided to conduct a focus group with the parents to assess where they are in the stage of change in order to develop a program that is specific to the needs of the audience. List 5–10 questions you would ask the group to determine the predominant stage of change.

Motivational Interviewing

The Theory **Motivational interviewing** (MI) is a counseling approach developed by Miller and Rollnick that builds upon the **client-centered counseling** model in order to "help clients build commitment and reach a decision to change."[16] It is a way of interacting with the client that actively facilitates the client's exploring and resolving his or her own uncertainty about change, building confidence, and enhancing his or her commitment to change. It is a style of counseling that shifts responsibility for identifying solutions to the "lifestyle expert"—the client. The process stresses the use of carefully crafted questions and reflective listening skills rather than the drive to provide information. **Table 3-3** shows examples of interaction techniques for motivational interviewing counselors.[17] The counselor listens carefully to client responses and provides information only when the client requests or desires it.[18] Four general principles guide this motivational approach: (1) "resisting the righting reflex"—or the urge to confront the client about the need for behavior change; (2) eliciting and understanding the client's own motivations; (3) listening with empathy; and (4) empowering the client, encouraging hope and optimism. These four principles can be remembered by the acronym RULE: Resist, Understand, Listen, and Empower.[19]

1. **Resist.** Resist the urge to confront the client about the need to change. Ask the client how he or she feels about making a change and what the pros and cons related to the change would be. The goal of MI is to help clients work through their ambivalence to change using key questions and reflective listening.
2. **Understand.** Proceed in a nonjudgmental way that evokes and explores the client's own perceptions about his or her current situation and motivations for change.

TABLE 3-3 Motivational Interviewing Interaction Techniques

COUNSELOR DIALOGUE	TECHNIQUE	RATIONALE
"John, you say that changing some of your current eating patterns is a 9 out of 10 for importance."	Importance ruler	Provides counselor information on how the client perceives the importance for change. Follow up question elicits response in support of change (change talk).
"What makes this so important for you?"	Open-ended question	Elicit the client's own motivation for change (change talk).
"It sounds like you have identified behaviors, such as skipping meals during the day and then overeating at night, as something you have concerns about. You also mentioned that your wife has expressed concern about your recent weight gain because you have a family history of diabetes and heart disease."	Reflective listening	Counselor paraphrases the client's comments with emphasis on client's change talk to keep the momentum moving toward change.
"What I am hearing is that there are some changes you have already made. That is great. It seems like you really care about this."	Affirmation	Supportive, recognizes client's attempt at behavior change to support self-efficacy
"John, based on our discussion today, it seems you are very committed to doing what you can to stay healthy. You recognize that there are some specific behaviors you would like to change and we have come up with a plan to help you be more consistent with the timing of your meals and snacks. You've also downloaded the phone app so you can have quick access to the nutrition information for specific foods. How are you feeling about this?"	Summarizing	In ending a session, this provides the counselor the opportunity to draw attention to the important elements of the session. Summaries can also help move the conversation from one topic to another, or to reflect client's ambivalence.

3. **Listen.** Express empathy; use reflective listening skills by paraphrasing what the client says to determine the meaning of the client's statements.
4. **Empower.** Support self-efficacy by exploring how the client *can* make a difference in his or her own health using his or her own ideas and resources (e.g., how the client could successfully build time for physical activity into his or her daily routine). Reinforce the client's hope that change is possible and can make a difference in his or her health.

The Application In response to program evaluation, a research team from Minneapolis tested the feasibility of an intervention program enhancement incorporating motivational interviewing into a classroom-based program called New Moves targeted to adolescent girls who are overweight or at risk to become overweight.[20] Program feedback from the original New Moves study was received from participants, school staff, and the research team and indicated the need for a more intense intervention involving individualized attention beyond what could be provided in a group classroom setting. This school-based obesity prevention intervention is designed as a nine-week, all-girl high school class that students can elect to take for physical activity credit. The class meets three days a week for physical education and two days per week for a one-hour classroom lesson on nutrition or social support (taught by a registered dietitian and health educator). The motivational interviewing enhancement included seven individual sessions and two face-to-face meetings (20–25 minutes each) during the nine-week intervention, and five individual sessions scheduled every two to three weeks during the maintenance phase. Two of these follow-ups were done telephonically (10- to 15-minute duration). The registered dietitian and health educator each served as a "coach," and each student was assigned a specific coach to follow them through the program. The feasibility study assessed whether 20 of the teens (1) would attend the sessions, (2) were interested in face-to-face meetings, (3) would adhere to a meeting schedule, and (4) would prefer phone or face-to-face follow-up.

Motivational interviewing was used to assess each student's readiness to change and assist the student in setting concrete and realistic goals. Written scripts utilizing motivational interviewing techniques were provided. Participants were encouraged to identify aspects of their behavior that they would like to change and identify benefits and barriers to making that change. Coaches would facilitate the discussion, eliciting from the client potential strategies that may work to overcome barriers, providing education as needed, and guiding the students to set realistic behavior change goals.

The motivational interviewing enhancement was well received by the teens. Among the students, 81% completed all seven sessions and 100% set behavior change goals. All participants completed the first two individual sessions held during the intervention phase, 70% completed the phone follow-up, and 85% completed the five face-to-face sessions. The students reported liking the face-to-face sessions better than the phone sessions and met at lunch, during study hall, or after school. The teens responded well to the motivational intervention approach, and the research team felt that the coach–participant (rather than expert–student) relationship resonated with the adolescents' desire for independence. Researchers concluded that motivational interviewing was a feasible addition to a classroom-based obesity prevention program.

The Health Belief Model

The Theory The health belief model was developed in the 1950s by social psychologists with the U.S. Public Health Service as a way to explain why people, especially those in high-risk groups, failed to participate in programs designed to detect or prevent disease.[21] The study of a tuberculosis screening program led G. M. Hochbaum to propose that participation in the program stemmed from an individual's perception of both his or her susceptibility to tuberculosis and the benefits of screening. Furthermore, an individual's "readiness" to participate in the program could be triggered by any number of environmental events, such as media advertising. Since Hochbaum's analysis, the health belief model has been expanded to include all preventive and health behaviors, from smoking cessation to complying with diet and drug regimens.

The health belief model has three components.[22] The first is the perception of a threat to health, which has two dimensions. An individual perceives that he or she is at risk of contracting a disease and is concerned that having the disease carries serious consequences, some of which may be physical or clinical (e.g., death or pain), whereas others may be social (e.g., infecting family members or missing time at work). The theory is of limited value for primary prevention but can be effective when used with populations with nutrition-related risk factors, such as high cholesterol or diabetes, where diet change can be linked to tangible risk reduction.[23] Nutrition assessment would include the population's or client's perceived susceptibility (Do you feel at risk for cardiovascular disease?) and perception of the severity of that risk (How do you think this will affect your life?). The second component is the expectation of certain outcomes related to a behavior. In other words, the individual perceives that a certain behavior (e.g., choosing high-fiber foods to facilitate weight loss) will have benefits. Bound up in the perception of benefits is the recognition that there are barriers to adopting a behavior (e.g., choosing high-fiber foods requires skill in label reading and knowledge of food composition). The third component is self-efficacy, or "the conviction that one can successfully execute the behavior required to produce the outcomes."[24] A key tenet of losing weight, for example, is the belief that one can lose weight. Even if the individual were convinced that weight loss would keep him healthier longer, if he does not have confidence in his ability to implement a weight-loss diet, he may not even try. **Table 3-4** identifies strategies appropriate for the various components of the health belief model.[25] Other variables—such as education, income level, sex, age, and ethnic background—influence health behaviors in this model, but they are believed to act indirectly.

TABLE 3-4

Intervention Strategies Appropriate for the Various Components of the Health Belief Model

THEORY COMPONENTS TO ASSESS	INTERVENTION STRATEGIES
Perceived susceptibility	• Ask client if he or she thinks that he or she is at risk or has the disease/condition • Educate on disease risk and link to diet • Explore ambivalence about change (motivational interviewing) • Tailor information on disease/condition risk factors to promote accurate perception of risk
Perceived severity	• Explore ambivalence related to risk (motivational interviewing) • Discuss potential impact on client's lifestyle • Educate on consequences of the disease/condition (show graphs, statistics)
Perceived benefits and barriers	• Motivational interviewing • Explore pros and cons of change • Summarize and affirm the positive • Role models, testimonials
Cues to action	• How-to education • Incentive programs • Link current symptoms to disease/condition • Discuss media information • Reminder phone calls/mailings/texting • Social support
Self-efficacy	• Skill training and demonstration • Coach on alternatives and choices • Behavior contracting; small, incremental goals • Verbal reinforcement

The Application The American Cancer Society (ACS) recommends choosing foods and drinks in amounts that help achieve and maintain a healthy weight, eating five or more servings of a variety of vegetables and fruits every day, choosing whole grains over processed grains, and limiting intake of processed and red meats as a means of lowering cancer risk.[26] Since these recommendations were first published in 2006, Americans have increased their fruit and vegetable intake slightly, but their intake of saturated fat is still above the recommended level and obesity is a widespread public health problem. The key question for community nutritionists and other practitioners in health promotion remains: Which factors promote dietary change in the general population?

> ▸ **THINK LIKE A COMMUNITY** NUTRITIONIST
>
> The Cancer Risk Behavior Study discussed in this section indicates that knowledge about fat and fiber was not enough to motivate behavior change. Rather, a strong belief in the link between diet and cancer, and knowledge of nutrition-related health recommendations, were important in improving behaviors. In light of this, what key messages would you include in a class on cancer risk reduction through healthy eating? What nutrition education elements would you include to improve self-efficacy related to the messages?

Researchers in Washington state sought an answer to this question. They surveyed adults aged 18 years and older about their beliefs and health practices using the Cancer Risk Behavior Survey, which consists of questions on risk factors for cancer, including dietary habits, alcohol consumption, sun exposure, smoking behavior, and preventive cancer screening. The researchers found that adults who believed strongly in a connection between diet and cancer, and who were knowledgeable about health recommendations, made a greater number of positive dietary changes than those who had little belief. Having knowledge of the fat and fiber content of foods and perceiving social pressure to eat a healthful diet did not predict who made behavioral changes in dietary patterns or weight.[27]

Knowing that beliefs play a key role in motivating people to make lifestyle changes, the community nutritionists with the Mississippi affiliate of the American Cancer Society increased the funding for their public awareness campaign. They designed three posters and a public service television announcement that reinforced the message that smoking, sun exposure, and certain dietary patterns are linked with increased cancer risk. This strategy was designed to influence the beliefs of people in high-risk groups.

The Theory of Planned Behavior

The Theory The theory of planned behavior, sometimes called the theory of reasoned action, was developed by Icek Ajzen and Martin Fishbein. It "predicts a person's intention to perform a behavior in a well-defined setting."[28] The theory is a fundamental model for explaining social influence and can be used to explain virtually any health behavior over which the individual has control. According to the model, behavior is determined directly by a person's intention to perform the behavior. **Intentions** are the "instructions people give to themselves to behave in certain ways."[29] They are the scripts that people use for their future behavior. In forming intentions, people tend to consider the outcome of their behavior and the opinion of significant others before committing themselves to a particular action. In other words, intentions are influenced by attitudes and **subjective norms**. Attitudes are determined by the individual's belief that a certain behavior will have a given outcome, by an evaluation of the actual outcome of the behavior, and by a perception of his or her own ability to control the behavior. Subjective norms are determined by the individual's normative beliefs. In forming a subjective norm, the individual considers the expectations of various other people. According to this theory, if people evaluate a recommended behavior as positive (attitude), and if they think their significant others want them to do it (subjective norm), the result is a higher intention (motivation), and they are more likely to perform the behavior.[30]

Intentions A determination to act in a certain way.

Subjective norms The perceived social pressure to perform or not to perform a behavior.

A modification of the theory, called the theory of trying, was proposed by Richard P. Bagozzi, who argued that an expression of intention is insufficient to produce a behavior change.[31] In the new model, shown in **Figure 3-2**, such factors as past experience (success or failure) with the behavior, the existence of mechanisms for coping with the behavior outcome (e.g., having a strategy for dealing with not meeting a weight-loss goal), and emotional responses to the process all influence the intention to try a behavior. Bagozzi and his colleagues hypothesized that when intentions are well formed, they are strong mediators of behavior; when intentions are poorly formed, however, their influence on behavior is diminished and that of attitudes grows stronger.[32]

We know that just providing information is frequently not adequate to precipitate diet change. Understanding a population's or an individual's intentions, attitudes, subjective norms, barriers, self-efficacy, and perceived behavioral control can facilitate tailoring of the nutrition intervention strategy to achieve the desired outcome. Campaigns targeting attitudes and perceived norms can be highly effective.

The Application and Infant Feeding Practices

The infant and maternal health benefits associated with breastfeeding have been well documented (see Chapter 11). The American Academy of Pediatrics recommends exclusive breastfeeding for approximately six months, followed by the continuation of breastfeeding as complementary foods are introduced for at least one year.[33] Although there has been continued progress made in the percentage of infants in the United States who are breastfed, the rates fall short of the *Healthy People 2020* objectives. Understanding factors influencing women's breastfeeding practices is an important step in developing interventions to support the behavior.

The theory of planned behavior (TPB) has been applied to research examining a variety of health behaviors such as healthy eating and exercise.[34] A study funded by the California Department of Health Services Special Supplemental Nutrition Program for Women, Infants and Children (WIC) used TPB to examine the factors impacting low-income women's infant-feeding practices.[35] A total of eight focus groups (four English-speaking and four Spanish-speaking) comprised of 64 mothers who were participants in the WIC

FIGURE 3-2

The Theory of Trying

Source: R. P. Bagozzi, "The Self-Regulation of Attitudes, Intentions, and Behavior," *Social Psychology Quarterly* 55 (1992): 179. Used with permission of R. P. Bagozzi and the American Sociological Association.

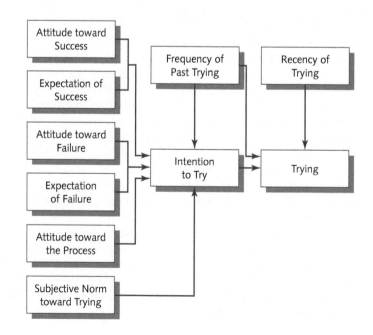

program and had infants aged 4–12 months participated in a facilitated discussion of their beliefs and intentions regarding infant feeding. The topics discussed were:

- Type of foods and fluids fed to infants up to six months of age and how they were given
- Reasons to choose breastfeeding or bottle-feeding
- Prior to the birth of their babies, how did the women believe they would feed their baby (breastfeed, bottle-feed, when to introduce solid food) and how does that compare to their actual feeding practices after their babies were born
- What influenced their actual feeding practices after the baby was born

The intent was to explore the women's attitudes (the extent that performing the behavior is positively or negatively valued), subjective norms (social pressure from others to engage or not engage in the behavior), and perceived behavioral control (sense of self-efficacy in performing the behavior).

The participants reported that medical providers and the staff at WIC provided information on infant-feeding guidelines. The majority of the participants understood the health benefits of breastfeeding and prior to the birth of their babies had intentions to breastfeed, although 60% of the mothers reported they provided formula within the first few weeks after birth or introduced solid food earlier than four months. Many communicated the perception of the inability to control circumstances that interfered with their ability to breastfeed exclusively. Conditions that impacted their intentions to breastfeed included concerns about adequate milk supply, initial breastfeeding difficulties, appeasing a "fussy" infant, the desire for the infant to sleep through the night, lack of support from childcare facilities, and returning to work. A common assumption was that infant waking and crying indicated hunger. Mothers expressed concern that the infant was not "full" or "satisfied" with breastfeeding alone; some mothers described giving additional food if they felt the infant may not be full for a sufficient time. Worried that their health care providers would not understand their inability to follow feeding guidelines, mothers relied on advice from family and friends.

This study demonstrates the usefulness of examining the influences on the infant-feeding intentions within the construct of the theory of planned behavior. Influences reported by the focus group participants included their belief about the importance of breastfeeding and the modifiers that made breastfeeding difficult, their perception of their lack of ability to comply with infant-feeding guidelines in light of challenges, and their response to opinions of family, friends, and health care providers. The investigators recommend using this information to develop targeted education interventions and provide specific tools to promote appropriate infant-feeding practices.

The Application and Weight Management

Dieting is a common method of trying to achieve an acceptable body shape. Young boys and girls often express the same dissatisfaction with their body shapes that older adolescents and adults do. Girls, in particular, express intentions to diet more frequently than boys express such intentions.[36] Research has shown, however, that even when the intention to diet is high, people have difficulty sticking with a weight-loss program.[37]

The community nutritionist at the Fairlawn Weight Management Center was experiencing a high dropout rate among adolescents participating in the center's Get Fit Now program, which included sessions on the principles of balanced eating, controlling eating impulses, and physical activity. Drawing on the principles of the theory of planned behavior, he decided to survey the program participants about their intentions to lose weight, their attitudes about their body shapes, their level of self-esteem, their expectations related to success, their support from family and friends, and their perception of their ability to control eating and lose weight. He used the survey results to add certain components to the Get Fit Now program. For example, he added two sessions: one to help participants

▶ **THINK LIKE A COMMUNITY NUTRITIONIST**

Suppose you are developing a breastfeeding promotion campaign for low-income women. If you were to use the theory of planned behavior as a framework for this intervention, list the audience (in addition to pregnant women) you would target with this effort.

clarify whether the time was right to lose weight and one to boost their coping skills so they could handle lapses. And he paired some participants who had not been successful losing weight in the past with others who had reached previous weight-loss goals. These actions were meant to improve the participants' intentions to master their eating habits and lose weight.

The Application Using Two Theories

Frequently, practitioners will incorporate concepts from more than one theory into an intervention design. Preventing osteoporosis is an important public health initiative. One of the *Healthy People 2020* objectives is to "increase the consumption of calcium in persons aged 2 years and older."[38] A community nutritionist sought to determine whether an eight-week, community-based education program designed using the health belief model and theory of planned behavior would be effective in improving calcium intake of study participants. Components of these theories were used to develop the program content and evaluation tool for the education program. Each class included a short lecture and a hands-on activity to increase self-efficacy.

Dietary calcium intake was quantified using a food frequency questionnaire. Health belief model constructs were measured using the validated Osteoporosis Health Belief Scale. Survey items were developed and tested to assess attitudes (about milk and dairy foods and the role of calcium in health), subjective norms (whether significant others liked dairy foods; health care providers' positions on calcium intake), and intention to change calcium intake. Lesson topics addressed severity and susceptibility to osteoporosis, benefits of increasing calcium intake, overcoming barriers, discussion of facts and fallacies, label reading, recipe sharing, taste testing, and serving-size games.

An active learning approach was included in each lesson not just to affect knowledge acquisition but to increase self-efficacy and influence attitudes and intentions to increase calcium intake. Assessment of theory constructs helped tailor the delivery of the program (addressing specific barriers and perceptions) and helped evaluate what components of the program worked well (e.g., label-reading skills) and where further program improvements could be made.[39]

Post-intervention calcium intake increased from a mean of 644 mg/day to a mean of 821 mg/day. Statistically, significant improvements were found for health belief model constructs related to beliefs about benefits of increasing calcium intake, susceptibility to developing osteoporosis, and three tasks associated with self-efficacy (I can find the calcium content of foods by reading food labels, I am sure I can increase the amount of calcium in my diet, and I use food labels to make shopping decisions). The intervention significantly improved the theory of planned behavior construct associated with attitude and intent to increase calcium intake, but there was no significant relationship between intention to increase calcium intake and calcium intake.

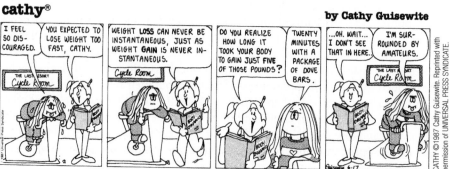

Social-Cognitive Theory

The Theory Social-cognitive theory (SCT) explains behavior in terms of a model in which behavior, personal factors such as cognition, and the environment interact constantly, such that a change in one area has implications for the others (known as reciprocal determinism). For example, a change in the environment (say, the loss of a spouse's support for a weight-loss effort) produces a change in the individual (a decrease in the incentive to lose weight) and consequently a change in behavior (abandonment of a regular exercise routine). This theory, which is also known as social learning theory, was developed to explain how people acquire and maintain certain behaviors.

An individual's confidence (self-efficacy) and ability to perform a particular behavior (behavioral capacity) and his or her perception of the probable outcome influence the amount of effort he or she will invest in a behavior change. The major concepts in SCT, many of which were formulated by Albert Bandura, and their implications for interventions are given in **Table 3-5**. In this context, the environment includes both the social realm (family, friends, peers, coworkers) and the physical realm (the workplace, the layout of a kitchen). A strength of SCT is that it focuses on certain target behaviors rather than on knowledge and attitudes.[40]

The Healthy Hunger-Free Kids Act of 2010 (HHFKA) provides funding and sets policy for the USDA's federal school meal and child nutrition programs and increases access to healthy food for low-income children. At a time when approximately one-third of U.S. children are overweight or obese and 20% live in poverty, the goal of this legislation is to provide the support needed to improve the health and well-being of our children.[41] The HHFKA authorizes the USDA to set nutrition standards for all foods sold in schools, including à la

TABLE 3-5 Key Concepts in Social-Cognitive Theory and Their Implications for Behavioral Interventions

COMPONENT TO ASSESS	DEFINITION	IMPLICATIONS FOR INTERVENTION STRATEGIES
Environment	• Factors that are physically external to the person	• Provide opportunities and social support
Reciprocal determinism	• Dynamic interaction of the person, the behavior, and the environment in which the behavior is performed	• Consider multiple behavior change strategies targeting motivation, action, the individual, and the environment • Motivational interviewing • Behavioral therapy (e.g., self-monitoring, stimulus control) • Social support
Self-regulation (control)	• Personal regulation of goal-directed behavior or performance	• Provide opportunities for decision making, self-monitoring, goal setting, problem solving, and self-reward
Behavioral capability	• Knowledge and skill to perform a given behavior	• Comprehensive education • Skill development training/coaching
Expectations	• A person's beliefs about the likely outcomes or results of a behavior	• Motivational interviewing • Model positive outcomes of diet/exercise
Self-efficacy	• The person's confidence in performing a particular behavior and in overcoming barriers to that behavior	• Skill development training/demonstrations • Small, incremental goals; behavioral contracting • Monitoring and reinforcement • Problem-solving discussions
Observational learning	• Behavioral acquisition that occurs by watching the actions and outcomes of others' behavior	• Demonstrations/peer modeling • Group problem-solving sessions
Reinforcement	• Responses to a person's behavior that increase or decrease the likelihood of its recurrence	• Affirm accomplishments • Encourage self-initiated rewards and incentives

Source: T. Baranowski et al., "How Individuals, Environments, and Health Behavior Interact: Social Learning Theory," in *Health Behavior and Health Education*—Theory, Research, and Practice, 3rd ed., eds. K. Glanz et al.

carte menus, vending machines, and school stores. Schools participating in the National School Lunch Program and/or School Breakfast Program are required to develop a wellness policy that includes specific goals for nutrition promotion and education, physical activity, and other school-based activities that promote student wellness. Members of the school community—such as parents, students, school foodservice personnel, health professionals, and administrators—are encouraged to participate in the wellness policymaking process. The USDA supports the implementation of the HHFKA standards by providing a series of grants to provide training and technical assistance for child nutrition foodservice professionals, encouraging locally sourced foods through "Farm to School" initiatives, and providing toolkits of evidence-based strategies to promote the consumption of healthier foods.

Consider the comprehensive nutrition services now provided in schools as a result of HHFKA within the framework of the social-cognitive theory of behavior change:

- *Environment.* The physical environment has been changed in terms of the composition and quality of the meals provided.
- *Self-efficacy.* Even small changes that increase the convenience and attractiveness of healthy foods can influence students' choices.[42]
- *Behavioral capability.* Comprehensive nutrition education develops students' knowledge and skills related to healthy eating.
- *Observational learning.* The influence of observing friends, peers, and school personnel making healthier choices impacts students' own motivations to change their behavior.
- *Reinforcement.* Partnerships with schools, families, and community members provide further reinforcement, sometimes utilizing incentives to encourage the students to adopt and maintain healthy eating patterns.

Results of the HHFKA school-based interventions are encouraging. Recent studies show that changes in the school food environment have a positive impact on eating behaviors.[43] One study concluded that children were eating 16% more vegetables and 23% more fruits at lunch.[44] Clearly, comprehensive school nutrition services can have an integral role in improving the dietary behaviors of students.

The Application Telephone-based counseling is an excellent strategy for connecting with clients who are homebound or located in geographically remote regions. A community nutritionist used a telephone-based intervention that incorporated a computer-assisted protocol based on social-cognitive theory that targeted increased consumption of fruits and vegetables in 94 healthy adults consuming fewer than five servings of fruits and vegetables per day. The nutrition prescription was three to five servings of vegetables; two to four servings of fruit; and three servings of whole grains, beans, or legumes per day. Average daily intake of fruits, vegetables, whole grains, beans, legumes, fiber, and fat was assessed at baseline and at six months, using a set of three 24-hour recalls, along with a measure of blood carotenoid levels in a subset of clients as an objective biomarker for fruit and vegetable intake. The intervention consisted of eight telephone counseling sessions planned over a three-month time period. Phase 1 consisted of four telephone calls, one every three to four days, that focused on education and enhancement of self-efficacy to set realistic, short-term goals. Phase 2 consisted of three phone calls at 10-day intervals, that focused on overcoming diet change barriers, modifying the environment, recipes, portion sizes, cooking, and encouraged goal setting. Phase 3 consisted of one call to assess progress and reinforce positive action. The intervention was successful at significantly increasing daily vegetable intake at six months by 67%, fruit intake by 71%, and whole grain and bean intake by 40%. These increases were corroborated by a significant increase in the biomarker of total blood carotenoids.[45] This study drew on the SCT concepts of environment, behavioral capabilities, expectations, self-efficacy, and reinforcement.

PROGRAMS IN **ACTION**

EatFit Intervention Program

Guided goal setting is an approach that presents individuals with a set of preformatted goals that can help facilitate behavior change. The process allows people to choose those goals that are most important to them. Through guided goal setting, a person can define success in self-fulfilling ways, come up with strategies for success, and divide behavior change into attainable steps. EatFit—an initiative of the Expanded Food and Nutrition Education Program (EFNEP) administered by the University of California, Davis—is based on this approach to goal setting in a comprehensive program for young teens.

EatFit is a goal-oriented intervention designed to challenge middle school students to improve their eating and fitness choices. This program uses computer technology to assist adolescents with diet assessment and "guided" goal setting for making healthy lifestyle choices. The program provides skill-building experiences and social support to promote dietary self-efficacy and goal attainment.

EatFit's audience was middle school students in various settings: low-income classrooms, after-school programs, 4-H Youth Development Programs, EFNEP, and other youth programs. EatFit staff conducted focus groups with middle schoolers and identified three factors that were motivators for behavior change: increased energy, improved appearance, and greater independence. The nine-lesson curriculum addressed these three factors rather than focusing on disease prevention, a difficult concept for middle school students. Student feedback influenced development of the program. Students were included in focus groups, individual interviews, pilot testing, and field testing. They recommended the workbook's magazine format as a tool that would be attention-getting.

The EFNEP Evaluation and Reporting System was adapted for the EatFit personalized assessment. Culturally diverse foods likely to be eaten by adolescents were added. The development of portion-size photographs allowed more accurate depiction of serving size. The assessment database was expanded to include "added sugar" to help students evaluate their sugar consumption. Students were aided in setting their dietary goals. Areas for which students could set guided goals included increasing calcium intake, increasing iron intake, reducing fat intake, reducing added sugar intake, increasing fruits and vegetables, and improving general eating habits. Using the computerized assessment package, they assessed their daily eating habits and were guided to set goals based on the assessment. EatFit encouraged community and family participation. Its website, *www.eatfit.net*, offers resources to staff for expanding the EatFit program into the community. Bilingual brochures encourage parent participation in the program.

EatFit is a Cooperative Extension program. Cooperative Extension offices throughout the United States, its territories and military bases, and several countries outside the United States can use the program with their English-speaking populations. Resources needed to replicate the program include print materials, Internet access, and supplies for food demonstrations. Online training is available 24 hours a day, seven days a week.

Theory Base/Rationale

Three major constructs of the social-cognitive theory—self-efficacy, outcome expectancies, and self-regulation—were applied to the development, implementation, and evaluation of EatFit. Lessons support self-efficacy by allowing students to practice skills, receive encouragement, and establish social support. Practice in cooking and physical skills in the classroom increases self-efficacy so that students are more likely to repeat these activities on their own. Students are informed of clear, meaningful results that will occur if they improve their dietary and physical activity choices: increased energy, independence, and improved appearance. The curriculum promotes self-regulation through the guided goal-setting process. Students have the opportunity to assess their dietary and physical activity behaviors, and then set goals and monitor their progress in achieving those goals, with prizes awarded for goal attainment.

Outcomes/Evaluation Data

Pilot testing of the program was conducted on 155 middle school students. Field testing was conducted with approximately 10,000 students throughout California by Cooperative Extension staff. In a crossover controlled field trial, EatFit was evaluated for effectiveness in 46 students. Some 44–73% of participants improved in dietary and/or physical activity for self-efficacy and behavior. Significant improvement was observed in dietary behaviors and in physical activity self-efficacy. When students set a dietary goal, they significantly increased positive dietary behaviors specific to that goal. Close to 75% of students rated themselves as having made at least one lasting improvement in dietary choices; 69% reported making at least one lasting improvement in physical activity choices. A randomized controlled field trial of 94 students was conducted to investigate the effect of the program's guided goal setting. Participants in the "treatment" group (intervention with goal setting) made significant improvements in dietary practices (73%), compared to the control group receiving intervention without guided goal setting (54%). The treatment group also improved significantly compared to controls on the physical activity self-efficacy variable (44% vs. 29%).

Lessons Learned

The success of this program reflects the inclusion of motivators and goals that are relevant to middle school students. The entire program reinforces the synergistic relationship among nutrition, physical activity, and overall physical fitness as a way to increase energy, improve appearance, and attain greater independence.

Source: From *Community Nutritionary* (White Plains, NY: Dannon Institute, Fall 2001). Used with permission. For more information about the Awards for Excellence in Community Nutrition, go to *www.dannon-institute.org*.

Cognitive-Behavioral Theory

The Theory There is strong evidence that behavioral therapy facilitates modification in dietary habits, weight, and cardiovascular and diabetic risk factors.[46] The theories discussed thus far have targeted attitudes, beliefs, and intentions. The cognitive-behavioral theory is best applied when people are actively ready to make a change. Cognitive-behavioral theory is based on the assumption that all behavior is learned and directly related to internal factors (e.g., thoughts and thinking patterns) and external factors (e.g., environmental stimuli and feedback). Clients are taught to use a variety of behavioral and cognitive strategies to recognize behaviors that lead to inappropriate eating and replace them with more rational thoughts and actions. The process is highly process oriented, goal directed, and facilitated through a variety of problem-solving tools. Strategies include goal setting, self-monitoring, problem solving, social support, stress management, stimulus control, cognitive restructuring, relapse prevention, rewards, and contingency management. It is frequently incorporated into self-help materials, group education, computer-based interventions, and nutrition counseling.

For diet change, effective strategies include self-monitoring, goal setting, problem solving, stimulus control, and cognitive restructuring. **Table 3-6** describes application tips for incorporating these behavioral strategies.[47]

The Application The Diabetes Prevention Program (DPP) Research Group used an intensive lifestyle-modification program based on cognitive-behavioral theory. This landmark study assessed the effect of lifestyle modification on the prevention or delay of development of diabetes in 3,234 nondiabetic persons as compared to drug therapy (850 mg metformin,

TABLE 3-6

Application Tips for Incorporating Behavioral Strategies of Cognitive-Behavioral Theory into Behavioral Interventions

BEHAVIORAL	APPLICATION TIPS
Self-monitoring	• Provide tools and instruction—tailor monitoring to improve compliance. • Coach client to review and identify eating patterns. • Assist with goal setting.
Goal setting	• Client identifies potential goal (self-monitoring may help). • Discuss pros and cons of goal and sources of support and barriers. • Track progress toward long- and short-term goals. • Encourage strategies to build confidence and reinforce success.
Problem solving	• Define the problem. • Brainstorm solutions. • Weigh pros and cons of potential solutions. • Select/implement strategy. • Evaluate outcomes/adjust strategy.
Stimulus control	• Review self-monitoring records for triggers. • Assist client in deciding how to modify the environment to eliminate the trigger. • Assist client in establishing rewards for success. • Reinforce only if criteria met.
Cognitive restructuring	• Self-monitor thoughts and feelings. • Help client replace irrational thoughts with more rational ones. • Coach client on replacing negative self-talk.

twice per day) or a placebo.[48] The lifestyle intervention was goal based, with a goal of 7% weight loss and physical activity of at least 150 minutes per week. Participants were assigned an individual case manager and met with their case manager 16 times over the first six months of the program and completed a core behavior therapy curriculum covering diet, exercise, and behavior-modification principles. Participants were seen in person at least once every two months. Participants were instructed to self-monitor minutes of physical activity and fat grams consumed every day during the core curriculum and then one week per month over the remainder of the trial. Outcome measures were taken at three years. Lifestyle intervention based on cognitive-behavioral theory reduced incidence of diabetes by an astounding 58% and drug therapy reduced the incidence by 31%, as compared to placebo. Lifestyle intervention was significantly more effective than drug therapy.

The Diffusion of Innovation Model

The Theory People often cannot or will not change their behavior, and many do not adopt innovations easily (recall the story about shopping carts at the beginning of this chapter). Even so, some people are more daring than others. Such people are the vanguard in the diffusion of innovation, the process by which an innovation spreads and involves an ever-increasing number of individuals within a population.[49] The diffusion of innovation model was developed by E. M. Rogers and F. F. Shoemaker in the 1970s to explain how a product or idea becomes accepted by a majority of consumers. The model consists of four stages:[50]

- **Knowledge**—The individual is aware of the innovation and has acquired some information about it.
- **Persuasion**—The individual forms an attitude either in favor of or against the innovation.
- **Decision**—The individual performs activities that lead to either adopting or rejecting the innovation.
- **Confirmation**—The individual looks for reinforcement for his or her decision and may change it if exposed to counter-reinforcing messages.

Innovations spread throughout a population largely by word of mouth. The speed of diffusion is a function, in part, of the number of people who adopt the innovation. Consumers can be classified according to how readily they adopt new ideas or products. Innovators adopt an innovation quite readily, usually without input from significant others. Innovators perceive themselves as popular and are financially privileged. This group is small. Like innovators, early adopters are integrated into the community and are well respected by their families and peers. Opinion leaders are often found in this group. Members of the early majority tend to be cautious in adopting a new idea or product, and persons in the late majority are skeptical and usually adopt an innovation only through peer pressure. Finally, the laggards are the last to adopt an idea or product, although they usually adopt it eventually. Members of this group tend to come from small families, to be single and older, and to be traditional.[51]

The Application A community nutritionist with Nutrition in Action, a company owned and operated by three registered dietitians, was concerned about several participants in her Heart-Healthy Living program. She perceived their lack of interest in making the kinds of dietary changes that would help lower their risk of having another heart attack. To boost their interest and enthusiasm for heart-healthy eating and cooking, she hit on the idea of contacting a popular local chef who had recently been interviewed on local television about the challenges he faced after surviving a heart attack. During the interview, the chef had indicated that he was just learning how to prepare heart-healthy foods and that he expected his new skills to make their way to his restaurant's menu. His comments agreed with those made by chefs who were surveyed about their food science

ENTREPRENEUR
IN ACTION
· · · · · · · · · · · · · · · ·

As a community health volunteer with the Peace Corps in West Africa, David Strefling, RD, witnessed the vital role of nutrition education in the lives of the women and children he worked with. Today, he works with an HIV/AIDS population in New York City for a nonprofit agency. Many of his clients have low levels of education, poor knowledge of nutrition, and other behavioral issues. The key, he says, is to provide basic education aimed at the education level of the client. Even the smallest change, such as walking 15 minutes more a day, can improve health and result in the desire to make other small changes leading to tangible, impressive changes over time. For David, seeing clients change their habits and improve their health condition remains the most rewarding endpoint in the profession. Find out more about David and his work online at *www.cengagebrain.com*.

knowledge and practice; that is, many chefs want to provide good nutrition to their customers but often lack the necessary knowledge and skills.[52] Believing the chef was a good early adopter, the community nutritionist persuaded him to join the group and expand his heart-healthy cooking repertoire. She believed his enthusiasm would be catching and would influence participants who resisted adopting innovations related to cooking.

Findings Regarding Applications of Theory to Nutrition Interventions

The Evidence Analysis Library of the Academy of Nutrition and Dietetics hosts a systematic analysis of the impact of behavior change theories on nutrition counseling in adults. In short, a plethora of evidence exists to support the use of cognitive-behavioral theory and strategies targeting weight loss, diabetes prevention and management, and cardiovascular disease. The addition of motivational interviewing to cognitive-behavioral programs has shown a significant boost in desired outcomes. Improved documentation of behavior change theories used to implement nutrition interventions is needed to build the body of evidence describing their effect.[53]

Put It All Together: Case Study 1
· ·

Chapter 4 introduces Case Study 1 (see page 106), which describes an assessment aimed at obtaining information about women and heart disease to determine if an intervention should be developed. As a result of the needs assessment, a team of nutritionists chose to develop several intervention activities, including healthy cooking and smoking cessation courses (see Table 5-5 on page 160).

The team of community nutritionists decided to conduct formative evaluation research to obtain information about the target population's skills. As discussed in Chapter 5, formative evaluation is the process of testing and assessing certain elements of a program before it is implemented fully. In focus group sessions, they asked women whether they had participated in cooking and smoking cessation courses, whether these programs had worked, and what they had found valuable about the course materials. The team asked about their expectations related to reducing the risk of coronary heart disease. The results of these focus group discussions led them to consider adding an innovative element to their intervention strategy: a smoking reduction course, in which the goal would not be to get people to quit smoking but rather to help them cut down on the number of cigarettes smoked daily and adopt positive lifestyle behaviors (e.g., eating less solid fat and getting moderate exercise). Before finalizing the intervention strategy, the team planned to conduct a review of the literature related to smoking and health behaviors, develop a course outline, and then evaluate this element of the intervention strategy.

As the overall intervention strategy began to take shape, the team could see how their health promotion activities had been influenced by the theories of consumer behavior. The website, posters, and brochures were aimed at people in the contemplation and preparation stages of change. The proposed activities in the policy arena—namely, advocating for legislation calling for smoke-free restaurants and a ban on advertising sponsored by tobacco companies at athletic events—were aimed at people in the maintenance stage. Some aspects of the Heartworks for Women cooking course, particularly those related to helping participants make simple dietary changes, reinforce healthful eating habits, and cope with setbacks, drew on the principles of the health belief model and social-cognitive theory. And the team could envision forming partnerships with other organizations, such as the local affiliates of the lung and cancer associations, to achieve some of their goals. The next step would be to develop the nutrition education component (described in Chapter 16).

PROGRAMS IN **ACTION**

Intrapersonal and Interpersonal Health Education

Five levels of influence for health education have been identified: intrapersonal/individual, interpersonal/group, institutional/organizational, community, and public policy. Programs can be targeted at just one level, or at two or more levels. It is thought that a multilevel approach employing a combination of different strategies can be most effective.

The Theory of Reasoned Action explains behavior at the intrapersonal level by examining the relationship between an individual's beliefs, attitudes, intentions, and behavior. It assumes that the most important determinant of behavior is a person's intention regarding that behavior. A person who believes that behavioral outcomes will be positive is likely to have a positive outlook on a change in behavior. Furthermore, a person who believes that others think he or she should perform certain behaviors will likely have a more positive attitude toward those behavioral changes. The Theory of Reasoned Action assumes that underlying reasons motivate people toward particular behaviors. In planning education at the intrapersonal level, one can influence healthy eating by affecting personal attitudes and increasing awareness of subjective norms related to healthy eating. On a practical level, individuals can be given activities and suggestions for applying health messages.

Intervention at the interpersonal level is predicated on the assumption that the thoughts, advice, examples, assistance, and emotional support of others affects one's own feelings, behavior, and, therefore, health. People are influenced by and influential in their social environments. Social-cognitive theory (SCT) explains the interactions among behavior, personal factors as discussed, and environmental influences, including the opinions of others. SCT states that people learn through their own experiences and by observing others. One aspect of SCT is observational learning or modeling; one's beliefs are based on observing the behaviors of others and their behavioral outcomes. Observational learning is most effective when the role model is perceived to be powerful or respected; for example, when the role model is a parent and the target is a child. Group interventions at the interpersonal level can foster peer support and positive behavioral change.

The case that follows exemplifies the use of both intrapersonal and interpersonal education to improve the nutritional health of low-income families.

Eat Healthy. Your Kids Are Watching

The Michigan Nutrition Support Network is a public–private partnership to improve the nutritional health of Michigan's low-income families. The network's pilot partnership in Kent County included more than 40 active representatives from local business, health care, private practice, nonprofit agencies, and schools. "Eat Healthy. Your Kids Are Watching" was the network's focus group–tested message designed to prompt awareness in parents that they are role models for their children.

Goals and Objectives

The primary goal of the campaign was to improve the nutritional health of Kent County's low-income families through collaborative efforts among partners. The objectives were to develop and implement "awareness-building" activities promoting healthy eating to the target audience and to the public in general, and to construct a public–private partnership with businesses and agencies to assist with specific programs for the campaign.

Methodology

Potential partners were located through personal contacts and written invitations to public agencies, commodity groups, food retailers, and others who work with community food and nutrition programs. Individual partners, once they became interested in the project, suggested others they believed would benefit from the collaborative effort. The activities of the four-week campaign were categorized into two groups: awareness building and partnership programming. Awareness-building activities included 30-second cable spots, campaign newsletters in English and Spanish, signs on and in transit buses, a logo and slogan program with grocery stores and school districts, and a toll-free telephone number with messages in English and Spanish. Information on grocery store tours, cooking demonstrations, and a WIC module for nutrition education were among the materials and activities available for partners. The extensive partner kit included an events schedule, lesson plans, activity sheets, and recipes.

Results

The program reached an estimated 49,000 residents, including close to 7,000 low-income households. A random sample of 800 adults in households with children were surveyed to test awareness of the campaign and acceptance of its core message. Campaign awareness was 52% in households with children and 67% in the target population of low-income households. Approximately two-thirds of respondents indicated that they understood and agreed with the message when they heard it. An additional 20% indicated that they would adopt the message. School lunch menus, billboards, and television commercials were seen as most effective for reaching the target audience.

Source: Adapted from *Community Nutritionary* (White Plains, NY: Dannon Institute, Spring 2000). Used with permission. For more information about the Awards for Excellence in Community Nutrition, go to *www.dannon-institute.org.*

PROFESSIONAL **FOCUS**

Being an Effective Speaker

Public speaking ranks number one on many people's list of most dreaded activities. If you feel this way about public speaking, take heart. You are not alone. More important, you can master the art of public speaking. There are several models of communication that can be applied to the process of public speaking. The transactional model of communication is based on the premise that both the speaker and the listener are simultaneously sending and receiving messages.[1] In public speaking, whether it is a formal presentation at a scientific meeting or an informal update for your colleagues at a staff meeting, you are communicating verbally and through gestures. Your audience is processing the communication and may simultaneously respond by nodding their head yes or no or by asking a question. Thinking in terms of public speaking as a "dialogue" rather than a "monologue" may make the experience feel more collegial for the presenter.

Being well prepared can help reduce apprehension. Tips for making an effective presentation are presented here.

Things to Do before Your Presentation

Public speaking is a skill just like any other skill. Even so, you may find that you expect more of yourself when it comes to public speaking than you do in other settings. If you are learning to downhill ski, you don't expect to be skiing the double black diamond trails and moguls at the end of your first season. If you are learning to speak Spanish, you don't expect to converse fluently after only a few lessons. So why should you expect to be a first-rate public speaker after a handful of presentations? Just like any other skill, public speaking requires practice and evaluation, and more practice and evaluation. It is an ongoing process. Even when you become skilled at public speaking, there will be room for improvement. In the beginning, try to remove a little pressure by remembering that you are working toward acquiring a skill that can be gained only by doing. You will improve over time. To accelerate your competency curve, follow these rules:

1. Organize your presentation around this basic principle of effective speaking. First, tell your audience what you are going to tell them; then tell them what you have to tell them; and finally, tell them what you told them! This strategy lets your audience know precisely what your presentation will cover and helps them remember the main points.

2. Prepare your visual aids so that they present your ideas effectively. Here are a few suggestions on preparing PowerPoint (or other presentation software) slides or other visual aids:[2]

   - **Clear purpose.** An effective slide should have a main point or central theme.

   - **Readily understood.** The slide's main point should be readily understood by the audience. If it is not, the audience will be trying to figure out what the slide has to say and will not be listening to the speaker.

   - **Simple format.** The slide should be simple and uncluttered. Avoid slides that present large amounts of data, such as columns of numbers or many lines of text. Avoid long sentences: Use generally no more than six words per line and no more than six lines per slide. Limit bullets to six per slide; bulleted items should be one or two lines in length. A slide's text should contrast with its background. Design templates can help you achieve standardization in your choice of colors, styles, and positioning of text and graphics. Strive for consistency in your use of special effects.

   - **Free of nonessential information.** Information not directly related to the slide's main point should be omitted.

- **Digestible.** The audience is capable of assimilating only so much information from a slide. It is better to have only a small amount of information (even just one sentence) than to cram numerous points onto a single slide.
- **Graphical format.** Some information is best presented graphically. In addition, the use of graphs and charts provides a visual change from slides containing only text.[3] Graphics and clip art can enhance and complement slide text. Balance their placement on the slide and use no more than two graphics per slide.
- **Visible.** Because most meeting rooms were not designed for projection, some people sitting in the back of the room may not be able to view the slides over the heads of those in front. For this reason, horizontal slides are more appropriate than vertical slides.
- **Legible.** Studies of projected image size and legibility show that the best slide template is about 42 spaces wide (9 centimeters) by 14 single-spaced lines (6 centimeters). The best type for slides is at least 5 millimeters, or 14 points. A larger font indicates more important information. Font size generally ranges from 18 to 48 points. Remember that decorative fonts can be hard to read.
- **Integrated with verbal text.** Slides should support and reinforce the verbal text. Conversely, the verbal text should lay a proper foundation for the slide.

3. Rehearse your presentation out loud several times. If the presentation is formal, use a table or desk to simulate a podium. Time the presentation from start to finish, including your opening and closing remarks, and adjust your presentation as needed. A general rule of thumb is that you should plan to spend about one minute per slide. If the presentation is informal, write down the key points you want to make and practice saying them. Rehearsing your presentation ensures that you will know your material and how you want to present it.

4. Use mental imaging to boost your self-confidence. What is mental imaging? It's a technique used by many successful businesspeople, politicians, actors, and athletes to develop and strengthen a positive mental picture of their performance. On several occasions before your presentation, walk yourself mentally through the speech from beginning to end. Picture being introduced, standing up and walking to the podium, adjusting the microphone, smiling, giving your opening remarks, asking for the first slide, and so on, right down to the very end of your presentation. Picture giving your presentation and handling questions at the end with complete confidence. The key to using mental imaging successfully is to use it whenever a negative thought about your presentation intrudes. If a mental picture of you passing out behind the podium surfaces suddenly, use mental imaging to squash it. Force yourself instead to picture a confident, in-control YOU. Allow no negative thoughts about your presentation to take form. Encourage only positive thoughts. Mental imaging takes a little practice, but it is worth the effort. You will find that because you think you are more confident, you *are* more confident.

Things to Do during Your Presentation

Use the following techniques to ensure that you give a first-rate presentation:

- **Smile.** A smile will go a long way toward helping you relax and making you appear accessible to your audience. This is especially important when dealing with the general public.
- **Use eye contact.** Regardless of the size of the audience, select one person with whom to establish eye contact. Let your eyes dwell on this one individual a few moments, and then move on to another person. This gives the appearance of a one-on-one interactive discussion, which engages the audience in your presentation and helps ensure that they are listening to you.
- **Use gestures.** Gestures give energy to your presentation and provide additional emphasis for key points. Practice making them during your rehearsals. Exercise a little common sense here—wild arm movements and pirouettes will detract from your presentation.
- **Control the pace.** Although maintaining a steady pace will ensure that you complete your speech on time, it may make your audience sleepy. Vary the pace to keep the audience interested in what you are saying.
- **Use pauses.** Pauses, like gestures, can be used for emphasis. A well-timed pause keeps your audience engaged and allows them a moment to process what you've just said.
- **Vary the volume and pitch.** Changing the volume and pitch of your voice has more auditory appeal for the audience than speaking in a monotone.

Finally, two other points deserve mention. First, remember that the purpose of your presentation is to share information with your audience. Your listeners will generally be much less critical of your performance than you are. Being an effective speaker simply means that your audience is listening to your messages and absorbing the material you present. Second, despite all the tips and techniques listed here, you will want to develop your own style. Learn to be a relaxed, confident speaker and to be yourself.

CHAPTER **SUMMARY** ....

Draw from Current Research on Consumer Behavior

▶ Researchers have developed and tested numerous behavior change theories and models that attempt to explain why and how people make behavior changes (see Table 3-1). Some strategies target changes in attitudes and beliefs, while others more directly target behavior change (i.e., goal setting and problem solving).

▶ Improved outcomes can be achieved if community nutrition experts understand the target population and are able to skillfully select relevant theory-based strategies to facilitate diet-related behavior change. A thorough nutrition assessment includes concepts from relevant behavior change theories (e.g., readiness to change, self-efficacy, perceived benefits, and barriers to change).

▶ **The transtheoretical model (stages of change)** describes an individual's motivation and readiness to change a problem behavior. The model is founded on three assumptions: (1) Behavior change involves a series of different steps or stages; (2) there are common stages and processes of change across a variety of health behaviors; and (3) tailoring an intervention to a person's current stage of change is more effective than not considering which stage the person is in (see Table 3-2). The five stages through which people move include precontemplation, contemplation, preparation, action, and maintenance.

▶ **Motivational interviewing** (MI) is a counseling approach that builds upon the client-centered counseling model. It is a way of interacting with the client that actively facilitates the client's exploring and resolving his or her own uncertainty about change, building confidence, and enhancing his or her commitment to change. The process stresses the use of carefully crafted questions and reflective listening skills rather than the drive to provide information (see Table 3-3).

▶ Four general principles guide this approach: (1) resisting the urge to confront the client about the need for behavior change; (2) understanding and exploring the client's own motivations; (3) listening with empathy; and (4) empowering the client.

▶ **The health belief model** was developed to explain why people, especially those in high-risk groups, fail to participate in programs designed to detect or prevent disease (see Table 3-4). The health belief model has three components: (1) the perception of a threat to health, (2) the expectation of certain outcomes related to a behavior, and (3) self-efficacy.

▶ **The theory of planned behavior** is sometimes called the *theory of reasoned action*. According to the model, behavior is determined directly by a person's *intention* to perform the behavior. Intentions are influenced by attitudes and subjective norms. A modification of the theory is called the *theory of trying*.

▶ **Social-cognitive theory** (SCT), also known as *social learning theory*, explains behavior in terms of a model in which behavior, personal factors such as cognition, and the environment interact constantly, such that a change in one area has implications for the others (known as *reciprocal determinism*). A strength of SCT is that it focuses on certain target behaviors rather than on knowledge and attitudes (see Table 3-5).

▶ **Cognitive-behavioral theory** is best applied when people are actively ready to make a change. Cognitive-behavioral theory is based on the assumption that all behavior is learned and directly related to internal factors (e.g., thoughts and thinking patterns) and external factors (e.g., environmental stimuli and feedback). Clients are taught to use a variety of behavioral and cognitive strategies to recognize behaviors that lead to inappropriate eating and replace them with more rational thoughts and actions (see Table 3-6).

▶ **The diffusion of innovation model** is the process by which an innovation spreads and involves an ever-increasing number of individuals within a population. The model consists of four stages: knowledge, persuasion, decision, and confirmation. Consumers can be classified according to how readily they adopt new ideas or products: innovators, early adopters, early majority, late majority, and laggards.

SUMMARY **QUESTIONS** . . . .

1. What are the stages of change in the transtheoretical model? Describe an intervention strategy related to weight loss for clients in each stage of the model.
2. Describe the four general principles that guide the motivational interviewing approach to counseling.
3. What are intentions and subjective norms, as defined by the theory of planned behavior, and how might they predict a client's future behavior regarding membership at a local gym?
4. Describe how a community nutritionist might use each of the following social-cognitive theory concepts in

classes designed to teach the principles of the USDA's "MyPlate" regarding fruits and vegetables.

a. Environment
b. Behavioral capability
c. Expectations
d. Self-efficacy
e. Observational learning

5. What are the basic principles of the cognitive-behavioral theory? Apply this theory to an intervention designed to improve calcium intakes in adolescent girls.

INTERNET **RESOURCES** . . . .

Applications of Behavior Change

Guide to Community Preventive Services
www.thecommunityguide.org

Theory at a Glance: A Guide for Health Promotion Practice
www.sbccimplementationkits.org/demandrmnch/wp-content/uploads/2014/02/Theory-at-a-Glance-A-Guide-For-Health-Promotion-Practice.pdf

Agency for Healthcare Research
www.ahrq.gov

HealthMedia Solutions
www.wellnessandpreventioninc.com

National Center for Chronic Disease Prevention and Health Promotion
www.cdc.gov/chronicdisease/index.htm

National Cancer Institute
www.cancer.gov

Other Nutrition and Health-Related Sites

▶ Find timely information from the following sites, which serve as major directories of links:

Academy of Nutrition and Dietetics
www.eatright.org

Evidence Analysis Library
www.adaevidencelibrary.com

FitDay (weight-loss journal)
www.fitday.com

MyPlate SuperTracker
www.choosemyplate.gov/supertracker-tools/supertracker.html

NHLBI Health Information
www.nhlbi.nih.gov/health

Weight-Control Information Network
www.niddk.nih.gov/health-information/health-communication-programs/win/Pages/default.aspx

Kansas State Research and Extension
www.ksre.k-state.edu

Food and Nutrition Information Center
www.nal.usda.gov/fnic

Links to Government Sites Related to Nutrition and Databases

Healthfinder® or Healthfinder® Español
www.healthfinder.gov or www.healthfinder.gov/espanol

National Institutes of Health (NIH)
http://health.nih.gov

MEDLINEplus
www.nlm.nih.gov/medlineplus

CHAPTER 4

Community Needs Assessment

Chapter Revision by Virginia B. Gray, PhD, RD

LEARNING **OBJECTIVES**

After you have read and studied this chapter, you will be able to:

- Describe the importance of conducting a community needs assessment.
- Describe seven steps in conducting a community needs assessment.
- Describe three categories of data that can be collected as part of a community needs assessment, and indicate how to obtain these data.
- Use available community and national data to investigate demographic, environmental, health behavior, and health status variables.
- Develop a plan for conducting a needs assessment of a defined community.
- List a minimum of eight methods for obtaining data about the target population.

- Discuss cultural issues that are considered when choosing a method for obtaining data about the target population.
- Discuss the issues of validity and reliability as they apply to data collection.
- Interpret community data and set priorities for action.

This chapter addresses such issues as needs assessment, evolving methods of assessing health status and screening individuals for nutrition risks, collecting pertinent information for comprehensive nutrition assessments, and exploring current information technologies, which have been designated by the Accreditation Council for Education in Nutrition and Dietetics (ACEND) as Foundation Knowledge and Learning Outcomes for dietetics education.

CHAPTER **OUTLINE**

Something to think about...

"Many people responsible for planning health education programs [have] more or less predetermined what intervention strategy they were going to employ. . . . In some instances, there was no apparent reason for choosing either the health issue to be addressed or the target population to be reached."

—*L. GREEN AND M. KREUTER*[1]

For a complete list of references, please access the MindTap Reader within your MindTap course.

Introduction

Imagine you are hired into a new position at your local city department of health. One of your roles in your new position is to lead a community assessment in a high-need neighborhood. The findings of your assessment will direct the nutrition-related work of your agency: which needs to address and how to address them. You have some ideas about who lives in your community, the foods they eat, and their needs. The city leaders you interact with also have their ideas about the priorities and needs of the community. Although these perspectives are important, the members of a community may hold different values and perceive their strengths, weaknesses, and needs differently. Collecting data that provide an accurate picture of both community needs and values is a priority. With this in mind, where would you start in planning the assessment? Who would you involve? What types of information would you want to gather? How would you learn about the values, beliefs, and lifestyle factors that might impact food choices? What would you do to learn about assets and barriers in the community that may impact nutrition? How would you decide which segment of the population to target?

The community needs assessment is a critical piece in the program planning process. Community needs assessments involve asking many questions, talking to a variety of stakeholders, and using multiple methods to gain understanding of your community before deciding how to move forward. The work of collecting data, opinions, and environmental characteristics helps to ensure that the program is matched to the needs of the audience and their environment.

Food insecurity Limited or uncertain ability to acquire or consume an adequate quality or sufficient quantity of food in socially acceptable ways (e.g., not knowing where one's next meal is coming from constitutes food insecurity).

A community needs assessment requires a strong plan. Consider the challenge of capturing a picture of **food insecurity** among Hispanics living in the United States. The Hispanic population is composed of about 54 million people, or nearly 17% of the U.S. population, making this population the nation's largest minority group.[2] Furthermore, this population group is rapidly growing, with Hispanics projected to be 31% of the population by 2060.[3] Food insecurity in Hispanic communities is believed to derive from poverty, racism, and high unemployment,[4] factors that directly or indirectly limit access to nutritious foods. Community nutritionists who aim to improve the food intake of Hispanics in a local community begin by working with local community leaders, state and federal agencies, and other groups to determine why the Hispanic population experiences food insecurity. They ask many questions:

- How many Hispanics in our community experience food insecurity?
- How does the rate of unemployment among Hispanics compare to other ethnic groups in the community?
- Are they more likely than other groups to have low-paying jobs?
- What is the mean income of Hispanic families?
- How many Hispanic families participate in food assistance programs?
- What are the barriers and facilitators to their participation in these programs?
- Are existing community programs and services reaching Hispanics? If not, why?

The answers to these and other questions fill in some pieces of the puzzle of why some Hispanics experience food insecurity. Then, it is important to consider the dietary habits, values, attitudes, and beliefs of the target population, as a community needs assessment is intended to suggest ways of intervention that resonate with community values, motivations, and needs. Also, the assessment will identify resources available at the national, state, and local levels to support healthy eating; determine where existing services and programs can be improved; and suggest areas where new programs and services are needed.

This chapter describes a process for planning and carrying out a needs assessment. You learn about the types of data to collect about your community, its environment, and your target population. Several methods used commonly to obtain such data and several issues to consider when choosing a method of data collection are also discussed. At the end of the chapter, you learn how to analyze and interpret needs assessment data, determine priorities, share findings, and set a plan for action.

Community Needs Assessment

Community needs assessment is the process of evaluating the health and nutrition status of a community, determining what the community's health and nutrition needs are, and identifying places where those needs are not being met.[5] It involves systematically collecting, analyzing, and making available information about the health and nutrition status of the community or some subgroup of it. The term **health status** refers to the condition of a population's or individual's health, including estimates of quality of life and of physical and psychosocial functioning.[6] **Nutrition status** is defined as the condition of a population's or individual's health as affected by the intake and utilization of nutrients and nonnutrients.[7] The assessment is undertaken to find answers to basic questions: Who has nutrition needs that are not being addressed? What programs and services exist to address these needs? Why do existing programs and services fail to address these needs? How do the community environment, background factors, and culture affect the ease and desirability of making healthy food choices? What can be done to improve the health and nutrition status of the population?

The assessment process is sometimes called "community analysis and diagnosis," "health education planning," or "**asset mapping**."[8] Its overall purpose is to provide a better understanding of how the community functions and how it addresses the public health and nutrition needs of its citizens. In some respects, the process is much like the clinical assessment of a patient's health, except that the community is the patient. The assessment is like a snapshot of the community that identifies areas where it performs well (e.g., local hospitals and clinics have good data on infant morbidity and mortality) and areas where it does not (e.g., although two food banks and several food assistance programs are available in the community, some families go without food). Going into a community needs assessment with an asset-based perspective will help you to identify both the strengths and weaknesses of the community.

What triggers a community needs assessment? Any number of factors may compel a city health department, state or federal agency, nonprofit organization, or other group to seek information about a community's health and nutrition status. There may be a need for new data on the community's health because existing data are several years old and may no longer accurately reflect a population's health and/or because data have never been collected on some segment of a population. Often a government agency at the state or federal level has a mandate to carry out such activities. Sometimes research findings are the impetus for taking action. For example, an article published in the *Journal of the Academy of Nutrition and Dietetics* reported that the infants of teenage mothers who participated in the Higgins Nutrition Intervention Program weighed more and were less likely to have low birthweights than infants whose mothers did not participate in the program.[9] These study findings may prompt municipal health clinics to determine the number of low-birthweight infants born to adolescents and to study the feasibility of implementing the Higgins program in their communities. In other cases, a community leader or community action group may raise awareness about a health or nutrition issue and prompt action to undertake a community needs assessment. The availability of funds may also stimulate the collection of data on the community's health and nutrition problems. As you can see, a variety of factors can trigger the decision to gather information about nutrition needs in a community.

Community needs assessment An evaluation of the community in terms of its health and nutrition status, its needs, and the resources available to address those needs.

Health status The condition of a population's or individual's health, including estimates of quality of life and physical and psychosocial functioning.

Nutrition status The condition of a population's or individual's health as influenced by the intake and utilization of nutrients and nonnutrients.

Asset mapping A community assessment that documents existing assets and resources; a community inventory of groups and group assets including the associations (business, cultural, religious, fraternal), private and nonprofit organizations (colleges, hospitals, social service agencies), and public institutions (libraries, schools, recreation departments) that are a fundamental part of community life and that can be mobilized for community improvement and problem solving.

Organizations approach the community needs assessment by first determining its purpose and then planning how it will proceed. The amount of time and money available to conduct the needs assessment, the staff members responsible for conducting it, and the scope of the assessment must all be specified. The scope deserves special mention. In some cases, the assessment is designed to identify the health and nutrition concerns of a large population, such as all residents of a community, which might be a nation, state, province, or city. The assessment cuts across all income, educational, and geographical sectors, and it aims to identify the major causes of disease, disability, and death among the community's residents. The most recent Behavioral Risk Factor Surveillance System (BRFSS), for example, identified increases in overweight and diabetes as two nutrition-related problems in all demographic and geographical segments of the U.S. population.[10] Blacks had the highest rates of both obesity and diabetes among all races and ethnic groups, and people with less than a high school education had higher rates of both obesity and diabetes than those with a high school education. Large-scale assessments tend to be expensive, time-consuming projects that may enlist the efforts of hundreds of people with expertise in public health, nutrition, epidemiology, statistics, management, and survey design and analysis. The team is pulled together from various departments within several agencies, all acting under the leadership of a single agency. Because they are costly and labor-intensive, such assessments may be undertaken only once every five or 10 years.

More often than not, the community needs assessment is limited in scope, focusing on a particular subgroup of the community. The small-scale assessment is relatively inexpensive to conduct and can be undertaken by a small team of community nutritionists and other professionals from several organizations and agencies. For example, an assessment of the nutrition status of school children may involve experts from the municipal departments of public health and education, a local dietitian who directs the National School Lunch Program, members of the hospital's community health department, and graduate students from the local university. In today's fiscal environment, where money for personnel, equipment, and other resources is scarce, the small-scale assessment is often the better—and sometimes the only—choice. It focuses on a high-risk group about which community nutritionists and other health professionals have some knowledge and concern. Another advantage of small-scale assessments is that they focus on a more specific population, and this allows for better tailoring of programs to unique needs.

Target population The population that is the focus of an assessment, study, or intervention.

Regardless of its scope, the purpose of the community needs assessment is to obtain information about the health and nutrition status of a particular group—namely, the **target population**. In the case of the large-scale assessment, the target population may be all residents of a nation. Because it is not practical or feasible to obtain information about every resident, large-scale assessments use statistical methods to select a sample of people whose age, sex, race, and other characteristics reflect the demographic profile of the entire population. The National Health and Nutrition Examination Survey (NHANES), for instance, is conducted annually on a nationally representative sample of about 5,000 persons.[11] Small-scale assessments evaluate every member of a significantly more limited population. The target population might be, for example, low-birthweight infants born between December 1 and March 31 to mothers living in the state of Missouri, lactating women with type 1 diabetes living in Chicago, or adults with lactose intolerance who present to three city hospitals.

Another important note about community needs assessments is that there is not one "correct" way to go about the process. In some cases, an organizational mandate may indicate that an assessment of a particular concern or group of people must be carried out. For example, imagine you are conducting a needs assessment focused on a local agency participating in the Special Supplemental Program for Women, Infants, and Children (WIC). Data collected by your agency indicate that your program has been successful in improving enrollment and retention of Hispanic clients, but that retention of African American participants has declined. You know that infants and children who are withdrawn from the WIC program are more likely to be at increased nutrition risk than those who participate fully in the program.[12] Therefore, the director of your agency asks you to conduct an assessment to learn how to effectively enhance enrollment and retention of WIC-eligible African Americans in your service area. In this case, the target population and issue are clearly defined from the beginning. Now imagine you are conducting a needs assessment for a local public health agency to help determine the direction of the five-year plan for the agency. In this case, you have geographic boundaries based on the service area of the agency, but you do not know which issues or which subset of the service area you will target. Thus, it is important to be flexible in how you plan a needs assessment, and to keep in mind that "one size does not fit all."

Basic Principles of Needs Assessment: Developing a Plan and Collecting Data

Certain basic principles apply, no matter what the scope of the needs assessment. In this chapter, we describe these principles and the process of conducting a community needs assessment. In this book, the community nutritionist is given primary responsibility for conducting it. She or he begins by setting the parameters of the assessment and determining what types of data must be collected to develop an understanding of the nutrition needs of the community and target population. The steps are diagrammed in **Figure 4-1** and described in the sections that follow.

In the course of living and working within the community and networking with colleagues, the community nutritionist probably has a notion about the community's nutrition needs. For example, the community nutritionist may have observed the following:

▶ **Obesity.** The prevalence of obesity more than doubled for men and women aged 20 years and over between 1988 and 2008. In 2013, no state had a prevalence of obesity less than 20%. Forty-three states had a prevalence of 25% or more, and 20 states (Alabama, Arkansas, Delaware, Georgia, Indiana, Iowa, Kansas, Kentucky, Louisiana, Michigan, Mississippi, Missouri, North Dakota, Ohio, Oklahoma, Pennsylvania, South Carolina, Tennessee, Texas, and West Virginia) had a prevalence of 30% or more according to data from the BRFSS, a telephone survey of health behaviors conducted among adults in 50 states.[13] Obesity contributes to increased morbidity, including increased risk of hypertension and diabetes mellitus. People who are successful at losing weight

Step 1	Set the parameters of the assessment.
Step 2	Develop a data collection plan.
Step 3	Collect data: about the community. about the community environment and background factors. about individuals who represent the target population.
Step 4	Analyze and interpret the data.
Step 5	Share the findings of the assessment.
Step 6	Set priorities.
Step 7	Choose a plan of action.

FIGURE 4-1 Steps in Conducting a Community Needs Assessment

and maintaining the weight loss report using a combination of diet, physical activity, and behavior modification to achieve their goals.[14] The prevalence of obesity in Johnson County is not known, nor is information available about strategies used by overweight people in Johnson County to lose weight successfully. (*Note:* See Chapter 8 for a detailed discussion of the obesity epidemic.)

▶ **Inadequate food intake of immigrants.** Results of the Ontario Health Survey indicate that only one-fifth of all immigrants consumed at least 75% of the minimum recommended number of servings of each food group in the *Eating Well with Canada's Food Guide.*[15] Routine consumption of less than the minimum recommended number of servings of each food group may cause inadequate intakes of essential nutrients. No information is available on the food group intake of immigrants in this province.

▶ **Poor quality of diets of high school students.** A survey conducted by the Heart and Stroke Foundation found that one-third of students in 11 of the city's secondary schools eat mainly french fries for lunch and that only 1 in 20 students consumes a lunch containing foods from all food groups.[16] It is not known whether students in other secondary schools have similar eating patterns, and no information about the factors that influence the food choices of secondary school students in the region is available.

As these examples illustrate, the community nutritionist beginning a needs assessment probably knows many of the issues that are most pressing in a community. However, the community nutritionist should be aware of preconceived ideas she or he may have about the needs, attitudes, and motivations of the community members and approach the process of planning a needs assessment ready to observe, listen, and learn from the community. Also, maintaining an "asset-based" perspective can help the community nutritionist not only focus on what can be improved in a community, but also to look for community strengths that may help improve the nutrition status of community members. Consider the following scenarios:

- Imagine you are planning a program to improve child nutrition in a low-income area. You are developing a school-based intervention and plan to offer workshops to parents as well. As a part of your needs assessment, you conduct focus groups with parents and find that many of them prefer heavier children, expressing concerns about bullying of children who are "thin." Thus, you learn that messages on helping children attain a healthy body weight may not be relevant to this population, and you need to focus on learning which nutrition messages would be meaningful, relevant, and motivating to your audience.
- You are planning a walk to school initiative as an adjunct to school nutrition programming in your area. You think that parent concerns regarding traffic safety will be a barrier to your program. You also believe that many parents drop off their children enroute to work, and believe this will serve as a barrier. Interviews with parents indicate that a major barrier to walking to school is fear of unrestrained dogs in the neighborhood. Without talking to parents, you would not have known to address this issue.

These two scenarios show the importance of observing the community and listening to its members prior to developing a program. Sometimes the priorities of those planning programs do not match the needs of the target population. Other times there are key messages that seem relevant to the program planners but are not motivating to change behaviors in the target population. For example, the national "5 a Day for Better Health Program" was initiated in 1991 by the National Cancer Institute and Produce for Better Health Foundation, and was successful in raising awareness that fruit and vegetable intake should be at least five servings per day. However, this increased awareness was not accompanied by changes in fruit and vegetable consumption. Interviews with consumers, industry, and government and nonprofit organizations indicated that a compelling emotional benefit and a focus on "small steps" rather than the end goal of "5 a Day" was needed.[17] This is a great illustration of the importance of gaining key insights into the target population's attitudes, beliefs, priorities, and motivations. Now, let's turn to looking at the steps in a community needs assessment.

Step 1: Set the Parameters of the Assessment

Before the community needs assessment is undertaken, certain parameters or elements must be determined. These parameters, which are described here, set the direction for the assessment. As you read the following material, consult **Table 4-1**, which describes the parameters for two assessments in the fictional city of Jeffers (population 612,000). One assessment (Case Study 1) focuses on the issue of women and coronary heart disease (CHD). The other (Case Study 2) focuses on issues surrounding the nutrition status of older adults living at home. These case studies illustrate two assessments that differ in scope and complexity. Case Studies 1 and 2 are discussed in this chapter and revisited in other chapters in the book.

Define the "Community"

The scope of the community to be assessed must be specified. Sometimes the community is a geographical region, state, nation, province, or group of countries. Other times it may be a group of people served by a particular program, such as elementary school students attending schools in a defined area. As discussed above, there are times when a subset of the community, known as the target population, is specified when you are planning the assessment. Other times, data will be collected to describe a defined community and then the target population will be selected. In the case studies described in Table 4-1, the community is a typical municipal unit, referenced as the fictitious city of Jeffers.

Determine the Purpose of the Needs Assessment

A needs assessment is undertaken to gather information about the social, political, economic, environmental, and personal factors that influence a community. The community needs assessment may have one or more of the purposes listed here:[18]

- Identify groups within the community who are at risk nutritionally.
- Identify the community's or target population's most critical nutrition needs and set priorities among them.
- Identify the factors that affect nutrition status (positively and negatively) within the community.
- Determine whether existing resources and programs meet the community's nutrition needs.
- Provide baseline information for developing action plans to address the community's nutrition needs and for evaluating the program.
- Plan actions to improve nutrition status in a community or target population, using methods that are feasible and focus on established health priorities.
- Tailor a program to a specific population.

Set Goals and Objectives for the Needs Assessment

This is an essential step because the goals and objectives determine the types of data collected and how they will be used. **Goals** are broad statements that indicate what the assessment is expected to accomplish. **Objectives** are statements of outcomes and activities needed to reach a goal. Statements of objectives use a strong verb, such as *identify, assess, determine,* or *measure,* that describes a measurable outcome. Each objective should state a single purpose.[19]

Goals Broad statements of what an activity or program is expected to accomplish.

Objectives Statements of outcomes and activities needed to reach a goal.

TABLE 4-1 Parameters for Two Community Needs Assessments in the Fictional City of Jeffers, Population 612,000

PARAMETER	CASE STUDY 1: WOMEN AND HEART DISEASE	CASE STUDY 2: NUTRITION STATUS OF OLDER ADULTS
Lead Organization	State affiliate of the American Heart Association or, in Canada, provincial Heart & Stroke Foundation	City of Jeffers Health Department
Focus of the Assessment	Coronary heart disease (CHD) is a leading cause of death among U.S. and Canadian women. Most women apparently do not realize that they are more likely to die from CHD than from cancer. There are no data on knowledge and awareness of CHD risk factors among women living in Jeffers or about existing CHD prevention programs and services in Jeffers.	The number of independent, non-institutionalized older adults (75+ years) has increased nationally. In Jeffers, this population has increased 12% since the 1995 assessment. Several community-based social service agencies have perceived an increased demand for nutrition services among this population, but there are no data on the availability of such services or on the nutrition status of these persons.
Definition of Community	The metropolitan area of Jeffers, including the adjoining municipalities of Oakdale, Chambers, Kastle, and Morgan	City of Jeffers, bounded by the city limits as of July 31, 2015
Purpose of the Assessment	To obtain information about women and heart health to help determine whether a program or other intervention should be developed	To obtain information about the nutrition status of independent older adults > 75 years of age and their needs for nutrition services
Target Population	Females over 18 years of age	Older adults > 75 years of age living independently
Overall Goal of Assessment	Identify women's knowledge, attitudes, and practices related to CHD risk and existing programs and services designed to reduce CHD risk	Determine the nutrition status of independent older adults (> 75 years) and their use of and attitudes regarding nutrition services available through community-based agencies
Objectives of Assessment	On a sample of 250 women over the age of 18 years, within 3 months: • Assess women's knowledge and awareness of the leading causes of death and CHD risk factors • Assess women's practices and attitudes related to CHD risk reduction • Identify existing services offered to women to help reduce their CHD risk • Assess women's use of existing services designed to reduce risk • Identify gaps in the delivery of such programs and services	On a sample of 150 older adults aged 75 years and older, within one year: • Assess the nutrition status of independent older adults (> 75 years) • Determine which community services are available for this population • Identify the existing community services used by this population • Identify attitudes of older adults regarding use of existing community services • Identify gaps in program and service delivery
Types of Data Needed: Community Data	• Mortality data for women (50+ years) • Morbidity data for women (50+ years) • Existing programs and services: Hospitals, medical clinics Fitness/sports centers Offered by health professionals in private practice • Educational materials available from doctors' offices, health professionals in private practice, food/pharmaceutical companies, bookstores, other	• Types of services offered by community organizations, including personal-care services, homemaker services, adult daycare, home-delivered meals, hospice, and home health care services • Number of older adults who use these services • Number of older adults who participate in federal/state assistance programs, such as Supplemental Nutrition Assistance Program (SNAP), Social Security, Medicare, Medicaid, Supplemental Security Income, Veteran's Benefits, assistance for housing and home heating, and home-delivered meals • Types of medical and social services offered by health professionals
Types of Data Needed: Community Environment and Background Factors	• Advertising related to smoking • Health messages about CHD in magazines, newspapers, etc. • Food availability • Social and cultural food norms • Physical activity opportunities	• Changes in eligibility for Medicare, Medicaid • Current funding of Older Americans Act
Types of Data Needed: Target Population Data	• See Table 4-12 on page 133.	• See Table 4-13 on page 135.

The assessments described in Table 4-1 specify one overall goal and several objectives. Assessments may have two, three, or more goals and 10–15 objectives. The needs assessment cannot proceed without clearly defined goals and objectives. More about writing goals and objectives is found in Chapter 5.

Step 2: Develop a Data Collection Plan

The types of data required in a needs assessment depend on the scope, purpose, goals, and objectives of the assessment. In developing a plan for data collection, remember that the assessment's overall purpose is to paint a picture of the many factors that are affecting food choices in a community and what might be done to improve food selection. Begin collecting data about the "big picture"—namely, the community, environment, and background factors. Then, when you have begun to get a sense of the big picture, you can decide on a population to target and collect data about individuals who make up the target population. (Again, in some cases, your target population will be specified from the beginning of the assessment.)

In this section, three categories of data are described: (1) community data (such as demographics, economic factors, and health indicators); (2) community environment and background factors (social and cultural norms, food availability, policies, etc.); and (3) target population data (food preferences and attitudes, health beliefs and knowledge, lifestyle factors, etc.). You will want to collect data to help you to understand the nutrition status of the community and the multiple factors that influence it. Recall the discussion of the social–ecological model in Chapter 1. It is a good idea to review this model to revisit the multiple layers of influence on individual behavior. This perspective will help you to develop a plan that considers the many factors that impact food choices and health status in communities. **Figure 4-2** provides a broad look at the types of data that might be collected over the course of the assessment and represents another way of thinking about the determinants of health shown in Table 1-2 on page 10.

Specify the Types of Data Needed There are three basic categories of data to collect: community data, community environment and background conditions, and target population data. Tables 4-2 to 4-4 portray summaries of the types and sources of data within each of these three categories. Both qualitative and quantitative data help describe the community and its values, health status, and needs. Community data are quantitative

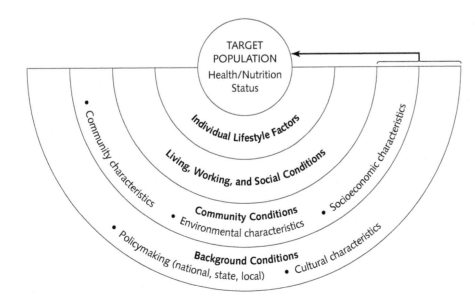

FIGURE 4-2 Types of Data to Collect about the Community

The focus of the community needs assessment is the target population, whose health and nutrition status are affected by many community and background factors, as well as by individual characteristics such as lifestyle, living and working conditions, and social networks.

Source: Adapted from M. Whitehead, "Tackling Inequalities: A Review of Policy Initiatives," in *Tackling Inequalities in Health: An Agenda for Action*, eds. M. Benzeval, K. Judge, and M. Whitehead (London: King's Fund, 1995), 23.

Quantitative data Numerical data (such as serum ferritin concentration, birth rate, and income) that can be measured and are considered objective.

Vital statistics Figures pertaining to life events, such as births, deaths, and marriages.

Qualitative data Data (such as opinions) that describe or explain, are considered subjective, and can be categorized or ranked but not quantified.

Key informants People who are "in the know" about the community and whose opinions and insights can help direct the needs assessment.

Stakeholders People who have a vested interest in identifying and addressing the nutrition status of a target population.

in nature. Quantitative and qualitative data can be collected to describe the community environment, background conditions, and target population. **Quantitative data** may be derived from a variety of databases, including registries of **vital statistics** (e.g., age at death and cause of death), published research studies, hospital records, and local health surveys.[20] **Qualitative data** such as opinions and insights may be derived from interviews with **key informants**—people who are knowledgeable about the community, its history, and its past efforts to promote healthy eating—and with **stakeholders**—the people and organizations with vested interest in promoting and achieving optimal nutrition status. Members of the community itself can also provide information about the community. It is important to include both quantitative and qualitative data, as numerical data often leave out details of the community "story" and may lack insights on how to address needs. On the flip side, qualitative data will not always portray an accurate picture of which issues are most prevalent, and may not show trends over time. Keep this in mind as you consider the three categories of data. Let's take a look at types of information to collect within the three categories.

Community Data Collecting community data will help you learn more about the people within your community of interest. These data are outlined in **Table 4-2**. Some community data may already be available ("existing data"), and you will need to collect other pieces of information. Let's take a look at the different types of community data.

TABLE 4-2 Types and Sources of Community Data

TYPE OF DATA	SOURCE OF DATA
Community Health	
• Mortality statistics (e.g., death rates according to age, sex, cause, location, and so on)	Census Bureau, FedStats[a], NCHS[b], Public Health Service, state and municipal health departments
• Morbidity statistics (e.g., frequency of symptoms and disabilities, distribution of disease conditions)	Census Bureau, NCHS, FedStats, Public Health Service, state and municipal health departments
• Fertility and natality statistics (e.g., age and parity of mother, duration of pregnancy, percentage of mothers who get prenatal care, number of unmarried mothers, infant's birthweight, type of birth [i.e., single, twin], fertility rate, infant mortality)	Census Bureau, FedStats, state data centers, data archives
• Communicable diseases (e.g., incidence, distribution)	FedStats, CDC, published studies
• Occupational diseases (e.g., incidence, distribution)	FedStats, National Institute for Occupational Safety and Health, published studies
• Leading causes of death	FedStats, NCHS, published studies
• Life expectancy	FedStats, NCHS, published studies
• Determinants and measures of health (e.g., vaccinations, disability days, cigarette smoking, use of selected substances [i.e., alcohol, marijuana, cocaine], hypertension, obesity, serum cholesterol concentrations, exposure to lead, occupational injuries, incidence of food-borne disease)	FedStats, CDC's *Vital and Health Statistics* series and the *Morbidity and Mortality Weekly Report*, NNMRRP surveys (e.g., NHANES, BRFSS)
• Food and nutrient intake (e.g., food group intake, nutrient and energy intakes, nutrient adequacy of diets compared with the DRI)	Agriculture Research Service, Older Americans Act (OAA) Nutrition Program
• Use of health resources (e.g., frequency of patient contact with physicians, number of office visits to physicians and dentists)	State Department of Community Health Services
• Health care resources (e.g., persons employed in service, number of active physicians and other health personnel)	FedStats, Health Resources and Services Administration
• Inpatient care (e.g., days of care and average length of stay in hospitals, number and types of operations, number of nursing home residents)	Hospitals, nursing homes, etc.
• Facilities (e.g., short-stay and long-term hospitals, community hospital beds)	Internet
Community Organizational Power and Structures	
• Organization of government (city, state, etc.)	Directory of municipal, state, etc., government
• Organization of health department (city, state, etc.)	Directory of municipal, state, etc., health department

TABLE 4-2 Types and Sources of Community Data—*continued*

TYPE OF DATA	SOURCE OF DATA
• Local, state, and national organizations with a health mandate (e.g., American Heart Association, American Cancer Society, Academy of Nutrition and Dietetics, American Public Health Association)	National or state directories, Internet
• Community groups and their leaders (e.g., United Way)	Internet, key informants
• Reporters and other people with the media	Local/national newspapers and magazines, television and radio stations
• Members of the Chamber of Commerce	Local Chamber of Commerce
Demographic Data and Trends	
• Total population by age, sex, race, marital status, etc.	Census Bureau, FedStats, state data centers, data archives, libraries
• Distribution of population subgroups (e.g., percentage of population that is black, Hispanic, Asian, and so on; percentage that is foreign born)	Census Bureau, FedStats, state data centers, data archives
• Size and composition of households (e.g., number of family members in households, number of children in households, percentage of all households consisting of two-parent families, percentage of single-parent families)	Census Bureau, FedStats, state data centers, data archives
Economic Data and Trends	
• Income of families and unrelated persons living in households	FedStats, Census Bureau
• Median incomes of families	FedStats, Census Bureau
• Percentage of families with incomes below the poverty level	FedStats, Census Bureau
• Number of families receiving Temporary Assistance for Needy Families	Administration for Children and Families (DHHS)
• Number of participants in the WIC, National School Lunch, and National School Breakfast programs	USDA, FedStats
• Number of individuals receiving SNAP benefits	Supplemental Nutrition Assistance Program (SNAP)
• Number of individuals receiving public assistance	Welfare office
• Unemployment statistics (e.g., percentage of households with one or more unemployed members)	FedStats, Census Bureau
• Tangible wealth (e.g., ownership of land and livestock, ownership of items such as personal computers and cellular phones)	Municipal, county, state records
Existing Community Services and Programs	
• Government-funded food assistance programs (e.g., number of referrals)	Related government agency
• Health and nutrition services and programs offered by hospitals, clinics, community health centers, sports/fitness centers, YMCA/YWCAs, the public health department, voluntary health organizations, schools, universities, colleges, civic groups	Hospitals, clinics, sports/fitness centers, directory of nutrition services (if available from state associations)
• Primary care services (e.g., location, accessibility)	Local hospitals, clinics, etc.
• Soup kitchens, food pantries	Internet, municipal community services department
• Programs and services offered by nutritionists, dietitians, and other health practitioners	Key informants, state associations
Sociocultural Data and Trends	
• Labor force characteristics (e.g., occupation, industry, class of workers, hours worked)	Census Bureau, Bureau of Labor Statistics
• Language spoken at home	FedStats
• Education (e.g., median school years completed by individuals 25 years of age and older, individuals who completed high school)	FedStats, Census Bureau
• Literacy levels of school children and adults	FedStats, Census Bureau

[a] The Internet address for FedStats is *http://fedstats.sites.usa.gov.*

[b] The following abbreviations appear in this table: BRFSS, Behavioral Risk Factor Surveillance System; CDC, Centers for Disease Control and Prevention; DHHS, Department of Health and Human Services; NCHS, National Center for Health Statistics; NHANES, National Health and Nutrition Examination Survey; NNMRRP, National Nutrition Monitoring and Related Research Program; DRI, Dietary Reference Intake; WIC, Special Supplemental Nutrition Program for Women, Infants, and Children; USDA, U.S. Department of Agriculture; YMCA/YWCA, Young Men's/Women's Christian Association.

▶ **Community health data.** A variety of health statistics are used to paint a picture of the community's health. Some health data describe the causes and rates of disease, disability, and death within the community; others focus on key life stages or events. Community health data help the community nutritionist describe the population's health and nutrition problems and identify persons who are malnourished. Some common health measures and related terms are listed in Table 2-1 on page 46.[21] For example, the infant mortality rate is an important measure of a nation's health and is used worldwide as an indicator of health status. The infant mortality rate in the United States has declined steadily over the past decades and was 6.0 per 1,000 live births in 2013. Even so, the infant mortality rate for blacks was 11.2 per 1,000 live births, or more than double that of the U.S. national average. American Indians and Alaska Natives also had infant mortality rates higher than the national average, signaling an urgent need to address this basic health issue.[22]

▶ **Community organizational and power structures.** Information is needed about how the community operates, how its population is distributed, and how healthy it is. Information about existing health services provides clues to the community's perception of its leading health and nutrition problems. The organizational charts for government agencies and city hall provide information about how the community delivers health services and develops health policy. Also, knowing the key players in local health organizations and community, business, and media groups helps the community nutritionist identify community leaders to involve in qualitative assessments of the community background.

▶ **Demographic data and trends.** Demographic data help define the people who live in the community by sex, age, race/ethnicity, education level, marital status, employment, socioeconomic characteristics, and household characteristics. Changes in the demographic profile of a community often serve as an early warning signal about potential gaps in services or undetected nutrition problems. For example, in an assessment of the nutrition and health status of persons aged 65 years and older in a rural community, the assessment team learned that the number of persons more than 85 years old who were living alone at home had increased significantly since the 2005 assessment. This trend suggested a need to increase home care services for the 85-plus age group.

▶ **Economic data and trends.** Information about the income of families and the number of families receiving public assistance provides a benchmark for comparing the target population's income with the community's mean or median family income.

▶ **Existing community services and programs.** Obtaining data on the community's existing health and nutrition services helps pinpoint gaps where services are needed. An inventory of the community's nutrition services and programs can be built by: (1) identifying the nutrition services and programs available through government agencies, health organizations, and civic groups; (2) cataloging the educational services and materials offered by voluntary health organizations such as the American Red Cross, the National Council on Alcoholism, the American Heart Association, and the American Cancer Society in the United States and, in Canada, the Canadian Diabetes Association, the Canadian Arthritis and Rheumatism Society, and the Heart and Stroke Foundation of Canada, among others; and (3) identifying the programs and services delivered by local nutritionists, dietitians, and other health professionals. The United Way of America is a network of volunteers and local charities that also maintains directories of local community services and programs.[23] In addition, national information centers such as the U.S. National Health Information Center can be contacted for general information about the availability of educational materials, programs, and referral services.

▶ **Sociocultural data and trends.** Information about the community's educational level, language use, literacy rate, and major industries and occupations helps identify factors that may affect the health and nutrition status of the target population.

Sources of Community Data Many demographic and socioeconomic data can be located in publications of the U.S. Bureau of the Census, Bureau of Labor Statistics, Department of Agriculture, and Department of Health and Human Services. The decennial Census of Population and Housing, for example, which is conducted by the Bureau of the Census, provides data on states, counties, local units of government, school districts, and congressional districts.[24] Census data typically describe age and sex distributions, births and deaths, labor force characteristics (e.g., occupation, industry, hours worked), income, housing characteristics (e.g., year built, number of rooms, plumbing, heating, kitchen facilities), and other demographic variables.

Additional investigative work helps locate health statistics and related health reports from local, county, and state health departments; social welfare agencies; birth, death, marriage, and divorce registries; and courts. The annual reports of local hospitals, clinics, and health centers provide information on the types of health problems within the community, the existence of screening programs for detecting health and nutrition problems, and the resources available to deal with them.[25]

It is sometimes necessary to resort to secondary data sources such as data archives, which serve as repositories for thousands of surveys conducted at a national and/or international level. Data archive services have collected and cataloged the surveys of many communities. These services usually charge a fee for data and supporting documentation, and may offer training and support related to survey design, data management, and analysis. Examples of data archive services include the University of Michigan's Institute for Social Research, the world's largest university-based social science survey and research organization,[26] and the University of North Carolina's Odum Institute for Research in Social Science, which is a source of national and international economic, electoral, demographic, financial, health, and public opinion data.[27]

The *Community Health Status Indicators Reports (CHSI)* also may provide helpful community data. These reports provide a health status snapshot of all 3,141 U.S. counties that includes causes of death, life expectancy, infectious diseases, teen mothers, and other indicators. You can compare your county with similar "peer counties," with the nation, or with the *Healthy People 2020* national objectives. In addition to the CHSI webpages, community profiles can be displayed on maps or downloaded in a brochure format. The CHSI mapping capability allows users to visually compare similar counties.[28]

In the case of international needs assessments, international agencies such as the Food and Agriculture Organization (FAO) and the World Health Organization (WHO) may provide useful data. These organizations have regional offices that can furnish relevant population health data. Since 1954, for example, the Pan American Health Organization has published a series of quadrennial reports that document the health progress achieved by its members. Entitled *Health in the Americas*, these reports provide general information on the region's social and political climate, primary demographic characteristics, mortality data, and health conditions, focusing on women, children, and older adults.[29]

It is seldom necessary, expedient, or possible to collect and use all data available about the community. Consider a situation where the local health department is aware of the high prevalence of type 2 diabetes in American Indians.[30] The department's health and wellness office wants to increase its initiatives to reduce type 2 diabetes risk among American Indians, especially children. It perceives a need to develop a wellness program specifically for American Indian children, but it needs information about type 2 diabetes in this population. The department's community nutritionist reviews the spectrum of community data that could be collected and decides to collect data about the structure of the tribal council, the distribution of type 2 diabetes among American Indians by sex and age, the types of health care and medical services available to the population, its use of health care and medical services, the availability of diabetes education programs and the population's participation in these programs, food patterns of American Indians, mean family income and education level, and literacy rate. Data are not needed on housing, the water supply, recreation facilities, labor force characteristics, tangible wealth, or transportation systems.

In this example, the focus of the assessment is fairly narrow, dealing with only one health condition (type 2 diabetes) experienced by a particular population (American Indian children and their caregivers living on a reservation). In contrast, consider the types of data required to evaluate the health and nutrition status of homeless people living in your community. Because homelessness cuts across all age and ethnic groups, a broad spectrum of data on homeless people and the community's resources for addressing their health and nutrition problems is needed. In the next section, we describe how to locate information about the community environment and background conditions.

Community Environment and Background Factors In this phase, you will collect information about the physical, political, social, and cultural environment in which the community is positioned. Certain aspects of the community environment, described in **Table 4-3**, can affect community health and nutrition status. In addition, many social, cultural, and political factors operate in the background but have the potential to affect how the community members live, the food choices they make, and where they obtain medical services. Community opinion is also an important part of the community environment. Thus, the values and priorities of community leaders and community members are important factors to consider when conducting a needs assessment. If you undertake an effort to promote a health behavior that does not align with community values, the effectiveness of the effort may be affected. Learning about the social and cultural climate of the community may help you to use techniques to promote a health behavior within the value system of your community, or to focus on an issue that is highly important to the community. Following is a description of how each of these types of data may be relevant to a community needs assessment.

▶ **Food systems and food availability.** Food availability is influenced by the community's geography and climate, which affect the length of the food-growing season; by the type of foods grown in commercial and family gardens; by the types of food storage systems needed to keep foods fresh; and by the location and types of grocery stores, convenience stores, and farmers' markets. The USDA's Food Environment Atlas allows one to get a spatial overview of a community's ability to access healthy food and its success in doing so (see Chapter 10 for more information).[31]

TABLE 4-3 Types and Sources of Data about the Community Environment and Background Factors

TYPE OF DATA	SOURCE OF DATA
Food Systems and Food Availability	
• National, regional, and local food distribution networks; extent of emergency and supplemental feeding systems; food wholesale and retail systems; and amount of food grown locally	Census Bureau, data archives, crop reports by county or state agencies (can be accessed through FedStats[a])
• Location, type, and number of grocery stores, supermarkets, convenience stores, health food stores, and farmers' markets; food availability within stores and markets	Internet; USDA Food Environment Atlas and Food Desert Locator; observation
• Location, type, and number of restaurants (e.g., family style, fast food, and so on)	Internet; USDA Food Environment Atlas and Food Desert Locator

TABLE 4-3 Types and Sources of Data about the Community Environment and Background Factors—*continued*

TYPE OF DATA	SOURCE OF DATA
Geography and Climate	Observation, state department of agriculture
Health Systems	
• Location, type, and number of hospitals, clinics, health maintenance organizations, long-term-care facilities	Internet
• Types of ambulatory care	Annual reports of hospitals, clinics
Housing	
• Type of housing (e.g., percentage of year-round housing that is single dwelling units; housing characteristics, such as units in structure, year built, number of rooms, plumbing, heating, and kitchen facilities)	Census Bureau, FedStats
• Condition of housing (e.g., percentage of standard housing with an exterior frame made of brick, wood, or concrete block)	Census Bureau, FedStats
National Policy	
• General information	Articles published in journals, magazines, newspapers; commentary on TV, radio, Internet
• Agriculture	USDA[b]
• Economics	Department of Commerce
• Education	Department of Education
• Health	DHHS[b]
• Housing	Department of Housing and Urban Development
• Labor	Department of Labor
• Nutrition	DHHS (FDA, CDC, NIH, etc.); USDA (CNPP, FNS)[b]
• Social Security	DHHS[b]
Recreation	
• Location and number of fitness centers, sports facilities	Internet
• Types of recreation available (swimming, golf, tennis, cross-country skiing, walking trails, etc.)	Observation, Internet, Chamber of Commerce
Social and Cultural Conditions	
Advertising	Television, radio, billboards, printed matter, Internet
Health messages	Television; radio; printed matter; Internet; educational materials available from government, food companies, nonprofit groups, etc.
Roles of women	Television, radio, printed matter, Internet
Belief systems	Television, radio, printed matter, Internet, family, friends, other social contacts
Community Values	
• Perceptions of community values, interests, and needs	Key informants in health departments, government, non-governmental organizations, industry, faith-based organizations, etc.; community members
• Perceptions of community strengths and weaknesses	
• Organizational values and needs	
Transportation Systems	
• Access to public transportation	Municipal/state/federal department of transportation
• Walkability by pedestrians	*http://safety.fhwa.dot.gov*
• Safe routes to school	*www.saferoutesinfo.org/*
• Bike paths	DOT Federal Highway Administration Bike and Pedestrian Program
Water Supply	
• Source of water, distance from residence, water quality	Municipal/state department of water works and water quality

[a] The Internet address for FedStats is *http://fedstats.sites.usa.gov.*

[b] The following abbreviations appear in this table: USDA, U.S. Department of Agriculture; CDC, Centers for Disease Control and Prevention; DHHS, Department of Health and Human Services; FDA, Food and Drug Administration; NIH, National Institutes of Health; CNPP, Center for Nutrition Policy and Promotion; FNS, Food and Nutrition Service.

▶ **Geography and climate.** This may be important if you are planning a program that involves growing food. Geography and climate also affect food access.

▶ **Health systems.** Access to medical clinics and ambulatory care services, which provide screening, diagnosis, counseling, follow-up, and therapy, influence health and nutrition status. You may consider looking at use of available services, which may vary by demographic segment.

▶ **Housing.** The type and condition of housing may affect health.

▶ **Policies.** National policy, for example, affects eligibility for food assistance programs, minimum-wage levels, and the distribution of commodity foods—all factors that may influence the target population's health and nutrition status. If the community consists of tribes of American Indians, the assessment team may review the health care policy of the Bureau of Indian Affairs, the federal agency charged with providing personal and public health services to American Indians and Alaska Natives. The assessment team may learn that the agency's policies have inadvertently created competition among tribes for money for health care services. This unexpected situation may result in less money being distributed to tribal communities to pay for expensive medical services,[32] an outcome that may affect the target population's health and nutrition status.

▶ **Recreation.** Availability and use of recreational facilities and parks shed light on potential for physical activity as well as community culture.

▶ **Social and cultural conditions.** The social and cultural fabric in communities can influence food norms, health beliefs, and values for food and nutrition. All of these factors impact food choices and, thus, nutrition status. **Social factors** include social norms and attitudes, safety of neighborhoods, social support and interactions, exposure to mass media, socioeconomic conditions, quality of education, and so on.[33] By **culture**, we mean the integrated pattern of human knowledge, beliefs, and behaviors that are learned and transmitted to succeeding generations.[34] Many of our food habits, attitudes, and practices arise from the traditions, customs, belief systems, technologies, values, and norms of the culture in which we live. For instance, in an assessment of the nutrition status of students with bulimia, certain background conditions—such as advertising, society's emphasis on leanness, and cultural expectations about weight and body size—are likely to influence the students' food patterns and body image. Furthermore, children who grow up seeing their peers choosing packaged snacks rather than fresh, whole foods learn to define a "snack" by what they see around them in society. Teens may feel pressured to choose fast-food items after school when spending time with peers who prefer these foods. A decision to breastfeed may be influenced by important people in a mother's social circle. In sum, we often feel compelled to follow the norms and expectations we see around us.[35] Social and cultural norms can create expectations that drive behavior. This background information should be evaluated as part of the assessment.

▶ **Transportation systems.** Ready access to transportation, whether in the form of personal car, bus, or commuter train, improves the target population's access to medical services and supermarkets.

▶ **Water supply.** Information to describe the source and quality of public drinking water may be included.

Sources of Data about the Community Environment and Background Factors

Table 4-3 includes potential sources of data for community environment and background factors. Many sources of data can be accessed via the Internet. A true understanding of a community is best developed, however, by spending time in it. Visiting

Social factors Social norms and attitudes; resource availability; access to health care; neighborhood safety; exposure to crime, violence, and social disorder; social support and interactions; exposure to mass media; socioeconomic conditions; quality of education; transportation options.

Culture The knowledge, beliefs, customs, laws, morals, art, and any other habits and skills acquired by humans as members of society.

the community—its leaders, its members, its food establishments and grocery stores—is a great way to learn about its values and priorities. You can learn about community opinion by conducting key informant interviews with formal leaders of the community, such as the mayor, who have a broad knowledge of the community. You may also talk with informal leaders, such as the owner of a community center or grocery store, whose opinions and connections provide valuable information about the community. Religious leaders, physicians, teachers, volunteers with nonprofit agencies, heads of social services, and members of the media are among those who can provide insights into how the community operates. Lastly, community members themselves provide key insights into the values of the community. Focus groups and interviews are helpful for learning from community members and leaders, and are discussed in the next section.

Target Population Data The community data, community environment, and background data provide a great framework for either: (1) deciding which population to target or (2) developing a plan to learn about a specified target population in more detail. Some data related to the audience may be existing, and some will need to be collected. When conducting an assessment, the community nutritionist can ask broad questions about the target population: What effect does a particular lifestyle choice have on the target population's nutrition status? Why does the target population behave this way? How can this behavior be changed? Alternatively, she or he can ask specific questions: Do people who begin an exercise program also make other positive lifestyle choices? Do people who routinely have their blood pressure checked also consume low-sodium diets? Do people who consume excessive amounts of alcohol also smoke and eat high-fat and salty foods? The point of these questions is to learn about the many factors that affect food choice, so that an intervention can be crafted that considers lifestyle, priorities, attitudes, and motivations of the target population.

Observing the target population in its community setting—doing a walkabout to learn about where people live, work, eat, and spend leisure time—provides essential information. If your target population is institutionalized older adults, then visit local nursing and residential homes, senior centers, and other facilities where this population lives. If the population you are interested in is Muslim, visit local grocery stores where this group shops and find out about Halal food. If it is athletes, visit fitness centers, sports facilities, and schools with sports programs. Observe the target population in the community and ask questions: Where do people shop for food? What kind of transportation is required for them to reach the supermarket or grocery store where they shop? What are the main occupations of this group? Do they live near a hospital or clinic? Which medical services do they use? Is a food bank, soup kitchen, or other emergency food assistance facility located near where they live? Do they grow some of their own food? What has the nutrition status of this group been in the past? Take time to ask members of the target population how they perceive their nutrition status. The important thing is to listen to what the target population has to say about their nutrition status, factors that affect it, and what they believe can be done to improve it. **Table 4-4** lists types of data you may collect about the target population and suggested sources. Let's take a look at the categories of data.

▶ **Food preferences and attitudes.** Learning about your target population's food preferences and attitudes helps you to understand why they select the foods they do. You may also assess their attitudes toward nutrition messages they have heard in the past. Also, taking a look at how confident your audience is in purchasing, preparing, and consuming healthy foods will help you to know where to focus your intervention.

▶ **Health beliefs and knowledge.** As nutrition professionals, we believe strongly in the link between diet and health outcomes. However, you will find some audiences who do not embrace this association. For example, some traditional cultural groups may believe

Visit grocery stores and supermarkets where your target population shops to learn about its food consumption and shopping practices. Observing that few members of your target population drive cars and most walk to the grocery store gives you important information about their lifestyle and needs.

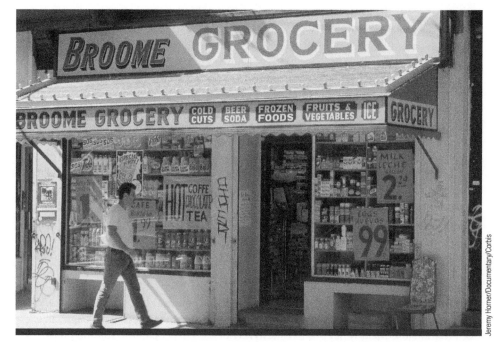

Jeremy Horner/Documentary/Corbis

fate determines their health, and that personal actions do not impact health outcomes. This is important to know. Furthermore, assessing the audience's knowledge and skill level related to food purchasing (e.g., label reading), preparation, and general nutrition is helpful for determining where to focus a program. For example, if you find that your audience already knows that they should eat a variety of colorful fruits and vegetables every day but they are not doing so, you need to work to understand the barriers they are experiencing to fruit and vegetable consumption and address those.

▶ **Lifestyle factors.** Lifestyle factors include such areas as physical activity level, leisure activities, stress management techniques, smoking status, and drug and alcohol usage; knowledge about your target population's lifestyle is important because it can influence health and nutrition status. For example, people who are physically active have lower blood cholesterol concentrations and a lower risk of coronary heart disease (CHD) than sedentary people.[36] Women who become pregnant unexpectedly are less likely to breastfeed their infants than women whose pregnancies are planned.[37] People who are convinced that eating fruits and vegetables protects against cancer are more likely to consume these foods than people who see no positive consequences to eating them.[38] People who smoke have higher body levels of oxidized products, including oxidized ascorbic acid, than nonsmokers.[39] The effects of these and other lifestyle choices on health and nutrition status are complex.

▶ **Nutrition status.** Nutrition status data include anthropometric, laboratory, clinical, and dietary data. Dietary data include food and nutrient intakes and dietary patterns. You can often gather general information about the target population's nutrition status from the research literature and/or existing survey data. Still, collecting data specific to your audience is often helpful. Moreover, collecting data specific to your target population will allow you to track changes over time associated with programs you implement.

▶ **Social and cultural factors.** In collecting community environment data, you get a good understanding of social and cultural factors in your community. Now you can focus on your specific target population and learn the social and cultural norms around what your population eats at home, on the go, and in social settings. Religion may affect food

TABLE 4-4 Types and Sources of Target Population Data

TYPE OF DATA	METHOD OF OBTAINING DATA
Nutrition Status	
• General information about target population's nutrition status	NNMRRP[a] surveys, literature review
• Anthropometric data: height, weight, weight change, skin folds, circumference measurements	Anthropometry
• Laboratory data: cholesterol, vitamin status, etc.	Phlebotomy
• Clinical data: medical history, physical exam data	Survey, direct assessment
• Dietary data: food and nutrient intakes, dietary patterns	NNMRRP surveys
	Methods of collecting data of target audience: survey, food diary, 24-hour recall, food frequency questionnaire, diet history (see Table 4-8 for more information on each of these dietary assessment tools)
Food Preferences and Attitudes	
• Preferred foods when eating at home, eating on the go, and eating at restaurants	NNMRRP surveys, direct survey of target audience, focus groups, interviews
• Perceptions of nutrition messages	
• Attitudes toward food	
• Confidence/self-efficacy in ability to purchase, plan, and consume healthy foods	
Health Beliefs and Knowledge	
• Belief in link between diet and health	NNMRRP surveys (e.g., Health and Diet Survey), direct survey of target audience, focus groups, interviews
• Knowledge of basic nutrition concepts, label reading, how to select healthy foods in grocery stores, restaurants, etc.	
Lifestyle Factors	
• Physical activity level	Survey, focus groups, interviews
• Leisure activities	
• Stress management techniques	
• Smoking status	
• Drug/alcohol usage	
Sociocultural Factors	
• Social and cultural norms around food purchase, preparation, and consumption patterns	Observation, key informant interviews, surveys, focus groups, interviews with target audience
• Food expectations in social settings: schools, sporting events, parties, events held by faith-based organizations and other community organizations, etc.	
• Religiosity	
Priorities and Motivation	
• Priorities that affect food purchase, preparation, and consumption patterns	Focus groups, interviews, surveys
• Motivations for food and health choices	

[a] NNMRRP, National Nutrition Monitoring and Related Research Program; information on NNMRRP surveys is found in Chapter 7.

practices for some people as well. Endeavor to understand the desirable and customary food choices for members of your target population.

▶ **Priorities and motivation.** Lastly, to create a program that is relevant to your population, it is critical to understand their priorities and motivation. What is important to your audience? Do they have a group orientation and strong value for family? If so, involving the family in interventions will improve success. Are they living fast-paced lifestyles? If so, looking for ways to promote healthy eating that are also convenient will be important.

Developing an understanding of the audience's values and desires will help you to develop messages and programs that motivate change.

Sources of Target Population Data Data about the target population may be available on a national scale or at the community level. Collecting data about your specific population can give you detailed information to guide development of your program plan according to the unique needs of your population. Let's take a look at ways of obtaining existing and new data about the target population.

▶ **Existing data.** Data related to the target population's nutrition status can often be gathered from large-scale population surveys, such as those conducted by the National Nutrition Monitoring and Related Research Program (NNMRRP) or from small surveys of special populations conducted in the immediate community or region. It is usually desirable to have both types of data on hand. NNMRRP survey data provide a national perspective on the target population and the factors that contribute to its nutrition needs in other regions of the country. In most cases, NNMRRP survey data can be obtained from the National Technical Information Service. Some data files and publications are available from the sponsoring agency (e.g., the U.S. Department of Agriculture or the National Institute of Child Health and Human Development) or from the U.S. Government Printing Office. The Internet Resources on pages 145–147 address key data sources online. Check the government websites for compilations of vital health statistics and reports on public health issues related to the community. Local historical records can be useful. Information available in newspaper archives, old maps, parish or county records, and other documents can provide a history of a local public health problem and the public attention given to it. In addition, many health and nutrition data are published in periodicals such as the *Journal of the Academy of Nutrition and Dietetics*, the *American Journal of Public Health*, *Public Health Reports*, and the *New England Journal of Medicine*. Consult the Public Health Service's publication *Nutrition Monitoring in the United States: The Directory of Federal and State Nutrition Monitoring and Related Research Activities* for a list of NNMRRP surveys and pertinent journal publications of survey findings and for a description of where NNMRRP survey data can be obtained.[40] Information about the availability of some nutrition monitoring and survey data is provided on the Centers for Disease Control and Prevention's website.[41] The decision whether to use NNMRRP survey data will be influenced by the level of detail needed about the target population, the personnel and facilities available for sorting and analyzing the data, and budget constraints. (*Note:* See Chapter 7 for more about the activities of the National Nutrition Monitoring and Related Research Program.)

▶ In some situations, data related to the target population are not readily available. National survey data do not always reflect the nutrition status or food intake of the target population in a particular community. Consider this scenario: National data from a recent NHANES survey found that 27% of women aged 50 years and older met recommended intakes of calcium;[42] however, a 2010 survey of women living in your community found that only 19% of women aged 50 years and older met current calcium recommendations. In this situation, the national data do not reflect your community particularly well, but they may be a good benchmark against which to compare your target population. The question for a community nutritionist is why some women in your community have a calcium intake lower than the national average. Thus, small surveys carried out locally provide insights about your particular community. Furthermore, they tend to be more relevant to defining your community's needs, priorities, and values than large, national surveys.

▶ **New data.** Once you have identified existing community data, you must then identify those data elements that are still needed and choose one or more methods for obtaining them. The method selected for assessing nutrition needs must be simple, cost-effective, and able to be completed within a reasonable time frame. You will find that community nutritionists have various strategies for going about this process. Many community nutritionists will start by making a list of what they want to know about the target population. Consider the factors listed in Table 4-4.

Step 3: Collect Data

After developing the data collection plan, you are ready to collect data. Having a good system for managing data and a plan for analyzing it are important considerations here. Developing data collection protocols and training those who will be collecting data to ensure consistency in collection methods are key. Although management functions are beyond the scope of this chapter, Chapter 18 covers several aspects of managing community nutrition programs.

Let's take a look at methods available for learning about the target population.

Methods of Obtaining Data about the Target Population

A variety of methods exist for collecting data about the target population. The methods range from simple surveys and screening tools to interviews with key informants. As you read about methods for obtaining target population data in this section, you will see that each method provides a different type of information about the population of interest.

Survey A **survey** is a systematic study of a cross-section of individuals who represent the target population. It is a relatively inexpensive way to collect information from a large group of people. Surveys can be used to collect qualitative or quantitative data in formal, structured interviews; by phone, by mail, or online; or from individuals or groups. Some survey instruments (such as questionnaires) are self-administered, whereas a trained interviewer administers others.[43]

Designing a questionnaire and conducting a survey involve more than heading out with a clipboard and a list of questions to interview people as they come into your clinic, office, or community center. Survey design and analysis is a discipline in itself, and the process of conducting a survey usually requires a team of experts with knowledge of survey research, statistics, epidemiology, public health, and nutrition. Although a detailed discussion of survey methodology is beyond the scope of this book, a few comments are in order about the issues to consider when designing a **nutrition survey** or adapting an existing survey for your own purposes.

> ▶ **THINK LIKE A COMMUNITY** NUTRITIONIST
>
> Imagine you are undertaking a needs assessment to develop a school-based nutrition program for elementary school–age children in a low-income, urban, Latino neighborhood. You have reviewed existing data about your population, and you know that childhood diabetes and obesity rates in the zip code are higher than state and national averages. You also learn that 95% of children in the zip code are eligible for free or reduced-price school meals. National data on energy and nutrient intakes for this age group are available from the most recent National Health and Nutrition Examination Survey (NHANES). However, you still want to gain a more intimate understanding of your audience's daily food choices and the factors that affect them. To do so, you decide it would be best to start by observing the neighborhood. You ask an administrator at a local school if you can sit in the cafeteria to observe lunchtime. You also take some walks in the neighborhood, paying close attention to food outlets near schools. You observe what children are buying and eating on their way to and from school. In this process, you notice that many children are stopping at corner stores (bodegas) on the way to school to buy processed snack foods and sugary drinks. Furthermore, you notice that those children share their food in the school cafeteria with their friends. You also notice that younger children are more likely to eat school lunches, and older children are more likely to bring food from home or from corner stores. You notice that the most common lunch brought from home is a bag of chips and a sugary drink. On the positive side, you see the school lunch program offers a salad bar with fresh fruits and vegetables, and a cafeteria worker is encouraging the children to take them. At the end of the school day, you also notice vendors selling churros to children as they are leaving school. This process of observation helps you begin to develop an understanding of what children are eating. Now, you need to work to understand a bit more about *why* they are eating what they are eating. You decide to develop a focus group guide to use with upper elementary school children to explore their food purchasing habits in the school vicinity. Make a list of questions you might use to learn about the children's current behavior and what motivates it, and to explore potential avenues for intervention. You may refer to the section on focus groups on page 123 to help you plan the questions. After you are finished developing a list of questions, take a look at Figure 4-4 on page 124 to see a set of focus group questions used by researchers to explore corner-store purchases among low-income, urban youth.

Survey A systematic study of a cross-section of individuals who represent the target population.

Nutrition survey An instrument designed to collect data on the nutrition status and dietary intake of a population group.

"Planning a survey consists of making a series of scientific and practical decisions."[44] The first step is to determine the purpose of the survey. Most food consumption surveys are carried out to assess the food patterns in households or among individuals, evaluate eating patterns, estimate the adequacy of the food supply, assess the nutritional quality of the food supply, measure the nutrient intake of a certain population group, study the relationship of diet and nutrition status to health, or determine the effectiveness of an education program.[45] Surveys can also investigate health beliefs, knowledge, self-efficacy, and nutrition-related attitudes that may impact food selection. A nutrition survey does not have to be complex and gargantuan to be meaningful, but it must have a well-defined purpose.

Next, decisions must be made about who will design the survey, who will conduct it, and how it will be carried out. The survey instrument must be designed and pretested, and the sample must be chosen. The personnel responsible for conducting the survey and analyzing data must be trained. Numerous other decisions must be made about the feasibility of the survey; the quality of data obtained by the survey; the costs of carrying it out; the readability of the survey; literacy issues; and the manner in which data will be analyzed and used. At every step in the planning process, there are practical constraints related to time and money.[46]

Surveys are important tools in assessing the health and nutrition status of individuals, but they must be designed and carried out carefully to provide valid and reliable information. One important consideration is the reading level of your target population. Readability can be assessed by formulas such as the SMOG formula (see Appendix C) and the Fog Index or by computer programs designed for this purpose. Another consideration is the method of delivery: written or oral, by phone or face to face, or electronically. For cases in which electronic surveys are appropriate, *SurveyMonkey* enables you to create professional online surveys quickly and easily. You can send your survey link by e-mail and download a summary of your results in multiple formats. For more information, go to SurveyMonkey at *www.surveymonkey.com.*[47] It is also very helpful to look at existing survey questions that are in use and have been shown to provide valid responses. BRFSS is the world's largest ongoing telephone health survey system, tracking health conditions and risk behaviors in the United States yearly since 1984. You can view sample questionnaires at *www.cdc.gov/brfss/.*[48] Consult **Table 4-5** for a list of questions to ask when designing a survey for your community needs assessment.

TABLE 4-5 Questions to Ask When Designing a Survey

- **Is the survey valid and reliable?** Will it measure what it is intended to measure and, assuming that nothing changed in the interim, will it produce the same estimate of this measurement on separate occasions?
- **Are norms available?** That is, are reference data or population standards available against which the data from your target group can be compared?
- **Is the survey suitable for the target population?** A survey designed to obtain health and nutrition data on free-living older adults may not be appropriate for institutionalized older adults.
- **Are the survey questions easy to read and understand?** Survey questions must be geared to the target population and its level of literacy, reading comprehension, and fluency in the primary language. Having a readable survey is especially important if it is to be self-administered.
- **Is the format of the questionnaire clear?** If the questionnaire is not laid out carefully, respondents may become confused and inadvertently skip questions or sections.
- **Are the responses clear?** A variety of scales and responses may be used in designing a survey. Some questions may require filling in blanks or providing simple yes/no or true/false answers. Others may ask respondents to rank-order their responses from "seldom/never use" to "use often/always." The trick when selecting such scales is to choose one that allows you to discriminate between responses but doesn't provide so many categories that respondents are overwhelmed.
- **Is the survey comprehensive but brief?** Often the length of the survey must be limited to ensure that respondents complete it within a reasonable time frame. With long questionnaires, respondents are likely to answer questions hurriedly and mark the same answer to most questions.
- **Does the survey ask "socially loaded" questions?** Each survey question should be evaluated for how it is likely to be interpreted. Questions that imply certain value judgments or socially desirable responses should be rewritten. This is especially important when dealing with respondents from cultures other than your own.

Source: Adapted from L. Fallowfield, *The Quality of Life* (London: Souvenir, 1990), 40–45.

Health Risk Appraisal The health risk appraisal (HRA) is a type of survey instrument used to characterize a population's general health status. We mention it here in a separate category because it is widely used in worksites, government agencies, universities, and other organizations as a health education or screening tool. The HRA is a kind of "health hazard chart" that asks questions about the lifestyle factors that influence disease risk,[49] and it has been used successfully to improve health behaviors.[50]

The HRA instrument consists of three components: a questionnaire, certain calculations that predict risk of disease, and an educational message or report to the participant.[51] A typical HRA asks questions about age, sex, height, weight, marital status, size of body frame, exercise habits, consumption of certain foods (e.g., fruits and vegetables) and ingredients (e.g., sodium), intake of alcohol, job satisfaction, hours of sleep, smoking habits, and medical checkups or hospitalizations. An HRA has been developed and tested for people aged 55 years and older.[52] A portion of the Healthier People Network's questionnaire is shown in **Figure 4-3**.

HRAs are used to alert individuals to any risky health behaviors that they engage in and to inform them how such behaviors might be modified, usually through a lifestyle modification program.[53] For example, a health risk questionnaire was used at a trucker

The HEALTHIER PEOPLE NETWORK, Inc.

. . . linking science, technology, & education to serve the public interest . . .

IDENTIFICATION NUMBER

The health risk appraisal is an educational tool, showing you choices you can make to keep good health and avoid the most common causes of death (for a person of your age and sex). This health risk appraisal is **not** a substitute for a check-up or physical exam that you get from a doctor or nurse; however, it does provide some ideas for lowering your risk of getting sick or injured in the future. It is NOT designed for people who already have HEART DISEASE, CANCER, KIDNEY DISEASE, OR OTHER SERIOUS CONDITIONS; if you have any of these problems, please ask your health care provider to interpret the report for you.

DIRECTIONS:
To get the most accurate results, **answer as many questions as you can**. If you do not know the answer leave it blank.

The following questions must be completed or the computer program cannot process your questionnaire:

1. SEX 2. AGE 3. HEIGHT 4. WEIGHT 15. CIGARETTE SMOKING

Please write your answers in the boxes provided. **(Examples: ☒ or 98)**

1. **SEX**	1 ☐ Male 2 ☐ Female
2. **AGE**	Years
3. **HEIGHT** (Without shoes) (No fractions)	Feet Inches
4. **WEIGHT** (Without shoes) (No fractions)	Pounds
5. Body frame size	1 ☐ Small 2 ☐ Medium 3 ☐ Large
6. Have you ever been told that you have diabetes (or sugar diabetes)?	1 ☐ Yes 2 ☐ No
7. Are you now taking medicine for high blood pressure?	1 ☐ Yes 2 ☐ No
8. What is your blood pressure now?	
★38. Do you eat some food every day that is high in fiber, such as whole grain bread, cereal, fresh fruits or vegetables?	1 ☐ Yes 2 ☐ No
★39. Do you eat foods every day that are high in cholesterol or fat, such as fatty meat, cheese, fried foods, or eggs?	1 ☐ Yes 2 ☐ No
★40. In general, how satisfied are you with your life?	1 ☐ Mostly satisfied 2 ☐ Partly satisfied 3 ☐ Not satisfied

FIGURE 4-3 A Portion of a Health Risk Appraisal Form

Source: Used with permission of The Healthier People Network, Inc.

Screening is one method of identifying people with high blood pressure. People whose screening value indicates high blood pressure are referred for medical diagnosis and treatment, which may include nutrition counseling.

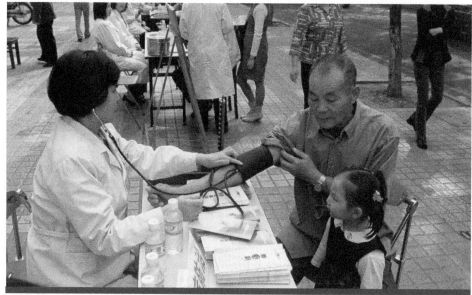

David Butow/News Archive/CORBIS SABA

trade show to assess the health status of truck drivers. Truckers who stopped at the trade show enjoyed free food, music, raffles, and other events. At one booth, truckers received free blood pressure measurements and health education materials and were asked to complete a survey of their health risk factors, health status, and driving patterns. An analysis of the survey results showed that truck drivers tend to smoke cigarettes, to be sedentary and overweight, and to be unaware if they have high blood pressure.[54]

Screening Screening is an important preventive health activity designed to reverse, retard, or halt the progress of a disease by detecting it as soon as possible. Screening occurs in both clinical practice and community settings, and it entails procedures that are safe, simple, and cheap. **Table 4-6** lists some common screening procedures. In community screening programs, people from the community are invited to have an assessment made

TABLE 4-6 Common Screening Procedures in Clinical Practice and Community Settings

SCREENING PROCEDURE	TARGET POPULATION
Clinical Practice	
Taking a medical history	All ages, both sexes
Height and weight	All ages, both sexes
Phenylketonuria (PKU)	Newborn infants
Posture (for detection of scoliosis)	Children over 3 years of age
Vision	Children over 3 years of age
Hearing	Children over 3 years of age
Tuberculin test	Children over 1 year of age
Community Settings	
Health risk appraisal	Primarily adults over 18 years of age
Blood pressure	Adults over 18 years of age
Blood cholesterol level	Adults over 18 years of age

Sources: Adapted from J. M. Last, *Public Health and Human Ecology*, 2nd ed. (New York: McGraw-Hill Professional, 1998); *The Merck Manual*, eds. M. Beers and R. Berkow, 17th ed. (Whitehouse Station, NJ: Merck Research Laboratories, 1999).

of a health risk or behavior. Their screening value is then compared with a predetermined cutpoint or risk level. For example, during Heart Month, a popular shopping mall sponsors a health fair that offers screening for high blood cholesterol concentrations. People who come through the screening booth give a fingerstick blood sample, which is analyzed on-site by a machine designed for this purpose. Their blood cholesterol concentrations are classified as high, borderline-high, or desirable, on the basis of the classification scheme developed by the National Cholesterol Education Program. Individuals whose screening value suggests an elevated risk are referred for medical diagnosis and treatment. Screening programs are not meant to substitute for a health care visit or routine medical monitoring for people already receiving treatment, but they do have educational value and serve to identify high-risk persons and refer them for treatment.[55]

Screening programs abound. One example is the Mini Nutritional Assessment (MNA®), a screening tool used—especially among older adults—to identify persons at increased risk of poor nutrition status. It is composed of 18 items encompassing anthropometry, dietary and clinical assessments, lifestyle, number of medications used, mobility, ability to eat without assistance, chewing and digestive problems, and self-perception of health and nutrition status. Recently, the MNA screening tool was used to measure the nutrition status of a group of older adults participating in government nutrition programs. Researchers reported that the seniors who were enrolled in a congregate dining site and a tai chi class scored better for overall nutrition status than those in the comparison group—suggesting that those who participate in government-sponsored programs may have better nutrition status than those who do not.[56] The MNA tool is included in Chapter 13.

Focus Groups

One method of obtaining information about the target population is to hold **focus group** interviews. Focus groups can be conducted before, during, and after program planning and are helpful for assessing needs, generating information, developing plans, testing new programs and ideas, improving existing programs, and evaluating outcomes. Focus groups usually consist of 5 to 12 people who meet in sessions lasting about one to three hours. The group members are brought together to talk about their concerns, experiences, or beliefs. Focus groups have traditionally been used to obtain advice and insights about new products and services, research qualitative information about key variables used in quantitative studies, and gather opinions about products or creative concepts such as advertising campaigns or program logos.[57]

Focus group An informal group of about 5 to 12 people who are asked to share their concerns, experiences, beliefs, opinions, or problems.

A trained moderator who is skilled at putting people at ease and promoting group interaction leads focus group sessions. Listening is the most important skill used during focus group interviews. Like a good teacher, the focus group leader must be able to listen on several levels, concentrating on what participants say—and do not say—*and* on the progress being made during the interview. A good session leader explores a topic without making participants feel guilty or defensive, avoids asking leading questions, does not interrupt participants when they are talking, pays attention to nonverbal cues such as body language, and keeps participants focused on the session's topic. Asking open-ended questions—for example, "How do you make decisions about buying milk, cheese, and other dairy products?"—allows participants to take any direction they want and to reconstruct particular experiences.[58] The information obtained from focus group interviews is then used to provide direction for the needs assessment or to change a marketing strategy, product, or existing program.[59] Key focus group questions used by researchers to assess perspectives of low-income, urban youth related to corner-store food purchases are listed in **Figure 4-4**.

Focus group interviews provide qualitative information that helps community nutritionists understand food and nutrition-related beliefs, attitudes, and practices among

FIGURE 4-4 Key Focus Group Questions A focus group guide was developed for learning about the corner-store experiences of low-income, urban youth (kindergarten through eighth grade). The results of the focus group were used to guide development of corner-store interventions to promote availability and selection of healthier products. The focus group questions are listed here. **Source:** S. Sherman, G. Grode, T. McCoy, S. S. Vander Veru, A. Wojatnowski, B. A. Sandoval, and G. D. Foster, "Corner Stores: The Perspective of Urban Youth," *Journal of the Academy of Nutrition and Dietetics* 115 (2015); 242–48.

Opening questions
- How often do you shop at corner stores?
- Why do you usually shop at these stores?
- What kind of snacks or drinks do you usually buy there?
- Do you remember what grade you were in when you started buying snacks at the corner stores near here?

Key questions
- Why do you think kids go to some stores and not others?
- What do you like about the stores you and your friends go to?
- Using the information from the answers that you just provided, if you could create your own store, what would it be like?
- Who usually gives you money to buy snacks at the corner stores?
- From the money that you receive, about how much do you spend in a day at the store? So on average, how much do you spend a day at a store, including both morning and afternoon purchases?

Debriefing
- Do you have any additional comments and/or questions?

members of a target population. They are less expensive to conduct than face-to-face interviews, and they help community nutritionists obtain information of a sensitive nature or information that might otherwise be difficult or costly to get.[60] The Johns Hopkins Hospital staff, for example, used focus groups to help them understand why some clients were not complying with cardiovascular health promotion programs to control hypercholesterolemia. Participants were asked questions about health, high blood cholesterol, current diet, food preferences, grocery shopping, and the types of education programs and materials they usually used. The staff learned that clients preferred to be taught by professionals in small groups and liked to hear from individuals who had successfully lowered their blood cholesterol. The focus group interviews helped the assessment team understand why a certain behavior developed; they also suggested ways to address the problem.[61]

Interviews with Key Informants Recall that key informants are people who interact with or whose positions affect the target population and may be able to shed light on factors that shape the target population's behaviors, beliefs, attitudes, lifestyle factors, and so on. Key informants may have worked with or conducted research related to the population's health status, beliefs, or practices and may thus be familiar with its attitudes and opinions. For example, if the target population is obese persons, then interviews with physicians in family practice, internal medicine, and endocrinology will provide information about how this group is managed medically, what advice it is given about weight management, and whether it follows advice received from physicians.[62] If the target population is teenagers with a high risk of HIV/AIDS, then interviews with teenagers who work in peer education programs will provide valuable information about how these high-risk teenagers perceive risky behavior, what they know about preventing and transmitting HIV/AIDS, how susceptible they are to peer pressure, and what their overall health beliefs are.[63]

When arranging interviews with key informants, develop a short list of open-ended questions (i.e., questions that require more than a simple yes-or-no answer); identify a few key informants whose opinions would be most useful to you; contact these informants for permission to interview them; conduct the interview in person, by mail, by e-mail, or by telephone; and summarize the results for other members of the assessment team.[64] It is always appropriate to thank the key informants for their time.

Another way to learn from key informants is to post queries on listservs to learn about the experiences of other professionals who have worked with similar groups or issues. Also, networking with colleagues who have worked in the community to develop, implement, and evaluate programs is a great way to learn about community needs and values. They may also be aware of similar needs assessments done in other cities, states, provinces, or regions. Networking with colleagues can be a great way to identify other potential key informants.

Direct Assessment of Nutrition Status: An Overview of Methods

Another method of determining nutrition needs is to conduct a direct assessment of individuals. Direct assessment methods use dietary, laboratory, anthropometric, and clinical measurements of individuals to identify those with malnutrition or a nutrient deficiency. These methods may be used alone or in combination.

In her comments at the Second International Conference on Dietary Assessment Methods, Elizabeth Helsing, of the World Health Organization Regional Office for Europe, remarked that "we still have a lot to learn from one another in the area of dietary assessment about the slow and arduous process of collecting vast amounts of data, the battle to mold them into some shape, and finally the wrestling of meaning from them."[65] Her comments allude to the challenge of collecting meaningful information about what people eat and why they make the food choices they do.

Dietary methods are used to determine an individual's or population's usual dietary intake and to identify potential dietary inadequacies. Dietary inadequacies represent stage 1 of the nutrient depletion scheme shown in **Table 4-7**. The primary methods of measuring the food consumption of individuals include the 24-hour recall method, the food diary or daily food record, the diet history interview, and the food frequency questionnaire. At the household level, food records and inventory methods are used to estimate food consumption; population dietary intakes are estimated using food balance sheets and market databases (discussed in Chapter 2).[66] The method chosen depends on many factors, some of which are shown in footnote *a* in **Table 4-8**. All have strong and weak points—and advantages and disadvantages. Table 4-8 provides a summary of dietary assessment tools. The trick is to choose the most valid method, given the financial resources and personnel available to collect and analyze the dietary intake information.[67]

TABLE 4-7 General Scheme for the Development of a Nutrient Deficiency

DEPLETION STAGE	METHOD(S) USED TO IDENTIFY
1. Dietary inadequacy	Dietary
2. Decreased level in reserve tissue store	Biochemical
3. Decreased level in body fluids	Biochemical
4. Decreased functional level in tissues	Anthropometric/biochemical
5. Decreased activity in nutrient-dependent enzyme	Biochemical
6. Functional change	Behavioral/psychological
7. Clinical symptoms	Clinical
8. Anatomical sign	Clinical

Source: Reprinted with permission from D. E. Sahn, R. Lockwood, and N. S. Scrimshaw, *Methods for the Evaluation of the Impact of Food and Nutrition Programmes* (Tokyo: United Nations University, 1984).

Fran Galasyn Miller

ENTREPRENEUR IN ACTION

Frances Galasyn Miller, MPH, RD, works for a coastal Northwest Indian tribe. A typical day for her can involve everything from individual nutrition counseling and teaching classes, to planning policy and environmental approaches to improve community health. Fran has led the effort to conduct a community nutrition and physical activity assessment involving data collection, key stakeholder interviews, and focus groups. As a result, the tribe's community health program is now planning environmental and policy interventions to make it easier for community members to eat healthy foods and live active lifestyles, with a long-range goal of reducing the incidence of childhood obesity. Future interventions will be guided by a workgroup comprised of tribal members, with input from health program staff. Find out what she has to say about entrepreneurship online at *www.cengagebrain.com*.

TABLE 4-8 Summary of Methods, Strengths, and Limitations of Selected Dietary Assessment Tools[a]

METHOD	STRENGTHS	LIMITATIONS
Client assessment questionnaire/ historical data form: A preliminary nutrition assessment form usually divided into sections for administrative data, medical history, medication data, psychosocial history, and food patterns	Provides clues to strengths and potential barriers	May seem invasive, may not be culturally sensitive
Food diary/food record/diet record: A written record of the food and beverages consumed by an individual over a period of time, usually three to seven days	Does not depend on memory Provides accurate intake data Provides information about food habits	Requires literacy Requires a motivated client Recording process itself may influence food intake Requires ability to measure/judge portion sizes Time-consuming
24-hour recall:[b] A retrospective dietary assessment method in which an individual is requested to recall all food and beverages consumed in a 24-hour period	Quick Easy to administer No burden for respondent Does not influence usual diet Literacy not required	Relies on memory May not represent usual diet or seasonal variations Requires ability to judge portion sizes Under/overestimation of food intake occurs Interviewer skill may affect outcome
Food frequency questionnaire: A method of analyzing a diet using a standardized form to assess how often foods are consumed (i.e., servings per day/week/month/year)	Furnishes overall picture of diet Not affected by season Useful for screening	Relies on memory Requires ability to judge portion sizes No meal pattern data Food lists often include common foods only
Diet history interview: An in-depth conversational assessment method in which clients are asked to review their normal day's eating pattern. Clients may be led through a series of questions to describe the foods and beverages consumed.	Provides clarification of issues	Relies on memory Requires interview training

[a] When selecting dietary assessment tools, consider: (1) the program objectives, including degree of accuracy needed and type of data needed (food intake, nutrient intake, dietary patterns, and food patterns); (2) study population characteristics (sample size needed, ability of respondents, age, literacy/language skills, willingness to cooperate, and time constraints); (3) financial issues (cost of software and staff for analyzing records, cost of training staff for analysis, cost of intake forms); (4) implementation requirements (time for completing intake forms; ease of completing intake forms; need for support materials such as instructions, scales, measuring cups, etc.; and training and skill of interviewers); and (5) analysis requirements (quality of nutrient database and/or software, training and skills of food coder, and level of quality control).

[b] See Figure 7-4 on page 243 for a description of the *multiple-pass* 24-hour dietary recall, which is designed to limit the extent of underreporting of food intake in national surveys.

Sources: Adapted from J. M. Karkeck, "Improving the use of dietary survey methodology," *Journal of the American Dietetic Association* 87 (1987): 869–71; K. Bauer, D. Liou, and C. Sokolik, *Nutrition Counseling and Education Skill Development*, 2nd ed. (Belmont, CA: Wadsworth/Cengage Learning, 2012), 110.

Diet History Method Bertha Burke, with the Department of Child Hygiene of the Harvard School of Public Health, reported one of the earliest descriptions of diet analysis. In studies of pregnant women and their infants and children conducted during the 1930s, Burke and her colleagues developed a diet history questionnaire to assess usual dietary intake. Their studies showed statistically significant relationships between a mother's diet during pregnancy and the condition of her infant at birth. In addition, there was a correlation between the dietary ratings of the children's diets and objective measures of nutrition status, such as hemoglobin concentration.[68]

The diet history method has the advantage of being easy to administer, although it is time-consuming and requires a trained interviewer. For these reasons, it is not practical for large population studies. A true validation of the diet history method is probably not possible, although the method allows for reasonable confidence in classifying respondents according to some preset dietary criteria (e.g., the Dietary Reference Intakes).[69] When undertaken repeatedly at different times, this method is fairly reliable. It is perhaps best used to provide qualitative, not quantitative, data.

Twenty-Four-Hour Recall Method The 24-hour dietary recall method is one of the most widely used diet assessment methods. It is easy to administer in person or by phone and lends itself to large population studies, mainly because it requires little time from either the respondent or the interviewer. Its appropriateness for assessing the intake of individuals—what is called **validity**, or the ability of the instrument to measure what it is intended to measure—has repeatedly been questioned, however.[70] There are indications that 24-hour recall data are subject to recall bias (i.e., respondents cannot accurately recall the foods they ate during the previous 24-hour period and thus either overestimate or underestimate their dietary intakes). Gender differences in recalling dietary intakes have also been reported. Thus, a single 24-hour recall does not provide an accurate estimate of an individual's usual dietary intake.

The validity of the 24-hour recall can be improved by administering repeated recalls. Seven or eight 24-hour recalls of an individual's dietary intake over a period of two or three weeks are more likely than a single recall to provide a reasonable estimate of that person's usual intake. Even so, 24-hour recall data are best suited to describing the intakes of populations, not individuals.[71] See Figure 7-4 on page 243 for a description of the *multiple-pass* 24-hour dietary recall, which is designed to limit the extent of underreporting of food intake in national surveys.

Diet Record Method Diet records or food records have been considered the "gold standard" of diet assessment methods. Completed over a period of three, four, or seven days, or even as long as a year, they have the advantage of providing detailed information about food products, including brand names and methods of food preparation, and they eliminate the uncertainty that goes with trying to recall the foods eaten. The amount of food consumed can be estimated or calculated by weighing. If the respondents are properly trained, diet records give a reasonably accurate picture of usual dietary intake. However, the diet record method replaces errors in recall with errors in recording, and the possibility always exists that the act of recording food intake changes the actual foods chosen for recording (e.g., choosing meals that are easy to record or not snacking in order to ease the task of recording). Accurate food records can be obtained if the respondents are highly motivated, literate, and well trained.

Food Frequency Method One of the first large-scale uses of the food frequency questionnaire was in the Nurses' Health Study, a study of a cohort of more than 95,000 female registered nurses being followed for the occurrence of coronary heart disease and cancer. A semi-quantitative food frequency questionnaire—sometimes called "Willett's FFQ" after the study's principal investigator, Dr. Walter C. Willett—was developed to categorize individuals by their intake of selected nutrients (e.g., vitamin A, vitamin C, and animal fat). The validity and precision of this instrument were evaluated using four sets of seven-day food records and a one-year diet record.[72]

Other standardized food frequency questionnaires are also available. Most have been tested and used with large groups of people participating in epidemiologic studies, where the use of more labor-intensive instruments such as food records is not practical. A few food frequency questionnaires have been used with varying success among minority populations in the United States.[73]

Validity The accuracy of the diet assessment instrument. Validity reflects the ability of a diet assessment instrument to measure what it is intended to measure; that is, a valid instrument accurately measures an individual's usual or customary dietary intake over a period of time.

The food frequency questionnaire offers several advantages: It is self-administered, requires only about 15 to 30 minutes to complete, and is analyzed at a reasonable cost. Thus it has been used in a variety of population studies where no other instrument could have been administered practically. It suffers, however, from the same limitations as any other recall method, in that the accurate reporting of intake depends on memory. In addition, the food list must necessarily be short and thus may fail to include some foods commonly consumed by the population being surveyed. Controversy over the appropriate uses of the food frequency questionnaire continues.[74]

Other Diet Assessment Methods One innovation in the diet assessment arena is the use of photography to record dietary intake. Photography reportedly has provided more valid and precise results than food records.[75] Today, numerous diet and nutrition apps are available for smartphones and tablets that feature a classic food diary and physical activity tracker.[76] Another method of estimating food intake is the picture-sort approach; in this method, participants sort into categories cards with pictures or drawings of various foods. The method was developed for use with a diverse population of older adults with low education or literacy levels. It can be self- or interviewer-administered. When tested among participants in the Cardiovascular Health Study, the method was an easy and quick way to obtain data on food patterns.[77] **Table 4-9** shows questions for exploring cultural food behavior when completing a dietary assessment.

Laboratory Methods Laboratory methods can be used to identify individuals at risk of a nutrient deficiency (stages 2 to 5 in Table 4-7) because tissue stores of nutrients gradually become depleted over time. The depletion may result in alterations in the level or activity of some nutrient-dependent enzymes or in the levels of metabolic products. Thus laboratory methods are used to detect subclinical deficiencies. Static biochemical tests measure a nutrient in biological tissues or fluids or the urinary excretion rate of the nutrient. Examples of static tests include the platelet concentration of α-tocopherol and urinary 3-hydroxyproline excretion. Functional biochemical tests measure the biological importance of a nutrient and the consequences of the nutrient deficiency. Functional biochemical tests include taste acuity, a measure of zinc status; dark adaptation, a measure of vitamin A status; and capillary fragility, a measure of vitamin C deficiency. Functional tests are generally too invasive and expensive to employ in most field surveys of nutrition status.[78]

Anthropometric Methods Measurements of the body's physical dimensions and composition are used to detect moderate and severe degrees of malnutrition and chronic imbalances in energy and protein intakes. The most common growth indices are measurements of stature (height or length), weight, and circumference of the head. Measurements of skin folds, mid-upper-arm circumference, and waist circumference are used to derive equations that predict muscle and fat mass. The body mass index (BMI) is a commonly used indirect measure of overweight and obesity in adults.[79] Anthropometric measurements are useful in large-scale community assessment programs because they involve simple, safe, noninvasive procedures; require inexpensive and portable equipment; and produce accurate and precise data when obtained by trained personnel. Such measurements are used to estimate an individual's long-term nutrition history. They do not provide data on short-term nutrition status, nor can they provide information about specific nutrient deficiencies.[80]

Clinical Methods Clinical assessment of health status consists of a medical history and a physical examination to detect physical signs and symptoms associated with malnutrition. The medical history includes a description of the individual and his or her living

Questions to aid in understanding of food habits and to assist in completing a dietary assessment:	**TABLE 4-9** Questions to Explore Cultural Food Behavior

Traditional Foods

What traditional foods do you eat?
What is your favorite cultural or traditional food?
How often do you eat traditional foods?
If you do not eat them, why not?

Foods and Health

Are there foods you won't eat? Why?
Can what you eat help cure your sickness? Or make it worse?
Are there foods you eat to keep healthy? To make you strong?
Are there foods you avoid to prevent sickness?
Do you balance eating some foods with other foods?

New Foods

What new foods have you tried since coming to this community?
Do you eat them regularly?
Which foods do you dislike, and why?

Food Acquisition

Where do you get most of your family's food (e.g., neighborhood supermarket, convenience store, open market)?
How do you get to the market? Does anyone go with you? Do they speak English?

Amount and Quality of Food

How do you describe the quality of the food you buy?
Do you have enough food to feed your family each day?
How do you divide up the food among family members if you do not have enough?
Are you able to get the types of foods and beverages needed by everyone in your family?

Food Preparation

Do you have enough time to prepare the kinds of foods your family enjoys?
Do you have the equipment you need for cooking and preparing the kinds of foods your family likes to eat?
Do you have any trouble preparing food?

Family Interaction around Food

Do the children in your family like the foods enjoyed by the adults?
Do your school-age children like the school meals?
Do you have recipes that your family enjoys?

Source: Adapted from D. E. Graves and C. W. Suitor, *Celebrating Diversity: Approaching Families Through Their Food* (Arlington, VA: National Center for Education in Maternal and Child Health, 1998).

situation (e.g., married or single, number of children, and nature of employment). It typically obtains information about existing clinical conditions, previous bouts of illness, presence of congenital conditions, smoking status, existence of food allergies and intolerances, use of medications, and usual levels of physical activity. In the physical examination, the clinician evaluates the major organ systems: skin, muscular and skeletal, cardiovascular, gastrointestinal, and nervous. The hair, face, eyes, lips, tongue, teeth and gums, and nails are also examined for signs associated with malnutrition.[81]

Issues in Data Collection

The choice of method for obtaining information about the target population is influenced by practical, scientific, and cultural considerations. These issues are described in this section.

Practical Issues The choice of assessment method is influenced by practical issues such as the number of staff available to collect and analyze data, the cost of administering the test, and the amount of time needed to identify and interview or sample members of the target population. For example, it may be impractical to use food records to collect data about the food patterns of low-income, immigrant women and their children who live in a city's public housing. This particular population may read English poorly, be uncomfortable with record keeping, and lack transportation to the clinic for training on how to keep food records. An interviewer-administered 24-hour dietary recall is a better choice of diet assessment method with this group.

The assessment method chosen should be simple to administer, take only a few minutes to complete, be inexpensive, and be safe. Blood pressure measurements are ideal screening tests, for example, because they are cheap, quick, need little advance preparation and setup, and are not uncomfortable or unsafe for participants.

Scientific Issues Scientific issues such as the validity and reliability of the assessment method and the nature of dietary variation also influence the choice of assessment method. Key scientific issues to consider when choosing an assessment method are described here.

Sensitivity The proportion of individuals in the sample with the disease or condition who have a positive test for it.

Sensitivity versus Specificity Two issues to consider when choosing an assessment method are sensitivity and specificity. **Sensitivity** is the proportion of subjects with the disease or condition who have a positive test result. A sensitive test rarely misses people with the disease or condition, and it is often used in screening situations in which the purpose of the test is to detect a disease or condition in people who appear to be asymptomatic.[82] For example, a screening test that uses phlebotomy to detect high blood cholesterol concentrations is more sensitive—that is, it is more likely to identify an individual's true blood cholesterol concentration and to yield a positive result in the presence of a high blood cholesterol concentration—than a finger-prick cholesterol test.

Specificity The proportion of individuals in the sample without the disease or condition who have a negative test for it.

Specificity is the proportion of subjects without the disease or condition who have a negative test. Specific tests are used to confirm a diagnosis, and they are important tests to administer when not properly identifying a disease or condition might harm the patient or subject. The oral glucose tolerance test is a highly specific test for diagnosing diabetes mellitus.

Ideally, it is desirable to have an assessment method that is both highly sensitive and highly specific, but this is seldom possible in practice. The trick is to choose a method that correctly classifies subjects into a particular group and misclassifies few of them.

Validity and Reliability Two questions arise when evaluating assessment methods: one concerns the instrument's validity and the other its reliability, or reproducibility. An assessment instrument's validity is its ability to measure what it is intended to measure. Another word for validity is *accuracy*. In the case of a diet assessment tool, a valid instrument accurately measures an individual's usual or customary dietary intake over a period of time—one day, three days, seven days, one month, one year. An instrument's validity can be affected by many factors:[83]

- Characteristics of the respondent—literacy level, education level, conscientiousness in completing the instrument, ability to follow instructions
- Questionnaire design—difficulty of instructions, ease of recording intake, number and types of foods listed, portion sizes given (if any)
- Adequacy of reference data—obtaining a sufficient number of days of intake data to estimate the "true" nutrient intake; completeness of the nutrient database used to calculate nutrient intake
- Accuracy of data input and management—quality control of data processing or coding of food items

Consider the validity of a survey instrument used during a telephone interview or mailed to respondents. One threat to the survey's validity is ambiguous language in the survey questions.[84] Writing a survey question that is easy for respondents to understand *and* that yields the health or nutrition information you want is no simple task. Examine the questions in **Table 4-10.** The first two questions are fairly straightforward. Most consumers know what fruits are, and they can estimate their fruit intake with a reasonable degree of accuracy. Furthermore, consumption of regular soda is fairly simple to estimate. The third question is more difficult to answer. Respondents must know what a fat is and must recognize butter, stick margarine, tub margarine, lard, fatback, bacon fat, and vegetable oils and shortening as fats used in cooking. They must then estimate how frequently they use one or more of these fats in cooking, a complex calculation for most consumers. The fourth question likewise presents a problem. Respondents must decide what the survey question means by mayonnaise and salad dressing. Is the question asking about all such products, be they low-fat, full-fat, or fat-free, or is it asking only about regular, full-fat mayonnaise and salad dressings? This fourth question thus illustrates that some survey instruments used to assess dietary intake are not valid because only full-fat foods are indicated on the survey form, and respondents cannot indicate that they usually consume reduced-fat or low-fat foods. These survey instruments tend to overestimate fat intake.

An individual's true usual diet cannot be known with certainty. It is not possible to follow respondents around all day and night and surreptitiously record every morsel they consume. And the very act of recording food intake can have a subtle influence because the respondents may make choices they might not have made otherwise. (Although people's food and beverage intake can be monitored with precision on a metabolic ward, their dietary intake cannot be considered "usual" under these circumstances.) However, doing everything possible to create and/or use an instrument high in validity ensures that respondents can be placed with great accuracy along a distribution of intake, from low to high consumption.

The second concern is the **reliability** of an assessment instrument—that is, its ability to produce the same estimate of dietary intake, for example, on two separate occasions, assuming that the diet did not change in the interim. (Other words for reliability are

Reliability The repeatability or precision of an assessment instrument.

SURVEY QUESTION	RESPONSE
During the past month, not counting juice, how many times per day, week, or month did you eat fruit? Count fresh, frozen, or canned fruit.	_____ times per _____ day, week, month
During the past 30 days, how often did you drink regular soda or pop that contains sugar? Do not include diet soda or diet pop. You can answer times per day, week, or month (e.g., twice a day, once a week, etc.).	_____ times per _____ day, week, month
How often do you use fat or oil in cooking?	_____ times per _____ day, week, month
How many servings, on average, do you eat of mayonnaise or salad dressing (serving size = 2 tablespoons)?	never or < 1 per month 1–3 per month 1–4 per week 5–7 per week 2 or more per day

TABLE 4-10

Examples of Survey Questions Designed to Obtain Information about Fruit, Soda, and Fat Intake

Sources: The first two questions were taken from the Centers for Disease Control and Prevention's 2013 Behavioral Risk Factor Surveillance System (BRFSS) Questionnaire (Atlanta, Georgia: U.S. Department of Health and Human Services, Centers for Disease Control and Prevention, 2012), 25, 40. The third question was taken from the National Cancer Institute's Health Habits and History questionnaire (Bethesda, MD: National Cancer Institute, 1987), 4. The fourth question was adapted from the University of Minnesota Healthy Worker Project questionnaire (Minneapolis: University of Minnesota, 1987), 3.

precision, repeatability, and *reproducibility.*) This issue is different from validity. It is possible for an instrument to give reproducible results that are also incorrect! An instrument's reliability can be affected by the respondents' ability to estimate their dietary intake reliably, by real dietary changes that occurred between the two assessment periods, and by inaccuracies in the coding of dietary data.

Cultural Issues A cultural assessment of the target population is needed before data collection begins. The cultural assessment is undertaken to identify culturally-specific food practices and health beliefs within the target population's culture. This is especially important if the assessment involves one-on-one interviews with members of the target population conducted in their home. Issues to consider during the cultural assessment are listed in **Table 4-11.** The manner in which strangers greet each other, the types of questions that are appropriate to ask, body language during interviews, and other customs differ among cultures.[85] In Japan, for example, a visitor who crosses her legs and shows the bottom of her shoe is being disrespectful. On the Canadian prairie, it is impolite for a guest to wear street shoes in someone's home. The people of North Africa value hospitality and time-honored rituals of eating, including handwashing, clapping, and eating with one's fingers. Visitors to the home of a North African are prepared to eat, whether they are hungry or not, for to refuse food would be insulting.[86]

Survey questions must also be culturally appropriate. For instance, a questionnaire designed to obtain information about the health attitudes and beliefs of Canadian aboriginal adults of the Mi'kmaq First Nation might have included a question that asked, "Do you worry about your diabetes?" If most aboriginal people responded no to this question, a researcher who was unfamiliar with the belief system and culture of the Mi'kmaq people might have concluded that aboriginal people were apathetic about their health. In fact, the question is culturally inappropriate, for in the traditional Mi'kmaq culture, the word *worry* has no meaning. A native person who gave a negative response to the question

TABLE 4-11 Factors to Consider during a Cultural Assessment[a]

Religion
- **Belief system**—Do this population's religious beliefs affect their food choices, use of alcohol, or other lifestyle decisions?
- **Food rituals**—Are particular foods consumed only during religious events/periods? Are certain foods taboo?

Etiquette and Social Customs
- **Typical greeting**—What is a proper form of address? Is a handshake appropriate? Are shoes worn in the home?
- **Social customs**—Should certain social exchanges occur before the interview or other assessment is undertaken? Are refreshments offered?
- **Direct and indirect communications**—Should a senior household member be expected to answer a question before a junior member does? Are some questions considered taboo by this ethnic population?

Nonverbal Communications
- **Eye contact**—Is eye contact considered polite or rude?
- **Tone of voice**—Does a soft voice have a particular meaning in this culture? A hard voice?
- **Facial expressions**—What do smiles and nods mean?
- **Gestures**—Are certain hand gestures considered rude and offensive? Is it acceptable to cross your legs?
- **Personal space**—Is the realm of personal space wider or narrower than in the North American culture?
- **Touch**—Is touch appropriate? If so, when, where, and by whom?

[a] See also Table 15-11: Communication Styles of Various Cultural Groups in Chapter 15.

Source: Adapted from M. C. Narayan, "Cultural Assessment in Home Healthcare," *Home Healthcare Nurse* 15 (1997): 665.

would probably be saying, "I pay attention to my diabetes, but it is a part of my life. I take it day by day." This meaning is far different from what an uninformed researcher might have concluded.[87] Cultural context is important when survey questionnaires are being designed. (Refer to Chapter 15 to learn more about how culture can affect community nutrition practice.)

Case Study 1: Women and Coronary Heart Disease

In this section, we return to Case Study 1 summarized in Table 4-1 on page 106. We consider this case study as an example of how to tie the assessment's objectives to particular questions about the target population, and then choosing methods for answering them. Table 4-1 specifies the main types of data needed for the two assessments in the city of Jeffers.

Recall that Case Study 1 described an assessment aimed at obtaining information about women and coronary heart disease (CHD). The community consisted of the city of Jeffers and four adjoining municipalities. The target population was women over 18 years of age. In the assessment's community phase, data were collected about community morbidity and mortality associated with CHD; types of educational materials available from non-profit organizations, doctors' offices, and other sources; and existing programs and services designed to reduce CHD risk. The community nutritionist now reviews the assessment's objectives and, for each objective, develops a list of questions about this population's knowledge, attitudes, and practices related to CHD risk. These questions are shown in **Table 4-12**.

There are two things we should consider when we examine this table. First, not all of the data that might be collected about the target population are shown. Some data, particularly demographic data such as age, education level, and income, are collected as a matter of course. These data allow the community nutritionist to compare the findings

TABLE 4-12 Case Study 1: Women and Coronary Heart Disease (CHD)

OBJECTIVE (REFER TO TABLE 4-1)	QUESTION(S) ASKED[a]	TYPES OF DATA (REFER TO FIGURE 4-2)	METHOD OF OBTAINING THE ANSWER
• Assess women's knowledge and awareness of the leading causes of death and CHD risk factors.	1. Do women know that CHD is the leading cause of death among women in the United States?	Knowledge/awareness (cognitions)	Survey, focus groups
	2. Can women identify four major risk factors for CHD?	Knowledge/awareness (cognitions)	Survey
	3. Where do women obtain information about health? About CHD?	Health practices	Survey
• Assess women's practices and attitudes related to CHD risk reduction.	1. Are women eating a heart-healthy diet?	Health practices	24-hour recall
	2. Do women exercise regularly?	Health practices	Survey
	3. Do women smoke? If yes, how many packs/day?	Health practices	Survey
	4. What are women's attitudes and beliefs related to CHD risk reduction? How do they prioritize heart-healthy habits?	Attitudes	Survey, focus groups
• Assess women's use of existing services designed to reduce CHD risk.	1. Which community services related to CHD do women use?	Community conditions	Survey
	2. What aspects of these services are most important to women?	Attitudes	Survey, focus groups

[a] The population in this case study is women over 18 years old living in the fictional city of Jeffers and four adjoining municipalities.

of this assessment with those of other assessments or studies. Decisions about which demographic data to collect are made with the help of a statistician. Second, the questions posed in column 2 of the table are asked about the target population as a whole—in this case, all women over 18 years of age who live in the fictional city of Jeffers and four adjoining municipalities. The answers, however, are obtained from individuals—called the **sample**—who represent the target population. Once again, the advice of a statistician is required to ensure that the individuals who are sampled represent the target population.

In this case study, the community nutritionist has developed a list of questions, each one tied to an objective. She then considers the types of data that might be collected to answer the question (e.g., knowledge, awareness, and health practices) and chooses a method for obtaining them. Her choices include a survey, a 24-hour recall, and focus group discussions. What is the purpose for placing this information in a table? The main purpose is to help organize data collection. She sees, for example, that a survey can be used to obtain answers to eight of the questions. In other words, a single survey instrument or questionnaire can be designed to answer all eight questions. The 24-hour recall method should be a separate tool. This approach is part of the planning process, and it helps streamline data collection.

Next, consider a second case study that focuses on assessing the nutrition status of an older adult population in the fictional city of Jeffers.

Case Study 2: Nutrition Status of Independent Older Adults

The target population for Case Study 2 is people older than 75 years of age who live at home in the city of Jeffers. (Review Table 4-1 on page 106.) The community phase of the assessment obtained information about the types of existing community services aimed at addressing the needs of this group and how many members of the target population used these services. As with the first case study, the community nutritionist is now positioned to collect data about the target population. He first reviews the purpose, goals, and objectives of the assessment and then develops a set of questions aimed at measuring the nutrition status of this target population. These questions are listed in **Table 4-13**.

This needs assessment is more complex, requires a larger data set, and involves more people than the first case study. The nutrition status assessment methods in this case study include measurements of laboratory, clinical, anthropometric, and dietary outcomes, plus measures of functional status and other risk factors for poor nutrition status. More data about the population's use of community services are also needed. Remember, the assessment's purpose is to (1) obtain data about the nutrition status of these independent older adults and (2) link these outcomes with the services described in the community phase of the assessment to determine where services can be improved.

As in the first case study, each group of questions is tied to a specific objective, and the material in the table helps the community nutritionist plan the data collection. How does the community nutritionist make a decision about the assessment method, given the important factors described in this chapter? Several strategies can be used in decision making. First, he might turn to the medical or nutrition literature for information about accepted, standard assessment tests, such as serum retinol for vitamin A status and serum ferritin for iron deficiency. Or he might conduct a search of MEDLINE or other databases for articles that describe studies of the method's validity, reliability, and sensitivity. (Consult the Internet Resources on pages 145–147.) Next, he might speak with colleagues who are working with similar populations to learn about their approach to the assessment of the target group.

Sample A group of individuals whose beliefs, biological characteristics, or other features represent those of a larger population.

TABLE 4-13 Case Study 2: Nutrition Status of Independent Older Adults

OBJECTIVE (REFER TO TABLE 4-1)	QUESTION(S) ASKED[a]	TYPES OF DATA	METHOD OF OBTAINING THE ANSWER
• Assess the nutrition status of independent older adults (> 75 years).	1. Has this population experienced a significant weight loss over time?	Anthropometric data (height, weight)	Scale
	2. Is their weight low or high for their height?	Anthropometric data (height, weight)	Scale
	3. Have they experienced a significant change in skin fold measurement?	Anthropometric data (skin folds)	Calipers
	4. Has this population experienced a significant reduction in serum albumin?	Laboratory data	Phlebotomy
	5. Does this population have nutrition-related disorders (e.g., osteoporosis, arthritis)?	Clinical data	Medical chart
	6. Does this population have an inappropriate food intake?	Dietary data	24-hour recall, focus groups
	7. Does this population use any dietary supplements?	Dietary data	24-hour recall, survey, and focus groups
	8. Does this population use nutrition support?[b]	Dietary data	Survey
	9. What is the functional status[c] of this population?	Clinical data	Survey
	10. What kinds of medications does this population take?	Clinical data	Survey
• Determine which community services are used by this population.	1. How many members of this population use: social services? mental health services? nutrition support services? home health care? home-delivered meals? federal/state assistance programs? housing and home heating assistance programs? other?	Community conditions	Survey
	2. How many members use services provided by dietitians and other health professionals?	Community conditions	Survey

[a] The population about which questions are asked consists of older adults over 75 years old who live at home in the fictional city of Jeffers.

[b] Nutrition support refers to enteral and total parenteral nutrition support.

[c] Functional status refers to the individual's ability to bathe, dress, groom, use the toilet, eat, walk or move about, travel (outside the home), prepare food, and shop for food or other necessities.

He might consider a standard measure of health or nutrition status. These measures, called **nutrition status indicators**, are quantitative measures that serve as guides "to screen, diagnose, and evaluate interventions in individuals."[88] Nutrition status indicators are often used to estimate the magnitude of a nutrition problem, its distribution within the population, its cause, and the effects of programs and policies designed to alleviate the problem. Researchers, program planners, health professionals, and policymakers use them for analyzing problems in health and nutrition.

Because there is no single "best" indicator, several may be used in the nutrition-focused needs assessment. For example, major indicators of poor nutrition status in older U.S. adults include a weight loss of 5% or more of body weight in one month; being underweight or overweight; and having a serum albumin below 3.5 grams per deciliter, an

Nutrition status indicators
A quantitative measure used as a guide to screen, diagnose, and evaluate interventions in individuals.

inappropriate food intake, a midarm muscle circumference below the 10th percentile, and folate deficiency, among others.[89] Several of these nutrition status indicators were used in this case study. Nutrition status indicators exist for vitamin, mineral, and protein status and for energy intake. Screening tools have been developed to assess risk among older adults; recall discussion of the MNA in the discussion of screening on page 123. See also Figure 13-9 in Chapter 13 for questions included in the MNA tool.

After assessing the nutrition status of the target population, services targeted at older adults in the community would need to be identified. Key informant interviews would be helpful in this effort. Local government offices (Departments of Health and/or Departments of Aging) would also be great resources. Table 4-13 indicates means of identifying use of such services. Lastly, the community nutritionist would devise a strategy for assessing attitudes of older adults regarding use of these services. Speaking with members of the target audience to learn about their needs, values, and priorities; use of services; and factors that impact their participation in existing services would be an important part of the assessment.

Basic Principles of Needs Assessment: Analyzing Data and Developing a Plan of Action

Step 4: Analyze and Interpret the Data
The next step in the community needs assessment process is to analyze and examine the data collected about the community and target population. This requires first collating the data collected about the community itself and any background conditions that may have influenced the target population. Then, data collected about the target population are coded, entered into the computer, checked for errors, and analyzed using accepted statistical methods. Working carefully during the data collection process is important and ensures that the assessment's findings will be valid.[90] Once the data are analyzed, a new issue arises: the choice of reference data against which the assessment's outcomes can be compared. For example, if the nutrition status of children whose mothers participate in the WIC program is being investigated, and the nutrition status indicators are height, weight, and hemoglobin, the community nutritionist might choose reference growth data for children published by the U.S. National Center for Health Statistics (NCHS) to evaluate the children's growth and development. The NCHS growth charts for evaluating the physical growth of children are based on a large, nationally representative sample of U.S. children. For evaluating the iron status of children, the community nutritionist might use reference data for hemoglobin from the most recent NHANES survey for children of the same age and sex.[91] The values obtained for the target population during the community needs assessment can be compared against the reference data. In Case Study 2 on page 134 (see also Table 4-13), reference data for evaluating skin fold measurements among the sample of independent older adults could be compared with skin fold standards derived from NHANES.[92]

Nutrient intake data are usually compared with the dietary reference intakes (DRIs). Reference data for comparison purposes can also be obtained from countries where national surveys of dietary intakes have been carried out. In situations in which no reference data for a country exist, the FAO and/or WHO requirements for nutrient intake can be used.[93] Statements drawn from the data collected about the target population and from comparisons with reference data are then organized and merged with the community and background data to form a comprehensive report. In this manner, the final report contains information about the target population and about the community in which it lives and works.

Data derived from the assessment are then used to diagnose the community. Four steps are involved in making the community diagnosis: (1) interpreting the nutrition status of the target population within the community, (2) interpreting the pattern of health care services and programs designed to address the target population's nutrition status, (3) interpreting the relationship between the target population's nutrition status and community characteristics, and (4) summarizing the evidence linking the target population's nutrition status to their community environment. The summary describes the dimensions of the nutrition need to be addressed, including its severity, extent, and frequency; its distribution across the urban, rural, or regional setting and across age groups; its causes; and the mortality and morbidity associated with it. The summary should specify the major strengths of existing community resources and health care services as they relate to the target population's nutrition status, the areas where nutrition problems seem to be concentrated, and the areas where delivery of nutrition services for the target population can be improved.[94] The summary may also indicate how the cost of treating the nutrition need compares with the cost of preventing it and provide information about the social consequences of not intervening in the target population.[95]

The final step is to prepare an executive summary that captures three or four key points that emerged from the assessment. The executive summary can be given to stakeholders and other interested parties who request information about the assessment outcomes. It can also be reformatted as a press release for the media.

Step 5: Share the Findings of the Assessment The results of the community needs assessment are often useful to agencies and organizations that were not directly involved in it. Sharing the assessment results with these other groups and stakeholders is cost-effective, prevents duplication of effort, and promotes cooperation among organizations and agencies. It also enlarges the sphere of awareness about nutrition in the community and increases the likelihood that more than one community group will choose to be involved in addressing nutrition concerns. However, releasing the results of an assessment to the community at large without seeking the support and approval of key stakeholders can create ill will. When in doubt, go back to the stakeholders and ask for permission to release sensitive material about the target population.

Step 6: Set Priorities Setting priorities involves deciding who is to get what at whose expense.[96] When several nutrition concerns are identified by the assessment—as often happens—the question asked by the community nutritionist is "Which health outcome is most important?" The term **health outcome** refers to the effect of an intervention on the health and well-being of an individual or population.[97] This outcome may result in a change in the knowledge, beliefs, attitudes, behaviors, or health status among members of the target audience. The change may be distinct, such as a drop in blood pressure or an increase in fiber intake, or it may be somewhat subjective, such as an increase in awareness of a health risk.[98] In other words, the community nutritionist is asking, "Given the several nutrition needs of the target population, where should my organization direct its efforts to achieve the best health outcome?" In most cases, the best health outcome is an improvement in the nutrition status of the target population. However, changes in knowledge, beliefs, attitudes, and behaviors are often needed to stimulate a change in nutrition status.

The challenge for the community nutritionist is deciding which of several nutrition needs of the target population deserves immediate attention. Considering the fierce competition for scarce resources, how do the community nutritionist, the assessment team, and community leaders decide where to put their efforts and money? No one method exists for ranking problems or needs, although various scoring systems that rank risk

Health outcome The effect of an intervention on the health and well-being of an individual or population.

factors by relative importance have been proposed. A few principles that provide guidance in identifying problems of the highest priority are listed in **Table 4-14**.

The priority-setting process begins with a review of the summary prepared in Step 4 (described previously). To determine where improvements in health services should be made, the findings of the community assessment can be compared with the *Healthy People 2020* topic areas of nutrition and weight status; physical activity; maternal, infant, child, and adolescent health; older adults; or other new and relevant objectives. The seriousness of each nutrition need relative to other nutrition and health concerns within the target population is considered. Members of the assessment team rank existing health and nutrition needs and make recommendations about where the community's resources should be directed. Perhaps only 10% of physician offices include nutrition education and counseling for clients with heart disease or diabetes, whereas the *Healthy People 2020* objective is 23%; or perhaps 67% of teenage girls consume 900 milligrams or less of calcium, whereas the *Healthy People 2020* target is 1,300 milligrams. Key stakeholders or community leaders help determine which needs of the target population deserve immediate attention.

Healthy People 2020 lists some 600 national health objectives that cover 42 topic areas. These can be useful in forming a basis for program design, monitoring, and evaluation. The objectives can also help you convince funders, administrators, and other key personnel that your program is worthwhile.[99] The Community Toolbox can be consulted for guidance on building community coalitions, creating a vision, measuring results, and forging partnerships for improving the health of the community.[100] Likewise, the *Healthy People 2020* Map It Toolkit offers guidance on helping the community translate the *Healthy People 2020* objectives into state-specific action plans.[101]

In a perfect world, ample personnel, money, and other resources would be available to spend on each of the target population's needs. Setting priorities would not be necessary. In reality, however, there are never enough resources to address all public health needs, and the decisions about which issues receive attention are not always rational, right, or fair. The process of setting priorities is influenced by the community's political power base, federal and state public health priorities, public opinion, and the beliefs of key stakeholders. The final decisions about which areas to address generally reflect the community's ranking of the importance of public health needs and its assessment of the probable impact of its interventions.

Step 7: Choose a Plan of Action

The community nutritionist is now ready to make a decision. She or he has on hand the results of the needs assessment and a ranking of the nutrition needs that most deserve attention. Now what? As shown in **Figure 4-5**, there are any number of options, but the most important thing is to do *something* based on the collected data. After all, the assessment required planning, team effort, and precious resources. Its findings are too valuable to ignore.

But what should be done? At the very least, remember that the key findings of the assessment should be shared with community leaders and other people who are interested

TABLE 4-14 Principles Involved in Setting Priorities

- Community priorities, preferences, and concerns should be given priority.
- Higher priority should be given to common problems than to rare ones.
- Higher priority should be given to serious problems than to less serious ones.
- The health problems of mothers and children that can easily be prevented should have a higher priority than those that are more difficult to prevent.
- Higher priority should be given to health problems whose frequencies are increasing over time than to those whose frequencies are declining or remaining static.

Source: Adapted from D. B. Jelliffe and E. F. P. Jelliffe, *Community Nutritional Assessment* (Oxford, UK: Oxford University Press, 1990), 452.

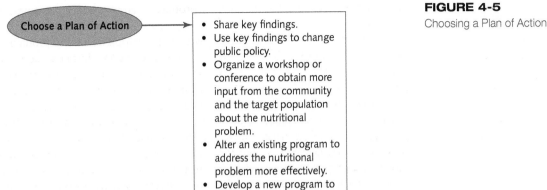

FIGURE 4-5

Choosing a Plan of Action

in the health and well-being of the target population. These people may use the findings within their own organizations to support interventions aimed at improving the target population's health and nutrition status. For example, the results of an assessment of the dietary changes made by pregnant teenagers can be shared with physicians, nurses, and other health care providers who need to know how and why teenagers change their food patterns during pregnancy.

Another action is to use the assessment's findings to advocate for a change in legislation or public policy that will ultimately improve the health potential of the target population. The term **advocacy** means building support for an idea, cause, or change. (Advocacy is discussed in Chapter 6.) Releasing the assessment's findings to the media is one way of increasing awareness of the nutrition need and building support for policy changes that address it.

Advocacy Building support for an idea, cause, or change.

The community nutritionist and other team members may elect to organize a workshop or conference to obtain additional data or pull together community leaders and stakeholders to explore future actions. Or they might decide to alter an existing program by developing new educational materials, enlarging a marketing campaign, or changing the mechanism for delivering the program. They may develop a new program to address the nutrition needs of the target population, in which case they may write a grant proposal to apply for money to pilot-test the new idea. (Grant writing is discussed in Chapter 19.) In reality, the community nutritionist and her or his team will probably take several actions simultaneously. Certainly, one or more actions should be taken to improve the target population's health and nutrition status through program planning and other activities. (The process of planning and evaluating programs is described in Chapter 5 and the process of marketing programs is described in Chapter 17.)

Entrepreneurship in Community Needs Assessment

Recall from Chapter 1 that entrepreneurship is the creation of something of value through the creation of organization.[102] In the case of the community needs assessment, that "something of value" is the snapshot of the nutrition status of the community. Obtaining this valuable commodity, this snapshot, requires organization, vision, and new ideas—all aspects of the entrepreneurial process. Community nutritionists can apply the principles of entrepreneurship to community needs assessment by developing new strategies for collecting information about hard-to-reach populations such as new immigrants and the homeless; by forging new partnerships with food producers, retailers, distributors, and marketers to collect

Christine Carroll

ENTREPRENEUR IN ACTION

Christine Carroll, MPH, RD, works as a wellness educator in both the corporate and community settings through her own business, Inspired Wellness Solutions. With previous positions as a nutrition educator in the Boston school setting and a wellness program coordinator at a transitional homeless shelter, she learned the importance of adequately assessing the health issues of your participants and the barriers to improving those issues. Her advice: Listen to the opinions of your target population, rather than just examining the raw assessment data. By learning as much as possible about your target population, you may discover that the barriers that you think hold people back are very different from those that actually do. Find out what she has to say about entrepreneurship online at *www.cengagebrain.com*.

information about dietary patterns and beliefs at the local level; and by developing new methods of assessing nutrition needs and problems.

The Centers for Disease Control and Prevention's Healthy Communities Program is an example of entrepreneurship in community needs assessment. The program reaches beyond public health and requires the concerted efforts of a wide range of disciplines, such as business, transportation, and city planning, to help improve the health of communities. The Healthy Communities Program provides funding to communities to support local efforts in schools, work sites, communities, and health care settings that address obesity, diabetes, asthma, physical inactivity, poor nutrition, and tobacco use.[103] As a result of the program, communities nationwide are promoting safe routes to school, developing new walking trails, and advocating for healthier school food options. Look at your own community for examples of organizations or people who recognized an opportunity and took the initiative to improve the community's quality of life. For more information about CDC's Healthy Communities Program, go to *www.cdc.gov/healthycommunitiesprogram/*.

PROFESSIONAL **FOCUS**

Getting Where You Want to Go

Imagine for a minute that circumstances require you to travel from Kansas City to Chicago. You might check recommended routes on Google Maps or MapQuest or, spreading a map across your lap, you might plot your own course. You could take an interstate highway all the way, following I-35 north to Des Moines and then turning east toward Chicago on I-80. Or you might take I-70 to St. Louis and turn due north onto I-55, a course that would take you right into the Chicago Loop. Or you might decide to bypass the interstate highways altogether and stick to the so-called blue highways, those tiny threads on the map that snake along from town to town. Your decision about which route to take depends on many factors, including the purpose and urgency of your trip and how much time you can allocate for traveling.

In many respects, deciding what you do in life is much like plotting a journey by car to a distant city. Many choices confront you, and there is always the possibility that circumstances may compel or entice you to change your route along the way. Right now, you might be asking yourself the following

questions: How can I get where I want to go? More important, how do I determine where I want to go in the first place? The answers to these questions are unique to each of you because each of you is unique. As you read through this discussion, write down your thoughts to help clarify your vision.

Square 1: Know Yourself

The first step in determining where you want to go is to know yourself. Hold yourself up to the light (so to speak) so that you can see yourself from every angle. Evaluate both your strong points and the areas marked for improvement. (The "To Be Improved" areas are sometimes called weaknesses. Weaknesses are not personality defects or deficits. They are areas of personal development that you have not had the time or inclination to explore and strengthen.) Consider your personality, your view of the world, and what you want out of life. Do you like working with people? Do you enjoy tinkering with gadgets and gizmos? Do you value public service? Are you an optimist or a cynic? Would you describe yourself as impulsive, dependable, driven, funny, unfocused, inquisitive, task-oriented, theatrical, or lazy? Write down the words that describe all aspects of your personality and character. There are no right or wrong answers.

Square 2: Define Your Dreams

Knowing who you are (and who you are not) will help you move to the next tier: defining your dreams. Your vision of your future lies in your dreams. What do you see yourself doing? To help you define your dreams, answer the following questions:[1]

- What would you most like, ideally, to be?
- What would you most like, ideally, to do?
- What kinds of experiences help you feel complete?
- In what kinds of situations do you most want and tend to share yourself?

Let yourself dream freely and without constraints. Do not be concerned at this point about finances or family obligations. Give your dreams room to grow.

Square 3: Set Goals

Having dreams won't get you very far if you don't add some structure to them. As Henry David Thoreau stated so eloquently, "If you have built castles in the air, your work need not be lost; that is where they should be. Now put the foundations under them."[2] Setting specific goals for your future is one of the most challenging tasks you will undertake. There are many areas in which goal setting is desirable: economic, spiritual, social, physical, mental, emotional, educational, personal, and vocational.

For this exercise, set at least one goal for your personal life. The goal should be achievable but broad enough to accommodate your dreams. Joe D. Batten, author of the book *Tough-Minded Leadership*, wrote his personal goal as follows:

An Example of a Personal Mission Statement*

1. Succeed at home first.
2. Never compromise with honesty.
3. Be sincere yet decisive.
4. Develop one new proficiency a year.
5. Plan tomorrow's work today.
6. Maintain a positive attitude.
7. Keep a sense of humor.
8. Do not fear mistakes—fear only the absence of creative, constructive, and corrective responses to those mistakes.
9. Help subordinates achieve success.
10. Concentrate all abilities and efforts on the task at hand; do not worry about the next job or promotion.

---

*Adapted from S. R. Covey, *The 7 Habits of Highly Effective People* (New York: Simon & Schuster, 1989), 106.

"I will make the lives of others richer by the richness of my own."[3] Your personal goal might be similar or entirely different.

Another way to approach this exercise is to write your personal mission statement. A personal mission statement is much like a nation's constitution; it is a set of principles to live by. In his best-selling book *The 7 Habits of Highly Effective People*, Stephen R. Covey cites the personal mission statement developed by a friend. A portion of it appears at the bottom of this page.

Square 4: Develop an Action Plan

To paraphrase a Chinese proverb, if you don't know where you are going, then any road will take you there. To get where you want to go, you must develop an action plan. Action is the essence of achievement. Stephen Covey calls this "beginning with the end in mind." You must begin your journey with a clear picture of your destination. Use the following steps to develop an action plan for your personal life:

- Develop a picture in your mind's eye of what you want to do with your life. You may see yourself having a family and a career position with a major food company, or helping an isolated community in a developing country improve its standard of living, or starting your own business. The technique of mental imaging enables you to fine-tune your picture so that when opportunities present themselves, you can determine whether they fit your action plan.
- Pretest your mental picture. If your mental picture shows you working with small animals as part of a research project, then find a way to test your decision before you commit yourself to this path. You may discover that you don't like working with rats or hamsters! Pretesting your decisions saves time and allows you to discard opportunities that are not useful or don't fit your action plan.
- Predetermine your alternatives. Have a backup plan to help you maximize your opportunities and forestall any crises. Explore your alternatives by talking to people who have pursued a similar dream.

Learn to Manage Yourself

Shirley Hufstedler, a lawyer who became the secretary of education, remarked, "When I was very young, the things I wanted to do were not permitted by social dictates. I wanted to do a lot of things that girls weren't supposed to do. So I had to figure out ways to do what I wanted to do and still show up in a pinafore for a piano recital, so as not to blow my cover. You could call it manipulation, but I see it as observation and picking one's way around obstacles. If you think of what you want and examine the possibilities, you can usually figure out a way to accomplish it."[4]

Getting where you want to go is nearly impossible if you don't learn to manage yourself—your goals, your time, your work. Aristotle observed that the hardest victory is the victory over self. Successful people have mastered themselves through discipline. For some people, *discipline* is a dirty word, but in truth, discipline means training. Any athlete will attest to the power of training, which builds, molds, and strengthens the body and mind for strong performance. Discipline is as important to life as it is to athletic competition. Without it, little can be accomplished. Acquiring discipline, the mastery of self, is a lifelong process for most of us, and there is no simple pattern by which it can be attained. The process involves developing a vision, setting goals, and following through on an action plan to reach those goals. The first step in acquiring discipline begins at square one: know yourself.

case study

Planning a Needs Assessment Focused on School Children

by Virginia B. Gray, PhD, RD

Scenario

You are the nutrition programming coordinator at the local department of health in a large, urban setting. In 2015, your agency began a needs assessment in one of the high-need neighborhoods within your service area to direct future programming. Local data indicated low consumption of fruits and vegetables among children as a high priority for programming. Your review of national data also indicated that children in the United States are consuming about two-thirds of the *Healthy People 2020* total fruit target and about half of the *Healthy People 2020* total vegetable target, with about 30% of total vegetables consumed being white potatoes (primarily as fried potatoes and potato chips).[1] Furthermore, you conducted focus groups with community leaders and parents in the neighborhood, and found that concern for child health related to eating habits is growing. Many participants expressed desire for a changed food environment and thought increasing consumption of fruits and vegetables would be an excellent programming priority. You also reviewed policies affecting child nutrition, and you learned that recent changes to the National School Lunch Program (NSLP) have increased availability of fruits, vegetables, and whole grains, with a requirement that students select at least one fruit or vegetable as a part of the reimbursable meal.[2] At this point,

you have selected the target population for your program: school children. The remainder of your needs assessment will be focused on collecting data about your target population so you know how to best intervene.

Learning Outcomes

- Link appropriate data collection strategies with the goal and objectives of a needs assessment.
- Develop a plan for collecting data on a selected target population.
- Develop a simple focus group instrument for use among a selected audience.

Foundation: Acquisition of Knowledge and Skills

1. Investigate school strategies for increasing fruit and vegetable intakes. You may consider wellness policies, farm-to-school programming, school nutrition policies, etc.
2. Investigate recent changes to nutrition in schools, such as those brought about by the Healthy, Hunger Free Kids Act of 2010 and by wellness policy requirements. The USDA Food and Nutrition Service (FNS) website provides information on school nutrition policies and programs.

Step 1: *Identify Relevant Information and Uncertainties*

1. Brainstorm about the target population. What are the needs, priorities, and values that might impact food choices? Consider the social–ecological framework for food and physical activity decisions and health (found on page 13).

Step 2: *Interpret Information*

1. The goal of your needs assessment will be to collect data to guide development of a school-based intervention to increase fruit and vegetable intake among children. Objectives to guide the assessment include:
   a. Assess current consumption of fruits and vegetables among children in the local school setting.
   b. Assess policies and practices currently in use to influence fruit and vegetable consumption in the local school setting.
   c. Investigate children's perceptions of fruits and vegetables and factors that motivate their consumption in the local school setting.
   d. Investigate foods that compete with fruits and vegetables for consumption among children and factors that motivate their consumption in the local school setting.
   e. Assess teacher/administrator support for school nutrition policies.
   f. Assess parent support for school nutrition policies.
   g. Investigate effective practices used in previous programs aimed at increasing fruits and vegetables via school interventions.

Make a chart to indicate how you will accomplish each of the objectives listed above. Include the following items in your chart: (1) objectives, (2) question(s) you intend to answer to meet each objective, (3) types of data needed, and (4) method(s) of obtaining the answer.

For example:

1. OBJECTIVE	2. QUESTIONS ASKED	3. TYPES OF DATA	4. METHOD(S) OF OBTAINING THE ANSWER
Objective: Assess teacher/administrator support for school nutrition policies.	1. To what degree do teachers enforce nutrition-related wellness policies in place? 2. To what degree do teachers view themselves as nutrition role models for their students?	Practices/attitudes	Focus group with teachers

Step 3: *Draw and Implement Conclusions*

1. Develop a simple focus group guide to assess teacher/administrator support for school-based nutrition efforts. Consider using the tips provided for writing a focus group guide available at: *http://www.eiu.edu/~ihec/Krueger-FocusGroupInterviews.pdf.*

Step 4: *Engage in Continuous Improvement*

1. Review the *CDC Guide to Strategies to Increase the Consumption of Fruits and Vegetables*[3] available at: *http://www.cdc.gov/obesity/downloads/fandv_2011_web_tag508.pdf.* Identify evidence-based strategies for increasing consumption of fruits and vegetables that may be effective in the school setting.

CHAPTER **SUMMARY** ....

Community Needs Assessment

▶ Community needs assessment is the process of evaluating the health status of a community, determining what the community's health needs are, and identifying places where those needs are not being met. A needs assessment is undertaken to gather information about the social, political, economic, environmental, and personal factors that influence nutrition status in a given community. It involves systematically collecting, analyzing, and making available information about the health status of a particular group—namely, the target population.

Basic Principles of Needs Assessment: Developing a Plan and Collecting Data

▶ **Step 1: Set the parameters of the assessment.** Specify the scope of the community to be assessed. Determine the purpose of the needs assessment. Set goals and objectives for the needs assessment.

▶ **Step 2: Develop a data collection plan.** Review the purpose, goal, and objectives of the needs assessment. Considering the three categories of data (community data, community environment and background factors, and target population data), develop a list of data needs. Choose a method for obtaining each item (using existing data, conducting a literature review, reviewing existing programs, networking with colleagues, and/or collecting data). When developing a plan for collecting data about the target population, it is helpful to write a list of questions you intend to answer in your effort to understand the nutrition needs of your audience and factors that influence their needs.

▶ **Step 3: Collect data.** Collect community data, community environment and background data, and target population data. Both qualitative and quantitative data help describe the community and its values, health problems, and needs.

Methods of Obtaining Data about the Target Population

▶ Methods range from simple surveys and screening tools to interviews with key informants.

▶ A survey is a systematic study of a cross-section of individuals who represent the target population. Surveys can be used to collect qualitative or quantitative data in formal, structured interviews or by phone, by mail, or online (see Table 4-5).

▶ Screening is designed to reverse, retard, or halt the progress of a disease by detecting it as soon as possible.

▶ Focus group interviews provide qualitative information from people who are brought together to talk about their concerns, experiences, or beliefs.

▶ Key informants—the people "in the know" about the community—can also be interviewed to provide information about the target population.

Direct Assessment of Nutrition Status: An Overview of Methods

▶ Direct assessment methods use dietary, laboratory, anthropometric, and clinical measurements to identify people with malnutrition or a nutrient deficiency.

▶ The primary methods of measuring the food consumption of individuals include the 24-hour recall method, the food diary or daily food record, the diet history interview, and the food frequency questionnaire (see Table 4-8).

Issues in Data Collection

▶ The choice of method for obtaining information about the target population is influenced by practical, scientific, and cultural considerations.

▶ An assessment instrument's validity is its ability to measure what it is intended to measure. An instrument's validity can be affected by many factors, such as characteristics of the respondent, questionnaire design, and accuracy of data input and management of data processing.

▶ The reliability of an instrument is its ability to produce the same estimate of dietary intake, for example, on two separate occasions, assuming that the diet did not change in the interim. An instrument's reliability can be affected by the respondents' ability to estimate their dietary intake reliably, by real dietary changes that occurred between two assessment periods, and by inaccuracies in the coding of dietary data.

Basic Principles of Needs Assessment: Analyzing Data and Developing a Plan of Action

▶ **Step 4: Analyze and interpret the data.** Data are used to diagnose the community by (1) interpreting the nutrition status of the target population within the community, (2) interpreting the pattern of health care services and programs designed to address the target population's nutrition status, (3) interpreting the relationship between the target population's nutrition status and community characteristics, and (4) summarizing the evidence linking the target population's nutrition status to their community environment.

▶ **Step 5: Share the findings of the assessment.** Sharing the assessment results with other groups is cost-effective, prevents duplication of effort, promotes cooperation among organizations and agencies, and enlarges the sphere of awareness about nutrition needs in the community.

▶ **Step 6: Set priorities.** Set priorities by asking: Which needs of the target population deserve immediate attention, and where would efforts achieve the best health outcome?

▶ **Step 7: Choose a plan of action.** Plan actions to improve the community's or target population's nutrition status, using methods that are feasible and focus on established health priorities.

Entrepreneurship in Community Needs Assessment

▶ Apply the principles of entrepreneurship to community needs assessment by developing new strategies for collecting information about hard-to-reach populations, by forging new partnerships to collect information about dietary patterns and beliefs at the local level, and by developing new methods of assessing nutrition needs.

SUMMARY **QUESTIONS**

1. Describe the seven steps involved in conducting a community needs assessment.
2. Name the sources of data in the community that you would utilize in a nutrition-focused community needs assessment in order to be able to describe the following:
   a. A community's socioeconomic characteristics
   b. A community's health status
   c. Existing community services and programs
   d. A community's environmental characteristics
   e. Community cultural characteristics
   f. Social norms around food selection
   g. Target population attitudes and values related to food habits
3. As a community nutritionist, what questions would you ask about the design of a survey in order to ensure that it will provide valid and reliable information for your nutrition-focused needs assessment?

4. As a community nutritionist seeking to evaluate the nutrition status of older adults participating in the local congregate meals program, list three nutrition status indicators you might include and the reference data you would use for each indicator.
5. Differentiate between qualitative and quantitative data and list examples of each type of data.
6. Discuss factors to consider during a cultural assessment and why it is beneficial to conduct a cultural assessment prior to beginning data collection for a target population.
7. Compare and contrast the strengths and limitations of three dietary assessment tools.
8. Discuss the principles involved in ranking community nutrition concerns in terms of highest priority for receiving community attention, efforts, and money.

INTERNET **RESOURCES**

Access data on vital statistics, income, unemployment, demographic characteristics, and other variables.

FedStats
http://fedstats.sites.usa.gov
More than 70 agencies provide data for this site. Search the site by keyword or alphabetically by topic.

U.S. Department of Agriculture

Agricultural Research Service (ARS)
www.ars.usda.gov

Community Nutrition Mapping Project
www.ars.usda.gov/Services/docs.htm?docid=15656

Economic Research Service (ERS)
www.ers.usda.gov

Current Population Survey Food Security in the United States
http://www.ers.usda.gov/data-products/food-security-in-the-united-states.aspx

Food Environment Atlas
www.ers.usda.gov/FoodAtlas/

Food Access Research Atlas
www.ers.usda.gov/Data/FoodDesert/

Food and Nutrition Service (FNS)
www.fns.usda.gov/fns/data.htm

National Agricultural Statistics Service
www.nass.usda.gov

State and Local Governments
www.loc.gov/rr/news/stategov/stategov.html
Use this homepage to access information about your state and local governments.

U.S. Bureau of Labor Statistics
www.bls.gov
Provides data on major economic indicators, wages, employment, unemployment, and other statistics.

U.S. Census Bureau
www.census.gov
This site provides national, state, and some city/county statistics. The site can be searched by word, place name, zip code, or map (geographical location). Browse the alphabetical listing of topics. Key features of the site include:

- Census State Data Centers (Click on your state's name to access information.)
- Health statistics
- Household statistics (e.g., American Housing Survey data)
- Household economic statistics
- Disability; Income; Labor force; Occupation; Poverty
- Population topics (e.g., estimates and projections for the nation, states, and households and families)
- State profiles

DataFerrett System
http://dataferrett.census.gov
DataFerrett is a unique data-mining and extraction tool. It allows you to select a data basket full of variables and then develop and customize tables and charts.

Community Health Status Indicators Report
http://wwwn.cdc.gov/communityhealth
Community profiles can be displayed on maps or downloaded in a brochure format.

County Health Rankings
www.countyhealthrankings.org
Provides access to 50 state reports, ranking each county within the 50 states according to its health outcomes.

Food Research and Action Center (FRAC)
www.frac.org
Access FRAC's database of demographic and nutrition assistance program measures to analyze how states are using the key public food and nutrition assistance programs. Users may compare up to three years of data in any state.

Kaiser Family Foundation State Health Facts
http://kff.org/statedata/
Offers individual state health profiles and comparisons of the 50 states.

Kids Count Data Center
http://datacenter.kidscount.org
Profiles the status of children and ranks states on measures of well-being.

MEDLINE
www.nlm.nih.gov
Search MEDLINE and other health databases from this website.

National Health Information Center
www.health.gov/nhic
Provides general information about the availability of educational materials, programs, and referral services.

Centers for Disease Control and Prevention
Chronic Disease Indicators (CDI)
http://www.cdc.gov/cdi
CDI is a set of indicators that allows states and large metropolitan areas to collect chronic disease data that are important to public health and provides links to data resources.

Health Data Interactive
www.cdc.gov/nchs/hdi.htm
Health Data Interactive presents tables with national health statistics for infants, children, adolescents, adults, and older adults. Tables can be customized by age, gender, race/ethnicity, and geographic location.

National Center for Health Statistics
www.cdc.gov/nchs
Check out the new releases, fact sheets, and publications.

Data Warehouse for NCHS public use data
www.cdc.gov/nchs/surveys.htm
Provides links to national survey data about numerous health topics.

Morbidity and Mortality Weekly Report
www.cdc.gov/mmwr
Provides state health statistics and surveillance summaries.

Vital Signs
www.cdc.gov/VitalSigns
CDC offers recent data and calls to action for important public health issues.

WONDER Database
http://wonder.cdc.gov
WONDER provides a single point of access to a wide variety of public health reports and data systems.

National Institute for Occupational Safety and Health
www.cdc.gov/niosh
NIOSH offers data on hundreds of workplace safety and health topics.

University of Michigan's Institute for Social Research
www.src.isr.umich.edu
Research programs include organizational behavior, survey methodology, life course development, social environment and health, urban and environmental studies, and others.

University of North Carolina's Odum Institute for Research in Social Science
www.irss.unc.edu
The Institute maintains one of the country's largest archives of social science data. The archive includes national and international economic, demographic, health, public opinion, and other types of data.

To locate published studies about the target population or diet assessment methods:

Current Bibliographies in Medicine
http://www.nlm.nih.gov/archive/20120907/pubs/resources.html

Risk Factor Monitoring and Methods
http://epi.grants.cancer.gov/rfab

Dietary Survey Questionnaire Validity References
www.nutritionquest.com

Health Literature References
www.nlm.nih.gov/medlineplus

Food Composition Resource List for Professionals
http://ndb.nal.usda.gov

Community Assessment Resources

The Community Toolbox
http://ctb.ku.edu

Community Health Assessment Clearinghouse
www.health.state.ny.us/statistics/chac

Washington State Community Nutrition Education Assessment Project
http://depts.washington.edu/commnutr/home

CHAPTER 5

Program Planning
for Success

LEARNING **OBJECTIVES**

After you have read and studied this chapter, you will be able to:

- Describe six factors that can trigger program planning.
- Describe seven steps in designing, implementing, and evaluating nutrition programs.
- Describe three levels of intervention.
- Discuss three reasons for conducting evaluations of programs.

- Discuss three major principles to consider when preparing an evaluation report.
- Describe the steps of the nutrition care process.

This chapter addresses such issues as needs assessment; program planning, the nutrition care process, and program evaluation; and current information technologies, which are designated by the Accreditation Council for Education in Nutrition and Dietetics (ACEND) as Foundation Knowledge and Learning Outcomes for dietetics education.

CHAPTER **OUTLINE**

Something to think about...

"One should get as many new ideas as possible."

—*ISABEL ARCHER*
in *Henry James's* The Portrait of a Lady

For a complete list of references, please access the MindTap Reader within your MindTap course.

Introduction

In the early 1990s, the state of Arizona foresaw a gap in services. Data obtained from the National Health Interview Survey on Child Health showed that at least two-thirds of children between the ages of one week and five years were placed in childcare. Some of these children had special health care needs. Arizona's own data predicted that by the year 2010, more than 25,000 children would have developmental delays and other special needs in Arizona and that many of these children would participate in childcare programs. The problem was that only limited training in providing quality nutrition services was available for childcare workers.

The Arizona Department of Health Services was determined to find a solution to the problem. It organized a team to develop a course that would make childcare workers more aware of the challenges involved in feeding children with special health care needs.[1] The team was composed of health professionals with expertise in pediatric medicine, occupational therapy, speech therapy, childcare programs, and community nutrition. A parent of a child with special needs was included on the team. The Office of Nutrition Services in the Arizona Department of Health Services obtained funding for the project through a Maternal and Child Health Improvement Project Field Grant and collaborated with the Office of Women's and Children's Health to develop the program.

The community nutritionists assigned to the project had a leadership role in designing and evaluating the course. They reviewed research studies and other technical material related to feeding children with special needs, determined who would use the course materials, assessed the knowledge and skill levels of childcare workers, and determined what types of nutritional problems childcare workers were likely to encounter in daycare and other settings. They evaluated the course and made adjustments in course materials. The end product was Project CHANCE, a course designed and tested by health professionals to meet the training needs of childcare workers.[2]

This chapter presents an overview of program planning—the process of designing a program to meet a nutritional need or fill a gap in services. It describes the factors to consider when designing an intervention: program elements such as goals and objectives, and the levels and types of interventions. It describes the process of program evaluation, explaining why evaluation is important, who conducts the evaluation, how evaluation findings are used, and how to prepare an evaluation report. Topics such as developing the marketing plan, choosing nutrition messages, managing personnel and data, and identifying funding sources are discussed in the chapters of Section Three.

Factors That Trigger Program Planning

The decision to develop a nutrition program or modify an existing program is usually made in response to some precipitating event. Perhaps the community needs assessment revealed that some older adults were not taking advantage of the community's Meals-on-Wheels program or that a large number of children living in an inner-city neighborhood had low intakes of vitamins A and C. In other cases, as shown in **Figure 5-1**, the stimulus for program planning may be a mandate handed down from an organization's national office. For example, when the national office of the American Heart Association (AHA) chose nutrition and physical activity as the organization's national health promotion initiatives for one year, state AHA offices then determined whether their existing programs met the organization's mandate in these areas.

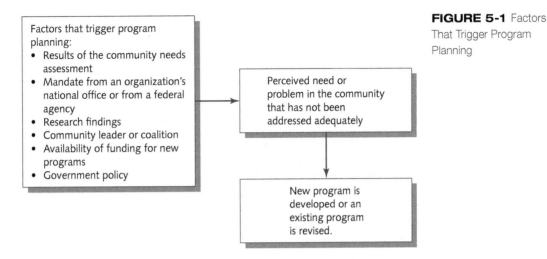

FIGURE 5-1 Factors That Trigger Program Planning

Research findings sometimes trigger the planning process. The report of the National Cholesterol Education Program (NCEP) on the detection, evaluation, and treatment of high blood cholesterol in adults described the findings of major studies that linked high blood cholesterol levels to coronary heart disease (CHD) risk. Two additional NCEP reports described population strategies for reducing total blood cholesterol. These reports led some hospitals and municipal health departments to review their programs for reducing CHD risk within their communities and, in some cases, to develop new programs to promote cardiovascular health.[3] Findings from the Bogalusa Heart Study, an epidemiologic study begun in Louisiana, led to development of the Heart Smart Family Health Promotion program, a school-based program that targeted high-risk elementary school children and their families. The program was designed to involve parents in improving the eating and activity patterns of school children.[4]

The concerns of a well-known community leader or coalition may stimulate program planning, as when a community activist helps state agencies plan innovative approaches to prevent obesity by increasing access to healthy foods through community gardens, farmers' markets, and local grocery stores. Government policy and the availability of new funding can also spur program planning. When the U.S. Department of Agriculture increased its funding for the WIC Farmers' Market Program, the National Commission on Small Farms called for expansion of the program to every state—an action that continues to motivate states where the program has not been implemented to offer the program to eligible mothers and children.[5] Regardless of the impetus, the community nutritionist considers developing a program when there is a nutritional or health problem in the community that has not been resolved adequately.

Steps in Program Planning

The community nutritionist reviews her organization's mission statement before developing or modifying a program. A **mission statement** is a broad declaration of the organization's purpose and a guideline for future decisions. It provides an identity and proclaims, "This is what this organization is all about."[6] The community nutritionist ensures that all programs fulfill her organization's mandate. If the match between the mission statement and the program concept is good, then she has a reasonable level of confidence about gaining senior management's support for it. If the match is not good, it will be difficult to justify the resources, time, and expense of a new program and to secure funding for it.

Mission statement A broad statement or declaration of an organization's purpose or reason for being.

Consider, for example, the First-Rate Spa and Health Resort mentioned in Chapter 1 (see Table 1-7 on page 27). Its mission statement reads, "The First-Rate Spa and Health Resort works to enhance the health and fitness of its members by promoting physical activity, healthy eating, and self-care." The director of health promotion will have difficulty obtaining internal support for a new program whose participants are not spa clients.

The program planning process consists of several steps, as shown in **Figure 5-2**. The first step is to review the results of the community needs assessment. In Step 2, goals and objectives that specify the expected outcomes of the program are defined. Step 3 is to develop a program plan that describes the intervention, the appropriate nutrition messages for the target population, and how the program will be marketed. In Steps 4 and 5, decisions are made about the management system, budgeting, and potential funding sources for program activities. The program is implemented in Step 6 and evaluated in Step 7. Evaluation focuses on program elements such as the nutrition education and marketing materials and the program's effectiveness—in other words, evaluation activities are designed to determine whether the program accomplished what it was designed to accomplish. Finally, after the program's effectiveness has been verified, colleagues, community leaders, and the community at large are notified of its success.

Step 1: Review the Results of the Community Needs Assessment

The community needs assessment provides information about the target population's nutritional problem or need. It is a major impetus for program planning. Consider the needs assessment undertaken by Project MANA, a program that provides emergency food relief to Hispanics, Caucasians, and migrant workers in the Incline Village area of Nevada. Project MANA staff were alerted to a problem with the Thanksgiving basket's food items, which traditionally included turkey, stuffing, and cranberry sauce. Some Spanish-speaking families were not familiar with cranberry sauce and did not know how to cook with it. The outcome of the needs assessment was to change an existing program so that families were offered a choice, the traditional Thanksgiving basket or a new basket containing chicken, salsa, and tortillas.[7]

When the community assessment identifies a gap in services, a new program may be developed to fill the gap. A needs assessment of the food and nutrition situation of low-income Hispanic children living in inner-city Hartford, Connecticut, found that about

FIGURE 5-2 Steps in Program Planning

		Discussed in...
Step 1	Review the results of the community needs assessment.	This chapter
Step 2	Define program goals and objectives.	This chapter
Step 3	Develop a program plan. • Design the intervention. • Design the nutrition education component. • Develop the marketing plan.	This chapter This chapter This chapter and Chapter 16 Chapter 17
Step 4	Develop a management system.	Chapter 18
Step 5	Identify funding sources.	Chapter 19
Step 6	Implement the program.	Chapter 18
Step 7	Evaluate program elements and effectiveness.	This chapter and Chapters 16–18

53% of caregivers did not breastfeed their infants. The assessment report called for the development of culturally sensitive campaigns that promote breastfeeding and inform caregivers about the appropriate times for introducing weaning foods in this population. An education program called Lactancia: Herencia y Orgullo (Breastfeeding: Heritage and Pride), based at the Hispanic Health Council, was designed to increase breastfeeding among low-income Hispanic women.[8]

Some results of the community needs assessments for Case Studies 1 and 2, first described in Chapter 4, are shown in **Tables 5-1** and **5-2**. The tables summarize key findings of the assessments and indicate areas where interventions are needed. (The tables are not meant to be comprehensive, and other information could have been presented.) The results of the needs assessment for Case Study 1 indicate a low level of awareness of CHD risk factors among women and a typical pattern of low activity levels and high intakes of saturated fat—factors that contribute to CHD risk and could serve as points for intervention. The results for Case Study 2 reveal several nutritional problems among the city's older adult population. Note the language and organization of the summaries. They were written for a broad audience, which is likely to include policymakers, community leaders, and the general public. See Table 4-1 on page 106, Table 4-12 on page 133, and Table 4-13 on page 135 to review the needs assessment results and objectives for Case Study 1, on women and coronary heart disease, and Case Study 2, on the nutrition status of older adults living at home.

Step 2: Define Program Goals and Objectives

The next step in the program planning process is to define the program goals and objectives. Goals are broad statements of desired changes or outcomes. They provide a general direction for the program. Objectives are specific, measurable actions to be completed within a specified time frame. An objective has four components: (1) the action or activity

---

TABLE 5-1 Results of the Community Needs Assessment for Case Study 1: Women and Coronary Heart Disease (CHD)

Results of Needs Assessment

The city of Jeffers and its four adjoining municipalities have a population of 612,000. The city's economic base is light manufacturing and service industries. Many residents have moved from traditional ethnic neighborhoods near downtown to the independent "bedroom" communities outside the city.

Jeffers is an ethnically diverse city. A majority (46%) of the population is non-Hispanic white, but there are several major ethnic groups: black (17%), Hispanic (22%), Portuguese (7%), and Asian (6%).

A survey of women aged 18–72 years, conducted at five medical clinics in the major metropolitan area, found that about two-thirds (64%) do not know that CHD is the leading cause of death among women. Three out of four cannot identify two major CHD risk factors. About one-third (32%) of women smoke cigarettes—a figure higher than the state average of 27%.

Although women claim to be eating a healthful diet and exercising regularly, 35% of all women surveyed are obese (BMI $\geq$ 30). This figure is similar to the national average of 35.7%, but higher than the state average of 33%. About 50% of black women and 42% of Hispanic women are obese.

Women's mean intake of saturated fat is 14% of total energy. This intake is above the recommended intake level of < 10% of total energy. (Mean intake of saturated fat reported in the National Health and Nutrition Examination Survey [NHANES] was 12% of total energy.)

Weight management programs and classes are available through private health/fitness clubs and dietitians in private practice. Nearly two-thirds (64%) of women report that they are trying to lose weight, but only 8% of women participate in organized classes and programs.

The local affiliate of the heart association offers some programming for the general public. Brochures describing the leading risk factors for CHD are available at a majority of hospitals and medical clinics. Only 14% of women were aware that some local restaurants feature "heart-smart" meals on their menus.

Women indicate that they want to do more to reduce their CHD risk and improve their health. No current programs are designed specifically to help women reduce their CHD risk.

TABLE 5-2 Results of the Community Needs Assessment for Case Study 2: Nutrition Status of Independent Older Adults (> 75 years)

Results of Needs Assessment

The city of Jeffers has a population of 434,000. This is 71% of the total metropolitan area population (i.e., Jeffers plus its four adjoining municipalities). The number of older adults > 75 years living in the city of Jeffers is 60,760 (14%), an increase of 12% since 2000. More than half (56%) of these older adults are living independently, typically in their own homes or apartments.

The overall nutrition status of the 34,025 independent older adults is fairly good, but several key nutritional problems emerged:

- About 2% of older adults (680), mostly black and Hispanic women, had serum vitamin A concentrations < 20 µg/dL. At these low levels, impairment of immune function and dark adaptation and development of ocular lesions are likely.

- Approximately 20% of white women and 38% of white men had low hemoglobin concentrations. Among non-Hispanic black men, 62% had low hemoglobin levels. (CDC criteria for low hemoglobin are < 13.5 g/dL in men and < 12.0 g/dL in women.)

- One in four older men and one in five older women had serum LDL-cholesterol concentrations ≥ 160 mg/dL.

- About two-thirds (64%) of independent older adults had hypertension.

- More than half (56%) reported using laxatives for the relief of constipation.

- About 12% of independent older adults reported having difficulty performing two or more personal care activities (e.g., bathing, dressing, using the toilet, getting into and out of a bed or chair, eating).

Fewer than one in five (18%) use community-based services such as personal care services, homemaker services, and adult daycare.

The numbers of independent older adults living in Jeffers who participate in federal assistance programs are shown below:

Program	Number (%) of Participants
SNAP[a]	3,240 (32%)
Social Security	8,912 (88%)
Medicare/Medicaid	7,190 (71%)
Supplemental Security Income	1,215 (12%)
Veterans Benefits	810 (8%)

Delivery of health care and nutritional services has traditionally occurred through the state Department of Social Services.

[a] SNAP = Supplemental Nutrition Assistance Program (previously known as the Food Stamp Program).

to be undertaken, (2) the target population, (3) an indication of how success will be measured or evaluated, and (4) the time frame in which the objective will be met.

Develop objectives by first asking yourself the following questions:[9]

- **WHAT** are we going to do?
- **WHY** is it important for us to accomplish this activity?
- **WHO** is going to be responsible for the activities?
- **WHEN** do we want this to be completed?
- **HOW** are we going to do these activities?

Once you have answered the questions listed above, define your objectives to move those ideas into action. SMART objectives are specific, measureable, achievable, relevant, and set within a time frame.

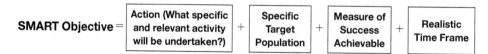

SMART Objective = Action (What specific and relevant activity will be undertaken?) + Specific Target Population + Measure of Success Achievable + Realistic Time Frame

Table 5-3 lists questions to guide you through the steps needed to translate objectives into SMART ones. There are three types of objectives:[10]

▶ **Outcome objectives**—These are measurable changes in a health or nutritional outcome, such as an increase in knowledge of folate-rich food sources, a decrease in total blood cholesterol concentration, an increase in serum ferritin concentration, or a change in functional status. An outcome objective might state, "By the year 2020, increase calcium intakes so that at least 75% of females aged 9 to 19 years consume recommended calcium intakes" or "By 2020, reduce iron deficiency to less than 5% among low-income children

TABLE 5-3 Developing SMART Objectives

SPECIFIC	MEASURABLE	ACHIEVABLE	RELEVANT	TIME FRAME
What exactly are we going to do? Who will be involved?	How will we know that change has occurred?	Can the objective be achieved in the proposed time frame?	Will the data or information collected be relevant to the goals?	When will this objective be accomplished?
What strategies will we use? Is the outcome specified?	Are we able to gather these measurements?	Can we achieve this objective with the resources available?	Will this objective lead to the desired results?	What is the stated deadline?
Is the objective clear and described with strong action verbs?				

THE CHART BELOW CAN GUIDE YOU THROUGH THE STEPS NEEDED TO DEFINE SMART OBJECTIVES.

List your goal: Provide healthy nutrition and physical activity environments in schools to increase the percentage of adolescents who are at a healthy weight in my home state.

Key components for one of the possible outcome objectives:[a]

Specific—What is the specific task or activity to be undertaken; who is the target population?	Increase consumption of fruits and vegetables by high school students by improving food choices in school cafeterias and vending machines Target = high school students in my home state
Measurable—What are the standards or parameters to measure or evaluate success?	Yes (e.g., baseline data available from CDC Chronic Disease Indicators: 20% of hometown state's youth consumed the recommended servings of fruits and vegetables daily in 2013; *www.cdc.gov/cdi*)
Achievable—Is the task realistic? Are sufficient resources available?	• Yes; nutrition education to be closely linked with school foodservice so that children are able to make healthy food choices in a timely manner • Grant money available for state department of public health's new Move More and Eat More Fruits and Vegetables campaign for schools and families • School wellness policies are available for implementation • 25% of schools have a Farm-to-School Program in place in the state
Relevant—Is it relevant to the goal of the group?	Yes—Increasing fruit and vegetable consumption may decrease consumption of higher calorie, less nutritious foods and thus decrease total energy intake and help adolescents achieve and/or maintain a healthy weight
Time frame—What are the start and end dates?	Beginning and end of 2016–2017 academic year

Write your SMART objective: By July 2016, increase the proportion of adolescents in my home state consuming a minimum of five servings of fruits and vegetables per day from 20% of students to 30% of students.

---

[a] Additional outcome objectives and process objectives are needed to achieve the stated goal.

Source: Adapted from Centers for Disease Control and Prevention, Office for State, Tribal, Local and Territorial Support, Communities of Practice Program, Resource Kit, May 2011.

CASE STUDY 1: WOMEN AND CHD RISK

Goals	Outcome Objectives
Reduce death from CHD among women	1. Decrease the number of CHD deaths among women to a rate of no more than 115 per 100,000 within five years. 2. Decrease the number of women who smoke by 33% within two years. 3. Decrease the mean saturated fat intake of women by 3% (from their current intake of 14% of total energy) within one year.
Increase women's awareness of CHD	1. Within one year, increase by 50% the number of women who can specify CHD as the leading cause of death in the city of Jeffers. 2. Increase the number of women who can specify two major CHD risk factors by 25% within one year.

under 2 years."[11] When writing outcome objectives, choose action verbs such as *achieve, choose, decrease, increase, maintain, identify, list,* and so on.

▶ **Process objectives**—These are measurable activities carried out by the community nutritionist and other team members in implementing the program. They specify the manner in which the outcome objectives will be achieved. A process objective might state, "Each community nutritionist will conduct two nutrition lectures per week over the course of the three-month program." When writing process objectives, choose action verbs such as *advise, assess, build, conduct, counsel, demonstrate, develop, instruct, screen, train,* and so on.

▶ **Structure objectives**—Structure objectives help achieve the process objectives. These are measurable activities surrounding the budget, staffing patterns, management systems, use of the organization's resources, and coordination of program activities. A structure objective might read, "On the last day of each month for the next 12 months, each community nutritionist will submit an itemized statement of expenses related to conducting the program."

The community nutritionists who participated in Case Study 1 developed two broad goals and several outcome objectives (see the box above) for a program designed to help women in the city of Jeffers reduce their CHD risk. See also Chapter 16 for more about writing goals and objectives for educational lessons.

These goals and objectives are the framework on which the program elements such as the type of intervention, the nutrition messages, and the marketing campaign are built. The goals and outcome objectives are the basis for determining whether the program was effective—that is, whether the program was successful in raising women's awareness of CHD risk factors and in reducing death from CHD among women.[12]

Step 3: Develop a Program Plan

The first step in designing an intervention is to review the program's goals and objectives, which specify the program outcomes. At this point in the design process, your overall goal is to have a rough outline of what the intervention might look like. The details will come later.

Using the goals and objectives as a guide, the community nutritionist develops a program plan, which consists of a description of the proposed intervention, the nutrition

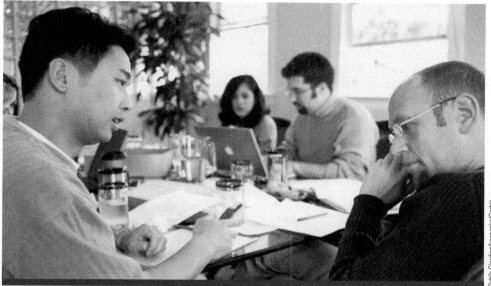

Program planning is best done in teams composed of people with different skill sets, ideas, opinions, and perspectives. The more extensive the program planning, the greater the chance that the program will succeed.

Patrik Giardino/keepsake/Corbis

education component, and the marketing plan. Other factors may also be described in the program plan: the number of clients expected to use the program; the staff, equipment, and material resources required to administer the program; the facilities available for staff offices and teaching rooms; and the level of staff training required prior to implementing the program. The community nutritionist plans how the program will work after asking many questions: What criteria determine a client's eligibility for the program? What federal, state, and/or local regulations must be considered in administering the program? What educational materials are needed to convey important nutrition messages? What provisions should be made for follow-up? Who will be responsible for implementing the program and assessing its effectiveness? How much money is required to administer the program? Well-designed programs are scrutinized before being made available to the target population.

The program plan is usually developed after reviewing existing programs and talking to colleagues and other professionals who have worked with similar programs or with the target population. One easy way to network with colleagues and stay informed about new programs and services is to join one or more listservs. Listservs are types of electronic discussion groups to which people subscribe, much like a magazine or newspaper.[13] They are convenient, electronic bulletin or message boards for exchanging ideas and information. Some popular listservs for community nutritionists are given in the list of Internet Resources on page 190.

Design the Intervention
Remember, the intervention or **intervention strategy** is the approach for achieving the program's goals and objectives. It addresses the question of *how* the program will be implemented to meet the target population's nutritional need. The intervention strategy can be directed toward one or more target groups: individuals, communities, and/or systems. Systems are the large, integrated environments in which all of us live and work. Targeting a system for intervention usually involves changing a public, corporate, or school policy, although it can include reorganizing a department to improve the manner in which a program is delivered.

Intervention strategy
An approach for achieving a program's goals and objectives.

The intervention strategy can also encompass one or more levels of intervention. That is, it can be designed to (1) build awareness, (2) change lifestyles, and/or (3) create a supportive environment.[14] At any one level, interventions may target individuals in small groups such as families, schools, worksites, and health clinics; people in social networks such as churches and bridge clubs; entire organizations; or the community at large, which can be a city, province, state, or nation. Level I interventions focus on increasing awareness of a health or nutritional topic or problem. Awareness programs can be very successful in helping change attitudes and beliefs and increasing knowledge of risk factors, but they seldom result in actual behavior changes. Level II interventions are designed to help participants make lifestyle changes such as quitting smoking, being physically active, eating more fruits and vegetables and less saturated fat, and managing stress. These interventions can be successful when they call for small changes over time and when they use a combination of behavior modification and education. Level III interventions work toward creating environments that support the behavior changes made by individuals. Thus, a company's policy to promote heart-healthy and high-fiber foods in the company cafeteria makes it easier for employees who are trying to lose weight or lower their blood cholesterol concentration to make healthy food choices at work.

An intervention may be as simple as providing a brochure describing the benefits of breastfeeding to clinic clients or distributing a fact sheet listing the fat content of snack foods to grocery store shoppers. An intervention may be fairly complex, such as a mass media campaign that targets health writers across the nation or adolescents with low calcium intakes. Some interventions are full-service programs, complete with training manual, lesson plans, reproducible handouts, videos, and interactive websites.

Examples of intervention strategies are shown in **Table 5-4**. Intervention activities that increase awareness among individuals include health fairs, screenings, flyers, posters, table tents, newsletters, and Internet sites. Special events, websites, radio advertising, and television public service announcements promote awareness across the entire community. An example of a special event that increased awareness about heart disease risk among women is the Mother/Daughter Walk sponsored by the Heart and Stroke Foundation of

TABLE 5-4 Examples of Intervention Strategies

TARGET GROUP	LEVEL OF INTERVENTION		
	Level I: Build Awareness	Level II: Change Lifestyles	Level III: Create a Supportive Environment
Individuals	• Health fairs • Health screenings • Flyers, posters, table tents, brochures • Internet websites • Special events	• One-on-one counseling • Small-group sessions	• Worksite cafeteria programs • Peer leadership
Communities	• Media announcements • Internet websites • Special events	• Fitness programs in schools • Health promotion programs for city employees	• Municipal policy that supports farmers' markets • Point-of-purchase labeling • Tax incentives for companies with health promotion programs
Systems	• Health claims on food labels • Restaurant menu labeling • Legislation	• Company incentives for employees to join local fitness clubs • Formation of a community-based wellness committee	• Medicare coverage of medical nutrition therapy • School policy that restricts access to candy and soft drink machines • Legislation

Manitoba. Food labeling is an example of a system intervention that can increase awareness. When the Food and Drug Administration authorized a health claim for folate on food product and dietary supplement labels, it recognized the ability of product labels to inform women of childbearing age about the relationship between adequate folate intake and reduced risk of neural-tube defects.

Level II interventions reach individuals through one-on-one counseling and small-group meetings. These interventions usually involve a formal program of assessing the individual's current attitudes, beliefs, and behaviors; setting goals for behavior change; developing the skills needed to change behavior; providing support for change; and evaluating progress. Examples of Level II interventions for communities are fitness programs in primary and secondary schools and health promotion programs for all city employees—activities that cut across broad sectors of the community. System interventions at this level include company incentives for employees to join local fitness clubs and the formation of a wellness committee composed of community and business leaders.

Examples of Level III interventions that target individuals include worksite health promotion and cafeteria programs. Identifying peer leaders who can model behavior change and talk about how they changed their lifestyles is another way of creating a supportive environment. In the community at large, supportive environments are created through policies that encourage local farmers' markets, "point-of-purchase" labeling, and tax incentives for companies with health promotion programs. At the system level, supportive environments occur as a result of Medicare coverage for medical nutrition therapy, when school policy restricts access to candy and soft drink machines, and when eligibility requirements for food assistance programs are broadened.

Design the Nutrition Education Component

This section describes the development of a nutrition education plan for the Heartworks for Women Program to Reduce CHD Risk: Case Study 1, a health promotion activity designed to help women reduce their CHD risk. Consider the following activities related to developing a nutrition education plan as you read this section:

- Assess needs.
- Set goals and objectives.
- Specify the format.
- Develop a lesson plan.
- Specify nutrition messages.
- Choose program identifiers.
- Develop a marketing plan.
- Specify partnerships.
- Conduct evaluation research.

The senior manager responsible for developing, implementing, and evaluating the intervention for reducing CHD risk among women (Case Study 1) reviews the proposed intervention levels and activities outlined in **Table 5-5**. The senior manager's goal is to develop a coordinated plan for carrying out the intervention and evaluating its effectiveness. She begins by reviewing the proposed intervention activities and the expertise and time commitments of her staff. She decides to organize intervention activities into two areas: smoking, which she assigns to team 1, and nutrition, which she assigns to team 2. Team 1 members have expertise in health promotion, medicine, and epidemiology; team 2 consists mainly of community nutritionists and a health educator. The margin list on this page shows how the manager divided the intervention activities. The manager expects the teams to collaborate on some activities, such as developing content for the website, and

Case Study 1: Assignment of Responsibility for Carrying Out Intervention Activities
• • • • • • • • • • • • •

TEAM 1 (Smoking)

Individuals:
- Smoking cessation course
- Smoking reduction course

Community:
- Special media events
- Public service announcements
- Antismoking campaigns in schools/worksites

Systems:
- Legislative activities

TEAM 2 (Nutrition)

Individuals:
- "Heartworks for Women" course
- Smoking reduction course

Community:
- Special media events

Systems:
- Legislative activities

TABLE 5-5 Case Study 1: Intervention Strategies for a Program Designed to Reduce Coronary Heart Disease Risk among Women

	LEVEL OF INTERVENTION		
TARGET GROUP	**Level I Intervention: Build Awareness**	**Level II Intervention: Change Lifestyles**	**Level III Intervention: Create a Supportive Environment**
Individuals	• Internet site • Posters, brochures	• "Heartworks for Women" course • Smoking cessation course • Smoking reduction course	
Communities	• Special media events • Public service announcements • Antismoking campaigns in schools/worksites		• Seek legislation prohibiting smoking in public venues
Systems			• Seek legislation prohibiting tobacco-related advertising at sporting events

to take leadership on others.[15] Some activities, such as creating education materials (e.g., flyers and brochures) will be developed by each team for its respective programs. The senior manager designates a leader for each team.

The community nutritionist assigned to lead team 2 is given responsibility for developing the nutrition component of three intervention activities: the Heartworks for Women program, the nutrition content of the website, and the smoking reduction program. Her team will work with team 1 to develop the smoking reduction program, which will probably include messages and activities in the areas of nutrition and physical activity. The teams will work together to secure antismoking legislation. The team leader maps a strategy for the activities she's been assigned, breaking each major activity into smaller ones. For the Heartworks for Women program, for example, she indicates that goals and objectives must be developed, a format chosen, nutrition messages specified, and evaluation research conducted. Next, she reviews the interests, skills, and current assignments of her staff and assigns a staff member to take responsibility for each of the major activities. The sections on page 162 describe how the Heartworks for Women program was developed.

▶ THINK LIKE A COMMUNITY NUTRITIONIST

Connecting program objectives with appropriate activities is an important program planning skill. Consider the following tips for linking objectives with activities (strategies for accomplishing objectives):

- Think of the three levels of intervention when linking objectives and activities. Ask yourself if each objective is intended to build awareness, change lifestyles, or create a supportive environment. Then refer to Table 5-4 for examples of activities at each level of intervention.
- Another way to test the fit between your objectives and activities is to develop an evaluation plan. Identifying a means of assessing each objective is an important part of program planning, and will help you to design activities that foster the accomplishment of each objective.
- Consider steps along the way toward accomplishing a behavior change. These steps may include changes in knowledge, attitudes, motivation, self-efficacy, and skills (preceding a change in behavior). Including objectives and strategies aimed at these intermediate outcomes can be helpful in fostering behavior change (see examples on the next page in the "Type of Change" columns).

In the first chart below, you will find examples of well-coordinated objectives and activities related to the goal "build skills related to heart-healthy cooking and eating." Note that this goal and objectives intend to build skills and change behaviors, and the activities align with skill building and behavior change. In addition, knowledge and motivational changes are included in the objectives.

OBJECTIVE	TYPE OF CHANGE	ACTIVITY FOR MEETING OBJECTIVE
At least 75% of Heartworks for Women participants will be able to use food labels to identify foods that are low in saturated and *trans* fats.	Skill change	Nutrition education class and grocery store tour focusing on label reading
At least 75% of Heartworks for Women participants will be able to identify at least three sources of heart-healthy fats.	Knowledge change	Nutrition education class focusing on fats and oils
At least 75% of Heartworks for Women participants will be able to plan and prepare a meal that includes a fruit, vegetable, whole grain, lean protein, low-fat dairy, and healthy oil.	Skill change	Nutrition education and cooking class focusing on heart-healthy meal planning and preparation
Heartworks for Women participants will be able to write a daily goal and develop a plan for accomplishing the goal related to heart-healthy eating.	Motivational change	Motivational activity related to goal setting and self-monitoring, as a part of the nutrition education and cooking class.

Well-Coordinated Objectives and Activities to Meet the Goal "Build Skills Related to Heart-Healthy Cooking and Eating"

In this next chart, you will find objectives and activities related to the goal "improve consumption of fruits and vegetables among school children." The italicized activities in this chart, however, are poorly linked with the objectives. Review the chart, and then suggest appropriate activities for fostering accomplishment of each listed objective.

OBJECTIVE	TYPE OF CHANGE	ACTIVITY FOR MEETING OBJECTIVE
At least 50% of school children in Anytown School District will be able to list at least three benefits of consuming fruits and vegetables.	Knowledge change	*Pricing incentive to increase accessibility of fruits and vegetables.*
At least 50% of school children in Anytown School District will be able to list at least one strategy for increasing motivation to eat fruits and vegetables.	Motivational change	*Legislation to improve access to fruits and vegetables*
At least 50% of school children in Anytown School District will be able to list at least one positive outcome they expect to experience by eating more fruits and vegetables.	Attitude change	*Legislation to improve access to fruits and vegetables*
At least 50% of school children in Anytown School District will be able to plan a meal that includes at least one fruit and one vegetable.	Skill change	*Health fair that focuses on benefits of fruit and vegetable consumption*
Increase by 25% the number of school children participating in the school lunch program in Anytown School District who consume at least ½ cup of fruits and vegetables at lunch time.	Ultimate outcome	*Health fair that focuses on benefits of fruit and vegetable consumption*

* Activities are poorly coordinated with listed objectives.

Poorly Coordinated Objectives and Activities Related to the Goal "Improve Consumption of Fruits and Vegetables among School Children"

Heartworks for Women Program: Assessing Participants' Needs

The community nutritionist responsible for developing the Heartworks for Women program first identifies the target population's educational needs. She asks these questions: What learning style is best suited for the potential program participants? What kinds of instructional tools (e.g., DVDs or printed handouts) will have the greatest impact with this group? Can Internet activities be incorporated into lesson plans? Will participants be comfortable in group settings? Should some individual nutrition counseling be provided? Where should group sessions be taught? The answers to these questions can be found by reviewing the data obtained during the community needs assessment and by conducting formative evaluation research. For instance, focus groups can be organized to gather information not obtained previously from members of the target population.[16] Focus group participants might be asked about suitable locations for group activities, whether they have access to the Internet, and what they would like to learn about diet and CHD risk. See Chapter 4 for more about focus groups.

Set Goals and Objectives

The next step is to develop goals and objectives for the Heartworks for Women program. Recall that the program is a Level II intervention, which means that it is a skills-building program. It will be designed to address three of the outcome measures specified on page 156: (1) decrease women's mean saturated fat intake to 11% from their current intake of 14% of total energy within one year, (2) increase the percent of women who can specify CHD as the leading cause of death in the city of Jeffers by 50% within one year, and (3) increase the percent of women who can specify two major CHD risk factors by 25% within one year. The Heartworks for Women program is not the only means of achieving these objectives; some Level I activities are designed to address these objectives at the individual and community levels. See Chapter 16 for more about nutrition education.

After reviewing the larger goals and objectives (described earlier in this chapter), the community nutritionist determines that the Heartworks for Women program has two goals: (1) to educate individuals about the contributions of diet to CHD risk and (2) to build skills related to heart-healthy cooking and eating. Specific objectives are as follows:

- Increase awareness of the relationship of diet to CHD risk so that by the end of the course, the percentage of participants who can name two dietary factors that raise total blood cholesterol will increase to 75% from 25%.
- Increase knowledge of dietary sources of saturated and *trans* fat so that by the end of the course, the percentage of participants who can name three major sources of dietary fat that contribute to heart disease will increase to 75% from 30%.
- Increase knowledge of heart-healthy cooking methods so that by the end of the course, the percentage of participants who can describe and use five heart-healthy cooking methods will increase to 75% from 60%.
- Increase label-reading skills so that by the end of the course, the percentage of participants who can specify accurately the fat content of foods using the nutrition information provided on food labels will increase to 75% from 20%.

Using these objectives as a guide, the community nutritionist sketches a rough outline of the program sessions, as shown in **Table 5-6**. The outline shows the link between the program objectives and the individual sessions. Session 1, for example, will provide general information about the major CHD risk factors and the contribution of diet to CHD risk. In this manner, the community nutritionist can be certain that any information that must be imparted to participants to meet the program objectives has been included in the program outline.

PROGRAM OBJECTIVE	PROPOSED SESSION TO MEET OBJECTIVE	
Increase awareness of the relationship of diet to CHD risk so that by the end of the course, 75% of participants can name two dietary factors that increase total blood cholesterol.	• Introduction to course	**TABLE 5-6** Case Study 1: Rough Outline Showing the Link between the Objectives and Proposed Sessions for the Heartworks for Women Program
Increase knowledge of dietary sources of saturated and *trans* fats as well as more healthy fats so that by the end of the course, 75% of participants can name three major sources of dietary fat that contribute to heart disease.	• Major food sources of various types of fats • Low-fat meats and meat alternatives • Low-fat dairy products and soy products • Shopping for heart-healthy fats	
Increase knowledge of heart-healthy cooking methods so that by the end of the course, 75% of participants can describe and use five heart-healthy cooking methods.	• Low-fat meats and meat alternatives • Low-fat dairy products and soy products • Fruits and vegetables • Reading restaurant menus	
Increase label-reading skills so that by the end of the course, 75% of participants can accurately specify the saturated fat and *trans* fat content of foods using the nutrition information provided on food labels.	• How to read food labels • Shopping for heart-healthy foods	

Specify the Program Format Program formats vary, depending on what the program is intended to accomplish and what resources are available to implement it. Choosing a format is much like choosing an intervention strategy: Begin with the big brushstrokes. The format might consist of only three didactic lectures, or it might require six lectures and two cooking demonstrations, or it might involve three individual counseling sessions and 10 group sessions. The community nutritionist chooses a format that suits the topic and the amount of information that must be presented. She anticipates making some changes to the program format after analyzing the results of evaluation research and estimating projected program costs.

The results of the community needs assessment and focus group sessions showed that most potential participants for the Heartworks for Women program have at least a high school education. Many have participated in group classes (e.g., weight management classes). About 75% of those surveyed in focus groups have access to the Internet. The community nutritionist considers these and other factors when choosing a format. She decides on an eight-week program designed to fulfill the goals and objectives outlined previously. The program will consist of 90-minute sessions in which participants will have an opportunity to set target dietary goals, try new behaviors, and assess their success. The key strategy will be to seek small behavioral changes. The participants' skill level at entry and readiness to learn will be evaluated at the beginning of the program. The sessions are organized as follows:

Session 1: Getting Started
Session 2: Looking for Fat in All the Right Places
Session 3: Choosing Heart-Healthy Protein Foods
Session 4: Dairy Goes Low-Fat
Session 5: Focus on Fruits and Vegetables
Session 6: Reading Food Labels
Session 7: Grocery Shopping Made Easy
Session 8: Reading Restaurant Menus

When choosing a format, the community nutritionist considers many details related to implementing the program. If the format calls for individual counseling, the facility must have private rooms for this activity. Likewise, if the format calls for small-group sessions, there should be conference rooms or classrooms for teaching groups. If cooking demonstrations are included in the format, the facility should have counters, sinks, electrical outlets, and other equipment. Her decision about the final program format is influenced by the availability of facilities, equipment, and staff. Lesson plans for the first two sessions of the Heartworks for Women program are described in Chapter 16—see Table 16-7.

Choose Program Identifiers The community nutritionist and her teammates choose program identifiers such as the program name, a logo, an action figure, or a **tag line**. Tag lines are short, simple messages that convey a key theme of the program. They are typically used in promotional materials such as flyers and brochures. The tag line "Good Food for Good Health" might appear on departmental stationery, along with the program name and logo. These elements give the program its own identity and foster a sense of ownership among participants. The program name is important. It is usually selected after consultation with colleagues and members of the target population.

Develop a Marketing Plan "If you don't exist in the media, for all practical purposes you don't exist," National Public Radio's Daniel Schorr once remarked.[17] The community nutritionist develops a marketing plan to promote the Heartworks for Women program to the target population. Details about this plan are presented in Chapter 17, and the marketing strategy for the Heartworks for Women program is shown in Figure 17-6.

Specify Partnerships Forming partnerships with grocery stores, local farmers, retail establishments, government agencies, nonprofit organizations, and other groups is one way of controlling the cost and increasing the reach of programs.[18]

Consider creative ways to build partnerships with:

- Businesses
- Cooperative extension offices
- Fitness and recreational facilities
- Food and pharmaceutical companies
- Hospitals, HMOs, and health departments
- Food and nutrition assistance programs
- Nonprofit and civic organizations
- Parent, church, and community groups
- Schools and universities

The community nutritionist with the Heartworks for Women program established a partnership with a local grocery store chain that enabled her to use one of its stores as the setting for one session on shopping for heart-healthy foods and reading labels. (The benefits to the store are obvious.) She also networked with a national food company and the local affiliate of the American Heart Association to obtain complimentary nutrition education materials for the course.

Step 4: Develop a Management System

In this context, the term *management* refers to two types of structures needed to implement the program: personnel and data systems. The personnel structure consists of the employees responsible for overseeing the program and determining whether it meets its

Tag line A simple, short message that conveys a key intervention message and is used on promotional materials.

objectives. The structure of the data management system is the manner in which data about clients, their use of the program, and the outcome measures are recorded and analyzed.

An important part of program planning is calculating the management costs of the program. Both direct costs (such as the salaries and wages of program personnel, materials needed, travel expenses, and equipment) and indirect costs (such as office space rental, utilities, and janitorial services) must be determined to identify the true cost of a program.

Step 5: Identify Funding Sources

Community nutritionists in nonprofit organizations and government agencies face many challenges in securing funding for all aspects of a program. Money may be available in the current year's budget for staff time to develop the program's format, choose nutrition education messages, and plan a marketing campaign, but there may not be enough money to print educational materials or to allocate personnel to pretest a survey instrument. Information about the projected budget for a program is presented in Chapter 18. The search for extramural funding is the subject of Chapter 19.

At this point in the program planning process, the community nutritionist reviews the program elements (e.g., educational materials and marketing campaign) and considers whether outside funding in the form of cash grants or in-kind contributions from partners can be found. He or she identifies the area where financial support is needed, reviews possible funding sources, and prepares and submits a grant application for funding. The grant-writing process requires the community nutritionist to be clear about the purpose of the funding request, demonstrate a specific need, and explain how the funds will be used to enhance the program's effectiveness. Chapter 19 provides details for the grant-writing and grant-management processes.

The Logic Model: A Framework for Planning, Implementing, and Evaluating Programs
The logic model[19] provides a framework for planning, implementing, managing, and evaluating community nutrition programs.[20] It can be very useful for grant proposal writers because, like a road map, it graphically shows where you are and what you'll need to get to where you want to be. In addition, some grant sponsors now require proposals to include a planning model like the logic model. This chapter's Programs in Action feature illustrates the use of a logic model. See also the Programs in Action feature in Chapter 13.

As you can see in **Figure 5-3**, the main components of the logic model are situation, inputs, activities, outputs, outcomes, and influential factors (assumptions and external factors).[21] The *situation* describes the current state of affairs, including needs and available assets. For most programs, needs outweigh assets; hence, needs need to be narrowed to identify those that are most pressing (i.e., *priorities*). *Inputs* are the resources that are invested to achieve the desired outputs and outcomes. These resources include the time and expertise of project personnel (staff, volunteers, partners), money, materials, equipment, technology, and space for conducting the program (e.g., office and classroom space). *Outputs* are the activities performed (e.g., classes, events, services) and products developed (e.g., fact sheets, television commercials, websites, podcasts) to address the priorities and reach the target audience. *Outcomes* are the ultimate goal. They describe the changes that occur in the target audience or broader community and help answer the question, "What difference is the program making?" Short-term outcomes focus on the target audience learning, including their awareness, knowledge, attitudes, beliefs, and motivations. Medium-term outcomes

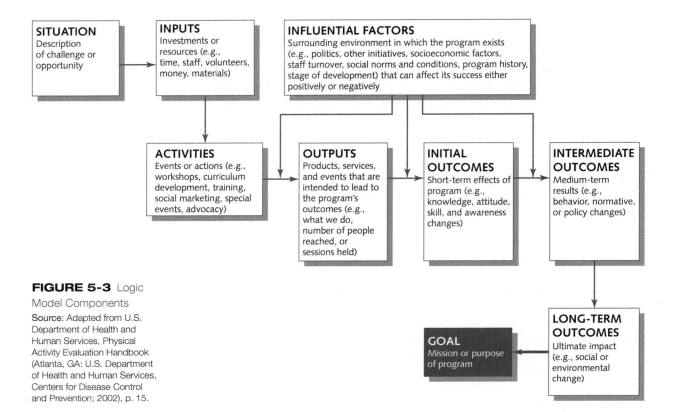

FIGURE 5-3 Logic
Model Components
Source: Adapted from U.S.
Department of Health and
Human Services, Physical
Activity Evaluation Handbook
(Atlanta, GA: U.S. Department
of Health and Human Services,
Centers for Disease Control
and Prevention; 2002), p. 15.

are action oriented and include behaviors, decisions, and policies. Long-term outcomes are social, economic, civic, environmental, and regulatory or legislative changes. *Assumptions* are the beliefs we have about inputs and outputs. For instance, assumptions include our thoughts regarding the target audience and how they will learn and change, how the program will work, likely program outcomes and benefits, the allocation of program resources, and the effect external environmental factors will have on program success. *External factors* are environmental conditions that interact with and influence the program's outcomes. External factors include media, economic and political circumstances, and participants' demographics (e.g., occupation, educational level, cultural/racial background).

After a proposal is funded, the logic model will help you stay on track and achieve the goals that were proposed. By regularly updating the project's logic model and sharing it with project personnel, everyone will know how the project is progressing and see the importance of their role in achieving its goals. To develop your skills, try completing the logic model in Figure 19-15 in Chapter 19. Also, visit *www.uwex.edu/ces/pdande* to learn more about this planning model.

Step 6: Implement the Program

Implementation The set
of activities directed toward
putting a program into effect.

After the program has been designed and tested, it is ready for **implementation**. This is the action phase of the program planning process. Implementation is "the set of activities directed toward putting a program into effect."[22] The format of the program has been finalized, educational materials developed, the marketing plan prepared, and staff trained. Now it is time to put the program into operation—to link the program goals with the plan of action.

The goal of this phase of the planning process is to deliver as faithfully as possible the program laid out in the nutrition education plan. Implementing the program as conceived is challenging, and glitches in program delivery are inevitable. Perhaps no one on the team thought about modifying handouts for Portuguese-speaking clients who participate in the program, or no one was aware of cultural barriers to teenage girls' participation in an inner city's after-school fitness program. Perhaps an ingredient or cooking utensil was omitted from the list of materials needed for a cooking demonstration, no projection screen was available at the facility, or a program flyer featured the wrong time for the session. Anything can happen. The key to successful implementation is to observe all aspects of program delivery and consider ways in which delivery can be improved.

Make a record of any unexpected problems so that you can devise a strategy for preventing them in future programs. Once the program is underway, the community nutritionist and her team work to keep it running smoothly. Two questions arise during this phase: How can program participation be increased? And how can the program be improved?

Enhancing Program Participation Let's state the obvious: The higher the level of participation in a program, the better. High participation increases the likelihood that a program will be effective and that people will be involved with it long enough to make a behavior change. But what is participation? And how do program planners maximize participation in their programs? **Participation** is the number of people who take part in a health promotion activity. If the health promotion activity is a group education program, participation consists of the number of people involved at the end of each educational session. If the activity is a newsletter, participation is the number of people who receive the newsletter times the number of newsletter editions per year. Participation rates vary, depending on how new the activity is and whether an incentive for participating is offered. For group education sessions offered on a voluntary basis and without incentives, the participation rate may range from 5–35% of the target population. A newsletter may have a much higher participation rate of 85–95%.[23]

> **Participation** The number of people who take part in a health promotion activity.

What can be done to improve participation rates? First, understand the target population and their needs and interests. Second, use evaluation research to improve the program design. Make the activity enjoyable and relevant to the target population's needs. Remove barriers to participation. Remember, people participate in health promotion activities for different reasons: to have fun, be with friends or family, learn something new, be challenged, fulfill a goal, or seek support. Find ways to help them see the immediate benefits of participating. Make it easy for people to sign up for or attend the activity. Schedule the activity at a convenient time. Third, use incentives for participating. Incentives range from formal recognition for achieving goals to raffle prizes and treats such as T-shirts, magnets, and cookbooks. Fourth, build "ownership" of the program among participants by using slogans, action figures, and logos to enhance the program's identity. Finally, promote, promote, promote—in other words, make the program highly visible for the target population.

Step 7: Evaluate Program Elements and Effectiveness

Evaluation is the use of scientific methods to judge and improve the planning, monitoring, effectiveness, and efficiency of health, nutrition, and other human service programs. The purpose of program evaluation is to gather information for making decisions about redistributing resources, changing program delivery, or continuing a program.[24] It takes the guesswork out of planning and implementing programs and occurs throughout the program planning process. Some Internet Resources that are useful for the program evaluation process are included in the list on page 190. The next sections describe the purposes and uses of evaluations.

> **Evaluation** The measurable determination of the value or degree of success in achieving specific objectives.

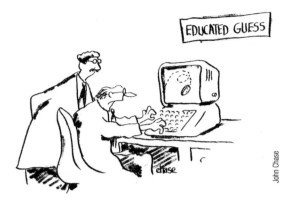

John Chase

Why Evaluation Is Necessary Although the immediate purpose of program evaluation is to help managers make decisions about the short- and long-term operation of their programs, evaluations also serve to inform the community at large about a program's success or failure. When a community-based nutrition program succeeds, nutritionists in other locations across the country want to know how the lessons can be used in their communities. Likewise, when a program fails, community nutritionists want to examine its flaws and figure out how to avoid them in the future.

However beautiful the strategy, you should occasionally look at the results.

—Winston Churchill

Program evaluations force community nutritionists to determine whether they are progressing toward their initial goals and whether these goals are still appropriate. Evaluations may be used for administrative purposes: to determine whether some elements of a program should be changed, to identify ways in which interventions can be improved, to pinpoint weaknesses in program content, to meet certain accountability requirements of the funding agency or senior management, to ensure that program resources (such as supplies, equipment, personnel, and facilities) are being used properly, or to conduct a cost–benefit analysis. They may be undertaken to test innovative approaches to a nutrition or public health problem, to fulfill policy or planning purposes, or to support the advocacy of one program over another. Finally, evaluations may be undertaken to determine whether objectives have been met or whether priorities need to be changed.[25] The finding that a program is not accomplishing its objectives signals a need to consider whether the program is worthwhile or whether its goals can be accomplished in some other fashion.[26] Consult **Table 5-7** for a list of reasons for undertaking evaluations.[27]

How Evaluation Findings Are Used Evaluation findings have many uses. Sometimes they are used to influence an executive or politician who has the authority to distribute resources and shape public policy. For example, in preparing its position on medical nutrition therapy, the Academy of Nutrition and Dietetics reviewed the literature on the economic benefits of nutrition services in acute, outpatient, home, long-term, and preventive care and in the care of pregnant women, infants, children, and older adults. Its evaluation of the impact of nutrition services led to the development of a platform on the benefits of nutrition services in health care. The platform was used in the Academy's

Evaluation to Improve Your Program

- To improve methods of placing clients in various activity programs
- To measure the effect of your program or the extent of client progress in your program
- To assess the adequacy of program goals
- To identify weaknesses in the program content
- To measure staff effectiveness
- To identify effective instructional, leadership, or facilitation techniques
- To measure the effectiveness of resources (such as materials, supplies, equipment, or facilities)

Evaluation to Justify Your Program or to Show Accountability

- To justify the budget or expenditures
- To show the need for increased funds
- To justify staff, resources, facilities, etc.
- To justify program goals and procedures
- To account for program practices
- To compare program outcomes against program standards

Evaluation to Document Your Program in General

- To record client attendance and progress
- To document the nature of client involvement and interaction
- To record data on clients who drop out and those who complete the program
- To document the major program accomplishments
- To list program weaknesses expressed by staff or others
- To list leader/therapist functions and activities
- To describe the context or atmosphere of the treatment setting
- To file supportive statements and testimonies about the program

TABLE 5-7 Reasons for Undertaking Evaluations

Source: A. D. Grotelueschen and coauthors, *An Evaluation Planner* (Urbana: Office for the Study of Continuing Professional Education, University of Illinois at Urbana–Champaign, 1974). Permission to reprint granted by Arden D. Grotelueschen.

grassroots lobbying campaign to inform members of Congress and state legislatures about the value of medical nutrition therapy.[28] Chapter 6 describes the complexities of the legislative process and lists opportunities for influencing public policy at the grassroots level (see Table 6-3 on page 205).

Evaluation findings alert managers and policymakers to the need for expanding or refining programs. For instance, in the United States, the Food Research and Action Center (FRAC) conducts an annual evaluation of the efforts of each state and the District of Columbia to provide nutritious summer meals to children of low-income families. Evidence of a decline in participation in any state is a signal that this state should develop innovative ways of increasing children's participation in the program.

Generally, evaluation findings are used at two levels. Of course, they are applied to an immediate problem and hence are used by managers and program staff who are focused on that problem. But they are also used to shape policies and services beyond the scope of the original problem. In other words, evaluations have many different audiences, some of whom may be directly involved in the program, whereas others are not involved at all or may be concerned with the program at some future date.

Who Conducts the Evaluation?

Evaluations may be carried out by program staff, other agency staff, or outside consultants. The evaluator may be intimately familiar with all aspects of a program because he or she manages or is involved with it, or the evaluator may have a limited knowledge of the program. Regardless, the evaluator is responsible for all aspects of the evaluation, from negotiating the evaluation focus to collecting data and preparing the final report. Because evaluations often occur in a politically charged atmosphere in which program stakeholders fret about the evaluation's outcome and its ramifications, the evaluator must be sensitive to this environment. In the final analysis, the evaluator must be able to recognize what has to be done and must remain objective about the evaluation and its findings.[29]

The Program Evaluation Process The purpose and scope of an evaluation depend on the questions being asked about the program. An evaluation may focus on one particular program element—for example, determining whether screening every client for high blood cholesterol concentration is cost-effective or whether a significant portion of the target population is aware of the nutrition messages appearing in posters placed in city buses. Or the evaluation may be comprehensive and examine the design of the program, how it is delivered, and whether it is being used properly. Evaluation occurs across all areas of program planning, from design to implementation, and no one method is always most effective for carrying out an evaluation. Rather, each evaluation must be tailored to the organization or department in which it is conducted.

When evaluating their programs, community nutritionists begin by asking the following questions:[30]

- Did the intervention reach the target population?
- For which participants was the program most effective?
- For which participants was the program least effective?
- Was the intervention implemented according to the original program plan?
- Was the program effective—that is, did it accomplish what it was supposed to accomplish?
- How much does the program cost?
- What are the program's costs relative to its effectiveness and benefits?

The answers to these and other questions help the community nutritionist design a better, more effective program and formulate recommendations for colleagues and community leaders. Recommendations can be made about the suitability of program goals and objectives, whether the objectives should be changed, whether the program can be applied successfully in another setting or among a different group of participants, and how the program should be changed to improve delivery.[31]

Evaluation as a Planning Tool Evaluation is fundamental to every step of community assessment and program planning. Recall from Chapter 4 that the community needs assessment itself is an evaluation of a population's health or nutrition status. It is designed to find answers to questions about who in the community has a nutritional problem, how the problem developed, what programs and services exist to address the problem, and what can be done to alleviate the problem. The evaluation tools of the community needs assessment are the health risk appraisal, focus group discussions, screenings, surveys, interviews, and direct assessments of nutrition status, as we saw in Chapter 4. During program planning, evaluation occurs at every step. In the design stage, managers develop goals and objectives for the program to determine its impact and effectiveness.

They conduct formative evaluation to achieve a good fit between the program and the target population's needs, to develop appropriate nutrition messages for the target population (Chapter 16), and to design a marketing plan for the program's target market (Chapter 17). In this section, we describe evaluations that occur during the implementation of the program and when the program is completed. Managers use evaluation findings to plan changes in programs, interventions, and staff activities.

Formative Evaluation Evaluation occurs right from the beginning of the design phase. It is often necessary and prudent to pilot-test certain design elements during the development phase. This process, called **formative evaluation**, helps pinpoint and eliminate any kinks in the proposed delivery system or intervention before the program is implemented fully. Formative evaluation can be used to assess educational materials in terms of the appropriateness of language used, accuracy and completeness of the contents, and readability.[32]

Formative evaluation The process of testing and assessing certain elements of a program before it is implemented fully.

For example, program planners in an inner-city district of Philadelphia found that most pregnant women don't consider breastfeeding their newborns and that those who do breastfeed do so for only a few weeks. They decided to conduct a formative evaluation before settling on the final intervention design. They surveyed potential program clients about their family's support for breastfeeding. The planners learned that few new mothers had a close female relative living nearby who could help explain how to breastfeed an infant and that many new mothers in the younger age groups had boyfriends or husbands who had negative attitudes about breastfeeding. The results of this formative evaluation led the planners to add two pieces to the program intervention: (1) the provision of an experienced mother to befriend the new mother prior to the infant's birth and (2) sessions with husbands and boyfriends to help change their attitudes about breastfeeding.

Process Evaluation Monitoring how a program operates helps managers answer questions and make decisions about what services to provide, how to provide them, and for whom. This **process evaluation** involves examining program activities in terms of (1) the age, sex, race, occupation, or other demographic variables of the target population; (2) the program's organization, funding, and staffing; and (3) its location and timing.[33] Process evaluation focuses on program *activities* rather than on outcomes.

Process evaluation A measure of program activities or efforts—that is, of how a program is implemented.

Process evaluation is gaining recognition as a tool to help managers make good decisions. Through process evaluation, managers can systematically exclude various explanations that may arise for a given outcome. If the program appears to have had no effect, process evaluation can determine which, if any, of the following problems was the reason:[34]

- The program was not properly implemented (in other words, program staff were not fully effective in implementing the program).
- The program could not be implemented properly in some participants (which suggests that compliance with the program protocol was a problem for some participants).
- Some participants had difficulty accessing the program.

Alternatively, if the program has had a beneficial effect, process evaluation can determine whether that effect was due, in fact, to the program or to one of the following:

- The greater receptivity of some participants or target groups compared with others
- Competing interventions

Process evaluation focuses on how a program is delivered. In the course of conducting a process evaluation, the evaluator examines the target population to determine how individuals were attracted to the program and to what extent they participated. In addition, the program is evaluated for bias in terms of how participants were served—that is, whether the target group received too much or too little coverage by the program. Such information can be obtained by examining the records kept on program participants and by conducting surveys of the target population and the program participants. The participant records should reveal which services were used and how often. Surveys help define the characteristics of clients who used the program, compared with those who dropped out or refused to use the program.

Process evaluation deals with activities that are planned to occur. In Case Study 1, an intervention strategy was designed to increase women's awareness of CHD risk factors and to reduce their deaths from CHD. Several process objectives were developed, including the following three:

- Provide the eight sessions of the Heartworks for Women program over a 12-week period at each participating worksite.
- Administer a CHD risk factor knowledge test to each participant at the beginning and end of the program.
- Obtain an estimate of usual saturated fat intake using a 24-hour dietary recall completed by each participant at the beginning and end of the program.

We might examine the third process objective listed above—to obtain an estimate of usual saturated fat intake using a 24-hour dietary recall of all participants at the beginning and end of the program—and consider how the planned activity compared with the actual results. If 66 employees entered the program and 24-hour recalls were obtained on 57 of them as planned, we can calculate the percentage of activities attained, using the following formula:

$$\frac{\text{Actual activities}}{\text{Planned activities}} \times 100 = \text{Percentage of activities attained}$$

$$\frac{57}{66} \times 100 = 86.4\%$$

Thus 86.4% of the planned 24-hour recalls were actually obtained during the specified time period. A number of questions arise immediately: Why weren't recalls obtained from all participants? Was there a problem scheduling employees to see the dietitian and, if so, why? Were the instructions to participants unclear? The information obtained through process evaluation signals the program manager that additional planning is required to improve the program's delivery.

Another example of process evaluation comes from the Child and Adolescent Trial for Cardiovascular Health (CATCH), an intervention that targeted the school environment, staff, students, and students' families in four centers located in California, Louisiana, Minnesota, and Texas. CATCH was designed to assess the effectiveness of school foodservice programs, physical education, classroom instruction, and family activities to reduce CHD risk in elementary school children. Process evaluation was used to assess the level of standardization of teacher instruction, the number of CATCH classroom activities completed out of the total number expected for each school session, the number of promotional activities sponsored by the foodservice operation, and the number of support visits made by CATCH staff to schools over the course of the year. Process evaluation determined that the fourth-grade classes had the lowest rate of completion of classroom activities, whereas third-grade classes had the highest rate of completion. The number of cafeteria promotional events ranged from about 6 to 14, and the number of support visits by CATCH staff ranged from 2.5 to 19.7. The overall findings of the process evaluation provided information that helped intervention planners improve the intervention.[35] See the Programs in Action feature in Chapter 8 for more about the CATCH program.

Impact evaluation The purpose of **impact evaluation** is to determine whether and to what extent a program or an intervention accomplished its stated goals. It describes the specific effect of program activities on the target population. In the Heartworks for Women program, the skills-building intervention in Case Study 1, the impact of the program

Impact evaluation The process of determining whether the program's methods and activities resulted in the desired immediate changes in the client.

would be the knowledge about CHD risk, and about major sources of saturated and *trans* fats, acquired by women who participated in the program. The impact evaluation would assess whether women had learned the key risk factors for heart disease and whether they could describe the types of fats in the diet, among other things. In the CATCH intervention, described previously, one unexpected finding of impact evaluation was that students in classes where teachers modified the CATCH sessions to suit their needs learned more about diet, health, and heart disease than students in classes headed by teachers who did not modify their sessions. Perhaps these teachers were more motivated, confident, and creative and had better communication skills than teachers who made no changes in the lesson plans. The finding led the intervention planners to consider changing the model on which the intervention was based.[36]

Impact evaluation focuses on immediate indicators of a program's success. Depending on the program's goals and objectives, it might examine variables such as beliefs, attitudes, decision-making skills, self-esteem, self-efficacy, and knowledge.[37]

Outcome Evaluation The purpose of **outcome evaluation** (also referred to as summative evaluation) is to determine whether the program or intervention had an effect on the target population's health status, food intake, morbidity, mortality, or other outcomes. Outcome evaluations are a challenging managerial activity, for they require technical skills in survey design and analysis. The problems associated with outcome evaluations arise from the difficulty of determining whether a particular effect was "caused" by the intervention and was not due to some extraneous factor. It is possible that factors beyond the control of the program staff influenced the outcome significantly. Such confounding factors might include secular trends within the community, the occurrence of unexpected events such as a natural catastrophe, or certain characteristics of clients (such as their tending to "self-select" for the program).[38]

Case Study 1 included a skills-building program, the Heartworks for Women program, and nutrition messages directed at women in the community at large. Did the intervention strategy accomplish its goals and objectives? The intervention manager plans outcome evaluations that target the three time frames (one, two, and five years) specified in the objectives. (Refer to the program objectives described on page 156.) The first evaluation will be undertaken 12 months after the startup of the intervention and program. Data will be collected from women who enrolled in the Heartworks for Women program and from women in the broader community. The purpose of the evaluation will be to determine whether the nutrition and smoking messages delivered through the intervention resulted in a behavior change in the target population. In other words, did women who participated in the Heartworks for Women program reduce their intake of saturated fat by 3%? Did the number of women who smoke decrease by 33%? The findings of the outcome evaluation will be used to modify the intervention strategy, nutrition messages, marketing plan, and other program elements.

Outcome evaluation, like impact evaluation, is tied to the program's goals and objectives. It is designed to account for a program's accomplishments and long-term effectiveness in terms of a health change in the target population. Outcome evaluation measures are associated with factors relevant to the particular program. Such measures can include serum ferritin levels, percent body fat, calcium intake, stroke prevalence, blood pressure, and use of home food services, depending on the nature of the program.

Structure Evaluation Here, structure consists of personnel and environmental factors related to program delivery, such as the training of personnel; the adequacy of the facility; the use of equipment such as laptop computers, overhead projectors, and skin-fold calipers; and the storage of participant records.[39] In preparing a **structure evaluation** of the Heartworks for Women program in Case Study 1, the senior manager specifies several structure objectives, three of which follow.

Outcome evaluation The process of measuring a program's effectiveness in changing one or more aspects of nutrition or health status.

Structure evaluation The process of determining adequacy of the internal processes and resources needed to deliver a program, including personnel (staff training) and environmental factors (supply of instructional materials, adequacy of facility and equipment).

- The 12-month operating budget for the program is $274,500.
- Monthly operating budgets for the next 12 months will not show a variance exceeding 0.02% of the total operating budget.
- In-house educational materials will be used at a monthly rate that does not exceed 10% of the total stored supply.

These and other structure objectives provide targets that regulate the resources needed to deliver the program. The third objective, for example, helps staff members plan for the use of educational materials. It guides session instructors in monitoring their use of the materials, and it helps the staff member who coordinates the supply and storage area maintain an adequate supply of materials for the program. The manager uses the findings from structure evaluation to make changes in the internal processes that support the staff and program activities.

Fiscal evaluation or efficiency The process of determining a program's benefits relative to its cost.

Fiscal or Efficiency Evaluation The purpose of **fiscal evaluation** is to determine how program outcomes compare with their costs. There are two types of efficiency evaluations: cost–benefit analysis and cost-effectiveness analysis. In performing a cost–benefit analysis, managers estimate both the tangible and intangible benefits of a program and the direct and indirect costs of implementing that program, as summarized in **Table 5-8** for the Heartworks for Women program. Once these have been specified, they must be translated into a common measure, usually a monetary unit. In other words, the cost–benefit analysis examines the program outcomes in terms of money saved or reduced costs. A prenatal program that costs $200 per participant to produce and results in reduced medical costs of $800 can be expressed as a cost–benefit ratio of 1:4. For every one dollar required to produce the program, there is a $4 savings in medical costs.[40] Refer to Chapter 11 for a discussion of a cost–benefit analysis of the Special Supplemental Nutrition Program for Women, Infants, and Children (WIC).

The second type of fiscal evaluation is cost-effectiveness analysis. Unlike cost–benefit analysis, which reduces a program's benefits and costs to a common monetary unit, cost-effectiveness analysis relates the effectiveness of reaching the program's goals to the monetary value of the resources going into the program. With this type of evaluation, similar programs can be compared to one another or ranked in order of their cost per program goal. A cost-effectiveness analysis would be done, for example, to determine which of two methods of intervention—individual dietary counseling or group nutrition education classes—produces a desired outcome for less cost.

TABLE 5-8 Costs and Benefits Considered in a Cost–Benefit Analysis of the Heartworks for Women Program

TYPE	COSTS	BENEFITS
Direct	Personnel—salaries Utilities (telephone, Internet) Travel (to/from worksites) Office supplies Postage Equipment Instructional materials Design Printing Promotion and advertising	Revenue from program
Indirect	Personnel—benefits Rental of office space Utilities Equipment depreciation Maintenance and repairs Janitorial services	Increased exposure for the program and the organization within the community Reduced use of health care services by employees of participating worksites

PROGRAMS IN **ACTION**

A Learn-and-Serve Nutrition Program: The Food Literacy Partners Program

An individual's health literacy has a direct effect on health status and outcomes.[1,2] The *Healthy People* initiative defines health literacy as "the degree to which individuals have the capacity to obtain, process, and understand basic health information and services needed to make appropriate health decisions."[3] The Food Literacy Partners Program (FLPP) focuses on food and nutrition information to help individuals make appropriate eating decisions. It was designed to deliver evidence-based nutrition information in a rural community with limited access to nutrition education professionals.[4]

The FLPP is a "learn-and-serve" program that provides 12 hours of food and nutrition education to volunteers in exchange for several hours of community volunteer service. The program appeals to a wide range of individuals, including nurses and other health professionals, exercise specialists and personal trainers, teachers and school volunteers, college students, child nutrition program managers, retirees, chefs, lay health advisors, church wellness committee members, and individuals with a chronic nutrition-related condition. Completion of the FLPP course involves 12 hours of self-instruction or group didactic sessions; three hours of practice talking about food and nutrition information to standardized patients representing underserved populations in Pitt County, North Carolina; two hours of group workshop on cultural competence and selection and design of materials appropriate for individuals with low literacy; and three hours of basic food safety and food preparation skills practice. The class can be taken in person or online through East Carolina University's online distance education system.

Two of the modules, an interactive healthy food preparation session and a simulated health fair, require in-person participation as a graduation requirement. Recently, a third in-person, optional supermarket tour was added to practice decision making based on the Nutrition Facts label. Six core modules focus on healthful eating and weight management information that can be taught by unlicensed individuals. Volunteers use this information to assist professionals at community and business health fairs, conduct demonstrations and samplings at farmers' markets, and teach healthful eating sessions in classrooms and churches. When volunteers encounter nutrition misinformation, they encourage audiences to seek information from their health care providers.

Because of the high rates of chronic nutrition-related diseases in this rural community and widespread misinformation about diet and disease, the FLPP advisory committee recommended the course include information about physical activity and dietary strategies to prevent and manage high blood pressure, type 2 diabetes, selected cancers, osteoporosis, and cardiovascular disease. Modules on these topics are offered to increase personal knowledge rather than for application in volunteer settings. Volunteers are instructed to use this information to be informed consumers, not teach the content.

At graduation, participants receive a cookbook, food thermometer, and other items to add to the up-to-date materials and references from credible organizations and sources that are provided with each module. Many of these materials can be accessed and downloaded from reputable websites that enable volunteers to provide sound educational information as needed. They remain enrolled in the online course, in which modules are updated at least annually, receive a monthly newsletter listing volunteer opportunities and testimonials, and are offered a yearly update session. As resources allow, volunteers are offered assistance by the FLPP coordinator.

An FLPP logic model[5] was generated to aid in program evaluation (see box that follows). This was an effective tool to help describe the program's potential impact on participants' nutrition and physical activity behaviors, their knowledge and comfort talking with others about food and nutrition, and volunteerism.[6] Tools used for the evaluation included key informant interviews; individual course evaluations; the Physical Activity and Nutrition Behaviors (PAN) questionnaire[7]; and an original 31-item survey with questions about motivation for taking the course, use of the online distance education site after graduation, value of the supermarket tour, and FLPP as a volunteer experience. All of the participant evaluation tools were completed anonymously in an effort to reduce social desirability bias.

The PAN questionnaire was administered to a subset of more recent participants, both before (baseline) and after completing the training. The survey was e-mailed to 186 graduates with active e-mail addresses, and 39% completed the questionnaire posted on SurveyMonkey.[8] The respondents reported behavior changes: 51% ate more vegetables, 49% ate more fruit, 31% consumed less soda and sweetened beverages, and 36% engaged in more physical activity. These self-reported behavior changes were complemented by survey responses that indicated increased knowledge and attitudes about the nutrition and physical activity topics covered in the FLPP. Graduates reported using the information they learned at work (62%) and

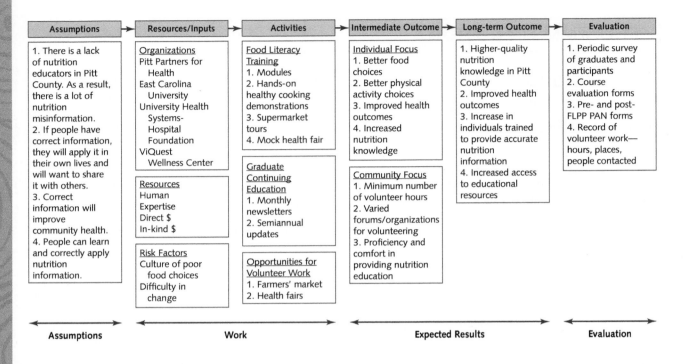

Assumptions	Resources/Inputs	Activities	Intermediate Outcome	Long-term Outcome	Evaluation
1. There is a lack of nutrition educators in Pitt County. As a result, there is a lot of nutrition misinformation. 2. If people have correct information, they will apply it in their own lives and will want to share it with others. 3. Correct information will improve community health. 4. People can learn and correctly apply nutrition information.	**Organizations** Pitt Partners for Health East Carolina University University Health Systems- Hospital Foundation ViQuest Wellness Center **Resources** Human Expertise Direct $ In-kind $ **Risk Factors** Culture of poor food choices Difficulty in change	**Food Literacy Training** 1. Modules 2. Hands-on healthy cooking demonstrations 3. Supermarket tours 4. Mock health fair **Graduate Continuing Education** 1. Monthly newsletters 2. Semiannual updates **Opportunities for Volunteer Work** 1. Farmers' market 2. Health fairs	**Individual Focus** 1. Better food choices 2. Better physical activity choices 3. Improved health outcomes 4. Increased nutrition knowledge **Community Focus** 1. Minimum number of volunteer hours 2. Varied forums/organizations for volunteering 3. Proficiency and comfort in providing nutrition education	1. Higher-quality nutrition knowledge in Pitt County 2. Improved health outcomes 3. Increase in individuals trained to provide accurate nutrition information 4. Increased access to educational resources	1. Periodic survey of graduates and participants 2. Course evaluation forms 3. Pre- and post-FLPP PAN forms 4. Record of volunteer work— hours, places, people contacted

Assumptions	Work	Expected Results	Evaluation

in day-to-day conversations (75%). They met their volunteer commitments at work (46%) and other venues. Overall, the graduates highly recommended the training and supermarket tours. Graduates found that both online training and in-person class training were effective delivery modes. There has been a dramatic increase in use of the online modules in recent years as more people have become comfortable with online learning and have more limited time to attend classes in person. More than 3,500 hours of volunteer service were completed, which was, on average, more than double the number of required hours. Many graduates chose not to report hours beyond their requirement.

It is possible for a learn-and-serve nutrition program to prepare volunteers to deliver nutrition education to consumers in rural areas. Graduates find that they are quickly able to find ways to pass on their newly acquired nutrition knowledge at home and in the community.

Source: R. Rawl, K. M. Kolasa, J. Lee, and L. M. Whetstone, "A Learn and Serve Nutrition Program: The Food Literacy Partners Program," *Journal of Nutrition Education and Behavior*, 40 (2008): 49–51. © 2008 SOCIETY FOR NUTRITION EDUCATION. Published by Elsevier Inc. All rights reserved; and the Food Literacy Partners Program available at *http://www.ecu.edu/dph/*.

Communicating Evaluation Findings Because the primary purpose of evaluations is to provide information for decision making, you do not want your findings to go unused. If they are stored away in a filing cabinet or dumped into the "circular file," a program may continue missing the mark or a success story may go unnoticed. With careful planning and work, you can ensure that the main findings of your evaluation get the attention they deserve.

Even as you begin the evaluation, you should be thinking about the final report! As the evaluation progresses, make notes on how problems were handled and which documents or materials were used. Retain copies of survey instruments and computer printouts as reference items or for use in the report's appendix. When you begin preparing your report, keep these three rules in mind:[41]

- Communicate the information to the appropriate potential users.
- Ensure that the report addresses the issues that the users perceive to be important.
- Be sure that the report is delivered in time to be useful and in a form that the intended users can easily understand.

With these issues in mind, prepare your report, which may be either informal (e.g., a short memorandum) or formal (e.g., a full report). Even if the report is only a three-page memorandum, it should be concise and understandable and should give the user what he or she needs to make a decision. Our focus in this discussion is on the formal report, which tends to be organized as follows:[42]

1. **Front cover.** The front cover should provide (a) the title of the program and its location, (b) the name of the evaluator(s), (c) the period covered by the report, and (d) the date the report was submitted. The front cover should be neat and attractively formatted.

2. **Summary.** Sometimes called the executive summary, this section of the report is a brief overview of the evaluation, explaining why and how it was done and listing its major conclusions and recommendations. Typically, this section is prepared for the individual who does not have time to read the full report. Therefore, it should not be longer than one or two pages. And even though the summary appears first in the report, it should be written *last*.

3. **Background information.** This section places the program in context, describing what the program was designed to do and how it began. The amount of detail provided in this section will depend on the needs and knowledge of the users. If most readers are unfamiliar with the program, it should be described in some detail; if most readers are involved with the program, this section can be kept short. A typical outline for this section might include the following:

- Origin of the program
- Goals of the program
- Program's target population
- Characteristics of program materials, activities, and administrative procedures
- Staff involved with the program

4. **Description of the evaluation.** This section states the purpose of the evaluation, including why it was conducted and what it was intended to accomplish. Here you define the scope of the evaluation and describe how it was carried out. This section establishes the credibility of the evaluator and the evaluation findings (much like the methods section of a research paper). Technical information about the evaluation design and analysis is presented here. Technical language should be kept to a minimum, however. Refer readers to appendices for specific technical information and for copies of any instruments used in the evaluation study. A general outline for this section might include the following headings:

- Purposes of the evaluation
- Evaluation design
- Outcome measures
     Instruments used
     Data collection and analysis procedures
- Process measures
     Instruments used
     Data collection and analysis procedures

5. **Results.** This section presents the results of the outcome or process evaluation. It is appropriate here to present data or summarize findings in tables, figures, graphs, or charts. Before you begin writing this section, you should have already analyzed the data, tested for statistical significance (if appropriate), and prepared the tables, figures, and other illustrations.

6. **Discussion of results.** This section interprets the results of the evaluation study and should address two key issues: How certain is it that the program caused the results? How good were the results? The results section explores some of the reasons why a certain

outcome was reached and how the program compares to similar programs. Any strengths and weaknesses of the program are described here.

7. **Conclusions, recommendations, and options.** This section is an influential part of the report because it outlines the major conclusions that can be drawn from the evaluation and suggests a course of action for enhancing the program's strengths and remedying its flaws. The recommendations should address specific aspects of the program and should follow logically from your interpretation of the evaluation findings. Preparing a list of recommendations about the program's delivery or impact is especially important when the actual results differ from the predetermined objectives.

Once your report is written, you must decide how best to distribute it. Several options are available. You may send the full report to your immediate supervisor, division director, and board of directors and provide a copy of the executive summary to interested community groups. You may inform the media and general public by distributing a press release and posting key findings on the organization's website. In some cases, the strategies for publishing the evaluation findings will have been specified up front by the primary client; if not, you may suggest the formats that best communicate the findings to various audiences. **Figure 5-4** shows how the findings of the evaluation study might be distributed.

FIGURE 5-4 Forms of Communicating Evaluation Findings to Various Audiences

Source: Adapted from L. L. Morris and coauthors, *How to Communicate Evaluation Findings*, pp. 9–10.

Possible Communication Form	Media	Organizations Interested in the Program Content	Program Service Providers (e.g., Nutritionists, Health Educators)	Political Bodies (e.g., City Councils, Legislatures)	Potential Clients	Current Clients	Community Groups	Funding Agencies	Advisory Committees	Board Members, Trustees, Other Management Staff	Program Administrators
Technical Report								X	X		X
Executive Summary			X	X			X	X	X	X	X
Technical Professional Paper		X							X		X
Popular Article		X	X	X		X	X			X	X
News Release, Press Conference	X										X
Public Meeting	X					X	X				
Media Appearance					X	X					
Staff Workshop			X								X
Brochure			X								
Memorandum			X								X
Personal Presentation			X						X		X
Internet Website/E-mail/Social Media	X	X	X	X	X	X	X	X	X	X	X

The Challenge of Multicultural Evaluation Multiculturalism poses some unique and difficult problems for program evaluation. Conducting a fair and democratic evaluation in a multicultural environment requires striking a balance between the rights of minority culture groups and the rights of the larger culture—a complex policy issue.

What does multiculturalism mean for the evaluator? First, the evaluator must strive to remain neutral in the face of competing minority interests. This is especially true when stakeholders have strong views about the evaluation outcome, try to influence the outcome, or downplay the possible contribution of the evaluation process.[43] Second, the evaluator must search out and define the views and interests of the minority groups to ensure that their needs are being met. When the minority group is defined as "poor" or "powerless," the evaluator has a compelling obligation to recognize the views and interests of this group.

Finally, the evaluator must be sensitive to the cultural differences that make implementing the evaluation difficult. The manner in which questions are asked, or the questions themselves, may be barriers to obtaining reliable data about the program's impact. Muslims, for example, are not comfortable answering personal questions about health and diet from a member of the opposite sex.[44] The Inuit of Nunavik, Quebec, are reluctant to answer questions about diet because they believe that thinking or talking too much about beluga whales and geese—traditional foods harvested by the Inuit—may result in their disappearance.[45] Perhaps the best message about multiculturalism was given by E. R. House at the University of Colorado at Boulder: "Treat minority cultures as you would be treated. Sooner or later, everyone may be a minority."[46] See Chapter 15 for more about cross-cultural communication and developing culturally appropriate intervention strategies.

" Learning to affirm differences rather than deny them is the essence of what multiculturalism is all about. "

—As cited in Kappa Omicron Nu's *Dialogue*, February 1997, p. 5

Spreading the Word about the Program's Success

In her book *The Popcorn Report*, Faith Popcorn describes the importance of developing a vision of the future. One of her book's chapters bears the title "You Have to See the Future to Deal with the Present."[47] These are apt words for community nutritionists, who are responsible for identifying a community's nutritional needs and developing programs to meet those needs. A good, effective nutrition program is achieved not by accident but by planning today to meet the needs of tomorrow.

The state of Arizona was following Popcorn's advice when it determined that existing training programs could not help childcare workers acquire the skills needed to provide proper nutrition for the state's children with special health care needs. Its response to this needs assessment was to develop a program—Project CHANCE—to provide the necessary training. But the department's work didn't end with the publication of the course manual. The final step in the program planning process was to let stakeholders, community leaders, community nutritionists, childcare program directors, and other interested parties know that the course was available. To do this, the department listed information about the course in national newsletters. It helped community colleges incorporate the course into their curricula. It had the course materials translated into Spanish to increase their

ENTREPRENEUR IN ACTION

Nicole Geurin, MPH, RD, is a nutrition consultant in the field of corporate wellness—designing, implementing, and evaluating wellness programs for employees. Nicole believes policy and environment have the biggest impact on behavior change and recommends that you build programs around changing these highly influential areas whenever possible. When working directly with target groups, she advises you to remember that community nutrition is something we do with and for people. It is not something we do to them. Nicole's presence in social media has provided several career opportunities, too. Learn to network effectively, says Nicole, as your peers can be your best source of information and referrals. Find out more about her sage advice regarding growing trends in the field of community nutrition at *www. cengagebrain.com*.

dissemination. The course was listed as a resource for schools in the USDA's Healthy School Meals Program on the Internet and was described in a presentation at an annual meeting of the Academy of Nutrition and Dietetics.[48] All of these activities served to get the word out to community nutritionists and other experts across the country that the Project CHANCE program had been designed, implemented, and tested and was ready for use in other states.

Use Entrepreneurship to Steer in a New Direction

Program planning is one of the most exciting aspects of the community nutritionist's job. It requires a great deal of creativity and offers opportunities to learn new skills and work with people in public relations, marketing, design, and communications. Go back to Chapter 1 and review the entrepreneurial activities listed on page 29. Three-quarters of the activities listed there are essential aspects of the planning process. You might be the first community nutritionist in your area to link clients in your weight management program with support groups and sound nutrition information on the Internet. Or maybe you convince a popular local television personality to help raise awareness of the need for healthy school environments. Perhaps you forge a partnership with a local company that has never supported health promotion activities in the past. Perhaps your team introduces inner-city school children to the new Apple Jane and the Cucumber King board game, a program designed to encourage children to eat several fruits and vegetables daily. The possibilities for being an entrepreneur in this area are boundless.

The challenge comes in thinking of new ways of delivering health messages and services to vulnerable populations. What is needed to ensure the success of community interventions? Manning Feinleib, a former associate editor of the *American Journal of Public Health*, writes that we need a better understanding of the community factors that influence change and of the reasons that consumers resist change.[49] When you plan community interventions, think of new ways to reach your target audience. Plan strategies for finding out why your clients are resisting a behavior change. Apply your creativity to influencing people to achieve behavior change. And when you are successful, consider helping other community nutritionists by publishing a carefully documented account of your own efforts and outcomes.

PROFESSIONAL **FOCUS**

The Nutrition Care Process: A Road Map to Quality Care

by Joanne M. Spahn, MS, RD, FAND

The Academy of Nutrition and Dietetics developed a comprehensive model called the **nutrition care process and model** (NCP) to standardize the *process* of nutrition care delivery and enable food and nutrition practitioners to compete successfully in a rapidly changing environment.[1] The model defines the standardized process "that food and nutrition practitioners use to think critically and make decisions" across all practice settings.[2] The model is designed to guide delivery of high-quality nutrition care to a specific client or target group, consistently produce positive outcomes, and document effectiveness of care. **Figure 5-5** illustrates the four distinct yet cyclical and interrelated steps of the nutrition care process: assessment, diagnosis, intervention, and monitoring and evaluation. Each NCP step will be more fully described in the sections that follow.

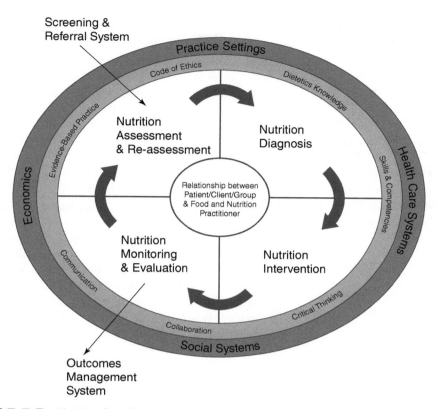

FIGURE 5-5 The Nutrition Care Process: A Road Map to Quality Care

The NCP incorporates four components:

1. *Central core:* Relationship between the client or target group and the food and nutrition practitioner.
2. The *nutrition care process* is a four-step process of nutrition care. Use the acronym ADIME to remember the four steps: **A**ssessment, **D**iagnosis, **I**ntervention, and **M**onitoring and **E**valuation.
3. *Middle and outer rings:* Middle ring shows characteristics of the food and nutrition practitioner (such as nutrition knowledge, skills, and competencies and skills in communication, critical thinking, and collaboration). Outer ring shows characteristics of the environment (e.g., economics, health care system) that influence the ways groups and clients receive nutrition services.
4. *Supporting systems:* Screening and referral (identifies clients and groups needing access to nutrition care) and the outcomes management system (supports collection of data describing outcomes achieved to demonstrate results and assess quality of care).

Source: K. Lacey and E. Pritchett, "Nutrition care process and model: ADA adopts road map to quality care and outcomes management," *Journal of the American Dietetic Association*, 103 (2003): 1061–72; Writing Group of the Nutrition Care Process/Standardized Language Committee, "Nutrition Care Process and Model Part I: The 2008 Update," *Journal of the American Dietetic Association*, 108 (2008): 1113–17. See also Nutrition Care Process Model Resources at *www.eatright.org/HealthProfessionals/content.aspx?id=7077.*

A standardized dietetics language or vocabulary has been developed to complement the NCP.[3] This language is necessary to clearly and consistently describe the unique services provided by food and nutrition practitioners across the spectrum of care.[4] Depending on the role they play, the community or public health nutritionist may utilize the NCP to design and deliver nutrition care, use the standardized language (SL) as part of community assessment, or use outcome data to advocate for new policy development.

The Nutrition Care Process: Step 1—Nutrition Assessment

During a nutrition assessment, as discussed in Chapter 4, the food and nutrition practitioner collects and interprets relevant types of data from various sources (such as interviews, observations, medical records, screening and referral forms, focus groups, and surveys) to identify nutrition-related problems and their underlying causes. The five categories of data are listed in **Table 5-9**. Critical thinking skills utilized in this step of the NCP include[5] determining appropriate data to collect (relevant vs. irrelevant data), selecting relevant norms and standards for comparing the data, and organizing and categorizing the data in a meaningful way to make nutrition diagnoses.

The Nutrition Care Process: Step 2—Nutrition Diagnosis

The purpose of the nutrition diagnosis step is to clearly identify, label, and describe an existing nutrition problem that can be resolved or improved through nutrition intervention.[6] The nutrition diagnosis is labeled using the dietetic profession's standardized terminology published in the *electronic Nutrition Care Process Terminology (eNCPT) Reference Manual*—formerly called the *International Dietetics and Nutrition Terminology (IDNT) Reference Manual*.[7]

The Academy of Nutrition and Dietetics endorses the use of a structured sentence called the PES statement to document the nutrition diagnosis. "PES" stands for the three component parts of the statement, which link the **P**roblem with the **E**tiology and **S**igns and symptoms (S/S).[8] Components are linked using the standard phrases *related to* and *as evidenced by* in the following manner:

> Nutrition problem label (using nutrition diagnosis terminology) *related to* etiology (root cause of the problem) *as evidenced by* signs and symptoms (observable indicators that the problem exists) within a target population.

In community and public health nutrition, the target population must be identified. A sample PES statement might read:

> Older homebound citizens in Higgins Township, Missouri (target population), have an "impaired ability to prepare meals" (problem) related to an inability to access food due to lack of transportation and distance to grocery stores (etiology) as evidenced by a township waiting list for meal delivery service exceeding 12 months and survey data indicating that access to groceries is a barrier for 20% of the population currently receiving meal support or on the waiting list (signs and symptoms).

The PES statement clearly and concisely defines the focus of the nutrition problem specific to the target population or client. Frequently, multiple nutrition problems exist. Critical thinking is required on the part of the nutrition expert to isolate the specific problem that nutrition intervention will most likely improve. Critical thinking skills routinely used in this step of the NCP include[9] clustering and finding patterns and relationships among available data, stating the problem clearly, and prioritizing and ruling in/out a specific diagnosis based on available evidence.

The use of nutrition diagnosis terminology distinguishes the nutrition problem from the health and/or medical problem. For example, "inappropriate intake of fat" is more specific than "elevated cardiovascular risk"; "inconsistent carbohydrate intake" is a more precise diagnosis than "elevated HbA$_{1c}$ level." The PES statement provides the foundation for linking the components of nutrition assessment, intervention, and monitoring and evaluation. It is the foundation of the NCP.

TABLE 5-9 Nutrition Assessment Data Categories and Examples

TYPE OF DATA	EXAMPLES
Food/nutrition history	• Food intake • Nutrition knowledge, beliefs, and practices, including readiness to change lifestyle behaviors • Food availability • Physical activity
Biochemical data, medical tests, and procedures	• Laboratory data such as hemoglobin, glycosylated hemoglobin (HbA$_{1c}$), lipid profile, bone density
Anthropometric measurements	• Weight • Height • Body mass index • Waist circumference
Physical examination findings	• General physical appearance • Oral health • Muscle and fat wasting
Client history	• Medical/health history • Personal/family/social history (age, occupation, etc.) • Medication and supplement use

Source: Adapted from *International Dietetics and Nutritional Terminology (IDNT) Reference Manual, 4th Edition* (Chicago: Academy of Nutrition and Dietetics), 2012.

Standardized Language for Nutrition Diagnosis

There are over 60 nutrition diagnoses recognized by the Academy of Nutrition and Dietetics, and these can be divided into three major domains or categories: intake, clinical, and behavioral–environmental. **Table 5-10** lists the domains and classes of nutrition diagnosis terminology and gives an example of one specific nutrition diagnosis in each class. **Table 5-11** gives examples of PES statements.

Frequently, more than one nutrition diagnosis may describe a single nutrition problem. If in doubt, consider taking the intake-related nutrition diagnosis, since that is most related to the food and nutrition practitioner's role. The NCP can accommodate more than one nutrition diagnosis targeting a patient or target population, but there must be nutrition assessment parameters, an intervention plan, and monitoring and evaluation plans to support each diagnosis statement.

The Nutrition Care Process: Step 3—Nutrition Intervention

Nutrition intervention, the third step of the NCP, is a client-driven method used to resolve or improve the nutrition problem or the underlying cause of the problem (e.g., lack of education, lack of access to services, lack of awareness of a problem, or lack of desire to change).[10] There are four categories of intervention strategies provided by nutrition experts:[11]

- *Food and/or nutrient delivery*—a tailored approach for providing food and nutrients including meals and snacks, food vouchers, supplements, and enteral and/or parenteral feeding
- *Nutrition education*—a process to instruct or train the target population in a skill or to impart knowledge to promote awareness and improve eating patterns
- *Nutrition counseling*—a collaborative process involving a counselor and client in exploring a nutrition problem, identifying priorities, setting goals, and creating an action plan designed to foster self-care to treat an existing condition and promote health
- *Coordination of nutrition care*—involves referral, consultation, or coordination of nutrition care with other health care providers, institutions, or agencies that can assist in treating or managing nutrition-related problems

Critical thinking skills required for this step include the ability to prioritize nutrition care goals, clearly define intervention goals in terms of measurable outcomes, match intervention strategies with client needs and nutrition diagnosis, and choose from among alternatives to determine a course of action.[12]

DOMAIN	CLASS	EXAMPLE OF NUTRITION DIAGNOSIS TERMINOLOGY
Intake	• Energy balance • Fluid intake • Bioactive substances • Nutrient • Fat and cholesterol • Protein • Carbohydrate and fiber • Vitamin • Mineral	• Inadequate energy intake • Inadequate fluid intake • Excessive alcohol intake • Malnutrition • Excess fat intake • Inadequate protein intake • Inconsistent carbohydrate intake • Inadequate vitamin intake (specify) • Increased calcium needs
Clinical	• Functional • Biochemical • Weight	• Swallowing difficulty; breastfeeding difficulty • Food–medication interaction • Overweight/obesity
Behavioral–Environmental	• Knowledge and beliefs • Physical activity and function • Food safety and access	• Undesirable food choices; disordered eating pattern • Impaired ability to prepare meals; physical inactivity • Limited access to food

TABLE 5-10 Nutrition Diagnosis Domains, Classes, and Examples of Nutrition Diagnoses[a]

[a] *The International Dietetics and Nutritional Terminology Reference Manual* contains reference sheets for each nutrition diagnosis, which provide a definition and list common etiologies and signs and symptoms for each nutrition diagnosis term. The Academy of Nutrition and Dietetics website (*www.eatright.org*) provides access to Web-based tutorials and other materials.

Source: Adapted from *International Dietetics and Nutritional Terminology (IDNT) Reference Manual*, 4th Edition (Chicago: Academy of Nutrition and Dietetics), 2012.

TABLE 5-11

Examples of Nutrition Diagnosis (PES) Statements

TARGET POPULATION	NUTRITION DIAGNOSIS	ETIOLOGY *"RELATED TO"*	SIGNS AND SYMPTOMS *"AS EVIDENCED BY"*
Clients with diabetes enrolled in Clinic X with a HbA$_{1c}$ > 8 mg/dL	Inconsistent carbohydrate intake	Food- and nutrition-related knowledge deficit regarding carbohydrate counting	Wide variations in blood sugar levels; inability to demonstrate carbohydrate-counting skills
Women > 18 years of age residing in McKee Housing Unit	Inappropriate intake of fat	Frequent consumption of meals and snacks high in saturated fat content	Food frequency questionnaire indicating saturated fat intake > 15% of total calorie intake
High school students enrolled at Lincoln High School	Undesirable food choices	Limited access to desirable healthy foods	42% of students with BMI > 27
WIC client	Breastfeeding difficulty	Decreased feeding frequency/duration	Poor infant weight gain and mother reports infant eating approximately every 4 hours for a 10-minute duration
Students in kindergarten through third grade (K–3)	Food and nutrition knowledge deficit regarding recommended fruit and vegetable intake	Lack of exposure to accurate information	Mean pretest scores of 60%

Planning an Intervention

The key steps in program planning were outlined earlier in this chapter. The community nutritionist uses needs assessment data to identify and describe the *etiology* and *signs and symptoms* of a *nutrition problem* (PES statement) and prioritizes the nutrition-related problem to be targeted. The intervention, whenever possible, is targeted to the cause or etiology of the problem identified in the PES statement. For example, consider the PES statement used earlier:

> Older homebound citizens in Higgins Township, Missouri, have an "impaired ability to prepare meals" related to an inability to access food due to lack of transportation and distance to grocery stores, as evidenced by a township waiting list for meal delivery service exceeding 12 months and survey data indicating that access to groceries is a barrier for 20% of the population currently receiving meal support or on the waiting list.

An intervention would be targeted to the "inability to access food due to lack of transportation and the distance to the grocery store." The intervention could be designed to deliver groceries to clients, or transportation services could be contracted with a private entity, depending on the resources available in the community.

During the planning phase, community nutritionists frequently access **evidence-based guidelines** to design effective intervention programs.* The Academy of Nutrition and Dietetics Evidence Analysis Library (*www.andeal.org*) and the National Guideline Clearinghouse (*www.guideline.gov*) are excellent sources of guidelines for various population groups (e.g., children, homeless persons), targeting various health and disease conditions (e.g., overweight, hypertension, cardiovascular disease) and intervention styles (e.g., nutrition counseling).

A **nutrition prescription** is a common component of a nutrition intervention and defines the community nutritionist's food and nutrient intake recommendations, which guide intervention design and monitoring and evaluation plans. For example, the nutrition prescription for a school nutrition education program targeting third graders may be the *consumption of three servings of fruits and vegetables at lunch and snack*. The prescription for individuals enrolled in an osteoporosis prevention class targeted to postmenopausal women may be an *intake of 1,200 milligrams of calcium per day from food and supplement sources*. A program targeting reduction in saturated fat intake may advocate (prescribe or recommend) *no more than 10% of calories from saturated fat*. The purpose of the nutrition

* See also the Centers for Disease Control and Prevention's *Guide to Community Preventive Services: What Works to Promote Health?* available at *www.thecommunityguide.org.*

prescription is to communicate clearly the individual's or target group's diet/nutrition recommendation based on a thorough nutrition assessment.

Nutrition Intervention Implementation

As outlined earlier in this chapter, implementation is the phase in which the nutrition intervention is communicated to involved personnel, the plan is carried out, and data is collected to assess progress and evaluate outcomes. The standardized language of the Academy of Nutrition and Dietetics, published in the *electronic Nutrition Care Process Terminology (eNCPT) Reference Manual*, defines the terminology used by food and nutrition practitioners to describe and document nutrition interventions. **Table 5-12** describes the main categories of interventions and gives specific examples of each. Community nutrition programs may incorporate multiple strategies to resolve the nutrition problem. For example, a WIC dietitian may provide nutrition education or nutrition counseling along with food vouchers tailored to the needs of a pregnant or breastfeeding client. The director of a Head Start Program or child nutrition program may begin an

TABLE 5-12 Types, Definitions, and Examples of Nutrition Interventions

TYPES OF INTERVENTION	DEFINITION	EXAMPLES OF INTERVENTION TYPES
Food and/or Nutrient Delivery		
Meal and Snack	Individualized approach for provision of meals/snacks	Meals on Wheels; Head Start; School Lunch Program; food vouchers
Supplements	Foods or nutrients not intended as a sole item or a meal or diet, but intended to provide additional nutrients	Provision of vitamin/mineral supplements by WIC program; provision of a high-energy and protein supplement by a home health care agency
Feeding Assistance	Accommodation or assistance in eating to support adequate nutrient intake and/or restore eating independence	Feeding assistance provided to clients; recommendation for adaptive equipment; implementation of a feeding assistance training program or texture-modified menu
Feeding Environment	Adjustment of the physical environment (e.g., seating arrangements, table height, meal schedule, minimization of distractions) to influence food consumption	Adjustments made to accommodate individuals in schools, long-term care, developmentally disabled facilities, or individual homes
Nutrition Education		
Initial/Brief Nutrition Education	Instruction intended to provide information or build and reinforce basic nutrition-related knowledge until further instruction can be provided	Brief instruction provided as part of a multidisciplinary class, health fair, screening program
Comprehensive Education	Instruction intended to lead to in-depth nutrition-related knowledge and/or skills in given topics	WIC group education classes, school curriculum, diabetes self-management training class
Nutrition Counseling[a]		
Theoretical Basis/Approach	Defines the theoretical framework used in counseling (e.g., cognitive-behavioral theory, transtheoretical model, health belief model, and/or social-cognitive theory)	Behavioral therapy or lifestyle change programs; tailored counseling based on "stage of change" or other theoretical construct
Strategies	Identifies the evidence-based strategies used in counseling (e.g., motivational interviewing, self-monitoring, goal setting, problem solving)	Self-monitoring, goal setting, problem solving, motivational interviewing
Coordination of Nutrition Care		
Coordination of Other Care during Nutrition Care	Interventions with other professionals, institutions, or agencies on behalf of the patient/client prior to discharge from nutrition care	Coordination of care with mental health professionals, social workers, or medical services

[a] For more information regarding behavior change theories and models, see Chapter 3.

Source: *International Dietetics and Nutritional Terminology (IDNT) Reference Manual*, 4th Edition (Chicago: Academy of Nutrition and Dietetics), 2012.

educational campaign related to fruits and vegetables using nutrition education and reinforce the message during delivery of meals and snacks.

The Nutrition Care Process: Step 4—Monitoring and Evaluation

Monitoring and evaluation (M&E) is the fourth step in the NCP and is routinely done to determine whether nutrition intervention goals and objectives are being achieved. The NCP is not linear (refer to Figure 5-5). The groundwork for the M&E step is laid during program planning, when intervention goals and objectives relevant to the desired outcomes are defined. The following steps are involved in monitoring and evaluation:[13]

- *Nutrition monitoring*. Periodic evaluation of the effectiveness of the nutrition intervention.

- *Evaluating outcomes against criteria*. A judgment must be made about the degree of progress achieved toward a nutrition-related outcome, based on a comparison of current measures of one or more nutrition care indicators with intervention goals and objectives. As you will recall, the program objectives indicate how program success will be measured or evaluated. Outcomes may reflect a change in such things as a client's nutrition-related knowledge, attitude, food or nutrient access and/or intake, lab values, or anthropometric measures.

Examples of Monitoring and Evaluation in the Community

A three-month telephone counseling intervention program promoted the following nutrition prescription: daily intake of three vegetable servings, 16 ounces of vegetable juice, and three fruit servings per day. The community nutritionist assessed interim and final nutrition intervention effectiveness using periodic 24-hour recalls. An individual's mean daily intake of vegetable and fruit servings and vegetable juice consumption in ounces was compared to the prescription. In this example, a program goal was the criteria for evaluation.

A WIC dietitian provided nutrition counseling to a young mother with a child with a medical diagnosis of obesity. The nutrition diagnosis was excessive energy intake *related to* lack of meal planning, *as evidenced by* a BMI-for-age percentile greater than the 95th percentile and an estimated calorie intake of 2,000 calories, primarily from high-fat snack foods. The dietitian counseled the client on meal-planning strategies and keeping a food record for her child. The dietitian and client will monitor calorie intake, adherence to meal-planning goals, and the child's growth parameters to assess progress related to pre-established goals.

Conclusions

Broad adaptation of nutrition practice to incorporate the nutrition care process is expected to facilitate improved nutrition care outcomes by carefully focusing limited resources on clearly identified nutrition problems. Clear linkage between nutrition assessment, intervention, and monitoring and evaluation will enhance measurement and communication of outcomes within and across practice settings. **Table 5-13** provides examples of applying the nutrition care process for heart disease in different practice settings.

The NCP terminology is currently being incorporated in various commercial electronic health record systems, making building of these systems easier and more standardized across the country. Use of NCP has enhanced the interconnectivity of nutrition practitioners, researchers, and academics by providing a common vocabulary and approach to nutrition care.

TABLE 5-13 Examples of Applying the Nutrition Care Process and Model for Heart Disease in Different Practice Settings	**NUTRITION CARE PROCESS AND MODEL**	**GROUP NUTRITION EDUCATION FOR DISEASE PREVENTION**	**COMMUNITY HEALTH PROMOTION**
	NCP Support System: Nutrition Screen/ Referral (provides access to NCP)	Advertise heart-healthy cooking class to local media and physician offices. People self-refer or are referred by primary care provider.	Public health statistics and health care utilization data show high population prevalence of coronary heart disease (CHD) and CHD risk factors
	Step 1 Nutrition Assessment	Nutrition educator asks audience to identify their concerns/questions that brought them to class (e.g., pretest)	Community nutritionist evaluates community assessment, verifying that there is a good opportunity to reach adults through worksites

NUTRITION CARE PROCESS AND MODEL	GROUP NUTRITION EDUCATION FOR DISEASE PREVENTION	COMMUNITY HEALTH PROMOTION
Step 2 Nutrition Diagnosis	Nutrition educator makes diagnosis: knowledge deficit of heart-healthy cooking techniques	Community nutritionist makes nutrition diagnosis: inadequate access to healthy food choices and environmental barriers to exercise
Step 3 Nutrition Intervention	Nutrition educator teaches heart-healthy cooking class, with emphasis on participants' identified needs	Community nutritionist recommends new vending machines with fruits, yogurt, etc.; addition of walking path; and nutrition and physical activity education program
Step 4 Monitoring and Evaluation of Nutrition Outcomes	At end of class, check whether needs met (e.g., posttest); contact two to four weeks later to see whether using new cooking techniques; rate satisfaction	Changes in types of food choices and more healthy foods purchased; usage of walking path; program participation
Support System: Outcomes Management System	Aggregate data from all groups; analyze data; report to funding agency	Merge and analyze data and combine for all worksites to determine outcomes of the intervention

TABLE 5-13

Examples of Applying the Nutrition Care Process and Model for Heart Disease in Different Practice Settings—*continued*

Note: Documentation is an ongoing process that supports all of the steps in the nutrition care process. Quality documentation should be relevant, accurate, and timely.

Source: Adapted from *International Dietetics and Nutritional Terminology (IDNT) Reference Manual*, 4th Edition (Chicago: Academy of Nutrition and Dietetics), 2012.

Miniglossary

Nutrition care process and model A systematic problem-solving method that food and nutrition practitioners use to evaluate and address nutrition-related problems and provide safe, effective, high-quality nutrition care.

Nutrition intervention A purposefully planned program or action designed to change a nutrition-related behavior, risk factor, environmental condition, or aspect of health status for an individual (including family members and caregivers), target groups, or the community at large.[14]

Evidence-based guidelines Guidelines that incorporate the best available research evidence in guiding the best course of action for practitioner and client in order to improve intervention outcomes; an approach based on scientific proof.

Nutrition prescription A tailored recommendation for energy, nutrient, or food intake (e.g., fruits and vegetables), based on current reference standards and dietary guidelines and the needs of the individual or target group.

Monitoring and evaluation (M&E) The process used to quantify the amount of progress the target group or client has made as a result of a specific nutrition intervention designed for their needs.

case study

Program Planning

by Alessandra Sarcona, MS, RD, CSSD, Alice Fornari, EdD, RD, and Alison Barkman, MS, RD, CDN

Scenario

A large accounting firm in an industrial park employs 212 workers who include certified public accountants, administrators, secretaries, and information technologists. The ratio of males to females is 3:1. The human resource department invited the company's main insurance carrier to hold a health fair on-site. Trained personnel conducted screenings for cholesterol, blood pressure, and body mass index. Attendance was mandatory for all employees. The screening showed that 34% of the employees are obese (BMI ≥ 30), 30% have a waist circumference ≥ 35 inches (female) and ≥ 40 inches (male), 24% of the employees not treated for high cholesterol (i.e., not on medication) have a blood cholesterol level ≥ 200 mg/dL (7% of employees are taking cholesterol-lowering medication), and 18% of the employees not treated for high blood pressure have a blood pressure ≥ 120/80 mmHg (4% of employees are taking blood pressure medication). A survey given to employees revealed that 60% are physically inactive and 48% did not correctly answer questions that related to diet, blood lipids, and heart disease. The insurance carrier offered the accounting firm a discount on health insurance premiums if a wellness program is instituted. The accounting firm has agreed to hire a registered dietitian to design and conduct the wellness program on-site. There is a conference room available for meetings and a "game room" that could be converted into a gym.

Learning Outcomes

- Identify the steps needed for planning a program.
- Classify information to complete a needs assessment.
- Describe the components of a program plan.
- Summarize an evaluation process to determine whether the goals and desired outcomes of a program are met.

Foundation: Acquisition of Knowledge and Skills

1. Review the *Steps in Program Planning* in the chapter text.
2. Define "metabolic syndrome" as from the National Heart, Lung, and Blood Institute, *www.nhlbi.nih.gov*.

Step 1: *Identify Relevant Information and Uncertainties*

As you begin to conduct a needs assessment for your target group, you have noted the nutritional parameters that the insurance company has provided and you suspect that the employees with obesity, high cholesterol, and high blood pressure have metabolic syndrome. Outline additional information that you need from the insurance carrier to have a complete needs assessment prior to setting up a wellness program.

Step 2: *Interpret Information*

1. After getting more medical information, your needs assessment has determined that 27% of the employees have metabolic syndrome. Write a nutrition diagnosis as a problem, etiology, signs and symptoms (PES) statement that would classify someone with metabolic syndrome.
2. Review the National Heart, Lung, and Blood Institute and/or the American Heart Association websites and outline the treatment program for metabolic syndrome. From this information, formulate goals and desired outcomes for your program.

Step 3: *Draw and Implement Conclusions*

1. The insurance company wants you to send it the program goals and objectives, a description of your wellness program plan that includes your proposed intervention activities (how you intend to set up the wellness program), the nutrition education component, the marketing plan, and any other additional information, such as resources (educational materials) and staff needed to implement the program, equipment, costs, and so on.
2. Link the proposed intervention activities with a level of intervention: Do the activities impact individuals, communities, or systems? Connect the program activities with national goals and objectives, if applicable (e.g., to illustrate coordination with *Healthy People 2020* or the *Dietary Guidelines for Americans*).

Step 4: *Engage in Continuous Improvement*

1. What type of data will you collect to determine whether your program has met its desired outcomes, and what is the purpose of this type of evaluation?

2. Explain how you will evaluate the program elements and program effectiveness. Include several types of evaluations and specify exactly how you will evaluate various aspects of the wellness program.

CHAPTER **SUMMARY**

Factors That Trigger Program Planning

▶ The stimulus to develop a program or modify an existing program is usually made in response to a need identified in a community needs assessment; a mandate handed down from an organization's national office or a federal agency; new research findings; the concerns of a well-known community leader or coalition; a new government policy; or the availability of new funding.

Steps in Program Planning

▶ Step 1: Review the organization's mission statement and the results of the community needs assessment.

▶ Step 2: Define program goals and objectives. Goals are broad statements of desired changes or outcomes. Objectives are specific, measurable actions to be completed within a specified time frame.

▶ Step 3: Develop a program plan that describes the intervention, the appropriate nutrition education component for the target population, and how the program will be marketed.

▶ The intervention strategy can encompass one or more levels of intervention. Level I interventions build awareness of a health or nutritional topic or problem. Level II interventions help participants make lifestyle changes. Level III interventions work toward creating environments that support the behavior changes made by individuals.

▶ In Step 4, decisions are made about the management system—the two types of structures needed to implement the program: personnel and data systems. Both direct costs and indirect costs must be determined to identify the true cost of a program.

▶ Step 5 identifies program areas where financial support is needed, reviews possible funding sources, and prepares and submits a grant application for funding.

▶ Step 6 is the action phase of the program planning process and involves program implementation—the set of activities needed to put a program into effect.

▶ In Step 7, program elements and effectiveness are evaluated to determine whether the program accomplished what it was designed to accomplish. Types of evaluation include: formative, process, impact, outcome, structure, and fiscal evaluation.

The Nutrition Care Process: A Road Map to Quality Care

▶ The nutrition care process (NCP) is a four-step process of nutrition care. Use the acronym ADIME to remember the four steps: assessment, diagnosis, intervention, and monitoring and evaluation.

SUMMARY **QUESTIONS**

1. Describe four of the factors that can trigger program planning.
2. Describe the seven steps in the program planning process.
3. The goal of your program is to "improve the physical activity status and food choices of employees in participating worksites." Define outcome and process objectives and write both an outcome and a process objective relevant to your program goal. Identify the various levels of change that may be needed to elicit behavior change in the employees (e.g., changes in knowledge, attitudes, self-efficacy, and so on).
4. Discuss two reasons for conducting evaluations of programs.
5. Describe the four distinct, interrelated steps of the nutrition care process.

INTERNET **RESOURCES** ....

Evaluation Working Group at CDC
www.cdc.gov/eval/resources/index.htm
Lists resources about evaluation or conducting an
evaluation. You can receive CDC e-mail updates and/or
RSS feeds[a] and select from a list of subscription topics at:
www.cdc.gov/Other/emailupdates.

Guide to Community Preventive Services
www.thecommunityguide.org
Systematic reviews and evidence-based recommendations.

**The Academy of Nutrition and Dietetics Evidence
Library (EAL)**
www.andeal.org
EAL provides a number of resources, including
bibliographies and evidence summaries of major research
findings.

National Guideline Clearinghouse (NGC)
www.guideline.gov
Comprehensive database of evidence-based clinical
practice guidelines and related documents on a variety
of topics.

Cochrane Database of Systematic Reviews
www.cochrane.org/cochrane-reviews
Evidence-based reviews that explore the evidence for
and against the effectiveness and appropriateness of
interventions.

Academy of Nutrition and Dietetics
www.eatright.org
The Academy supports several e-newsletters, blogs,[b]
social network websites, RSS feeds, podcasts, videos, and
electronic mailing lists (EMLs) as a member benefit to
promote networking and sharing of expertise.

Food and Nutrition Information Center (FNIC)
http://fnic.nal.usda.gov/
Find numerous professional and career resources,
databases, and electronic discussion groups and blogs.

Healthy People 2020
www.healthypeople.gov/2020/healthy-people-in-action/
Sign up for e-mail, follow *Healthy People 2020* on Twitter,
connect on LinkedIn, or join the Consortium and stay up-to-
date with the latest *Healthy People* information and events.

National Institutes of Health
www.nih.gov/news-events/social-media-outreach
Site for subscribing to several food and nutrition
newsletters and RSS feeds.

USDA's Economic Research Service (ERS)
Announcements of new food assistance program items;
subscribe to RSS feeds or e-mail updates at:
www.ers.usda.gov/Updates.

[a] RSS (Really Simple Syndication) feed or Web feeds is an easy way for you to be alerted when content that interests you
appears on your favorite websites.

[b] Blog (Weblog): A type of social media website. Bloggers post new content frequently and interact with their readers.

CHAPTER 6

The Art and Science of Policymaking

LEARNING **OBJECTIVES**

After you have read and studied this chapter, you will be able to:

- Describe the policymaking process.
- Explain how laws and regulations are developed.
- Describe the federal budget process.
- Identify emerging policy issues in the food and nutrition arena.
- Communicate with elected officials.
- Identify different strategies for influencing policy and regulatory changes.

- Communicate effectively when working with the media.

This chapter addresses such issues as public policy development, food and nutrition laws and regulations, advocacy and communication skills, and current information technologies, which have been designated by the Accreditation Council for Education in Nutrition and Dietetics (ACEND) as Foundation Knowledge and Learning Outcomes for dietetics education.

CHAPTER **OUTLINE**

Something to think about...

"Each of the great social achievements of recent decades has come about not because of government proclamations but because people organized, made demands and made it good politics to respond. It is the political will of the people that makes and sustains the political will of governments."

—*JAMES P. GRANT,*
Former Executive Director, UNICEF

For a complete list of references, please access the MindTap Reader within your MindTap course.

Introduction

In bold letters, the newspaper headline proclaimed, "Little Ones Doomed: Child Malnutrition a 'Silent Emergency.'"[1] According to Stephen Lewis, deputy executive director of UNICEF, who was quoted in the accompanying article, "The silent emergency of malnutrition is so shocking and simultaneously unnecessary that it must be brought to public attention." His comments coincided with the release of one of UNICEF's *State of the World's Children* reports, which indicated that more than 200 million children in developing countries under the age of five years are malnourished. Two weeks after the newspaper article appeared, *Time* magazine featured a two-page column, donated jointly by *Time* and Canon, that called attention to UNICEF's message about the silent emergency of malnutrition.[2]

What relevance do these documents have for community nutritionists? What do they have to do with policy, the topic of this chapter? The answer to both questions is "A great deal." The newspaper article and magazine column are examples of how an organization (UNICEF) used a particular strategy (a press release to the media and partnerships with two companies, *Time* magazine and Canon) to help convince people that a serious problem (global childhood malnutrition) exists. As a result, strategies addressing global malnutrition increased dramatically. In 2013, an estimated 6.3 million children worldwide died before five years of age—down from 9.9 million in 2000, showing that countries have made progress in improving child survival since the turn of the millennium.[3] Nevertheless, to end preventable child deaths, more substantial policy efforts are needed, as more than 90 million children under age five—one in seven children worldwide—remain underweight and at greater risk of dying from common infections.[4] Chapter 14 discusses strategies aimed at further reducing child malnutrition worldwide.

Addressing problems is the core activity of the policymaking process. Whether the issue is regulating agricultural practices, controlling air and water pollution, or providing quality health care for all citizens, policymaking is an ongoing process that affects our lives daily. As a community nutritionist, you will find that both local and national policy issues affect the way you work, how you deliver nutrition services, and the dietary messages you give to clients in your community. Consider how you would respond to the following issues in the nutrition policy arena:

- In order to assist consumers in understanding the relative significance of the amount of added sugars in a serving of a product in the context of a total daily diet, should the Food and Drug Administration (FDA) establish a Daily Reference Value (DRV) for total energy intake from added sugars (e.g., 10% of total energy intake from added sugars)? Should the FDA also require the declaration of the percent DV for added sugars on Nutrition and Supplement Facts labels?
- Should U.S. manufacturers of baby formula be allowed to sell their products in developing countries where the use of such products may undercut breastfeeding practices?
- Should television stations be required to run public service announcements that feature healthful food messages for children to balance current food-related advertising, which tends to promote empty-calorie, high-sugar foods? Or should media advertisers be prohibited from marketing foods of low nutritional value to children?
- Should mandatory labeling of foods be required of manufacturers who include genetically modified foods or food ingredients in their products so that consumers can know the source of the foods they choose? Or should the labeling of genetically modified foods be required only when a specific health concern—such as an allergy to specific proteins—needs to be communicated to consumers?

- Because overweight and obesity are viewed as public health problems, should states and cities levy taxes on less nutritious foods, including soft drinks, candy, and snack foods (such as potato chips), in order to raise tax revenues to help fund healthful eating and nutrition education campaigns? Or does such a tax penalize the wrong target because it affects consumers and not manufacturers, who may be more to blame for the preponderance of the many low-nutrient-density foods.
- Should lower health insurance premiums be made available to employees who maintain a healthy weight and participate in worksite wellness programs on a weekly basis?
- Should the costs incurred by people losing weight in order to achieve a healthy weight be tax deductible?
- Should penalties be imposed on makers of both exercise equipment and supplements that claim their products melt away pounds effortlessly?
- In order to feed an expanding population with shrinking natural resources while also putting a cap on greenhouse gas emissions, should a role of public health professionals be to educate the public regarding the benefits of moving from meat-centered diets to more plant-based diets in order to sustain a healthy population and a healthy planet?[5] Does the USDA MyPlate food guidance system serve as a policy tool for directing the public to a more plant-based diet?
- Should the FDA—rather than the food industry itself—develop a standardized front-of-package (FOP) nutrition labeling system for all food and beverage products to help consumers use point-of-purchase information to make more nutritious choices for themselves? Should the FOP symbol be based on calories, sodium, solid fats, and added sugars because these components of the diet are most linked to chronic diseases—even though it would make "good food/bad food" distinctions as opposed to the "all foods can fit" approach to a healthy diet?

There are no simple answers to these difficult policy questions. This is not surprising, for public policy is complex and ever-changing. The purpose of public policy is to fashion strategies for solving public problems. In the nutrition arena, the strategies for solving problems typically include food and nutrition assistance programs, dietary recommendations, and reimbursement mechanisms for nutrition services. This chapter describes the policymaking process, examines emerging policy issues, and discusses the policymaking activities of community nutritionists.

The Process of Policymaking

You may not think of yourself as a political animal. You may think of politics as being confined to Senate hearings, city council meetings, and elections. But if you have ever lobbied a professor to allow you to take an exam at a later date or signed a petition calling for increased funding for a local food bank, then you have walked onto the political stage. You have tried to get something you want by presenting compelling reasons why an existing policy should be changed.

> *" If dietetics is your profession, politics is your business. "*
>
> —Academy of Nutrition and Dietetics

Recall that policy was defined in Chapter 1 as the course of action chosen by public authorities to address a given problem. A **problem** is a "substantial discrepancy between what is and what should be."[6] When public authorities state that a problem exists, they are recognizing the gap between current reality and the desired state of affairs. Policies, then, are guides to a range of activities designed to address a problem.[7]

Problem A significant gap between current reality (the way things are) and the desired state of affairs (the way things should be).

Policymaking The process by which authorities decide which actions to take to address a problem or set of problems.

Policymaking is the process by which authorities decide which actions to take to address a problem or set of problems, and it can be viewed as a cycle, as shown in **Figure 6-1**.[8] This diagram has the advantage of simplifying the policymaking process but also makes it a little too simple and neat. In reality, the various stages often overlap as a policy is fine-tuned. Sometimes the stages occur out of sequence, as when agenda setting leads directly to evaluation. For instance, when the issue of hunger became a part of the national policy agenda in the 1960s, as discussed in Chapter 10, existing nutrition and welfare programs were evaluated to discover why they were not reaching hungry children, and this approach effectively bypassed the policy design and implementation stages. Nevertheless, viewing the policymaking process as a cycle enables us to see how policies evolve over time.

The discussion that follows focuses on policymaking at the national level because the laws that arise from federal policy may affect some aspects of community nutrition practice. As you study this section, think of ways in which the policy cycle can be applied to lower levels of government, such as your state or municipal government, and to institutions, such as your college, university, or place of employment. As a student, for example, your life is affected by your school's policies on course requirements for graduation, residency, use of campus library electronic databases, and many other activities. Consider how the policy cycle described here reflects the process by which your school formulated its policies.

FIGURE 6-1 The Policy Cycle

Source: Adapted from W. Lyons, J. M. Scheb II, and L. E. Richardson, Jr., *American Government: Politics and Political Culture* (Eagan, MN: West, 1995), 468. Copyright © 1995 West Publishing Company. Used by permission of Wadsworth Publishing Co.

1. **Problem definition and agenda setting.** The first step in the policy process is to convince other people that a public problem exists. For example, the fact that more than 42 million people in the United States do not have medical insurance could be seen as either a public problem or a private (individual) problem.[9] Before a problem can be addressed, then, a majority of people must be convinced that it is a public issue. A clear statement of the problem is derived by asking questions: Who is experiencing the problem? Why

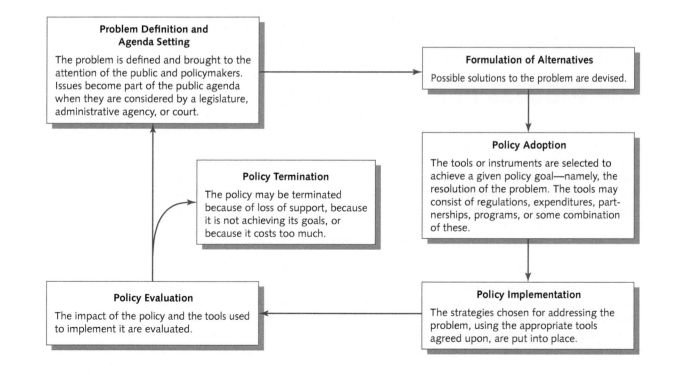

did this problem develop? How severe is the problem? What actions have been taken in the past to address the problem? What action can be taken now to solve the problem? What resources exist to help alleviate the problem?[10] The manner in which the problem is defined will probably determine whether it succeeds in capturing the public's attention and whether action is taken to address it.

Once a problem is defined and gains attention, it is placed on the **policy agenda**. This agenda is not a written document or book but a set of controversial issues that exist within society. Agenda setting is a process in which people concerned about an issue work to bring the issue to the attention of the general public and policymakers. Getting policymakers to place a problem on the official agenda can be difficult. An issue may be so sensitive that policymakers or public attitudes work to keep it from reaching the agenda-setting stage. Consider, for example, the question of whether gay couples should be allowed to marry legally or adopt children. In the absence of widespread public support, some gay couples have taken this issue to the courts as a means of accessing the policy agenda. In other situations, an issue may be perceived as a problem only by a small number of people who lack the political clout required to get the issue onto the agenda. Sometimes a major catastrophe, such as an earthquake, assassination, riot, or unusual human event, triggers a public outcry and pushes an issue onto the policy agenda. When CBS aired its television report "Hunger in America" in May 1968, the problem of malnutrition and the failure of major government feeding programs for families became vividly real. Millions saw the televised images of starving and dying American children. The public reaction was swift and angry, pushing Congress to form the Senate Select Committee on Nutrition and Human Needs to investigate hunger and malnutrition among America's poor.[11]

> " *Public opinion in this country is everything.* "
>
> —Abraham Lincoln

How are issues placed on the policy agenda? The first step is to build widespread public interest for the issue that deserves government attention. One of the most effective ways to build public interest and support for an issue is to work through the media—radio, television, newspapers, and the Internet. Because the media can both create and reflect public issues, they are one of the most powerful tools for setting the public policy agenda. For example, the publication in 1962 of Rachel Carson's book *Silent Spring* opened the public's eyes to environmental dangers and launched the modern environmental movement.[12] UNICEF's success at getting newspapers and magazines to carry the message about childhood malnutrition is another example of using the media to increase public awareness of an issue and seek support for efforts to address it. UNICEF also uses the Internet to keep the issue in the public eye. Its website (*www.unicef.org*) provides information about its annual *State of the World's Children* reports. The Professional Focus at the end of this chapter offers tips on developing media skills and enhancing your image and visibility as a professional. The more that food and nutrition practitioners succeed in developing a media presence, the better the chances of gaining support for issues critical to nutrition and public health.

However, it is not enough merely to bring the issue to the attention of policymakers and the public through the media. The issue must get onto the **institutional agenda** defined by each legislative body of the government (e.g., Congress, state legislatures, city councils). This is accomplished by winning support for the issue among what some political scientists have called the "iron triangles," because they often exert enormous control over the policymaking process. An iron triangle is made up of three powerful participants in the policymaking process: interest groups, congressional committees or subcommittees, and administrative agencies. These groups are not formal, recognized units of government; rather, they consist of anyone interested in policy issues and outcomes, such as

Policy agenda The set of problems to which policymakers give their attention.

Institutional agenda The issues that are the subject of public policy.

A photograph such as this one can be an effective method of bringing an urgent issue to the public's attention. Convincing people that a problem exists is the first step in the policy process.

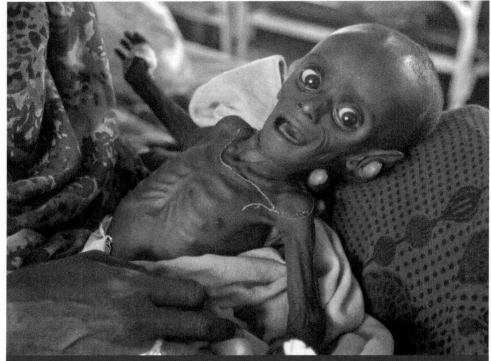

AP Images/Schalk van Zuydam

government administrators, members of Congress and their staffs, bureau chiefs, interest groups, professionals (e.g., dietitians, physicians, bankers, real estate agents), university faculty members, governors, and members of state and local governments, coalitions, and networks.

2. **Formulation of alternatives.** Possible solutions to the problem are devised in this, the most creative phase of the policymaking process. How can the WIC program be modified to meet the needs of working women? How can school food programs be improved to feed more children and teenagers? Should families experiencing food insecurity be given greater access to food banks and food programs? Or should they receive job training to help them increase their income?

Discussion of possible solutions to public problems—what is sometimes called "policy formulation"—often begins at the grassroots level. **Interest groups**, **coalitions**, and **networks** of experts and people interested in the issue craft a set of possible solutions and bring them forward to policymakers, who continue the discussion of solutions in legislative assemblies, government agencies, other institutions, congressional hearings, town hall meetings, and even focus groups. These forums give the general public an opportunity to express its opinions about possible solutions, potential costs and benefits of various alternatives, and the "best" course of action. A key consideration is whether the best proposed solution—in other words, the action that will become policy—is reasonable. The act of making policy needs to be coupled with the process of implementing it. Policies designed to address food- and nutrition-related problems are nearly always workable, although they change as circumstances, information, and priorities change.

In the United States, policy is formulated by the legislative, executive, and judicial branches of the government at the national, state, and local levels. Three examples of national policies formulated by Congress are the Federal Food, Drug, and Cosmetic Act, the legislation

Interest groups A body of people acting in an organized manner to advance shared political interests.

Coalitions (alliance) A group of individuals or organizations working together in a common effort toward a common goal to make more effective and efficient use of resources.

Networks Individuals or organizations who share information, ideas, resources, or goals to accomplish individual or group goals.

that regulates the U.S. food supply;[13] the Nutrition Labeling and Education Act (NLEA), the legislation that specifies national uniform food labels and mandatory nutrition labeling information on nearly all foods marketed to U.S. consumers;[14] and the Dietary Supplement Health Education Act (DSHEA), the legislation that severely restricts the FDA's authority over dietary and herbal supplements. The DSHEA legislation is discussed later in this chapter.

3. **Policy adoption.** In this step, the tools or instruments for dealing with the problem are chosen. Examples of policy "tools" include regulations, cash grants, loans, tax breaks, certification, fines, price controls, quotas, public promotion, public investment, and government-sponsored programs.[15] These tools are wielded by federal, state, and municipal departments and agencies that are responsible for implementing policy.

At the federal level, two departments are important for our purposes: the Department of Health and Human Services (DHHS) and the U.S. Department of Agriculture (USDA). The mission of the DHHS is to protect the health of all Americans and provide essential human services, especially for those who are least able to help themselves. Its organizational chart is shown in **Figure 6-2**. The DHHS includes more than 300 programs covering a broad spectrum of activities from conducting health and social science research and preventing outbreaks of infectious disease to ensuring food and drug safety and providing financial assistance for low-income families and older Americans. The DHHS works closely with state and local governments, and many of its services are provided by state or county agencies. The Public Health Service operating division of the DHHS includes the National Institutes of Health, which houses 27 separate health institutes and centers such as the National Library of Medicine and supports about 38,000 research projects worldwide; the Food and Drug Administration, which works to ensure the safety of the food supply and cosmetics, and the safety and efficacy of pharmaceuticals; and the Centers for Disease Control and Prevention, which collects national health data and works to prevent and control disease. The Human Resources operating division includes the Centers for Medicare and Medicaid Services (CMS), which administers the Medicare and Medicaid programs; the Administration for Children and Families, which administers some 60 programs for low-income children and families, including the Head Start program; and the Administration for Community Living (including the Administration on Aging), which provides services to older adults.[16]

The USDA is also concerned with some important aspects of public health and policymaking. Its overall mission is to provide leadership on food, agriculture, natural resources, and related issues. The USDA seeks to enhance the quality of life for all Americans by working to ensure a safe, affordable, nutritious, and accessible food supply; reducing food insecurity in America; and supporting the production of agriculture. Its organization is illustrated in **Figure 6-3**. The USDA's food safety mission strives to make sure that the nation's meat and poultry supply is safe for consumption, wholesome, and packaged and labeled properly. The agency responsible for carrying out this mission is the Food Safety and Inspection Service.

The mission of the USDA's Food, Nutrition, and Consumer Services is to ensure access to nutritious, wholesome food and healthful diets for all Americans and to provide dietary guidance to help them make healthful food choices. Two agencies within this division are important to community nutritionists. The Food and Nutrition Service administers food and nutrition assistance programs such as the Supplemental Nutrition Assistance Program (SNAP—formerly the Food Stamp Program) and the National School Lunch Program (described along with other programs in Section Two of this book). The Center for Nutrition Policy and Promotion coordinates nutrition policy within the USDA and provides national leadership in educating consumers about nutrition. This center works with the Department of Health and Human Services to review, revise, and disseminate the *Dietary Guidelines for Americans* (described in Chapter 7).

The mission of the USDA's Research, Education, and Economics division is to develop innovative technologies that improve food production and food safety. This area includes

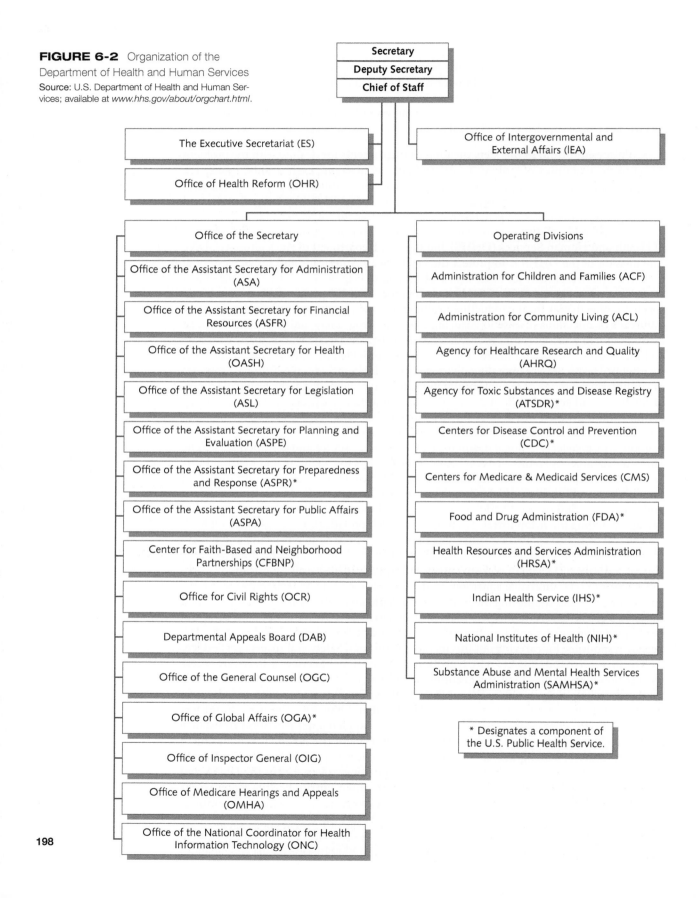

FIGURE 6-2 Organization of the Department of Health and Human Services

Source: U.S. Department of Health and Human Services; available at *www.hhs.gov/about/orgchart.html*.

Secretary
Deputy Secretary
Chief of Staff

The Executive Secretariat (ES)

Office of Intergovernmental and External Affairs (IEA)

Office of Health Reform (OHR)

Office of the Secretary

Office of the Assistant Secretary for Administration (ASA)

Office of the Assistant Secretary for Financial Resources (ASFR)

Office of the Assistant Secretary for Health (OASH)

Office of the Assistant Secretary for Legislation (ASL)

Office of the Assistant Secretary for Planning and Evaluation (ASPE)

Office of the Assistant Secretary for Preparedness and Response (ASPR)*

Office of the Assistant Secretary for Public Affairs (ASPA)

Center for Faith-Based and Neighborhood Partnerships (CFBNP)

Office for Civil Rights (OCR)

Departmental Appeals Board (DAB)

Office of the General Counsel (OGC)

Office of Global Affairs (OGA)*

Office of Inspector General (OIG)

Office of Medicare Hearings and Appeals (OMHA)

Office of the National Coordinator for Health Information Technology (ONC)

Operating Divisions

Administration for Children and Families (ACF)

Administration for Community Living (ACL)

Agency for Healthcare Research and Quality (AHRQ)

Agency for Toxic Substances and Disease Registry (ATSDR)*

Centers for Disease Control and Prevention (CDC)*

Centers for Medicare & Medicaid Services (CMS)

Food and Drug Administration (FDA)*

Health Resources and Services Administration (HRSA)*

Indian Health Service (IHS)*

National Institutes of Health (NIH)*

Substance Abuse and Mental Health Services Administration (SAMHSA)*

* Designates a component of the U.S. Public Health Service.

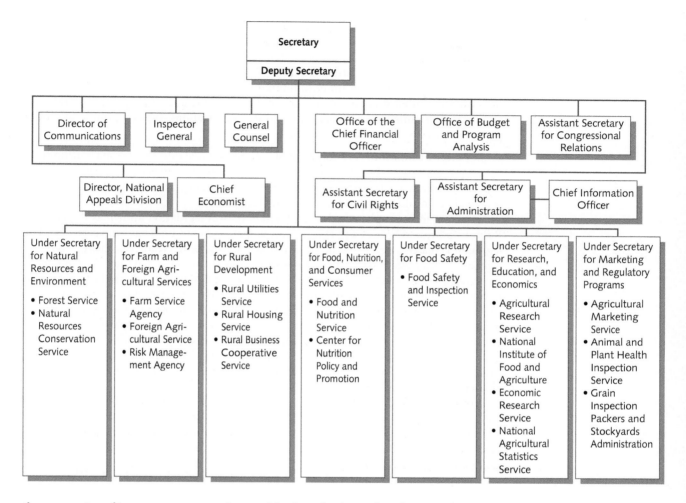

FIGURE 6-3

Organization of the U.S. Department of Agriculture

Source: U.S. Department of Agriculture; available at *www.usda.gov.*

three agencies of interest to community nutritionists: the Agricultural Research Service, which works to solve broad agricultural problems and ensure an adequate supply of food for all consumers; the National Institute of Food and Agriculture (NIFA—formerly the Cooperative State Research, Education, and Extension Service), which strives to develop national priorities in research, extension services, and higher education; and the Economic Research Service, which produces economic and social science data to help Congress make decisions about the practice of agriculture and rural development. The main research division of the USDA is the Agricultural Research Service. It oversees research related to nutrient needs throughout the life cycle, food trends, the composition of the diet, nutrient interactions, and the bioavailability of nutrients. It compiles data on the nutrient composition of foods through its Nutrient Databank; the food values are published electronically in the USDA National Nutrient Database for Standard Reference series.

Policy adoption also occurs at the state level. States are the basic unit for the delivery of public health services and the implementation of health policies. They determine the form and function of local health agencies, select and appoint local health personnel, identify local health problems, and guarantee a minimum level of essential health services. State and federal public health services have a similar organization.

4. **Policy implementation.** After the best solution to the problem has been agreed upon and the tools for dealing with the problem have been chosen, the policy is modified to fit the needs, resources, and wants of the implementing agencies and the intended clientele.

Implementation is the process of putting a policy into action. In Tacoma, Washington, for example, the Tahoma Food Policy Coalition, a nonprofit organization, implemented a policy to promote a sustainable food system. Its policy supported a community coalition called the Bridging Urban Gardens Society (BUGS), which helps create "greening" projects such as organic gardens on unused, littered vacant lots.[17] The implementers of public policy in the United States number in the millions and include employees of federal, state, and local governments who work with private organizations, interest groups, and other parties to carry out government policy.

5. **Policy evaluation.** As soon as public policies move into the agenda-setting stage, the evaluation process begins. The purpose of policy evaluation is to determine whether a program is achieving its stated goals and reaching its intended audience, what the program is actually accomplishing, and who is benefiting from it.

Consider, for example, whether the welfare reform legislation known as the Personal Responsibility and Work Opportunity Reconciliation Act of 1996 has been a success. This legislation created a new program—Temporary Assistance to Needy Families (TANF)—to replace the old welfare "safety net" system and dramatically changed the requirements for receiving assistance. To measure TANF's success, the Children's Defense Fund and other nonprofit social justice organizations have conducted a number of post-welfare-reform surveys.[18] Surveys of former welfare recipients indicate that many working parents had been unable to pay rent, buy food, or afford medical care and had had their telephone and electric service disconnected. As a result, hunger advocacy groups now seek legislation guaranteeing a living wage, access to health care, and affordable housing, along with the assistance that enables people to move successfully from welfare to work (e.g., help with childcare, transportation, and education).

From almost the moment of their conception, public policies undergo both formal and informal evaluations by citizens, legislators, administrative agencies, the news media, academicians, research firms, auditors, and interest groups. Ideally, public policies should be evaluated *after* they have been implemented, using the best available research methods and according to a systematic plan. In the real world, policy evaluation seldom works this way. Instead, it is often undertaken without a preconceived plan and before the strategy chosen to solve a problem has been fully implemented.

6. **Policy termination.** A policy or program may be terminated for any of several reasons: the public need was met, the nature of the problem changed, government no longer had a mandate in the area, the policy lost political support, private agencies relieved the need, a political system or subgovernment ceased to function, or the policy was too costly. Determining when a policy should be terminated is somewhat subjective. At what point do you decide that the public's need has been met? What measures do you use to conclude that the problem was solved? Typically, policy termination represents a process of adjustment in which the policymakers shift their focus to other policy concerns. Whereas some policy systems go out of existence, others survive and expand, bringing the policy cycle full circle to a redefinition of the public problem.[19]

The People Who Make Policy

The stages of the policy cycle outlined in Figure 6-1 do not correspond directly to the agencies and institutions involved in making government policy. We tend to assume that policy is formulated by legislatures and implemented by administrative agencies, such as the Public Health Service. In fact, administrative agencies sometimes formulate policy and legislatures become involved in policy implementation. **Table 6-1** lists roles of various levels of government in food policymaking.

TABLE 6-1 Role of Various Levels of Government in Food Policymaking

ISSUE	FEDERAL LEVEL	STATE LEVEL	LOCAL LEVEL
Food Safety	The Food and Drug Administration (FDA) creates the FDA *Food Code*, which recommends (but does not require) food safety provisions for retail stores and restaurants. It is not mandatory but has been adopted in some form by most states.[a] The federal government oversees food safety for products moving in interstate commerce, as well as regulating poultry and meat processing, monitoring general food safety, and exercising its food recall authority.[b]	State governments implement laws and regulations affecting restaurants and retail stores, based on federal guidance. Most states adopt a modified version of the FDA *Food Code*. States can create their own meat and poultry processing inspection regime, but it must be at least as stringent as the federal regime.	Local public health departments are often tasked with enforcing state food safety requirements. Some local governments also have their own set of food safety ordinances applicable to local restaurants or grocery stores.
Food Labeling	The federal government regulates ingredient and nutrition labeling for all packaged foods that travel in interstate commerce.[c] However, state and local governments can choose to require menu labeling or other labeling for items not included in the federal laws. Federal law also regulates nutrition labeling of certain chain retail food establishments and chain vending machine operators.[d]	States are preempted from enacting labeling laws for packaged foods or certain chain restaurants/vending machines, as these are regulated by federal law. However, states may: require labeling for non-packaged foods, require labeling for non-chain restaurants, pass labeling rules for foods that do not cross state lines, and require other label information (e.g., Alaska requires the labeling of farm-raised salmon products).[e]	If allowed under state law, local governments can pass some food labeling rules for foods not covered under federal law. For example, local governments can require labeling for non-chain restaurants.
Food Assistance Benefits	Most food assistance programs, like SNAP, WIC, etc., are authorized and funded at the federal level, though states may contribute funds for program administration or to increase the amount of benefits available to participants.	State governments are responsible for administering food assistance programs in terms of authorizing participants and, in some cases, vendors. States sometimes contribute additional funds to the programs.	Local governments generally do not play a role in administering food assistance programs, but they can encourage their residents to participate in the programs, which are often underutilized, or provide incentives to those who purchase healthy options with their benefits.
Geographic Preference in Food Procurement	Food purchased using federal dollars, such as meals under the National School Lunch Program (NSLP), must follow federal procurement guidelines. Federal law now authorizes schools using NSLP dollars to prefer food grown locally.[f] Programs using state or local dollars do not need to follow federal rules.	State agencies or institutions using state funds must follow state procurement guidelines. An increasing number of states have tailored their procurement regulations to encourage local purchasing by state agencies/institutions.[g] When using federal money, federal rules still apply.	Local agencies, schools, and institutions may prefer local food when spending federal funds, as authorized under federal law.[f] When using state funds or local funds, they may give preference to local food if authorized under the relevant state or local authority.

[a] *Real Progress in Food Code Adoptions*, FDA (July 1, 2011).

[b] Three government agencies share responsibility for federal food safety. The USDA's Food Safety and Inspection Service (FSIS) inspects meat and poultry processing and reviews product labels. The FDA monitors the safety and labeling of most non-meat and processed foods, and licenses food-use chemicals other than pesticides. The EPA registers pesticides and sets pesticide tolerances that are enforced by the FDA or the FSIS.

[c] Nutrition Labeling and Education Act of 1990, 21 U.S.C. § 343-1 (2012).

[d] The nutrition-labeling provision was initially enacted as section 4205, Pub L. No. 111-148, § 4205, 124 Stat. 119, 573 (2010), and was codified at 21 U.S.C. § 343(q)(5).

[e] Alaska Food, Drug, and Cosmetic Act, ALASKA STAT. § 17.20.040(a)(12) (2012).

[f] Geographic Preference Option for the Procurement of Unprocessed Agricultural Products in Child Nutrition Programs, 7 C.F.R. §§ 210, 215, 220, 225, 226 (2012).

[g] At least twelve states have passed legislation allowing purchasing preferences for in-state agricultural products. *State Farm to School Legislation*, National Farm to School Network, (Nov. 2, 2010).

Source: Adapted from E. B. Leib, A. Condra, and coauthors, *Good Laws, Good Food: Putting state food policy to work for our communities*, Harvard Law School Food Law and Policy Clinic and Mark Winne Associates, November 2012.

This point leads us to ask, "Who makes policy?" The authorities who "make policy" may be executives, administrators, or committees of an organization or company; elected officials; officers and employees of municipal, state, or federal agencies; members of Congress and state legislatures; and even **street-level bureaucrats**: welfare workers, public health nutritionists and nurses, police officers, schoolteachers, housing authority managers, judges, and many other people working in government agencies. In the course of carrying out their jobs, these street-level bureaucrats make policy decisions daily by interpreting government laws and regulations for citizens. For example, as a community nutritionist, you will find yourself making policy decisions when you tailor a program to meet a particular client's needs or when you recommend a calcium supplement for a client on the basis of your interpretation of the dietary reference intakes (DRIs).

Street-level bureaucrats
Individuals within government who have direct contact with citizens.

Legitimizing Policy

Once it has been decided that a policy should be put into effect, a choice must be made about *how* it will be implemented. This is not a trivial decision. Consider, for example, the decision by the FDA to allow food product labels to carry health claims such as those listed in **Table 6-2**. Some consumers, scientists, and food companies objected to this policy, believing that some health claims on food product labels might distort research findings or be extravagant in presenting evidence of a link between food components and health. Others believed that the policy would help the public make healthful food choices. Thus, a policy may be perceived as benefiting some citizens and working to the detriment of others. Because it is impossible to achieve universal agreement on a policy and its effects, careful attention must be given to the process by which policy decisions are made. This is the point at which legitimizing policy is important.

Legitimacy is "the belief on the part of citizens that the current government represents a proper form of government and a willingness on the part of those citizens to accept the decrees of that government as legal and authoritative."[20] In this sense, legitimacy is mainly in the mind, for it depends on a majority of the population's accepting that the government has the right to govern. In the case of the FDA's health claim policy, the appearance of health claims on food labels indicates that consumers and food companies accept the FDA's *authority* to allow this action.[21]

TABLE 6-2

A Sampling of Health Claims Currently Authorized by the U.S. Food and Drug Administration under the Nutrition Labeling and Education Act of 1990

DIET–DISEASE RELATIONSHIP	MODEL CLAIM
Dietary saturated fat and cholesterol and risk of coronary heart disease	While many factors affect heart disease, diets low in saturated fat and cholesterol may reduce the risk of this disease.
Fruits and vegetables and cancer	Low-fat diets rich in fruits and vegetables may reduce the risk of some types of cancer, a disease associated with many factors.
Folate and neural tube birth defects	Healthful diets with adequate folate may reduce a woman's risk of having a child with a brain or spinal cord birth defect.
Foods that contain fiber from whole oat products and coronary heart disease	Diets low in saturated fat and cholesterol that include soluble fiber from whole oats may reduce the risk of heart disease.
Whole-grain foods and risk of heart disease and certain cancers	Diets rich in whole-grain foods and other plant foods and low in total fat, saturated fat, and cholesterol may reduce the risk of heart disease and some cancers.

Source: U.S. Food and Drug Administration, Center for Food Safety and Applied Nutrition, *A Food Labeling Guide*, Appendix C, available at *www.fda.gov/Food/IngredientsPackagingLabeling/default.htm*.

Government, then, must somehow legitimize each policy choice. Several mechanisms exist for legitimizing policies: the legislative process; the regulatory process; the court system; and various procedures for direct democracy, such as referenda, which put sensitive issues directly before the people. In the next section, we explore the legislative and regulatory processes in greater detail because most policies in the areas of health, food, and nutrition arise through these mechanisms.*

The Legislative and Regulatory Process

Governments can use any number of instruments to influence the lives of their citizens: taxes and tax incentives, services such as defense and education, use of subsidies to support commodity production, unemployment benefits, and laws, to name only a few. Laws are a unique tool of government. In the United States, we traditionally associate lawmaking with Congress, the primary legislative body. It is Congress that sets policy and supplies the basic legislation that governs our lives.

Laws and Regulations

The laws passed by Congress tend to be vague. A law defines the broad scope of the policy intended by Congress. For example, the Special Supplemental Nutrition Program for Women, Infants, and Children (WIC) was authorized by Public Law 92-433 and approved on September 26, 1972. This law authorized a two-year, $20 million pilot program for each of the fiscal years 1973 and 1974. It gave the secretary of agriculture the authority to make cash grants to state health departments or comparable agencies to provide supplemental foods to pregnant and lactating women, infants, and children up to four years of age who were considered at "nutritional risk" by competent professionals. (The WIC program presently covers children up to five years of age.) As written, this law, like most others, was too vague to implement. It did not define or specify which professionals would determine the eligibility of clients. It did not define the concept of "nutritional risk" and other eligibility requirements, the method by which clients would obtain food products, or other aspects of the proposed program. Sorting out these details was left to the USDA.

Thus, once a law is passed, it is up to administrative bodies such as the USDA to interpret the law and provide the detailed regulations or rules that put the policy into effect. These regulations are sometimes called "secondary legislation." The total volume of this activity is enormous, as is apparent in the size of the *Federal Register*, a weekly publication that contains all regulations and proposed regulations, and the *Code of Federal Regulations (CFR)*, a compendium of all regulations currently in force. When the WIC program was started, the details of the regulations were not published in the *Federal Register* until July 11, 1973, nearly nine months after Congress passed the law. Over time, new laws and amendments to the existing law were enacted to increase the amount of money allocated for the WIC program, specify the means by which the program should be implemented, and authorize the continuation of the program for additional budget years.[22] (A detailed discussion of the WIC program appears in Chapter 11.)

---

* The use of the court system for legitimizing policy in the nutrition arena is not discussed in this chapter, although it is important in formulating food and nutrition policy. Regulations are challenged through the court system. When the FDA issued a final rule establishing nutrition labeling regulations in 1973, a portion of the regulations dealing with special dietary foods was challenged in the courts by the National Nutritional Foods Association (see *National Nutritional Foods Association v. FDA* and *National Nutritional Foods Association v. Kennedy*, as cited in the *Federal Register* 1990 [July 19]: 29476–77).

How an Idea Becomes Law

All levels of government pass laws. (At the local level, laws are sometimes called ordinances or bylaws.) The process by which an idea becomes law is complicated. It may take many months, or even years, for an idea or issue to work its way onto the policy agenda. Then, once it reaches the legislative body empowered to act on it, the formal rules and procedures of that body can delay decision making on a proposed bill or scuttle it altogether, especially at the end of the legislative sessions. Lewis Carroll, writing in *Alice in Wonderland*, could have been speaking of the U.S. Congress when he wrote, "I don't think they play at all fairly, and they quarrel so dreadfully one can't hear oneself speak—and they don't seem to have any rules in particular: at least, if there are, nobody attends to them—and you've no idea how confusing it is."[23]

The general process by which laws are made is outlined in **Figure 6-4**, which shows the path a bill would take on its way through Congress. The process is much the same for bills introduced into state legislatures. The process begins when a concerned citizen, a group of citizens, or an organization brings an issue to the attention of a legislative representative at the local, state, or national level. Typically, the issue is presented to private attorneys or the staff of the legislative counsel, who draft the bill in the proper language and style. A bill is introduced by sending it to the clerk's desk, where it is numbered and printed. It must have a member as its sponsor. Simple bills are designated as either "H.R." or "S.," depending on the house of origin. For instance, the Healthy, Hunger-Free Kids Act of 2010 was designated S. 3307, indicating that the bill was introduced into the U.S. Senate. When the bill is introduced, the bill's title is entered in the *Congressional Journal* and included in the *Congressional Record*.[24]

FIGURE 6-4 How a Bill Becomes Law

When a bill is introduced in the Senate (or House), it is assigned to a committee. The committee usually refers the bill to a subcommittee for hearings, revision, and approval. The subcommittee sends the bill back to the full committee, which may write revisions or amendments to the bill. The full committee (or Rules Committee in the House) decides whether to send it to the floor of its chamber for approval. The leaders of the chamber then schedule the bill for debate and vote. The bill is debated, amendments may be offered and voted on, and a final vote is taken.

Note: If the two chambers pass different versions of the bill, then a conference committee, composed of members of each chamber, will work out a compromise bill. The bill is returned to each chamber for a vote on the revised bill. The president signs or vetoes the bill. If signed, the bill becomes a law; if the president vetoes the bill, it cannot become law unless it is passed by a two-thirds vote of both chambers.

Source: Adapted from W. Lyons, J. M. Scheb II, and L. E. Richardson, Jr., *American Government: Politics and Political Culture* (Eagan, MN: West, 1995), 360.

Copyright © 1995 West Publishing Company. Used by permission of Wadsworth Publishing Co.

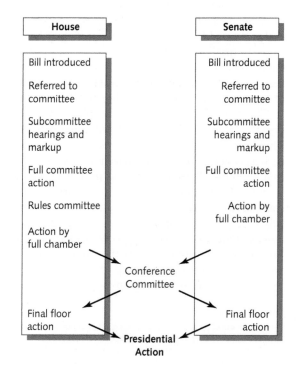

As bills work their way through the House and Senate, they are considered by several committees and subcommittees, which may hold public hearings and seek the testimony of interested persons or experts before deciding whether to move the bill forward. The bill is revised during a **markup session**. If the bill approved by the Senate is identical to the one passed by the House, it is sent to the president to be signed. If the two versions differ, a joint House–Senate conference committee is formed to modify the bill by mutual agreement. Once both houses agree on the compromise bill, it is sent to the president, who may sign it into law, allow it to become law without his or her signature, or veto it. When Congress overrides the president's veto by a two-thirds majority vote in both houses, the bill becomes law without the president's signature.[25] (In state legislatures, of course, the bill is sent to the governor.) When the bill is signed into law by the president, it becomes an act and is given the designation "P.L.," which stands for Public Law, and a number: the first two or three digits indicate the number of the congressional session in which the law was enacted, and the remaining digits represent the number of the bill. Recall that the bill authorizing the WIC supplemental feeding program became Public Law 92-433 (i.e., bill number 433, enacted by the 92nd Congress). **Table 6-3** lists the typical opportunities for input in the legislative process.

Before a law enacted by Congress goes into effect, it is reviewed by the appropriate federal agency, which is responsible for issuing guidelines or regulations that detail

Markup session A congressional committee session during which a bill is put into its final form before being reported out of committee.

BILL INTRODUCTION/SPONSORSHIP

State or federal legislators can be encouraged to introduce a bill to address a specific issue or to co-sponsor a bill introduced by another legislator. Obtaining a large number of co-sponsors on a bill is one strategy for gaining attention and credibility for an issue.

SUBCOMMITTEE

The most important time for constituent involvement is the subcommittee stage. Legislators are not yet committed to specific bills or legislative language. Grassroots advocates can communicate their positions on the issue and suggest specific provisions or language. Action by constituents of subcommittee members can be very effective at this point.

COMMITTEE

Grassroots advocacy at the committee stage is also important. Communications may focus on supporting or opposing specific language developed by the subcommittee; encouraging legislators to sponsor amendments; and asking committee members to vote for or against the bill. Again, action by constituents of committee members can be effective.

FLOOR

Constituent communication with all senators and representatives is important when it comes to the floor vote. Grassroots efforts at this stage focus on encouraging a legislator to vote either for or against the bill, to sponsor a floor amendment, or to vote for or against a floor amendment offered by another legislator.

CONFERENCE

Opportunities are more limited at the conference stage. The conference committee works out the differences between similar bills passed by the House and Senate. Communication at this point may influence whether the House or the Senate provision is accepted in the compromise bill.

FLOOR

Once a conference committee has worked out differences, passage of a bill is normally routine and is not affected by further constituent communication.

TABLE 6-3

Opportunities for Input in the Legislative Process

Sources: Data from "The Legislative Process," *Influencing Public Policy at the Grassroots, A Guide for Hospital and Health System Leaders* (American Hospital Association, 1999), 14; and E. Winterfeldt, "Influencing Public Policy," *Topics in Clinical Nutrition* 16 (2001): 10.

how the law will be implemented and what penalties may be imposed if the law is violated. These regulations, such as the final rule shown in **Figure 6-5**, are published in the *Federal Register*. Because federal law requires that the public have the opportunity to comment on an agency's proposed guidelines, the agency first issues "proposed or interim regulations" (**Figure 6-6**). During the comment period that follows the publication of proposed regulations, the general public, experts, companies, and interested organizations submit their written comments and, in some cases, present their views at public hearings. Comments are taken for 30 to 120 days, depending on the type and complexity of the regulations. At the end of the comment period, the agency reviews all comments, both positive and negative, before issuing its final regulations, which are incorporated into the *CFR*. The *CFR* and the *Federal Register* are available at most local libraries and county courthouses; recent rules and regulations can be found on the Internet. (See the list of government Internet addresses at the end of this chapter.)

As an example of the interplay between state and federal government, California passed a menu-labeling law in 2008 that required chain restaurants of a certain size to include calorie and other nutritional information on their menus and display boards.[26] At that time, this was an area of law in which the Nutrition Labeling and Education Act (NLEA) did not preempt states from taking this kind of action. Two years later, in the Patient Protection and Affordable Care Act of 2010, Congress included provisions to require the same kind of menu labeling of chain restaurants on a national scale.[27] Now that Congress has passed a law on this issue, states are preempted from regulating menu labeling at the chain restaurants that fall under the federal law. However, states may still require menu labeling at other types of restaurants within the state. California's lead on menu labeling is a good example of how policy change on a state level can lead to national policy change, but it also shows a place where state rules can be preempted by federal ones.[28]

FIGURE 6-5 A Portion of a Final Rule Published by the Food and Drug Administration in the *Federal Register*
The Patient Protection and Affordable Care Act of 2010 requires restaurants and similar retail food establishments with 20 or more locations to list calorie content information for standard menu items on restaurant menus and menu boards, including drive-through menu boards. Other nutrient information—total calories, fat, saturated fat, cholesterol, sodium, total carbohydrates, sugars, fiber, and total protein—has to be made available in writing upon request. This mandate also requires vending machine operators who own or operate 20 or more vending machines to disclose calorie content for certain items.
Source: *Federal Register*.

DEPARTMENT OF HEALTH AND HUMAN SERVICES

Food and Drug Administration

21 CFR Part 11 and 101

[Docket No. FDA–2011–F–0172]

RIN 0910–AG57

Food Labeling: Nutrition Labeling of Standard Menu Items in Restaurants and Similar Retail Food Establishments

AGENCY: Food and Drug Administration, HHS.

ACTION: Final rule.

SUMMARY: To implement the nutrition labeling provisions of the Patient Protection and Affordable Care Act of 2010 (Affordable Care Act or ACA), the Food and Drug Administration (FDA or we) is requiring disclosure of certain nutrition information for standard menu items in certain restaurants and retail food establishments. The ACA, in part, amended the Federal Food, Drug, and Cosmetic Act (the FD&C Act), among other things, to require restaurants and similar retail food establishments that are part of a chain with 20 or more locations doing business under the same name and offering for sale substantially the same menu items to provide calorie and other nutrition information for standard menu items, including food on display and self-service food. Under provisions of the ACA, restaurants and similar retail food establishments not otherwise covered by the law may elect to become subject to these Federal requirements by registering every other year with FDA. Providing accurate, clear, and consistent nutrition information, including the calorie content of foods, in restaurants and similar retail food establishments will make such nutrition information available to consumers in a direct and accessible manner to enable consumers to make informed and healthful dietary choices.

DATES: *Effective date:* December 1, 2015.

DEPARTMENT OF AGRICULTURE

Food and Nutrition Service

7 CFR Parts 210 and 220

[FNS–2011–0019]

RIN 0584–AE09

National School Lunch Program and School Breakfast Program: Nutrition Standards for All Foods Sold in School as Required by the Healthy, Hunger-Free Kids Act of 2010

AGENCY: Food and Nutrition Service, USDA.

ACTION: Interim final rule.

SUMMARY: This interim final rule amends the National School Lunch Program and School Breakfast Program regulations to establish nutrition standards for all foods sold in schools, other than food sold under the lunch and breakfast programs. Amendments made by Section 208 of the Healthy, Hunger-Free Kids Act of 2010 (HHFKA) require the Secretary to establish nutrition standards for such foods, consistent with the most recent Dietary Guidelines for Americans, and directs the Secretary to consider authoritative scientific recommendations for nutrition standards; existing school nutrition standards, including voluntary standards for beverages and snack foods; current State and local standards; the practical application of the nutrition standards;

and special exemptions for infrequent school-sponsored fundraisers (other than fundraising through vending machines, school stores, snack bars, à la carte sales and any other exclusions determined by the Secretary). In addition, this interim final rule requires schools participating in the National School Lunch Program and School Breakfast Program to make potable water available to children at no charge in the place where lunches are served during the meal service, consistent with amendments made by section 203 of the HHFKA, and in the cafeteria during breakfast meal service. This interim final rule is expected to improve the health and well-being of the Nation's children, increase consumption of healthful foods during the school day, and create an environment that reinforces the development of healthy eating habits.

DATES: *Effective date:* This rule is effective August 27, 2013.

Implementation dates: State agencies, local educational agencies and school food authorities must implement the provisions of this rule as follows:

1. The *potable water* provisions in §§ 210.10(a)(1)(i) and 220.8(a)(1) must be implemented no later than August 27, 2013.

2. All other provisions of this interim final rule must be implemented beginning on July 1, 2014.

Comment Date: Written comments on this interim final rule must be received on or before October 28, 2013 to be assured of consideration.

FIGURE 6-6

A Portion of an Interim Final Rule Published by the USDA in the *Federal Register* with a Comment Period of 120 Days
On June 28, 2013, the USDA published an interim final rule establishing healthier nutrition standards for competitive foods. The "Smart Snacks in School" standards require schools to provide snacks and beverages with more whole grains, low-fat dairy, fruits, vegetables, and lean protein. They also set limits on fat, sugar, and salt. The USDA Smart Snacks nutrition standards apply to all competitive foods sold on school campus during the school day in public schools, private schools, and residential childcare institutions participating in the National School Lunch Program and School Breakfast Program.
Source: *Federal Register*.

The Federal Budget Process

Laws and regulations will have no effect unless there are funds to enforce them. Congress must enact bills to fund the programs and services mandated by federal legislation. The federal budget process has been described as "fractured, contentious, and chaotic," mainly because it forces the president and Congress to negotiate and agree on the problems that deserve top priority.[29] Budgets are designed to count and record income and expenditures, to demonstrate the government's intention regarding the funding (and, more important, the priority) of programs, and to control and shape the activities of government agencies. In its simplest form, the budget process has two stages: The president proposes a budget, and then Congress reacts to the president's proposal. The actual budget process is complex and cumbersome, with the final budget reflecting the distribution of power among competing concerns and groups within the current political system.[30]

The Language of the Budget
The budget is the president's financial plan for the federal government. It indicates how government funds have been raised and spent, and it proposes financial policy choices for the coming fiscal year and sometimes beyond. Financial policy, or fiscal policy, consists of the government's plan for taxation and spending on the economy in general.[31] The budget describes the government's **receipts or revenue**, **budget authority**, and **budget outlays**.

Receipts or revenue Amounts that the government expects to raise through taxes and fees.

Budget authority Amounts that government agencies are allowed to spend in implementing their programs.

Budget outlays Amounts actually paid out by government agencies.

Entitlements Programs that require the payment of benefits to all eligible people as established by law.

The budget allocates funds to cover two types of spending. *Mandatory spending* is required by law for **entitlements**—that is, programs that require the payment of benefits to any person who meets the eligibility requirements established by law.[32] For these programs, Congress provides whatever money is required from year to year to maintain benefits for eligible people. Many of these programs are indexed to the cost of living or similar measures, resulting in steady increases in benefits with inflation. Entitlements such as Social Security, Medicare, SNAP, agricultural subsidies, and veterans' benefits—so-called "uncontrollable expenditures"—command a major portion (about two-thirds) of the federal budget. The remainder of the federal budget consists of *discretionary spending*—that is, the budget choices that can be made in such areas as defense, energy assistance, nutrition assistance (e.g., the WIC program and nutrition programs for seniors), and education after the mandatory allocations have been made.[33]

Principles of Federal Budgeting The federal fiscal year begins on October 1 and runs through September 30 of the following year. The fiscal year is named for the year in which it ends; thus fiscal year 2017, or FY17, begins October 1, 2016, and ends September 30, 2017. (States and municipalities differ in terms of fiscal years; some follow a calendar year [January–December], some start on July 1, and others have two-year fiscal cycles.[34]) The fiscal year is the year in which money allocated in the budget is actually spent, but important steps must be taken both before and after the fiscal year that can affect the government's or an agency's programming. These steps form the budget cycle and include budget formulation, approval, implementation (sometimes called execution), and audit.

Figure 6-7 shows the federal budget cycle for FY17. The first step—budget formulation—begins 15 to 18 months before the start of the fiscal year. (For FY17, the budget process began in March 2015). During this phase, the Office of Management and Budget (OMB), the central budget office at the federal level, works with federal agencies to outline their funding projections for new and ongoing programs. After this consultation process, a single budget document is prepared and released, usually in September. This document is revised by the president in November and December and becomes the basis of his budget message—the most important statement of the administration's priorities and concerns—submitted to Congress in late January or early February.

Congress can approve, disapprove, or modify the president's budget proposal, adding or eliminating programs or altering methods of raising revenue. After the president's budget

FIGURE 6-7 Federal Budget Cycle for 2017 (FY17)

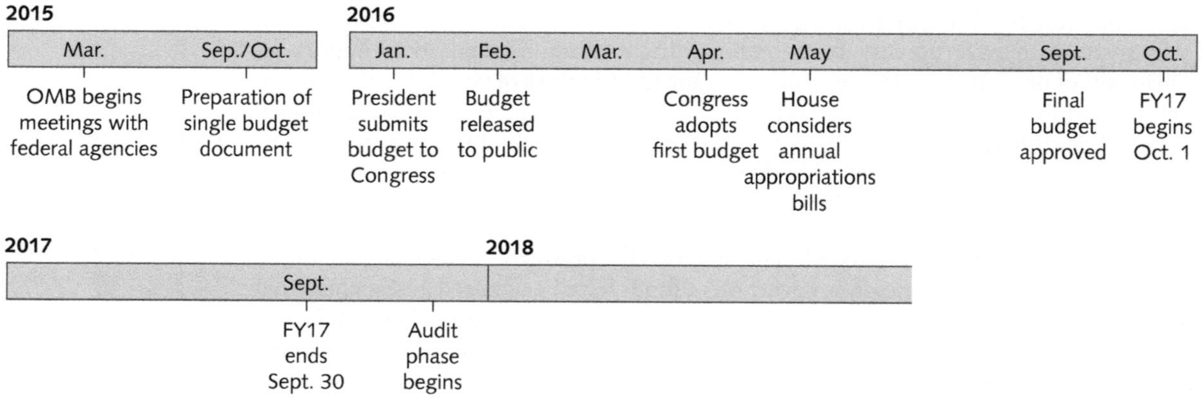

2015

Mar.	Sep./Oct.
OMB begins meetings with federal agencies	Preparation of single budget document

2016

Jan.	Feb.	Mar.	Apr.	May	Sept.	Oct.
President submits budget to Congress	Budget released to public		Congress adopts first budget	House considers annual appropriations bills	Final budget approved	FY17 begins Oct. 1

2017 / **2018**

Sept.	
FY17 ends Sept. 30	Audit phase begins

is submitted to Congress, it is reported to committees and subcommittees that must make decisions about budget authority, taxes, appropriations, and the reconciliation of the budget. In this process, Congress passes revenue bills that specify how funds to support the government's activities will be raised. In the House, the Ways and Means Committee has jurisdiction over revenue bills, a responsibility that makes it one of the most powerful committees in Congress. In terms of spending, congressional committees must pass bills to authorize government programs. An **authorization** defines the scope of a program and sets a ceiling on how much money can be spent on it. Before money can be released to a program, however, an **appropriation** bill must be passed. The appropriation for a program may cover a single year, several years, or an indefinite period of time.

Authorization A budget authorization provides agencies and departments with the legal ability to operate.

Appropriation A budget appropriation is the authority to spend money.

All revenue and appropriations bills passed by the House are forwarded to the Senate for consideration. Differences between the two houses are worked out in *conference committee*, and ultimately a *reconciliation bill* is passed. The end result of the authorization and appropriations work is that Congress adopts its version of the budget in a *budget resolution*. The first budget resolution is usually passed by May 15, and the second, after all spending bills have been passed, by September 15. If Congress is unable to pass a budget by the beginning of the fiscal year, it may adopt *continuing resolutions*, which authorize expenditures at the same level as in the previous fiscal year, until a budget agreement can be reached.

The fiscal year 2017 start date of October 1, 2016, marks the implementation stage of the budget cycle when government agencies execute the agreed-upon policies and programs. At the end of FY17, the audit phase begins, during which time the agencies' operations are examined and verified. In recent years, the audit phase has come to include performance auditing, or determining whether the agency's goals and objectives were met and whether the agency made the best use of its resources.

The Political Process

The complexities of the legislative and policymaking process present many challenges, and years may be required to reach a critical mass in public support for a policy change. As a case in point, consider that until 1906 no *federal* legislation regulated the nation's food supply and protected consumers against food adulteration, mislabeling, and false advertising. Even then, more than 25 years of persistent pressure from consumers and the agricultural community had been required to achieve this legislative milestone.[35] Check the box on the next page for a description of the imperfect process leading to the passage of the Food and Drugs Act.

A more recent example of the legislative process is the campaign by the Academy of Nutrition and Dietetics supporting medical nutrition therapy (MNT). MNT is a service provided by a registered dietitian or food and nutrition practitioner that includes counseling, nutrition support, and nutrition assessment and screening to improve people's health and quality of life. The Academy launched its MNT campaign in 1992 with the publication of a position paper on health care services and a report on the importance of including reimbursable nutrition services as part of any health care reform legislation.[36] It organized a grassroots campaign among its members to raise the visibility of the nutrition and dietetics profession on Capitol Hill and to lobby Congress to support MNT,[37] and it formed coalitions with other health-oriented organizations to develop a uniform position on health care reform.[38] Members of the Academy of Nutrition and Dietetics wrote letters to legislators, met with Washington lobbyists and key members of Congress,[39] and testified at a hearing held by the Health Subcommittee of the House Ways and Means Committee.[40]

> ## The Legislative Process in Real Life

Between 1880 and 1906, nearly 200 bills designed to protect consumers against food adulteration, misbranding, and false advertising were introduced into Congress without success. One such bill was submitted to the House and passed in 1904; the Senate began debating and eventually passed a similar bill, with amendments, in 1906. During the debates on the bill, Dr. Harvey W. Wiley, who was the chief chemist of the Department of Agriculture, testified about adulterated foods, bringing examples to show before Congress. At his urging, women who were concerned about food safety also lobbied Congress to pass the bill. When the bill went to the conference committee to iron out differences between the two houses, tensions were high. At one point, President Theodore Roosevelt felt compelled to lean on Congress and express his support for the pure foods bill. Finally, the bill passed both the House and Senate on June 27, 1906, and was signed into law by President Roosevelt on June 30, 1906. The Food and Drugs Act became law effective January 1, 1907.

Unfortunately, the law was defective. In the beginning, Congress failed to pass appropriation bills to provide the funds to enforce the law. Congress also failed to authorize the development of standards of food composition and quality, an omission that made it difficult for authorities to prove in court that a food was an imitation and not the genuine food product. Thus, because the Food and Drugs Act lacked teeth, food adulteration remained a threat to public health. Attempts to strengthen the law failed until 1938, when Congress passed the Federal Food, Drug, and Cosmetic Act, which was signed into law by President Franklin D. Roosevelt in 1938. It became effective one year later and is the primary legislation by which our food supply is regulated today.

Source: Adapted from H. W. Schultz, *Food Law Handbook* (Westport, CT: Avi, 1981), 3–21.

Advertisements, such as the one shown in **Figure 6-8**, helped educate consumers and policymakers about the importance and potential impact of MNT. The Academy's efforts resulted in the introduction of the Medical Nutrition Therapy Act (H.R. 2247 and S. 1964) during the 104th Congress. Although the House version had 91 co-sponsors and the Senate version had four co-sponsors, both bills expired when Congress adjourned.[41] Even so, the bills' support encouraged the Academy of Nutrition and Dietetics to continue its efforts. On April 17, 1997, the Medicare Medical Nutrition Therapy Act of 1997 (H.R. 1375 and S. 597) was introduced in the 105th Congress,[42] and the Academy launched a new effort, the Majority by March Campaign, to secure a majority of congressional members as co-sponsors of the legislation by March 1998.[43] During the following two years, the Academy of Nutrition and Dietetics continued to work for passage of legislation that, in the words of the Honorable John E. Ensign, who introduced the bill in the House, "will help to save Medicare, and most importantly, to save lives."[44]

After eight years of effort, victory was finally achieved on December 21, 2000, when President Bill Clinton signed legislation (Public Law 106-554) that included the provision for creating a new Medicare MNT benefit for patients with diabetes or kidney disease (predialysis). The MNT benefit was part of a package of Medicare provisions (H.R. 5661) that was incorporated into a massive omnibus bill (H.R. 4577) approved by Congress on December 15. Academy president Jane White acknowledged the tangible importance of the MNT victory: "As we consider the significance of this victory, we can say without reservation that our work to bring recognition to dietetic professionals working in all settings is producing results. The ability of dietetic professionals to serve in the food and health care systems is growing in meaningful ways." With Clinton's signature, the implementation process for the MNT benefit began. The final rules developed by the Centers for Medicare and Medicaid Services (CMS) of DHHS to govern the application

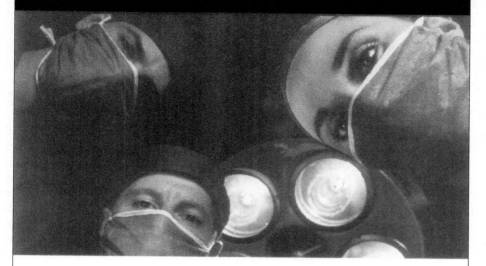

Medicare will pay more than $80,000 for this quadruple bypass surgery. Why won't it pay $66 a visit for treatment that's proven to prevent heart disease?

After years of high cholesterol and poor eating habits, George Anderson's arteries have become dangerously clogged. So today, surgeons are performing a quadruple bypass operation. George's medical bills for this procedure will be more than $80,000. Medicare will pay for almost all of it. Yet, it doesn't pay a penny for treatment that could have helped delay or even avoid surgery—office visits to a **Registered Dietitian** for Medical Nutrition Therapy.

Research shows that patients with heart disease and diabetes who regularly receive Medical Nutrition Therapy have a much better chance of managing their disease. They require fewer hospitalizations, surgeries, medications and have fewer complications. So, over the course of a long-term condition like George's, Medicare could save millions.

Increase coverage now, save millions later.

This year Medicare will spend $113 billion to treat patients with diabetes and heart disease. By covering office visits to R.D.s for Medical Nutrition Therapy now, the savings will offset additional costs by $26 million in just 5 years. And the savings would grow each year thereafter.

But, it's not just the money. Medical Nutrition Therapy could help millions to live longer, more productive lives with less pain and suffering.

Medical Nutrition Therapy
A Solution That Saves.

ACADEMY OF NUTRITION AND DIETETICS • THE VOICE OF NUTRITION

FIGURE 6-8 An Advertisement for Medical Nutrition Therapy

Source: Academy of Nutrition and Dietetics. Reprinted with permission.

© Academy of Nutrition and Dietetics. Reprinted with permission.

of the benefit were published in the *Federal Register* in November 2001 and took effect on January 1, 2002. This process determined the payment levels, provider qualifications, and other coverage details.

The Affordable Care Act of 2010 authorizes CMS to add coverage of "additional preventive services" for Medicare recipients. As a result, in 2011, Medicare began covering screening and behavioral counseling for obesity and cardiovascular disease by primary care providers in primary care settings for Medicare beneficiaries. Registered Dietitians/Nutritionists (RD/RDN) can be reimbursed (when working with primary care providers) by Medicare for preventing and treating risk factors for cardiovascular disease and obesity.[45] The Academy continues to work to expand medical nutrition therapy and position RDs/RDNs as direct providers and billers for behavioral therapy services for obesity and other conditions.[46] See Chapter 9 for more discussion of MNT benefits and health care reform.

Current Legislation and Emerging Policy Issues

In this chapter, we have seen that policies, and the laws and regulations derived from them, are the means by which public problems are addressed. Like the discipline of community nutrition itself, policies are dynamic. In the food and nutrition arena, existing policies are constantly being challenged by market forces, scientific knowledge, and consumer practices and attitudes. Current legislation and emerging issues have the potential to affect the delivery of food and nutrition programs and the way in which community nutritionists work. The *Eat Right Weekly* is a free weekly e-newsletter providing members of the Academy of Nutrition and Dietetics with weekly updates on public policy, continuing education, career resources, and research, and is available from *www.eatright.org.*

The Academy of Nutrition and Dietetics is currently addressing the following three priority areas: disease prevention and treatment, life-cycle nutrition, and quality health care.[47]

- *Disease Prevention and Treatment.* Develop appropriate and effective prevention and treatment techniques to reduce the risk for and severity of chronic disease. This includes focusing on cancer, cardiovascular health, diabetes and prediabetes, HIV/AIDS, obesity and weight, and access to health care. Put food and nutrition practitioners on the front lines in addressing overweight and obesity in all populations. See Chapter 8 for a detailed discussion of the obesity epidemic and descriptions of current public health policies, as well as proposed policies and legislation to prevent obesity and overweight.
- *Life-Cycle Nutrition.* Support programs and policies, such as the Special Supplemental Nutrition Program for Women, Infants, and Children (WIC), the National School Lunch Program, and the Older Americans Act, that help keep Americans healthy throughout their lives. Focus on various programs including prenatal and maternal health, early childhood nutrition, school-age children, and nutrition for older adults.
- *Quality Health Care.* Promote health policy choices that ensure that sufficient resources are available for optimal health. Encourage a comprehensive health care system that is patient-centered and addresses health care equity, consumer protection and licensure, workforce demand, research and monitoring, lowering health care costs, and quality measures.

State Licensure Laws Licensure is a state regulatory action that establishes and enforces minimum competency standards for individuals working in regulated professions such as dietetics. Licensure is designed to help the general public identify individuals qualified by training, experience, and testing to provide nutrition information and medical nutrition therapy. Forty-four states currently have statutory provisions regarding professional regulation of dietitians and/or nutritionists. Enacting licensure laws in those states that still do not have such a law remains a high priority of the Academy of Nutrition and Dietetics in the area of state affairs. State legislatures are charged with protecting the health and safety of the public, so every state regulates occupations that have an impact on the public's health and safety.

According to the Academy of Nutrition and Dietetics, licensing of dietitians and nutritionists ensures that individuals disseminating nutrition advice have the appropriate education and experience.[48] Because medical nutrition therapy is used in the treatment of various diseases, individuals seeking nutritional advice deserve assurance that the individual treating them has the requisite education and experience. Licensure laws protect the public from unqualified individuals who portray themselves as nutrition experts.

Bioterrorism and Food Safety Within hours of the September 11, 2001, attacks on the United States, the nation's food and water supplies were identified as likely targets of terrorists. The term *food safety* refers to foods free of foodborne pathogens and a food supply free of contamination via bioterrorism.[49] The Centers for Disease Control

► **THINK LIKE A COMMUNITY NUTRITIONIST**

Imagine you are meeting with a state legislator to talk about the importance of licensing for dietitians. Prepare a list of talking points to guide your conversation.

and Prevention estimate that 48 million people suffer from foodborne illness each year, resulting in 128,000 hospitalizations and 3,000 deaths. Recent outbreaks—such as those that occurred from tainted spinach, the salmonella outbreak linked to peanut products, and a multistate outbreak of listeriosis from contaminated cantaloupe melons—can easily exceed $100 million in damages to both victims and the food industry.[50] Currently, 12 agencies are involved in regulating the food supply. **Table 6-4** lists them and identifies each agency's responsibilities in ensuring the safety of the nation's food. The FDA Food Safety Modernization Act—the first major reform of food safety laws in more than 70 years— was signed into law by President Obama on January 4, 2011. The law aims to ensure the U.S. food supply is safe by changing the focus from a tradition of government inspectors responding to contamination to placing significant responsibilities on farmers and food processors to prevent contamination. The FDA will address the hazards from farm to table, including the producing, processing, transporting, and preparation of foods.*

Biotechnology The introduction of biotechnology-derived foods and crops has created challenges for scientists, regulatory agencies, and consumers worldwide. Early applications of food biotechnology included the production of vinegar, alcoholic beverages,

AGENCY	FOOD SAFETY RESPONSIBILITIES
FDA Center for Food Safety and Applied Nutrition (CFSAN)	Ensures safety of domestic and imported food products (except meat, poultry, and processed egg products), animal drugs, and animal feed
CDC	Conducts surveillance for foodborne diseases; develops new methods to enhance surveillance and detection of outbreaks; assists local, state, and national efforts to identify, characterize, and control foodborne hazards
USDA's Food Safety and Inspection Service (FSIS)	Ensures that meat, poultry, and some eggs and egg products are safe, wholesome, and correctly marked, labeled, and packaged
USDA's Animal and Plant Health Inspection Service	Ensures the health and care of animals and plants to protect them against pathogens or diseases that pose a risk for humans
USDA's Grain Inspection, Packers and Stockyards Administration	Reports to FDA any grain, rice, or food products that are considered objectionable for consumption
USDA's Agricultural Marketing Service	Establishes quality standards for grading dairy, fruit, vegetable, livestock, meat, poultry, and egg products
USDA's Agricultural Research Service	Conducts food safety research
National Marine Fisheries Service	Conducts voluntary safety and inspection programs for seafood products meant for human consumption
Environmental Protection Agency	Regulates all pesticide products and sets maximum allowed residue levels for pesticides on food and animal feed
Federal Trade Commission	Prevents representations about food that are meant to deceive consumers
U.S. Customs Service	Assists FDA and FSIS in carrying out their regulatory roles in food safety
Bureau of Alcohol, Tobacco, and Firearms	Administers and enforces laws covering the production, use, and distribution of alcoholic beverages

TABLE 6-4 Federal Agencies Involved in Food Safety

Source: General Accounting Office report GAO-02-47T, "Food Safety and Security: Fundamental Changes Needed to Ensure Safe Food."

---

* In response to heightened awareness of bioterrorism threats, the FDA has created a special website that links to information about bioterrorism, as well as to other information sources. See *www.fda.gov/food/fooddefense/default.htm.*

sourdough, and cheese. Today, biotechnology has many applications in the dairy, baking, meat, enzyme, and fermentation industries.[51] In the last decade, plant biotechnology has been applied to producing plants that are resistant to viruses, insects, fungi, and herbicides. From a regulatory standpoint, the development and testing of genetically modified plants are monitored by the FDA, the USDA, the Environmental Protection Agency (EPA), and most state governments.[52] The FDA has approved as safe several genetically engineered crops, including herbicide-resistant soybeans, beetle-resistant potatoes, and virus-resistant squash.[53] Future biotechnology goals are to improve the nutritional quality of plants, increase harvest yield, and produce special oils, carbohydrates, and proteins.[54] However, new advances in this area will continue to challenge existing regulations, and public concern about the safety and environmental impact of genetically engineered foods remains. Some consumers and advocacy groups urge mandatory labeling that discloses the use of genetic engineering. Others advocate more stringent testing of these products before marketing. Still others want a ban on all genetically engineered foods.[55] See Chapter 14 for more about the debate over genetically engineered foods and crops.

Sustainable Food Systems and Public Health
The involvement of public health professionals in food and agricultural policy provides many opportunities for advancing the public's health.[56] A growing coalition of public health professionals is advocating for food and agriculture policies that promote public health as a means to address a range of issues such as the societal costs of diet-related chronic diseases, the fact that the per-calorie cost of fresh fruits and vegetables has become considerably higher than the per-calorie cost of many highly processed foods, insufficient access and consumption of fruits and vegetables by consumers, and increasing outbreaks of foodborne illnesses nationwide.[57] **Food policy councils (FPCs)** are an effective tool, particularly at the local and state level, for food and nutrition practitioners to become involved in developing comprehensive food system policies that advance public health.[58] See the Professional Focus on Moving Toward Community Food Security in Chapter 10.

Table 6-5 provides a few examples of food system policy options that foster healthier food environments and improvement in the public's health. As one food policy analyst has indicated:[59]

> The food system presents a "wicked problem," where the complex interdependencies between socioeconomic and policy forces create a thicket of poorly understood drivers and unclear policy options for advancing public health. Faced with these food system complexities, most food and agriculture issues are discussed in silos and without adequate consideration for the ancillary impacts on other food system issues or the public's health. The resulting political reality is that it is easier to create a USDA program to support nutrition education in some low-income schools than to ensure that all public school children have adequate access to healthy school food environments, including comprehensive programs in nutrition and culinary education, school gardens, farm-to-school connections, and health-promoting school food.

Complementary and Alternative Medicine
Complementary and alternative medicine (CAM) is commonplace in many parts of the world, where it is accepted as appropriate therapy. In North America, CAM has emerged more recently as a potential adjunct approach to traditional Western medicine, mainly owing to its adoption by consumers who have embraced it as an alternative to the invasive treatments typical of Western medical practice today. The National Institutes of Health defines CAM as "those treatments and health care practices not taught widely in medical schools, not generally

Food policy councils (FPCs) A group of citizens and government officials that convene for the purpose of examining a state or local food system to determine how the food system is operating, identify assets and gaps, and develop recommendations on how to improve it. FPC initiatives have included publicizing of local food resources; creating new transit routes to connect underserved areas with full-service grocery stores; persuading government agencies to purchase from local farmers; and organizing community gardens and farmers' markets.

TABLE 6-5 Examples of Food System Policies Designed to Advance Public Health

FOOD SECTOR	FEDERAL POLICY	STATE POLICY	LOCAL POLICY
Food Production	Authorize and appropriate agricultural legislation that provides incentives to increase production of foods that promote health (e.g., fruits, vegetables, whole grains).	Require gardening and food preparation programs integrated into school curriculums.	Enforce land-use protections for urban agriculture, community gardens, and farmers' markets.
Food Processing, Distribution, and Marketing	Prohibit the marketing of foods of low nutritional value to children.	Offer tax incentives for small to mid-sized industries that process, store, and distribute perishable foods grown in the state.	Implement standards and secondary labels/logos for foods produced within a specific geographic region.
Food Distribution and Transportation	Establish procurement policies that give priority to locally produced foods in federal food programs.	Establish cooperative transportation and warehousing opportunities for local producers.	Develop zoning requirements that create transit routes (sidewalks, pedestrian malls, bicycle paths) from all neighborhoods to grocery stores.
Food Access and Food and Nutrition Security	Expand farm-to-school efforts through the Child Nutrition Act; appropriate funds to fully support WIC and Senior Farmers' Market Nutrition Programs in all states.	Establish zoning restrictions limiting fast-food outlets within a specified distance of schools and youth-centered facilities.	Establish a city ordinance allowing mobile fruit and vegetable vendors in low-income neighborhoods.
Food Consumption	Ensure that food and nutrition programs (SNAP, School Lunch, WIC) provide foods that meet current dietary guidelines.	Establish and expand education and training programs for culinary arts and sciences.	Limit the soft drink and snack industry's access to schools and other institutions.

Source: Adapted with permission from M. Muller, A. Tagtow, S. Roberts, and E. MacDougall, "Aligning Food Systems Policies to Advance Public Health," *Journal of Hunger and Environmental Nutrition*, 4 (2009): 225–40. Copyright © 2009 by Taylor & Francis.

available in hospitals, and not usually reimbursed by medical insurance companies."[60] CAM practices include acupuncture, homeopathy, herbal therapy, manual healing methods such as reflexology and chiropractic, methods of controlling the mind and body such as meditation and biofeedback, pharmacological and biological treatments such as chelation therapy, and dietary therapies such as macrobiotics and nutritional supplements. The main objection to CAM is that additional controlled, clinical studies of its safety and efficacy are needed.[61] The growth in CAM practices is likely to challenge existing policies related to health care delivery and the practice of dietetics.

The National Center for Complementary and Alternative Medicine (NCCAM), a division of the National Institutes of Health, is devoted to conducting and supporting basic and applied research and training, and it disseminates information on complementary and alternative medicine to practitioners and the public. Some of the herbs that are currently undergoing research investigations in the United States are garlic, St. John's wort, *Ginkgo biloba*, saw palmetto, echinacea, hawthorn, and cranberry. Appendix B provides more information about complementary nutrition and health therapies.

Functional Foods and Nutraceuticals in the Mainstream Functional foods—foods that may provide health benefits beyond basic nutrition—are increasingly evident on grocery store shelves. The Reuters news agency reported that health-conscious baby boomers see links between diet and health and are increasingly buying functional foods or nutraceuticals.[62] The term *nutraceutical* is used to describe food products created by new technologies and scientific developments. A proposed definition for *nutraceutical* is "any substance that may be considered a food or part of a food and provides medical or health benefits, including the prevention and treatment of disease."[63] Under this definition, nutraceuticals would include nutrients, dietary supplements, herbal products, genetically engineered "designer" foods, and some processed foods. The wide range of foods and ingredients classified as nutraceuticals has stimulated some controversy over whether they are really "healthful" or "healing" foods.

The Growing Dietary and Herbal Supplement Markets The dietary and herbal supplement markets continue to grow despite minimal government oversight and a profusion of questions regarding the quality and reliability of the products available in today's marketplace. In 1994, Congress passed the Dietary Supplement and Health Education Act (DSHEA), which severely restricted the FDA's authority over virtually any product labeled "supplement" so long as the product made no claim to affect a disease.[64] DSHEA allowed herbal medicines to be marketed without prior approval from FDA. What DSHEA did allow manufacturers to state on a label is a description of how the product affects a structure or function of the body, such as the claim that the herbal product can "support," "promote," or "maintain" health. DSHEA states that a product cannot claim that it affects disease, and a manufacturer cannot state on the label that the herbal product will "prevent," "treat," "diagnose," "mitigate," or "cure" disease. A disclaimer must always be included on the label stating that "This product has not been evaluated by the Food and Drug Administration. This product is not intended to diagnose, treat, cure, or prevent any disease." Therefore, herbal products are not obliged to meet any standards of effectiveness or safety that have been established for other medicines, which require extensive laboratory and clinical trials before approval. Today a supplement is presumed safe until the FDA receives well-documented reports of adverse reactions. The Office of Nutrition, Labeling, and Dietary Supplements hosts a website developed to help consumers sort through the increasing amounts of information about dietary supplements by providing tips for searching the Internet and evaluating research.

Consumers and public interest groups have been lobbying for the regulation of herbal supplements. DSHEA did give the FDA the power to require that supplement makers follow "good manufacturing practices." This specifies standards for sanitation, but not necessarily for efficacy or purity.

Genome A term that combines the words *gene* and *chromosome*; the genetic material in the chromosomes of the cell that contains the complete set of instructions (DNA) for making an organism.

Genetic disorders A disease caused in whole or in part by a variation or mutation of a gene.

The Human Genome and Genetic Screening The Human Genome Project was an international effort to locate and identify the sequencing of all of the human genes—together known as the human **genome**—a blueprint that we now know consists of about 20,000 to 25,000 genes that encode the templates for thousands of proteins.[65] **Genetic disorders** can be passed on to family members who inherit a genetic variation or abnormality. When inherited, these variations can cause alterations in nutrient absorption, digestion, metabolism, and other individual differences. A small number of rare disorders (such as sickle cell disease and cystic fibrosis) are caused by a mistake in a single gene. But most disorders involving genetic factors—such as heart disease and most cancers—arise from a combination of small variations in genes, often in concert with environmental influences.

Advances in genetics research have identified more than 1,400 disease-associated genes.[66] These advances are likely to alter disease management. For example, it will become possible to complete a series of genetic tests to determine your susceptibilities to certain diseases and receive counseling tailored to your genetic characteristics. Nutrition and health practitioners must update their knowledge of genetics in order to meet the coming challenges of counseling clients affected by genetic disorders.[67]*

---

* For more information on genetics, visit the Human Genome Research Institute at *www.genome.gov*; see also *www.cdc.gov/genomics/hugenet/default.htm* and *www.ornl.gov/sci/techresources/Human_Genome/home.shtml*.

Policies in the food and nutrition arena will continue to evolve as our knowledge of foods and their relationship to health expands and the issues of public concern change. The broad scope of food and nutrition policy provides ample opportunity for you to become involved in the policy process.

The Community Nutritionist in Action

Whether the issue is food safety legislation, health care reform, licensure of registered dietitians, or funding of the School Lunch Program, there are many ways in which you, as a community nutritionist, can influence the policymaking process. Whether you are new to this effort or not, consider which category of involvement shown in the grassroots pyramid in **Figure 6-9** best describes your current level of involvement.[68] Are you a fence sitter who doesn't think about the big issues in community nutrition? Or are you a "banner carrier" who has strong opinions about issues but would rather talk about them than take action? What kind of player will you be in the future? No matter where you fall on the grassroots pyramid, there are opportunities in community nutrition for you to move up a level of involvement—or even two! Some strategies for influencing and becoming involved in the political process are described next.

Make Your Opinion Known

Expressing your opinion about an issue is one way of influencing the political process. When the issue is important to you, present your ideas and opinions at a public meeting or write a letter to the editor of a newspaper, magazine, or scientific journal.

Use basic principles of letter writing when responding to proposed rules and regulations. When writing the FDA, for example, refer to the proposed rule's publication in the *Federal Register*, outline your concerns, and keep your comments as short and direct as possible.

FIGURE 6-9

Grassroots Pyramid
Source: Adapted from the Academy of Nutrition and Dietetics' Grassroots Targeting (1997).

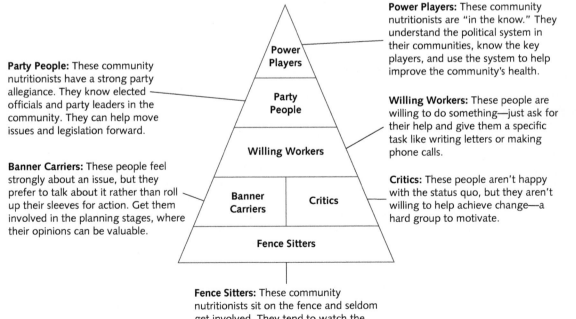

Power Players: These community nutritionists are "in the know." They understand the political system in their communities, know the key players, and use the system to help improve the community's health.

Party People: These community nutritionists have a strong party allegiance. They know elected officials and party leaders in the community. They can help move issues and legislation forward.

Willing Workers: These people are willing to do something—just ask for their help and give them a specific task like writing letters or making phone calls.

Banner Carriers: These people feel strongly about an issue, but they prefer to talk about it rather than roll up their sleeves for action. Get them involved in the planning stages, where their opinions can be valuable.

Critics: These people aren't happy with the status quo, but they aren't willing to help achieve change—a hard group to motivate.

Fence Sitters: These community nutritionists sit on the fence and seldom get involved. They tend to watch the policymaking process from the sidelines. They *can* be motivated for a specific issue.

Become Directly Involved

When you become directly involved in policymaking, *you* become a political actor and run for political office, sponsor a referendum, or initiate a campaign to bring an issue to the attention of the general public or policymakers. For example, you might seek an elected position within your state or the national dietetic association as one means of influencing the practice of dietetics, or you might participate on a local advisory board that is in a position to influence the political process in your community. You might organize the collection of signatures for a petition to be sent to your state legislature or city council, or you might work to elect a candidate to political office. Perhaps you help raise campaign funds for a local politician. Getting involved directly in the political process requires time and energy, but it is rewarding.

Join an Interest Group

Joining an interest group is another way of becoming involved in policymaking. Interest groups are pressure groups that try to influence public policy in ways that are favorable to their members. They consist of people who work together in an organized manner to advance a shared political interest.[69] Interest groups may exert pressure by persuading government agencies and elected officials to reach a particular decision, by supporting or opposing certain political candidates or incumbents, by pursuing litigation, or by trying to shape public opinion. Although interest groups are sometimes accused of being bureaucratic and power-hungry and not always representing their constituents fairly, they do contribute to the political process. Among other things, they encourage political participation and strengthen the link between the public and the government. In addition, they provide government officials with valuable technical and policy information that may not be readily obtained elsewhere.[70]

There are different types of interest groups. Business, for example, is well represented on Capitol Hill by lobbyists from food companies, such as Kellogg's, Procter & Gamble, and the Coca-Cola Company, and from trade associations, such as the American Meat Institute, the Sugar Association, and the American Beverage Association. Professional groups, such as the Academy of Nutrition and Dietetics and the American Medical Association, also have certain policy concerns. "Public interest" groups are a special category, in that they work to achieve goals that do not directly benefit their membership but serve to inform, educate, and influence the legislative process.[71] The Sierra Club, Common Cause, Bread for the World, and the Food Research and Action Center are well-known public interest groups. Still other interest groups may represent particular segments of the population, such as blacks (for instance, the National Association for the Advancement of Colored People) and women (such as the National Organization for Women). Activities to influence the political process even occur within the government itself. The National Governors' Association and the Hall of the States, for example, have been active in trying to set and direct the policy agenda.

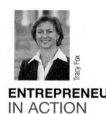
Tracy Fox

ENTREPRENEUR IN ACTION

As president of Food, Nutrition & Policy Consultants, Tracy Fox, MPH, RD, has extensive experience in federal nutrition policy and the legislative and regulatory process. Her areas of expertise include child nutrition and school health; nutrition education; food labeling and marketing; federal, state, and local nutrition policy; advocacy; and government relations. Whether helping a client decipher the complexities of legislation and regulations, drafting testimony and press releases, or advocating for nutrition policies that promote health, Tracy knows that high-quality work and a passion for what you do are essential skills for an entrepreneur. While Tracy is passionate about making sure that food and nutrition practitioners get recognized for their contributions, it is also important to realize that in addition to being rewarding, volunteering may arm you with important skills and contacts that lead to other, more "profitable" opportunities down the road. Find out more about Tracy's career as a food and nutrition policy consultant at *www.cengagebrain.com*.

Work to Influence the Political Process

Interest groups and their memberships use a number of tactics to influence the political process. Litigation is increasingly being used to change policy through the court system. Filing a class action suit in court on behalf of all persons who might benefit from a court action is one example. Another tactic is the public relations campaign, in which interest groups try to influence public opinion favorably. Three other common tactics are political action committees, lobbying, and building coalitions.

Political Action Committees (PACs)

A political action committee, or PAC, is the political arm of an interest group. It has the legal authority to raise funds from its members or employees to support candidates or political parties. The purpose of a PAC is to help elect candidates whose views are favorably aligned with the group's mission or goals. PACs also work to keep the lines of communication open between policymakers and the interest group's membership.[72] The PAC of the Academy of Nutrition and Dietetics strives to influence the policymaking process and its outcome. Academy member contributions support a special fund that makes contributions to the election or reelection campaigns of selected candidates. The Academy PAC is run by a board of directors appointed by the Academy president. The PAC Board selects candidates for contributions on the basis of whether they are in a position to assist the Academy on priority issues, what committee assignments or leadership positions they hold, and whether they are supportive of the Academy's positions.

ENTREPRENEUR IN ACTION

Dawn Crayco was unsure about her career path *until* she took a class in community nutrition. Today she is the deputy director of End Hunger Connecticut!, whose mission is to eliminate hunger in the state through legislative and administrative advocacy, outreach, and public education. She is involved in shaping legislation and policy at the state level, working to make sure children and low-income families are represented and heard in discussions of policy that will affect their lives. Her passion lies in grassroots advocacy and community organizing, which can truly impact food security for families and communities. It's highly rewarding, says Dawn, to see a community come together on a project. She knows the value in creating and maintaining relationships with community partners over time. "It's a small world, so you'd be surprised how a successful partnership with one person leads to other connections and opens more doors." Find out more about Dawn's advocacy work at *www.cengagebrain.com*.

Lobbying

Lobbying is often the method of choice when trying to influence the political system. "It is probably the oldest weapon, and certainly one of the most criticized."[73] Lobbying has acquired a negative connotation, giving rise to images of backdoor, professional power brokers who bend the political process through large campaign contributions. Although this image may be appropriate in some situations, it does not apply to all lobbyists. Remember, **lobbying** means talking to public officials and legislators to persuade them to consider the information you provide on an issue you believe is important.[74] Lobbyists' experience, knowledge of the legal system, and political skills make them an important part of the political process. They provide technical information to policymakers, help draft laws, testify before committees, and help speed (or slow) the passage of bills.

Lobbying Providing information to elected officials.

When this tactic is used, three issues are important: deciding how to lobby, knowing whom to lobby, and determining when to lobby. One of the first decisions is whether to lobby directly or to hire a registered lobbyist. In some cases, you or your organization may not need a registered lobbyist to achieve your goal; in other situations, you may not be successful without the knowledge of the political machine and its players that a registered lobbyist offers.

Knowing whom to lobby and when is also critical. To lobby successfully, identify the politicians or elected officials who are in a position to act on your concern by studying the formal structure of the government and its agencies, reading the newsletters of interest groups, and talking with policymakers who share your concerns. Sometimes, reporters who cover certain events can help you identify the proper authority figures. Once you know whom to lobby, choose the right time. You will accomplish little if you lobby a legislator when a bill is up for the final reading instead of when it is being considered in subcommittee. Use a triggering event to bring an issue to a politician's attention. If possible, turn the triggering event into an opportunity for placing the issue on the policy agenda. Above all, remember that you will have to lobby for as long as it takes, even if that means years. Establishing rapport and building recognition for your concern among elected officials take time.

Having determined where and when to lobby, you must consider how to do it most effectively. Four points are helpful when trying to influence public officials:

1. Show that you are concerned about the official's image. You want to make it easy for the politician to give you what you want, and *at the same time*, you want to make the politician look good. You must not appear to be applying force directly. Instead, provide compelling reasons why the politician should support your proposal.
2. Accept the constraints under which elected officials work. Politicians must deal daily with many pressing issues and diverse groups, including their constituents and staff, lobbyists, party politics, committee leadership, fundraising, campaigning, and the media. All of these place demands on officials' time. Effective lobbyists recognize the cross pressures that politicians face and, when possible, develop strategies for reducing those pressures.
3. Consider reaching elected officials indirectly. Politicians can be influenced through their staff, campaign workers, former colleagues, financial contributors, business associates, and friends. Approaching someone among these groups may enhance your ability to refine your proposal and avoid creating a problem for the politician.
4. Provide information for the official through letters, phone calls, and meetings. Ralph Nader, a consumer advocate, once remarked, "Talking frequently to legislators is the best way to persuade them of your position; the importance of this simple method cannot be overstated."[75]

Building Coalitions An organization is sometimes too small or isolated to influence the political system effectively. It can better achieve policy changes by working with other organizations toward a common goal. Depending on the scope or depth of the cooperative effort, the joint venture may be a formal coalition or a more informal network.[76] Formal coalitions tend to arise in geographical areas where problems affect many people across different communities. Coalitions may bring together social service organizations, church groups, professional associations, neighborhood groups, and businesses to develop a long-term, joint commitment to solving problems. The challenge is getting such diverse groups to agree on which problems deserve immediate attention.*

Networks tend to arise when different organizations across the country share a variety of problems. A network may support a permanent staff in one location and have a common training and information system, but individual members of the network may pursue different problems. In general, network members share a common philosophy about how to mobilize people for action.

Coalitions and networks are often formed to increase the pressure on the political system. By joining forces, organizations can launch more effective public information and media campaigns to mobilize public support for an issue and bring it to the attention of policymakers. The Academy of Nutrition and Dietetics, for example, has more than 200 partners in government, industry, and health care, and is a member of several coalitions to help leverage its legislative efforts. Examples include:

- *National Alliance for Nutrition and Activity (NANA)*—a collection of 230 groups who advocate for national policies and programs to promote healthy eating and physical activity; *www.cspinet.org/nutritionpolicy/nana.html*

---

* For more information, see *Developing Coalitions: An Eight Step Guide* at *www.preventioninstitute.org*.

- *National Fruit and Vegetable Alliance (NFVA)*—a group of public and private partners working to increase access to and demand for all forms of fruits and vegetables for improved public health; *http://nfva.org*
- *National Coalition of Food and Agriculture Research (National C-FAR)*—an organization that seeks enhanced federal funding for food, nutrition, and agricultural research, extension, and education; *www.ncfar.org*

In Manitoba, Canada, the Alliance for the Prevention of Chronic Disease was formed to improve the health of Manitobans, prevent chronic disease, and reduce total spending on health care. The coalition consists of six nonprofit health charities that focus on five major chronic diseases: cancer, diabetes, and heart, kidney, and lung diseases. As the first organization of its kind in Canada, the coalition works with regional health authorities to help shift the emphasis from the traditional medical model to disease prevention and health promotion.[77]

Take Political Action Community nutritionists *are* lobbyists at the local, state, and national levels. Here are a few strategies to keep in mind when trying to influence the political process.

Write Effective Letters A personal letter to an elected official from a constituent can be a powerful instrument for change. Public opinion is important to politicians, and they take note of the number of letters received on a particular issue. Consider the following points when writing to your elected official:[78]

- Get the elected official's name right! Misspelling his or her name detracts from your credibility.
- Limit your letter to one page. Letters should be typed or handwritten legibly.
- Write about a single issue.
- Refer to the legislation by bill number and name. Note the names of sponsors, and refer to hearings that have been held.
- Explain how a legislative issue will affect your work, your organization, or your community.
- Use logical rather than emotional arguments in support of your position. Let the facts speak for themselves.
- Ask direct questions and request a reply.
- Be cooperative. Offer to provide further information. Do not seek confrontation, but don't hesitate to ask for your legislator's position on the issue.
- Follow up. Congratulate your legislator for a positive action or express concern again if the legislator acted contrary to your view on the issue.
- Whenever possible, use an example from your local community to draw attention to the issue.
- Write as an individual rather than as a member of the Academy of Nutrition and Dietetics (although you should identify yourself as a registered dietitian or dietetic technician, registered).

Many state dietetic associations prepare sample letters to send to elected officials. The letter in **Figure 6-10**, for instance, was prepared by the Academy of Nutrition and Dietetics as a sample letter to a legislator seeking support of the Preventing Diabetes in Medicare Act, which seeks to expand Medicare coverage for medical nutrition therapy to include people with prediabetes. An identical letter could be sent to a member of the House of Representatives, except that the salutation should be changed to read "Dear Congressman [or 'Congresswoman']." In either case, use the sample letter as your guide, but change it to make it more personal. Elected officials do not enjoy getting dozens of form letters online or in the mail!

> ► **THINK LIKE A COMMUNITY NUTRITIONIST**
>
> Imagine you are writing a letter to a legislator asking him or her to support a bill to increase the number of hospitals participating in the Baby Friendly Hospital Initiative. How would you try to persuade the legislator to vote for the bill? What data would you include in your letter, and why? (*Hint:* Remember that to vote for this bill, the legislator will want to be convinced not only of the health and economic benefits of breastfeeding, but also that this particular initiative is effective at increasing breastfeeding rates.)

FIGURE 6-10 Sample Letter to a Senator Asking for Support of Expanded Medicare Reimbursement for Nutrition Services

Source: Used with the permission of the Academy of Nutrition and Dietetics.

August 17, 2015

Sen. Susan Collins
Dirksen Senate Office Building
Constitution Avenue and 1st Street, NE
Washington, DC 20510-1904

Dear Senator Susan Collins:

I am writing to urge you to cosponsor H.R. 1686, the bipartisan Preventing Diabetes in Medicare Act. As you may be aware, 29 million Americans have diabetes. More than 8 million of those individuals have undiagnosed diabetes. Another 86 million have prediabetes and are at high risk for developing type 2 diabetes within 10 years. The prevalence of chronic conditions and risk factors for these conditions in the Medicare population is dangerously high and growing. Two-thirds of all Medicare beneficiaries have at least two or more chronic conditions. Nearly 11 million seniors, or 26.9% of the Medicare population, have diabetes and half of all seniors over age 65 have prediabetes. Interventions targeted at preventing or delaying the onset of serious and debilitating illnesses like diabetes must be a national priority.

Currently, 1 in 3 Medicare dollars is spent on people with diabetes. Given the escalating numbers in diabetes, this disease continues to be one of the largest health care threats to our nation's economy. The cost of diabetes has continued to increase significantly, with the true total cost of diabetes rising to $322 billion per year in 2012, up 48% ($100 billion) in just five years, from $218 billion in 2007.

According to a recent study, medical nutrition therapy provided by a registered dietitian nutritionist can result in weight loss and improved blood glucose, which are key outcomes for diabetes prevention programs. Medicare now covers MNT provided by an RDN for people with diabetes or renal disease. The Preventing Diabetes in Medicare Act would expand this to include people with prediabetes, helping to reduce health care costs and improve health outcomes of the ever-growing Medicare population.

Given the potential to make a difference in the lives of millions of people with diabetes and prediabetes, your support of this bill is critical. I look forward to receiving your reply about this important issue. To cosponsor, please contact Tommy Walker with Congresswoman Dianna DeGette at tommy.walker@mail.house.gov. Thank you again for your prompt attention to this matter.

Best regards,

Jesse B James

Jesse B. James, R.D.
196 Briarcliff Lane
Naples, ME 04071

IDENTIFYING MEMBERS OF CONGRESS
www.congress.org
Find your senators:
www.senate.gov
Find your House
representative(s):
www.house.gov

MAKING CONTACT BY PHONE
For the Senate:
www.senate.gov
For the House:
http://clerk.house.gov

MAKING CONTACT BY MAIL
For the Senate:
www.senate.gov
For the House:
http://clerk.house.gov

MAKING CONTACT BY E-MAIL
For the Senate:
www.senate.gov
For the House:
www.house.gov/representatives/

Make Effective Telephone Calls   Getting through to a legislator or other elected official can be difficult. When the opportunity presents itself, remember the following points when phoning an elected official:

- Write down the points you wish to make, your arguments supporting them, and the action you want the legislator to take.
- Don't expect to speak directly with the legislator. Contact the staff person responsible for the issue you want to address.
- Request a written response so that you will have a record of the legislator's position on the subject.

Use E-mail Effectively   E-mail is an acceptable way to communicate with your elected officials.[79] Be sure to use the same rules as for letter writing, including formality in salutations and content. Try to limit your message to two or three brief paragraphs. Be specific about the issue or bill number and about what you are asking the member of Congress to do. Make sure you include your name and street address on all correspondence to confirm that you are a constituent of the member of Congress.

Work with the Media   Reporters and journalists with radio and television stations and newspapers can help build support for your position on an issue. Get to know the key media representatives in your community. When they call about an issue, be prepared to answer their questions about the issue and its impact on the community. When appropriate, prepare a press release to alert them to activities related to an issue. Press releases should be short (no longer than two pages, double-spaced) and concise, and they should provide one or two quotes by a key spokesperson on the issue and give a contact's name, address, and phone number. The Professional Focus feature on page 225 offers tips for working with the media.

Political Realities

Reread the quotation at the beginning of this chapter. What does it mean? In the political realm, it means that an issue isn't important on Capitol Hill until it is important back home. It means that constituents can have more influence over elected officials than party officials have. It means that a local example of a problem carries more weight with policymakers than a national statistic. It means that elected officials measure the importance of an issue by the number of messages they receive about it—which explains why your letters and political activities count.

> *Never doubt that a small group of thoughtful, committed citizens can change the world; indeed, it's the only thing that ever has.*
>
> —*Margaret Mead*

Getting involved in the policymaking process is one way to strengthen your connections with other people and with your community. It can be chaotic at times, but knowing that your effort as an individual has improved the health or well-being of people in your community can also provide great personal satisfaction. You *can* make a difference in your community by understanding the policymaking process, taking time to express your opinion, and being persistent and patient.

case study

Food Safety as a Food Policy Issue
by Alice Fornari, EdD, RD, Alessandra Sarcona, MS, RD, CSSD, and Alison Barkman, MS, RD, CDN

Scenario

There has been a series of articles in the local newspaper asserting that food pantries have empty shelves and soup kitchens do not have enough meals to feed the number of patrons who need their services. The president of the dietetics club at a nearby college decides to ask the professor in charge of the foods laboratory what is done with the leftover prepared and unprepared food from all the food courses (basic foods, cultural foods, and experimental foods). Unfortunately, the response indicates all leftover food is discarded daily and that leftover nonperishable food is discarded at the end of the semester.

This is astonishing to the student, who is very moved by the articles that she has read recently regarding hunger among local residents. She decides she must mobilize her fellow nutrition students to promote a new policy for the foods courses that would result in distributing leftover food, perishable and nonperishable, to the local food pantries or soup kitchens.

This seems to the student to be a simple task to accomplish. She proposes that all recipes be doubled to ensure that there are perishable leftovers to be distributed. All leftovers can be wrapped and refrigerated. Leftover nonperishables will be collected in a box or crate for distribution to either pantries or soup kitchens. Deliveries would be three times per week, and students would be required to assume this responsibility on a rotating schedule. It would be a service learning activity required in the program. The club would make the delivery schedule and distribute the schedule in classes and electronically.

Our idealistic student is very diligent and prepares a written proposal, which she submits to the head of the Foods and Nutrition Department. This individual is impressed with the proposal and arranges a meeting with the student to congratulate her on her increasing awareness of the connection between dietetics and hunger—but also to raise the following questions with the student:

- What are the food safety issues associated with distribution of prepared and nonperishable food items?
- Do the food pantries and soup kitchens have an existing written policy on accepting food?
- Does the Department of Health have a policy on accepting prepared food?
- Does the government have a policy or guidelines on recycling food? Which government agency addresses this issue? Is it a federal or a state body?
- Is there a written policy in the departmental foods laboratory manual on this issue? If not, are you prepared to write one?
- Where will funds come from to double recipes? Are there ways that the dietetics club could fund the increase in ingredient purchases?

The student is overwhelmed that a "simple" idea could generate so many questions. She needs to begin the process of answering the questions in preparation for a follow-up meeting with the entire faculty.

Learning Outcomes

- Identify how a community nutritionist can influence the policymaking process.
- Communicate food safety issues specific to food distribution.
- Link food safety issues to policy.
- Develop a written policy, specific to the department food courses, that addresses the food safety issues relevant to food distribution of prepared and nonperishable food items.

Foundation: Acquisition of Knowledge and Skills

1. Access the latest position papers of the Academy of Nutrition and Dietetics on food insecurity in the United States, nutrition insecurity in developing nations, and food and water safety. As a member, you can access position papers at *www.eatright.org*.
2. Access government documents on the Internet related to food safety, such as
   - Consumer Research Studies: *www.fightbac.org*
   - Food Safety Research Information Office: *http://fsrio.nal.usda.gov*
   - Food Safety and Inspection Service: *www.fsis.usda.gov*
   - National Food Safety Programs: *www.foodsafety.gov*
   - Centers for Disease Control and Prevention Food Safety Office: *www.cdc.gov/foodsafety*
3. Identify why food safety is a critical issue to food distribution in a community setting.
4. Outline the basic steps involved in the process of policymaking—this task can vary at different levels of an organization.
5. On the basis of your reading of this chapter, identify components of the policymaking cycle.

Step 1: *Identify Relevant Information and Uncertainties*

1. Consult experts and/or explore literature, online and offline, to create a list of food safety issues that may arise from food distribution in a community setting.
2. Explain how commodity-based food distribution—of both raw and prepared food—can violate food safety parameters.

Step 2: *Interpret Information*

With the goal of distributing food to hungry individuals, and to ensure that food safety is an integral component of any food distribution plan, include a description of food safety measures that are required. If applicable, prioritize the measures.

Step 3: *Draw and Implement Conclusions*

Prepare a written policy for food distribution.

Step 4: *Engage in Continuous Improvement*

1. Identify any limitations of the new policy, consider budget implications to the department, and determine how the dietetics club could be involved.
2. Devise an implementation plan or procedure for the new policy to make sure that all faculty teaching food courses are aware of the food distribution guidelines.
3. Identify three indicators to assess whether the food being distributed is appropriate and usable to the community.

PROFESSIONAL **FOCUS**

Building Media Skills

In America the President reigns for four years, and journalism governs for ever and ever.

—*Oscar Wilde*

Louis Pasteur said, "Chance favors the prepared mind." When working with the media, always be prepared to provide credible nutrition information. Besides keeping current with the various scientific and trade journals and the popular press, you'll need to consider radio and television news and talk shows. (The Professional Focus feature in Chapter 2 offers tips for becoming a media monitor.) When you provide accurate information, everyone benefits—the media by providing valuable information to the audience, the public by receiving accurate information, and you as a community nutritionist by enhancing your image and visibility as a professional.

The Academy of Nutrition and Dietetics' latest survey of consumers' attitudes about nutrition tells us that although food and nutrition practitioners are among the most valued resources of nutrition information, consumers get the majority of their nutrition and health information from various media outlets.[1] This Professional Focus offers tips on developing media skills. The more that food and nutrition practitioners succeed in developing a media presence, the better the access that consumers have to positive, science-based messages. As you work with the media, consider the following tips:[2]

- Be sure that the information you supply is accurate—check and recheck all names, dates, facts, and figures. This helps establish your credibility with the media.
- Become familiar with the types of coverage of the various media—television and radio news and talk shows, newspapers, newsletters and local publications, trade publications and magazines, and online magazines and websites. Adapt your messages to the format of the media you choose. Identify how a particular audience will benefit from the information you provide. Know what the media cover in your area, who covers it, when they cover it, why they cover it, and how they cover it. This will help you to pitch your ideas to the appropriate media market.[3]
- Present scientific information in a concise, understandable manner so that your audience can readily use and remember it. Avoid technical language. Be able to communicate a *single overriding communications objective* (SOCO).[4] For

example, in a news story on osteoporosis prevention, the SOCO might be: for the audience to know that healthy bones require calcium. Next, develop three key points that will support the SOCO and provide the foundation for the news story. These points represent the key messages that you want your audience to retain. In this example, the key points might be: (1) Diet can make a difference in lowering your risk of osteoporosis, (2) weight-bearing exercise can enhance the benefits of a calcium-rich diet, and (3) consider calcium supplements if dietary changes cannot or will not be made.

- Be consumer-oriented. Keep your audience in mind as you prepare your media information. Be both an authority on nutrition information and (when appropriate) an entertainer. Get the audience involved with your message. Consider using visuals to support your messages.

General Guidelines for Working with the Media

- Nurture good press relations with the media contact people (reporters, editors, program directors, and producers) in your area. Keep a list of the names, e-mail addresses, phone and fax numbers, and deadlines of the media in your community. They are the "gatekeepers" to your target audiences. Occasionally, you may send people on your contact list an FYI (for your information) piece about a research report or recently published article. This alerts them to newsworthy topics or events that they may find useful either now or at a later date. Make yourself available to them for follow-up information or assistance.
- When working with television or radio, consider your appearance—dress with professional style. Practice your presentation as much as possible beforehand. You'll want your facial expressions, body language, and voice to show animation and enthusiasm for your topic.

There are several things you can do to encourage media to cover nutrition issues. Here are some examples:[5]

- Send out a news release with a newsworthy local story.
- Write a letter "pitching" a story to a TV station, newspaper, or local magazine, including background information.
- Write a letter to the editor.
- Listen to call-in radio shows that cover current news or health issues, and call in to voice your opinion on nutrition-related topics.

Issuing a News Release

A well-written news release can generate significant publicity at relatively little cost by convincing a reporter or producer to cover a story.[6] Opportunities to issue a news release include tying into any major medical research announcement that involves a nutrition component; an RD visiting a legislator or a legislator visiting an RD's workplace; RDs receiving recognition from employers or patient groups; or a particular human-interest angle emerging from an RD–client relationship. Keep in mind the following tips when writing a news release:

- Write a gripping headline that conveys, "This is NEWS!"

- Writers learn to capture their readers' attention with a news "hook" or "spin" in the first paragraph, followed by answers to the five Ws: who, what, when, where, and why.

- Write the news release in the third person; keep it brief and to the point—usually around two pages in length.

▶ **THINK LIKE A COMMUNITY** NUTRITIONIST

Imagine you are being interviewed by a media representative to talk about the Baby Friendly Hospital Initiative. Take a look at the two interview scripts below. How is the "interview gone wrong" different from the "winning interview"?

INTERVIEW GONE WRONG

Interviewer: Thanks so much for being here with us today. The Baby Friendly Hospital Initiative has gained momentum in recent years, alongside advocacy for breastfeeding. Why is this?

Interviewee: This is an important initiative because breastfeeding gives babies the best start in life. Also, childhood obesity among U.S. children is an increasing concern among policymakers and health advocates; approximately 17.7% of children ages 6–11 years are obese. Childhood obesity is not only associated with risk of adult obesity and metabolic syndrome but also with health, social, and psychological risks during childhood. Breastfeeding helps reduce the risk of childhood obesity.

Interviewer: That is a concern. Aren't there other factors that contribute to the rates of childhood obesity besides breastfeeding?

(This interview is now off track. Rather than focusing on the Baby Friendly Hospital Initiative, you are now focusing on childhood obesity as a health and policy issue.)

A WINNING INTERVIEW

Interviewer: Thanks so much for being here with us today. The Baby Friendly Hospital Initiative has gained momentum in recent years, alongside advocacy for breastfeeding. Why is this?

Interviewee: This is an important initiative because breastfeeding gives babies the best start in life. Breastfeeding exclusively and then continuing on throughout at least the first year of life are recommended practices; however, only 14% of babies are breastfed exclusively for six months, while 23% are breastfed through the first year of life. Breastfeeding supports optimal growth, while also potentially reducing the risk of a variety of conditions, such as allergies, sudden infant death syndrome, and obesity.

Interviewer: Breastfeeding rates have increased in recent years, correct?

Interviewee: That is correct. Due to the hard work of many breastfeeding advocates, the rates have climbed. Efforts such as the Baby Friendly Hospital Initiative have been a part of this. Being exposed to the practices used in Baby Friendly hospitals, such as mother and babies staying in the same room, early initiation of breastfeeding after birth, supporting skin-to-skin contact between the mother and baby, and not routinely delivering formula to babies, are associated with higher breastfeeding rates. Even more, the effects of these early practices are not only effective in the hospital setting, but being exposed to all seven Baby Friendly practices is associated with about 50% higher rates of exclusive breastfeeding at three months of age, compared to breastfeeding rates among babies born at non-Baby Friendly hospitals.

(You have now linked the Baby Friendly Hospital Initiative with the desired outcome: increased, sustained rates of breastfeeding. Furthermore, you've shown that breastfeeding is important for giving babies the best start in life.)

- Make the opening statement strong to get the attention of the journalist.
- Include important quotations in the second or third paragraph to tie the story quickly to individuals who live in your area.
- List a contact name, telephone number, and e-mail address.
- Include extra information in an accompanying fact sheet or brief backgrounder.

Writing a Letter to the Editor or an Op-Ed Piece

A letter to the editor is most likely to be used when it is timed to respond quickly to events such as an article that appeared in the newspaper, remarks made by an elected official at a public event, or activities in the capital.[7] A letter to the editor is written to a newspaper editor expressing an opinion, issuing a call to action, or citing an issue or situation that needs attention or change (**Figure 6-11**). Here are some guidelines for writing to newspaper editorial pages:

- Look at similar pieces in the newspaper or magazine before writing to see what topics are covered, how similar pieces are written, and how long the average letter that is printed seems to be.
- Contact the newspaper or magazine to see whether it has specific guidelines for letters to the editor.
- Develop a strong news slant or a local angle, with examples of real individuals who are affected.
- Include your name and affiliation if you are writing on behalf of your state or student dietetic association; speaking for a group carries more weight.

Pitching Your Ideas Online

As a community nutritionist, you may have an opportunity to help develop your organization's website or contribute to existing websites, or you may want to design and post your own homepage on the World Wide Web. Whatever the case, there are basic questions to ask and issues to consider when contributing to or designing a website. Answer as many of the following questions as possible before designing a website.

FIGURE 6-11

A Sample Letter to the Editor

Source: From *Advocacy Guide: Food and Nutrition Matters: Effective Nutrition and Health Policy Begins with You* (p. 38). Used with the permission of the Academy of Nutrition and Dietetics.

---

xx/xx/xxxx

Dear (Editor's name):

Everyone agrees that the future of the Medicare Trust Fund is in jeopardy, while very few agree on how to fix it. While the Bipartisan Commission on the Future of Medicare and leaders in Congress investigate ways to fix the Medicare system, it makes sense to focus on solutions that save money over the long run and also improve the quality of care.

Medical nutrition therapy (MNT) is one solution. An important study from The Lewin Group, an independent health policy research firm, projects that savings to Medicare would be greater than cost after just three years. The study, conducted for the Academy of Nutrition and Dietetics, projected savings to grow steadily in following years. It just makes common sense to adopt this solution. If people who need medical nutrition therapy can get access to it regularly without having to worry about how they will pay for it, they can avoid more complicated, more expensive health problems.

Medical nutrition therapy is the service a registered dietitian (RD) provides in many medical cases. It begins with assessing a patient's overall nutrition status, followed by prescribing a personalized course of treatment. An RD may consider a range of factors including medications, food/drug interactions, physical activity, other complex therapies such as chemotherapy, and the patient's ability to feed himself or herself. MNT is a medically necessary and cost-effective way of treating and controlling life-threatening diseases and medical conditions, including diabetes, heart disease, cancer, AIDS, kidney disease, and severe burns. It saves money because it reduces the need for medicines, reduces hospital admissions, reduces the length of stay in the hospital, and reduces many painful and dangerous complications.

It's time to look at all possible solutions that can save Medicare for future generations, while also protecting the quality of health care to all Americans. Medical nutrition therapy is a solution that saves.

(name, RD)

The more time you spend thinking about what you want—and don't want—the easier the design process will be. Also go to *www.usability.gov* for more guidelines for writing for the Web and designing useful websites. See the Professional Focus in Chapter 17 for tips on using social media.

- *Who will develop the website?* If you are helping design a website for your organization, the chances are good that a webmaster has been hired to develop, test, update, and maintain the site. In this case, your role may be one of choosing the site's content. If it is your own website, you must decide whether to develop it yourself or hire a web-page designer to do it for you.
- *What is the purpose of the website?* Your site may be designed to sell a product or service, present information to a certain audience, or provide a collection of links to other websites. Perhaps it will do all three of these things. Specify the purpose of your site right from the beginning to help control costs and design time.
- *Who is the intended audience?* Your site may be designed to reach clients, customers, people who already know something about the subject matter, or people who are unfamiliar with the topic. Specifying the intended audience helps determine how much background information must be provided and the terminology that must be explained. When answering this question, consider the typical user of your website and the type of problem he or she is trying to solve. In other words, think about why this user accessed your site in the first place.
- *How long should the website pages be?* One frustrating aspect of web browsing is scrolling up and down long pages. A rule of thumb is to keep page lengths to one window. This translates to about one and one-half screenfuls of text.

Other Issues to Consider

The number one consideration in website design is ease of use. If a website is cluttered, disorganized, or takes several minutes to download, users may seek information elsewhere—and you will have lost an opportunity to get your message across. To prevent clutter, use graphics wisely. Use only those that are essential to the website's purpose. To help keep the site organized, use document and chapter headings and put a title heading on each page.

The second consideration is quality. A website should be as presentable as an educational brochure, journal article, or textbook. Check spelling. Write well. Test every link. Update the site's pages often and date the pages.

Finally, pay attention to "netiquette." Do not publish registered trademarks or copyrighted material without permission. Do not publish a link to someone else's website without permission. Take time to respond to the people who send you queries about the information on your website. Provide good customer service to ensure that users keep coming back.

A Final Word about Content

Whatever the format, keep these guidelines in mind when preparing your media information:[8]

- Make your message easy to understand and recall.
- Focus on the positive.
- Be certain your information is based on sound scientific research.
- Be practical: Zoom in on specific nutrition facts that can be easily applied.
- Be sure that your presentation exhibits cultural sensitivity and that your content is relevant.
- Tailor the information to your audience.

CHAPTER **SUMMARY** . . . .

The Process of Policymaking

▶ The purpose of public policy is to fashion strategies for solving public problems. Policymaking is the process by which authorities decide which actions to take to address a problem or set of problems, and it can be viewed as a cycle (see Figure 6-1):

- **Problem definition and agenda setting.** Once a problem is defined and gains attention, it is placed on the policy agenda by bringing the issue to the attention of the general public and policymakers.
- **Formulation of alternatives.** Possible solutions to the problem are devised in this, the most creative phase of the policymaking process.
- **Policy adoption.** In this step, the tools for dealing with the problem are chosen (i.e., regulations, cash grants, fines, programs) and used by federal, state,

and municipal departments and agencies that are responsible for implementing policy.

- **Policy implementation.** Implementation is the process of putting a policy into action.
- **Policy evaluation.** The purpose of policy evaluation is to determine whether a program is achieving its stated goals and reaching its intended audience.
- **Policy termination.** A policy or program may be terminated because the public need was met, the nature of the problem changed, government no longer had a mandate in the area, or the policy was too costly.

The Legislative and Regulatory Process

▶ Congress is the primary legislative body. A law defines the broad scope of the policy intended by Congress. Once a law is passed, it is up to administrative bodies such as the USDA or DHHS to interpret the law and provide the detailed regulations that put the policy into effect.

▶ **How an Idea Becomes Law.** When a bill is introduced in the Senate (or House), it is assigned to a committee and follows the process shown in Figure 6-4.

▶ **The Federal Budget Process.** Laws and regulations will have no effect unless there are funds to enforce them. Budgets are designed to count and record income and expenditures, to demonstrate the government's intention regarding the funding (and, more important, the priority) of programs, and to control and shape the activities of government agencies.

The Political Process

▶ Current legislation and emerging issues have the potential to affect the delivery of nutrition programs and the way in which community nutritionists work. The Academy of Nutrition and Dietetics is currently addressing three priority public policy areas: disease prevention and treatment, life-cycle nutrition, and quality health care.

The Community Nutritionist in Action

▶ Some strategies for influencing and becoming involved in the political process include expressing your opinion about an issue at a public meeting or writing a letter to the editor of a newspaper; getting involved directly in the political process; joining an interest group; lobbying; and joining a coalition or network.

SUMMARY **QUESTIONS**

1. Describe the usual steps of the policymaking cycle.
2. A state dietetic association was interested in introducing a restaurant menu labeling bill that would extend current federal food labeling requirements to non-chain restaurants in the state during the state legislative session. After two years, a menu labeling bill for non-chain restaurants was signed into law. Describe the probable sequence of events for such a bill from the time the local dietetic association first raised the extension of menu labeling as a policy issue to the day the governor signed the bill into law.
3. Discuss two of the emerging policy issues that have the potential to affect the delivery of food and nutrition programs and services.
4. Identify three ways in which the community nutritionist can influence policymaking.
5. What points should you keep in mind in order to write an effective letter to your elected official?

6. Imagine you work for a local health department, and it is part of your work assignment to provide assistance to schools working to improve their wellness policies. You notice varying levels of implementation of the policies that have been written for many of the schools. In some classrooms, the teachers are enforcing the policies and requiring healthy foods at classroom celebrations. In other classrooms, very little has changed since the policies went into place. What steps would you take to improve wellness policy implementation in schools?
7. One of the recent criticisms of changes in school meals brought about by the Healthy, Hunger-Free Kids Act of 2010 is that children may not change their eating habits simply because they are offered a greater variety of vegetables, more whole grains, and so on. How would you respond to this criticism? What can be done in schools to improve the chances that children's eating habits will be positively affected by changes in school meals?

INTERNET **RESOURCES**

Information Locators

Code of Federal Regulations
www.archives.gov/federal-register/cfr

Federal Register
www.federalregister.gov

FedWorld
http://fedworld.ntis.gov

Library of Congress, Thomas Legislative Information
www.congress.gov

GovTrack.us—a tool to track activities in Congress
www.govtrack.us

Kaiser Family Foundation State Health Facts
www.statehealthfacts.org

Library of Congress State and Local Government Information
www.loc.gov/rr/news/stategov/stategov.html

U.S. State and Local Government Gateway
www.usa.gov/states-and-territories

Federal Agencies

Office of Management and Budget
www.whitehouse.gov/omb

Department of Health and Human Services
www.hhs.gov

Administration for Children and Families
www.acf.hhs.gov

Administration on Aging
www.aoa.gov

Centers for Disease Control and Prevention
www.cdc.gov

Food and Drug Administration
www.fda.gov

Centers for Medicare and Medicaid Services
www.cms.gov

Health Resources and Services Administration
www.hrsa.gov

Indian Health Service
www.ihs.gov

National Institutes of Health
www.nih.gov

U.S. Department of Agriculture
www.usda.gov

Agricultural Research Service
www.ars.usda.gov

Center for Nutrition Policy and Promotion
www.usda.gov/cnpp

National Institute of Food and Agriculture
http://nifa.usda.gov

Economic Research Service
www.ers.usda.gov

Food and Nutrition Service
www.fns.usda.gov

Food Safety and Inspection Service
www.fsis.usda.gov

Canada

Agriculture and Agri-Food Canada Online
www.agr.gc.ca/index_e.phtml

Government of Canada
http://canada.gc.ca

CHAPTER 7

A National Nutrition Agenda for the Public's Health

LEARNING OBJECTIVES

After you have read and studied this chapter, you will be able to:

- Describe the relationship of nutrition research and nutrition monitoring to U.S. national nutrition policy.

- Describe key components of the National Nutrition Monitoring and Related Research Program.

- Discuss the Dietary Reference Intakes and explain how they are used to plan and assess diets.

- Describe appropriate uses of current dietary guidance systems.

This chapter addresses such issues as public policy development, the role of food in health promotion and disease prevention, current information technologies, and research methodologies, which have been designated by the Accreditation Council for Education in Nutrition and Dietetics (ACEND) as Foundation Knowledge and Learning Outcomes for dietetics education.

CHAPTER OUTLINE

Something to think about...

"Action is the proper fruit of knowledge."

—THOMAS FULLER, MD

For a complete list of references, please access the MindTap Reader within your MindTap course.

Introduction

There was a time when scientists investigating the role that diet plays in health zeroed in on the consequences of getting too little of one nutrient or another. Until the end of World War II in 1945, in fact, nutrition researchers concentrated on eliminating deficiency diseases such as goiter and pellagra. Since then, however, there has been a paradigm shift: The dietary recommendations now focus on preventing chronic disease. Although an abundant food supply and the practice of enriching and fortifying foods with essential nutrients have virtually eliminated deficiency diseases in North America, diseases related to dietary excess and imbalance are widespread. Many cases of cardiovascular disease, cancer, and diabetes are preventable, yet these diseases are among the most prevalent (and costly) diseases in the United States. Not only do these and other chronic diseases account for 7 out of every 10 deaths in the United States, but these diseases also account for more than 86% of the nation's $2.9 trillion health care costs.[1] Many thousands of preventable deaths result from overweight and obesity annually, and a recent study estimates their cost to be $190 billion in direct (health care) costs and indirect costs (e.g., lost wages).[2]

How do we know the prevalence of obesity, and how do we know that dietary imbalances exist in the United States? Likewise, what population subgroups are at risk of malnutrition? And having determined who is malnourished, what guidelines can community nutritionists and other health professionals use to address the nutritional needs of malnourished groups? The answers to these questions are found in the policy arena, for nutrition policy dictates the strategies used in national nutrition monitoring to determine who is malnourished and formulates the appropriate dietary guidance to improve nutritional intake.

National Nutrition Policy in the United States

National nutrition policy A set of nationwide guidelines that specify how the nutritional needs of the population will be met.

By **national nutrition policy**, we mean a set of nationwide guidelines that specify how the nutritional needs of the American people will be met and how the issues of food insecurity, malnutrition, food safety, food labeling, menu labeling, food fortification, sustainable agricultural practices, and nutrition research will be addressed.[3] Does the United States have a national nutrition policy? The answer is both yes and no. It is no in the sense that no one federal body or agency has as its sole mandate to establish, implement, and evaluate national nutrition policy. This deficiency in national policymaking and planning was recognized more than four decades ago, when the late George McGovern, the chairman of the Senate Select Committee on Nutrition and Human Needs, called for the formation of such a body:

> We need a Federal Nutrition Office. The White House Conference on Food, Nutrition and Health recommended such an Office more than five years ago. . . . We cannot continue to operate on the assumption that the increasingly complex threads affecting nutrition policy will automatically weave themselves together into a coherent plan.[4]

The function of such an entity would be to coordinate and direct federal nutrition policy. This federal nutrition office would follow through on the commitments made by federal agencies in implementing a national nutrition plan, help develop surveillance systems to monitor the population's overall health and nutrition status, and guarantee that any secondary nutritional implications of major policy decisions would be recognized and published in a "nutrition impact statement."[5]

Still, decades later, there is no Federal Nutrition Office, and nutrition policy in the United States is still fragmented. The problem with formalizing federal policy decisions in the nutrition arena lies in determining which agency should be the "power center" responsible for final decisions. This task is both complex and politically sensitive because nutrition policy cuts across several policy areas, including agriculture, exports, imports, commerce, foreign relations, public health, and even national defense. No one federal agency can claim exclusive jurisdiction over nutrition issues. It is interesting that the comments made by McGovern in 1975 are still relevant in today's health care and policy environment:

> Nutrition is . . . [the] neglected [component] of income maintenance programs, which themselves are woefully inadequate. This narrow conception virtually denies the nutrition dimension in comprehensive health care, or even that nutrition is a health issue. This parochial view ignores disturbing questions about misleading food advertising and other issues totally unrelated to income inequality. It fails to grapple with the reality that even wealthy Americans are often nutritionally illiterate, and that arteriosclerosis and other diseases associated with the aging process affect more than the poor. These and other issues germane to the health and well-being of the American people go far beyond the perils of poverty, and require a much broader Federal conception of the nation's nutritional policy requirements.[6]

And yet, even though the United States utilizes a more decentralized system with no single Federal Nutrition Office, the country can still be said to have a national nutrition policy. Palumbo remarked that "we can assume that no matter what was intended by government action, what is accomplished is policy."[7] Thus, national nutrition policy in the United States manifests itself in activities such as:

- Food assistance programs
- National nutrition and health objectives as found in the *Healthy People 2020* initiative
- Regulations to safeguard the food supply and ensure the proper handling of food products
- Dietary guidance systems such as the Dietary Reference Intakes, the *Dietary Guidelines for Americans*, and the MyPlate Food Guide
- Monitoring and surveillance programs
- Food labeling legislation and other activities in the nutrition arena

The activities that form the basis of the nation's agenda to improve the public's health are outlined in **Figure 7-1**.[8] Research results and data obtained from nutrition monitoring provide information that helps in decision making—and hence, policymaking—within the two main federal agencies that deal with food and nutrition issues, the U.S. Department of Agriculture (USDA) and the Department of Health and Human Services (DHHS). Some policy decisions affect the types of data collected during nutrition surveys and research related to human nutrient needs. Some aspects of nutrition policy, such as food assistance programs, are discussed in Chapter 10 and later chapters; this chapter focuses on three elements of U.S. nutrition policy: national nutrition monitoring and surveillance activities, nutrient intake standards, and dietary guidance systems.

National Nutrition Monitoring

As early as 1878, Congress authorized a systematic method of data collection to prevent the introduction and spread of disease in the United States.[9] Public health surveillance is "the ongoing, systematic collection, analysis, and interpretation of data essential to the

FIGURE 7-1

Relationships among
Nutrition Research,
Monitoring, and
Policymaking

Source: Adapted from R. Briefel, *Nutrition Monitoring in the United States, in Present Knowledge in Nutrition*, 8th ed. (Washington, D.C.: International Life Sciences Institute, 2001), 617.

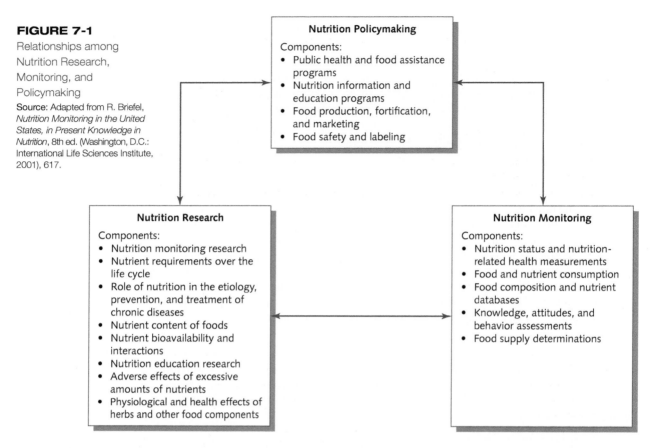

Nutrition Policymaking

Components:
• Public health and food assistance programs
• Nutrition information and education programs
• Food production, fortification, and marketing
• Food safety and labeling

Nutrition Research

Components:
• Nutrition monitoring research
• Nutrient requirements over the life cycle
• Role of nutrition in the etiology, prevention, and treatment of chronic diseases
• Nutrient content of foods
• Nutrient bioavailability and interactions
• Nutrition education research
• Adverse effects of excessive amounts of nutrients
• Physiological and health effects of herbs and other food components

Nutrition Monitoring

Components:
• Nutrition status and nutrition-related health measurements
• Food and nutrient consumption
• Food composition and nutrient databases
• Knowledge, attitudes, and behavior assessments
• Food supply determinations

Nutrition screening
A system that identifies specific individuals for nutrition or public health intervention, often at the community level.

Nutrition assessment The measurement of indicators of dietary status and nutrition-related health status to identify the possible occurrence, nature, and extent of impaired nutrition status (ranging from deficiency to toxicity).

Nutrition monitoring The assessment of dietary or nutrition status at intermittent times with the aim of detecting changes in the dietary or nutrition status of a population.

Nutrition surveillance The continuous assessment of nutrition status for the purpose of detecting changes in trends or distributions so that corrective measures can be taken.

planning, implementation, and evaluation of public health practice, closely integrated with the timely dissemination of these data to those responsible for prevention and control."[10] As part of public health surveillance, most nations monitor the health and nutrition status of their populations as a means of deciding how to allocate scarce resources, enhance the quality of life, and improve productivity. National nutrition policies are typically guided by the outcomes of food and health surveys, which are designed to obtain data on the distribution of foodstuffs, the extent to which people consume food of sufficient quality and quantity, the effects of infectious and chronic diseases, and the ways in which these factors are related to human health. Such information can be derived by any of several methods, including **nutrition screening**, **nutrition assessment**, **nutrition monitoring**, and **nutrition surveillance**.[11] These methods are sometimes treated together under the rubric "nutrition monitoring." Such activities provide, at regular intervals, information about nutrition in populations and the factors that influence food consumption and nutrition status. The objectives of any national nutrition monitoring system, as outlined by the United Nations Expert Committee Report, are shown in **Table 7-1**.[12] The U.S. Congress has defined nutrition monitoring and related research as "the set of activities necessary to provide timely information about the role and status of factors that bear on the contribution that nutrition makes to the health of the people of the United States."[13]

Background on Nutrition Monitoring in the United States The U.S. government has been involved in tracking certain elements of the food supply and food consumption for the last century, beginning with the USDA's Food Supply Series undertaken in 1909. In the 1930s, the first USDA Household Food Consumption Survey was conducted. In the late 1960s, concerns about the "shocking" nutrition status of Mississippi

- To describe the health and nutrition status of a population, with particular reference to defined subgroups who may be at risk.
- To monitor changes in health and nutrition status over time.
- To provide information that will contribute to the analysis of causes of disease and associated factors and permit selection of preventive measures, which may or may not be nutritional (e.g., smoking).
- To provide information on the interrelationship of health and nutrition variables within population subgroups.
- To estimate the prevalence of diseases, risk factors, and health conditions and of changes over time, which will assist in the formulation of policy.
- To monitor nutrition programs and evaluate their effectiveness in order to determine met and unmet needs related to target conditions under study.

TABLE 7-1 Objectives of a National Nutrition Monitoring and Surveillance System

Source: G. B. Mason and coauthors, *Nutritional Surveillance* (Geneva: World Health Organization, 1984). Used with permission.

school children and widespread chronic hunger and malnutrition led to the nation's first comprehensive nutrition survey, the Ten-State Nutrition Survey, conducted between 1968 and 1970 in California, Kentucky, Louisiana, Massachusetts, Michigan, New York, South Carolina, Texas, Washington, and West Virginia.[14] In the 1970s other surveys, such as the National Health and Nutrition Examination Surveys (NHANES I and II) and the Pediatric Nutrition Surveillance System, were added to the roster of methods used to obtain information about the nutrition status of the population.

In 1990, the U.S. Congress passed legislation (PL 101-445) that established the **National Nutrition Monitoring and Related Research Program (NNMRRP).**[15] The legislation specified that the USDA and the DHHS would jointly implement and coordinate the activities of the NNMRRP to obtain, through surveys, surveillance, and other monitoring activities, data about the nutrition status and nutrition-related health status of the U.S. population; the relationship between diet and health; and the factors that influence nutrition and dietary status. The NNMRRP takes a multidisciplinary approach to monitoring the nutrition and health status of Americans in general and of high-risk groups (such as low-income families, pregnant women, older adults, and minorities) in particular.[16] Today, the NNMRRP includes more than 50 surveillance activities that monitor and evaluate the health and nutrition status of the U.S. population.[17]

National Nutrition Monitoring and Related Research Program (NNMRRP) The set of activities that provides regular information about the contribution that diet and nutrition status make to the health of the U.S. population and about the factors affecting diet and nutrition status.

The National Nutrition Monitoring and Related Research Program

The NNMRRP includes all data collection and analysis activities of the federal government related to (1) measuring the health and nutrition status, food consumption, dietary knowledge, and attitudes about diet and health of the U.S. population and (2) measuring food composition and the quality of the food supply.[18] Overall, the NNMRRP has the following goals:[19]

- Provide the scientific foundation for the maintenance and improvement of the nutrition status of the U.S. population and the nutrition quality and healthfulness of the national food supply.
- Collect, analyze, and disseminate timely data on the nutrition and dietary status of the U.S. population, the nutritional quality of the food supply, food consumption patterns, and consumer knowledge and attitudes concerning nutrition.
- Identify high-risk groups and geographical areas, as well as nutrition-related problems and trends, to facilitate prompt implementation of nutrition intervention activities.
- Establish national baseline data and develop and improve uniform standards, methods, criteria, policies, and procedures for nutrition monitoring.
- Provide data for evaluating the implications of changes in agricultural policy related to food production, processing, and distribution that may affect the nutritional quality and healthfulness of the U.S. food supply.

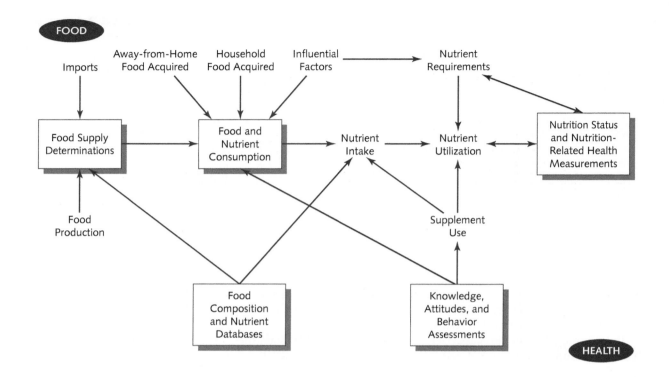

FIGURE 7-2

A Conceptual Model of the Relationships of Food to Health, Showing the Major Components of the National Nutrition Monitoring and Related Research Program

Source: Federation of American Societies for Experimental Biology, Life Sciences Research Office, prepared for the Interagency Board for Nutrition Monitoring and Related Research, *Third Report on Nutrition Monitoring in the United States*, Vol. 1 (Washington, D.C.: U.S. Government Printing Office, 1995), 6.

The NNMRRP surveys can be grouped into the five areas shown in **Figure 7-2**: nutrition status and nutrition-related health measurements; food and nutrient consumption; knowledge, attitudes, and behavior assessments; food composition and nutrient databases; and food supply determinations. The next sections, which describe the major surveys in each area, are based on the directory of federal and state nutrition-monitoring activities compiled by the Interagency Board for Nutrition Monitoring and Related Research.[20] Consult Figure 7-2 to see how the various surveys are used to obtain information about the relationship of food to health. The figure indicates that an individual's health and nutrition status is influenced by his or her food intake, which includes the food prepared and eaten at home and away from home. Food intake is influenced by the individual's knowledge about the relationship between diet and health, use of supplements, nutrient requirements, and attitudes about food and dietary and health practices. The composition and types of food available in the food supply also influence food choices. The boxes in the figure represent the five major component areas of the NNMRRP.

Refer to **Table 7-2** for a description of the major surveys described in the section that follows. Other major NNMRRP surveys not mentioned in this chapter are described in *The Directory of Federal and State Nutrition Monitoring and Related Research Activities*. Table 7-2 and the Internet Resources at the end of this chapter provide addresses for accessing online survey data and other documents. *The Directory of Federal and State Nutrition Monitoring and Related Research Activities* is a comprehensive summary of federal and state nutrition-monitoring activities and a resource for finding nutrition-monitoring data sources, as well as published research using these data. The summary is available at *www.cdc.gov/nchs/pressroom/00facts/nutrit.htm* and provides extensive links to other federal websites.

TABLE 7-2 Sources of Data from the Five Component Areas of the National Nutrition Monitoring and Related Research Program[a]

COMPONENT AREA AND SURVEY	SPONSORING AGENCY	DATE	POPULATION	DATA COLLECTED
Nutrition Status and Nutrition-Related Health Measurements				
Pediatric Nutrition Surveillance System (PedNSS) *www.cdc.gov/pednss/index.htm*	NCCDPHP, CDC (HHS)	1973–2012	Low-income, high-risk children, birth to 17 years of age, with emphasis on birth to five years of age	Demographic information; anthropometry (height and weight), birthweight, hematology, breastfeeding
Pregnancy Nutrition Surveillance System (PNSS) *www.cdc.gov/pednss/index.htm*	NCCDPHP, CDC (HHS)	1973–2012	Convenience population of low-income, high-risk pregnant women	Demographic information; pregravid-weight status, maternal weight gain during pregnancy, anemia, pregnancy behavioral risk factors (smoking and drinking), birthweight, breastfeeding and formula-feeding data
National Health Interview Survey *www.cdc.gov/nchs/nhis.htm*	NCHS, CDC (HHS)	1957, continuous	Civilian, noninstitutionalized household population in the United States. Oversampling of African Americans, Asians, and Hispanics	Household interview: demographic information, data on health trends and ability to perform daily activities, injuries, health care access and utilization, health insurance, immunizations, cancer screenings, complementary and alternative medicine
Continuous National Health and Nutrition Examination Survey (NHANES) *www.cdc.gov/nchs/nhanes.htm*	NCHS, CDC (HHS)	1999–present, annual	Civilian, noninstitutionalized population of all ages. Oversampling of adults ≥ 60 years, African Americans, and Hispanics	Survey elements resembling those of NHANES III and the National Health Interview Survey; includes the What We Eat in America Survey (WWEIA)
Third National Health and Nutrition Examination Survey (NHANES III) *www.cdc.gov/nchs/surveys.htm*	NCHS, CDC (HHS)	1988–1994	Civilian, noninstitutionalized population two months of age and older. Oversampling of non-Hispanic blacks and Mexican Americans, children < 6 years of age, and adults aged ≥ 60 years	Dietary intake (24-hour recall and food frequency), socioeconomic and demographic information, biochemical analyses of blood and urine, physical examination, body measurements, blood pressure, bone densitometry, dietary and health behaviors, and health conditions
Hispanic Health and Nutrition Examination Survey (HHANES) *www.cdc.gov/nchs/surveys.htm*	NCHS (HHS)	1982–1984	Civilian, noninstitutionalized Mexican Americans in five southwestern states; Cuban Americans in Dade County, FL; and Puerto Ricans in New York, New Jersey, and Connecticut. Ages six months to 74 years	Dietary intake, socioeconomic and demographic information, dietary and health behaviors, biochemical analyses of blood and urine, physical examination, body measurements, and health conditions
Food and Nutrient Consumption				
Consumer Expenditure Survey	U.S. Bureau of Labor Statistics	1980, continuous	Noninstitutionalized population and a portion of institutionalized population	Demographics, use of SNAP benefits, annual food expenditures
5-a-Day for Better Health Baseline Survey	NCI (HHS)	1991	Adults 18 years of age and older in the United States	Demographic information; fruit and vegetable intake; knowledge, attitudes, and behaviors regarding fruit and vegetable intake

continued

TABLE 7-2 Sources of Data from the Five Component Areas of the National Nutrition Monitoring and Related Research Program[a]—*continued*

COMPONENT AREA AND SURVEY	SPONSORING AGENCY	DATE	POPULATION	DATA COLLECTED
Food and Nutrient Consumption				
Total Diet Study (TDS) *www.fda.gov/Food/default.htm*	FDA (HHS)	1961, annual	Representative diets of specific age and gender groups	Chemical analysis of nutrients and contaminants in the U.S. food supply. Food composition data are merged with food consumption data to estimate daily intake of nutrients and contaminants.
What We Eat in America (WWEIA)—the dietary intake component of NHANES *www.ars.usda.gov/services/docs.htm?docid=13793*	NCHS (HHS), ARS (USDA)	1999–present, annual	Civilian, noninstitutionalized population of all ages. Oversampling of adults ≥ 60 years, African Americans, and Hispanics.	Two days of 24-hour dietary recall data with times of eating occasions and sources of foods eaten away from home. Day 1 interview is conducted in the Mobile Exam Center. Day 2 intake is collected by telephone. Data provide amounts of food energy and more than 60 nutrients consumed.
School Nutrition Dietary Assessment (SNDA I, II, III, IV) *www.fns.usda.gov*	Food and Nutrition Service (USDA)	1992, 1998, 2005, 2010	Part I: Public schools in the 48 contiguous states that participate in the National School Lunch and School Breakfast Programs	Demographics, plate waste, school and foodservice characteristics, nutrients by food group, relative to the DRIs and the *Dietary Guidelines*, by meals, source of meals, and nutrient content of USDA meals, availability of competitive foods, school wellness policies, food safety
Knowledge, Attitudes, and Behavior Assessments				
Behavioral Risk Factor Surveillance System (BRFSS) *www.cdc.gov/brfss/*	NCCDPHP, CDC (HHS)	1984, continuous	Adults 18 years of age and older residing in households with telephones in participating states	Demographic information; height; weight; smoking, alcohol use, weight control practices, diabetes, mammography, pregnancy, cholesterol-screening practices, and modified food frequencies for dietary fat, fruit, and vegetable consumption by telephone interview
Youth Risk Behavior Survey (YRBS) *www.cdc.gov/HealthyYouth/yrbs/index.htm*	NCCDPHP, CDC (HHS)	1990, annual	Youth attending school in grades 9–12 in the 50 states, the District of Columbia, Puerto Rico, and the Virgin Islands	Demographic information; smoking, alcohol use, weight control practices, exercise, and eating practices information
Health and Diet Survey *www.fda.gov/default.htm*	FDA's Center for Food Safety and Applied Nutrition (HHS)	1980s to present, ongoing household survey	Respondents are randomly selected noninstitutionalized adults in the 50 states and the District of Columbia	Telephone survey tracks demographic data and consumer self-perceptions of relative nutrient intake levels, awareness of diet–health relationships, use of food labels, knowledge of fats and cholesterol, attitudes and practices related to health and diet issues, and prevalence of supplement use.

COMPONENT AREA AND SURVEY	SPONSORING AGENCY	DATE	POPULATION	DATA COLLECTED
Food Composition and Nutrient Databases				
Health and Diet Survey: *Dietary Guidelines* Supplement *www.fda.gov/Food/FoodScienceResearch/ConsumerBehaviorResearch/ucm188571.htm*	ODPHP and FDA (HHS)	2004, 2005	Computer-assisted telephone interview of noninstitutionalized adults 18 years of age or older in households in the 50 states and the District of Columbia	Tracks national change of Americans' attitudes, awareness, knowledge, and behavior regarding various elements of nutrition and physical activity
USDA National Nutrient Database (NNDB) *http://ndb.nal.usda.gov*	ARS (USDA)	1892, continuous	U.S. food supply	This database includes data on the nutrient content of 9,000 food items and up to 150 components. It serves as the foundation of most food and nutrition databases in the United States.
Food Label and Package Survey (FLAPS) *www.fda.gov/Food/default.htm*	FDA (HHS)	1977–present, triennial	All brands of processed, packaged foods regulated by FDA and distributed through grocery stores	Use of nutrition labeling; declaration of selected nutrients and ingredients; nutrition claims; label statements and descriptors; nutrient analysis of a representative sample of packaged foods with nutrition labels
Food Supply Determinations				
U.S. Food and Nutrient Supply Series *www.cnpp.usda.gov/USFoodSupply*	ERS/CNPP (USDA)	1909, annual	U.S. total population	Quantities of foods available for consumption on a per capita basis; quantities of food energy, nutrients, and food components provided by these foods (calculated)
A.C. Nielsen SCANTRACK	ERS (USDA)	1985, monthly	~3,000 U.S. supermarkets	This survey measures supermarket sales of all scannable packaged food products; for each item, the sales, physical volume, selling price, and percent of stores selling the product are recorded

a Within each component area, entries are listed in reverse chronological order. NCCDPHP, National Center for Chronic Disease Prevention and Health Promotion; CDC, Centers for Disease Control and Prevention; HHS, Department of Health and Human Services; NCHS, National Center for Health Statistics; USDA, U.S. Department of Agriculture; NCI, National Cancer Institute; HNIS, Human Nutrition Information Service; FDA, Food and Drug Administration; ODPHP, Office of Disease Prevention and Health Promotion; ARS, Agricultural Research Service; NHLBI, National Heart, Lung, and Blood Institute; CNPP, Center for Nutrition Policy and Promotion; ERS, Economic Research Service.

Source: Interagency Board for Nutrition Monitoring and Related Research, Nutrition Monitoring in the United States: *The Directory of Federal and State Nutrition Monitoring and Related Research Activities* (Hyattsville, MD: National Center for Health Statistics, 2000). Additional nutrition-monitoring activities can be found at *www.cdc.gov/nchs/data/misc/direc-99.pdf.*

Nutrition Status and Nutrition-Related Health Measurements The surveys that form the basis of the health and nutrition status component of the NNMRRP target a variety of specific population groups, including noninstitutionalized civilians over the age of 55 years, children ages two to six years, women of reproductive age, and individuals residing in nursing homes. The surveys collect data on diverse issues, such as family structures, community services, risk factors associated with cancer, and the causes of low birthweight among infants. The NHANES series is included in this component.[21]

The following surveys are among the most important of the health and nutrition status measurements. The NHANES series uses a sample that is representative of the civilian, noninstitutionalized population, and it has a good **response rate**. Consequently, it has dramatically influenced several aspects of health, including development of the 2000 CDC Growth Charts; awareness of dietary and lifestyle strategies associated with high cholesterol; and evidence related to high lead levels among Americans, evidence largely responsible for the current use of lead-free gasoline.[22]

Response rate The value obtained by multiplying the participation rates for each survey component.

National Health and Nutrition Examination Survey (NHANES I) Conducted in 1971–1974, the NHANES I was designed to collect and disseminate data that could be obtained best or only by direct physical examination, laboratory and clinical tests, and related measurements. The target population was civilian, noninstitutionalized persons aged 1–74 years. The measures included dietary intake (one 24-hour recall), body composition, hematologic tests, urine tests, X-rays of the hand and wrist, dental examinations, and other measurements.

NHANES II Conducted in 1976–1980, this program targeted civilian, noninstitutionalized persons aged six months to 74 years. It collected the same types of data as the NHANES I.

Hispanic Health and Nutrition Examination Survey (HHANES) This survey, conducted in 1982–1984, was designed to collect and disseminate data obtained from physical examinations; diagnostic tests; anthropometric measurements; laboratory analyses; and personal interviews of Mexican Americans, Puerto Ricans, and Cubans. Dietary intake was assessed by one 24-hour recall and a food frequency questionnaire. The target population consisted of "eligible" Hispanics aged six months to 74 years. "Eligible" Hispanics were limited to Mexican Americans living in five southwestern states; Cubans living in Dade County, Florida; and Puerto Ricans living in New York, New Jersey, and Connecticut.

NHANES III The NHANES III was conducted in 1988–1994 on a nationwide sample of about 34,000 persons aged two months and over. The survey was divided into two three-year surveys (phase 1 and phase 2) so that national estimates could be produced for each three-year period and for the entire six-year period.[23] Its target population was civilian, noninstitutionalized persons aged two months and over. Dietary intake was assessed by one 24-hour recall and a food frequency questionnaire. The examination components vary by age. Infants aged 2–11 months underwent a physician's exam, body measurements, and an assessment of tympanic impedance; a dietary interview was conducted with the child's caregiver or parent. Between the ages of one and 19 years, additional assessments were added, including a dental exam, vision test, cognitive test, allergy skin test, and spirometry (a measurement of lung capacity). Participants over 20 years of age underwent these assessments, plus an oral glucose tolerance test, bone density test, fitness test, electrocardiogram, and other tests.[24] NHANES III data were used to develop new, nationally representative equations to predict stature for non-Hispanic white, non-Hispanic black, and Mexican American adults aged 60 years and older.[25]

Compared with other surveys, the response rate for the NHANES III was good. In NHANES III, 100% of households were screened, and 86% of those screened were later interviewed. The survey's overall response rate was 73%. NHANES III also investigated the effects of the environment on health. Data were gathered to measure the levels of pesticide exposure, the presence of certain trace elements in the blood, and the amounts of carbon monoxide present in the blood.[26] For example, NHANES III found that nearly 9 out of 10 nonsmoking Americans were exposed to smoke either at home or on the job.

NHANES Today NHANES is considered a keystone in national nutrition policy-making decisions (**Figure 7-3**). Results of NHANES benefit people in the United States in various ways, as listed in **Table 7-3**. Facts about the distribution of health problems and risk factors in the population give researchers important clues to the causes of disease.[27] Information collected from the current survey is compared with information collected in previous surveys to detect the extent that health problems and risk factors have changed over time. By identifying the health care needs of the population, government agencies and other organizations can establish policies and plan research and health promotion programs that may improve public health and prevent future health problems.[28] For example, overweight and obesity prevalence data from NHANES have led to development of programs, research initiatives, and policies to decrease obesity rates. NHANES data help track prevalence of chronic diseases, such as hypertension and diabetes. NHANES data indicate a need for increasing awareness of diabetes risk, particularly targeting minority populations and the undiagnosed.

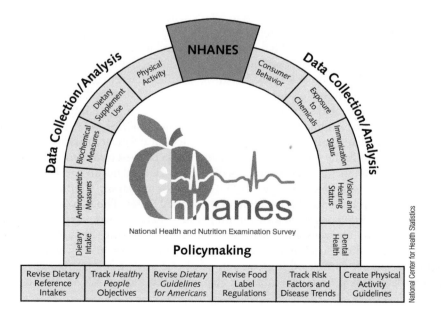

FIGURE 7-3 NHANES Serves as a Keystone of Twenty-First-Century Nutrition Policy

The National Health and Nutrition Examination Survey (NHANES) is a keystone for nutrition policy-making. NHANES collects and analyzes information on the health and nutrition status and health-related behaviors of the U.S. population. NHANES data have been used to influence policy and improve the health of Americans in many ways, including getting lead removed from gasoline and revising food labeling regulations and the *Dietary Guidelines for Americans*.

TABLE 7-3 NHANES
Data Contribute to Public
Health

- Past surveys have provided data to create the growth charts used nationally by pediatricians to evaluate children's growth.

- Blood lead data were instrumental in developing a policy to eliminate lead from gasoline and in food and soft drink cans.

- Overweight prevalence figures have led to the proliferation of programs emphasizing diet and physical activity, stimulated additional research, and provided a means to track trends in obesity.

- NHANES provides essential nutrition and health data for revising the Dietary Reference Intakes (DRIs), tracking the *Healthy People* objectives, and revising the *Dietary Guidelines for Americans.*

- NHANES data have continued to indicate that undiagnosed diabetes is a significant problem in the United States. Efforts by government and private agencies to increase public awareness, especially among minority populations, have been intensified.

- NHANES information helps the Food and Drug Administration decide if there is a need to change vitamin and mineral fortification regulations for the food supply.

- National programs to reduce hypertension and cholesterol levels continue to depend on NHANES data to steer education and prevention programs toward those at risk and to measure success in curtailing risk factors associated with heart disease.

- NHANES physical activity data are used in the *Healthy People* initiative and to evaluate compliance with current physical activity guidelines.

- NHANES provided the first U.S. population-based assessment of mercury exposures in women and children; data was essential for making dietary recommendations on fish consumption for pregnant women.

Source: Adapted from Centers for Disease Control and Prevention, *NHANES: 50 Years of Contributions to Public Health, www.cdc.gov/nchs/video/nhanes50th_contributions/nhanes_contributions.htm.*

Beginning in 1999, the NHANES program took a new direction as a continuous survey that can be linked to related government surveys of the U.S. population—specifically, the National Health Interview Survey (NHIS), a nationally representative study conducted by the U.S. Census Bureau on a broad range of health topics, including health status and health care access.[29] NHANES is linked to NHIS, with regard to questionnaire content of the household interview, for selected topics.

Early in 2000, the USDA and the DHHS announced a decision to integrate NHANES and the Continuing Survey of Food Intakes by Individuals (CSFII) into a single, more cost-effective survey.[30] The merger is viewed as the most efficient use of the limited government funding available for nutrition-monitoring purposes. As of January 2002, the dietary portion of the new integrated survey—"What We Eat in America"—is administered as part of the NHANES. The National Center for Health Statistics (NCHS) of DHHS is responsible for sample design and survey operations. The Agricultural Research Service (ARS) of the USDA has responsibility for processing the dietary data derived from two-day food recalls.

The integrated nutrition survey collects data about diet and health annually rather than periodically, as it was done in the past.[31] The sample for the survey is representative of the civilian, noninstitutionalized population of the United States. The survey interviews and examines about 5,000 people in a 12-month period. There are two parts to the NHANES survey: the home interview and the health examination. During the in-home interview, participants are asked questions about their health status, disease history, and diet. Dietary 24-hour recalls are completed in person or by phone using a research-based, multiple-pass approach. **Figure 7-4** reviews the five-step approach used in NHANES. Community

- Computerized
- Interviewer-administered, in person or by phone
- Used in NHANES
- Five-step approach designed to enhance complete and accurate food recall and reduce respondent burden
- Uses research-based strategies
    Respondent-driven, allowing initial recall to be self-defined (as opposed to starting with "breakfast," for example)
    Association with a 24-hour day's events
    Probes for frequently forgotten foods
- Companion Food Model Booklet for portion size estimation
- Utilizes Food and Nutrient Database for Dietary Studies
- Five steps of the multiple-pass approach
    Quick list. Collect a list of foods and beverages consumed the previous day.
    Forgotten foods. Probe for foods forgotten during the quick list.
    Time and occasion. Collect time and eating occasion for each food.
    Detail cycle. For each food, collect detailed description, amount, and additions. Review 24-hour day.
    Final probe. Final probe for anything else consumed.

FIGURE 7-4 Overview of the Automated Multiple-Pass Method (AMPM) for 24-Hour Dietary Recalls

Source: USDA Automated Multiple-Pass Method; available at *http://www.ars .usda.gov/Services/docs. htm?docid=7710.*

nutritionists can use aspects of this approach to improve the quality of dietary information gathered in practice.

The health examination is performed in a mobile exam center (MEC). **Table 7-4** is a summary of the health exams that are part of NHANES. As in NHANES III, the examinations that a participant will have depend on that participant's age and gender. In the current NHANES, there is oversampling of older persons (60 years and over), African Americans, Asians, and Hispanics. The oversampling allows greater precision for estimates of food and nutrient intakes for these groups. The sample design allows for limited estimates to be produced annually and for more detailed estimates to be determined on three-year samples (e.g., 2011–2014).

TABLE 7-4 A Sampling of NHANES Health Exam Tests and Measurements

HEALTH MEASUREMENTS	LABORATORY MEASUREMENTS
• Physician's exam	• Anemia
• Blood pressure	• Cholesterol
• Body fat	• Glucose measures
• Bone density	• Markers of immunization status
• Dentist's oral health exam	• Kidney function tests
• Vision test	• Lead
• Hearing test	• Cadmium
• Fitness test	• Mercury
• Height, weight, and other body measures	• Liver function tests
• Balance	• Nutrition status
• Leg circulation and sensation	• Exposure to environmental chemicals
• Skin conditions (hand dermatitis and psoriasis)	• Infectious diseases

Source: Health Exam Tests. See complete list of NHANES tests by participant age and gender; available at *wwwn.cdc.gov/nchs/nhanes/search/datapage.aspx?Component=Laboratory.*

The annual NHANES provides estimates of the health of Americans by examining a representative sample of people. To accomplish this, survey teams travel to approximately 15 sites per year across the United States in specially equipped mobile examination centers (MECs). Each MEC consists of four large, interconnected trailer units. Each survey team consists of one physician, one dentist, two dietary interviewers, three medical technologists, five health technicians, one phlebotomist, two interviewers, and one computer data manager. To take a virtual tour of the MEC, go to *www.cdc.gov/nchs/nhanes/. mec_tour/mectour.htm*.

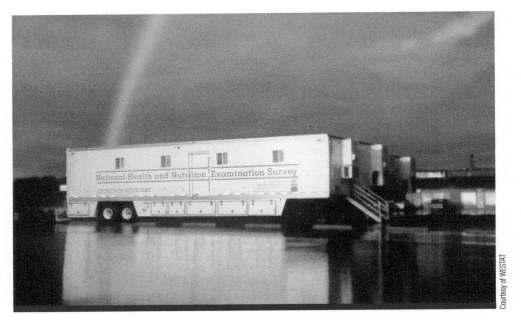

Courtesy of WESTAT

Food and Nutrient Consumption These surveys collect data that are used to describe food consumption behavior and to evaluate the nutritional content of diets in terms of their implications for food policies, marketing, food safety, food assistance, and nutrition education. Over the years, a variety of surveys have been conducted, including the 5-a-Day for Better Health Baseline Survey, the Nationwide Food Consumption Survey, and the Vitamin and Mineral Supplement Survey. The following are the current major surveys of this NNMRRP component.

What We Eat in America Survey (WWEIA) As summarized previously, this is the dietary interview component of NHANES. It is conducted annually through a DHHS and USDA partnership.[32] This survey replaced the CSFII conducted from 1985 to 1998.

Total Diet Study (TDS) This survey, conducted annually by the FDA, is designed to assess the levels of various nutritional components and organic and elemental contaminants of the U.S. food supply. The Selected Minerals in Food Survey, a component of the TDS, estimates the levels of 11 essential minerals in representative diets. The target population is eight specific age and gender groups: infants, young children, male and female teenagers, male and female adults, and male and female older persons. The design includes collecting 234 foods from retail markets in urban areas, preparing them for consumption, and analyzing them for nutritional elements and contaminants four times a year.

Knowledge, Attitudes, and Behavior Assessments Surveys in this component of the NNMRRP gather a variety of data related to behavior and disease risk. Previously, studies have also been conducted on weight loss practices and diet–health relationships. The Weight Loss Practices Survey was administered in 1991, and the Diet and Health Knowledge Survey (DHKS) was used by the USDA as a follow-up to the CSFII to measure consumers' awareness of diet–health relationships and dietary guidance, knowledge of food sources of nutrients, use of food labels, and beliefs about food safety from

1989 until 1996. Currently, the Behavioral Risk Factor Surveillance System (BRFSS) is a unique system active in all 50 states. It is the main source of information on risk behaviors among adult populations. The BRFSS collects data related to health status; access to health care; tobacco and alcohol use; injury control (e.g., use of seat belts); use of prevention services such as immunization and breast cancer screening; HIV and AIDS; weight management practices; treatment for high blood cholesterol; and frequency of intake of dietary fat, fruits, and vegetables. The BRFSS surveys adults by telephone interview.[33] To find data about risk factors and health behaviors of U.S. adults for one or all 50 states, the District of Columbia, or Puerto Rico, go to *www.cdc.gov/brfss*. You can choose the way you want to see the behavior data (e.g., How many people eat the recommended five fruits and vegetables a day?) or risk factor data (e.g., How many people lack health insurance?) by selecting among the following options.

- Grouped by age, gender, race, income, or education
- Comparisons of different states
- Comparisons of different years

The high-risk behaviors of teenagers, such as smoking, alcohol use, eating practices, and weight management practices, are assessed in the Youth Risk Behavior Survey (YRBS).

Food Composition and Nutrient Databases Information about the nutrient content of foods is provided by various activities. The Food Label and Package Survey (FLAPS), undertaken triennially by the FDA in the DHHS, is designed to monitor the labeling practices of U.S. food manufacturers; it analyzes about 300 foods to check the accuracy of nutrient values on food labels. Other USDA activities are part of the Nutrient Data Laboratory, which houses a variety of database products. The Nutrient Data Laboratory is responsible for developing the USDA's National Nutrient Database for Standard Reference, the foundation of most food and nutrition databases in the United States, and is used in food policy, research, and nutrition monitoring.

Food Supply Determinations Food available for consumption by the U.S. civilian population is determined by the USDA's Center for Nutrition Policy and Promotion through its Food Supply Series surveys. These food supply data or **food disappearance data** have been available annually since 1909.[34] The nutrient content of the available food supply is determined using food composition data and then used to estimate the nutrient content of the food supply on a per capita basis.

Uses of National Nutrition-Monitoring Data
The primary purpose of national nutrition-monitoring activities is to obtain the information needed to ensure a population's adequate nutrition. The collected data are used in health planning, program management and evaluation, and timely warning and intervention efforts to prevent acute food shortages.[35] Data related to the population's nutrition status and dietary practices, obtained through national nutrition-monitoring activities, are then used to direct research activities and make a variety of policy decisions involving food assistance programs, nutrition labeling, and education. For instance, the BRFSS allows for comparisons among states and between individual states and the nation. BRFSS data are also used to help states set priorities among health issues; develop strategic plans; monitor the effectiveness of public health interventions; measure the achievement of program goals; and create reports, fact sheets, press releases, and other publications to help educate the public, health professionals, and policymakers about disease prevention and health promotion. National policymakers use BRFSS data to monitor the nation's progress toward the *Healthy People 2020* objectives.[36] Specific uses of NNMRRP surveys are listed in **Table 7-5**. Congress, in

Food disappearance data The amount of food remaining, from the total available food supply, after subtracting nonfood uses such as exports and industrial uses. These data represent the food that "disappears" into the marketing system and is available for human consumption.

TABLE 7-5 Uses of Data from the National Nutrition Monitoring and Related Research Program

Assessment of Dietary Intake

- Provide detailed benchmark data on food and nutrient intakes of the population

- Monitor the nutritional quality of diets

- Determine the nature of populations at risk of having diets low or high in certain nutrients

- Identify socioeconomic and attitudinal factors associated with diets

Monitoring and Surveillance

- Identify high-risk groups and geographical areas with nutrition-related problems to facilitate implementation of public health intervention programs and food assistance programs

- Evaluate changes in agricultural policy that may affect the nutritional quality and healthfulness of the U.S. food supply

- Assess progress toward achieving the nutrition and health objectives in *Healthy People 2020*

- Evaluate the effectiveness of nutritional initiatives for military feeding systems

- Recommend guidelines for the prevention, detection, and management of nutrition and health conditions

- Monitor food production and marketing

Regulatory

- Develop food labeling policies

- Document the need for food fortification policies and monitor such policies

- Establish food safety guidelines

Food Programs and Guidance

- Develop food guides and dietary guidance materials that target nutritional problems in the U.S. population

- Identify educational strategies to increase the knowledge of nutrition and to improve the eating habits of Americans

- Identify factors affecting participation in some food programs and estimate the effect of participation on food expenditures and diet quality

- Identify populations that might benefit from intervention programs

- Identify changes in food and nutrient consumption that would reduce health risks

- Develop food guides and plans that reflect food consumption practices and meet nutritional and cost criteria

- Determine the amounts of foods that are suitable to offer in food distribution programs

Scientific Research

- Establish nutrient requirements (e.g., Dietary Reference Intakes)

- Study diet–health relationships and the significance of knowledge and attitudes toward dietary and health behavior

- Conduct national nutrition monitoring research

- Conduct food composition analysis

Historical Trends

- Correlate food consumption and nutrition status with incidence of disease over time

- Follow food consumption through the life cycle

- Predict changes in food consumption and nutrition status as they may be influenced by economic, technological, and other developments

- Track use and understanding of food labels and their effect on dietary intakes

Source: Adapted from Food Surveys Research Group, Beltsville Human Nutrition Research Center, Agricultural Research Service, U.S. Department of Agriculture website at *https://fnic.nal.usda.gov/food-composition/ars-food-surveys-research-group*.

particular, needs the data from nutrition-monitoring activities to formulate nutrition and health policies and programs, assess the consequences of such policies, oversee the efficacy of federal food and nutrition assistance programs, and evaluate the extent to which federal programs result in a consistent and coordinated effort (a significant activity, considering that no Federal Nutrition Office exists at the present time).[37]

Nutrient Intake Standards

Merely collecting data on a population's nutrient intake and eating habits is not enough. Such data are meaningless on their own; to be valuable, they must be compared with some national standard related to nutrient needs. In the United States, the Food and Nutrition Board was established in 1940 to study issues of national importance pertaining to the safety and adequacy of the nation's food supply; to establish principles and guidelines for adequate nutrition; and to render authoritative judgment on the relationships among food intake, nutrition, and health, at the request of various agencies. The Food and Nutrition Board (FNB), a unit of the Institute of Medicine (IOM), is part of the National Academies, a private, nonprofit corporation created by an Act of Congress, with a charter signed in 1863 by President Abraham Lincoln. The IOM, chartered in 1970, acts as an adviser to the federal government on issues of medical care, research, and education.[38]

The major focus of the FNB is to evaluate emerging knowledge of nutrient requirements and relationships between diet and the reduction of risk of common chronic diseases, to relate this knowledge to strategies for promoting health and preventing disease in the United States and internationally, and to assess aspects of food science and technology that affect the nutritional quality and safety of food and thereby influence health maintenance and disease prevention. The inside front cover of this text summarizes the Dietary Reference Intakes (DRIs), which can be used in assessing and planning diets. The next section reviews the DRIs.

Dietary Reference Intakes (DRIs) The DRIs are nutrient goals to be achieved over time.[39] They can be used to set standards for food assistance programs and for licensing group facilities such as daycare centers and nursing homes, to design nutrition education programs, and to develop new food products.[40]

The DRIs consist of reference values developed by Health Canada and the Food and Nutrition Board of the Institute of Medicine to be used in planning and assessing the diets of individuals and groups.[41] The DRIs include the Estimated Average Requirement, Recommended Dietary Allowance, Adequate Intake, Estimated Energy Requirement, Acceptable Macronutrient Distribution Range, and Tolerable Upper Intake Level. These terms are defined on the inside front cover of this book.

Both the Institute of Medicine and Health Canada's Office of Nutrition Policy and Promotion have information about the DRIs available. The DRIs are a good example of policymaking in action. Compared with the former policies related to nutrient intake recommendations, the DRIs represent a major shift in thinking about nutrient requirements for humans—a shift from prevention of nutrient deficiencies to prevention of chronic disease.[42] They also herald new thinking about the role of dietary supplements in achieving good health. Overall, the DRIs represent a new approach to dietary guidance and have the potential to influence the dietary messages provided to clients and communities, affect food fortification policy, and stimulate the development of new food products by industry. DRIs for all age groups are listed on the inside front cover of this book. The DRI reports can be accessed via *www.nap.edu.*

Dietary Recommendations of Other Countries and Groups Various nations and international groups have published sets of standards similar to the DRIs. Among the most widely used recommendations are those of the Food and Agriculture Organization (FAO) and the World Health Organization (WHO). The FAO/WHO recommendations are considered sufficient for the maintenance of health in nearly all people. They differ from the DRIs because they are based on slightly different judgment factors and serve different purposes. The FAO/WHO recommendations take into consideration people worldwide; for the most part, however, the various recommendations fall within the same general range.

Measuring Health Risks among Adults: CDC's Unique Surveillance System

In the early 1980s, the CDC worked with states to develop the Behavioral Risk Factor Surveillance System (BRFSS). Now active in all 50 states, the District of Columbia, Guam, Puerto Rico, and the U.S. Virgin Islands, the BRFSS is the primary source of information on the health-related behaviors of Americans. States use standard procedures to collect data through a series of monthly telephone interviews with adults. Questions are related to chronic diseases, injuries, and infectious diseases that can be prevented. A strong focus has been on the following behaviors, which are linked with heart disease, stroke, cancer, diabetes, and injury—the nation's leading killers:

- Not consuming enough fruits and vegetables
- Being overweight
- Not using seat belts
- Using tobacco and alcohol
- Not getting preventive medical care, such as flu shots, Pap smears, mammograms, and colorectal cancer screening tests

The surveys have given us a wealth of knowledge about these and other harmful behaviors—how common they are, whether they are increasing over time, and which people might be most at risk. Such information is essential to public health agencies at the national, state, and local levels.

State and local health departments rely heavily on data from the BRFSS to:

- Determine priority health issues and identify populations at highest risk for morbidity
- Develop strategic plans and target prevention programs
- Monitor the effectiveness of interventions and progress in meeting prevention goals
- Educate the public, the health community, and policymakers about disease prevention
- Support community policies that promote health and prevent disease

BRFSS data also help public health professionals monitor progress in meeting the nation's health objectives outlined in *Healthy People 2020*. BRFSS information is used by researchers, voluntary and professional organizations, and managed-care organizations to target prevention efforts.

- The BRFSS data can be analyzed according to age, sex, education, income, race, ethnicity, and other variables. This enables states to find groups at highest risk for health problems and make better use of scarce resources to prevent these problems.
- The BRFSS is designed to examine trends over time. For example, state-based data from the BRFSS have revealed a national epidemic of obesity.

- States can readily address urgent and emerging health issues. Questions may be added for a wide range of important health issues, such as diabetes, indoor air quality, anxiety and depression, folic acid consumption, and natural disasters.
- You can learn about and view questionnaires at *www.cdc.gov/brfss/questionnaires/index.htm.*

The BRFSS is flexible in that it allows states to add timely questions specific to their needs. Yet standard core questions enable health professionals to make comparisons between states and reach national conclusions. BRFSS data have highlighted wide state-to-state differences in key health issues. In 2010, for example, the percentage of adults who smoked ranged from a low of 9% in Utah to a high of 28% in West Virginia.

BRFSS data can also be used to examine smaller geographic areas within states. For example, the CDC has analyzed BRFSS data for more than 200 metropolitan and micropolitan statistical areas (MMSAs). For example, in areas analyzed in 2008, the prevalence of having no health insurance ranged from 3.1% in the Cambridge–Newton–Framingham, Massachusetts MMSA to 39.5% in the El Paso, Texas MMSA. Data are available on a searchable website called Selected Metropolitan/Micropolitan Area Risk Trends (SMART) BRFSS. The BRFSS Maps interactive website can graphically display the prevalence of behavioral risk factors at state and MMSA levels. This tool is available at *www.cdc.gov/brfss.*

Source: Centers for Disease Control and Prevention; available at *www.cdc.gov/brfss.*

Nutrition Survey Results: How Well Do We Eat?

What do the results of national surveys tell us about the nutrition status and dietary patterns of Americans? How well do we eat? The answers to these questions are mixed. Although we are well nourished, we are also generally overfat, underexercised, and beset to some extent with nutrient deficiencies. Chapter 8 reviews the obesity epidemic in the United States, but what else do we know about the health and nutrition of people in the United States, according to NHANES data?

Caution must be exercised in interpreting the NHANES data. On the one hand, when average nutrient intakes are examined, severe deficiencies in individuals can be missed. On the other hand, findings based on one or two days of dietary intake can overestimate the extent of undernutrition.[43] What do survey results indicate about U.S. dietary patterns? The following section examines the current status of the *Healthy People* nutrition and weight status objectives.

The National Agenda for Improving Nutrition and Health

As discussed in Chapter 1, almost no progress was made toward the *Healthy People 2010* targets for objectives in the nutrition and overweight focus area. The proportion of persons with healthful eating patterns (regarding consumption of fruits, vegetables, whole grains, sodium, saturated fat, total fat, and iron) showed little change.[44] Only one objective (calcium intake) showed improvement. Obesity in the population has increased among all age groups (see Chapter 8). In addition, statistically significant health disparities were observed among racial and ethnic populations, as well as by sex, income, and disability status.

The focus of the nutrition and weight status objectives for *Healthy People 2020* was expanded to include a broader range of policies and environmental factors that support eating a healthful diet and maintaining a healthy body weight in settings such as schools, worksites, health care organizations, and communities.[45] **Table 7-6** lists selected objectives from the Nutrition and Weight Status, Physical Activity, and Food Safety topic areas of *Healthy People 2020*.[46] To evaluate and track the nation's progress in reaching the *Healthy People 2020* nutrition and weight status objectives, visit the *Healthy People 2020* website at *www.healthypeople.gov/2020/How-to-Use-DATA2020*.

TABLE 7-6 A Selection of *Healthy People 2020* Objectives from the Nutrition and Weight Status (NWS), Physical Activity, and Food Safety Topic Areas[a]

OBJECTIVE NUMBER AND OBJECTIVE	BASELINE (YEAR)[b]	*HEALTHY PEOPLE 2020* TARGET
Nutrition and Weight Status		
NWS-3 Increase the number of states that have state-level policies that incentivize food retail outlets to provide foods that are encouraged by the *Dietary Guidelines for Americans*.	8 states (2009)	18 states
NWS-4 (Developmental) Increase the proportion of Americans who have access to a food retail outlet that sells a variety of foods that are encouraged by the *Dietary Guidelines for Americans*.	TBD[c]	TBD[c]
NWS-5 Increase the proportion of primary care physicians who regularly measure the body mass index of their patients.	48.7% (2008)	53.6%[d]
NWS-6.2 Increase the proportion of physician office visits made by adult patients who are obese that include counseling or education related to weight reduction, nutrition, or physical activity.	28.9% (2007)	31.8%[d]
NWS-7 (Developmental) Increase the proportion of worksites that offer nutrition or weight management classes or counseling.	TBD[c]	TBD[c]
NWS-8 Increase the proportion of adults who are at a healthy weight.	30.8% (2005–2008)	33.9%[d]
NWS-13 Reduce household food insecurity and in so doing reduce hunger.	14.6% of households were food-insecure (2008)	6%[e]
NWS-14 Increase the contribution of fruits to the diets of the population age two years and older.	0.5 cup equivalents of fruits per 1,000 calories (2001–2004)	0.9 cup equivalents per 1,000 calories
NWS-15.1 Increase the contribution of total vegetables to the diets of the population age two years and older.	0.8 cup equivalents of total vegetables per 1,000 calories (2001–2004)	1.1 cup equivalents per 1,000 calories
NWS-15.2 Increase the contribution of dark green vegetables, orange vegetables, and legumes to the diets of the population age two years and older.	0.1 cup equivalents of dark green or orange vegetables or legumes per 1,000 calories (2001–2004)	0.3 cup equivalents per 1,000 calories
NWS-16 Increase the contribution of whole grains to the diets of the population age two years and older.	0.3 ounce equivalents of whole grains per 1,000 calories (2001–2004)	0.6 ounce equivalents per 1,000 calories
NWS-17.1 Reduce consumption of calories from solid fats.	18.9% (2001–2004)	16.7%

OBJECTIVE NUMBER AND OBJECTIVE	BASELINE (YEAR)[b]	*HEALTHY PEOPLE 2020* TARGET
NWS-17.2 Reduce consumption of calories from added sugars.	15.7% (2001–2004)	10.8%
NWS-18 Reduce consumption of saturated fat in the population age two years and older.	11.3% (2003–2006)	9.5%
NWS-19 Reduce consumption of sodium in the population age two years and older.	3,641 milligrams of sodium (2003–2006)	2,300 milligrams
NWS-20 Increase consumption of calcium in the population age two years and older.	1,118 milligrams (2003–2006)	1,300 milligrams
NWS-21 Reduce iron deficiency among young children and females of childbearing age.		
NWS-21.1 Children age 1–2 years.	15.9% (2005–2008)	14.3%[d]
NWS-21.2 Children age 3–4 years.	5.3% (2005–2008)	4.3%
NWS-21.3 Females age 12–49 years.	10.4% (2005–2008)	9.4%[d]
Physical Activity		
PA-1 Reduce the proportion of adults who engage in no leisure-time physical activity.	36.2% of adults engaged in no leisure-time physical activity (2008)	32.6%[d]
PA-2.4 Increase the proportion of adults who meet the objectives for aerobic physical activity and for muscle-strengthening activity.	18.2% (2008)	20.1%[d]
PA-10 Increase the proportion of the nation's public and private schools that provide access to their physical activity spaces and facilities for all persons outside of normal school hours (i.e., before and after the school day, on weekends, and during summer and other vacations).	28.8% (2006)	31.7%[d]
Food Safety		
FS-5 Increase the proportion of consumers who follow key food safety practices.		
FS-5.1 Clean: wash hands and surfaces often.	67.2% (2006)	74%[d]
FS-5.2 Separate: don't cross-contaminate.	89% (2006)	92%
FS-5.3 Cook: cook to proper temperatures.	37% (2006)	50%
FS-5.4 Chill: refrigerate promptly.	88.1% (2006)	91.1%

[a] See Chapter 8 for more objectives related to obesity. See also Chapters 11, 12, and 13 for specific maternal, child, and adult-related objectives.

[b] Data sources include CDC State Indicator Report on Fruits and Vegetables, National Survey on Energy Balance Related Care among Primary Care Physicians, National Health and Nutrition Examination Survey (NHANES), Supplement to the Current Population Survey (Bureau of the Census), National Health Interview Survey, School Health Policies and Programs Study, and Food Safety Survey (FDA).

[c] Proposed data source: To be determined.

[d] Target setting method: 10% improvement.

[e] Retain *Healthy People 2010* target.

Source: *Healthy People 2020: Improving the Health of Americans; www.healthypeople.gov.*

Dietary Guidance Systems

One approach to improving the public's knowledge about healthful eating involves the dissemination of dietary guidance in the form of dietary guidelines and food group plans. In his report to the American Society for Clinical Nutrition on "The Evidence Relating Six Dietary Factors to the Nation's Health," former Assistant Secretary for Health and Surgeon General Julius Richmond commented, "Individuals have the right to make informed choices, and the government has the responsibility to provide the best data for making good dietary decisions."[47] Dietary guidance systems are methods by which the federal government helps the American people make prudent dietary decisions.

Dietary Guidelines
Dietary guidelines are typically broad plans that focus on goal statements related to overall nutrient intake and daily eating patterns. The first attempt to formulate national dietary guidelines was undertaken in 1977, with the publication of the "Dietary Goals for the United States," a report of the U.S. Senate Select Committee on Nutrition and Human Needs.[48] In the 1980s and 1990s, so many dietary guidelines were published that consumers were overwhelmed by the dietary advice, not knowing which group to listen to.[49] In this section, we describe the major dietary guidelines published by government agencies and non-government organizations.

Government Guidelines While no single office coordinates nutrition policy in the United States, the basis of nutrition policy is the *Dietary Guidelines for Americans*, which serves as the foundation for all federal nutrition guidance in food assistance programs, nutrition education efforts, and decisions about national health objectives.[50] Although the federal government's decision to promote a set of dietary guidelines to improve the public's health would seem to be a straightforward matter of setting national nutrition policy, there has been much discussion about whether the government should establish such guidelines for the entire population. Concerns have focused on whether scientists could achieve a consensus on research outcomes and the relationship of diet to disease processes. Other questions also arose: What obligation do nutrition scientists and educators have to the general public to explain study outcomes and the differences that sometimes arise in interpreting study results? Who decides when research results are firm enough to warrant incorporating them into dietary guidance systems for the public? Is it appropriate to make general dietary recommendations for the entire population, when only a portion may be at risk for a specific disease condition? In what ways will the availability of national dietary guidelines—or the lack of them—affect the delivery of health care and educational efforts in the public health arena?[51]

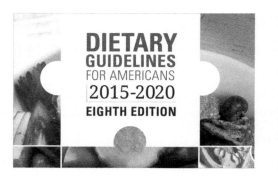

Dietary Guidelines for Americans By law (P.L. 101-445), the *Dietary Guidelines for Americans* must be revised every five years, beginning in 1995.[52] A short history of the development of this policy tool can be found at the Internet address shown in this chapter's list of Internet Resources. The eighth edition of the *Dietary Guidelines for Americans* was released jointly by the USDA and the DHHS for 2015–2020. The principles of healthful eating promoted by the 2015 edition of the *Dietary Guidelines*, illustrated in **Table 7-7**, are science-based advice to promote health and reduce the risk for major chronic diseases through diet and physical activity; these principles grew out of a variety of reports indicating the need for improved eating and physical activity patterns in the U.S. population.

TABLE 7-7 The *2015–2020 Dietary Guidelines for Americans*

The *2015–2020 Dietary Guidelines for Americans* are built around five *Guidelines*. *Key Recommendations* for healthy eating patterns provide further guidance on how individuals can follow the five *Guidelines*.[a]

The Guidelines:

1. **Follow a healthy eating pattern across the lifespan.** All food and beverage choices matter. Choose a healthy eating pattern at an appropriate calorie level to help achieve and maintain a healthy body weight, support nutrient adequacy, and reduce the risk of chronic disease.

2. **Focus on variety, nutrient density, and amount.** To meet nutrient needs within calorie limits, choose a variety of nutrient-dense foods across and within all food groups in recommended amounts.

3. **Limit calories from added sugars and saturated fats and reduce sodium intake.** Consume an eating pattern low in added sugars, saturated fats, and sodium. Cut back on foods and beverages higher in these components to amounts that fit within healthy eating patterns.

4. **Shift to healthier food and beverage choices.** Choose nutrient-dense foods and beverages across and within all food groups in place of less healthy choices. Consider cultural and personal preferences to make these shifts easier to accomplish and maintain.

5. **Support healthy eating patterns for all.** Everyone has a role in helping to create and support healthy eating patterns in multiple settings nationwide, from home to school to work to communities (see the accompanying box).

Key Recommendations:

• Consume a healthy eating pattern that accounts for all foods and beverages within an appropriate calorie level.

  A healthy eating pattern includes:

  • A variety of vegetables from all of the subgroups—dark green, red and orange, legumes (beans and peas), starchy, and other

  • Fruits, especially whole fruits

  • Grains, at least half of which are whole grains

  • Fat-free or low-fat dairy, including milk, yogurt, cheese, and/or fortified soy beverages

  • A variety of protein foods, including seafood, lean meats and poultry, eggs, legumes (beans and peas), and nuts, seeds, and soy products

  • Oils

• A healthy eating pattern limits saturated fats and *trans* fats, added sugars, and sodium:

  • Consume less than 10% of calories per day from added sugars.[b]

  • Consume less than 10% of calories per day from saturated fats.[c]

  • Consume less than 2,300 milligrams (mg) per day of sodium.[d]

  • If alcohol is consumed, it should be consumed in moderation—up to one drink per day for women and up to two drinks per day for men—and only by adults of legal drinking age.[e]

• Meet the *Physical Activity Guidelines for Americans* (see the inside back cover of this book).[f]

[a] The *2015–2020 Dietary Guidelines for Americans* are intended for adults and children age two years and older, including those who are at increased risk of chronic disease. By 2020, the *Dietary Guidelines* are expected to expand to include dietary guidance for infants and toddlers from birth to 24 months and for women who are pregnant. To learn more about the Birth to 24 Months and Pregnancy project, visit *www.cnpp.usda.gov/birthto24months*.

[b] The recommendation to limit intake of calories from added sugars to < 10% per day is a target based on the need to meet food group and nutrient needs within calorie limits. For most calorie levels, there are not enough calories available after meeting food group needs to consume 10% of calories from added sugars and 10% of calories from saturated fats and still stay within calorie limits.

[c] The recommendation to limit intake of calories from saturated fats to < 10% per day is a target based on evidence that replacing saturated fats with unsaturated fats is associated with reduced risk of cardiovascular disease.

[d] The recommendation to limit intake of sodium to less than 2,300 mg per day is based on the UL for individuals ages 14 years and older (see the inside front cover of this book).

[e] It is not recommended that individuals begin drinking or drink more for any reason. There are many circumstances in which individuals should not drink, such as during pregnancy.

[f] Currently, only 20% of adults meet the *Physical Activity Guidelines*, and would benefit from increasing the amount of physical activity they do each week.

Source: U.S. Department of Health and Human Services and U.S. Department of Agriculture, *2015–2020 Dietary Guidelines for Americans*, 8th edition, December 2015.

> ## Recommendations for Supporting Healthy Eating Patterns for All
>
> Everyone has a role to play in encouraging easy, accessible, and affordable ways to support healthy choices at home, school, work, and in the community. Strategies to support healthy choices include the following:
>
> - At home, **individuals and families** can try out small changes to find what works for them, like adding more veggies to favorite dishes, planning meals and cooking at home, and incorporating physical activity into time with family or friends.
> - **Schools** can improve the selection of healthy food choices in cafeterias and vending machines, provide nutrition education programs and school gardens, increase school-based physical activity, and encourage parents and caregivers to promote healthy changes at home.
> - **Workplaces** can offer healthy food options in the cafeteria, vending machines, and at staff functions; provide health and wellness programs and nutrition counseling; and encourage walking or activity breaks.
> - **Communities** can increase access to affordable, healthy food choices through community gardens, farmers' markets, shelters, and food banks and create walkable communities by developing and maintaining safe public spaces for physical activity.
> - **Food retail outlets** can inform consumers about making healthy changes and provide healthy food choices.
>
> Source: Dietary Guidelines Digital Press Kit: Frequently Asked Questions about the *Dietary Guidelines for Americans*. U.S. Department of Health and Human Services and U.S. Department of Agriculture, *2015–2020 Dietary Guidelines for Americans*, 8th edition, December 2015.

The work of the 2015 Dietary Guidelines Advisory Committee (DGAC) was guided by two realities:[53] (1) Some 117 million individuals (half of all U.S. adults) have one or more preventable, chronic diseases, and nearly 155 million individuals (about two-thirds of U.S. adults) are overweight or obese; and (2) eating behaviors of individuals are shaped by complex but modifiable factors, including personal, household, social/cultural, community/environmental, systems, and policy-level factors. Making healthful changes in individual diet and physical activity behaviors, as well as in the environmental factors that affect them, could improve health outcomes (**Figure 7-5**). For example, strategies to reduce sodium intake could include providing education on how to interpret sodium information on food labels or restaurant menus, reformulating foods and meals to reduce sodium content in retail and foodservice establishments, and conducting public health campaigns to promote the importance of reducing sodium intake.[54]

The *Dietary Guidelines for Americans* incorporate several general themes as listed in the box on page 256. The DGAC compared average U.S. dietary intakes with DRI recommendations and identified nutrients that are over-consumed and under-consumed. Americans currently consume too much sodium and too many calories from saturated fats, added sugars, and refined grains. These replace nutrient-dense foods and beverages and make it difficult for people to achieve recommended nutrient intakes without exceeding their

FIGURE 7-5 A Social–Ecological Model for Food and Physical Activity Decisions

A dynamic interplay exists among individuals' nutrition, physical activity, and other lifestyle behaviors and their environmental and social contexts. The Social–Ecological Model demonstrates how various factors overlap and influence food and beverage intake, physical activity patterns, and ultimately health outcomes.

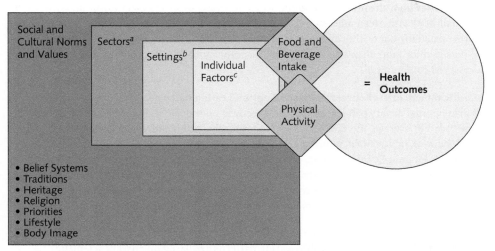

[a] *Sectors* include systems (e.g., government, education, health care, and transportation), organizations (e.g., public health, community, and advocacy), and businesses and industries (e.g., planning and development, agriculture, food and beverage, retail, entertainment, marketing, and media). These sectors either influence the degree to which people have access to healthy food and/or opportunities to be physically active, or they influence social norms and values.

[b] *Settings* include away-from-home settings such as childcare, schools, worksites, community centers, and food retail and foodservice establishments. These settings determine what foods are offered and what opportunities for physical activity are provided. Strategies to align with the *Dietary Guidelines* that are implemented in these settings can influence food and physical activity choices. In combination, sectors and settings can influence social norms and values.

[c] *Individual factors* include age, sex, socioeconomic status, race/ethnicity, the presence of a disability, as well as other influences, such as physical health, knowledge and skills, and personal preferences.

Sources: Adapted from Centers for Disease Control and Prevention, *Addressing Obesity Disparities: Social Ecological Model*; Institute of Medicine, *Preventing Childhood Obesity: Health in the Balance* (Washington, DC: The National Academies Press; 2005, p. 85); M. Story and coauthors, Creating Healthy Food and Eating Environments: Policy and Environmental Approaches, *Annual Reviews Public Health* 29 (2008): 253–72; and U.S. Department of Health and Human Services and U.S. Department of Agriculture, *2015–2020 Dietary Guidelines for Americans*, 8th edition, December 2015.

energy needs. For this reason, the *Dietary Guidelines* emphasize major goals for building healthy **eating patterns:**

- Balance calories from food and beverage choices with physical activity to manage weight and reduce the risk of chronic disease.
- Consume more nutrient-dense foods such as fruits, vegetables, whole grains, fat-free and low-fat dairy products, seafood, lean meats and poultry, eggs, beans and peas, and unsalted nuts and seeds.
- Consume fewer foods with sodium (salt), saturated fats, *trans* fats, added sugars, and refined grains.[55]

The *Dietary Guidelines for Americans* provide a consistent science base for nutrition policymaking. For example, both the National School Lunch Program and the Congregate Meals Program for older adults incorporate the *Dietary Guidelines* in menu planning.

Eating pattern The combination of foods and beverages that constitute an individual's complete dietary intake over time; may describe a customary way of eating or a combination of foods recommended for consumption. Specific examples include USDA Food Patterns and the Dietary Approaches to Stop Hypertension (DASH) Eating Plan.

Overarching Themes of the *2015–2020 Dietary Guidelines for Americans*

The nation has high chronic disease rates.
About half of all American adults—117 million people—suffer from one or more preventable diseases related to poor quality dietary patterns and physical inactivity. High chronic disease rates have persisted for more than two decades and disproportionately affect low-income people and underserved communities.

A significant gap exists between actual and optimal eating patterns.
Less than optimal dietary patterns contribute directly to poor population health and high chronic disease risk. On average, the U.S. diet is low in vegetables, fruit, and whole grains, and high in sodium, calories, saturated fat, refined grains, and added sugars. Underconsumption of the essential nutrients vitamin D, calcium, potassium, and fiber are public health concerns for the majority of the U.S. population, and iron intake is of concern among adolescents and premenopausal females. The current food environment is abundant in highly processed, convenient, low-cost, energy-dense, nutrient-poor foods, making it challenging to implement diet-related behavior changes.

The common characteristics of healthy eating patterns are based on current scientific evidence.
Evidence demonstrates that a healthy dietary pattern is higher in vegetables, fruits, whole grains, low- or non-fat dairy, seafood, legumes, and nuts; moderate in alcohol (among adults); lower in red and processed meat; and low in sugar-sweetened foods and drinks and refined grains.

Healthy lifestyle changes are possible at the individual and population level.
Sound behavioral interventions and resources, like the *Dietary Guidelines for Americans* and the *Physical Activity Guidelines for Americans*, can help individuals achieve healthy diet and physical activity patterns.

Public policy impacts population-wide outcomes.
Research from early childcare settings, schools, and worksites demonstrates that policy changes can influence population-wide eating patterns by increasing healthy food choices and overall dietary quality, and improve weight outcomes, particularly when combined with other programs, such as nutrition education, food labeling, and behavioral interventions.

Food choices impact the environment.
Access to sufficient, nutritious, and safe food is an essential element of food security. A sustainable diet ensures this access for both the current population and future generations. The major findings regarding sustainable diets were that a diet higher in plant-based foods, such as vegetables, fruits, whole grains, legumes, nuts, and seeds, and lower in calories and animal-based foods is more health promoting and is associated with less environmental impact than is the current U.S. diet.

Source: U.S. Department of Agriculture and U.S. Department of Health and Human Services, *Scientific Report of the 2015 Dietary Guidelines Advisory Committee* (2015), available at *www.health.gov.*

The *Dietary Guidelines* are implemented by school nutrition policies such as the ruling that all grains offered must be whole-grain rich, defined as at least 51% whole grain (in coordination with the *Dietary Guidelines for Americans* recommendation to make at least half of grains whole grain). The Special Supplemental Nutrition Program for Women, Infants, and Children (WIC) applies the *Dietary Guidelines* in its educational materials; and the *Healthy People 2020* objectives for the nation include objectives based on the *Dietary Guidelines*.[56]

Non-Government Dietary Recommendations
Dietary recommendations are also issued by a variety of nonprofit health organizations, such as the American Heart Association and the American Cancer Society. These groups are motivated to provide dietary guidance for the public because of the growing scientific evidence linking certain dietary patterns to increased risk for heart disease and some types of cancer. These recommendations, which are listed in **Table 7-8**, represent attempts to create broad, noncontroversial recommendations for dietary patterns in the United States.

TABLE 7-8 Guidelines from Nonprofit Health Organizations

THE AMERICAN HEART ASSOCIATION'S DIET AND LIFESTYLE RECOMMENDATIONS

- **Use up at least as many calories as you take in.**
  - Start by knowing how many calories you should be eating and drinking to maintain your weight. Nutrition and calorie information on food labels is typically based on a 2,000-calorie diet. You may need fewer or more calories depending on several factors, including age, gender, and level of physical activity.
  - Aim for at least 150 minutes of moderate physical activity or 75 minutes of vigorous physical activity—or an equal combination of both—each week.
  - If you would benefit from lowering your blood pressure or cholesterol, the American Heart Association recommends 40 minutes of aerobic exercise of moderate to vigorous intensity three to four times a week.
- **Eat a variety of nutritious foods from all the food groups.**
  - One of the diets that fits this pattern is the DASH (Dietary Approaches to Stop Hypertension) eating plan (see Table 7-10). Most healthy eating patterns can be adapted based on calorie requirements and personal and cultural food preferences.
- **Eat less of the nutrient-poor foods.**
  - Limit foods and beverages high in calories but low in nutrients. Also limit the amount of saturated fat, *trans* fat, and sodium you eat.
- **As you make daily food choices, base your eating pattern on these recommendations:**
  - Eat a variety of fresh, frozen, and canned vegetables and fruits without high-calorie sauces or added salt and sugars. Replace high-calorie foods with fruits and vegetables.
  - Choose fiber-rich whole grains for most grain servings.
  - Choose poultry and fish without skin and prepare them in healthy ways without added saturated and *trans* fat. If you choose to eat meat, look for the leanest cuts available and prepare them in healthy and delicious ways.
  - Eat a variety of fish at least twice a week, especially fish containing omega-3 fatty acids (e.g., salmon, trout, and herring).
  - Select fat-free (skim) and low-fat (1%) dairy products.
  - Avoid foods containing partially hydrogenated vegetable oils to reduce *trans* fat in your diet.
  - Limit saturated fat and *trans* fat and replace them with the better fats, monounsaturated and polyunsaturated. If you need to lower your blood cholesterol, reduce saturated fat to no more than 5 to 6% of total calories. For someone eating 2,000 calories a day, that's about 13 grams of saturated fat.
  - Cut back on beverages and foods with added sugars.
  - Choose foods with less sodium and prepare foods with little or no salt. To lower blood pressure, aim to eat no more than 2,400 milligrams of sodium per day. Reducing daily intake to 1,500 mg is desirable because it can lower blood pressure even further. If you can't meet these goals right now, even reducing sodium intake by 1,000 mg per day can benefit blood pressure.
  - If you drink alcohol, drink in moderation. That means no more than one drink per day if you're a woman and no more than two drinks per day if you're a man.
  - Follow the American Heart Association recommendations when you eat out, and keep an eye on your portion sizes.
- **Also, don't smoke tobacco—and avoid secondhand smoke.**

continued

TABLE 7-8 Guidelines from Nonprofit Health Organizations—*continued*

STRATEGIES TO MAKE IMPLEMENTATION OF AHA GUIDELINES EASIER

Improve consumer access to nutrition information.

- Front-of-package food labeling should be streamlined to provide shoppers easy-to-read, at-a-glance information to inform them as to which foods and beverages are healthy options within product categories.

Government

- Provide subsidies that encourage agricultural production of more whole-grain products, *trans* fat-free oils, low-fat dairy, fruits, and vegetables.
- Provide greater funding and prioritize government and nonprofit consumer education campaigns (such as Fruits & Veggies—More Matters) around nutrition and healthy foods and beverages.
- Regulate food and beverage industry marketing and advertising; require healthy food advertising.

The Health Care System

- Hospital systems should offer healthy nutrition choices throughout hospital foodservice for patients, providers, families, and visitors; just as many hospital campuses are going smoke-free, health care systems should model healthy food and beverage offerings.
- Health care providers should model healthy behaviors; they should commend parents who are modeling healthy behaviors; and they should encourage and give guidance to parents who want to be effective role models.
- Health care providers should incorporate weight screening and BMI calculation into all health care visits for adults and children.

AMERICAN CANCER SOCIETY'S NUTRITION AND PHYSICAL ACTIVITY GUIDELINES FOR CANCER PREVENTION

Recommendations for Individual Choices

- **Be as lean as possible throughout life without being underweight.**
  - Avoid excess weight gain at all ages. For those who are overweight or obese, losing even a small amount of weight has health benefits and is a good place to start.
  - Get regular physical activity and limit intake of high-calorie foods and drinks as keys to help maintain a healthy weight.
- **Be physically active.**
  - *Adults:* Get at least 150 minutes of moderate-intensity or 75 minutes of vigorous-intensity activity each week (or a combination of these), preferably spread throughout the week.
  - *Children and adolescents:* Get at least one hour of moderate- or vigorous-intensity activity each day, with vigorous activity on at least three days each week.
  - Limit sedentary behavior such as sitting, lying down, watching TV, and other forms of screen-based entertainment.
  - Doing some physical activity above usual activities, no matter what one's level of activity, can have many health benefits.
- **Eat a healthy diet, with an emphasis on plant foods.**
  - Choose foods and drinks in amounts that help you achieve and maintain a healthy weight.
  - Eat *at least* 2.5 cups of vegetables and fruits each day.
  - Choose whole grains over processed (refined) grains.
  - Limit intake of processed and red meats.
- **If you drink alcoholic beverages, limit your intake.**
  - Drink no more than one drink per day for women or two per day for men.

Recommendations for Community Action

- **Public, private, and community organizations should work to create social and physical environments that help people adopt and maintain healthful nutrition and physical activity behaviors.**
  - Increase access to affordable, healthy foods in communities, places of work, and schools, and decrease access to and marketing of foods and drinks of low nutritional value, particularly to youth.
  - Provide safe, enjoyable spaces for physical activity in schools and worksites.
  - Provide for safe, physically active transportation (such as biking and walking) and recreation in communities.

Sources: American Heart Association (*www.americanheart.org*); *2013 ACC/AHA Guideline on the Treatment of Blood Cholesterol to Reduce Atherosclerotic Cardiovascular Risk in Adults;* and American Cancer Society, 2015 (*www.cancer.org*).

Food Intake Patterns/Food Group Plans Dietary guidance in the form of food intake patterns or **food group plans** have been provided to the U.S. population since the turn of the century. The early forms of dietary recommendations tended to focus on the consumption of adequate amounts of the foods needed to provide nutrients and energy intake for good health.[57] The USDA, for example, published its first dietary guidance plan in 1916. Between 1916 and the 1940s, a variety of food group plans, featuring anywhere from 5 to 12 food groups, were published by federal agencies and voluntary health organizations. In 1943, the Bureau of Home Economics published a food guide that promoted seven food groups as part of the USDA's National Wartime Nutrition Program. This guide served as the basis for nearly all nutrition education programs for more than a decade. Then, in 1955, the Department of Nutrition at the Harvard School of Public Health published a recommendation that these seven food groups be collapsed into four.[58] This format was adopted in 1956 by the USDA and promoted as the Four Food Group plan. The USDA added a fifth group (fats, sweets, and alcohol) to the Basic Four plan in 1979 to draw attention to foods targeted for moderation, but it did not offer specific limitations for the fifth group.

Since the publication of the Basic Four plan, however, the emphasis of nutritional guidance has expanded from just meeting nutrient needs to also eating a diet low in added sugars, saturated fat, and sodium and generous in fruits, vegetables, and whole grains. With the publication of the *Surgeon General's Report on Nutrition and Health* in 1988, the overconsumption of certain dietary constituents became a major concern. For this reason, the Food Guide Pyramid was introduced to reinforce our understanding of the nutrient composition of foods, human nutrient needs, and the relationship of diet to health. The Food Guide Pyramid conveyed five of the essential components of a healthful daily diet: adequacy, balance, moderation, energy control, and variety.[59] The MyPyramid food guidance system was released in 2005, after a revision of the 1992 food guide pyramid.[60] Similar to the development of the original food guide pyramid, a stepwise process was used to develop MyPyramid. First, the Estimated Energy Requirement (EER) formulas were used to set energy levels for MyPyramid. Next, nutrient goals were set, based on DRI standards. Food groupings were then established, based on nutrient content, use in meals, and familiarity. Finally, food intake patterns were determined to identify food group amounts that meet nutrient goals within recommended energy levels.[61]

In 2011, MyPlate replaced MyPyramid. MyPlate is designed to help consumers choose foods that supply a good balance of nutrients, and it aims to moderate or limit dietary components often consumed in excess, such as saturated fat, *trans* fat, refined grains and added sugars, and sodium, in keeping with the U.S. government's *Dietary Guidelines for Americans*. MyPlate illustrates the five food groups using a familiar mealtime visual, a place setting. The plate is split into four sections: red for fruits, green for vegetables, purple for protein foods, and orange for grains. A separate blue section, shaped like a drinking glass, represents dairy foods (refer to the inside back cover of this book). MyPlate provides a visual reminder of a key nutrition principle: Fruits and vegetables form the foundation of a healthy diet and should fill at least half of a plate at every meal.

Food group plans A diet-planning tool that sorts foods of similar origin and nutrient content into groups and then specifies that the individual eat a certain number of foods from each group.

Understanding the Nutrition Gap

The most recent data from the NHANES surveys show a considerable gap between current nutrition recommendations and consumers' practices. Undoubtedly, trends such as eating away from home and increased portion sizes in grocery and restaurant items negatively affect American eating habits. In the 1960s, an average fast-food meal of a hamburger, fries, and a 12-ounce cola provided 590 calories; today, many super-sized, extra-value fast-food meals deliver 1,500 calories or more.[62]

Figure 7-6 provides insights into how the typical American diet compares to recommended intakes or limits. In general, we do not meet recommendations for vegetables, fruit, dairy, oils, or whole grains, and exceed recommendations, leading to overconsumption of sodium, saturated fat, refined grains, solid fats, and added sugars. As shown in Figure 7-6, three-fourths of the population has an eating pattern that is low in vegetables, fruits, dairy, and oils, and half the population is not meeting the recommendation for whole grains. By eating fewer nutrient-dense foods from these food groups, consumers are at risk for lower than recommended levels of specific nutrients, including vitamin D, calcium, potassium, and dietary fiber.

Some 70% of consumers exceed the recommended limits—less than 10% of calories per day—for both added sugars and saturated fat.[63] Added sugars account for almost 270 calories, or more than 13% of calories per day in the average U.S. diet; average intake of saturated fat is 11% of calories. Most consumers also have sodium intakes above the Tolerable Upper Intake Level (2,300 milligrams). The average daily intake of sodium is 4,240 milligrams for men and 2,980 milligrams for women. **Figure 7-7** shows the major sources of added sugars, saturated fat, and sodium in typical U.S. diets.

Another way to rate the American diet is to use the USDA Healthy Eating Index (HEI). The HEI was developed jointly by the USDA and the National Cancer Institute to assess and score various components of the diet to give an indication of overall diet quality. The tool measures the degree to which a person's diet conforms to federal dietary guidelines. As noted in **Figure 7-8**, trends in food intake reveal that Americans are not consuming healthy eating patterns. As the prevalence of overweight and obesity has risen for the past two decades, HEI scores have remained low.

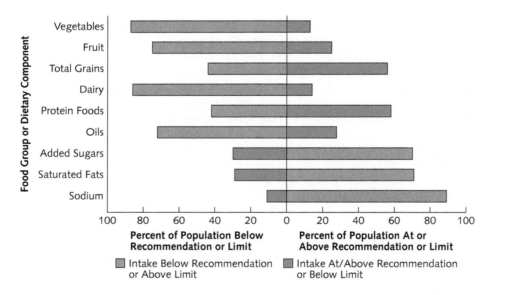

FIGURE 7-6 How the U.S. Diet Measures Up to Current Dietary Guidance

The figure shows the percentage of the U.S. population ages one year and older with intakes below the recommendation or above the limit for different food groups and dietary components.

Note: The center (0) line is the goal or limit. For those people represented by the gray sections of the bars, shifting toward the center line will improve their eating pattern.

Sources: What We Eat in America, NHANES 2007–2010 for average intakes by age–sex group. Healthy U.S.-Style Food Patterns, which vary based on age, sex, and activity level, for recommended intakes and limits; and U.S. Department of Health and Human Services and U.S. Department of Agriculture, *2015–2020 Dietary Guidelines for Americans*, 8th edition, December 2015.

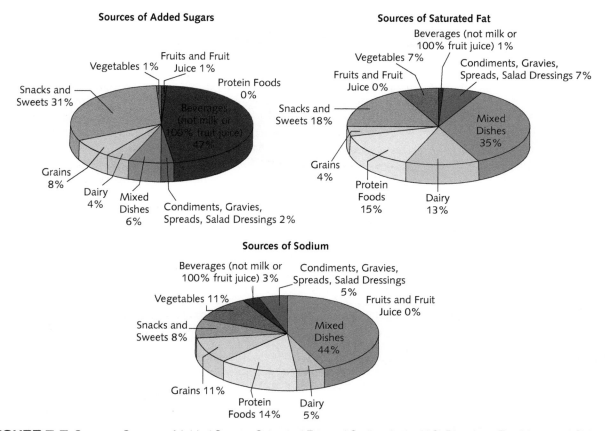

FIGURE 7-7 Common Sources of Added Sugars, Saturated Fat, and Sodium in the U.S. Diet, Ages Two Years and Older The major sources of added sugars in typical U.S. diets are snacks, sweets, and sugar-sweetened beverages, which include soft drinks, fruit drinks, sweetened coffee and tea, energy drinks, alcoholic beverages, and flavored waters. The mixed dishes food category is the major source of saturated fats, especially those dishes containing cheese and/or meat. These include burgers, sandwiches, and tacos; pizza; rice, pasta, and grain dishes; and meat, poultry, and seafood dishes. Most sodium consumed in the United States comes from salts added during commercial food processing and preparation. Mixed dishes—including burgers, sandwiches, and tacos; rice, pasta, and grain dishes; pizza; meat, poultry, and seafood dishes; and soups—account for almost half of the sodium consumed in the United States.

Sources: Data from What We Eat in America (WWEIA) Food Category analyses for the 2015 Dietary Guidelines Advisory Committee. Estimates based on dietary recalls from WWEIA, NHANES 2009–2010; and U.S. Department of Health and Human Services and U.S. Department of Agriculture, *2015–2020 Dietary Guidelines for Americans*, 8th edition, December 2015.

Implementing the Recommendations: From Guidelines to Groceries

The challenge today is to help consumers put the wide assortment of dietary recommendations into practice. This requires translating the recommendations into food-specific guides that consumers can implement in their homes, at the grocery store, and in restaurants.[64] For example, consider this dietary guideline recommendation: Consume less than 2,300 milligrams per day of sodium. This broad guideline must first be translated into food-specific behaviors for consumers, who must acquire the knowledge and skills to change their eating patterns. **Table 7-9** lists three food-specific behaviors that can be derived from the guideline and the knowledge and skill set required for each behavior. The Dietary Approaches to Stop Hypertension (DASH) diet shown in **Table 7-10** is an example

(Text discussion continued on page 264.)

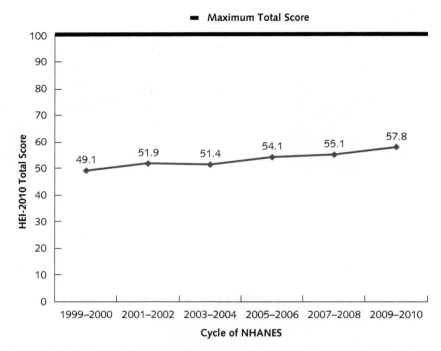

FIGURE 7-8 Adherence to the *Dietary Guidelines for Americans* as Measured by Average Healthy Eating Index Scores[a]
The Healthy Eating Index (HEI) gives a summary measure of people's overall diet quality. The tool measures the degree to which a person's diet conforms to recommended intakes from the USDA food guide's five major food groups: Grains, Vegetables, Fruits, Dairy, and Protein Foods. A high score for these components is reached by maximizing consumption of recommended amounts. The tool also measures compliance of intakes of sodium, saturated fat, and calories from solid fats and added sugars according to the *Dietary Guidelines for Americans*. A high score is reached by consuming at or below recommended amounts. Although the HEI scores have been increasing slightly since 1999, the overall score remains low.

[a] HEI total scores are out of 100 possible points. A score of 100 indicates that recommended intakes from food groups were met and limits for added sugars, saturated fat, and sodium were not exceeded. A higher total score indicates a higher quality diet.

Sources: Analyses of What We Eat in America, National Health and Nutrition Examination Survey (NHANES) data from 1999–2000 through 2009–2010; and U.S. Department of Health and Human Services and U.S. Department of Agriculture, *2015–2020 Dietary Guidelines for Americans*, 8th edition, December 2015. See also *www.cnpp.usda.gov/healthyeatingindex*.

TABLE 7-9 Translating a Dietary Guideline into Food-Specific Behaviors

DIETARY GUIDELINE	FOOD-SPECIFIC BEHAVIOR	KNOWLEDGE AND/OR SKILLS REQUIRED TO SUPPORT THE BEHAVIOR
Consume less than 2,300 milligrams per day of sodium.	• Purchase foods that are low in sodium.	• Identify major sources of sodium in the diet. • Analyze the Nutrition Facts label to compare the amount of sodium in processed foods, such as frozen dinners, cereals, soups, salad dressings, and sauces. • Choose reduced-sodium or no-salt-added products when possible.
	• Consume more fresh foods and fewer processed foods that are high in sodium.	• Choose fresh fruits or vegetables instead of salty snack foods. • Know how to read restaurant menus. • Be able to read food product labels.
	• Prepare foods with less salt.	• Know how to adapt recipes and add flavor with herbs, spices, lemon, or salt-free seasoning blends. • Know food preparation techniques for lowering sodium in meals (i.e., rinsing canned foods). • Avoid adding salt when cooking and/or eating.

TABLE 7-10 Eating Pattern to Reduce Daily Sodium Intake by Consuming More Fresh Foods[a]

FOOD GROUP	SERVINGS PER DAY 2,000 CALORIES	SERVING SIZES	EXAMPLES AND NOTES	SAMPLE MENU
Grains[b]	6–8	1 slice bread 1 oz dry cereal ½ cup cooked rice, pasta, or cereal	Whole-wheat bread and rolls, whole-wheat pasta, English muffin, pita bread, bagel, cereals, grits, oatmeal, brown rice, unsalted pretzels and popcorn	**BREAKFAST** 1 cup of cooked oatmeal or 1 cup ready-to-eat oat cereal *(choose brand with less sodium)* 1 cup low-fat milk or 1 cup plain nonfat yogurt ½ oz of walnuts 1 small banana Beverage: water, coffee, or tea[c]
Vegetables	4–5	1 cup raw leafy vegetable ½ cup cut-up raw or cooked vegetable ½ cup vegetable juice	Broccoli, carrots, collards, green beans, green peas, kale, lima beans, potatoes, spinach, squash, sweet potatoes, tomatoes	**LUNCH** Three-bean vegetarian chili on rice: ¼ cup each cooked kidney beans, navy beans, and black beans *(rinse under water to remove sodium)* ½ cup *low-sodium* tomato sauce ¼ cup chopped onion 2 Tbsp chopped bell peppers ½ tsp *salt-free* spice blend 1 tsp olive oil (to cook onion and peppers) 1 cup cooked brown rice *(no salt added to cooking water)* 1 medium fresh fruit Beverage: water, coffee, or tea[c]
Fruits	4–5	1 medium fruit ¼ cup dried fruit ½ cup fresh, frozen, or canned fruit ½ cup fruit juice	Apples, apricots, bananas, dates, grapes, oranges, grapefruit, mangoes, melons, peaches, pineapples, raisins, strawberries, tangerines	**DINNER** Roasted chicken: 3 ounces cooked chicken breast 1 large baked sweet potato ½ cup steamed zucchini or other vegetable Large green salad with 2 cups greens, ½ ounce *unsalted* pecans, ½ cup of fresh tangerine sections, and 2 Tbsp oil and vinegar dressing 1 oz whole-wheat roll 1 tsp tub margarine 1 cup fruit parfait made with ½ cup frozen chocolate yogurt and ½ cup sliced strawberries Beverage: water, coffee, or tea[c]
Fat-free or low-fat milk and milk products	2–3	1 cup milk or yogurt 1½ oz cheese	Fat-free (skim) or low-fat (1%) milk or buttermilk; fat-free, low-fat, or reduced-fat cheese; fat-free or low-fat regular or frozen yogurt	

continued

TABLE 7-10 Eating Pattern to Reduce Daily Sodium Intake by Consuming More Fresh Foods[a]—continued

FOOD GROUP	SERVINGS PER DAY 2,000 CALORIES	SERVING SIZES	EXAMPLES AND NOTES	SAMPLE MENU
Lean meats, poultry, and fish	6 or less	1 oz cooked meats, poultry, or fish 1 egg	Select only lean; trim away visible fats; broil, roast, or poach; remove skin from poultry	**Use snacks to fill in nutrient gaps in your overall diet:** ¼ cup dried apricots or 1 medium apple 1 cup raw green or red bell peppers and carrot sticks (instead of chips) 1 cup blueberry Greek-style yogurt
Nuts, seeds, and legumes	4–5 per week	⅓ cup or 1½ oz nuts 2 Tbsp peanut butter 2 Tbsp or ½ oz seeds ½ cup cooked legumes	Almonds, hazelnuts, mixed nuts, peanuts, walnuts, sunflower seeds, peanut butter, kidney beans, lentils, split peas	
Fats and oils[d]	2–3	1 tsp soft margarine 1 tsp vegetable oil 1 Tbsp mayonnaise 2 Tbsp salad dressing	Soft margarine, vegetable oil (such as canola, corn, olive, or safflower), low-fat mayonnaise, light salad dressing	
Sweets and added sugars	5 or less per week	1 Tbsp sugar 1 Tbsp jelly or jam ½ cup sorbet, gelatin 1 cup lemonade	Fruit-flavored gelatin, fruit punch, hard candy, jelly, maple syrup, sorbet and ices, sugar	

Abbreviations: oz, ounce; Tbsp, tablespoon; tsp, teaspoon.

[a] You might need to eat fewer or more calories, depending on your activity level and whether you are a man or a woman. For more menu planning help based on the *Dietary Guidelines*, go to *www.choosemyplate.gov*.

[b] Whole grains are recommended for most grain servings as a good source of fiber and nutrients.

[c] Beverages are unsweetened and without added cream or whitener.

[d] Fat content changes serving amount for fats and oils. For example, 1 Tbsp of regular salad dressing equals one serving; 1 Tbsp of a low-fat dressing equals one-half serving; and 1 Tbsp of a fat-free dressing equals zero servings.

Sources: In Brief: Your Guide to Lowering Your Blood Pressure with DASH, U.S. Department of Health and Human Services, National Institutes of Health, National Heart, Lung, and Blood Institute. Menu adapted from MyPlate Sample Menus for 2,000 Calorie Food Pattern; *www.nutrition.gov/smart-nutrition-101/myplate-food-pyramid-resources*.

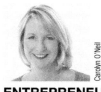

Carolyn O'Neil

ENTREPRENEUR IN ACTION
....

Noted nutrition expert, award-winning food journalist, author, and television personality Carolyn O'Neil, MS, RD, writes a weekly column for the *Atlanta Journal-Constitution*, "Healthy Eating Out," and appears on the Food Network regularly as "The Lady of the Refrigerator," a nutrition expert on Alton Brown's hit program *Good Eats*. She foresees a return to the basics of culinary arts as an important trend in dietetics. Her advice: "Learn to cook and learn how to read a recipe. Learn to write a recipe. Recipe writing is a craft, an art, and a science. A recipe to prepare nutritious dishes—that's the formula folks need for good health." Find out what she has to say about entrepreneurship online at *www.cengagebrain.com*.

of a recommended eating pattern for reducing sodium intakes and lowering blood pressure. Successfully choosing such foods means having some knowledge of food composition, recognizing major food sources of sodium, knowing how to boost flavor in meals without adding salt, knowing how to adapt recipes, and being able to read both a food label and a restaurant menu.

The process of breaking down a dietary guideline into specific behaviors can be carried a step further. The guideline can be translated into an actual eating pattern, as shown in Table 7-10. The eating pattern should reflect the basic principles of the dietary guidelines and should focus on variety—eating a selection of foods from all of the food groups; proportionality—eating appropriate amounts of foods to meet nutritional needs; moderation—enjoying food but avoiding eating patterns that are associated with chronic disease; and usability—being flexible and practical enough to accommodate individual food preferences and meet nutrient needs.

Policymaking in Action

It can be difficult to see the connection between policymaking and your work as community nutritionists. An example of this connection can be drawn from the job responsibilities of the director of health promotion for the First-Rate Spa and Health Resort (described in Chapter 1). The director decides to update a risk-reduction program that will help spa clients make more healthful eating choices. The new program will address eating strategies to reduce the risk of coronary heart disease, stroke, cancer, and osteoporosis.

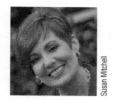

Susan Mitchell

ENTREPRENEUR IN ACTION

A 19-year radio veteran known for her smart, sassy straight talk about food and fitness, Susan Mitchell, PhD, RDN, LDN, FAND, helps thousands of her faithful followers navigate through the hype of conflicting nutrition information through her podcast, videos, and blog. She takes the science of nutrition and turns it into easy-to-follow health messages that people understand and want to live by. Her goal is to deliver a positive, empowering health message to the public instead of one that focuses on what *not* to do or what to *avoid*. She says, "The most rewarding part of my work is sharing the message of nutrition and health through a multimedia platform that reaches people globally. I love driving the nutrition messages from conception to delivery, and I am always looking for a way to keep them fresh." Find out more about her sage advice on starting your own private practice at *www.cengagebrain.com*.

In organizing the content of the program, the director realizes that clients need to be given information about healthful eating patterns; recommendations related to fat, calcium, and antioxidant vitamin intake; and instructions on how to read food product labels, among other topics. **Table 7-11** shows six decisions the director must make in developing the program's content, the policy "tool" to be used for each decision, and the source of each tool. The first decision is to choose a program instructor who is a registered dietitian.

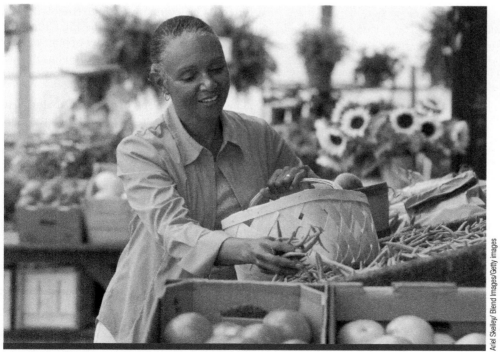

Consumers who follow the *Dietary Guidelines for Americans* eat plenty of fruits, vegetables, and whole grains and balance their food intake with physical activity.

Ariel Skelley/ Blend Images/Getty images

TABLE 7-11 Connection between Policy Tools and Policy Decisions

DECISION	POLICY TOOL	SOURCE OF POLICY TOOL
Instructor will be a registered dietitian (RD/RDN).	Credentials	Commission on Dietetic Registration
Program should include a discussion of healthful eating patterns.	*Dietary Guidelines for Americans*	U.S. Department of Agriculture; U.S. Department of Health and Human Services
Program segment on osteoporosis should include recommendations for obtaining calcium from foods, including fortified foods and dietary supplements.	Dietary Reference Intakes (DRIs)	Food and Nutrition Board of the National Academy of Sciences
Program should include a segment on reading food product labels.	Labeling regulations	Food and Drug Administration
All materials must show the company logo.	Company policy	First-Rate Spa and Health Resort
Program segment on dietary fats should include information about omega-3 fatty acids and alpha-linolenic acid.	Dietary Reference Intakes (DRIs)	Food and Nutrition Board of the National Academy of Sciences

▶ **THINK LIKE A COMMUNITY** NUTRITIONIST

Table 7-11 provides examples of policy decisions that the First-Rate Spa and Health Resort director must make in planning a new program focused on reducing chronic disease risk. Four of these decisions relate to program content, while the remaining two decisions indicate that an RD will teach the class and all materials will show the company logo. Choose one of the "content"-related decisions. Then review the listed policy tool for guidance. What other resources and tools would be helpful in developing the program content? Investigate other resources, and make a list of the titles and authors (or organization) for each.

This decision enhances the image of the program and ensures that accurate and timely information will be offered to clients.

Deciding to use the *Dietary Guidelines for Americans* is a fairly obvious choice because it is a widely accepted policy tool of the federal government. The company's requirement that all visual aids show the logo of the First-Rate Spa and Health Resort is also a matter of policy. Every organization, agency, and institution has its own policies that affect the practice of community nutritionists.

The decision about how much material to present to clients on the essential fatty acid, alpha-linolenic acid, and other omega-3 fatty acids—hot topics for consumers today—is more complex. A DRI for the intake of omega-3 fatty acids has been published but is not currently used in the spa's education materials. Should the DRI be used, in this situation, to justify the additional expense for developing educational materials on this topic? This is precisely where we see policymaking in action, for the director is making a policy decision when choosing to include the DRI for omega-3 fatty acids in program materials. Many decisions made by community nutritionists are opportunities for making and implementing policy.

Policymaking Does Not Stand Still This is an exciting time in community nutrition. Legislation related to health care reform, as discussed in Chapter 9;

third-party reimbursement for medical nutrition therapy; food and supplement labeling requirements; new evidence-based dietary guidelines; *Healthy People 2020* objectives with a focus on the social and environmental determinants of health; the increasing use of social media; and market forces in the health care field and the food industry promise many opportunities for community nutritionists to serve as liaisons between policymakers and the general public.[65] The one guarantee is that nutrition policy will continue to change.

The task of formulating a national nutrition agenda is daunting. Government must make a commitment to develop and promote a coordinated plan to improve the nation's nutrition and health status, scientists must reach a consensus on the interpretation of scientific findings and appropriate dietary advice for all Americans, and sufficient financial resources must be allocated to implementing the policy. As the 2015 Dietary Guidelines Advisory Committee noted:[66]

> It will take concerted, bold actions on the part of individuals, families, communities, industry, and government to achieve and maintain the healthy diet patterns and the levels of physical activity needed to promote the health of the U.S. population. These actions will require a paradigm shift to an environment in which population health is a national priority and where individuals and organizations, private business, and communities work together to achieve a population-wide "culture of health" in which healthy lifestyle choices are easy, accessible, affordable, and normative—both at home and away from home.

case study

From Guidelines to Groceries

by Alice Fornari, EdD, RD, Alessandra Sarcona, MS, RD, CSSD, and Alison Barkman, MS, RD, CDN

Scenario

As a nutrition consultant and public relations chair of your local district dietetic association, you are approached by the local health department to prepare a series of educational announcements for the adult clinic waiting room. It is up to you to determine whether the announcements should be communicated as a written document or as video clips.

The focus of the announcements is to acquaint consumers with current public health issues as determined by national databases and surveys. In addition, you are asked to translate the *Dietary Guidelines for Americans* into behaviors that consumers could adopt to implement the recommendations.

To further assess your audience, you decide it is important to meet clients who would be hearing or reading the announcements. A visit to the Department of Health indicates that communication with clients is achieved by written publications, video monitors, and a visible bulletin board.

You also notice that most of the clients are African American women of various ages and their children.

You take time during the visit to approach some of the clients waiting for services. These brief conversations reveal that the clients have no preliminary knowledge of the *Dietary Guidelines* and definitively do not apply these guidelines to personal food choices. Here are some comments by clients:

> *"I use sweetened iced tea as our beverage. All the kids like it."*
> *"Milk is not healthy; it gives everyone stomachaches."*
> *"Fresh fruits and vegetables are too expensive. I use canned ones."*

A sample recall from a middle-aged woman reveals the following:

> *Breakfast:* Donut or egg on a biscuit and sweetened coffee
> *Lunch:* Fast-food hamburgers with french fries and a sweetened soft drink
> *Dinner:* Fried chicken, potatoes or rice, peas or corn
> *Snacks:* Chips, ice cream, snack cakes, iced tea

These conversations reveal that your task is much more complex than you anticipated. You must begin by identifying a goal for your educational announcement. As a first attempt, you decide that the video monitor will be the most effective tool for communication.

Learning Outcomes

- Identify and access, via the web, USDA/Economic Research Service (ERS) food consumption survey data and the most recent *Dietary Guidelines for Americans*.
- Use survey data to identify at-risk groups that could be targeted for intervention by a department of health.
- Prepare an educational announcement translating data into positive food-specific behaviors for a target population.

Foundation: Acquisition of Knowledge and Skills

1. Outline the *2015–2020 Dietary Guidelines for Americans*: http://health.gov/dietaryguidelines.
2. What do Americans think about dietary guidance issues, and how does the American diet measure up to the *Dietary Guidelines*? These questions are addressed at the following sites:
   a. Go to *www.foodinsight.org/2015-food-health-survey-consumer-research* to access the International Food Information Council Foundation 2015 Food and Health Survey on Consumer Attitudes toward Food Safety, Nutrition, and Health.
   b. Access descriptive text on USDA surveys from the web: *www.ers.usda.gov/Briefing/DietQuality*

Step 1: *Identify Relevant Information and Uncertainties*

1. After your visit to the health clinic, and considering the *Dietary Guidelines for Americans*, create a list of priority nutrition issues for the population who would be accessing the educational announcements.
2. Explain why the clinic population may have difficulties following the *Dietary Guidelines for Americans*. That is, judging on the basis of your observations and interactions with the clinic clientele, identify barriers to following the guidelines.

Step 2: *Interpret Information*

1. Connect the nutrition issues identified for the target population to the survey data reported on the web by the USDA.
2. Identify knowledge and/or skills that this target population will need to support positive behavior changes.

Step 3: *Draw and Implement Conclusions*

1. Refer to the chapter discussion of translating a dietary guideline into food-specific behaviors. Identify a dietary guideline, not sampled in the text, that appears to be one that this clinic population is having difficulty following. Link the selected dietary guideline to positive food-specific behaviors; in addition, identify the knowledge and/or skills necessary to support positive behavior changes in the target population.
2. Outline an educational announcement to be viewed in the clinic, through the waiting room video monitor.

Step 4: *Engage in Continuous Improvement*

1. If you had the opportunity to continue working on publications for the clinic, how could you monitor the impact of your efforts?
2. For use on the clinic bulletin board, develop a shopping guide to be used as a resource for a hands-on tour of a local supermarket. The tour will help clients visualize healthy food and beverage purchases and strategies for incorporating the *Dietary Guidelines for Americans*.

Evaluating Research and Information on Nutrition and Health

Nutrition and health policy is based on sound research. However, at the same time that science has shown that to some extent we really are what we eat, many consumers are more confused than ever about how to translate the steady stream of new findings about nutrition into healthful eating.[1] Each additional nugget of nutrition news that comes along raises new concerns: Is caffeine bad for me? Does feverfew prevent headache? Should I take vitamin supplements? Will diet pills work? Can a sports drink improve my performance? Do pesticides pose a hazard? As a community nutritionist, you will find that many consumers turn to you as the resident expert on these questions and more.

Some manufacturers of food and nutrition-related products, as well as many members of the media, compound the confusion by offering a myriad of unreliable products and misleading dietary advice targeted to health-conscious consumers. Unfortunately, many consumers fall prey to this barrage of misinformation. Americans spend more than $30 billion annually on medical and nutritional health fraud and quackery, up from $1 billion to $2 billion in the early 1960s.[2] At the same time, the sale of weight-loss programs and products—not all of them sound—has become a $60 billion industry. Media attention to "hot" foods and nutritional supplements generally causes spending on those items to soar. This Professional Focus provides a sieve with which you can help consumers separate valid from bogus nutrition information.

Money down the drain is just one of the problems stemming from misleading dietary information. Some fraudulent claims about nutrition are harmless and make for a good laugh, but others can have tragic consequences. False claims about nutritional products have been known to bring about malnutrition, birth defects, mental retardation, and even death in extreme cases. Negative effects can happen in two ways. One is that the product in question causes direct harm. Even a seemingly innocuous substance such as vitamin A, for instance, can cause severe liver damage over time if taken in large enough doses. The other problem is that spurious nutritional remedies build false hope and may keep a consumer from obtaining sound, scientifically tested medical treatment. A person who relies on a so-called anticancer diet as a cure, for example, might forgo possible lifesaving interventions such as surgery or chemotherapy.

Part of the confusion stems from the way the media interpret the findings of scientific research. A good case in point is the controversy over whether a high-fiber diet protects against colon cancer, a disease that affects some 141,000 Americans each year. This issue dates back to the early 1970s, when scientists observed that colon cancer was extremely uncommon in areas of the world where the diet consisted largely of unrefined foods and little meat. The researchers theorized that dietary fiber may be protective against colon cancer by binding bile and speeding the passage of wastes and potentially harmful compounds through the colon. Since then, other studies have suggested that those who eat a high-fiber diet have a lower risk of colon and rectal cancers.[3]

However, in 1998 a flurry of headlines threatened to pull the pedestal out from under the popular fiber theory, asking, "Fiber: Is It Still the Right Choice?" A Harvard-based study published in the *New England Journal of Medicine* suggested that fiber did nothing to prevent cancer.[4] The 16-year trial of almost 90,000 nurses—called the Nurses' Health Study—found that the nurses who ate low-fiber diets (less than 10 grams daily) were no more likely to develop colon cancer than those who ate higher levels of fiber (about 25 grams daily). As a result, the researchers concluded that the study provided no support for the theory that fiber could reduce the risk of colon cancer.

This surprising news reinforces the need for research studies to be duplicated. All studies have their limitations, and a number of questions can be raised regarding the conclusions of the Nurses' Health Study. For example, the study relied on participants to recall their eating habits accurately. Is this type of self-reported dietary information reliable? Back in 1980, the nurses were asked for information about their intakes of "dark" breads. However, food labels at that time did not list the fiber content of breads, and some wheat breads on the shelf had amounts of fiber similar to those found in white bread. Did the nurses mistakenly consider "dark" bread the same as 100% whole-wheat bread?

Another question to ask is "What are the optimal levels of fiber intake for colon cancer protection?" Some experts believe that it may take more than 25 grams of fiber a day to show cancer-protective effects, which might explain the lack of effect noted in the Nurses' study.

This fiber story illustrates how news reports based on only one study can leave the public with the impression that scientists can't make up their minds. It seems as though one week scientists are saying that fiber is good, and the next week the word is that fiber doesn't do any good at all.

Contrary to what some headlines imply, reputable scientists do not base their dietary recommendations for the public on the results of one or two studies. Scientists are still conducting research to determine whether fiber does in fact help to prevent colon cancer, and if so, what types of fiber and in what amount. Scientists design their research to test theories, such as the notion that eating a high-fiber diet is associated with lower risk of cancer. Other factors, however, often confound the matter at hand. The study of fiber and colon cancer is complex because many other factors, such as inactivity, obesity, saturated fat intake, and low calcium or folate intake, are linked with the development of colon cancer.

You can critique the nutrition news you read by asking a series of questions. Consider the following points as a checklist for separating the bogus news stories from those worth your attention.

- *Where is the study published?*

The study being described in the news story should be published in a peer-reviewed journal—a journal that uses experts in the field to review research results. These reviewers serve to point out any flaws in the research design and can challenge the researcher's conclusions before the study is published.

- *How recent is the study?*

The science of nutrition continues to develop. New studies employ state-of-the-art methods and technology and benefit from the scrutiny of experts in the particular field of study.

- *What research methods were used to obtain the data?*

Are the results from an epidemiologic study or an intervention study? Epidemiologic studies examine populations to determine food patterns and health status over time. These population studies are useful in uncovering correlations between two factors (e.g., whether a high calcium intake early in life reduces the incidence of bone fractures later in life). However, they are not considered as conclusive as intervention studies. A correlation between two factors may suggest a cause-and-effect relationship between the factors but does not prove it.

Intervention studies examine the effects of a specific treatment or intervention on a particular group of subjects and compare the results to a similar group of people not receiving the treatment. An example is a cholesterol-monitoring study in which half the subjects follow dietary advice to lower their blood cholesterol and half do not. Ideally, intervention studies should be randomized and controlled—that is, subjects are assigned to either an experimental group or a control group by means of a random selection process. Each subject has an equal chance of being assigned to either group. The experimental group receives the "treatment" being tested; the control group receives a placebo, or neutral substance. If possible, neither the researcher nor the participants should know which group the subjects have been assigned to until the end of the experiment. A randomized, controlled study helps to ensure that the study's conclusions are a result of the treatment and minimizes the chances that the results are due to a placebo effect or to bias on the part of the researcher.

- *What was the size of the study?*

In order to achieve validity—accuracy in results—studies must generally include a sufficiently large number of people, such as 50 or more in intervention studies. This reduces the chances that the results are simply a coincidence and justifies generalizing the conclusions of the study to a wider audience.

- *Who were the subjects?*

Look for similarities between the subjects in the study and yourself. The more you have in common with the participants (age, diet pattern, gender, etc.), the more pertinent the study results may be for you.

- *Does a consensus of published studies support the results reported in the news?*

Even if an experiment is carefully designed and carried out perfectly, its findings cannot be considered definitive until they have been confirmed by other research. Testing and retesting reduce the possibility that the outcome was simply the result of chance or an error or oversight on the part of the experimenter. Every study should be viewed as preliminary until it becomes just one addition to a significant body of evidence pointing in the same direction.

When making dietary recommendations for the public, experts pool the results of different types of studies, such as analyses of food patterns of groups of people and carefully controlled studies on people in hospitals or clinics. Before drawing any conclusions, they then consider the evidence from all of the research. The bottom line is that if you read a report in the newspaper or watch one on television that advises making a dramatic change in your diet or lifestyle on the basis of the results of one study, don't take it to heart. The findings may make for a good story, but they're not worth taking too seriously.

Consumers sometimes ask why the government doesn't prevent the media from disseminating misleading nutrition information, but the government lacks the power to do so. The First Amendment guarantees freedom of the press, which means that people may express whatever views they like in the media, whether these opinions are sound, unsound, or even dangerous. By law, writers cannot be punished for publishing misinformation unless it can be proved in court that the information has caused a reader bodily harm.

Fortunately, most professional health groups maintain committees to combat the spread of health and nutrition misinformation. Remember, too, that although the Internet is an excellent source of health information, it has also become one of the fastest-growing outlets for health fraud.

As the Internet continues to grow and becomes integrated into community nutrition practice, community nutritionists will increasingly be expected to evaluate information obtained from the Internet. Perhaps your clients will have questions about information they found on the World Wide Web, or your organization may ask you to choose 5–10 sites to link to its own webpage, or you may wish to include websites on a handout for program participants. Whatever the reason, community nutritionists must have skills for evaluating Internet information.

Information is rampant on the Internet. In a sense, the Internet is information, and the information is continually being revised and created. Internet information exists in many forms (e.g., facts, statistics, stories, and opinions). This information is created for many purposes (e.g., to entertain, to inform, to persuade, to sell, and to influence), and it varies in quality from very good to worthless or even dangerous. One method for determining whether the information found on the Internet is reliable and of good quality is the CARS Checklist.[5] The acronym CARS stands for credibility, accuracy, reasonableness, and support.

- *Credibility.* Check the credentials of the author (if there is one!) or sponsoring organization. Is the author or organization respected and well known as a source of sound, scientific information? The lack of a posted author and the presence of misspelled words or bad grammar can be taken as evidence of a lack of credibility. A credible sponsor will use a professional approach to designing the website.
- *Accuracy.* Check to ensure that the information is current, factual, and comprehensive. If important facts, consequences, or other information is missing, the website may not be presenting a complete story. There being no date on the document, the use of sweeping generalizations, and the presence of outdated information are evidence of a lack of accuracy. Watch for testimonials masquerading as scientific evidence. This is a common method for promoting questionable products on the Internet.
- *Reasonableness.* Evaluate the information for fairness, balance, and consistency. Does the author present a fair, balanced argument supporting the ideas presented? Are the arguments offered rational? Has the author maintained objectivity in discussing the topic? Does he or she have an obvious—or hidden—conflict of interest? Evidence of a lack of reasonableness includes gross generalizations ("Foods not grown organically are all toxic and shouldn't be eaten") and outlandish claims ("Kombucha tea will cure cancer and diabetes").
- *Support.* Check to see whether supporting documentation is cited for scientific statements. Are there references to legitimate journals and publications? Is it clear where the information came from? An Internet document that fails to indicate the sources of its information is suspect.

It's not always easy to separate the nutrition wheat from the chaff, given that many misleading claims are supposedly backed by scientific-sounding statements, but you can offer your clients some tips to help them tell whether a product is bogus. The following red flags can help you spot a quack:

- *The promoter claims that the medical establishment is against him or her and that the government won't accept this new "alternative" treatment.*
  If the government or medical community cannot accept a treatment, it is because the treatment has not been proven to work. Reputable professionals do not suppress knowledge about fighting disease. On the contrary, they welcome new remedies for illness, provided that the treatments have been carefully tested.

- *The promoter uses testimonials and anecdotes from satisfied customers to support claims.*
  Valid nutrition information comes from careful experimental research, not from random tales. A few persons' reports that the product in question "works every time" are never acceptable as sound scientific evidence.

- *The promoter uses a computer-scored questionnaire for diagnosing "nutrient deficiencies."*
  Those programs are designed to show that just about everyone has a deficiency that can be reversed with the supplements the promoter just happens to be selling, regardless of the consumer's symptoms or health.

- *The promoter claims that the product will make weight loss easy.*

  Unfortunately, there is no simple way to lose weight. In other words, if a claim sounds too good to be true, it probably is.

- *The promoter promises that the product is made with a "secret formula" available only from this one company.*

  Legitimate health professionals share their knowledge of proven treatments so that others can benefit from it.

- *The treatment is offered only in the back pages of magazines, over the phone, or by mail-order solicited by ads in the form of news stories or 30-minute commercials (known as infomercials) in talk-show format.*

  Results of studies on credible treatments are reported first in medical journals and are administered through a physician or other health professional. If information about a treatment appears only elsewhere, it probably cannot withstand scientific scrutiny.

CHAPTER SUMMARY

National Nutrition Policy in the United States

▶ National nutrition policy is a set of nationwide guidelines and manifests itself in food assistance programs, national nutrition and health objectives as found in the *Healthy People 2020* initiative, regulations to safeguard the food supply and ensure the proper handling of food products, dietary guidance systems, monitoring and surveillance programs, food labeling legislation, and other activities in the nutrition arena.

National Nutrition Monitoring

▶ National nutrition policies are typically guided by the outcomes of nutrition and health surveys. The primary purpose of national nutrition-monitoring activities is to obtain the information needed to ensure a population's adequate nutrition. Such information can be derived by any of several methods, including nutrition screening, nutrition assessment, nutrition monitoring, and nutrition surveillance. The collected data are used in health planning, program management and evaluation, and timely warning and intervention efforts to prevent acute food shortages (see Table 7-5).

▶ The National Nutrition Monitoring and Related Research Program (NNMRRP) includes all data collection and analysis activities of the federal government related to (1) measuring the health and nutrition status, food consumption, dietary knowledge, and attitudes about diet and health of the U.S. population and (2) measuring food composition and the quality of the food supply.

▶ The NNMRRP surveys can be grouped into the five areas: nutrition status and nutrition-related health measurements; food and nutrient consumption; knowledge, attitudes, and behavior assessments; food composition and nutrient databases; and food supply determinations.

- The NHANES series forms the basis of the health and nutrition status component of the NNMRRP.

- The Food and Nutrient Consumption surveys collect data that are used to describe food consumption behavior and to evaluate the nutritional content of diets in terms of their implications for food policies, marketing, food safety, food assistance, and nutrition education. Current surveys include the What We Eat in America Survey, the dietary interview component of NHANES, and the Total Diet Study.

- The knowledge, attitudes, and behavior assessment surveys gather a variety of data related to behavior and disease risk and include the Behavioral Risk Factor Surveillance System and the Youth Risk Behavior Survey.

- Information about nutrient content of foods is provided by the Food Label and Package Survey and the USDA National Nutrient Database for Standard Reference.

- Food available for consumption by the U.S. civilian population is determined by the USDA's Food Supply Series surveys.

▶ **Nutrient Intake Standards.** Merely collecting data on a population's nutrient intake and eating habits is not enough. Such data are meaningless on their own; to be valuable, they must be compared with some national standard related to nutrient needs. The Dietary Reference Intakes (DRIs) are nutrient goals to be achieved over time.

Nutrition Survey Results: How Well Do We Eat?

▶ The most recent data from the NHANES surveys show a considerable gap between current nutrition recommendations and consumers' practices.

▶ The nutrition and weight status objectives for *Healthy People 2020* emphasize a broad range of policies and environmental factors that support eating a healthy diet and maintaining a healthy body weight in settings such as schools, worksites, health care organizations, and communities.

▶ One approach to improving the public's knowledge about healthful eating involves the dissemination of dietary guidance in the form of dietary guidelines and food group plans.

- The basis of nutrition policy is the *Dietary Guidelines for Americans*, which serves as the foundation for all federal nutrition guidance.

- Dietary recommendations are also issued by a variety of nonprofit health organizations, such as the American Heart Association and the American Cancer Society.

- Dietary guidance in the form of the MyPlate food guidance system is designed to help consumers choose foods that supply a good balance of nutrients, and it aims to moderate or limit dietary components often consumed in excess, such as saturated fat, *trans* fat, refined grains and added sugars, and sodium, in keeping with the U.S. government's *Dietary Guidelines for Americans*.

- The challenge today is to help consumers put the wide assortment of dietary recommendations into practice. This requires translating the recommendations into food-specific guides that consumers can implement in their homes, at the grocery store, and in restaurants.

SUMMARY **QUESTIONS**

1. How does nutrition research relate to nutrition monitoring in the United States?
2. List five nutrition-related components of the National Health and Nutrition Examination Survey.
3. Describe how you could use the results of the What We Eat in America Survey as a community nutritionist.
4. Differentiate among *nutrition screening, nutrition assessment, nutrition monitoring*, and *nutrition surveillance*.

5. Describe a strategy for using MyPlate in your community nutrition practice that focuses on adult wellness.
6. Translate one of the key recommendations of the *2015–2020 Dietary Guidelines for Americans* into food-specific behaviors for consumers and identify the knowledge and skill set required to support the behaviors.

INTERNET **RESOURCES** . . . .

Canada
Health Canada
www.hc-sc.gc.ca

Healthy Living
www.hc-sc.gc.ca/hl-vs/index-eng.php

Canada's Food Guide
www.hc-sc.gc.ca/fn-an/food-guide-aliment/index-eng.php

Nutrition Policy Reports
www.hc-sc.gc.ca/fn-an/nutrition/pol/index-eng.php

United States
Center for Nutrition Policy and Promotion
www.cnpp.usda.gov

Dietary Guidelines for Americans
www.cnpp.usda.gov/Dietaryguidelines.htm

Food and Nutrition Information Center
https://fnic.nal.usda.gov

Food Labeling Information
https://fnic.nal.usda.gov/food-labeling

Nutrition Surveys
Behavioral Risk Factor Surveillance System (BRFSS)
www.cdc.gov/brfss

National Health and Nutrition Examination Survey
www.cdc.gov/nchs/nhanes.htm

National Center for Health Statistics Data Briefs
www.cdc.gov/nchs/products/databriefs.htm

National Health and Nutrition Examination Survey: Survey Results and Products
www.cdc.gov/nchs/nhanes/nhanes_products.htm

U.S. Department of Agriculture: Agricultural Research Service
www.ars.usda.gov/main/main.htm

Government-Sponsored Websites for Public Information Regarding Lifestyle Habits
Nutrition and Dietary Guidance
www.nutrition.gov

National Heart, Lung, and Blood Institute Information
www.nhlbi.nih.gov/health

Smoking Cessation
www.cdc.gov/tobacco/data_statistics/sgr/2012/index.htm

Physical Activity Guidelines for Americans
http://health.gov/paguidelines

International Nutrition Recommendations
World Health Organization (WHO)
www.who.int/en/

Food and Agriculture Organization of the United Nations (FAO)
www.fao.org/home/en/

CHAPTER 8

Addressing the Obesity Epidemic: An Issue for Public Health Policy

Deanna M. Hoelscher, PhD, RD, LD, and Christine McCullum-Gómez, PhD, RD, LD

LEARNING **OBJECTIVES**

After you have read and studied this chapter, you will be able to:

- Define the terms *obesity* and *overweight* as they apply to adults and children, and discuss why the definitions differ.

- Describe the epidemiology of obesity and overweight among adults and children, including the changes during the last two decades and potential reasons for those changes.

- Explain how to assess and survey obesity and overweight in the population, and why this is important.

- List and discuss determinants of obesity and overweight within the context of the social–ecological model.

- Discuss various interventions, settings, and strategies for the prevention and treatment of obesity and overweight among adults and children, as well as the pros and cons of each approach.

- Describe potential public health strategies to prevent obesity, including examples of current and proposed policies and legislation, and elaborate on how these public health approaches differ from more individual, clinical approaches.

- List strategies, tools, and resources that a nutritionist can use for obesity prevention efforts in the community.

This chapter addresses such issues as the influence of socioeconomic and psychological factors on food and dietary behaviors, assessment of nutritional health risks, public policy, food and nutrition laws and regulations, and current information technologies, which have been designated by the Accreditation Council for Education in Nutrition and Dietetics (ACEND) as Foundation Knowledge and Learning Outcomes for dietetics education.

CHAPTER **OUTLINE**

For a complete list of references, please access the MindTap Reader within your MindTap course.

Introduction

During the past 20 years, obesity has emerged as a significant public health problem because of its increasing and high prevalence, as well as the morbidity and mortality attributed to it, both in the United States and in other countries.[1] This increase has been noted in both adults and children, although recent data from the United States show a slowing in the rate of increase among the general population.[2] Although the development of obesity is a clinical problem at the individual level, the increasing morbidity and mortality attributed to the metabolic abnormalities associated with excess body weight, as well as the increased health care costs, ultimately affect all of the population, making it a significant public health issue.[3]

Why are overweight and obesity so prevalent now? No one underlying cause has been determined, but because it takes extended periods of time to change the genetic makeup of an organism or population, it is unlikely that the increased rates of obesity are due only to heritable factors.[4] More likely, the rapid increases in obesity over the past three decades are due primarily to societal and environmental factors.[5] Factors in the environment that may contribute to the obesity epidemic include increased caloric intake due to innovations in food production and transportation, other technological changes, increased portion sizes, increased consumption of foods and meals away from homes, sedentary lifestyles and media influences, social inequities, urban sprawl and other changes in the built environment, and poverty. Because many factors contribute to obesity, the solutions must also be multifactorial and will likely involve both societal and environmental changes. Since obesity is linked with chronic diseases, such as type 2 diabetes, cardiovascular disease, and some forms of cancer, it can be projected that the increases in rates of obesity will lead to increased death and disability in the future.[6] Currently, the epidemic of obesity is among the most important public health challenges in the United States.

Body mass index (BMI) An index of a person's weight in relation to height that correlates with total body fat content. BMI = (weight in kg)/[(height in m)²], where kg = kilogram and m = meter.

Conversions:
1 kilogram = 2.2 pounds
1 inch = 2.54 centimeters
100 centimeters = 1 meter

BMI can be estimated using pounds and inches with the following equation:

[Weight in pounds/(height in inches × height in inches)] × 703

Defining Obesity and Overweight

The terms *obesity* and *overweight* both refer to the accumulation of excess adipose tissue; obesity is the more severe form.[7] Although many measures of excess body fat exist, the most common criterion for screening and monitoring at the population level is the **body mass index (BMI)**, with a BMI of 25–29.9 defined as *overweight* and a BMI of 30 or more defined as *obese* for adults. Obesity can be further divided into categories, such as *extreme obesity* (**Table 8-1**). A BMI of 30 translates into approximately 30 extra pounds

CLASSIFICATION	OBESITY CLASS	BMI (kg/m²)
Underweight		< 18.5
Healthy weight		18.5–24.9
Overweight		25–29.9
Obese	I	30–34.9
	II	35–39.9
Extreme obesity	III	≥ 40

TABLE 8-1

Classification of Overweight and Obesity by Body Mass Index in Adults

Source: From National Heart, Lung, and Blood Institute Expert Panel on the Identification, Evaluation, and Treatment of Overweight and Obesity in Adults, "Executive Summary of the Clinical Guidelines on the Identification, Evaluation, and Treatment of Overweight and Obesity in Adults," *Journal of the American Dietetic Association* 98: 1178–91. Copyright © 1998 by Elsevier. Reprinted with permission.

CLASSIFICATION	DEFINITION
Underweight	BMI-for-age < 5th percentile
Healthy weight	BMI-for-age ≥ 5th percentile to < 85th percentile between underweight and overweight
Overweight	BMI-for-age ≥ 85th percentile to < 95th percentile
Obese	BMI-for-age ≥ 95th percentile

TABLE 8-2

Classification of Overweight in Children and Adolescents by Body Mass Index

Source: CDC, 2009.

for an adult. For example, a woman 5 feet 6 inches tall who weighs 186 pounds would be considered obese (see the BMI chart on the inside back cover of this book).

Other measures of obesity exist, but most are expensive to use and not practical for large population-based studies. Although BMI has been shown to correlate highly with body fat, the measure may be inaccurate for persons with large muscle mass (such as weight lifters) or for those with low muscle mass, such as older adults. Body fat distribution is also important because **central obesity** (fat around the abdomen) is more highly associated with metabolic disturbances and health problems. Excessive fat is indicated by **waist circumference**, with measures of greater than 40 inches for men and greater than 35 inches for women considered risk factors for chronic diseases, such as cardiovascular disease.[8]

For children, the Centers for Disease Control and Prevention (CDC) have defined **obesity** as a BMI at or above the growth chart criterion of 95th percentile based on gender and age standards (**Table 8-2**).[9] **Overweight** reflects a BMI at or above the CDC growth chart criterion of 85th percentile, but lower than the 95th percentile based on gender and age standards.[10] For a fourth-grade child (9 years of age), obese is approximately 10 pounds over the maximum ideal or healthy weight, whereas for an eighth-grade child (13 years of age), obese is approximately 20 pounds over maximum ideal or healthy weight.*

Epidemiology of Obesity and Overweight

In the United States, data for adult obesity are generally obtained from two national surveys: (1) the National Health and Nutrition Examination Survey (NHANES) and (2) the Behavioral Risk Factor Surveillance System (BRFSS). NHANES is conducted by the National Center for Health Statistics and involves a nationally representative sample.[11]

Central obesity Characterized by an "apple-shaped" body with large fat stores around the abdomen; a strong risk factor for type 2 diabetes, heart disease, and other problems. Central fat is also known as *android fat* to distinguish it from fat deposition on thighs and hips (*gynoid*, or *peripheral, fat*).

Waist circumference A measure used to assess abdominal (visceral) fat. Substantially increased risk of obesity-related health problems is associated with waist circumference measures as follows:

Men: > 40 inches
Women: > 35 inches

Weight classifications in children:
Obesity BMI-for-age ≥ 95th percentile
Overweight BMI-for-age ≥ 85th to < 95th percentile

* The International Obesity Task Force (IOTF) has also set criteria for child overweight and obesity. For the IOTF criteria, excess weight in children and adolescents is classified as obese and overweight, but these values differ slightly from the values on the CDC growth charts because they are based on reference standards from several countries, including the United States, whereas the CDC National Center for Health Statistics (NCHS) growth charts are based on U.S. data only.

For NHANES data collection, traveling measurement trailers obtain subjective or self-reported information about dietary and physical activity behaviors, as well as objective measures on body size. NHANES staff members measure and weigh participants, so this is considered an *objective* measurement. Other data are collected for NHANES, including dietary recalls for intake data; physical activity information; and other anthropometric data, such as waist circumference (see Chapter 7).

Data from NHANES show that the prevalence of overweight and obesity in the United States has increased substantially during the last two decades. The most recent NHANES data from 2011–2012 show an age-adjusted prevalence of adult (age 20 years and over) obesity of 34.9%[12] compared with 22.9% in 1988–1994. In contrast, the percentage of overweight adults has remained stable during this time; 33.6% of U.S. adults were overweight in 2011–2012 compared to 33.1% in 1988–1994. Not only has the prevalence of obesity increased, the prevalence of people who are at Obese Grade 3 levels (BMI ≥ 40) has also increased; current data from 2011–2012 show that the prevalence of extreme (or morbid) obesity is 6.4%.[13] The prevalence of obesity varies by race/ethnicity: 32.6% for non-Hispanic whites versus 47.8% for non-Hispanic blacks and 42.5% for Hispanics.

In 2011–2012, the prevalence of overweight or obesity (BMI ≥ 25) was 71.3% and 65.8% for men and women over age 20, respectively, while the prevalence of obesity was 33.5% and 36.1%. In women, the prevalence of obesity was significantly higher in non-Hispanic black (56.6%) and Hispanic women (44.4%) compared to non-Hispanic white women (32.8%); in men, the prevalence of obesity was similar for non-Hispanic white (32.4%) and non-Hispanic black (37.1%), but marginally higher for Hispanic men (40.1%) compared to non-Hispanic men. Between 2003–2004 and 2011–2012, the prevalence of obesity increased significantly in adults aged 60 years and above; no other significant trends over time were seen in adults, indicating that, for the most part, the prevalence of adult obesity has been relatively unchanged during that time period.[14]

The increasing prevalence of obesity has been noted in children as well, with recent data showing obesity prevalence rates of 16.9% among children aged 2–19. Child obesity has increased dramatically in the United States, from 4% in the 1960s to 11% in 1988–1994 to 17.7% in 2011–2012 in children aged 6–11, and from 5% in the 1960s to 11% in 1988–1994 to 20.5% in 2011–2012 in children aged 12–19 years old (**Figure 8-1**).[15] For children aged 2–5,

FIGURE 8-1 Trends in Obesity (BMI ≥ 95th Percentile of the CDC Growth Charts) among Children and Adolescents

Sources: National Center for Health Statistics, *www.cdc.gov/obesity/childhood/data.html*; C. L. Ogden and coauthors, 2006, 2008, 2010, 2012, and 2014.

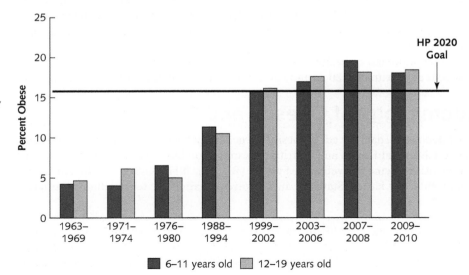

the prevalence of obesity in 2011–2012 was 8.4%, which was a significant decrease over time compared to 2003–2004; further monitoring is necessary to see if this trend continues, but these data are consistent with other regional data from preschool children.[16] Non-Hispanic black and Hispanic youth have higher rates of obesity compared to non-Hispanic white youth. As in adults, excess body weight in children is associated with increased morbidity and mortality and psychological disorders.[17]

For the BRFSS, data are collected from individual states through a random-digit dial telephone interview with adults age 18 and older. Thus, data on height and weight collected for the BRFSS constitute a *subjective* measurement, in which participants report their own measurements without objective confirmation. Weight is often underreported in self-reported surveys, so it can be assumed that the actual prevalence of overweight and obesity obtained from BRFSS data is lower than the actual, or objective, values. Because the data collected for the BRFSS are representative at the state level, trends in overweight and obesity among adults can be obtained for states beginning in the 1980s through 2010. As seen in **Figure 8-2A**, a rapid increase in the rates of obesity across the states was seen from 1990 to 2010.[18]

In 2011, the methodology for collection of data for BRFSS changed. Prior to that year, BRFSS data were collected using phone interviews conducted through landlines linked to selected addresses. Because of the widespread use of cell phones, certain segments of the population no longer had a landline linked to an address, which led to a change in the sampling techniques. Thus, these limitations should be noted when comparing data from 2011 forward with data from previous years.[19]

Data from the 2013 BRFSS are shown in **Figure 8-2B**. In 2013, two states (Mississippi and West Virginia) had a prevalence of obesity of 35.1%, which was the highest among all of the states; Colorado had the lowest prevalence of obesity at 21.3%, followed by Hawaii at 21.8%. Almost half (23) of the states had a prevalence of obesity between 25% and < 30%, and no state had a prevalence of obesity less than 20%.[20]

Although relatively good estimates of child obesity are available at the national level through NHANES, there are few monitoring systems at the state level. The Youth Risk Behavior Surveillance System (YRBSS) does provide the prevalence of youth BMI by state, but the data are self-reported and limited to high school students.[21] Of the 21 large urban school districts that reported data for students' obesity levels in the year 2013, five reported rates below 10%.[22] The highest obesity levels for high school students by state were in Kentucky (18.0%) and Arkansas (17.8%). The lowest prevalence of obesity for high school students was in Utah (6.4%), New Jersey (8.7%), and Montana (9.4%). The prevalence of obesity and overweight for high school students across all states in 2013 was 12.4% and 14.9%, respectively.[23]

Several states are conducting more extensive statewide sampling among different age groups to determine the prevalence of child overweight by grade or age for the state. For example, Texas conducted a statewide survey of children in grades 4, 8, and 11.[24] This survey, the School Physical Activity and Nutrition (SPAN) project, selected a random sample of children from Texas public schools and obtained measured height and weight to calculate BMI, as well as collecting self-reported information on diet and physical activity behaviors. Children in Texas had a higher prevalence of obesity (BMI ≥ 95th percentile) compared to national data, with the highest prevalence rates among fourth-grade children (25.6%), Hispanic/Latino boys in eighth grade (32.6%), and fourth-grade African American girls (30.8%).

The state of Arkansas has been conducting statewide surveys of BMI among public school children since 2003.[25] In 2011–2012, 21% of school-age children in Arkansas were obese, and 17% were overweight; these levels have remained relatively stable since the 2003–2004 school year.[26] More recently, data from children aged 5–14 enrolled in

FIGURE 8-2

Prevalence of Obesity
by State, 1990–2010
and 2013

Source: CDC, Obesity Prevalence
Maps, *www.cdc.gov/obesity/
data/prevalence-maps.html*.

New York public schools showed a significant decrease in the prevalence of obesity, from 21.9% to 20.7% from 2006–2007 to 2010–2011.[27]

The prevalence of obesity in infants and toddlers from birth to two years is determined using weight-for-recumbent length. In 2011–2012, the rate of high weight-for-recumbent length (≥ 95th percentile of CDC 2000 growth charts) was 8.1%. The prevalence of high weight-for-recumbent length was higher in girls compared with boys, but there were no racial/ethnic differences noted.[28]

A. Obesity Trends* among U.S. Adults, BRFSS, 1990, 2000, 2010
(*BMI ≥ 30, or about 30 lbs overweight for 5'4" tall person)

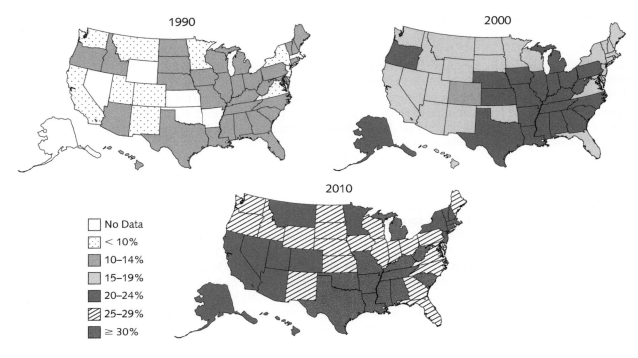

B. Prevalence* of Self-Reported Obesity** among U.S. Adults, BRFSS, 2013
(*Prevalence estimates reflect BRFSS methodological changes in 2011. These estimates should not be compared to prevalence estimates before 2011.
**BMI ≥ 30, or about 30 lbs overweight for 5'4" tall person)

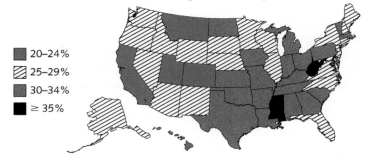

Medical and Social Costs of Obesity

The total cost of overweight and obesity in the United States has been estimated at $190 billion a year based on 2005 dollars, or approximately 21% of all medical costs.[29] A more recent analysis has found that persons with obesity have societal costs that are $92,235 more than a person without obesity, based on 2013 dollars.[30] Using this estimate, if all U.S. youth with obesity (currently 12.7 million) become obese adults, the costs to society could approach $1.1 trillion.[31] Compared to people of normal weight, obese people spent approximately 37% more on health care costs in 2001.[32] Of this increase, 38% was related to spending for diabetes, 22% was related to spending for hyperlipidemia, and 41% was related to spending for heart disease. Higher medical costs are also associated with obesity and obesity-related diseases in children and adolescents.[33]

Obesity is costly to society because it is associated with chronic diseases, including cardiovascular disease, type 2 diabetes, hypertension, stroke, dyslipidemia, osteoarthritis, selected cancers, gallbladder disease, sleep-breathing disorders, musculoskeletal disorders, and all-cause mortality (**Table 8-3**).[34] Obesity is associated with increased blood lipid levels, increased blood glucose levels, increased waist circumference, and hypertension; together, these risk factors can be characterized as **metabolic syndrome**.[35] The prevalence of metabolic syndrome (age-adjusted) in the United States was 36.3% in 1999–2004 based on American Heart Association/National Heart, Lung, and Blood Institute criteria, and this prevalence is higher among Mexican Americans, people ages 70–79, and those living in poverty.[36] Metabolic syndrome can also be found among youth, especially those who are overweight.[37]

Metabolic syndrome
A syndrome associated with development of type 2 diabetes and cardiovascular disease and is defined by abnormal values of three of the following indicators: waist circumference, serum triglycerides, HDL-cholesterol, blood glucose, and blood pressure:

- Central obesity as measured by waist circumference: Men: > 40 inches; Women: > 35 inches
- Fasting blood triglycerides greater than or equal to 150 mg/dL
- Blood HDL cholesterol: Men < 40 mg/dL; Women < 50 mg/dL
- Blood pressure greater than or equal to 130/85 mm Hg
- Fasting blood glucose greater than or equal to 110 mg/dL

TABLE 8-3 Problems Associated with Obesity in Children and Adults

CHILDREN	ADULTS
Accidents	Abdominal hernias
Complications with surgical procedures	Accidents
Decreased quality of life	Certain cancers: colon, rectum, prostate, breast, uterus, cervical, ovarian
Depression	Complications during pregnancy
Difficulties with pubertal development	Complications with surgical procedures
Gallbladder and liver disease	Decreased longevity
High blood cholesterol levels	Decreased quality of life
Hormonal imbalances	Depression
Hypertension	Fertility problems
Injury to weight-bearing joints	Gallbladder and liver disease
Kidney abnormalities	Gout
Metabolic syndrome	Heart disease
Poor self-esteem	High blood cholesterol levels
Respiratory problems	Hormonal imbalances
Sleep disturbances	Hypertension
Type 2 diabetes	Injury to weight-bearing joints
	Kidney abnormalities
	Metabolic syndrome
	Osteoarthritis
	Poor self-esteem
	Respiratory problems
	Sleep disturbances
	Type 2 diabetes
	Varicose veins

Sources: Adapted from A. Must and coauthors, "The Disease Burden Associated with Overweight and Obesity," *Journal of the American Medical Association* 282 (1999): 1523–29; A. Must and R. S. Strauss, "Risks and Consequences of Childhood and Adolescent Obesity," *International Journal of Obesity and Related Metabolic Disorders* 23 (1999): S2–S11; and M. Boyle, *Personal Nutrition*, 9th ed. (Belmont, CA: Wadsworth/Cengage Learning, 2016), 284.

Obesity and overweight can result in social costs as well, for both adults and children. Overall quality of life is often worse with increasing obesity, and obese people experience prejudice and discrimination.[38] Children who are overweight are often seen as lazy and unmotivated and can have lower self-esteem and depression.[39] Children who are overweight tend to have fewer friends and social networks; in addition, students who were overweight were more likely to be teased about their weight, and the teasing behavior was associated with depressive symptoms and low self-esteem.[40]

Determinants of Obesity

Basal metabolic rate The rate at which the body expends energy to support its basal metabolism.

Excess weight accumulation occurs with an imbalance in energy, caused by either a surplus of energy intake (calories from food) or a lack of energy expenditure (physical activity).[41] Energy needs depend on the individual's **basal metabolic rate (BMR)**, which is influenced by fat-free body mass (muscle and skeletal tissue), age, genetics, temperature, hormones, growth, and other factors. BMR is the largest influence on energy expenditure (60–65%), followed by volitional physical activity (25–35%) and the energy needed for digestion of food (the thermic effect of food, 5–10%). Theoretically, a small energy imbalance each day can result in a large weight gain over time. Mathematical modeling indicates that the maintenance of the obesity epidemic in adults can be potentially explained by an energy imbalance of approximately 220 calories/day/person.[42] For example, consuming just one 12-ounce sweetened soda per day in excess of a person's energy requirements would mean taking in 150 extra calories per day. *Provided that energy expenditures remain constant, these extra calories would result in a 16-pound weight gain over a year!*

Determinants of obesity can be related to either dietary intake or physical activity or to both, and they can be *genetic, psychosocial, behavioral,* or *environmental.* Although in the past much emphasis was placed on individual risk factors for obesity, recent reviews and recommendations have focused on the contribution of environmental factors to the development of obesity.[43] One way to frame this current thinking of obesity is using the social–ecological model (SEM). See Figure 1-3 on page 13, in which these factors are arranged by relative proximity to the individual; thus, interpersonal relationships such as family factors are more proximal to the individual, whereas structures, policies, and systems, such as changes in food supply or food costs, are more distal. **Figure 8-3** is a more

FIGURE 8-3

Child Obesity Influencing Factors

Source: Adapted from C. L. Perry, D. M. Hoelscher, and H. W. Kohl III, Research Contributions on Childhood Obesity from a Public–Private Partnership, *International Journal of Behavioral Nutrition and Physical Activity* 12 (2015), (Suppl 1): S1 doi:10.1186/1479-5868-12-S1-S1.

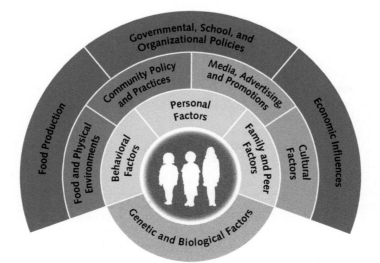

recent research model for child obesity that is based on the social–ecological model, but also includes genetic and biological factors.[44]

Genetic and Biological Risk Factors
With familial associations, it is sometimes difficult to disentangle the effects of the environment from the genetic influences. However, the variable response to diet that is found among humans in the same environment is likely due to differences in genetic risk factors.[45] The heritability of obesity has been shown to range from 40 to 70%, but environmental factors can significantly alter these percentages.[46] These genetic factors can range from relatively rare monogenic or syndromic (e.g., one gene mutation) forms of extreme obesity to more complex polygenic or common obesity, which results from a combination of variants in different genes in the general population.[47]

Mutations in the gene that codes for leptin, the "satiety hormone," was the first single monogenic form of obesity that was discovered; this variant leads to a deficiency in leptin, which in turn results in an inability to regulate appetite.[48] Other monogenic mutations that lead to obesity are found in the leptin receptor gene, the melanocortin 4 receptor gene (MC4R), and the pro-opiomelanocortin gene.[49] MC4R is the most common, with a prevalence ranging from 0.5 to 2% in adults with obesity, and a prevalence of up to 6% in children with obesity.[50] Syndromic mutations also lead to obesity, but are often accompanied by developmental abnormalities or cognitive impairments, such as observed in Prader–Willi syndrome.[51]

The identification of polygenetic or common obesity has advanced significantly since 2005, largely due to genome-wide association studies (GWAS), in which frequencies of millions of genetic variants, known as single-nucleotide polymorphisms (SNPs), are associated with different phenotypes or outcomes, such as obesity or cardiovascular risk factors.[52]* Most of the GWAS to date have been conducted in populations of European ancestry, but future work is focused on different racial/ethnic groups.[53]

Environmental interactions, such as dietary intake, can have a significant influence on gene expression, not only in the immediate future, but in a more lasting way. **Epigenetics** is a change in gene expression that occurs without changing the heritability of the gene. Epigenetics occurs through DNA methylation, histone modifications, or other chemical changes in the DNA structure; this process can be influenced by nutrient intake and status.[56] Although knowledge of epigenetics is limited at this time, it does provide potential for understanding diet–gene interactions and possible prevention efforts.

Epigenetics A change in gene expression that occurs without changing the heritability of the gene.

Recent work has shown an intriguing association between meal timing and energy balance.[57] Circadian rhythms are physiologic, metabolic, and behavioral oscillations that occur within a 24-hour period. These cycles are regulated by clock-controlled genes.[58] Consumption of food outside of the usual circadian cycle has been found to be associated with weight loss. A recent study in 420 adults in Spain who were overweight and obese[59] found that the timing of the main meal was predictive of weight loss, independent of 24-hour caloric intake. Those who ate later in the day lost less weight than those who ate early.

In addition to the meal timing, the timing and amount of sleep is associated with obesity. The amount of sleep Americans get every night has decreased over the years, and epidemiological studies in both children and adults have found a positive association between short sleep duration (SSD) and obesity, although most are based on self-reported data. The mechanism to explain the association between SSD and obesity is believed to be linked to low leptin and high ghrelin levels—two hormones that control appetite. Studies with children have found an association between bedroom media use and SSD.[60] Based

---

* As of 2014, a total of 32 established loci for BMI had been identified, and an additional 14 loci were associated with increased BMI-adjusted waist-to-hip ratio.[54] These loci include the fat-mass and obesity-associated FTO gene, and MC4R, MAF, PTER, NPC1, OLFM4, and HOXB5 genes.[55]

on research where sleep was assessed longitudinally, both shorter night-time sleep durations and later bedtime at four years of age were associated with increases in BMI values between four and five years of age.[61]

Psychosocial Risk Factors Research has begun to highlight the association between certain psychosocial risk factors (such as depression or stress) and the risk of obesity.[62] For example, one study showed that childhood depression was associated with an increased BMI in adulthood.[63] This association persisted after controlling for other socioeconomic factors. Other researchers found that "depressed adolescents are at increased risk for the development and persistence of obesity during adolescence." These researchers concluded that "the shared biological and social determinants linking depressed mood and obesity may inform the prevention and treatment of both disorders."[64] It has been postulated that in adults, overconsumption of high-fat, high-carbohydrate comfort foods, such as macaroni and cheese or baked goods, may be used as a way to reduce chronic stress. Individuals may eat comfort foods in an attempt to counter the body's response to stress and the resulting anxiety. These mechanisms may help explain how psychosocial factors (such as stress and depression) are contributing to obesity in society.[65] Social networks and social norms may also play a part in the recent increases in obesity. Recent studies have shown that people are more likely to be obese if their friends and family members are obese, and this relationship has been found in both adults and adolescents, especially in relationships between people of the same sex. This relationship points to the public health aspect of the obesity epidemic and indicates that obesity prevention programs can potentially be more effective if designed to address the social aspects of determinants of excess weight gain, such as social norms and supportive relationships.[66]

Behavioral/Lifestyle Risk Factors Various behavioral risk factors are determinants of obesity. These range from caloric intake to physical activity to other lifestyle behaviors such as media use.

Dietary Intake Although information on per capita energy consumption has shown that energy intake has increased during the past several decades,[67] recent data show a potential decrease in population energy intake from three separate sources of data. When examining national energy intake data in adults from 1971–1975 to 2003–2004, an increase was noted, from 1,955 kcal/day to 2,269 kcal/day; however, mean energy intake declined during 2009–2010, to 2,195 kcal/day. A downward trend in energy intake was noted between 1999–2000 and 2009–2010, and these decreases in energy intake were significant for young adults (aged 20–39), men, women, and participants with normal or obese BMI.[68] A similar study that examined food intake data from NHANES from 2003–2004 to 2009–2010, as well as food and beverage purchases by U.S. households using the Nielsen Homescan Panel from 2000–2011, found similar results. Analysis of NHANES data showed that energy intake decreased significantly among children, with greater decreases among Mexican American children, children from low-income families, and children with household heads who had a high school education. Overall, significant changes were not seen among adults during that same time period. Data from the Nielsen Homescan Panel showed decreases in daily per capita food and beverage purchases for households with either children or adults only. In both analyses, the decreases from consumption or purchase of beverages were greater than decreases from consumption or purchases of food.[69]

Sugar-sweetened beverages are the single largest source of added sugar and the top source of energy intake in the U.S. diet. Results of several recent meta-analyses in adults and children provide convincing data that reducing consumption of sugar-sweetened beverages will decrease the risk of obesity and related diseases such as type 2 diabetes.[70] Data from the National Health and Nutrition Examination Survey revealed that males consume more sugar drinks than females; teenagers and young adults consume more sugar drinks than other age groups; low-income persons consume more sugar drinks in relation to their overall diet than those with higher incomes; and non-Hispanic black children and adolescents consume more sugar drinks in relation to their overall diet than their Mexican American counterparts.[71] A study based on a review of data from 9,600 children aged 2–5 in the Early Childhood Longitudinal Survey found that regular consumption of sugary drinks—defined as one or more 8-ounce servings daily—was associated with higher BMI scores in 4- and 5-year-olds. In addition, these researchers reported that children who drink sugary beverages were less likely to drink milk and watch more than two hours of television daily than children who had sugary drinks infrequently or not at all.[72] Eliminating one can of soda per day, regardless of any other diet or exercise change, can reduce a child's risk of type 2 diabetes.[73]

Adults who drink one or more sodas per day are 27% more likely to be overweight than those who do not drink soda. They also have a 26% higher risk for developing type 2 diabetes and a 20% higher risk for a heart attack.[74] An analysis from 1999 to 2010 found that among a representative sample of adults in the United States, intake of sugar-sweetened beverages has trended downward, and several biomarkers of chronic disease significantly improved over the last 12 years.[75] A review of the long-term health outcomes associated with replacing sugar-sweetened beverages with alternative beverages found that substitution of sugar-sweetened beverages by alternative beverages was associated with long-term lower energy intake and lower weight gain. The authors concluded that "[a]lthough the studies on this topic are sparse, the available evidence suggests a potential benefit effect on body weight outcomes when sugar-sweetened beverages are replaced by water or low-calorie beverages."[76]

Emerging research has highlighted a possible role of dietary energy density with obesity and metabolic syndrome in U.S. adults. *Dietary energy density* is defined as the amount of energy able to be metabolized per unit weight or volume of food. Recent studies have reported that an "energy-dense, low-fiber, high-fat diet is associated with higher fat mass and greater odds of excess adiposity in childhood."[77] However, as noted by other researchers, it may not be prudent to recommend foods solely on their energy density values, since certain foods with a high energy density (e.g., nuts) are not necessarily associated with weight gain, but instead focus on lowering the overall dietary energy density value of the diet. One way to reduce dietary energy density is to decrease consumption of foods that are high in saturated fats and refined carbohydrates and to substitute increased consumption of fruits and vegetables.[78]

Physical Activity Data on trends in energy expenditure, or physical activity, are not as clear, largely because of lack of adequate surveillance. Although the 2008 U.S. Physical Activity Guidelines for Americans recommend increased physical activity, data suggest that neither adults nor children achieve recommended levels of physical activity, which may have a negative effect on weight status.[79] For example, one study found that failing to meet the guideline for 60 minutes per day of moderate to vigorous physical activity was associated with overweight status for both adolescent girls and boys aged 11–15 years.[80] An analysis of data from the National Human Activity Pattern Survey revealed that leisure-time physical activity contributed only 5% of the population's total energy expenditure. Not counting sleep, the largest contributor to energy expenditure was "driving a car," followed by "office work" and "watching TV."[81] Women, the majority of racial/ethnic minority populations in the United States, and older adults have the greatest prevalence of leisure-time physical inactivity.[82]

The first U.S. report card on physical activity was released in April 2014 by the National Physical Activity Plan Alliance and the American College of Sports Medicine. The report card found that only about a quarter of children ages 6–15 meet the physical activity recommendation (at least 60 minutes per day, most of which should be moderate to vigorous in intensity).[83] The 2008 U.S. Physical Activity Guidelines recommend that any physical activity is better than inactivity. For children, a total of 60 minutes of physical activity/day is recommended. For health benefits, adults should engage in 150 minutes a week of moderate-intensity physical activity or 75 minutes per week of vigorous-intensity physical activity, as well as at least two days per week of strength training; however, weight loss may not occur at these levels and may require higher levels of physical activity (see the inside back cover of this book).[84]

Other Lifestyle Behaviors A variety of other lifestyle behaviors may influence rates of overweight and obesity. Using data from the National Longitudinal Study of Adolescent Health (students in grades 7–12), one researcher found that the number of days in the past week that adolescents reported eating three balanced meals as well as their weekly inactivity levels (measured by how much time was spent watching television or playing video or computer games in an average week) were as great an influence on child overweight status as having a parent who was obese.[85]

Obesogenic Obesity-promoting, as in "obesogenic environment."

Toxic environment Modern eating and exercise environment that contributes to obesity; includes the wide availability of food and technological innovations that contribute to increases in sedentary activity and decreases in physical activity.

Environmental Risk Factors Researchers often refer to the environment in which we live as an **obesogenic** (obesity-promoting) or **toxic environment** because of the decrease in opportunities for physical activity; the increasing supply of highly palatable, energy-dense, low-nutrient foods; and a media environment that bombards certain populations, such as children, with food marketing messages.[86] Similarly, some researchers argue that increasingly obesogenic environments are probably the main driving force behind the obesity epidemic.[87]

Media and Media Use Data on media use in children suggest that children 8–18 years old report an average of 7 hours and 38 minutes of daily electronic media exposure, with 10 hours and 45 minutes of total media exposure, due to multitasking.[88] In a longitudinal study, television viewing between ages 5 and 15 years old remained a significant predictor of adult BMI, even after adjustment for childhood socioeconomic status.[89] Recently, a meta-analysis was conducted on media use and children's health. The meta-analysis included 73 studies that assessed the effect of various forms of media and technology (e.g., television, video games, films, computer or Internet use) on weight status in children. The majority of these studies (including 18 of 22 longitudinal studies) found a positive association between media exposure and weight status in children. For example, a longitudinal study of 5,493 children reported that those children who spent more than eight hours watching television per week at age three were significantly more likely to be obese at age seven.[90]

The effect of television use on child obesity is hypothesized to be mediated primarily through exposure to advertising; for each hour of television watched, a child consumes an average of 167 extra calories a day.[91] In a study of urban adolescents' technology use, non-Hispanic adolescents had stronger associations between television viewing and cravings for sweet snacks, salty snacks, and sweetened drinks. In contrast, being Hispanic was associated with stronger associations between phone messaging and cravings for sweet snacks, salty snacks, and sweetened drinks.[92] A recent study[93] found that television use and child obesity was mediated by social interactions and friendship dynamics: Children who spent more time with friends watched less television and engaged in more physical activity.

Food Production and Transportation Some researchers have hypothesized that an increase in calorie intake, not a decline in physical activity, is the major factor behind increased obesity in the United States, indicating that innovations in food production and transportation that have reduced the real cost of prepared foods are responsible for a major part of the obesity epidemic.[94] In particular, these researchers indict the mass production and preparation of ready-to-eat meals, which have replaced home food preparation.

Using multiple data sets, a recent analysis concluded that about 40% of the increase in weight over the last few decades may be due to expansion of the food supply, partly through agricultural innovation, which leads to a decline in food prices.[95] Technological change may lead to an expanding food supply, putting downward pressure on the price of food, which in turn stimulates consumption at the consumer level. However, the downward trend in food prices is more likely to be for energy-dense foods. One recent research study found that prices of the most energy-dense foods sold in Seattle supermarkets had dropped by 1.8% over a two-year period, while the prices of the least energy-dense foods had increased by 19.5% during the same time period.[96] More recently, a report titled "The Rising Cost of a Healthy Diet" found that fruit and vegetable prices had risen 2–3% on average per year since 1990 while for other foods the rate stood at around 1–2%. From 1990–2012, fruit and vegetable prices increased by 55–91% depending on the crop and region, while the cost of some processed foods such as ready-to-eat meals dropped by up to 20%. The authors noted that use of technologies such as fruits and vegetables that are cut, trimmed, bagged, and washed and available year-round could be one reason for the price hikes in fruits and vegetables. Based on the results, the authors concluded that governments in emerging economies (e.g., Brazil, Mexico, China) should consider introducing taxes and subsidies to offset these price changes.[97] (See Pricing Policies on pages 311–313.)

If agricultural technology—which enables large-scale production of highly processed foods—is determined to be a major factor driving the trend toward increases in obesity, then economic incentives, rather than nutrition education alone, may be important.[98] An example of a food intervention that is based on economic incentives includes subsidized employee meals in worksite cafeterias. Another example is the USDA's Fresh Fruit and Vegetable Program and "farm-to-school" and "farm-to-work" programs, which are based on partnerships between institutions and local farmers.[99] See the Programs in Action feature in Chapter 13 for a description of a farm-to-work program. All 50 states and Washington, D.C., have farm-to-school programs but only 35 states and Washington, D.C., have established mandatory programs.[100] A study by researchers at the University of California, Davis, found that farm-to-school programs not only increase consumption of fruits and vegetables but also change eating habits, leading students to choose healthier options at lunch. A more recent analysis of state-level farm-to-school policies found that fruit and vegetable availability in U.S. public elementary schools was highest in states with farm-to-school laws and in schools with farm-to-school programs. [101] Sourcing foods locally can also help avoid increases in food costs as energy costs increase.[102] The Farm to School Act of 2015 aims to continue and expand upon the successes of the USDA's Farm to School Grant Program (**Table 8-4**).

Portion Sizes Food portion sizes have increased over time in the United States. This trend toward larger marketplace portions has occurred in parallel with rising rates of obesity.[103] For example, some researchers have noted the expansion of large portions of snack items and fast food and the parallel increase in childhood obesity. Using data from the Children's Lifestyle and School Performance study, researchers observed that children from socioeconomically disadvantaged families or children who eat while watching

TABLE 8-4 Examples of Obesity-Related Legislation Introduced in the 114th Congress (2015–2016)

BILL TITLE	DESCRIPTION OF BILL
Community Parks Revitalization Act (H.R. 201)	Requires the Secretary of Housing and Urban Development (HUD) to carry out a community revitalization program of federal grants to eligible local governments located within standard metropolitan statistical areas for various park and recreation purposes, including grants for rehabilitation and construction, innovation and recreation programming, and recovery action programs.
Expanding Nutrition's Role in Curricula and Healthcare Act (ENRICH Act) (H.R. 1411)	Requires the Health Resources and Services Administration to establish a program of three-year competitive grants to accredited medical schools for the development or expansion of an integrated nutrition and physical activity curriculum. The curriculum must: (1) be designed to improve communication and provider preparedness in the prevention, management, and reversal of obesity, cardiovascular disease, diabetes, and cancer; and (2) address additional topics in high-risk populations, as practicable, including physical activity and training programs, food insecurity, and malnutrition.
Farm to School Act of 2015 (S. 569, H.R. 1061)	Continues and expands upon the successes of the USDA's Farm to School Grant Program by: • Fully including preschools, summer foodservice program sites, and after-school programs on the list of eligible entities • Increasing annual mandatory funding from $5 million to $15 million to better meet the high demand and need for this funding • Increasing access among tribal schools to farm-fresh and traditional foods, especially from tribal producers • Improving program participation from beginning, veteran, and socially disadvantaged farmers and ranchers
FIT Kids Act (S. 1075, H.R. 2013)	Amends the Elementary and Secondary Education Act of 1965 to reauthorize and amend the Carol M. White Physical Education Program, which is administered by the Department of Education. Of the funds appropriated for the program, the Department of Education must reserve a portion to award competitive grants for states to implement comprehensive programs based on: (1) scientifically valid research, and (2) an analysis of need that considers indicators in a state system measuring conditions related to physical fitness, physical education, student health, and nutrition.
Healthy Kids Outdoors Act of 2015 (S. 1078, H.R. 2014)	Authorizes the Department of Interior to issue an eligible entity a cooperative agreement for each state for the development, implementation, and updating of a five-year Healthy Outdoors State Strategy designed to encourage people in the United States (especially children, youth, and families) to be physically active outdoors.
Sugar-Sweetened Beverages Tax Act of 2015 (or the SWEET Act) (H.R. 1687)	• Amends the Internal Revenue Code to impose an excise tax on the sale or transfer of any specified sugar-sweetened beverage product by the manufacturer, producer, or importer thereof. Establishes the rate of such tax as 1 cent per 4.2 grams of caloric sweetener contained in such product. • Transfers revenues from such tax to the Prevention and Public Health Fund for the sole purpose of funding programs and research to reduce the human and economic costs of diabetes, obesity, dental caries, and other diet-related health conditions in priority populations.
Treat and Reduce Obesity Act of 2015 (S. 1509, H.R. 2404)	Amends Title XVIII (Medicare) of the Social Security Act to authorize the Department of Health and Human Services (HHS), in addition to qualified primary care physicians and other primary care practitioners, to cover intensive behavioral therapy for obesity furnished by: (1) a physician who is not a qualified primary care physician; (2) an evidence-based, community-based HHS-approved lifestyle counseling program; or (3) any other appropriate health care provider (including a physician assistant, nurse practitioner, clinical nurse specialist, a clinical psychologist, and a registered dietitian, or nutritional professional).

television and in fast-food restaurants preferred larger portions of french fries and potato chips. Consequences of eating larger portions of these foods included poor diet quality and increased energy intake.[104] Thus, larger portion sizes encourage people to eat and drink more, although consumers may not always understand this intuitive connection.[105] As one nutrition professor explained, "Many people seem to view a soft drink as a soft drink, no matter how big it is. When I explain that a 64-ounce soft drink container could provide as much as 800 kcal, audiences gasp."[106]

Foods Available at Restaurants Consumption of food prepared away from home plays an increasingly large role in the American diet. In 1970, 25.9% of all food spending was on food away from home; by 2012 that number rose to 43.1%. A number of factors have contributed to the trend of dining out since the 1970s, such as a larger share of women working outside of the home, more two-earner households, more affordable and convenient fast-food outlets, increased advertising and promotion by large food chains, and the smaller size of U.S. households.[107] Based on data from the BRFSS and restaurant data from the U.S. Economic Census, a 2008 study found that fast-food density and a higher ratio of fast-food to full-service restaurants were associated with higher individual-level weight status (for BMI and risk of being obese). Another study reported that prevalence of fast-food restaurants in the United States was associated with obesity on a statewide basis.[108] More recently, researchers found that a higher level of fast-food restaurant concentration was associated with increased levels of preschool-aged childhood obesity in both poor and urban areas, with the largest negative effect of fast-food availability on obesity occurring in more economically disadvantaged, urban areas.[109] In California, researchers found that the presence of fast-food restaurants near middle and high schools (within one-half mile) was associated with students' eating patterns (e.g., eating fewer fruits and vegetables, drinking more soda), overweight, and obesity.[110] In Arkansas, researchers reported that the number of fast-food restaurants within a mile from a school can significantly affect school-level obesity rates.[111] Further study is required to find out whether these results apply to other parts of the United States.

A study that examined dietary data from the NHANES between 2007 and 2010 for 4,466 children between 2 and 18 years old concluded that fast-food consumption may not be the major cause of rising childhood obesity rates, with an overall poor dietary pattern (e.g., Western diet) that includes few fruits and vegetables and relies instead on high amounts of processed food and sweetened beverages as the problem.[112] Still, the dietary quality of fast food has been shown to be consistently poor. In a review of the dietary quality of fast-food menu offerings at five popular fast-food chains, researchers found that the menus scored lower than 50 out of 100 possible points on the Healthy Eating Index (HEI). Scores for total fruit, whole grains, and sodium were particularly poor. Kids' menus scored 10 points higher (on average).[113] These authors concluded that "the poor quality of fast-food menus is a concern in light of increasing away from home eating, aggressive marketing to children and minorities, and the tendency for fast-food restaurants to be located in low-income and minority areas."[114]

Social Environment Examples of factors in the social environment that may influence the risk of childhood overweight include parental overweight; maternal smoking during pregnancy; cumulative stress experienced by a child's mother; parental depression, which is a stressor on parenting behavior; and low rates of breastfeeding.[115] Researchers found that cumulative stress experienced by a child's mother is an important determinant of childhood overweight. Such stress may have its roots in financial worries and other related factors such as insufficient health insurance coverage. Children in food-secure households may respond to environmental stress by consuming more energy-dense comfort foods—which are readily available.[116] Other researchers have reported that food insecurity influenced parental depression and parenting practices, which in turn were significantly associated with infant feeding practices and toddlers' overweight. Such results suggest the need to strengthen policies that ensure that families with infants and toddlers have access to a sufficient, predictable, and reliable food supply.[117]

Some investigators believe that low rates of breastfeeding among minority and disadvantaged women may partially explain why minority and disadvantaged children in the United States are at greater risk of becoming overweight. Recent research has shown that breastfed babies are less likely to be overweight and develop type 2 diabetes when they reach adolescence.[118] A recent evaluation of data from the National Survey of Children's Health found that in early childhood (i.e., children aged 2–5), breastfed children had an 8.9% lower probability of being obese compared to children who were never breastfed. Additionally, compared to children who were breastfed for more than three months, infants who were breastfed for less time had a 4.7% higher probability of being obese. These results indicate that the length of breastfeeding, whether exclusive or not, may be associated with lower risk of obesity in childhood.[119] Another recent two-year study that tracked 595 children in a health care system in central New York found that infants at risk for childhood and adult obesity had a better chance of not becoming overweight if breastfeeding continued for more than two months.[120] See Chapter 11 for more about breastfeeding practices and infant health.

Urban Sprawl and the Built Environment

Urban sprawl has been defined as "an overall pattern of development across a metropolitan area where large percentages of the population live in lower-density residential areas."[121] Various investigators have found an association between obesity and urban sprawl as well as other aspects of the built environment, such as **mixed land use** patterns and **walkability**, which is defined by residential density, mixed land use, and street connectivity.[122] The **built environment** encompasses a variety of community design elements such as street layout, zoning, transportation options, stairs, public and green spaces (walking paths, parks/recreation areas, playgrounds, community gardens), and business areas.[123]

The effect of the built environment on overnutrition in industrialized countries is only now beginning to be recognized.[124] One group of researchers found that after controlling for individual factors such as gender, age, race/ethnicity, and education, urban sprawl was associated with leisure-time walking, obesity, and hypertension, but not with overall physical activity, diabetes, or coronary heart disease.[125] Other researchers have reported that residents of high-walkability neighborhoods had a lower prevalence of obesity (adjusted for individual demographics) than residents of low-walkability neighborhoods.[126] More recently, researchers have found that neighborhoods built before 1950 are more walkable and have lower rates of overweight and obese people. For each decade older the neighborhood, the risk of obesity dropped by approximately 8% in women and 13% in men. These researchers concluded that walkability indicators, particularly certain land-diversity measures, are important predictors of body weight.[127] Because older neighborhoods have stores and businesses within walking distance, persons living in these neighborhoods may be more likely to do errands and other activities by foot (rather than by car) than persons living in more newly built neighborhoods.

Poverty

At the environmental level, it has been observed that obesity rates are higher in lower-income neighborhoods, states, and legislative districts. For example, differences in state-level obesity prevalence reported from the BRFSS (see previous section) may reflect socioeconomic differences across states with higher obesity rates in less-affluent states such as Mississippi and West Virginia.[128]

Some experts argue that the association between energy-dense diets and low energy costs (dollars per megajoule) may be contributing to the higher obesity rates in socioeconomically disadvantaged groups.[129] That is, energy-dense diets provide low-income households with inexpensive sources of concentrated energy from fat, sugars, potatoes, and high-fat meats but offer little in the way of whole grains, fruits, and vegetables.[130] For more about the paradox of poverty and obesity, see Chapter 10.

A recent analysis of NHANES data with corresponding prices from the USDA's Center for Nutrition Policy and Promotion's Food Prices Database found almost no statistical support for higher energy-dense foods being less expensive than low energy-dense foods.[131] However, a separate analysis conducted from 1990–2012 reported that fruit and vegetable prices had increased substantially during this time period, while the cost of

Mixed land use A layout of land that allows multiple types of use together, such as commercial and residential use. This is in contrast to single-use zoning, which allows land use for only one specific purpose.

Walkability A neighborhood characteristic defined by residential density, mixed land use, and street connectivity.

Built environment The built environment encompasses a variety of community design elements such as street layout, zoning, transportation options, stairs, public and green spaces, and business areas.

some processed foods (e.g., ready-to-eat meals, noodles, and cookies) had dropped by as much as 20%.[132] Numerous studies have indicated that neighborhoods that are poor, rural, or predominantly minority do not have ready access to supermarkets and more healthful foods.[133] It is estimated that more than 29 million Americans lack access to healthy, affordable foods.[134] These persons live in food deserts, defined by the USDA as "urban neighborhoods or rural towns without ready access to fresh, healthy, and affordable food." Low-income census tracts qualify as food deserts if "at least 33% of the census tract's population live more than one mile from a supermarket or large grocery store or 10 miles in non-metropolitan tracts."[135] In Mississippi, 70% of Supplemental Nutrition Assistance Program (SNAP) recipients live 30 miles away from the closest large grocery store.[136] Researchers in Baltimore found that supermarkets in predominantly black and low-income neighborhoods had lower availability of healthful foods than supermarkets in predominantly white and higher-income neighborhoods. The lower availability of healthful foods in black and low-income neighborhoods was due to differential placement of types of stores as well as differential offerings of healthful foods within similar stores.[137] In a separate study, availability of supermarkets was found to be associated with lower adolescent BMI. This association was larger for African American students and for students in households where the mother worked full time.[138] A review of neighborhood environments concluded that lower-income, ethnic/racial minority, and rural neighborhoods are most affected by poor access to supermarkets and healthful foods and greater availability of fast-food restaurants and energy-dense foods.[139] In a study evaluating food accessibility on 22 Native American reservations in the state of Washington, researchers observed both physical and financial barriers to accessing healthy food. Fifteen reservations did not have an onsite supermarket or grocery store; and the cost of shopping off reservations was approximately 7% higher than the national reference cost.[140]

Obesity Prevention and Treatment Interventions

In public health applications, interventions that address body weight are often preventive, rather than treatment-oriented. The goal of an *obesity prevention* program is to maintain a stable weight and not increase body size over time, in contrast to an *obesity treatment* program, in which the primary goal is to lose weight over time. Current recommendations for *obesity treatment* range from lifestyle changes, which include dietary therapy or prescriptions (low-calorie diets, very low-calorie diets, vegetarian diets, and other regimens designed to lower energy intake), increases in physical activity, and behavioral therapy (e.g., use of behavioral strategies such as goal setting) to clinical therapies such as pharmacotherapy and weight-loss surgery. Generally, pharmacotherapy is not recommended unless patients are obese (BMI > 30) with no related risk factors or have a BMI *greater than* 27 with related risk factors, such as hypertension or type 2 diabetes. Weight-loss or bariatric surgery, which includes gastric bypass procedures, is recommended for patients with severe obesity: BMI of 40 or greater, or BMI between 35 and 40 with related risk factors such as hypertension or type 2 diabetes.[141] For children, recommendations for obesity treatment should include family-based, developmentally appropriate intervention with strategies that include nutrition education, parenting skills, behavioral techniques, and physical activity; structured dietary approaches and pharmacological treatment should be reserved for youth who are obese with concomitant comorbidities. Weight-loss surgery may be considered for adolescents who are severely obese.[142] Public health approaches, or *primary prevention*, target lifestyle therapies, which are less invasive and more appropriate for population-level interventions. Other public health intervention approaches can include screening for high-risk patients, such as those with extreme obesity, and subsequent referral for clinical treatment.

For an effective intervention in the public health setting, the program has to have significant effectiveness in clinical settings, broad reach in the population of interest, and consistent implementation in real-life settings.[143] Many obesity prevention programs are oriented around a site where people congregate, such as churches, worksites, community settings, childcare centers, and schools. Because effectiveness and reach can vary depending on age, interventions can also be divided into adult-based programs and programs for children and adolescents.

The recidivism rate for obesity is high, and a significant number of patients regain weight within three to five years after the end of most obesity treatment interventions.[144] The National Weight Control Registry is a study that examines the habits of people who have lost 30 or more pounds and kept it off for at least a year.[145] As part of their weight-loss plan, most registry participants had made significant and consistent changes in dietary intake and physical activity, were engaged in regular exercise (predominantly walking), consumed a diet with limited variety within food groups, and ate breakfast regularly.[146]

Adult Interventions

Public health interventions tend to focus on lifestyle approaches, such as dietary changes and physical activity. In general, dietary interventions produce modest weight loss, and caloric content seems to be more important than macronutrient composition. Physical activity can also be useful in weight loss, but the most effective interventions include both dietary changes and increases in physical activity. Most environmental community-based studies in adults have not been rigorously evaluated.[147] One exception is a faith-based weight-loss intervention called The WORD (Wholeness, Oneness, Righteousness, Deliverance), which utilized a community-based participatory research approach. The program was developed to address obesity issues that are sensitive to the African American community. The treatment group participated in weekly small-group meetings (led by trained community members), which emphasized healthful nutrition practices, physical activity, and faith's connection to health. The mean weight loss in the treatment group was 3.60 pounds compared to a 0.59-pound weight loss in the control group.[148] The unique aspects of this randomized controlled trial are the focus on weight-loss maintenance and the use of a faith-based, community-based participatory approach in translating evidence-based obesity interventions.[149] In another study, researchers reported that use of a grocery list was associated with a healthier diet and lower BMI among household shoppers in low-income, primarily African American neighborhoods who had limited access to healthy foods.[150]

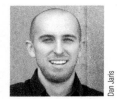
Dan Jaris

ENTREPRENEUR IN ACTION

Dan Jaris began his career in community nutrition with the desire to make a difference in the lives of others. He worked as a health coach for an established industry leader in the corporate wellness field. In this capacity, he engaged employee populations from many different companies, encouraging healthier lifestyle behaviors through nutrition and exercise. Dan later transitioned to his new role as Nutrition and Exercise Program Coordinator for the Include Program in Canada. There, he set the framework for facilitators to work with developmentally challenged individuals within the community to improve their health and quality of life. Successful implementation of entrepreneurship in community nutrition leads to individuals and community members who are motivated and empowered to not allow any obstacles to interfere with adopting healthy lifestyle behaviors. Says Dan: "Above anything else, be passionate about what you do, and everything else will follow naturally. Those that are passionate about their work easily distinguish themselves with their sincerity and interest in genuinely making a difference, which sets the foundation for a meaningful relationship built on trust. This level of rapport helps to inspire and motivate others to embrace healthy lifestyle behaviors." Find out more about what he has to say about entrepreneurship online at *www.cengagebrain.com*.

Many of the public health interventions for adults have been implemented through worksites.[151] A recent evaluation of worksite-based weight-loss programs assessed 11 studies lasting from 2 to 18 months. The programs included both education and counseling components (to promote more healthful dietary practices and increase physical activity). The evaluation found that those employees in the intervention groups lost significantly more weight than controls, with the mean difference in weight loss ranging from 0.2 to 6.4 kilograms. Whether or not these reported weight-loss results can be sustained in the long term is not known. Thus, there is a need for the development, implementation, and evaluation of worksite-based interventions that integrate educational, behavioral, environmental, and economic supports.[152]

Child and Adolescent Interventions

Most public health interventions for overweight prevention in children and adolescents have been conducted through the schools.[153] Public health interventions that include a component on decreasing television viewing have been shown to be effective.[154] School-based programs that increase physical activity also appear to have a significant effect on reducing body size, especially when physical activity is for an hour or more per day.[155] In the United Kingdom, a targeted, school-based education program produced a modest reduction in the number of carbonated drinks consumed, which was associated with a reduced number of overweight and obese children.[156]

Interventions that include multiple coordinated components, such as a school-based program enhanced by community programs and social marketing campaigns, also show much promise in the prevention of child obesity (see also the CATCH Programs in Action feature on page 317).[157] More recently, a multicomponent intervention titled the School Policy Nutrition Initiative was implemented in five urban public schools (in the Mid-Atlantic region) with a high proportion of children who were eligible for free and reduced-price school meals (in grades 4–6). The intervention included school self-assessment, nutrition education, social marketing, and family outreach. The intervention resulted in a 50% reduction in the incidence of overweight. In addition, significantly fewer children in intervention schools (7.5%) became overweight than children not attending intervention schools (15%).[158] However, the fact that 7.5% of children in the intervention group still gained weight over the two-year period suggests that stronger or additional intervention components may be needed.

Interventions that involve a family and other environmental components may be important, as it has been reported that growth in childhood BMI is typically faster and more variable in the summer, especially in high-risk groups (e.g., black children, Hispanic children, and children already overweight).[159] A recent study found that a reduced consumption of food away from home was associated with improved diet quality and greater reductions in BMI and body fat in 170 overweight and obese children ages 7–11 years who completed a 16-week family-based behavioral weight-loss treatment as part of a larger clinical research trial. Associations between food consumed away from home and anthropometric outcomes were mediated by changes in diet quality (e.g., changes in total energy intake and added sugars mediated the change in food away from home and standardized BMI).[160] Family involvement is important for young children; however, adolescents are often more interested in peer relationships and influences, so interventions for adolescents should include a peer component as well.[161]

For young children, the parents are often "gatekeepers" for diet and physical activity, inasmuch as they control the types of foods in the house, the access to and availability of those foods, opportunities for activity or inactivity, and meal patterns. In addition, parents often serve as role models for their children. The High 5 for PreSchool Kids (H5-KIDS) program tested the effectiveness of a home-based intervention that taught parents how to ensure a positive fruit and vegetable environment for their preschool-aged children, and to examine whether changes in parents' fruit and vegetable behavior was associated with improvements in their children's fruit and vegetable intake. The researchers found that parents in the H5-KIDS group increased their intake of fruits and vegetables, and the children's increased fruit and vegetable intake correlated with their parents' intake (except for children who were already overweight). Thus, parents may need to focus on preventing obesity in their young children by implementing appropriate infant and toddler feeding practices, including avoiding coercive "clean your plate" feeding practices; offering appropriate portion sizes of healthful foods from the basic food groups (e.g., fruits, vegetables, and grains); offering healthful foods numerous times; and allowing infants and toddlers to eat until satiated.[162]

With preschool-age children, obesity prevention efforts need to focus on multiple environments, including the home and early care and education (ECE) settings, and various stages of development (from the mother's pregnancy through the child's preschool years). This is because research has shown that smoking during pregnancy, parental overweight, and rapid weight gain during infancy (particularly the first five months) can influence risk of overweight in preschool-age children.[163] From a population-health perspective, interventions aimed at preventing early childhood obesity may need to educate mothers and their support systems during pregnancy (e.g., smoking cessation for smoking pregnant women and sustained breastfeeding).[164]

Recently, the Institute of Medicine (IOM) reviewed factors related to overweight and obesity from birth to age five, with a focus on nutrition, physical activity, and sedentary behavior. The report, titled *Early Childhood Obesity Prevention Policies* (2011), recommends a variety of actions that health care professionals can take to prevent obesity in children age five and younger. For example, it recommends that health care professionals measure weight, height, and length in a standardized way and also pay attention to obesity risk factors, such as rate of weight gain, during pediatric visits. In addition, the report recommends that parents and childcare providers keep children active throughout the day; provide them with a diet rich in fruits, vegetables, and whole grains and low in energy-dense, nutrient-poor foods; and support breastfeeding during infancy. Finally, the report recommends that caregivers should limit young children's screen time and exposure to food and beverage marketing and ensure that children sleep an adequate amount each day.[165]

The pediatrician and primary care offices are increasingly becoming involved in obesity prevention efforts. A recent clinical report by the American Academy of Pediatrics (AAP) details evidence-based steps for pediatricians and their offices, including promoting a diet with no sugary beverages; decreased consumption of high-energy, low-nutrient foods; and increased consumption of fruits and vegetables, as well as increased physical activity and reduced sedentary behaviors.[166] To promote brief counseling sessions and follow up for obesity prevention, the AAP has partnered with the National Institute for Children's Health Quality to develop a flipchart and guide called *Next Steps* to help physicians dialogue with their patients about obesity prevention–related behaviors.

Racial and Ethnic Disparities in Obesity

Because obesity rates remain higher among black and Hispanic communities than non-Hispanic white communities, racial and ethnic disparities should be addressed.[167] Based on a series of in-depth interviews with public health experts in black and Latino communities, policy recommendations were issued to develop and implement more effective obesity-prevention policies in these communities. These policy recommendations include: (1) involve local communities in all public and private investments, including partnering with black residents and organizations, and understand the assets and resources within each community to determine priorities and develop culturally relevant and sustainable solutions (black communities); (2) use equity as a grant criterion and measure to ensure that addressing disparities is a priority goal for a given project and program (black communities); (3) increase support to address racial and ethnic inequities in obesity at federal, state, and local levels (black and Latino communities); (4) use culturally sensitive community-based obesity prevention and control strategies (black and Latino communities); (5) develop strategies with community leaders and members, including the implementation of common practices, such as joint-use agreements to allow community members to use playgrounds and fields when schools are not in session and improving zoning rules for increased numbers of grocery stores in low-income communities (black communities); (6) increase grant programs to encourage minority business owners to open grocery stores in low-income communities and ensure that such initiatives are sustainable and include appropriate support (black and Latino communities); (7) limit advertising for unhealthy foods and encourage policies that increase marketing of healthy foods and beverages (black and Latino communities); (8) increase access and use of *promotores* (community health workers, peer leaders, and health advocates) (Latino communities); (9) educate Latino parents about childhood obesity (Latino communities); and (10) partner with local communities (e.g., government, businesses, faith-based groups, community organizations, schools) to promote increased access to healthy, affordable food and safe places for physical activity in Latino communities and neighborhoods (Latino communities).[168]

Salud America! conducted a national Delphi survey among researchers and stakeholders to yield the first-ever National Latino Childhood Obesity Research Agenda,[169] which provided a framework to stimulate research and collaboration and inform policymakers about the specific needs for priority funding to address prevention of obesity in Latino children. The agenda ranks family as the main ecological level to prevent Latino childhood obesity—followed by community, school, society, and individual (see Figure 1-3 on page 13 for the CDC's Social–Ecological Framework). A collection of research studies published as a special supplement in the *American Journal of Preventive Medicine* highlights guided grocery store trips, menu labeling at restaurants, community gardens, and video-based exercise programs as examples of culturally appropriate ways to prevent obesity among Latino children.[170]

Public Health Policy Options for Addressing the Global Obesity Epidemic

Obesity is a significant public health issue that will affect the entire population through increased health care costs and increased morbidity and mortality. As Dr. William Dietz of the Centers for Disease Control and Prevention acknowledged in his statement before the Subcommittee on Public Health of the Committee on Health, Education, Labor, and Pensions for the U.S. Senate on May 21, 2002,

> "Given the size of the population that we are trying to reach, we obviously cannot rely solely upon individual interventions that target one person at a time. Instead, the prevention of obesity will require coordinated policy and environmental changes that affect large populations simultaneously."[171]

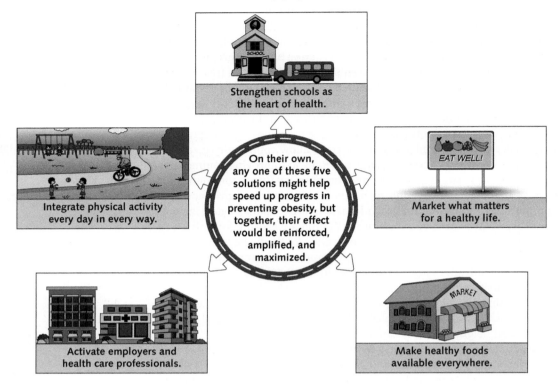

FIGURE 8-4 Major Goals Outlined in the IOM *Accelerating Progress in Obesity Prevention* Report, 2012

Source: Institute of Medicine (IOM), *http://iom.nationalacademies .org/Reports/2012/Accelerating -Progress-in-Obesity-Prevention .aspx.*

The most recent recommendations for obesity prevention at the population level can be found in the IOM report, *Accelerating Progress in Obesity Prevention: Solving the Weight of the Nation.*[172] For this report, close to 800 recommendations and strategies from other organizations and governmental entities were distilled to five major goals (**Figure 8-4**):

- Make physical activity an integral and routine part of life.
- Create food and beverage environments that ensure that healthy food and beverage options are the routine, easy choice.
- Transform messages about physical activity and nutrition.
- Expand the role of health care providers, insurers, and employers in obesity prevention.
- Make schools a national focal point for obesity prevention.

Table 8-5 describes the various recommendations and strategies that correspond to these goals. Many of these strategies can be addressed through policy options, which can include obesity surveillance and monitoring efforts; awareness building, education, and research; regulating environments; pricing policies, such as subsidies and taxation; and societal-level solutions.

Many of the policy initiatives address children rather than adults, for a number of reasons. First, because obesity is so intractable, it is preferable and more cost-effective to focus on prevention. The rates of overweight are increasing in children as well as in adults, so prevention of obesity at a young age can potentially attenuate the development of chronic disease, which develops over a long period of time. Food habits are still fairly malleable for children, so it makes sense to target policies and programs at this age group. Finally, it is easy to reach children because the majority of children attend schools, and school programs often include physical activity and nutrition elements that can be targeted.[173]

TABLE 8-5 Summary of Goals, Recommendations, and Strategies from the Institute of Medicine *Accelerating Progress in Obesity Prevention: Solving the Weight of the Nation*

GOAL	RECOMMENDATION	STRATEGY
Goal 1: Make physical activity an integral and routine part of life.	**Recommendation 1:** Communities, transportation officials, health professionals, and governments should make promotion of physical activity a priority by substantially increasing access to places and opportunities for physical activity.	**Strategy 1-1.** Enhance the physical and built environment. **Strategy 1-2.** Provide and support community programs designed to increase physical activity. **Strategy 1-3.** Adopt physical activity requirements for licensed childcare providers. **Strategy 1-4.** Provide support for the science and practice of physical activity.
Goal 2: Create food and beverage environments that ensure that healthy food and beverage options are the routine, easy choice.	**Recommendation 2:** Governments and decision makers in the business community/private sector[a] should make a concerted effort to reduce unhealthy food and beverage options and substantially increase healthier food and beverage options[b] at affordable, competitive prices.	**Strategy 2-1.** Adopt policies and implement practices to reduce overconsumption of sugar-sweetened beverages. **Strategy 2-2.** Increase the availability of lower-calorie and healthier food and beverage options for children in restaurants. **Strategy 2-3.** Utilize strong nutritional standards for all foods and beverages sold or provided through the government, and ensure that these healthy options are available in all places frequented by the public. **Strategy 2-4.** Introduce, modify, and utilize health-promoting food and beverage retailing and distribution policies. **Strategy 2-5.** Broaden the examination and development of U.S. agriculture policy and research to include implications for the American diet.
Goal 3: Transform messages about physical activity and nutrition.	**Recommendation 3:** Industry, educators, and governments should act quickly, aggressively, and in a sustained manner on many levels to transform the environment that surrounds Americans with messages about physical activity, food, and nutrition.	**Strategy 3-1.** Develop and support a sustained, targeted physical activity and nutrition social marketing program. **Strategy 3-2.** Implement common standards for marketing foods and beverages to children and adolescents. **Strategy 3-3.** Ensure consistent nutrition labeling for the front of packages, retail store shelves, and menus and menu boards that encourages healthier food choices. **Strategy 3-4.** Adopt consistent nutrition education policies for federal programs with nutrition education components.
Goal 4: Expand the role of health care providers, insurers, and employers in obesity prevention.	**Recommendation 4:** Health care and health service providers, employers, and insurers should increase the support structure for achieving better population health and obesity prevention.	**Strategy 4-1.** Provide standardized care and advocate for healthy community environments. **Strategy 4-2.** Ensure coverage of, access to, and incentives for routine obesity prevention, screening, diagnosis, and treatment. **Strategy 4-3.** Encourage active living and healthy eating at work. **Strategy 4-4.** Encourage healthy weight gain during pregnancy and breastfeeding, and promote breastfeeding-friendly environments.
Goal 5: Make schools a national focal point for obesity prevention.	**Recommendation 5:** Federal, state, and local government and education authorities, with support from parents, teachers, and the business community and the private sector, should make schools a focal point for obesity prevention.	**Strategy 5-1.** Require quality physical education and opportunities for physical activity in schools. **Strategy 5-2.** Ensure strong nutritional standards for all foods and beverages sold or provided through schools. **Strategy 5-3.** Ensure food literacy, including skill development, in schools.

[a] The business community/private sector includes private employers and privately owned and/or operated locations frequented by the public, such as movie theaters, shopping centers, sporting and entertainment venues, bowling alleys, and other recreational/entertainment facilities.

[b] Although there is no consensus on the definition of "unhealthy" foods/beverages, in the APOP report, the term refers to foods and beverages that are calorie-dense and low in naturally occurring nutrients. Such foods and beverages contribute little fiber and few essential nutrients and phytochemicals, but contain added fats, sweeteners, sodium, and other ingredients. Unhealthy foods and beverages displace the consumption of foods recommended in the *Dietary Guidelines for Americans* and may lead to the development of obesity.

Source: Institute of Medicine (IOM), *http://iom.nationalacademies.org/~/media/Files/Report%20Files/2012/APOP/APOP_insert.pdf.*

Obesity Surveillance and Monitoring Efforts

In an effort to align evaluation efforts with the goals outlined in the *Accelerating Progress in Obesity Prevention* report and to assess the progress in obesity prevention efforts, another report, *Evaluating Obesity Prevention Efforts: A Plan for Measuring Progress*, was developed by the Institute of Medicine.[174] This report included an outline for a National Obesity Evaluation Plan (with options for State Obesity Evaluation Plans), a how-to for Community Obesity Evaluation Plans, and evaluation tools and resources (**Table 8-6**).

TABLE 8-6 Summary of Goals and Recommendations from the Institute of Medicine *Evaluating Obesity Prevention Efforts: A Plan for Measuring Progress*

GOAL	RECOMMENDATION
Goal 1: Improve leadership and coordination for evaluation.	**Recommendation 1:** An obesity evaluation task force or another entity should oversee and implement the National Obesity Evaluation Plan and provide support for the Community Obesity Evaluation Plan and should coordinate with other federal, state, and local public- and private-sector groups and other stakeholders who support, use, or conduct evaluations. The task force/entity could be a new or existing entity or combination of existing entities.
Goal 2: Improve data collection for evaluation.	**Recommendation 2:** Using the recommended indicators and gaps identified in this report as guides (i.e., related to *Accelerating Progress in Obesity Prevention* report strategies), all federal agencies[a] and state and local health departments responsible for collecting data relevant to obesity prevention efforts, in coordination with relevant private partners, should identify, coordinate, and maximize current efforts for ongoing collection of recommended indicators and, according to the priorities identified, address existing evaluation gaps at the national and local levels.
Goal 3: Provide common guidance for evaluation.	**Recommendation 3:** Relevant federal agencies (e.g., in the U.S. Departments of Agriculture, Commerce, Health and Human Services, Labor, and Transportation) and state and local health departments, in collaboration with nonfederal partners, should standardize the collection and analysis of data, including common indicators, measures, methods, and outcomes used for assessment, monitoring, surveillance, and summative evaluation to ensure aggregation among localities and back to the National Obesity Evaluation Plan.
Goal 4: Improve access to and dissemination of evaluation data.	**Recommendation 4:** Relevant federal agencies (e.g., in the U.S. Departments of Agriculture, Commerce, Health and Human Services, Labor, and Transportation) in collaboration with academics, non-governmental organizations, and state and local health departments, should coordinate existing efforts to ensure the federal, state, and local assessment, monitoring, surveillance, and summative evaluation systems include a mechanism for feedback to users of evaluation data. In addition, local evaluations should continue to build the evidence base for the *Accelerating Progress in Obesity Prevention* report strategies; be stored, curated, synthesized, and shared to improve generalizable knowledge about implementation barriers and opportunities; and clarify "what works" in different contexts.
Goal 5: Improve workforce capacity for evaluation.	**Recommendation 5:** The Centers for Disease Control and Prevention, National Institutes of Health, and the U.S. Department of Agriculture, through the National Collaborative on Child Obesity Research and other non-governmental and professional organizations, should build on their existing evaluation resources to ensure support for the diverse and inter-disciplinary workforce engaged in conducting assessments, surveillance, monitoring, and summative evaluation activities.
Goal 6: Improve evaluations to address disparities and health equity.	**Recommendation 6:** The U.S. Department of Health and Human Services in collaboration with nonfederal partners should increase its capacity to address health equity by practicing participatory and culturally competent evaluation, and it should standardize the collection, analysis, and reporting of data targeting disparities and health equity, and improve the accessibility of tools and methods for measuring social determinants that put populations at elevated risk for obesity.
Goal 7: Support a systems approach in evaluation.	**Recommendation 7:** Evaluators, government, and private funders should incorporate a systems approach to evaluating obesity prevention efforts into their research-related activities through leadership, funding, and training support.

[a] Agricultural Research Service, Economic Research Service, and Food and Nutrition Service of the U.S. Department of Agriculture; Census Bureau of the U.S. Department of Commerce; Agency for Healthcare Research and Quality, Centers for Disease Control and Prevention, Health Resources and Services Administration, and National Institutes of Health of the U.S. Department of Health and Human Services; Bureau of Labor Statistics of the U.S. Department of Labor; and Federal Highway Administration of the U.S. Department of Transportation.

Source: Institute of Medicine (IOM), *Evaluating Obesity Prevention Efforts: A Plan for Measuring Progress.* Washington, DC: The National Academies Press, 2013.

Healthy People 2020 outlines a set of health objectives for the nation to achieve over the second decade of the twenty-first century.[175] Several objectives from *Healthy People 2020* are related to overweight and obesity in adults and children (**Table 8-7**). Targets for *Healthy People 2020* objectives on Nutrition and Weight Status (NWS) are set at a 10% improvement over baseline values, and data are obtained from NHANES, the CDC, and the NCHS. In 2010, the CDC conducted the National Youth Physical Activity and Nutrition Study to augment data collected from YRBSS and to expand our understanding of the diet and physical activity determinants of BMI.[176]

In its 2003 policy statement and the updated 2015 recommendations, the AAP recommended BMI monitoring and screening for children and adolescents to diagnose overweight and obesity, as well as to provide preventive care.[177] The IOM has also recommended that health care professionals routinely track BMI in children and youth and offer appropriate counseling and guidance to children and their families.[178] Although several states have school-level child obesity monitoring surveys in place, BMI screening is not viewed favorably, largely because schools and communities lack resources for families with children who have obesity or severe obesity.[179]

> ▶ **THINK LIKE A COMMUNITY** NUTRITIONIST
>
> What is the best way to identify children who have obesity? Should children be screened through physician offices or schools (or both)? What are the pros and cons of screening children for obesity and overweight through physician offices? Through schools?

TABLE 8-7 *Healthy People 2020* Objectives Related to Weight Status Compared to Current Data on Obesity and Overweight

HEALTHY PEOPLE (HP) 2020 OBJECTIVE NUMBER	HEALTHY PEOPLE 2020 OBJECTIVE	BASELINE (YEAR)	HEALTHY PEOPLE 2020 TARGET
NWS-8	Increase the proportion of adults who are at a healthy weight.[a]	30.8% of persons 20 years and older in 2005–2008	33.9%
NWS-9	Reduce the proportion of adults who are obese.[b]	33.9% of persons 20 years and older in 2005–2008	30.5%
NWS-10	Reduce the proportion of children and adolescents who are considered obese.[c]		
NWS-10.1	Children ages 2–5 years	10.4% in 2005–2008	9.4%
NWS-10.2	Children ages 6–11 years	17.4% in 2005–2008	15.7%
NWS-10.3	Adolescents ages 12–19 years	17.9% in 2005–2008	16.1%
NWS-10.4	Children and adolescents ages 2–19 years	16.1% in 2005–2008	14.5%
NWS-11 (Developmental)	Prevent inappropriate weight gain in youth and adults		
NWS-11.1	Children ages 2–5 years	N/A	N/A
NWS-11.2	Children ages 6–11 years	N/A	N/A
NWS-11.3	Adolescents ages 12–19 years	N/A	N/A
NWS-11.4	Children and adolescents ages 2–19 years	N/A	N/A
NWS-11.5	Adults ages 20 and over	N/A	N/A

[a] Healthy weight is defined as a BMI of 18.5 to 24.9.

[b] Obesity is defined as a BMI $\geq$ 30.

[c] Weight Classifications in Children: Obese, BMI-for-age $\geq$ 95th percentile; Overweight, BMI-for-age $\geq$ 85th to $<$ 95th percentile.

Source: Adapted from Nutrition and Weight Status Objectives for *Healthy People 2020* at *http://www.healthypeople.gov/2020/topics-objectives/topic/nutrition-and-weight-status/objectives*.

Awareness Building, Education, and Research

Numerous government programs, initiatives, and agencies are involved in federal obesity policy in the United States, including the U.S. Department of Health and Human Services, the U.S. Department of Agriculture, the Federal Trade Commission, and the Department of Transportation. A more detailed review of cabinet-level agencies and federal programs that affect obesity is detailed elsewhere.[180]

Let's Move! The most significant and widespread governmental public awareness campaign for prevention of childhood obesity is *Let's Move!*, championed by First Lady Michelle Obama. When Mrs. Obama launched the campaign in February 2010, President Obama appointed a White House Task Force on Childhood Obesity to guide the campaign. The program has since grown to include several initiatives, including *Let's Move Cities and Towns, Let's Move Salad Bars to Schools*, and *Let's Move Child Care*, as well as a new focus on faith-based communities. Recommendations for *Let's Move!* focus on five pillars: (1) creating a healthy start for children; (2) empowering parents and caregivers; (3) providing healthy foods in schools; (4) improving access to healthy, affordable foods; and (5) increasing physical activity.[181]

Department of Health and Human Services (DHHS) Most of the agencies and offices within DHHS are involved in obesity-related programs, including the CDC, the Centers for Medicare and Medicaid Services, the Food and Drug Administration, the National Institutes of Health, the Health Resources and Services Administration, the Office of Women's Health, the Administration on Aging, the Head Start Bureau, and the Indian Health Service.[182] Several obesity prevention programs within the CDC and National Institutes of Health are highlighted below.

Centers for Disease Control and Prevention (CDC) The National Center for Chronic Disease Prevention and Health Promotion (NCCDPHP) at the CDC has been leading the agency's obesity-related prevention and health promotion efforts. Within NCCDPHP, divisions that implement and oversee obesity prevention programs include the Division of Adolescent and School Health (DASH) and the Division of Nutrition, Physical Activity, and Obesity (DNPAO). The most notable obesity-related program administered by Adolescent and School Health is the Coordinated School Health (CSH) Program, which promotes healthful behaviors in schools by focusing on an integrated model involving eight components: health education, physical education, health services, nutrition services, counseling and social services, healthful school environments, health promotion for staff, and family and community involvement. This program has now been expanded to include the community and governmental entities in the Whole School, Whole Community, Whole Child (WSCC) model (see the Programs in Action feature on page 317).[183] DASH also developed and distributes the *School Health Index for Physical Activity and Healthy Eating*, a self-assessment guide for schools to measure progress in physical activity and nutrition initiatives against a series of benchmarks and goals, as well as published *School Health Guidelines to Promote Healthy Eating and Physical Activity*.[184] DNPAO supports a wide variety of obesity-related programs at the community level, which include prevention, applied research, tracking of health behaviors, health communication/social marketing, and partnership development.

One of the major CDC DNPAO obesity initiatives is the funding of State Public Health Actions to Prevent and Control Diabetes, Heart Disease, Obesity and Associated Risk Factors and Promote School Health (State Public Health Actions) at each of the 50 states. These funds are used to coordinate programs across obesity and other chronic diseases, with a work plan that includes focusing on environmental intervention, improving delivery of care, community–clinical linkages, and the use of data to guide work. Other priority strategies for this initiative include physical activity in ECE settings, nutrition standards for foods, increased access to healthy food and beverages, promotion of physical activity, and support for breastfeeding.[185] An additional $4.2 million was allocated to six land grant institutions to focus on obesity prevention programs in states with counties that have obesity prevalence rates of 40% or greater. As part of the program, several states have developed and updated state plans to address overweight and obesity. Examples of websites for these programs and state plans are shown in **Table 8-8**.

TABLE 8-8 Examples of State-Level Nutrition and Physical Activity Plans and Programs to Prevent Obesity and Related Chronic Diseases

STATE	WEBSITE	PLAN DATES
Alabama	http://adph.org/obesity/assets/ObesityPlan.pdf	2010
California	https://www.cdph.ca.gov/programs/COPP/Documents/COPP-ObesityPreventionPlan-2010.pdf.pdf	2010
Delaware	http://dhss.delaware.gov/dhss/dph/dpc/files/pano_comp_plan-09.pdf	2010–2014
Georgia	http://beproactivefoundation.org/media/6a9a857bc6e14cbdffff8020ffffd523.pdf	2011–2021
Hawaii	http://health.hawaii.gov/physical-activity-nutrition/files/2013/08/Hawaii-PAN-Plan-2013-2020.pdf	2013–2020
Illinois	http://www.idph.state.il.us/HealthWellness/IL_Existing_State_Plan.pdf	2007–2013
Kansas	http://healthykansans2020.org/KHAIP/Health-Assessment-Section2-4.pdf?v51	2015–2020
Louisiana	http://dhh.louisiana.gov/assets/docs/LegisReports/LA-Obesity-Council2008-2009.pdf	2008–2009
Maine	http://healthymainepartnerships.org/PANP/documents/226-701-05_PAN_Plan.pdf	2005–2010
Massachusetts	http://www.mass.gov/eohhs/docs/dph/mass-in-motion/action-plan.pdf	2008
Michigan	http://www.michigan.gov/documents/mdch/Mi_Healthy_State_Plan_353817_7.pdf	2010–2020
Montana	http://mtdh.ruralinstitute.umt.edu/blog/?page_id51337	2006–2010
New Hampshire	http://www.healnh.org/images/pdffiles/HPHP/HEAL_HPHP_plan_with_links_for_web.pdf	2014–2019
New Jersey	http://www.state.nj.us/health/fhs/shapingnj/library/ShapingNJ%20Obesity%20Prevention%20Plan-Final.pdf	2013
New Mexico	http://physicalactivityplan.org/resources/PA-Plans/NewMexicoPA.pdf	2006–2015
New York	http://www.health.ny.gov/prevention/prevention_agenda/2013-2017/docs/prevent_chronic_diseases.pdf	2012
North Carolina	http://www.eatsmartmovemorenc.com/ESMMPlan/Texts/NC%20Obesity%20Prevention%20Plan%20 2013-2020_LowRes_FINAL.pdf	2013–2020
Ohio	http://www.odh.ohio.gov/~/media/HealthyOhio/ASSETS/Files/Chronic%20Disease%20Plan/State%20Plan.pdf	2014–2018
Oregon	http://public.health.oregon.gov/DiseasesConditions/ChronicDisease/Documents/hpcdp-strategic-plan.pdf	2012–2017
Rhode Island	http://www.health.ri.gov/publications/actionplans/2010InitiativeForHealthyWeight.pdf	2010–2015
South Carolina	http://www.scdhec.gov/Agency/docs/NewsReleaseDocs/EXECUTIVESUMMARYObesityActionPlan.pdf	2014–2019
South Dakota	http://healthysd.gov/wp-content/uploads/2015/05/NPAStatePlan.pdf	2015–2020
Tennessee	http://www.nptinternal.org/productions/chcv2/healthupdates/pdf/TN%20Statewide%20Nutrition%20 and%20Physical%20Activity%20Plan.pdf	2010–2015
Utah	http://www.choosehealth.utah.gov/documents/pdfs/U-PAN_State_Plan.pdf	2010–2020
Washington	http://stage-linux.governor.wa.gov/sites/default/files/policy_briefs/pb_HealthiestNextGeneration2015F.pdf	2015
Wisconsin	https://www.dhs.wisconsin.gov/publications/p0/p00507.pdf	2013–2020

In addition to state funding, the CDC and its partners have developed the *HHS Blueprint for Action on Breastfeeding*, which establishes a comprehensive national breastfeeding policy.[186] Breastfeeding may protect against obesity and may increase the acceptability of fruits and vegetables among infants.[187]

CDC has made obesity prevention in ECE a high priority and provides funding, training, and technical assistance to a variety of state and community agencies.[188] CDC's framework for obesity prevention in the childcare and early education setting is known as the *Spectrum of Opportunities*. The Spectrum identifies ways that individual states, and to some extent communities, can support ECE facilities to achieve recommended standards and best practices for obesity prevention.[189]

The CDC also funds two major research initiatives that encompass obesity prevention: the Health Protection Research Initiative and the Prevention Research Centers. The Health Protection Research Initiative is a CDC program to generate research that can be used in outreach efforts to employers to inform them about the benefits of wellness programs and the cost-effectiveness of a healthy workplace.[190] The CDC also funds 26 academic research centers known as Prevention Research Centers that investigate ways to prevent and control chronic diseases, including obesity, at the community level.[191] Funding helps to support infrastructure and community-based research projects, especially those that target **translational research**.

Translational research The adaptation of more highly controlled, experimental health promotion interventions that are effective to less controlled, but more generalizable, community-based conditions.

Recently, the CDC has been charged with administration of new initiatives to promote obesity prevention in communities, most notably the Community Transformation Grants, the Childhood Obesity Research Demonstration projects, and the Communities Putting Prevention to Work (CPPW) grants. These projects are located in communities across the United States and are designed to decrease chronic disease, including obesity.[192] In addition to addressing individual-level changes, these programs target policy, systems-level, and environmental solutions to obesity prevention. One of those projects, conducted in King County, Washington, showed a significant decrease and change in the prevalence of obesity in youth in schools participating in CPPW activities compared to youth in comparison schools. The CPPW intervention activities included nutrition guidelines for school meals, healthy eating and active living promotion campaigns conducted by students, farm-to-school initiatives, quality physical education, and community health coalitions.[193]

National Institutes of Health (NIH)

NIH serves a dual function in the fight against obesity: It furthers obesity prevention awareness and supports research funding and treatment measures. The 2011 *Strategic Plan for NIH Obesity Research*—which was developed by the NIH Obesity Research Task Force—is framed around the following overarching themes:

1. Discover fundamental biologic processes that regulate body weight and influence behavior.
2. Understand the factors that contribute to obesity and its consequences.
3. Design and test new interventions for achieving and maintaining a healthy weight.
4. Evaluate promising strategies for obesity prevention and treatment in real-world settings and diverse populations.
5. Harness technology and tools to advance obesity research and improve health care delivery.
6. Facilitate integration of research results into community programs and medical practice.

Research to identify and reduce health disparities is considered essential to all themes of the *Strategic Plan*. Several additional topics span the themes of the *Strategic Plan*. One of these areas is translational research, whose goal is to bridge scientific discovery to improvements in public health.[194]

NIH also oversees several different government institutes that administer programs focused on obesity-related education and research, including programs within the National Heart, Lung, and Blood Institute (NHLBI); the National Cancer Institute; the National Institute of Diabetes and Digestive and Kidney Diseases; and the National Institute of Environmental Health Sciences.

One major initiative that targets childhood obesity through the NHLBI is We Can!, or Ways to Enhance Children's Activity and Nutrition.[195] We Can! focuses on family and community strategies to improve healthful nutrition choices, increase physical activity, and decrease screen time. The We Can! website includes intervention materials, evaluation tools, and program recognition and networks.

United States Department of Agriculture (USDA)

The USDA is responsible for a range of food and nutrition programs that affect obesity via (1) nutritional advice and guidance, (2) food labeling regulations, (3) food and obesity education campaigns, (4) distribution of food products to schools, and (5) oversight and protection of the nation's agricultural and dairy markets. The USDA's division of Food, Nutrition, and Consumer Services includes two departments that target obesity-related programs and policies: the Food and Nutrition Service and the Center for Nutrition Policy and Promotion. The Food and Nutrition Service administers food and nutrition assistance programs to needy and eligible populations through school lunch and school-based educational programs.[196] Examples of such programs include SNAP, the National School Lunch Program, and the Fresh Fruit and Vegetable Program. Chapter 10 provides a detailed discussion of the USDA food and nutrition assistance programs.

The Agriculture Act of 2014, also referred to as the 2014 Farm Bill, expands nutrition education and obesity prevention activities. For example, it added promotion of physical activity as a component of SNAP's nutrition education program (SNAP-Ed), which provides grants to state SNAP agencies for nutrition education and obesity prevention. It also requires that SNAP retailers carry healthier food options. In addition, the 2014 Farm Bill permits SNAP participants to purchase Community Supported Agriculture Shares, which allow consumers to pay in advance for a share of a farmer's harvest and, in return, receive a weekly share of fresh fruits and vegetables. Finally, the 2014 Farm Bill provided $100 million for the Food Insecurity Nutrition Program, which is designed to increase the purchase of fruits and vegetables by low-income consumers participating in SNAP by providing incentives at the point of purchase. A new program would award grants to farmers' markets and grocery stores that match SNAP dollars, if recipients buy fruits and vegetables. It also includes funding to help build grocery stores in low-income areas that don't have many retail outlets.[197]

The National School Lunch Program (NSLP), which is one of the largest food and nutrition assistance programs in the United States, feeds millions of children every day. Due to the constraint of needing to meet nutritional requirements while covering costs, schools around the country are implementing a wide variety of changes in their lunchrooms, including those that aim to increase revenues through higher student participation. The Berkeley Unified School District, through its School Lunch Initiative, has upgraded its kitchens to better handle fresh food and reheat meals made from scratch in a central kitchen; has started a salad bar in each school; and has given priority to locally produced organic food.[198] To recognize schools that are actively engaged in fostering healthy school environments, the USDA is implementing the HealthierUS School Challenge, a voluntary program that provides monetary incentives and certifications to schools that are promoting healthy food and physical activity.[199]

The Fresh Fruit and Vegetable Program is a program designed to increase fruit and vegetable availability to schools. The program provides schools with federal money, enabling them to serve fruits and vegetables as snacks to children free of charge. Research has shown that children who report a high preference for fruits and vegetables are less likely to be overweight or at risk of overweight than those who report a very low preference for fruits and vegetables.[200]

The Center for Nutrition Policy and Promotion (CNPP) develops nutrition education information and works to disseminate research findings via outreach materials to target populations.[201] CNPP developed the USDA Healthy Eating Index (HEI), a tool for measuring overall diet quality that enables users to compare their diets with USDA recommendations in the *Dietary Guidelines for Americans* and the MyPlate food guidance system. The HEI is an important tool for monitoring diet quality, given that research has indicated that a low HEI score is associated with overweight and obesity.[202] In December 2011, the CNPP released SuperTracker, an interactive computer program that allows individuals to plan, record, and analyze their food intake and physical activity.[203]

Federal Trade Commission (FTC) The FTC has an important role to play in ensuring that the marketplace is receptive to healthful lifestyles and nutrition. More specifically, the FTC oversees (1) claims of health effects and labeling of food (including dietary supplements), (2) disclosure of caloric information, and (3) deceptive marketing of foods and food-related products. The FTC has compiled a set of obesity-related consumer blogs and information to guide the general public in making better diet and health choices and in not falling for "too good to be true" claims on topics such as weight loss and fitness.[204] See this chapter's Professional Focus feature for tips on how to evaluate popular weight-loss diets.

Department of Transportation (DOT) The DOT's Transportation Alternatives Program provides grants to states and localities to fund walking and biking projects. However, overall funding levels for these projects including *Safe Routes to School (SRTS)* were reduced when Congress last reauthorized the surface transportation law—known as Moving Ahead for Progress in the 21st Century (MAP-21)—in 2012. Since then, lawmakers have not yet reauthorized MAP-21, which would reauthorize the Federal-Aid Highway Program for six years from FY 2015 through FY 2020.[205]

Recent Legislative Efforts Multiple pieces of legislation have been introduced into Congress with the goal of reducing the obesity epidemic through increased educational efforts. Table 8-4 details selected bills introduced during the 114th Congress in 2015. It is expected that similar bills will be introduced in current and subsequent legislative sessions. Details about legislation that includes mandates related to nutrition and/or physical activity can be found at the CDC legislative website or at the policy website maintained by the Center for Science in the Public Interest (see the Internet Resources at the end of this chapter).

Regulating Environments

Much emphasis has been placed on the "toxic environment" or "obesogenic" environment in the development of obesity. It is logical to conclude that regulation of environmental factors, such as food availability and opportunities for physical activity, can influence diet and exercise habits, which in turn lead to the decrease or increase of obesity rates in a population. From an economic perspective, increased rates of obesity lead to higher costs to society in a number of ways, including direct health care costs (e.g., increase in type 2 diabetes rates) or work productivity losses. Thus, because society bears some of the financial burden of the obesity problem, this is a population-level issue, which can justify population-level approaches, such as regulation.[206] Systematic change of environments has greater potential than education alone to affect overall diet and physical activity patterns in populations.[207] A number of proposed options for regulating food, school, worksite, and built environments are presented in the following sections.

The Food Environment Cohen has reflected that "it is incumbent upon society as a whole to regulate the food environment, including the number and types of food related cues, portion sizes, food availability, and food advertising." Such an approach may be needed to limit reflexive neurohormonal responses to food images, cues, and smells.[208] Examples of regulatory interventions that could help create more healthful food environments include mandatory food product labeling at restaurants and restrictions on food advertisements and other food marketing and media messages targeted to children. Other examples of regulatory approaches that can be used to influence the food environment are discussed under The ECE Environment (page 306), The School Environment (page 307), The After-School Environment (page 309), The Worksite Environment (page 309), and The Built Environment (page 309).

With regard to the food environment, it has been argued that mandating point-of-sale nutrition information in restaurants would enable consumers to make more informed dietary decisions. It might also encourage restaurants to modify their ingredients and menus to provide a greater number of healthful food and beverage options.[209] On March 23, 2010, President Obama signed health reform legislation into law. The Patient Protection and Affordable Care Act of 2010 requires restaurants and similar retail food establishments to list calorie content information on restaurant menus and menu boards, including drive-through menu boards. Other nutrient information—total calories, fat, saturated fat, cholesterol, sodium, total carbohydrates, sugars, fiber, and total protein—has to be made available in writing upon request. This mandate also requires vending machine operators who own or operate 20 or more vending machines to disclose calorie content for certain items.[210] Under the Act, the U.S. Food and Drug Administration (FDA) requires all restaurants and food vendors with 20 or more locations to post calorie counts on their menus by December 2016.[211] In addition to restaurants, the final menu labeling requirements also apply to restaurant-type establishments selling prepared foods such as movie theaters, bowling alleys, grocery stores, convenience stores, and other establishments.[212]

A recent study of restaurant calorie labels found that persons with higher income and educational levels were more likely to make food choices based on calorie information provided in restaurant menus than those with lower income and education levels. The authors concluded that nutrition education needs to start early in life, and that school-age children should be taught how to read labels.[213] Others have noted that additional work is needed to figure out how to make calorie menu labels more understandable to people with low literacy and numeracy skills, such as placing the information in context by indicating how many hours of exercise it would require to burn the calories.[214] A systematic review and meta-analysis of the influence of menu labeling on calories selected found that the addition of contextual or interpretive nutrition information on menus appeared to assist consumers in the selection of fewer calories.[215]

Various professional organizations have issued policy statements calling for a ban on food and beverage advertisements to children, particularly those children under the age of 12.[216] A report issued by the IOM titled *Food Marketing to Children and Youth: Threat or Opportunity* found that "there is strong evidence that television advertising influences the short-term consumption of children ages 2–11 years old." The IOM report recommended that if voluntary, industry-driven efforts do not work, Congress should enact legislation "mandating the shift of both broadcast and cable television away from advertising calorie-dense, low-nutrient dense foods to healthful foods and beverages."[217]

A 2008 study found that a ban on fast-food advertisements during children's television programming in the United States would reduce the number of overweight children age 3–11 by 18%.[218] More recently, a study found that for network and cable television shows aimed at children under age 12, the majority of television commercials were for food products with too much added sugar, saturated fat, and sodium. Ninety percent of the food ads met the guidelines for *trans* fat of the Interagency Working Group of Foods Marketed to Children (IWG), and 60–70% met the guidelines for sodium and saturated fat. However, only 20% complied with added sugar guidelines and fewer than 2% of commercials met all the IWG guidelines. The authors concluded that "child-targeted food advertising remains strongly biased toward less healthy options."[219]

In addition to television food advertisements, there are other venues for food and beverage marketing messages in the broader food environment that are targeted to children. A recent study examining marketing directed at children on the interior and exterior of fast-food restaurants found that the majority of black, rural, and middle-income communities are disproportionately exposed to such marketing tactics. Fast-food restaurants in predominantly black neighborhoods were about 67% more likely to use child-directed marketing than those in white neighborhoods. Restaurants in rural areas were 40% more likely to use these marketing tactics than urban areas. Finally, restaurants in middle-income neighborhoods (defined at the 25th–75th percentiles of median incomes) were 28–34% more likely to use interior and exterior marketing focused on children than restaurants in upper-income neighborhoods.[220] Food and beverage companies also reach children with marketing messages in schools through signs, posters, scoreboards, branded fundraisers, corporate incentive programs, scholarships, and educational materials. One analysis found that only 20% of school districts have a policy in place that addresses food marketing, and only half of those school districts specifically prohibit unhealthy food and beverage advertising.[221] In 2014, the industry's overall self-regulatory effort—the Children's Food and Beverage Advertising Initiative (CFBAI)—adopted new uniform nutrition criteria for the 17 participating companies.[222] However, because CFBAI standards only cover children up to age 11, older children may still be vulnerable, particularly because they are more independent and use more media.[223] Recent comprehensive guidelines for responsible food marketing to children may help close industry loopholes for food marketing practices directed to children. The recommendations address the food marketing practices aimed at children, and specify the preferred strategies, techniques, media platforms, and venues for use with children.[224]

The Early Care and Education (ECE) Environment

Over half of young children under the age of six spend time in care outside their homes,[225] making the ECE setting one of the best places to reach young children with obesity prevention efforts. It has been estimated that more than 11 million children under the age of six years spend an average of 30 hours in nonparental care, with children of working mothers spending almost 40 hours a week in such care. Hence, the use of ECE facilities—childcare centers, daycare homes, Head Start Programs, and preschool and prekindergarten programs—has become the norm in the United States.[226]

The amendments made by the Healthy, Hunger-Free Kids Act (HHFKA) of 2010 require the USDA through its Child and Adult Care Food Program (CACFP) to promote health and wellness in childcare and ECE settings through guidance and technical assistance that focuses on nutrition, physical activity, and limiting electronic media use.[227] Experts in public health have identified 50 components that all types of early care and educational settings should include in standards for infant feeding, nutrition, physical activity, and screen time.[228] An assessment of childcare providers' feeding practices compliance with the Academy of Nutrition and Dietetics benchmarks for nutrition in childcare programs found that Head Start providers, parents, and children received more nutrition education opportunities, more balance and variety of foods, more modeling of healthy eating, and more nutrition education compared with CACFP and non-CACFP providers.[229]

In 2011, the USDA began requiring that sites participating in the CACFP make drinking water available throughout the day and serve only low-fat or nonfat milk to children age two years and older. In 2012, the California Healthy Beverages in Childcare law additionally required that all childcare sites eliminate beverages with added sweeteners and limit 100% juice to one daily.[230] A recent assessment of this policy in California found that 60% of sites were aware of the beverage policies and 23% were fully compliant.[231] In Texas, a *Let's Move!* Farm to Child Care Program has been funded through the USDA's Food and Nutrition Service (FNS) Child Care Wellness Grants.[232] The program encourages centers and daycare homes to buy local produce and increase the appeal and nutrient quality of preschool meals. The farm-to-childcare lesson plans teach children and parents how to start their own gardens, which prompted children to consume more fruits and vegetables at home.[233] The Public Health Law Center has developed a Minnesota Child Care Toolkit, which includes the promotion of healthy eating, positive exercise habits, reduced screen environments, and tobacco-free environments.[234]

The School Environment Because children spend a significant percentage of their formative years in school, a healthful school environment is an important venue for shaping a child's future eating and physical activity habits.[235] Food is typically available for sale in most schools in two ways: (1) the USDA-regulated NSLP, School Breakfast Program (SBP), and after-school snack programs; and (2) "competitive foods," which include food sold from snack shops, school stores, and vending machines and in à la carte lines in the cafeteria, as well as through bake sales, fundraisers, and other school activities. State education departments receive subsidies from the USDA for school meals if the programs follow national nutritional guidelines and offer free or reduced-price meals to children from low-income households.[236]

The USDA published a proposed rule to update nutrition standards for meals served through the NSLP and SBP as part of the Healthy, Hunger-Free Kids Act of 2010, which was signed into law by President Obama.[237] The HHFKA directed the USDA to update the nutrition standards for school meals for the first time in a decade, and update standards for school snacks and drinks for the first time in more than 30 years. By the spring of 2014, 86% of schools across the country were certified as serving healthier meals that met the updated nutrition standards.[238] The HHFKA of 2010 also requires that schools provide easily accessible, clean water to students at no cost. Research shows that children who drink more water consume less sugar.[239] In 2013, the *Partnership for a Healthier America* launched a "Drink Up" campaign to support increased water availability and consumption, including in schools.[240]

In June 2013, the USDA published an interim final rule establishing healthier nutrition standards for competitive foods. The "Smart Snacks in School" standards require schools to provide snacks and beverages with more whole grains, low-fat dairy, fruits, vegetables, and lean protein. They also set limits on fat, sugar, and salt.[241] See Chapter 12 for more about "Smart Snacks" in schools.

> ▸ **THINK LIKE A COMMUNITY** NUTRITIONIST

A variety of public health policies have been enacted to increase availability of healthy food. Some have argued that changes in food availability alone will not result in improved eating, citing that food preferences are not easily changed. This brings to light an important issue: to change eating habits, healthy foods must be available *and* desirable. Within social and cultural settings, the "norms" (typical behaviors and expectations) can be powerful. Thinking about how to promote healthy norms is an important part of community nutrition interventions. Consider the Healthy, Hunger-Free Kids Act of 2010, which resulted in recent changes to the National School Lunch Program. Specifically, one new requirement is that every student participating in the program takes a fruit or vegetable with lunch. How might this requirement change the norms in school cafeterias? Will this process be quick? What strategies might be used in school nutrition programs to enhance *desirability* of and *consumption* of fruits and vegetables?

Until 2010, federal law restricted the sale of carbonated drinks, candies, and other "foods of minimal nutritional value" only in the cafeteria during meal service hours, leaving many nutrient-poor products available for sale with lax oversight.[242] However, the HHFKA of 2010 required the USDA to release new national standards for competitive foods. A recent analysis of state-level competitive food and beverage laws found that children living in states with weak competitive food laws for middle schools had over 20% higher odds of being overweight or obese than children living in states with strong competitive food laws.[243]

Another key regulatory opportunity at the state level lies in improving and encouraging physical and nutrition education programs. Physical education programs often fail to meet the recommendations for daily physical education for children.[244] Physical education standards often are not enforced at the state or local level because schools and districts have so many other mandated curriculum requirements that are evaluated in standardized tests and for which schools are accountable.[245] Ultimately, failure to fund nutrition and physical education could result in increased levels of obesity and, therefore, increased state and federal health care spending.

There are a number of types of physical activity that schools can support as part of a Comprehensive School Physical Activity Program, which encompasses physical education, interscholastic sports and physical activity clubs, classroom physical activity breaks, before-school access to physical activity opportunities or facilities, recess for elementary school students, walking and biking to school, sharing facilities with community physical activity organizations, and opening physical activity facilities to families outside school hours. The Carol W. White Physical Education Program (PEP) provides federal grants to school districts and community organizations that implement comprehensive physical fitness and nutrition programs for students designed to help reach state physical education standards.[246]

At the national level, the Child Nutrition and WIC Reauthorization Act of 2004 mandated that schools form wellness committees and develop local school wellness policies, which include goals for nutrition education, physical activity, and other school-based activities designed to promote student wellness and nutrition guidelines for all foods available on each school campus during the school day.

Wellness policies required by the Child Nutrition and WIC Reauthorization Act of 2004 were updated and strengthened by the HHFKA of 2010, which amended the Richard B. Russell National School Lunch Act of 1966 to establish a local school wellness policy for all schools participating in the National Lunch Program and/or School Breakfast Program. At a minimum, wellness policies must include specific goals for nutrition promotion, nutrition education, physical activity, and other school-based activities that promote student wellness. Local educational agencies are required to periodically measure and provide an assessment of the wellness program to the public, including implementation of the wellness policy, the extent to which the schools are in compliance with the policy, how well the policy compares to model policies, and a description of the progress made in attaining wellness policy goals.[247]

The After-School Environment A review of school district wellness policies from 2006–2007 through 2010–2011 found that no more than 5% of school districts nationwide have a wellness policy that requires the recommended amount of daily physical education time.[248] In addition, children at highest risk for obesity are the least likely to attend schools that offer recess.[249] Therefore, some public health organizations are recommending that school wellness policies address physical education and physical activity in after-school and out-of-school programs, including school partnerships with nonprofit organizations.[250] Starting in 2014, the Boys and Girls Clubs of America and the National Recreation and Park Association agreed to provide at least 30 minutes of physical activity during after-school and summer programs.[251] A recent study that assessed the impact of after-school physical activity programs over 20 years predicted that by 2032 after-school physical activity programs could reduce obesity in children 6–12 years of age by about 2 percentage points.[252]

The Worksite Environment Obesity in the workplace may result in higher health care costs for obese and sedentary employees because of poorer health among these individuals. One study found that obese employees cost private employers approximately $45 billion a year due to medical expenditures and absenteeism. Thus, in their capacity as health care insurance providers, employers may pay the high costs associated with increasing rates of obesity among their employees.[253] Employee worksite wellness programs are becoming an accepted and essential component of many organizations. Worksite wellness programs include promotion of physical activity and fitness, nutrition education, and healthy weight. In terms of weight management, multicomponent interventions that focus on both physical activity and nutrition behavior over single dietary programs are recommended.[254] The USDA Center for Nutrition Policy and Promotion has released a Worksite Wellness Toolkit, which focuses on helping employees implement SuperTracker—a personalized nutrition and physical activity planning and tracking tool—into their lives. The USDA's toolkit features an eight-week promotion plan to use with employees, encouraging employees to take control of their health and become familiar with SuperTracker.[255]

The Built Environment As noted earlier, the "built environment" encompasses a variety of community design elements such as street layout, zoning, transportation options, stairs, public and green spaces (walking paths, parks and other recreation areas, playgrounds, community gardens), and business areas (farmers' markets, supermarkets, and grocery stores).[256] Various investigators have found an association between obesity and urban sprawl, as well as other aspects of the built environment (e.g., lack of grocery stores in inner cities).[257] The IOM recommends that local governments, private developers, and community groups expand opportunities for physical activity, including recreational facilities, parks, playgrounds, sidewalks, and safe streets and neighborhoods, especially for populations at high risk of childhood obesity.[258] Regulatory options to enhance opportunities for physical activity and to increase access to affordable, nutritious food through the built environment include mixed-use zoning, improved bicycling and walking opportunities, and providing economic incentives to attract supermarket development in underserved areas.

Land use in local municipalities is determined through zoning. *Mixed-use zoning* regulations allow commercial and residential areas to be located together and can promote physical activity by making it possible to walk or bike from home to work, school, shopping, and entertainment. Examples of local jurisdictions using zoning to promote healthy nutrition include reducing the density of fast-food restaurants within a specified distance from schools, incentivizing farming in urban areas, and incentivizing development of large grocery stores in urban areas. In July 2008, the Los Angeles City Council passed a one-year moratorium on opening or expanding fast-food establishments. The purposes of the moratorium were to address a perceived overconcentration of fast-food restaurants in the South Los Angeles region and allow community planning to attract dining establishments, grocery stores, and other options to enhance quality of life for community members. Since the South Los Angeles moratorium, studies have suggested that the density of fast-food restaurants in the South Los Angeles area is not as critical a factor as the lack of supermarkets available to the area or the high number of small corner grocery stores that stock less healthy food choices. Strategies to attract supermarkets with healthier food choices to the area and educating the public about calories with restaurant menu labeling may be more effective to reduce obesity in the region.[259]

The CDC's *Recommended Community Strategies and Measurements to Prevent Obesity in the United States* [260] includes zoning strategies communities can implement to reduce obesity. For example, communities can use zoning to increase the number of full-service grocery stores, reduce the density of fast-food restaurants, and provide incentives for farmers' markets in underserved areas. The National Policy and Legal Analysis Network to Prevent Childhood Obesity (NPLAN)[261] provides model policies, fact sheets, toolkits, training, and technical assistance to explain legal issues related to the public health issue of obesity. The NPLAN website provides model zoning ordinances that local governments can use to establish and protect the number of community gardens and create healthy food zones, which strive to prohibit fast-food restaurants from locating near schools or in areas where they are extremely dense.[262]

A second regulatory option for enhancing the built environment is through *improved bicycling and walking opportunities*. Safety issues should be considered when increasing these opportunities because residents may be reluctant to walk or bike in areas with high rates of pedestrian accidents.[263] The Safe Routes to School (SRTS) programs operate in all 50 states and Washington, D.C., benefiting close to 15,000 schools nationwide; however, implementation and funding varies across states. Programs that identify and create bicycle routes to schools and provide safety education have been found to increase physical activity.[264] More than half of all states have adopted Complete Street policies,[265] which incorporate features such as sidewalks and bike lanes to encourage physical activity and green transportation, walking and cycling, and building or protecting urban transportation systems that promote healthy lifestyles. Specific environmental features with the strongest evidence for creating active-friendly environments included park proximity, mixed land use, trees/greenery, accessibility and street connectivity, building design, and workplace physical activity policies/programs.[266]

Another policy to improve the built environment is to *relocate supermarkets in urban and rural areas* that currently have few stores and high unemployment rates. One such strategy that has become a priority for policymakers is the Healthy Food Financing Initiatives (HFFI), a public–private partnership in which grants and loans are given to full-service supermarkets or farmers' markets in lower-income urban or rural communities. The most successful program to date is the Pennsylvania Fresh Food Financing Initiative (FFFI), which since 2004 has financed supermarkets and other fresh food outlets in 78 urban and rural areas serving 500,000 city residents.[267] In the process, FFFI has created or retained 4,860 jobs in underserved neighborhoods. An analysis of the economic impacts of five new stores that opened with FFFI assistance found that, for four of the stores, total employment surrounding the supermarket increased at a rate higher than city-wide trends.[268] This is an important outcome in that it helps address the underlying social and economic contributors to obesity, including poverty, unemployment, living and working conditions, poor housing quality, lack of access to healthy food, and unsafe neighborhoods.[269]

To date, HFFI has distributed more than $109 million in grants across the country, helping to support the financing of grocery stores and other healthy food retail outlets including farmers' markets, food hubs, and urban farms. The Agriculture Act of 2014, also known as the Farm Bill, passed in February 2014, authorized $125 million for the federal HFFI to provide grants and tax incentives to food retailers to operate in low-income communities and, for the first time, created a permanent home for the program in the USDA.[270]

Living closer to supermarkets and other food outlets that sell fresh foods may be a necessary but not sufficient condition to improve healthy food consumption among lower-income individuals. Additional factors that may need to be addressed include lack of transportation to food outlets; quality and variety of fruits and vegetables available at stores; convenience of purchasing and preparing fresh foods; lack of cooking skills; and insufficient nutrition knowledge.[271] Qualitative research has demonstrated that store environment (e.g., safety, cleanliness, customer service), quality and variety of food available, and cost are important factors in determining access to healthy foods in low-income communities.[272]

Another strategy for increasing access to healthy food in low-income communities is encouraging corner stores to increase their offerings of healthy food and beverage selections. Recent research found that an urban corner store intervention was associated with improvements of low-fat milk and some fruit and vegetable offerings, especially when infrastructure changes, such as refrigeration and shelving enhancements, are provided.[273] Other research on interventions conducted in small food stores (in rural and urban settings) reported significant effects for increased availability of healthy foods, improved sales of healthy foods, and improved consumer knowledge and dietary behaviors.[274] For more information on interventions that are targeted to offering more healthy foods and beverages through corner stores, see the Healthy Corner Stores Network at *www.healthycornerstores.org.*

Pricing Policies

Recently, researchers have begun to explore the connection among agricultural subsidies, economic policies, and the obesity epidemic.[275] The majority of these subsidies in the United States are targeted to a small number of agricultural crops such as corn, wheat, and soybeans.[276] A large percentage of these commodity crops is used as either animal feed for meat production and/or to provide ingredients for highly processed foods, such as the high-fructose corn syrup used in soft drinks. Consider the following argument:

> There are lots of subsidies for the two things we should be limiting in our diets, which are fat and sugar, and there are not a lot of subsidies for broccoli and Brussels sprouts. . . . What would happen if we took away the subsidies on the sugar and fat? Probably not much. They might go up a little bit, but the cost of food is not the cost of the final products. But if we're trying something political that might make a difference, try subsidizing fruit and vegetable growers so the cost is comparatively lower for better foods.[277]

In the 2014 Farm Bill, traditional commodity subsidies were cut by more than 30%, to $23 billion over 10 years, while funding for fruits and vegetables and organic programs increased by more than 50% over the same period, to about $3 billion.[278]

Taxation is another type of pricing policy measure that legislatures can employ to influence consumers' buying practices. Tax incentives could be used to encourage more healthful dietary and physical activity behaviors, by (1) encouraging employers to promote worksite wellness programs and (2) encouraging real estate developers to convert unused or abandoned spaces into physical activity–oriented facilities or to include green space and accessible sidewalks in their plans for residential development.[279] The National

Governors Association's Center for Best Practices and the World Health Organization have noted that taxes on less nutritious foods are tools that can be used to influence consumer food-buying behavior.[280] Federal and state governments currently impose taxes on alcohol and tobacco; such taxes raise revenue but also promote public health and discourage consumption of these products.

Although states and cities that choose to levy taxes on less nutritious foods, including soft drinks, candy, chewing gum, and snack foods (such as potato chips), may not appreciably alter food consumption patterns, these tax revenues could be used to help fund healthful eating and nutrition education campaigns.[281] Opponents argue that because these taxes are levied on the purchase of foods that all income groups consume, they disproportionately affect low-income people, who spend a greater percentage of their total income on food.[282] Others have argued that such a tax penalizes the wrong target because it affects consumers and not manufacturers, who may be more to blame for the preponderance of the many low-nutrient-density foods.[283] Public opinion is also divided on the issue of a "junk-food" tax. The largest American Indian reservation, the Navajo nation, approved a junk-food tax to fight obesity that took effect in 2015.[284] The tax results in a 2% increase in sales tax for food with little to no nutritional value. It has been estimated that about one-third of Navajos have diabetes or pre-diabetes, and the obesity rate for some age groups is as high as 60%. The $1 million per year additional tax that is expected to be generated will pay for projects such as farmers' markets, vegetable gardens, and wellness and exercise equipment in the tribe's 110 communities. Another bill to eliminate the tribe's 5% sales tax on fresh fruits and vegetables sold on the Navajo nation went into effect in 2014.[285]

> ► **THINK LIKE A COMMUNITY** NUTRITIONIST
>
> What are the pros and cons of a junk-food tax? For more information, see the article "The Navajo Nation's Tax on Junk Food Splits Reservation" at *www.npr.org/sections/ codeswitch/2015/04/08/398310036/the-navajo-nations -tax-on-junk-food-splits-reservation*.

To address the growing epidemic of obesity, one option is to combine programs that target individual behavior change with fiscal policy, such as an excise tax on sugar-sweetened beverages. A meta-analysis reviewed published articles that reported changes in diet or BMI, overweight, and/or obesity due to a tax on, or price change of, sugar-sweetened beverages between January 2000 and January 2013. Higher prices of sugar-sweetened beverages were associated with a lower demand for sugar-sweetened beverages. All six articles from the United States showed that a higher price on sugar-sweetened beverages could lead to a decrease in BMI, and decrease the prevalence of overweight and obesity.[286] Further research is needed to identify potential health gains and wider economic impacts in low- and middle-income countries.[287]

In 2014, voters in Berkeley, California, became the first U.S. city to pass a per-ounce tax on sodas and other sweetened beverages including iced tea and energy drinks, which is estimated to raise $1 million to $3 million annually.[288] Mexico passed a soda tax—roughly equivalent to a 10% price increase—which took effect in 2014. A year's worth of data show that the modest tax had a measurable difference in the consumption of sugar-sweetened drinks. The greatest changes occurred in the most vulnerable low-income households, where consumers were able to cut consumption by 17%.[289]

A systematic review of the potential effectiveness of food and beverage taxes and subsidies for improving public health found that studies that linked soda taxes to weight outcomes had minimal effects on weight. However, these taxes were based on existing state-level sales taxes that were relatively low. Higher fast-food prices were associated with lower weight outcomes, particularly among adolescents. Lower fruit and vegetable prices (e.g., subsidies) were generally found to be associated with lower body weight outcomes among both low-income children and adults.[290] More recently, a study that assessed the impact over 20 years of the effect of a 1 cent per ounce excise tax on sugar-sweetened beverages predicted that by the year 2032 such an excise tax on sugar-sweetened beverages could reduce obesity among adolescents ages 13–18 by 2.4 percentage points, and generate significant revenue for additional obesity prevention activities.[291] All three federal policies assessed in this analysis (e.g., after-school physical activity programs, a child-directed fast-food television advertising ban, and an excise tax on sugar-sweetened beverages) were predicted to reduce childhood obesity, but the excise tax ($0.01 per ounce) was predicted to reduce childhood obesity the most among 13- to 18-year-olds. In addition, the authors found that all three federal policies would reduce obesity more among blacks and Hispanics than among whites.[292] Another recent systematic review of the literature concluded that maximum success was achieved when food taxes/subsidies are at least 10–15%, and when subsidies and taxation are used together.[293]

Societal-Level Solutions

The World Health Organization (WHO) report *Obesity—Preventing and Managing the Global Epidemic* first highlighted obesity as a worldwide problem that now affects most countries.[294] More recently, the WHO has declared overweight one of the top 10 health risks in the world.[295]

Countries in Asia, the Middle East, and Latin America are already experiencing a double burden of undernutrition and nutritional disease, such as diabetes and heart disease, caused by obesity and poverty.[296] The rise in obesity on a global scale means that health systems (and thus government budgets) will face an ever-growing financial burden from chronic disease unless effective obesity prevention and treatment strategies are implemented.[297] A recent study found that while the prevalence of diabetes has been rising in developed countries for several decades, a more recent major shift is underway in developing countries, with rises in diabetes prevalence reported in countries such as Saudi Arabia, Mexico, China, and India.[298]

Examples of social and environmental trends that may be contributing to the global obesity epidemic include increased use of motor transport; increased traffic hazards for walkers and cyclists; fewer opportunities for recreational physical activity; greater quantities of food available; more frequent and widespread food-purchasing opportunities; rising use of soft drinks to replace water; multiple television channels available around the clock; and globalization of markets, which favors energy-dense foods of low nutritional value.[299]

A primary goal of public health initiatives addressing the global obesity epidemic is to increase the awareness of people in sectors outside the health care field (such as culture and education, commerce and trade, development, planning, and transport) of the potentially adverse effects of their various actions on the ability of people to maintain energy balance.[300] **Table 8-9** outlines a range of societal-level solutions that can be implemented for obesity prevention at the population level.

Where Do We Go from Here?

Awareness of obesity and overweight as a significant public health issue is in its beginning stages. The rapid increases in the prevalence of obesity and overweight are fairly recent, and current standards for child overweight were developed only since the early 2000s. With a multifactorial problem such as obesity, multiple approaches are necessary, and change may occur slowly. The progress of the obesity epidemic can be likened to another public health problem—smoking. As illustrated in **Figure 8-5**, smoking rates rose from the early 1900s through the 1960s. Awareness of the association between smoking and cancer arose during the 1950s, and public health initiatives were put into place as a result. These

TABLE 8-9 Potential Societal-Level Solutions for Obesity Prevention

National governments	• Provide economic incentives for supply of "healthy" foods and disincentives for supply of "unhealthy" foods.
Food supply	• Produce, distribute, and promote food products that are low in dietary fat and energy. • Introduce economic incentives for supermarkets to locate in low-income neighborhoods. • Introduce new and improved labeling schemes (covering fat and energy) that do not mislead the consumer.
Media	• Regulate television advertising aimed at children. • Incorporate positive behavior change messages into television programs and popular magazines.
Non-governmental and international organizations	• Develop and implement healthful eating, physical activity, and obesity prevention programs. • Provide training in obesity prevention for physicians and other health care providers.
Education sites	• Introduce and enforce nutrition standards for school meals. • Provide classes in food preparation and cooking; introduce school gardening curricula and "farm-to-school" programs. • Increase the range and number of physical activities offered at school throughout the day: before, during, and after school.
Worksites	• Provide healthful food and drink options in staff restaurants and vending machines. • Establish farmers' markets and "farm-to-work" programs. • Empower employees to integrate physical activity into the workday.
Neighborhoods, homes, and families	• Set up community gardening programs, farmers' markets, and food cooperatives. • Increase the walkability of city centers and residential areas, using programs such as Complete Streets. • Set up walking programs in shopping malls and parks, and open safe-cycling routes.

Source: Adapted from S. Kumanyika and coauthors, "Obesity Prevention: The Case for Action," *International Journal of Obesity* 26 (2002): 425–36.

FIGURE 8-5 Annual Adult Per Capita Cigarette Consumption and Major Smoking and Health Events—United States, 1900–1998

Source: United States Department of Agriculture and "Reducing Tobacco Use: A Report of the Surgeon General"; accessed at *www.cdc.gov/tobacco/data_statistics/sgr/2000.*

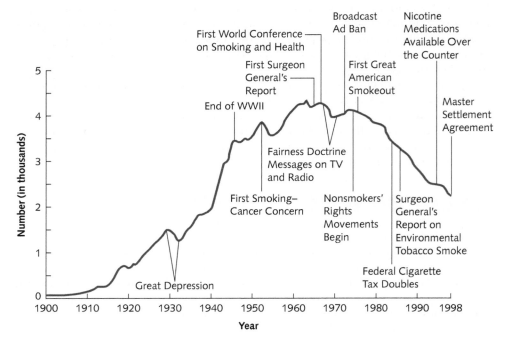

initiatives resulted in societal changes that occurred over a 30-year period. As these public health approaches began to be implemented, smoking rates reached a plateau and then started to drop in the United States.

Public health approaches and societal change must begin now, but it is likely to be several years before the surveillance data show decreases in the prevalence of obesity and obesity-related diseases. A public health approach to address the global obesity epidemic must apply the same kind of multifaceted and coordinated approach that reduced tobacco use in the United States in order to change individual behavior patterns and effectively address environmental barriers to physical activity and healthful food choices.[301]

In general, environmental changes will follow a strong lead from policy and/or social change. Before this can occur, however, a paradigm shift is needed—one that recognizes "toxic" or "obesogenic" environments as the main drivers of the obesity epidemic and that actively recruits sectors outside the field of health and nutrition (culture and education, commerce and trade, development, planning, and transport) as essential allies in tackling the obesity epidemic. Similarly, sectors such as local governments, schools, the food industry, and the media (through marketing and advertising practices) need a paradigm shift to recognize the significance of their contributions to reversing the obesity epidemic.[302] This paradigm shift involves encouraging these sectors to consider health effects as a major part of planning and decision making.

What can the community nutritionist do? As we have seen, the first step is to build an understanding of the magnitude of the problem, especially awareness of the chronic diseases associated with obesity and their ultimate financial costs to the taxpayer. A second step is to put into effect policies and practices that target both individual behavioral and environmental factors. Because it is difficult to change behavioral factors without a supportive environment, it is essential to bring together other interested stakeholders through community coalitions or groups devoted to a common goal. Legislators at all levels (local, state, and national) need to be made aware of this issue and to be included in these efforts. Funding for research should be increased, with special allocations for new and innovative pilot programs, studies to change environmental factors, and evaluation of obesity-related policies and their impact on the population. Finally, solutions for prevention of overweight and obesity need to be creative—perhaps by involving nontraditional partners or targeting less obvious determinants of obesity such as parenting skills, social and economic policies that may influence a family's access to a healthful food supply, or methods of transportation. Several good resources for the community nutritionist—including background information, model legislation, and other resources promoting healthful nutrition and physical activity—can be found at the Internet sites listed at the end of this chapter.

How can the community nutritionist get started? Current recommendations for obesity prevention, such as the Institute of Medicine's *Accelerating Progress in Obesity Prevention* report (see the recommendations listed in Table 8-5), or the recommendations in *The Surgeon General's Call to Action to Prevent and Decrease Overweight and Obesity*, provide an outline of activities and areas to target.[303]

Here are some examples of immediate steps that a community nutritionist can take:

- Develop and promote community awareness campaigns to highlight health risks associated with obesity.
- Organize a community coalition or partnerships to address obesity-related issues.
- Work with schools in the development, implementation, and evaluation of local school wellness policies or Coordinated School Health Programs that reflect the Whole School, Whole Community, Whole Child approach.
- Work with ECE centers, schools, and worksites to implement farm-to-childcare, farm-to-school, and farm-to-work programs.

- Implement evidence-based behavioral interventions through community-based clinics and organizations, ECE centers, schools, worksites, faith-based communities, and WIC centers.
- Provide environmental intervention strategies through opportunities for increased access to physical activity and healthful foods, such as encouraging funding for walking trails and community gardens and increasing the number of grocery stores and supermarkets in low-income neighborhoods; developing standards for foods sold in schools and at public venues; and encouraging healthful catering guidelines for child-care centers, school, community, and worksite functions.
- Encourage health care professionals to measure and track BMI and to provide counseling and referrals for patients who exceed current standards for overweight and obesity.
- Participate in local or national movements, such as First Lady Michelle Obama's *Let's Move!* campaign.
- Write to or educate local municipal officials, state legislators, and/or members of Congress about upcoming obesity-related legislation.
- Participate in evaluation of community programs to establish a further evidence base for obesity prevention. Examples of types of community evaluation can be found in the IOM *Evaluating Obesity Prevention Efforts: A Plan for Measuring Progress* report.[304]

Working with organizations such as the *Partnership for a Healthier America (PHA)* provides another option for the community nutritionist. PHA was created in 2010 to work in conjunction with, but independent from, First Lady Michelle Obama's *Let's Move!* effort. PHA brings together public, private, and nonprofit leaders to broker meaningful commitments and develop strategies to end childhood obesity. Recent accomplishments include:

- PHA partners nearly doubled the number of food stores in areas that lacked access to healthy, affordable food (from 372 to 602), serving more than 6.4 million individuals.
- Hospitals participating in PHA's Hospital Healthier Food Initiative are reporting year-over-year increases in sales of fruits, vegetables, and wellness meals.
- Drink Up, PHA's effort to encourage people to drink more water more often, resulted in a 4% lift in bottled water and water filter sales.
- More than 15,000 schools have joined *Let's Move!* Active Schools, and are reaching over 9 million children in all 50 states.
- More than 28,500 restaurants and hotels are now serving healthier children's meals.
- By the year 2020, PHA partners will reach nearly 6 million children in childcare and out-of-school programs with healthier food and increased physical activity.

PHA has also launched a multimedia campaign called "FNV" (fruit 'n' veggies) whose aim is to make eating fruits and vegetables as cool as owning an iPhone. The campaign has enlisted celebrities and athletes to help spread the campaign's message and will use multiple media outlets including television, radio, billboard advertising, in-store marketing, Facebook, Twitter, Instagram, and Tumblr.[305]

The development of a solution to the obesity epidemic is a complex issue that will likely involve a combination of societal and individual-level approaches. It is likely that the solution will include a coordinated, **systems-level approach** that includes targeting multiple levels within one comprehensive program or goal. Although the task of decreasing the epidemic of obesity seems formidable, it is also a challenge that will provide increasing employment and personal opportunities, especially for the field of nutrition and dietetics.

Systems-level approach
An approach that frames a problem in terms of different components contributing to that problem, as well as the relationships and interactions between these components. The focus is not directly on individuals and communities but on the systems that impact health. This viewpoint includes incorporation of the wider context into the solution, as well as acknowledging that persons affected by those problems are embedded within broader societal systems (e.g., political, social, economic, and so on).

PROGRAMS IN **ACTION**

Whole School, Whole Community, Whole Child Programs

Given that over 95% of children attend schools[1] and that most schools have nutrition resources and opportunities for physical activity, school systems are an excellent avenue for obesity prevention programs.[2] Schools can target obesity prevention through behaviorally based classroom education programs that target individual and cognitive factors, as well as environmental influences such as physical activity (through physical education classes) and diet (through cafeterias and vending sales of foods).

Adolescent and School Health at the CDC has expanded their previous model for health promotion programs at the school level to include a focus on the larger environment, which is consistent with the social–ecological model (SEM). This expanded model, known as WSCC (**Figure 8-6**), views the school in a multidimensional and systems-level fashion, in which all components at the school level work together to maintain consistent, healthful messages, including the surrounding community and environment.[3] Thus, messages about health are delivered to the students through different modalities that reinforce concepts and support healthful behaviors. Probably the best example of a program that addresses both nutrition and physical activity is the Coordinated Approach to Child Health, or CATCH, program.

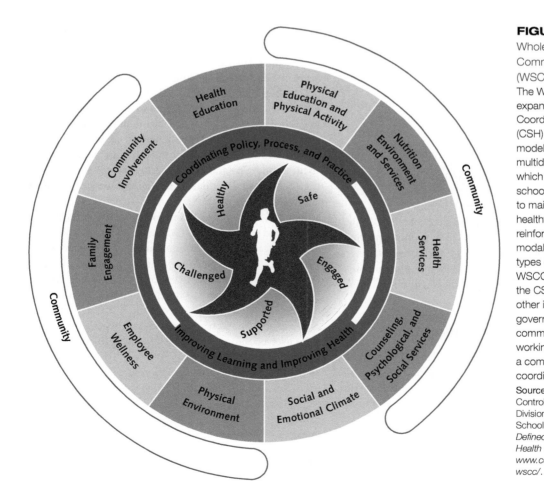

FIGURE 8-6 The Whole School, Whole Community, Whole Child (WSCC) Model
The WSCC model is an expansion of the CDC's Coordinated School Health (CSH) approach. The CSH model views the school in a multidimensional fashion in which all components at the school level work together to maintain consistent, healthful messages that are reinforced using different modalities and appeal to all types of learning styles. The WSCC approach expands the CSH model to include other influences, such as governmental agencies and community organizations working with schools in a comprehensive and coordinated fashion.
Source: Centers for Disease Control and Prevention (CDC), Division of Adolescent and School Health, *School Health Defined: Coordinated School Health Program*; available at *www.cdc.gov/healthyyouth/wscc/*.

Goals and Objectives

The overall goal of the CATCH program is to create healthy children and healthy school environments. The specific aims of the program are:

1. To encourage students to consume a diet that is moderate in fat (30% of energy); low in saturated fat (10% of energy) and energy-dense foods; and high in fruits, vegetables, and whole grains, emphasizing healthful meal patterns and whole foods.
2. To encourage students to participate in increased moderate to vigorous physical activity (MVPA), or activity that makes a child's heart beat quickly and/or makes a child breathe hard.
3. To increase MVPA in schools to 50% of the physical education class.
4. To provide food in school cafeterias that is lower in fat and saturated fat and higher in fruits, vegetables, and whole grains.
5. To encourage parental participation in the school health program.

CATCH was originally developed and evaluated as the Child and Adolescent Trial for Cardiovascular Health from 1991 to 1994.[4] The dissemination phase of CATCH was conducted beginning in 1996, shortly after the main trial. The goal of dissemination is to broadly promote the philosophy, materials, and methods of coordinated school health to school teachers and staff.[5]

Priority Population

CATCH targets several population groups. These include elementary school children and their parents, elementary school teachers, and school administration and staff.

The main trial of CATCH included a cohort of 5,106 third-grade students enrolled in 96 schools in four sites (San Diego, California; New Orleans, Louisiana; Minneapolis, Minnesota; and Austin, Texas).[6] The current dissemination phase of CATCH includes training school teachers and staff to implement the program at the school level.

Rationale for the Intervention

The original CATCH was funded by NHLBI to determine whether a school-based curriculum could affect cardiovascular risk factors, such as blood cholesterol levels, diet, and physical activity. Because children's diets were high in fat and saturated fat, and it has been shown that health behaviors track from childhood into adulthood,[7] it was reasoned that changes in children's diets and physical activity habits would benefit them in the future as well as in the present.

The dissemination efforts for CATCH began in Texas, and spread throughout the United States and internationally. Since CATCH had shown promise in changing diet and physical activity patterns in children, the Diabetes Council of the Texas State Department of Health Services began to fund dissemination of CATCH to schools in Texas as a program that targets behaviors that are precursors to chronic diseases such as obesity, type 2 diabetes, and cardiovascular disease. Later dissemination efforts have been focused in states such as Delaware, Illinois, New Mexico, and Florida.

Methodology

The main CATCH study was a randomized controlled trial in which each of 96 schools at four sites (24 schools per site) was assigned to one of three conditions: control (usual health program) ($n = 40$), school-based program ($n = 28$), or school-based program plus family component ($n = 28$).

Control schools implemented their usual health program, while intervention schools implemented behaviorally based classroom curricula for grades 3–5, a physical education component, and a cafeteria program. Schools with a family-based component also had a series of lessons designed to be completed at home with parents or guardians, as well as family-based health fairs at the schools.

The dissemination phase of CATCH was conducted after the main trial, with initial funding from the Texas Department of State Health Services.[8] CATCH was packaged into a set for schools, and the name was changed to "Coordinated Approach to Child Health" to better reflect the implementation of the program as opposed to the randomized clinical trial. Initially, *opinion leaders* (people who influence other people's attitudes about a program) and *change agents* (people who can influence decisions to implement a program) were contacted and familiarized with the program. As these people became better acquainted with it, they began to implement it in their own schools and school districts. Because these people were leaders in their organizations and communities, they began to influence others, who adopted the program or suggested legislative efforts to promote CATCH-type programs more widely. Partnerships between groups with the common goal of promoting school-based physical activity and nutrition programs to decrease obesity and related risk factors began; these partnerships evolved into a coalition. These dissemination efforts led to recognition of the program, especially in local communities and among Texas legislators. As a result, Texas Senate Bill 19 (now Texas Education Code 38.013) was passed in 2001. This legislation mandated daily physical education for kindergarten through grade 5 (through grade 6 if the school is K–6), formation of school health advisory councils (SHACs) for nutrition and physical activity, and implementation of coordinated school health programs in all elementary schools by 2007. Continued visits, training sessions, and presentations by CATCH staff further served to publicize the program.

CATCH dissemination was measured using both quantitative and qualitative methods to determine the reach of the program and subsequent implementation. These methods included enumeration of the schools that purchased CATCH materials or attended a training session, surveys mailed to training participants, and observations of physical education classes.

Results

The original CATCH trial resulted in significant changes in self-reported diet and physical activity levels of the children.[9] These changes were maintained for three years without additional intervention.[10] Although changes in rates of child overweight were not found in the CATCH main trial, it should be noted that decreasing the rate of child obesity was not a targeted goal of CATCH. During the time period for the main CATCH trial (1991–1994), rates of child overweight were not a significant public health priority, largely because the increase in the prevalence of child overweight was just beginning to be evident. More recent follow-up evaluations of CATCH have shown decreases in the prevalence of child obesity and overweight after implementation of CATCH in both the El Paso and Austin, Texas, areas.[11] Dissemination rates have been significant as well: As of October 2004, more than 1,600 schools had adopted part of the CATCH curriculum and more than 700 schools had been trained in coordinated school health.

Lessons Learned

The main CATCH trial demonstrated that it is possible to implement a school-based health promotion program to change child and adolescent diet and physical activity patterns; however, these changes in diet and physical activity do not necessarily result in changes in related physiologic risk factors. More recent data indicate that implementation of CATCH in schools is associated with significant decreases in BMI over time.[12] These results may be reflective of the increased rate of child overweight in today's society. With a larger population of overweight children, it may be that diet and physical activity behaviors have significantly changed over time, and thus, the changes targeted by CATCH may be more evident now compared to the early 1990s, when child overweight was not so prevalent.

CATCH is an excellent example of translational research, in which studies that are rigorously evaluated under controlled conditions and show promising results are "translated" into community-based interventions that are implemented in real-life situations.[13] CATCH was evaluated in a randomized clinical trial in which all the schools and measures were strictly monitored and differences between the schools were minimized. In the dissemination phase of CATCH, the program was individualized to each school setting. This means there was somewhat less control over implementation of the program, but a greater probability that the changes would be maintained over time. The goal of translational research is to maintain the effectiveness of the program while still providing for implementation in a variety of real-life settings.

The dissemination phase of CATCH presents new challenges and new learning opportunities. Implementing CATCH involves partnering with different organizations and groups to advance common goals, packaging the materials in an easy-to-follow program, and extensive training sessions and networking that highlight the compatibility and flexibility of the program.[*]

New Directions

Consistent with the concept of the WSCC approach, a new study is linking CATCH with a more intensive obesity prevention approach to get population-level changes in child obesity in low-resource communities.[14] The Childhood Obesity Research Demonstration (CORD) projects[15] were funded to test community-level interventions that address different levels of the social–ecological model, in particular linking primary care to public health approaches. In the Texas CORD project, obesity prevention involves both *primary prevention programs* such as CATCH that are aimed at entire populations and emphasize healthy behaviors that are relevant to any body size, with coordinated *secondary prevention programs* that include more intensive strategies focused on families with children who have overweight or obesity.[16] In the Texas CORD study, primary programs include CATCH for elementary schools, CATCH Early Childhood for early care and education centers, and the Next Steps program for physician offices, as well as community-level policy trainings. Children are screened for overweight and obesity at the pediatrician offices and are referred to a one-year intensive program including the Mind Exercise Nutrition Do It! (MEND) program paired with CATCH activities for three months, followed by cooking classes, reinforcement activities, and enrollment in YMCA sports programs for children. The theory behind this approach is that children and their families will be surrounded by consistent messages at different levels of the SEM in a systems-level approach that seeks to change the way that current organizations function to result in a healthy weight.

---

[*] Implementation of a Coordinated School Health program such as CATCH involves partnering with such groups as the department of state health services, state education agency (health and physical education, child nutrition services), state department of agriculture, area health education centers, community health agencies, parent–teacher associations, pediatric and state medical groups, the Centers for Disease Control and Prevention Texas Prevention Research Center, and state chapters of the American Heart Association and American Cancer Society.

case study

Worksite Health Promotion Program for Prevention of Overweight

Scenario

You are a consultant nutritionist who has recently been contacted by the headquarters of a large manufacturing plant in your city. This company has about 300 employees in one location, with large open outdoor spaces and sidewalks around the facility and an on-site cafeteria. In addition, there are several break rooms that contain vending machines. The employees are shift workers, 75% are blue-collar, and the majority are Latino and African American.

Six months ago, a group from your local university came to the company and measured heights and weights of the employees as part of a larger study. After calculating BMIs, the university researchers found that the majority (65%) of employees were either overweight or obese. The company president had recently had a heart attack and was appalled at the high rate of overweight among company employees, so he decided to take action. He has hired you to put together a one-year worksite health promotion program that targets obesity prevention for the employees. He has told you that he is willing to change company policies regarding food and physical activity and that you have a budget to develop some infrastructure and implement an intervention. Because the company president is investing a great deal of effort and resources in the program, he expects to see some success over time. On the basis of your previous experience in designing, implementing, and evaluating worksite-based programs, you know that you will need to obtain "buy-in" from the stakeholders (people who will be implementing and participating in the intervention) and set up appropriate goals for the program.

Learning Outcomes

- Identify program outcomes based on current *Healthy People* objectives for nutrition and physical activity.
- Identify individual and environmental determinants of obesity in the company. *Hint:* You might want to refer to the social–ecological model.

- Determine steps for implementation of a new worksite health promotion program.
- Outline a worksite health promotion program that targets obesity prevention and treatment in this company.

Foundation: Acquisition of Knowledge and Skills

1. Find the healthy weight goals for adults from the objectives of *Healthy People 2020* in this chapter.
2. List seven benchmarks of success for worksite health promotion from the Wellness Council of America at *www.welcoa.org*.
3. Review previous worksite health promotion programs developed for weight loss and obesity prevention. Several articles and reviews can be found in the references at the end of this section.
4. Access the Academy of Nutrition and Dietetics position paper "The Role of Nutrition in Health Promotion and Chronic Disease Prevention," *Journal of the Academy of Nutrition and Dietetics* 113 (2013): 972–79. Behaviorally based programs have been found to be the most effective, so review basic behavioral theories (see Theory at a Glance at *www.sneb.org/2014/Theory%20at%20 a%20Glance.pdf*). These theories are also discussed in Chapter 3. Note that several of these theories incorporate environmental factors (e.g., changes in the company cafeteria, addition of walking trails) in addition to psychosocial and behavioral factors.

Step 1: *Identify Relevant Information and Uncertainties*

1. Identify relevant psychosocial (e.g., self-efficacy, attitudes, and social norms) and behavioral (e.g., diet and physical activity) determinants of overweight and/or obesity in this population. Be sure that the determinants you target can be changed through a worksite health promotion program.
2. Determine appropriate weight-loss goals for this type of population and this type of program.

3. List different strategies for a worksite health promotion program that can be implemented at this particular site. Be sure to include both behavioral and environmental strategies.

4. Determine key stakeholders for implementation of the program and new company policies. (In other words, whom do you need to persuade to implement the program?)

Step 2: *Interpret Information*

1. Determine which behavioral- and/or environmental-oriented theory or theories could be used in a worksite setting with the strategies you proposed.

2. Formulate a plan to bring together key stakeholders for implementation of the program and convince them that they should implement the program.

3. List specific aims for behavioral objectives (diet and physical activity behaviors) and identify environmental-level factors (social or physical conditions) that will lead to prevention of weight gain or to weight loss in this population. Be sure to use SMART objectives: those that are Specific, Measurable, Attainable, Relevant, and Time-Bound (as discussed in Chapter 5).

4. Outline several strategies for the proposed worksite health promotion program. Be sure to include strategies for both nutrition and physical activity. If you are including environmental modifications in your program, include these strategies as well.

Step 3: *Draw and Implement Conclusions*

Develop a proposal for the company president that includes an account of any previous work that has been done in this area, specific goals or objectives for the program, a list of company employees who will help you implement the program, an outline of the program that includes specific strategies to be implemented, and a timetable for the program.

Step 4: *Engage in Continuous Improvement*

1. Create an evaluation plan to determine whether you have made a significant difference in the overweight/obesity problem. Remember to measure your primary outcome (such as body weight or BMI); behavioral outcomes such as diet and physical activity; psychosocial factors such as self-efficacy, attitudes, and social norms; and broader environmental-level changes.

2. What barriers do you anticipate during the implementation of this health promotion program? How do you intend to address these barriers?

3. What can you do to be sure that the program is institutionalized—that is, continues to be implemented—in the company after the initial year?

Recommended Reading

1. J. R. Strickland and coauthors, Enhancing Workplace Wellness Efforts to Reduce Obesity: A Qualitative Study of Low-Wage Workers in St Louis, Missouri, 2013–2014, *Preventing Chronic Disease* 12 (2015): 140405.

2. J. R. Strickland and coauthors, Worksite Influences on Obesogenic Behaviors in Low-Wage Workers in St Louis, Missouri, 2013–2014, *Preventing Chronic Disease* 12 (2015): 140406.

3. J. A. Hipp and coauthors, Review of Measures of Worksite Environmental and Policy Supports for Physical Activity and Healthy Eating, *Preventing Chronic Disease* 12 (2015): 140410.

4. J. M. Cairns and coauthors, Weighing Up Evidence: A Systematic Review of the Effectiveness of Workplace Interventions to Tackle Socio-Economic Inequalities in Obesity, *Journal of Public Health*, 2014; Pii: fdu077.

5. S. Schroer, J. Haupt, and C. Pieper, Evidence-Based Interventions in the Workplace—An Overview, *Occupuational Medicine* 64 (2014): 8–12.

6. M. A. Benedict and D. Arterbum, Worksite-Based Weight-Loss Programs: A Systematic Review of the Literature, *American Journal of Health Promotion* 22 (2008): 408–16.

7. J. Schaeffer, Workplace Wellness: Companies Make Employee Health Their Business, *Today's Dietitian* 10 (2008): 34–37.

8. L. H. Engbers and coauthors, Worksite Health Promotion Programs with Environmental Changes: A Systematic Review, *American Journal of Preventive Medicine* 29 (2005): 61–70.

9. D. L. Katz and coauthors, Public Health Strategies for Preventing and Controlling Overweight and Obesity in School and Worksite Settings: A Report on Recommendations of the Task Force on Community Preventive Services, *MMWR Recommendations and Reports* 54 (2005): 1–12.

Diet Confusion: Weighing the Evidence

Lose weight while you sleep! Lose 30 pounds in just 20 days! Eat the foods you love and lose weight! You will never be hungry! Do these claims look familiar to you? With the recent focus on the increase in obesity in the United States and the world, there are burgeoning efforts to promote diet books, products, and programs. The truth is that although most diets can provide weight loss in the short term, few people can lose weight and keep it off permanently, and some of these claims might actually be harmful. Dieting is big business in the United States. In 2013, one nationally representative survey found that 24% of American adults are on a diet, and the weight-loss industry is estimated to be worth more than $60 billion.[1]

How Do Diets Work?

Diets work because people limit their food consumption. Excess weight is the consequence of an energy imbalance, caused by either overconsumption of food or decreased physical activity relative to individual requirements. Limiting of dietary intake can occur through elimination or restriction of certain food groups, such as carbohydrates; portion control through prepackaged meals, snacks, or drinks; alteration of meal patterns or content; and control of food intake through point systems or monitoring. A comparison of the approximate caloric content and macronutrient distribution of several types of diets is provided in **Table 8-10**.

What Are Some Common Diets?

Although the current diet fad can change quickly, certain types of diets have appeared during the past few years. Here are some of the most common:[2]

- *DASH (Dietary Approaches to Stop Hypertension) Diet.* This diet was developed to combat hypertension, and includes eating ample servings of fruits and vegetables, whole grains, lean protein, and low-fat diary, with decreases in sweets and red meats, and a moderate or reduced amount of sodium.
- *The Atkins Diet.* In this diet, consumption of high-fat meats, cheeses, and fats is encouraged, while consumption of carbohydrates (such as fruit, breads, and cereals) is severely limited. The underlying premise of the diet is that elimination of these foods will produce a "benign dietary ketoacidosis," which leads to a decrease in hunger and slows excessive food consumption. Ketosis can be accompanied by bad breath, nausea, headaches, and fatigue. High intakes of protein may exacerbate gout and kidney disease, and high intakes of saturated fat can increase blood cholesterol levels.
- *The Zone Diet.* This rigid eating plan separates foods into "macronutrient blocks."
- *The South Beach Diet.* This regimen is a more permissive version of the Atkins high-protein, low-carbohydrate diet, with incorporation of lower-fat protein sources such as chicken and fish, whole grains, and vegetables and fruits. The plan does limit some foods, such as carrots, bananas, pineapple, and watermelon, and the first phase of the diet is more restrictive than later phases.
- *Dr. Ornish Eat More, Weigh Less.* Weight loss is based on consuming a very-low-fat diet (10% of its kilocalories from fat), with little meat, oils, nuts, butter, dairy (except nonfat), sweets, or alcohol. The original Ornish plan included diet together with exercise and stress reduction.
- *Jenny Craig.* Dieters can sign up for individual counseling sessions and meal plans at company outlets, either by telephone or online. The diet consists of Jenny Craig–prepared foods of single-serving entrees and snacks, supplemented by dairy, salads, and other vegetables you prepare. Vegetarian menu options are available. The diet requires minimal food preparation and meets dietary guidelines. On the negative side, a published study of actual clients revealed a high dropout rate. However, individuals who stuck with the plan lost a considerable amount of weight.
- *Eat, Drink, & Weigh Less.* Harvard researcher Dr. Walter Willett teamed up with cookbook author Mollie Katzen to write a book on the Mediterranean Diet. The authors' premise is that you can "mindfully" follow this diet while enjoying eating. The diet allows for only small amounts of red meat or full-fat dairy and one glass of wine per day.
- *Weight Watchers.* Weight Watchers is a weight-loss program that uses weekly meetings and weigh-ins for motivation and behavioral support for diet and exercise changes. Alternatively, members can sign up to receive similar support online. Dieters either earn or spend points with food or exercise. A vegetarian menu option is available. Recipes have been judged appetizing and fairly easy to prepare.

TABLE 8-10 Comparison of Diet Programs/Eating Plans to the Typical American Diet

TYPE OF DIET	EXAMPLE	GENERAL DIETARY CHARACTERISTICS	COMMENTS
Typical American diet		Carb.: 50% Protein: 15% Fat: 35% Average of 2,200 cal/day	• Low in fruits and vegetables, dairy, and whole grains • High in saturated fat and refined carbohydrates
Balanced nutrient, moderate-calorie approach	DASH diet or diet based on MyPlate food guide; commercial plans such as Diet Center, Jenny Craig, Nutrisystem, Physician's Weight Loss, Shapedown Pediatric Program, Weight Watchers, New Sonoma Diet, TOPS Clubs, Volumetrics	Carb.: 55–60% Protein: 15–20% Fat: 20–30% Usually 1,200–1,700 cal/day	• Based on set pattern of selections from food lists using regular grocery store foods or prepackaged foods supplemented by fresh food items • Low in saturated fat and ample in fruits, vegetables, and fiber • Recommend reasonable weight-loss goal of 0.5 to 2.0 lb/week • Prepackaged plans may limit food choices • Most recommend exercise plan • Many encourage dietary record-keeping • Some offer weight-maintenance plans/support
Very low-fat, high-carbohydrate approach	Ornish Diet (Eat More, Weigh Less), Pritikin Diet, Choose to Lose, Fit or Fat	Carb.: 65% Protein: 10–20% Fat: ≤ 10–19% Limited intake of animal protein, nuts, seeds, other fats	• Long-term compliance with some plans may be difficult because of low level of fat • Can be low in calcium • Some plans restrict healthful foods (seafood, low-fat dairy, poultry) • Some encourage exercise and stress-management techniques
Low-carbohydrate, high-protein, high-fat approach	Atkins Diet, Protein Power, Stillman Diet (The Doctor's Quick Weight Loss Diet), the Carbohydrate Addict's Diet, Scarsdale Diet	Carb.: ≤ 20% Protein: 25–40% Fat: 55–65% Strictly limits carbohydrates to less than 100–125 g/day	• Promote quick weight loss (much is water loss rather than fat loss) • Ketosis causes loss of appetite • Can be too high in saturated fat • Low in carbohydrates, vitamins, minerals, and fiber • Not practical for long term because of rigid diet or restricted food choices
Moderate-carbohydrate, high-protein, moderate-fat approach	The Zone Diet, Sugar Busters, South Beach Diet, Flat Belly Diet	Carb.: 40–50% Protein: 25–40% Fat: 30–40%	• Some diets are rigid and difficult to maintain • Enough carbohydrates to avoid ketosis • Can be low in carbohydrates; can be low in vitamins and minerals
Novelty diets	Immune Power Diet, Rotation Diet, Cabbage Soup Diet, Beverly Hills Diet, Paleo Diet	Most promote certain foods, combinations of foods, or nutrients as having unique (magical) qualities	• No scientific basis for recommendations
Very low-calorie diets	Health Management Resources (HMR), Medifast, Optifast	Less than 800 cal/day	• Require medical supervision • For clients with BMI ≥ 30 or BMI ≥ 27 with other risk factors; may be difficult to transition to regular meals
Weight-loss online diets	*Nutrio.com, SparkPeople.com, WeightWatchers.com, SouthBeachDiet.com*	Meal plans and other tools available online	• Recommend reasonable weight-loss goal of 0.5 to 2.0 lb/week • Most encourage exercise • Some offer weight-maintenance plans/support

Sources: Adapted from M. Boyle, *Personal Nutrition*, 9th ed. (Belmont, CA: Wadsworth/Cengage Learning, 2016), 297; "Weighing the Diet Books," *Nutrition Action Newsletter*, January/February 2004: 3–8; M. Freedman and coauthors, "Popular Diets: A Scientific Review," *Obesity Research* 9 (2001): 1S–39S; "A Guide to Rating the Weight-Loss Websites," *Tufts University Health and Nutrition Letter*, May 2001: 1–4.

- **The Volumetrics Eating Plan.** This eating plan aims to maximize the amount of food available per calorie, primarily by using reduced-fat products, liberal additions of vegetables, and low-fat cooking techniques. The plan encourages that a meal's first course be a broth-based soup or low-calorie salad to take the edge off a person's appetite. Recipes are appetizing but somewhat time-consuming to prepare.
- **The Paleo Diet.** The premise behind this diet is that we need to eat like our ancestors: animal protein (meat, fish, and poultry) and fruits and vegetables, but no sugar, dairy, legumes, and grains. This diet is very restrictive and high in protein.

A study published in the *Journal of the American Medical Association* evaluated four of these diets (the Atkins, Ornish, Weight Watchers, and Zone diets) and found that all four modestly reduced body weight and some cardiac risk factors at one year.[3] Adherence to each diet for the 12-month period varied, ranging from 50% for the Ornish diet and 53% for the Atkins diet to 65% for both the Weight Watchers and Zone diets. The subjects who had the best adherence to the diets had the best results, and cardiac risk factors were more closely associated with weight loss than with diet type. In general, the subjects had more difficulty following the more restrictive diets (the Ornish and Atkins diets). Although this is just one study with small sample sizes, it does suggest that there are many ways to lose weight, that people find it difficult to adhere to very restrictive diets for a long time, and that we need to find methods of keeping people motivated to stay on any new eating plan.

A two-year randomized controlled trial published in the *New England Journal of Medicine* compared weight loss with a low-carbohydrate diet, a Mediterranean diet, or a low-fat diet in moderately obese participants.[4] Among participants who completed the intervention ($n = 272$), the mean weight losses for the low-carbohydrate, Mediterranean, and low-fat groups were 5.5 kilograms (12.1 pounds), 4.6 kilograms (10.1 pounds), and 3.3 kilograms (7.3 pounds), respectively. Among participants with diabetes, changes in fasting plasma glucose and insulin levels were more favorable among those persons assigned to the Mediterranean diet than among those assigned to the low-fat diet ($p < 0.001$). The Mediterranean diet was rich in vegetables and low in red meat, with poultry and fish replacing beef and lamb. It also contained a goal of no more than 35% of calories derived from fat, with a high proportion of fat coming from monounsaturated fat. The main sources of added fat were olive oil and nuts. After the two-year period, adherence rates were 90% in the low-fat group, 85% in the Mediterranean group, and 78% in the low-carbohydrate group. Thus, one of the challenges of a low-carbohydrate diet is the difficulty some persons may have adhering to it over an extended period of time, especially in an obesogenic environment.

Most recently, *U.S. News and World Report* (2015) asked 22 nutrition experts to rate the diets. The DASH (Dietary Approaches to Stop Hypertension) diet was judged to be the best overall diet, with the Weight Watchers diet selected as the best commercial weight-loss diet (easiest diet to follow) and the Ornish diet selected as the best heart-healthy diet. The best plant-based diet was the Mediterranean diet.[5]

How Can You Evaluate a Diet to Determine Whether It Is Healthful?

Frequently, community nutritionists are asked to provide guidance on various diets or diet plans. What can you do to determine whether a particular diet plan is useful to a consumer? Use the checklist that follows.[6]

1. *Does the weight-loss program systematically eliminate one group of foods from a person's eating pattern?* For example, are all carbohydrates systematically eliminated from a person's diet? Are dairy products eliminated? In general, a diet that eliminates a certain food group is probably lacking in important nutrients and dietary variety, and it will be difficult for a person to adhere to that eating plan.
2. *Does the weight-loss program encourage specific supplements or foods that can be purchased only from selected distributors?* These supplements or foods often contain ingredients that may be harmful or unproven.
3. *Does the weight-loss program tout magic or miracle foods or products that burn fat?* The only way to burn fat is to increase your physical activity levels or decrease the amount of total food that you consume. You cannot "burn" fat with sauna belts, body wraps, thigh-reducing creams, or similar products.
4. *Does the weight-loss program promote bizarre quantities of only one food or one type of food?* Some diets include eating only one food each day, or unlimited amounts of certain foods, such as grapefruit or cabbage soup. Such advice runs counter to everything we know about the broad spectrum of human nutritional needs.
5. *Does the weight-loss program have rigid menus?* If a diet has specific meal plans and times to eat, it will be difficult to incorporate individual taste preferences. People are unique, so no one diet plan will work for everyone. A person who loves Thai food will not succeed on a diet if there is no way to incorporate Thai food into his or her eating plan.
6. *Does the weight-loss program promote specific food combinations?* Some diets provide combinations of foods that should or should not be eaten at the same time. These food combinations have no basis in fact and needlessly restrict the dieter's options for reasonable dietary intake and food choices.
7. *Does the weight-loss program promise a weight loss of more than 2 pounds per week for an extended period of time?*

If so, the initial weight loss will probably be due to water loss. A more realistic diet plan will aim for a weight loss of 0.5 to 2.0 pounds per week.

8. *Does the weight-loss program provide a warning to people with diabetes, high blood pressure, or other health conditions?* People with preexisting health conditions need to consult a physician or other health care provider before beginning any diet. Elimination of certain food groups or eating excessive amounts of certain foods can exacerbate these problems and interfere with the efficacy of certain medications.

9. *Does the weight-loss program encourage or promote increased physical activity?* Although people can lose weight by limiting food intake alone, research has shown that the most successful weight-loss plans include lifestyle changes, such as increased exercise.

10. *Does the weight-loss program encourage an intake that is very low in calories (below 800 kcal/day) without supervision of medical experts?* Very low-calorie diets are designed to be used for persons with severe obesity or obesity with other health-related problems. Because the energy level is so low, the diet must be supplemented with vitamins and minerals. In addition, the patient must be strictly observed for any adverse health effects. Finally, the person needs dietary counseling before the end of the diet to handle "real" food choices, or weight gain can quickly ensue.

What Can You Do?

Some of your clients may believe that weight loss is a lost cause, but tell them not to give up! Several strategies and diets have proven successful. The strategies supported by the most evidence are detailed in a recent analysis by the USDA and are backed up by data from the National Weight Control Registry, a study that examines people who have lost at least 30 pounds and have maintained that loss for at least a year.[7]

In your practice as a community nutritionist, there are several steps that you can take to prepare yourself for dealing with the public—and with fad diets:

1. Be familiar with the current fad diets. Before you can answer questions, you need to be familiar with the latest diet craze or diet book. Study the diet—these food plans often include scientifically based statements intermingled with inaccuracies, so you have to know the literature to refute any incorrect claims.

2. Recommend appropriate weight-loss strategies and programs. One evidence-based review indicates that most weight loss is associated with consumption of diets that contain about 1,400 to 1,500 calories per day, so it is essential to control energy intake for any weight-loss plan.[8] Weight

Watchers has been cited as a good option in many recent studies for the variety of foods offered and for principles based on scientific evidence. Internet-based programs may be good for people who like to keep records and need support but cannot attend group sessions. The DASH diet has been found to significantly affect hypertension and other chronic disease outcomes, and it is free on the NIH website. It is interesting to note that about half of the people in the National Weight Control Registry lost weight without any formal program, indicating that the more individualized a program, the more likely it is for people to adhere to it for longer periods of time. Finally, it should be noted that most successful weight-loss attempts include regular exercise of some type.

3. Refer the public to websites that list resources for determining whether a diet is a fad. The following websites contain good information or handouts that the public can use to determine whether following a diet will be harmful or not: the Federal Trade Commission website (*https:// www.consumer.ftc.gov/topics/health-fitness*), including Weighing the Evidence in Diet Ads at *www.ftc.gov/bcp/ edu/pubs/consumer/health/hea03.shtm*, and the American Heart Association *No Fad Diet Tricks* at *www.heart.org/ HEARTORG/GettingHealthy/WeightManagement/No-Fad-Diet-Tips_UCM_305838_Article.jsp*.

4. Report fraudulent or deceptive weight-loss claims. Any weight-loss claims that are distributed via the Internet, television, or print media can be reported at *www.ftc.gov*.

Websites

Choosing a Safe and Successful Weight-Loss Program
http://win.niddk.nih.gov/publications/choosing.htm

USDA Center for Nutrition Policy and Promotion
www.cnpp.usda.gov

Learning Tool for Fad Diets
Go to *www.wemarket4u.net/fatfoe/* to see an ad for FatFoe™ Eggplant Extract, and click on the Order Now button.

Aim for a Healthy Weight, National Heart, Lung, and Blood Institute
www.nhlbi.nih.gov/health/educational/lose_wt

Weight Loss and Nutrition Myths, National Institute of Diabetes and Digestive and Kidney Diseases
www.win.niddk.nih.gov/publications/myths.htm

Obesity and Physical Activity and Aim for a Healthy Weight Publications and Fact Sheets
www.nhlbi.nih.gov/health/resources/heart#obesity

CHAPTER **SUMMARY** ....

Defining Obesity and Overweight

▶ The body mass index is the most common criterion for screening and monitoring of obesity (BMI ≥ 30) and overweight (BMI 25–29.9). For children, obesity is defined as a BMI at or above the CDC growth chart criterion of 95th percentile based on gender and age standards. Overweight reflects a BMI at or above the CDC growth chart criterion of 85th percentile, but lower than the 95th percentile.

▶ **Epidemiology of Obesity and Overweight.** Data for adult obesity are generally obtained from two national surveys: the National Health and Nutrition Examination Survey and the Behavioral Risk Factor Surveillance System. Data from NHANES show a prevalence of adult obesity of 34.9%; an additional 33.6% of adults are overweight. Data show obesity prevalence rates of 16.9% among children ages 2–19.

▶ **Medical and Social Costs of Obesity.** Although the development of obesity is a clinical problem at the individual level, the increasing morbidity and mortality attributed to the metabolic abnormalities associated with excess body weight, as well as the increased health care costs, ultimately affect all of the population, making it a significant public health issue (see Table 8-3).

▶ **Determinants of Obesity.** Determinants of obesity can be related to either dietary intake or physical activity or both, and they can be *genetic, psychosocial, behavioral,* or *environmental.*

Obesity Prevention and Treatment Interventions

▶ Current recommendations for obesity treatment call for lifestyle changes, including dietary therapy, increases in physical activity, and behavioral therapy.

▶ Many obesity prevention programs are oriented around a site where people congregate, such as churches, worksites, community settings, childcare centers, and schools.

▶ Interventions that include multiple coordinated components, such as a family- or school-based program enhanced by community programs and social marketing campaigns, show promise in the prevention of child obesity.

▶ With preschool-age children, obesity prevention efforts need to focus on multiple environments, including the home and childcare settings, and on various stages of development.

Public Health Policy Options for Addressing the Global Obesity Epidemic

▶ Policy options for addressing the obesity epidemic include obesity surveillance and monitoring efforts; awareness building, education, and research; regulating environments; pricing policies, such as subsidies and taxation; and societal-level solutions.

▶ Researchers have begun to explore the connection among agricultural subsidies, economic policies, and the obesity epidemic. Taxation is another type of pricing policy to influence consumers' buying practices.

▶ Examples of trends that may be contributing to the global obesity epidemic include increased use of motor transport; increased traffic hazards for walkers and cyclists; fewer opportunities for recreational physical activity; greater quantities of food available; more frequent and widespread food-purchasing opportunities; rising use of soft drinks to replace water; multiple television channels available around the clock; and globalization of markets, which favors energy-dense foods of low nutritional value. Table 8-9 outlines a range of societal-level solutions.

Where Do We Go from Here?

▶ With a multifactorial problem such as obesity, multiple approaches are necessary. The first step is to build an understanding of the magnitude of the problem. A second step is to put into effect policies and practices that target both individual behavioral factors and environmental factors.

▶ Solutions for prevention of overweight and obesity need to be creative—perhaps by involving nontraditional partners or targeting less obvious determinants of obesity such as parenting skills, social and economic policies that may influence a family's access to a healthful food supply, or methods of transportation.

SUMMARY **QUESTIONS**

1. Define overweight and obesity for adults and children, and explain why different criteria are used for each.
2. List and discuss examples of the following determinants of obesity and overweight:
   a. Genetic and biological risk factors
   b. Psychosocial risk factors
   c. Behavioral/lifestyle risk factors
   d. Environmental risk factors
3. Discuss intervention strategies for the treatment of obesity and overweight among children, and enumerate pros and cons of each one.
4. Discuss ways that the food, worksite, and built environments might be regulated to prevent or reduce obesity among adults. Include specific policy examples where possible.
5. As a community nutritionist, how can you prepare yourself to offer evidence-based methods to clients seeking to prevent and/or treat overweight and obesity among their family members?

INTERNET **RESOURCES**

Data on Obesity and Overweight

National Health and Nutrition Examination Survey
www.cdc.gov/nchs/nhanes.htm

Behavioral Risk Factor Surveillance System
www.cdc.gov/brfss

Youth Risk Behavior Surveillance System
www.cdc.gov/HealthyYouth/yrbs/index.htm

Arkansas Center for Health Improvement
www.achi.net

General Information on Obesity/Overweight

Dietary Guidelines for Americans 2015–2020
http://health.gov/dietaryguidelines

2008 Physical Activity Guidelines for Americans
http://health.gov/PAGuidelines

CDC Overweight and Obesity
www.cdc.gov/obesity/index.html

CDC Obesity Trends
www.cdc.gov/obesity/data/index.html

The Community Guide: Obesity Prevention and Control
www.thecommunityguide.org/obesity/index.html

Academy of Nutrition and Dietetics
www.eatright.org

HBO Weight of the Nation Documentary
http://theweightofthenation.hbo.com

National Institute of Diabetes and Digestive and Kidney Diseases: Weight Loss and Control
www.niddk.nih.gov/health-information/health-topics/weight-control

NIDDK Weight-Control Information Network (WIN)
http://win.niddk.nih.gov/index.htm

The Obesity Society
www.obesity.org

USDA Food and Nutrition Information Center: Weight and Obesity
http://fnic.nal.usda.gov/weight-and-obesity

Health Equity Resource Toolkit for State Practitioners Addressing Obesity Disparities
www.cdc.gov/Obesity/Health_Equity/pdf/toolkit.pdf

Measurement and Evaluation of Obesity/ Overweight and Food Intake

School Physical Activity and Nutrition Survey
http://go.uth.edu/span

BMI Calculator
www.cdc.gov/healthyweight/assessing/bmi/index.html

SuperTracker
www.choosemyplate.gov/tools-supertracker

Nutrient Data Laboratory Food Composition Database
http://ndb.nal.usda.gov

National Collaborative on Childhood Obesity Research (NCCOR)
www.nccor.org

Evaluating Obesity Prevention Efforts: A Plan for Measuring Progress
http://iom.nationalacademies.org/Reports/2013/Evaluating-Obesity-Prevention-Efforts-A-Plan-for-Measuring-Progress.aspx

Built Environment Assessment for Obesity
www.ajpmonline.org/article/S0749-3797%2815%2900026-4/abstract

Programs and Research

CATCH Global Foundation
http://catchglobalfoundation.org

Harvard's Planet Health
www.planet-health.org

Stanford's Student Media Awareness to Reduce
Television (SMART)
http://notv.stanford.edu

USDA Team Nutrition
www.fns.usda.gov/tn

National Weight Control Registry
www.nwcr.ws

Let's Move!
www.letsmove.gov

Partnership for a Healthier America
http://ahealthieramerica.org/

HealthierUS School Challenge
www.fns.usda.gov/hussc/healthierus-school-
challenge-smarter-lunchrooms

Alliance for a Healthier Generation
https://www.healthiergeneration.org

Action for Healthy Kids
www.actionforhealthykids.org

PreventObesity.net
www.preventobesity.net

NIH We Can! Program
www.nhlbi.nih.gov/health/educational/wecan

NIH Strategic Plan for Obesity Research
http://obesityresearch.nih.gov/about/strategic-
plan.aspx

Mission Readiness
www.missionreadiness.org

Active Living Research
http://activelivingresearch.org

Healthy Eating Research
http://healthyeatingresearch.org

Salud America!
http://salud-america.org

African American Collaborative Obesity Research
Network (AACORN)
www.aacorn.org

Robert Wood Johnson Foundation
www.rwjf.org/en/our-topics/topics/childhood-
obesity.htm

Obesity, Physical Activity, and Nutrition Policy and Legislation

CDC Information on Legislation (Chronic Disease
State Policy Tracking System)
http://nccd.cdc.gov/CDPHPPolicySearch/Default.aspx

Center for Science in the Public Interest Policy
Information
www.cspinet.org/nutritionpolicy

National Policy and Legal Analysis Network to Prevent
Childhood Obesity
www.changelabsolutions.org/childhood-obesity

National Alliance for Nutrition and Activity
www.cspinet.org/nutritionpolicy/nana.html

Recommendations for Obesity Prevention

The Surgeon General's Call to Action
www.surgeongeneral.gov/library/calls/

Preventing Childhood Obesity: Health in the Balance
http://iom.nationalacademies.org/reports/2004/
preventing-childhood-obesity-health-in-the-balance.aspx

Progress in Preventing Childhood Obesity
http://iom.nationalacademies.org/Reports/2006/
Progress-in-Preventing-Childhood-Obesity--How-Do-
We-Measure-Up.aspx

Report on Measuring Progress in Obesity Prevention
http://iom.edu/Reports/2012/Measuring-Progress-in-
Obesity-Prevention.aspx

Food Marketing to Children and Youth: Threat or
Opportunity?
http://iom.nationalacademies.org/Reports/2005/
Food-Marketing-to-Children-and-Youth-Threat-or-
Opportunity.aspx

Early Childhood Obesity Prevention Policies
http://iom.nationalacademies.org/Reports/2011/Early-
Childhood-Obesity-Prevention-Policies.aspx

Nutrition Standards for Foods in Schools
http://iom.nationalacademies.org/Reports/2007/
Nutrition-Standards-for-Foods-in-Schools-Leading-the-
Way-toward-Healthier-Youth.aspx

Accelerating Progress in Obesity Prevention: Solving
the Weight of the Nation
http://iom.nationalacademies.org/Reports/2012/
Accelerating-Progress-in-Obesity-Prevention.aspx

World Health Organization (WHO): Obesity
www.who.int/topics/obesity/en/

CHAPTER 9

Health Care Systems and Policy

LEARNING **OBJECTIVES**

After you have read and studied this chapter, you will be able to:

- Describe factors affecting the cost and delivery of health care.
- Explain why health promotion is a major component of the rhetoric about health care reform at the national level.
- Differentiate between traditional systems of health care and managed forms of health care.
- Describe eligibility requirements for and services provided to recipients of Medicare and Medicaid.

- Identify consumer trends affecting health care.
- State the value of using medical nutrition therapy protocols to document client outcomes in various health care settings.

This chapter addresses such issues as health care policy and delivery systems, current reimbursement issues, policies and regulations, and the nutrition care process, which have been designated by the Accreditation Council for Education in Nutrition and Dietetics (ACEND) as Foundation Knowledge and Learning Outcomes for dietetics education.

CHAPTER **OUTLINE**

Something to think about... "The enjoyment of the highest attainable standard of health is one of the fundamental rights of every human being without distinction of race, religion, political belief, economic or social condition. . . . Governments have a responsibility for the health of their peoples, which can be fulfilled only by the provision of adequate health and social measures."

—*Preamble to the Constitution of the World Health Organization*

For a complete list of references, please access the MindTap Reader within your MindTap course.

Introduction

Prevention of disease makes sense, especially in light of the cost of health care. Health care expenditures in the United States continue to increase. In 1960 these costs totaled $27.5 billion, but in 2013 Americans spent $2.9 trillion for health care.[1] This hefty sum represents almost 18% of the gross domestic product (GDP)—compared with 9% in 1980.[2] By the year 2020, health care costs are projected to increase to $4.6 trillion.[3] Compared with other industrialized nations, U.S. per capita health spending exceeds that of other countries by significant margins.[4]

A strange paradox exists today in U.S. health care: It treats preventable illness rather than investing in prevention. A former secretary of health and human services observed that prevention "must become a national obsession."[5] He went on to say that health promotion and disease prevention offer perhaps the best opportunity to reduce the ever-increasing portion of resources spent treating preventable illness and functional impairment. Likewise, in the U.S. surgeon general's remarks before the Joint Economic Committee of Congress on October 1, 2003, Richard H. Carmona, MD, stated, "There is no greater imperative in American health care than switching from a treatment-oriented society to a prevention-oriented society. Right now we've got it backwards. We wait years and years, doing nothing about unhealthy eating habits and lack of physical activity until people get sick. Then we spend billions of dollars on costly treatments, often when it is already too late to make meaningful improvements to their quality of life or life span."[6]

Public policy is now attempting to direct the medical system toward health promotion, disease prevention, and the efficient use of scarce resources. *Healthy People 2020*, the U.S. health agenda designed to help reduce preventable disease, has four overarching goals: attain high-quality, longer lives free of preventable disease, disability, injury, and premature death; achieve health equity, eliminate disparities, and improve the health of all groups; create social and physical environments that promote good health for all; and promote quality of life, healthy development, and healthy behaviors across all life stages.[7] The Academy of Nutrition and Dietetics agrees with this paradigm shift and asserts that "primary prevention is the most effective, affordable course of action for preventing and reducing risk for chronic disease,"[8] rather than assigning health care only a curative or treatment role.

The Academy of Nutrition and Dietetics underscores that a healthful diet coupled with physical activity will promote and maintain health throughout the life cycle.[9] Many studies show that early detection and intervention, immunization, and behavior change could significantly reduce many of the leading causes of death and disability.[10] By investing in health maintenance through health promotion and disease prevention, many of the economic and social costs of disease and injury could be avoided. Good health could be preserved at a reduced cost if we made the "front end" (i.e., prevention) the primary concern, rather than waiting to devote substantial resources to illness and disability after they strike.[11] Yet, despite recommendations for both clinical and community services, the current health care system generally provides only limited reimbursement for prevention activities and/or intervention for conditions such as obesity, cardiovascular disease, osteoporosis, and other chronic conditions that contribute to increasing health care costs.[12] It seems that the most logical avenue, in light of the prevalence of chronic diseases among Americans, is chronic disease prevention. Not only are chronic diseases the leading causes of death in the United States,[13] but they also can limit everyday activities and alter the ability of community members to lead independent lives.[14]

This chapter introduces you to the challenges facing health care. One question, for example, is how we can balance the traditional medical model of health care with a wellness/preventive-medicine model. Other issues discussed here are resource allocation and cost containment, social justice and adequate access to health care resources, program account-ability and quality in health care, and funding for health promotion and disease prevention.

An Overview of the Health Care Industry

The pluralistic system of health care in the United States includes many parts: employment-based private insurance, direct-purchase private insurance, Medicare, Medicaid, workers' compensation, the Veterans Health Administration medical care system, the Department of Defense hospitals and clinics, the Public Health Service's Indian Health Service, state and local public health programs, and the Department of Justice's Federal Bureau of Prisons. Currently, the system is structured around the provision of health insurance. In 2013, 87% of the U.S. population were insured and 13% were not.[15] Some choose not to have health insurance because they can pay for their health care; however, many Americans are forced to make this choice due to income limitations. In a recent government survey, 68% of adults said that one of the reasons they are uninsured is that the cost is too high or that they lost their job and their employer-provided health insur-ance.[16] Characteristics of the uninsured are discussed later in the chapter.

In the United States, there are two general categories of **health insurance**: private and government/public health insurance.[17] A private health insurance plan is provided through an employer or a union, or it is purchased by an individual from a private company. On the other hand, government health insurance includes a variety of federal programs (Medicare, Medicaid, and the Military Health System), the Children's Health Insurance Program (CHIP), and individual state health plans. **Figure 9-1** shows the categories of health insurance and the percentage of people enrolled in each.[18]

Private Insurance

More Americans carry private insurance than are covered under a government health program. The following sections discuss a variety of plans within this privatized system.

Indemnity or Traditional Fee-for-Service Insurance
Private insurance can be in the form of traditional fee-for-service insurance or **group contract** insurance. The traditional fee-for-service plans include a billing system in which the provider of care charges a fee for each service rendered. This type of insurance is provided by both commercial insurance companies and not-for-profit organizations, such as Blue Cross and Blue Shield and independent employee health plans. While this type of insurance has become relatively

Health insurance
Protection against the financial burdens associated with health care services and assurance of access to the health care system.

Group contract A health insurance contract that is made with an employer or other entity and covers a group of persons identified as individuals by reference to their relationship to the entity.

FIGURE 9-1
Categories of Health Insurance and Percentage of U.S. Population Enrolled, 2013
[a] Medicaid also includes other public programs: CHIP and other state programs, military-related coverage. Numbers may not add to 100% due to rounding, and a person can be covered by more than one type of health insurance during the year.
Source: KCMU/Urban Institute Analysis of 2014 ASEC Supplement to the Current Population Survey of the U.S. Census Bureau.

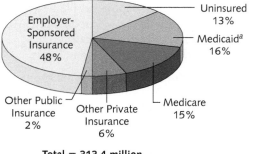

Employer-Sponsored Insurance 48%

Uninsured 13%

Medicaid[a] 16%

Other Public Insurance 2%

Other Private Insurance 6%

Medicare 15%

Total = 313.4 million

Managed-care system An approach to paying for health care in which insurers try to limit the use of health services, reduce costs, or both. These health plans are subject to utilization review (UR). That review aims to prevent unnecessary treatment by requiring enrollees to obtain approval for nonemergency hospital care, denying payment for wasteful treatment, and monitoring severely ill patients to ensure that they get cost-effective care.

Health maintenance organization (HMO)
A prepaid plan that both finances and delivers health care. HMOs enroll patients as members, charge a fixed fee per year, and provide all medical services deemed necessary. Enrollees generally must use the plan's providers or face financial penalties.

Preferred provider organization (PPO)
A group of providers, usually hospitals and doctors, who contract with private indemnity (fee-for-service) insurance companies to provide medical care for a discounted fee. PPOs are subject to peer review and strict use of controls in exchange for a consistent volume of patients.

Point-of-service plan (POS) Members have the option of using providers in the plan's network at a reduced cost or going outside the network—at a higher cost.

Exclusive provider organization (EPO) EPO plans generally limit coverage to care from providers (doctors, specialists, or hospitals) in the plan's network.

Capitation A predetermined fee paid per enrollee to the health care provider.

uncommon, proponents of fee-for-service systems prefer the greater flexibility and unrestricted access to physicians, tests, hospitals, and treatments. Critics of fee-for-service plans claim that it encourages physicians to provide more services than are necessary.[19]

Managed-Care Insurance
In the latter part of the twentieth century, the nation's health care system went through a major transition from the traditional unmanaged fee-for-service system to a predominantly **managed-care system**, represented by **health maintenance organizations (HMOs)**, **preferred provider organizations (PPOs)**, **point-of-service plans (POSs)**, and **exclusive provider organizations (EPOs)**. Generally, all are prepaid group practice plans that offer health care services through groups of medical practitioners. The presumed goal of managed care is improved quality of care with decreased costs. Considering job-based coverage, in 1988 only 27% of employees were enrolled in a managed-care plan, a figure that increased to 99% in 2013 (**Figure 9-2**).[20]

In HMOs, physicians practice as a group, sharing facilities and medical records. The physicians may either be salaried or provide contractual services. Finally, members must select a primary care physician (PCP). There are four general models of HMOs:

1. *Staff model:* The HMO owns and operates its own facility; is equipped for laboratory, pharmacy, and X-ray services; and hires its own physicians and other health care providers.
2. *Group model:* The HMO contracts with one or more multispecialty group practices that contract to provide health care services exclusively to its members.
3. *Network model:* Much like the group model, the HMO contracts with multiple group practices, hospitals, and other providers to provide services to its members, but in a nonexclusive arrangement.
4. *Independent practice association (IPA):* A decentralized model—or HMO without walls—in which the HMO contracts with individual physicians to care for plan members in their own private offices for a discounted fee. The physicians are free to contract with more than one plan and may provide care on a fee-for-service basis as well.

HMOs typically provide comprehensive services across the continuum of care. In some HMO programs, the provider receives a **capitation** payment, usually a specific amount per enrollee per month, to provide a defined group of health care services. Dietitians may be included under specialists or as part of the primary care provider portion of the payment, depending on the contractual agreement of the HMO.[21] Appropriate services must be delivered to the enrollee even if costs exceed the capitation payment.[22]

The HMO idea—a fixed cost to the consumer, with health care insurer and health care provider as one and the same—is viewed as a more cost-effective way of practicing medicine than the traditional fee-for-service systems. Because HMOs make money by keeping you healthy, they have a greater stake in your wellness than most fee-for-service doctors.[23] Prepaid group health plans emphasize health promotion because they provide health care services at a preset cost. By keeping people healthy, HMOs avoid the need for lengthy hospitalizations and costly services. Enrollees of HMOs are hospitalized less frequently than patients of fee-for-service physicians.[24]

Other managed-care plans include PPOs, POSs, and EPOs:[25]

- **Preferred Provider Organizations (PPOs):** PPOs are similar to HMOs, as they enter into agreements with health care providers, who form the provider network; however, a member is not required to select a PCP. PPOs give members the choice of getting care from in-network or out-of-network providers, but members pay less if they use providers that belong to the plan's network.
- **Point-of-Service Plans (POSs):** POSs allow members to get medical care from both in-network and out-of-network providers. Unlike PPOs, POSs encourage selection

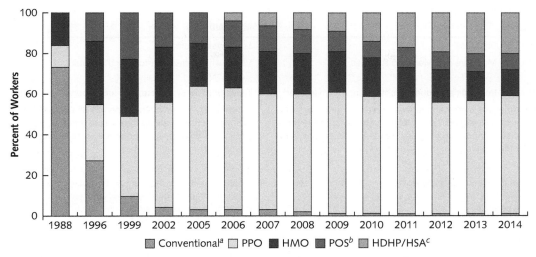

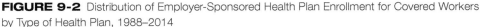

FIGURE 9-2 Distribution of Employer-Sponsored Health Plan Enrollment for Covered Workers by Type of Health Plan, 1988–2014

For employer-sponsored health plans in 2011, enrollment was highest in preferred provider organizations (PPOs, 55%), followed by HMOs (17%), high-deductible health plans combined with health savings accounts or health reimbursement account (HDHP/HSA or HRA, 17%), point-of-service plans (POSs, 10%), and conventional plans (1%). Note the decrease in conventional plan enrollments from 73% in 1988.

a Conventional plans refer to traditional fee-for-service (indemnity) insurance plans.

b Information was not obtained for POSs in 1988.

c HDHPs were added as a new type of health plan in 2006.

Source: Adapted from Kaiser Family Foundation/Health Research & Educational Trust Survey of Employer-Sponsored Health Benefits, 1999–2014; The Health Insurance Association of America, 1988.

of a PCP from a list of participating providers. The PCP can refer to other network providers when needed. To visit an out-of-network provider, members need a referral and may pay higher out-of-pocket costs.

- **Exclusive Provider Organizations (EPOs):** EPO plans generally limit coverage to care from providers (doctors, specialists, or hospitals) in the plan's network.

Consumer-Directed Health Plans Consumer-directed health plans constitute a growing market and define employer contributions while asking employees to be more responsible for health care decisions and cost-sharing. Essentially, these plans combine a high-deductible health plan (HDHP) with a tax-advantaged health reimbursement arrangement (HRA) or health savings account (HSA) that enrollees use to pay for a portion of their health expenses. Due to the high deductibles associated with HDHPs, premiums are typically low. Proponents of these plans contend that enrollees seek lower-cost health care services and only seek care when necessary. On the other hand, critics contend that only healthier individuals are attracted to these plans. In addition, employers may use these plans to shift the cost of coverage to employees.[26]

Government/Public Insurance

The Centers for Medicare and Medicaid Services (CMS) is the federal agency responsible for administering Medicare, Medicaid, CHIP (the Children's Health Insurance Program), and several other health-related programs, including HIPAA (the Health Insurance Portability and Accountability Act of 1996) and CLIA (Clinical Laboratory and Improvement Amendments). The two major public health insurance plans in the United States are **Medicare** and **Medicaid**. A comparison of their features is provided in **Table 9-1**.

Medicare A federally run entitlement program through which people 65 years of age or older and people in certain other eligible categories receive health insurance.

Medicaid A federally aided, state-administered entitlement program that provides medical benefits for certain low-income persons in need of health and medical care.

TABLE 9-1 A Comparison of Medicare and Medicaid Services

	MEDICARE	MEDICAID
Administration	Social Security office	Local welfare office
	Centers for Medicare and Medicaid Services	Varies within state, territory, or the District of Columbia
Financing	Trust funds from Social Security; contributions from insured	Taxes from federal, state, and local sources
Eligibility	People 65 years of age and older, people with end-stage renal disease, people eligible for Social Security/Railroad Retirement Board disability programs for 24 months; Medicare-covered government employees, possibly others	Individuals with low incomes, people 65 or older, the blind, persons with disabilities, all pregnant women and infants with family incomes below 133% of poverty level, possibly others[c]
Benefits[a]	Same in all states	Varies from state to state
	Hospital insurance (Part A) Helps pay for inpatient hospital care, skilled nursing facility care, home health care, and hospice care	**Hospital services:** inpatient and outpatient hospital services; other laboratory and X-ray services; physician services; screening, diagnosis, and treatment of children; and home health care services
	Medical insurance (Part B) Helps pay for physicians' services; outpatient hospital services; home health visits; diagnostic X-ray, laboratory, and other tests; necessary ambulance services; other medical services and supplies; outpatient physical or occupational therapy and speech pathology; partial coverage of mental health treatment; kidney dialysis; medical nutrition therapy services (e.g., for people with diabetes or kidney disease); and certain preventive services[b]	**Medical services:** Many states pay for dental care; health clinic services; eye care and glasses; prescribed medications; and other diagnostic, rehabilitative, and preventive services, including nutrition services.
	Medicare Part C (Medicare Advantage) Includes all benefits and services covered under Part A and Part B; run by Medicare-approved private insurance companies; usually includes Medicare prescription drug coverage (Part D) as part of the plan; may include extra benefits and services for an extra cost	
	Medicare Part D (Medicare Prescription Drug Coverage) Helps cover the cost of outpatient prescription drugs; run by Medicare-approved private insurance companies	
Typical Exclusions	Regular dental care and dentures, routine physical exams and related tests, eyeglasses, hearing aids and examinations to prescribe and fit them, nursing home care (except skilled nursing care), custodial care, immunizations (except for pneumonia, influenza, and hepatitis B), cosmetic surgery	Varies from state to state
Premium Costs (2015)	Part A: none if eligible, or up to $407/month	None (federal government contributes 50–80% to states to cover eligible persons)
	Part B: $105/month (higher premium if income is above a certain amount)	

[a] Medicare beneficiaries who have both Part A and Part B can choose to get their benefits through a variety of risk-based plans (e.g., HMOs, PPOs), known as the Medicare Advantage Plan, which may expand coverage. An additional premium may apply.

[b] Certain recipients are covered for bone mass measurements, colorectal cancer screening, diabetes self-management training and supplies, glaucoma screening, mammogram screening, Pap test and pelvic examination, prostate cancer screening, and certain vaccinations. The Medicare Modernization Act of 2003 expanded coverage. For more information, visit *www.medicare.gov*.

[c] In January 2014, due to the Affordable Care Act, Medicaid was extended to all adults under 65 years of age with income under 133% of the federal poverty level.

Source: Adapted from Centers for Medicare and Medicaid Services, *Medicare and You* (Baltimore: U.S. Department of Health and Human Services, 2015).

Workers' compensation, which pays benefits to workers who have been injured on the job, is another public-sector health benefit program. The Children's Health Insurance Program (CHIP) provides health coverage to uninsured children whose families earn too much money to qualify for Medicaid but too little to afford private coverage.[27] Health care services are also provided by the Department of Veterans Affairs (VA), the Public Health

Service (including the Indian Health Service), the Department of Defense (including TRI-CARE, formerly known as the Civilian Health and Medical Program of the Uniformed Services, or CHAMPUS), public hospitals and community health centers, and state and local public health programs.[28]

The Medicare Program In 2015, some 55 million individuals were enrolled in Medicare. Approximately 19 million additional people are expected to enroll in Medicare over the next 11 years as more members of the Baby Boom generation reach the Medicare eligibility age. This program was established in 1965 by Title XVIII of the Social Security Act and is administered by the **Centers for Medicare and Medicaid Services (CMS)** of the Department of Health and Human Services. The Social Security Administration provides information about program eligibility and handles enrollment.[29] Medicare is designed to assist:

- People 65 years of age or older
- People of any age with end-stage renal disease
- People eligible for Social Security or Railroad Retirement Board disability benefits for 24 months
- Individuals who are receiving or are eligible to receive retirement benefits from Social Security or Railroad Retirement Boards
- People who had Medicare-covered government employment

To obtain Medicare benefits, recipients are offered the Original Medicare Plan or a Medicare Advantage Plan. Basically, Medicare consists of two separate parts: hospital insurance (Part A) and medical insurance (Part B). No monthly premium is required for Medicare Part A if a person or his or her spouse is entitled to benefits under either Social Security or the Railroad Retirement System or has worked a sufficient period of time in federal, state, or local government to be insured because premiums were paid through payroll taxes while the individual or spouse was working.[30] Those who do not meet these qualifications (40 or more quarters of Medicare-covered employment) may purchase Part A coverage if they are at least age 65 and meet certain requirements.[31] For Medicare Part B, the premium is $105.00 per month. The Department of Health and Human Services announces these premiums annually.

Medicare Part A Medicare Part A provides hospital insurance benefits that include inpatient hospital care, care at a skilled nursing facility, hospice care, and some home health care. Deductible and **coinsurance** fees apply. Since 1983, the government has shifted a larger portion of health care costs to Medicare beneficiaries through larger **deductibles**, greater use of services with coinsurance, and use of services not covered by Medicare.

Medicare Part B Medicare Part B is an optional medical insurance program financed through premiums paid by enrollees and contributions from federal funds; it provides supplementary medical insurance benefits for eligible physician services, outpatient services, certain home health services, medical supplies, and preventive services.[32] Medicare pays qualified dietitians and nutrition professionals who enroll in the Medicare program as providers, regardless of whether they provide medical nutrition therapy (MNT) services in an independent practice setting, hospital outpatient department, or any other setting, except for patients in an inpatient stay in a hospital or skilled nursing facility.[33] Enrolled Medicare MNT providers are able to bill Medicare for MNT services provided to Medicare beneficiaries with type 1 diabetes, type 2 diabetes, gestational diabetes, nondialysis kidney disease, and post-kidney-transplant status using specified codes. A physician's referral for MNT is required.

Centers for Medicare and Medicaid Services (CMS) A federal agency that establishes guidelines and monitors Medicare, Medicaid, CHIP, HIPAA, and CLIA.

Coinsurance A cost-sharing arrangement in which the insured assumes a portion of the costs of covered services.

Deductibles The amount of expense that must be incurred by a person who is insured before an insurer will assume any liability for all or part of the remaining cost of covered services.

▶ **THINK LIKE A COMMUNITY** NUTRITIONIST

One of the policy-related priorities of the Academy of Nutrition and Dietetics is to expand Medical Nutrition Therapy (MNT) benefits for Medicare patients. Although Registered Dietitians are eligible providers of MNT for patients with diabetes or renal disease, expanded coverage of MNT to other conditions (such as heart disease and prediabetes) could reduce health care costs (see Medical Nutrition Therapy Providing Return on Investment on page 356)

Imagine you are advocating for extending this benefit to patients with prediabetes. You would need evidence that early intervention can reverse elevated blood glucose levels and prevent progression into diabetes. Visit the National Institute of Diabetes and Digestive and Kidney Diseases (NIDDK)'s website to learn about the results of the Diabetes Prevention Program at *www.niddk.nih.gov/about-niddk/research-areas/diabetes/diabetes-prevention-program-dpp/Pages/default.aspx#results*. What did the research trial indicate regarding early intervention? Make a list of talking points to use in speaking with a legislator to advocate for expanding coverage of MNT to prediabetic patients.

For more information, read the journal article reporting results of the Diabetes Prevention Program: W. C. Knowler, E. Barrett-Connor, S. E. Fowler, R. F. Hamman, J. M. Lachin, E. A. Walker, D. M. Nathan, and Diabetes Prevention Program Research Group, Reduction in the Incidence of Type 2 Diabetes with Lifestyle Intervention or Metformin, *New England Journal of Medicine* 346 (2002): 393–403.

Coverage Gaps The two most notable gaps in Medicare coverage have been prescription drug coverage and skilled nursing/long-term institutional care. Traditionally, most prescription drugs were not covered at all under the Medicare program. Only 100 days of skilled nursing/long-term care are covered annually. Thereafter, patients or their families must either pay the costs themselves or "spend down" their assets in order to reduce their net worth and be eligible for Medicaid coverage of long-term care. However, the Medicare Prescription Drug, Improvement, and Modernization Act of 2003 (Medicare Modernization Act) provides optional coverage to Medicare recipients, including drug discount cards/prescription drug plans and other preventive benefits (wellness physical exam, cardiovascular disease blood screening, and diabetes screening for those at risk) in addition to those preventive benefits already covered (cancer screening, bone mass measurements, and vaccinations).[34]

For those in the Original Medicare Plan, a Medigap policy may be purchased if the individual participates in both Medicare Part A and Part B. This is a supplemental insurance policy sold by private insurance companies to help pay the deductible, coinsurance fees, prescription drug costs, and certain services not covered by Medicare.[35]

Another option for individuals is to receive their Medicare benefits through a Medicare Advantage Plan (Medicare, Part C). These plans must cover at least the same benefits covered by Medicare Part A and Part B; however, the costs may vary among these Medicare Managed-Care Plans, Medicare Preferred Provider Organization Plans, Medicare Private Fee-for-Service Plans, or Medicare Specialty Plans.[36] To join, the individual must have Medicare Part A and Part B. The Part B premium is still paid, and a monthly premium may have to be paid to the Medicare Advantage Plan provider. Medicare participants can also get Medicare prescription drug coverage by adding a Medicare Prescription Drug Plan (Part D), or getting a Medicare Advantage Plan (Part C) such as an HMO or PPO that offers Medicare prescription drug coverage.

For additional benefits, Medicare recipients often explore other options. They may continue insurance coverage through a current or former employer. Individuals may also choose to purchase nursing home or long-term care insurance policies, which pay cash amounts for each day of covered nursing home or at-home care. Finally, individuals may qualify for full Medicaid (see the next section) benefits or at least to receive some state assistance in paying Medicare costs.

The Medicaid Program Medicaid, an entitlement program, insured nearly 70 million individuals in 2015.[37] From December 2007 to December 2010, Medicaid enrollment grew by almost 8.8 million, with children representing over half of the total growth during this recession period. Notable growth has also occurred in Medicaid enrollment since the Affordable Care Act coverage expansion went into effect in 2014. Medicaid was established as a joint state and federal program, the federal government paying 50% or more of the costs depending on a state's per capita income. ("States" include states, U.S. territories, and the District of Columbia.) It was established in 1965 by Title XIX of the Social Security Act. Medicaid provides assistance with medical care for:

- Eligible persons with low incomes
- Certain pregnant women and children with low incomes
- Older adults, the blind, and people with disabilities
- Members of families with dependent children in which one parent is absent, incapacitated, or unemployed

The individual states administer the program and define eligibility, benefits and services, and payment schedules. Typically, one must meet three criteria: income, categorical, and resource. Prior to the passage of the Affordable Care Act, income had to be below—sometimes significantly below—the federal poverty guidelines. The 2015 guidelines are summarized in Table 10-1 in Chapter 10. The new health care reform law expands Medicaid eligibility to 133% of poverty ($15,654 for an individual or about $32,253 for a family of four in 2015) to help reduce state-by-state variation in eligibility for Medicaid. Although the Medicaid expansion was intended to be national, a 2012 Supreme Court ruling made Medicaid expansion optional for states. To date, 31 states (including the District of Columbia) have adopted the expansion.[38]

Because states administer the program, an individual may qualify for Medicaid in one state but not in another. Generally, those eligible for Medicaid include the following:

- Those eligible for Temporary Assistance for Needy Families (TANF) or Supplemental Security Income (SSI)
- Children under age 19 living in a household at or below 200% of the poverty guidelines in most states
- Pregnant women (eligible only for services related to pregnancy/complications, delivery, and postpartum care)
- Recipients of adoption or foster care assistance under Title IV of the Social Security Act
- Special protected groups, including individuals who lose cash assistance as a consequence of work or increased Social Security benefits
- Medicare beneficiaries with low incomes

To meet the categorical requirements, one must be a member of a family with dependent children or be an older adult, blind, or a person with a disability. The 2010 Affordable Care Act extends program eligibility to income-eligible adults under age 65 without dependent children as well.[39] The resource test sets a maximum allowable amount for liquid resources and other assets. Standards for asset eligibility vary widely among the states, territories, and the District of Columbia.

Medicaid covers inpatient and outpatient hospital services; physician, pediatric/family nurse practitioner, and nurse–midwife services; selected health center and rural health clinic services; prenatal care and family planning services/supplies; vaccines for children and other services for those under 21 years; laboratory and X-ray services; and skilled nursing home and home health services, among others. Some states include other benefits, such as prescription drug coverage and dental services, but there is significant variability among states. In many states, Medicaid programs cover certain forms of nutrition services provided by dietitians.[40]

Historically, Medicaid has covered less than half of those below the poverty line.[41] The American Medical Association believes that the new expansion of Medicaid to provide acute-care coverage for all persons below 133% of the poverty line will improve access to health services and potentially decrease health care costs in the long run.[42]

The Children's Health Insurance Program President William J. Clinton signed into law the Balanced Budget Act of 1997, which included Title XXI, the **Children's Health Insurance Program (CHIP)**. CHIP was the largest single expansion of health insurance coverage for children in more than 30 years.[43] At the time, nearly 11 million American children—one in seven—were uninsured, largely due to fewer children being covered by employer-sponsored health insurance.[44] The CHIP initiative was designed to reach these children, many of whom were part of working families with incomes too high to qualify for Medicaid but too low to afford private health insurance.[45] States are able to use part of their federal funds to expand outreach and ensure that all children eligible for Medicaid and the CHIP program are enrolled. The initiative is a partnership between the federal and state governments that will help provide children with health coverage. Because Medicaid allows states flexibility in determining eligibility, states currently cover children whose family incomes range from below the poverty guidelines to as high as 300% of the poverty guidelines. Funds for the program became available to states in 1997. States receive federal matching funds only for actual expenditures to insure children. In 2014, more than 8 million children were covered by CHIP.[46] **Figure 9-3** summarizes the enrollment of children in CHIP since 1998.

Under the program, states have flexibility in targeting eligible uninsured children. States may choose to expand their Medicaid programs, design new child health insurance programs, or create a combination of both. States choosing a new children's health insurance program may offer one of the following benchmark plans: the standard Blue Cross/Blue Shield Preferred Provider Option offered by the Federal Employees Health Benefit Program, a health benefit plan offered by the state to its employees, or the HMO benefit plan with the largest commercial enrollment in the state. A state may also choose to offer the "equivalent" of one of the benchmark plans. If a state chooses this option, its plan's value must be at least equal to that of the benchmark plan, and it must include inpatient and outpatient hospital services, physicians' surgical and medical services, laboratory and X-ray services, and well baby/childcare services including immunizations. In addition, a benchmark-equivalent plan must include benefits similar to the benchmark plan coverage of prescription drugs, mental health services,

Children's Health Insurance Program (CHIP) Created under Title XXI of the Social Security Act; expands health coverage to uninsured children whose families earn too much income to qualify for Medicaid but too little to afford private coverage.

FIGURE 9-3

Percentage of Children under Age 18 Who Were Uninsured by Poverty Status: United States, 1997–2014
CHIP enrollment has increased steadily since the program's inception. Insure Kids Now is a website with eligibility and contact information for each state, each territory, and the District of Columbia. It also contains information about local and national outreach activities, including school-based outreach. Visit *www.insurekidsnow.gov*.
Source: Centers for Medicare and Medicaid Services, State Children's Health Insurance Program (CHIP) site portal, Enrollment Reports.

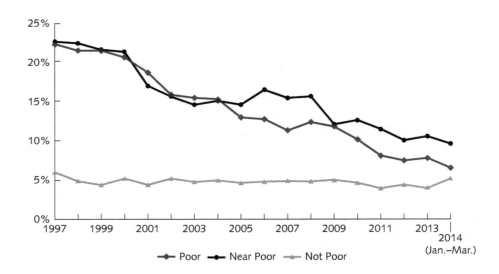

vision care, and hearing-related care. States choosing the Medicaid option must offer the full benefit package.

The Uninsured

In theory, health care coverage is available to virtually all U.S. citizens through one of four routes: Medicare for older adults and people with disabilities, Medicaid for low-income people and people with certain disabilities, employer-subsidized coverage at the workplace, or self-purchased coverage for those ineligible for the previous three.[47] Yet in 2013 an estimated 42 million people (13% of the population) with no insurance coverage at all lived in the United States, and perhaps an even larger number of people have coverage that is inadequate for any major illness.[48] Decreasing the number of uninsured was a key goal of the 2010 Patient Protection and Affordable Care Act (ACA), which provides Medicaid or subsidized coverage to qualifying individuals with incomes up to 400% of the poverty line. Data through early 2015 suggest that the ACA has helped expand coverage to 9 million previously uninsured people since 2013.[49]

Who, then, are the uninsured? Statistics show that they are not older adults, who have Medicare, or the very poor, who have Medicaid. Instead, those who lack coverage are primarily people in the middle (e.g., the working poor and those who work for small businesses). More than half are in families with incomes below 200% of the poverty guidelines.[50] They also include the self-employed, those who work part time, seasonal workers, the unemployed, full-time workers whose employers offer unaffordable insurance or none at all, and early retirees—age 55 through 64—who retired from companies that either offered no health insurance or have since dropped it.[51] **Figure 9-4** summarizes the characteristics of those without health insurance coverage in the United States in 2013.

When those without health insurance do get sick, they often wind up using the most expensive treatment available—hospital emergency room care—or they delay getting treatment and later require more expensive and prolonged medical services. These costs are shifted to the people who are insured.

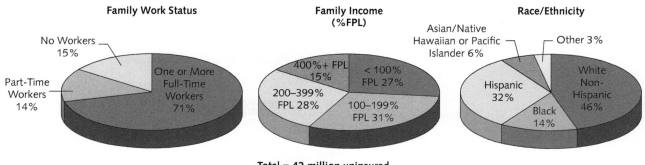

Total = 42 million uninsured

FIGURE 9-4 Percentage of Persons in the United States without Health Care Coverage, by Race/Ethnicity, Income, and Family Work Status, 2013

Notes: Data may not total 100% due to rounding. Federal Poverty Level (FPL) for a family of four in 2013 was $23,550/year. Children includes all individuals under age 19.

Source: Adapted from Urban Institute and Kaiser Commission on Medicaid and the Uninsured analysis of the March 2013 Current Population Survey; and Kaiser Commission on Medicaid and the Uninsured /Urban Institute analysis of 2014 ASEC Supplement to the Current Population Survey.

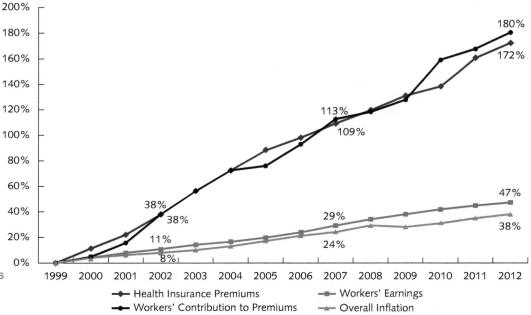

FIGURE 9-5

Cumulative Increases in Health Insurance Premiums, Workers' Contributions to Premiums, Inflation, and Workers' Earnings, 1999–2013

Sources: Kaiser/HRET Survey of Employer-Sponsored Health Benefits, 1999–2013; Bureau of Labor Statistics, Consumer Price Index, U.S. City Average of Annual Inflation, 1999–2013; Bureau of Labor Statistics, Seasonally Adjusted Data from the Current Employment Statistics Survey, 1999–2013.

All community members, including the employed and nonworking uninsured, the homeless, and others, should be able to obtain medical care when it is needed. However, cost is a barrier for health care access. From 1999 to 2011, family premiums for employer-sponsored insurance increased by 160%, while wages went up 50% and inflation went up 38% (**Figure 9-5**). In fact, between 2007 and 2013, increasing numbers of people reported cost as the reason for postponing needed health care, skipping recommended medical tests, not filling a prescription, skipping doses of medicine, and skipping dental care check-ups (**Figure 9-6**).[52]

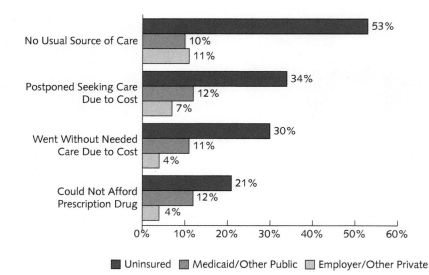

FIGURE 9-6 Barriers to Health Care among Adults < 65 Years of Age by Insurance Status, 2013

Source: CDC/NCHS, *Health, United States, 2013*, data from the National Health Interview Survey.

Demographic Trends and Health Care

Between 1946 and 1964, 78 million babies were born in the United States; these individuals—the baby boomers—now make up more than one-fourth of the population.[53] By the year 2030, the baby boom will become a senior boom, with 21% of the population over 65 years of age.[54] Not only will older adults be greater in number, but they may require care for a greater number of years, placing a heavier burden on the long-term care system (**Figure 9-7**). Because older Americans consume a disproportionate amount of medical care, the demand for such care, including pharmaceutical products and services, can be expected to rise.[55]

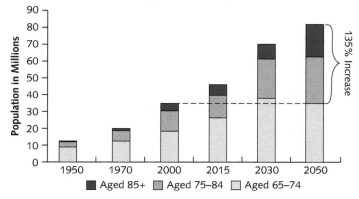

A. Population of Americans Aged 65 and Over, in Millions

135% Increase

■ Aged 85+   ■ Aged 75–84   □ Aged 65–74

FIGURE 9-7 Population of Americans Aged 65 and Over and the Increase in Older Adults Needing Long-Term Care

The number of individuals needing skilled nursing care is expected to rise as the baby boomers age.

Sources: Population Projections Program, *Projections of the Total Resident Population by 5 Year Age Groups, Race, and Hispanic Origin with Special Age Categories: Middle Series, 1999 to 2100* (Washington, D.C.: Population Division, U.S. Census Bureau), and *A Call for Action: Final Report of the Pepper Commission* (Washington, D.C.: U.S. Government Printing Office, 1990).

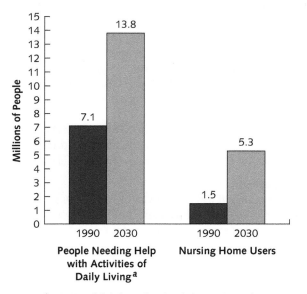

B. Number of Older Adults Needing Long-Term Care, 1990 and 2030

People Needing Help with Activities of Daily Living[a]   **Nursing Home Users**

[a]Activities of daily living (ADL) include activities such as bathing, dressing, toileting, continence, and feeding.

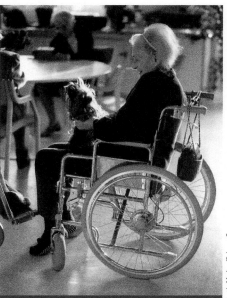

C. By the Year 2030, the Number of Older Adults Needing Nursing Home Care Will More Than Triple

Ursula Markus/Science Source

Racial and geographical factors in the population are also important to the shape of the future. In some parts of the United States, particularly the Southwest, the Hispanic population will dramatically increase. To the extent that such a population may exhibit differing utilization patterns for medical services or pharmaceuticals, such changes may significantly affect the marketplace. Geographical demographics will also be important, especially if the population drift from the Northeast to the Southwest and the Sun Belt continues.[56]

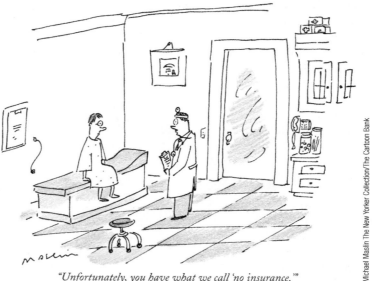

"Unfortunately, you have what we call 'no insurance.'"

Michael Maslin The New Yorker Collection/The Cartoon Bank

The Need for Health Care Reform

To determine the rating of a particular health care system, one must examine three crucial variables: cost, quality, and access.[57] At the zero end of the scale is no health care system. As we have seen, millions of Americans cannot afford to buy into or gain meaningful, ongoing access to any health care at all. At the other end of the scale is high-quality, reasonably priced, accessible health care. On such a scale, how does the U.S. health care system rate?

Before you respond, consider the following scenario:[58] Imagine that you are the decision maker in a large corporation, and I approach you and try to sell you a product. I say that I want to sell you a key piece of equipment that meets the following specifications:

- It will cost you $3,200 per employee per year.
- It will consume up to half of each profit dollar and will rise in price by 15 to 30% annually.
- There is a tremendous unexplained variation in this product depending on who uses it.
- There is no way to measure its quality in terms of appropriateness, reliability, or outcome.
- And you'll just have to take my word for it when I tell you that we adhere to the highest professional standards.

Would you buy this product? Many believe the U.S. health care system fits this description. Not only is it expensive, but we don't necessarily know what we are paying for or whether what we are paying for is worth it.[59]

The term "health care reform" refers to the efforts undertaken to ensure that everyone in the United States has access to affordable, quality health care. Among the challenges for health care reform are how to make health care accessible to everyone, how to control rising health care costs, how to provide nursing home care to those who need it, and how to ensure that Medicare and Medicaid can serve all who are eligible.

As we will see, cost, access, and quality are interrelated; manipulating one has an astounding impact on the others. For example, some people argue that we should abandon free enterprise and turn the system over to the government, as has been done in other countries, including Canada.

ENTREPRENEUR IN ACTION

Dr. Nancy Munoz, DCN, MHA, RD, FAND, LDN, is involved in the development, communication, and implementation of nutrition and foodservice protocols. She believes the possibilities for a successful and rewarding career in geriatrics are endless. The cost of providing health care services to this segment of the population is forcing payers to "get creative" and develop venues where health care services can promote health and well-being in an effort to reduce health care spending associated with the management of chronic disease. Many of the RDs working in long-term care today will have the opportunity to expand their practice into the community as the focus of nutrition services changes from intervention to prevention. Says Nancy: "It is time to showcase the unique set of skills RDs bring to the interdisciplinary team that is working toward improving community health." Find out more about her sage advice online at *www.cengagebrain.com*.

Critics of government-run health care systems say they appear promising at first but soon bog down in bureaucracy, unable to keep pace with advances in medical technology. Some point to the Canadians who travel to the United States to purchase treatment out of their own pockets rather than wait in line.[60] Is there a way to extend the scope of the system without sacrificing quality?

Health care policymakers have studied alternative models of delivery and financing in hopes of applying to the United States approaches that have been successful in other nations.[61] The U.S. health care system appears both to have higher costs (**Figure 9-8**) and

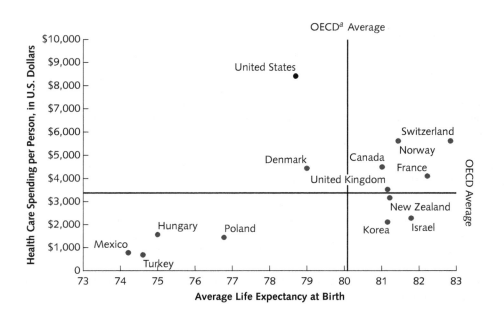

FIGURE 9-8 Total Health Expenditures Per Capita, U.S. and Selected Countries, 2013
Many people in countries spending far less than the United States on health care live longer than people in the United States.

[a] OECD = Organization for Economic Cooperation and Development.

Source: Organization for Economic Cooperation and Development (2010), "OECD Health Data," *OECD Health Statistics*.

to offer less access than the systems of other industrialized nations. During the last two decades, U.S. health care trends differed from those in other nations in a variety of ways, most notably in rising costs and erosion of access to health care services. Per capita health spending in the United States exceeds that of other industrialized countries by huge margins.[62] The following sections consider each of these issues.

The High Cost of Health Care

Health care inflation is well established. In 2013, $2.9 trillion was spent on health care services and products.[63] The level of health care activity is expected to grow. This growth is a result of various factors, including an aging population, technological advances requiring expensive equipment, increasing cost and dependence upon pharmaceutical products, increased demand (fostered in part by more consumer awareness of health issues), and continuing advances in medicine, which make it possible to offer more treatment options to people than ever before.[64]

A major contributor to health care expenditures in the United States is the administrative cost of the insurance process itself. Yet another factor contributing to the cost of our health care is the practice of defensive medicine and the associated phenomenon of ever-rising professional liability costs, which have skyrocketed.[65] Patient safety and the legal process remain at the forefront of the medical malpractice crisis, and in order to help curtail the cost of liability insurance, reforms are necessary.[66]

Efforts at Cost Containment

Efforts to curb soaring health care costs cover a broad spectrum: slowing hospital construction, modifying hospital and physician reimbursement mechanisms, reducing the length of hospital stays, increasing **copayments** and deductibles for insured employees and Medicare recipients, changing eligibility requirements for Medicaid, reducing unnecessary surgery by requiring patients to obtain second opinions, restricting access to new technology, encouraging alternative delivery systems, and emphasizing prevention.[67] Use of generic drugs has also been utilized to help contain the costs of health care.[68]

The cost-containment efforts of the past few decades is actually a fierce competition among *third-party* payers (government, insurance companies, and employers) to control their own costs. This effort has been characterized by three trends:[69]

1. A movement away from traditional fee-for-service health care to managed care, evident in the enrollments in HMOs, PPOs, and POSs, as well as consumer-directed health plans (refer back to Figure 9-2).
2. As more and more of their profits are siphoned off into health care coverage, companies are increasingly attempting to manage the health care of their employees themselves to reduce expenditures. In an effort to avoid **cost shifting**, many businesses are moving to **self-insured health plans**, thereby determining which benefits are covered and assuming the risks involved.[70]
3. The payers (government, insurance companies, and employers) have routinely set **reimbursement** restrictions and limitations.

Over two-thirds of national health care expenditures are hospital care, physician and clinical services, and prescription drugs as illustrated in **Figure 9-9**.[71] Efforts to contain costs have therefore largely been aimed at these items.

One example of cost containment is the **prospective payment system (PPS)** implemented by the federal government as a result of the 1983 Social Security Act Amendments. The purpose of the PPS was to change the behavior of health care providers by changing the incentives under which care is provided and reimbursed. Prospective payment means knowing the amount of payment in advance. The PPS uses **diagnosis-related groups (DRGs)** as a basis for reimbursement. Patients are classified according to their **principal diagnosis**, secondary diagnosis, sex, age, and surgical procedures.

Copayments The portion of the charge for medical services that the patient must pay.

Cost shifting A much-criticized aspect of the existing health care system in which hospitals and other providers bill indemnity (fee-for-service) insurers at higher rates to recover the costs of charity care and to make up for discounts given to HMOs, PPOs, Medicare, and Medicaid.

Self-insured health plan A health plan whereby the risk for medical costs of employees is assumed by the employer rather than an insurance company.

Reimbursement Payment made by a third party (e.g., government or private or commercial insurance).

Prospective payment system (PPS) A payment system under which hospitals are paid a fixed sum per case according to a schedule of diagnosis-related groups.

Diagnosis-related groups (DRGs) A method of classifying patients' illnesses according to principal diagnosis and treatment requirements, for the purpose of establishing payment rates.

Principal diagnosis The condition chiefly responsible for the patient's need for services. The principal diagnosis determines the payment the hospital or other provider receives from Medicare.

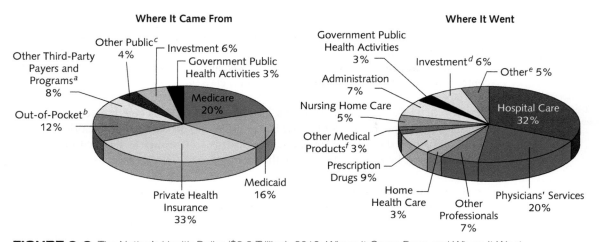

FIGURE 9-9 The Nation's Health Dollar ($2.9 Trillion), 2013: Where It Came From and Where It Went

[a] Includes worksite health care; other private revenues; Indian Health Service; workers' compensation; general assistance; maternal and child health; vocational rehabilitation; Substance Abuse and Mental Health Services Administration; school health; and other federal, state, and local programs.

[b] Includes copayments, deductibles, and any amounts not covered by health insurance.

[c] Children's Health Insurance Program (CHIP), VA, Department of Defense.

[d] Includes noncommercial research (2%) and structures and equipment (4%).

[e] Other spending includes expenditures for residential care facilities, ambulance providers, medical care delivered in nontraditional settings (such as community centers, senior citizens centers, schools, and military field stations), and expenditures for home and community waiver programs under Medicaid.

[f] Includes durable medical equipment (1%) and other non-durable over-the-counter medical products (2%).

Note: Totals may not add to 100% due to rounding.

Source: Centers for Medicare & Medicaid Services, Office of the Actuary, National Health Statistics Group, 2014.

The DRG approach is based on a system of classifying hospital admissions. The system begins with the *International Classification of Diseases: Clinical Modifications*, abbreviated **ICD-CM**, which contains approximately 10,000 possible reasons for a hospital admission, organized into 23 major categories. The 23 categories are subdivided into 490 DRGs. Tables compute average cost per discharge by state, region (rural or urban), hospital bed size, and other factors.[72] All DRGs have been assigned a *relative weight* that reflects the cost of caring for a patient in the particular category. **Table 9-2** shows a sample payment based on DRGs. Note that a patient with a complication or comorbidity (e.g., with malnutrition) is assigned a higher relative weight, reflecting the need for more intensive services.

One consequence of the PPS has been an increased focus on outpatient services as opposed to more costly inpatient care. This trend has significant implications for dietitians.

ICD-CM *(International Classification of Diseases: Clinical Modifications)* Codes used by health care providers on billing forms to classify diseases/diagnoses.

NAME OF DRG	DRG NUMBER	MEDICARE RELATIVE WEIGHT		BASE RATE		PAYMENT AMOUNT
Respiratory infections and inflammations without complication/comorbid condition	080	1.0404	×	$4,000	=	$4,162
Respiratory infections and inflammations with complication/comorbid condition	079	1.8144	×	$4,000	=	$7,258

TABLE 9-2 Sample Payment Based on DRGs, with and without Complication/Comorbid Condition[a]

[a] A comorbid condition is present at the time of admission to the hospital but is not the primary reason for treating that patient. For example, if a patient is admitted for a cholecystectomy and has diabetes, diabetes is a comorbidity.

Source: D. D'Abate Cicenas, *Increasing Medicare Reimbursement through Improved DRG Code, Reimbursement and Insurance Coverage for Nutrition Services* (Chicago: American Dietetic Association, 1991), p. 53. Used with permission of Ross Products Division, Abbott Laboratories, Columbus, OH 43216. © 1990 Ross Products Division, Abbott Laboratories.

Home health agency An agency that provides home health care. To be certified under Medicare, the agency must provide skilled nursing services and at least one additional therapeutic service (e.g., physical, speech, or occupational therapy).

It will continue to bring increased opportunities for consulting in outpatient settings, such as hospital outpatient clinics and **home health agencies**, and for private-practice counseling and consulting in physician or other health care provider offices, HMOs, health and fitness facilities, worksite wellness programs, weight loss programs, community health centers and clinics, and group patient education classes.

Equity and Access as Issues in Health Care

Is health care a basic right? The majority of people in the United States (54%) say that providing health insurance to the uninsured should be a top legislative priority.[73] In reality, as deVise has observed, health care may be more of a privilege than a right:

> If you are either very poor, blind, disabled, over 65, male, female, white, or live in a middle- or upper-class neighborhood in a large urban center, you belong to a privileged class of health care recipients, and your chances of survival are good. . . . But, if you are none of these, if you are only average poor, under 65, female, black, or live in a low-income urban neighborhood, small town, or rural area, you are a disenfranchised citizen as far as health care rights go, and your chances of survival are not good.[74]

In 1983, a presidential commission studying ethical issues in medicine reported, "Society has a moral obligation to ensure that everyone has access to adequate [health] care without being subjected to excessive burdens."[75] Proponents of this view argue that just as the federal government provides for defense, postal delivery, and certain other services, it should provide at least a *minimal* amount of basic health care.[76]

This debate leads to another question: Access to what? What *is* an acceptable level of health care? The states that have considered or passed health care plans for their uninsured have aimed at providing "basic" or "minimum" health care benefits, unlike the "comprehensive benefits" offered through the national health plans of other industrialized countries.

Providing comprehensive benefits, of course, does not necessarily mean providing unlimited care. The right to health care in Britain, Germany, and Canada does not mean the right to all treatments. Although most services provided in these countries are covered, the extent to which services are offered varies substantially across countries. Equity in health care in reality means a commitment to providing some common, adequate level of care. As yet, however, no country has explicitly determined what this level is.[77]

In countries with universal access, referral systems tend to restrict access to high-technology services while maintaining comprehensive coverage of services. This is different from the approach in the United States of providing open access to technological services but restricting the type and quantity of services that are covered under the various insurance plans.[78]

Racial and Ethnic Disparities in Health

Even though significant improvements in the health of racial and ethnic minorities have been reported, health disparities persist among different populations.[79] The *Healthy People* initiative is an effort to set health goals for each decade and then measure progress toward achieving them. Indicators reflect various aspects of health such as infant mortality, teen births, prenatal care, and low birthweight, as well as death rates for all causes and for heart disease, stroke, lung and breast cancer, suicide, homicide, motor vehicle crashes, and work-related injuries.

"In many ways, Americans of all ages and in every racial and ethnic group have better health today," former Surgeon General David Satcher said. "But our work isn't done until all infants have the same chance to thrive, all mothers have equal access to prenatal care, and all Americans are equally protected from cancer, heart disease, and stroke."[80] During the past two decades, one of *Healthy People*'s overarching goals has focused on disparities. In *Healthy People 2000*, it was to reduce health disparities among Americans. In *Healthy People 2010*, it was to eliminate, not just reduce, health disparities. In *Healthy People 2020*, that goal is expanded even further: to achieve health equity, eliminate disparities, and improve the health of all groups.[81] *Healthy People 2020* defines health equity as the "attainment of the highest level of health for all people."[82] Specific issues that *Healthy People* is monitoring during the current decade include: [83]

- Increasing and measuring access to appropriate, safe, and effective care, including clinical preventive services
- Decreasing disparities and measuring access to care for diverse populations, including racial and ethnic minorities and older adults
- Increasing and measuring access to safe long-term and palliative care services and access to quality emergency care

Throughout the decade, *Healthy People 2020* will assess health disparities in the U.S. population by tracking rates of illness, death, chronic conditions, behaviors, and other types of outcomes in relation to demographic factors, including race and ethnicity, gender, sexual orientation, disability status or special health care needs, and geographic location (rural and urban).[84] For more about health disparities, see Chapter 15.

Health Care Reform in the United States

Practically all industrialized countries except the United States have national health care programs.[85] Coverage is generally universal (everyone is eligible, regardless of health status) and uniform (everyone is entitled to the same benefits). Costs are paid entirely from tax revenues or by some combination of individual and employer premiums and government subsidization.

The concept of government-sponsored comprehensive health care is not new to the United States.[86] In 1934, President Franklin D. Roosevelt strongly supported national health insurance (NHI) and almost pushed to have it included with old age and unemployment insurance in the Social Security Act of 1935. Fearing that NHI might jeopardize passage of the Social Security Act, however, he decided to drop the proposal. As a result of World War II and the passage of the Hill-Burton Act of 1946, federal monies were diverted away from NHI and used for construction of new hospitals. Two decades later, the nation shifted its focus from NHI to providing for those without private insurance. Consequently, through the efforts of Presidents John F. Kennedy and Lyndon B. Johnson, Congress enacted the Social Security Amendments of 1965, which created Medicare (Title XVIII) and Medicaid (Title XIX).

Now, five decades later, increased health care costs and decreased patient satisfaction with the health care available in the United States have prompted consideration of a new approach to health care. Rather than proposing the comprehensive reform of health care, many suggest incremental reforms on broad issues, such as health insurance reform, physician malpractice reform, and incentives to induce businesses to include health promotion initiatives in their insurance plans.[87] Changes in medical education have also been discussed. Because medicine has its roots in the treatment of acute disease, the greatest emphasis is on training physicians in treating patients with chronic diseases, the most prevalent problem in health care today, through a coordinated management team, including nutrition professionals.[88]

Health care reform for the United States raises a formidable list of issues, including overall cost containment, universal access, emphasis on prevention, and reduction in administrative superstructure and costs (**Figure 9-10**). These issues require difficult decisions. Consider the following questions:[89]

- Who should be covered?
- How can coverage be expanded to reach all people?
- What services should be included in basic health care packages?
- Should health care cover both acute problems and prevention?
- Who should decide what constitutes preventive services?
- Who will pay for this coverage—consumers, employers, government?
- Where will government get the money to pay for it?
- How can health care costs be reduced or contained?
- What are the advantages and disadvantages of managed competition versus single-payer systems?

Health Care Reform: Challenges and Opportunities Ahead

While Congress continues to debate what kind of health care system is needed and how to pay for it, health care reform is beginning to evolve at an accelerating rate. On March 23, 2010, President Obama signed comprehensive health reform into law by signing the Patient Protection and Affordable Care Act of 2010 (P.L. 111-148), as amended by the Health Care and Education Recovery Act of 2010 (P.L. 111-152), together known as the Affordable Care Act (ACA). The law includes several measures

FIGURE 9-10

Conflicting Health Care Expectations

The triad of goals and desires depicted here reflect the struggle of the U.S. health care system to adapt to the conflicting expectations among consumers, health care providers, and public health and government policymakers. For example, the consumer's preference for choice of health providers with low out-of-pocket costs can be incompatible with insurers' goals for reducing costs. The challenge is to resolve these conflicting expectations between consumer desires, clinician interests, and social policy in order to achieve changes in health care delivery that favor improved outcomes and reduced expenditures.

Source: Adapted from H. Moses III and coauthors, The Anatomy of Health Care in the United States, *Journal of the American Medical Association* 310 (2013): 1960.

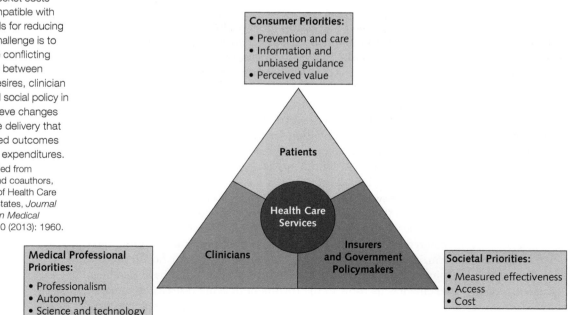

Consumer Priorities:
- Prevention and care
- Information and unbiased guidance
- Perceived value

Patients

Health Care Services

Clinicians

Insurers and Government Policymakers

Medical Professional Priorities:
- Professionalism
- Autonomy
- Science and technology

Societal Priorities:
- Measured effectiveness
- Access
- Cost

that fundamentally change the health care system in the United States.[90] Some of the law's major provisions include: [91]

- Requiring that most U.S. citizens and legal residents have health insurance
- The creation of state-based health benefit insurance exchanges through which individuals can purchase coverage, with subsidies available to lower-income individuals
- A major expansion of the Medicaid program for the nation's poorest individuals
- Requiring employers to cover their employees or pay penalties, with exceptions for small employers
- New regulations on health plans in the private market requiring them to cover all individuals, regardless of health status
- Greater support for prevention, wellness, and public health activities

Table 9-3 summarizes provisions in the law that expand coverage, provide preventive services at lower cost, and improve health care access.[92] The new health reform law provides many opportunities to improve health care in this country by:[93]

- Reducing the number of people who are uninsured as noted in **Figure 9-11**
- Making the health insurance system work better for all consumers
- Transforming delivery and payment systems to get better value
- Reorienting health care to focus on prevention and primary care

TABLE 9-3 How the Affordable Care Act Reforms Health Care

FOR PEOPLE WITH MEDICARE	FOR PEOPLE WHO ARE UNINSURED OR BUY THEIR OWN COVERAGE	FOR PEOPLE WITH INSURANCE	FOR PEOPLE PLANNING LONG-TERM CARE NEEDS
• Expands coverage for wellness and preventive care under Medicare; eliminates cost-sharing (copayments and deductibles) for preventive services recommended by the U.S. Preventive Services Task Force • Allocates extra resources to fight fraud and abuse in Medicare • Provides funds to help improve access to primary care doctors • Provides older adults with a rebate to fill the so-called doughnut hole in Medicare drug coverage, which severely limits prescription medication coverage expenditures over $2,700 • Closes the Medicare Part D coverage gap by 2020	• Helps people with preexisting conditions who have been uninsured to obtain temporary insurance coverage • Allows some young adults to be covered by their parent's insurance plan until they turn 26 • Expands Medicaid eligibility to include all individuals and families with incomes up to 133% of the poverty line along with a simplified CHIP enrollment process • Creates Insurance Exchanges[a] where individuals and small businesses can buy private health insurance • Creates a standard set of essential benefits for all plans offered by exchanges • Provides help for those with limited incomes up to 400% of the poverty line to pay premiums for plans offered by exchanges	• End of rescissions: prohibits insurance companies from dropping health coverage due to illness, and from denying coverage to children because of a preexisting condition • Restricts insurers from placing annual dollar caps on health coverage • Reduces out-of-pocket costs for certain preventive care services • Bans insurers from placing lifetime dollar limits on health coverage • Prohibits insurance companies from denying anyone health coverage because of a preexisting condition	• Funds some states to promote independent living by expanding home- and community-based services • Makes it easier to file complaints about the quality of care in nursing homes • Expands protections for spouses of people on Medicaid who are receiving care at home

[a] The Health Benefit Insurance Exchange program sets up a new competitive private health insurance market, giving tens of millions of Americans and small businesses access to affordable coverage. Exchanges allow individuals and small businesses to pool their purchasing power and compare health plan options.

Source: Adapted from AARP, Health Care and You: The Health Care Law at a Glance, 2011. For more information, go to *www.hhs.gov/healthcare/facts-and-features/key-features-of-aca/index.html*.

FIGURE 9-11 Effects of the Affordable Care Act on Health Insurance Coverage, 2024

Notes: The nonelderly population consists of residents of the 50 states and the District of Columbia who are younger than 65. ACA, Affordable Care Act; CHIP, Children's Health Insurance Program.

a "Other" includes Medicare; the changes under the ACA are almost entirely for nongroup coverage.

b The uninsured population includes people who will be unauthorized immigrants and thus ineligible either for exchange subsidies or for most Medicaid benefits; people who will be ineligible for Medicaid because they live in a state that has chosen not to expand coverage; people who will be eligible for Medicaid but will choose not to enroll; and people who will not purchase insurance to which they have access through an employer, an exchange, or directly from an insurer.

Source: Congressional Budget Office; staff of the Joint Committee on Taxation. *Updated Estimates of the Effects of the Insurance Coverage Provisions of the Affordable Care Act,* April 2014, p. 5.

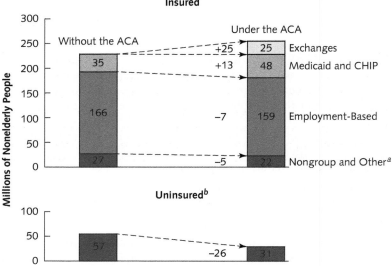

According to the Academy of Nutrition and Dietetic's Legislative and Public Policy Committee Chair, "President Obama signed into law the single most significant piece of federal legislation in the history of the Academy. It sweeps across all areas of practice and opens doors to new opportunities for our members. Congress has finally recognized the full value of preventive nutrition in communities in addition to the value of the dietetics profession."[94] How will the health reform law affect nutrition and dietetics professionals? **Table 9-4** highlights specific provisions of the Affordable Care Act that pertain to expansion of preventive care services in health care delivery systems with potential implications for providers of nutrition services.

The challenge ahead lies in the details of implementing the provisions of the new health reform law.[95] The focus of the Academy and its members must be to ensure that RDs and DTRs are represented in new state and community wellness initiatives and included in new health reform regulations as providers of reimbursable nutrition services for maintaining health and wellness; disease prevention; and chronic care management throughout the continuum of life—preconception to end-of-life care.[96]

Nutrition as a Component of Health Care Reform

Community health care systems must include provision of nutrition services to preserve health and prevent disease. As previously noted, the Academy of Nutrition and Dietetics believes that "primary prevention is the most effective, affordable course of action for preventing and reducing risk for chronic disease."[97] In fact, realizing the importance of nutrition in overall health, the Academy posits that "application of medical nutrition therapy (MNT) and lifestyle counseling as part of the nutrition care process is an integral component of the medical treatment for management of specific disease states and conditions and should be the initial step in the management of these situations."[98] Gro Harlem Brundtland, MD, MPH, the former director-general of the World Health Organization, has said, "Nutrition is a cornerstone that affects and defines the health of all people, rich and poor. It paves the way for us to grow, develop, work, play, resist infection and aspire to realization of our fullest potential as individuals and societies. . . . Putting first things first, we must . . . realize that resources allocated to preventing and eliminating disease will

TABLE 9-4 How the Affordable Care Act Impacts Providers of Nutrition Services[a]

- **Prevention Services:** Establishes a preventive services task force and an investment fund with funding up from $2.4 billion in 2010 to $4.6 billion by 2019.

- **Healthy Aging:** Establishes a grant program for state and local health departments and Indian tribes for public health interventions, community preventive screenings, and referral and treatment for chronic diseases for individuals between 55 and 64 years old. Intervention activities include improving nutrition and increasing physical activity.

- **Employee Wellness:** Allows discounts up to 50% of insurance premiums if the wellness program is determined beneficial for employees.

- **Health Care Workforce:** Analyzes current health care workforce to determine gaps in delivery of care in underserved communities.

- **School-Based Health Clinics:** Establishes grants to launch school-based clinics. Optional services include nutrition counseling.

- **Medicare Preventive Services:** Adjusts current law to allow the Centers for Medicare and Medicaid to expand current and new preventive services. Medical nutrition therapy (MNT) is included in the list of possible services to be expanded. • Provides for an annual wellness visit. RDs are listed as providers for screening and counseling.

- **Medicaid:** Establishes a five-year grant program to incentivize healthy lifestyles, including weight reduction, reducing cholesterol, preventing the onset of diabetes, and diabetes self-management. • Covers preventive services recommended by the U.S. Preventive Services Task Force and eliminates cost-sharing for preventive services (copayments and deductibles).

- **Home Health Care:** Establishes a demonstration program that would provide direct, home-based care. RDs are listed as possible providers under this program.

- **Medical Homes:**[b] Allows for medical home waivers for state-coordinated Medicaid programs that focus on diabetes treatment and prevention, treat cardiovascular disease, and treat those considered overweight. Nutritionists are listed among providers under this program, allowing for inclusion of RDs. Establishes the medical home model in community public health programs and includes the dietitian as part of the medical home team.

- **Child Obesity Demonstration Project:** Fully funds $25 million for a demonstration project aimed at reducing childhood obesity in community-based settings and schools through educational, counseling, and training activities.

- **Nutrition Labeling of Menu Items at Chain Restaurants:** Requires chain restaurants and food sold from vending machines to disclose the nutritional content of each item.

[a] These provisions may pertain to you as a registered dietitian or dietetic technician, registered.

[b] Medical home models provide accessible, continuous, coordinated, and comprehensive patient-centered care and are managed centrally by a primary care physician with the active involvement of various nonphysician providers to facilitate the provision of recommended services, eliminate redundancies or unnecessary care, and engage patients. The physician receives supplementary payments (e.g., per patient per month) for coordinating patient care.

Source: From Academy of Nutrition and Dietetics, "Health Care Reform: What the Final Bill Means to You as a Provider of Nutrition Services, 2010." Copyright © 2010 Academy of Nutrition and Dietetics. Used with permission. Check for updates at *www.eatright.org/advocacy* or in the Eat Right Weekly.

be effective only if the underlying causes of malnutrition—and their consequences—are successfully addressed. This is the 'gold standard': health and human rights. It makes for both good science and good sense, economically and ethically."[99]

One cannot have good health without proper nutrition. Conversely, poor nutrition contributes substantially to infant mortality; retarded growth and development of children; premature death, illness, and disability in adults; and frailty in older adults, causing unnecessary pain and suffering, reduced productivity in the workplace, and increased health care costs.[100]

Many believe that nutrition services are the cornerstone of cost-effective prevention and essential to halting the spiraling cost of health care.[101] Any health care reform legislation needs to recognize the expertise of the registered dietitian as the nutrition expert of the health care team, with a scope of practice that is guided by a logical framework. While the scope of dietetics practice is not rigid, due to the breadth of the profession, it includes:[102]

- *Nutrition assessment* for the purpose of determining individual and community needs and recommendations of appropriate nutrient intake to maintain, recover, or improve health

- *Nutrition counseling and education* of individuals, families, community groups, and health professionals

- *Research, development, and evaluation* of appropriate nutrition practice guidelines

- *Administration* through *management* of time, finances, personnel, protocols, and programs
- *Consultation* with patients, clients, and other health professionals
- *Evaluation* of the effectiveness of nutrition counseling/education and community nutrition programs

Cost-Effectiveness of Nutrition Services

Cost-effectiveness An approach to evaluation that takes into account both costs and outcomes of intervention for a specific purpose. The analysis is especially useful for comparing alternative methods of intervention.

The **cost-effectiveness** of nutrition services has been well documented.[103] The Academy encourages all its practitioners to document the cost-effectiveness of nutrition services. Community nutritionists need to compete successfully for a fair share of the health care dollar. To do so, they must document the demand for and effectiveness of nutrition services so that they can market those services to health care officials, providers, payers, and the public.

Obviously, no payer in the health care system wants additional costs. For a new technology or service, including nutrition services, to be a reimbursable benefit, it must prove its cost-effectiveness. Only services that have a proven impact on the quality of patient care will be funded. As Simko and Conklin have said, no expenditure of resources is justified for a service that fails to achieve its intended outcome.[104]

Cost-effectiveness studies compare the costs of providing health care against a desirable change in patient health outcomes (e.g., a reduction in serum cholesterol in a patient with hypercholesterolemia).[105] **Figure 9-12** shows increasing opportunities for testing the costs and benefits of nutrition services. As this model shows, effective nutrition therapy can produce economic benefits as a result of altered risk factors.

Practice guidelines Guidelines used by doctors and other health professionals for treating various conditions in order to ensure cost-effective care.

Protocols Detailed guidelines for care that are specific to the disease or condition.

To promote improved health care and nutrition-related outcomes, among other reasons, the Academy of Nutrition and Dietetics has created Standards of Practice in Nutrition Care (SOP) and Standards of Professional Performance (SOPP) for registered dietitians and dietetic technicians, registered.[106] In an effort to enhance the quality, efficiency, and effectiveness of the health care system, policymakers are urging physicians and other health professionals to develop **practice guidelines** or **protocols** that clearly specify appropriate care and acceptable limits of care for each disease state or condition. **Table 9-5** lists guidelines from the American Heart Association regarding lifestyle interventions for the prevention of heart disease in women.[107]

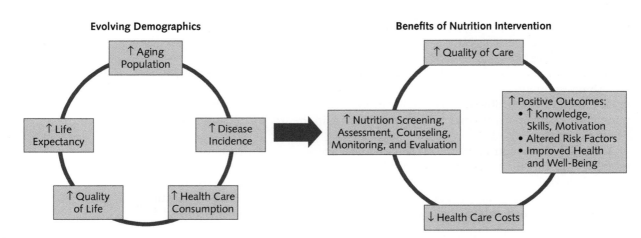

FIGURE 9-12 Benefits of Nutrition Intervention

Current trends in aging and life expectancy provide an opportunity to showcase the role of nutrition in improving health outcomes. A healthy diet and optimal nutrition status can reduce the risk and improve outcomes for several chronic conditions, such as heart disease, type 2 diabetes, and obesity. Evidence-based nutrition interventions can achieve long-term health benefits and reduced health care expenditures for individuals, organizations (e.g., worksites), and communities.

Source: Adapted from Abbott Nutrition, Quality Outcomes and Financial Benefits of Nutrition Intervention, September 2015.

TABLE 9-5 Evidence-Based Lifestyle Guidelines for the Prevention of Cardiovascular Disease in Women

1. Dietary Strategies
- Women should be advised to consume a diet rich in fruits and vegetables; to choose whole-grain, high-fiber foods; to consume fish, especially oily fish, at least twice a week; to limit intake of saturated fat, cholesterol, alcohol, sodium, and sugar; and to avoid *trans* fatty acids.
- Consumption of omega-3 fatty acids in the form of fish or in capsule form (EPA 1,800 mg/day) may be considered in women with hypercholesterolemia and/or hypertriglyceridemia for primary and secondary prevention.

Specific Dietary Intake Recommendations for Women

NUTRIENT	SERVING[a]	SERVING SIZE
Fruits and vegetables	≥ 4.5 cups/day	1 cup raw leafy vegetable, ½ cup cut-up raw or cooked vegetable, ½ cup vegetable juice; 1 medium fruit, ¼ cup dried fruit, ½ cup fresh, frozen, or canned fruit, ½ cup fruit juice
Fish	2/week	3.5 oz cooked (preferably oily types of fish)[b]
Fiber	30 grams/day[c]	Oatmeal, raw fruits and vegetables, etc.
Whole grains	3/day	1 slice bread, 1 oz dry cereal, ½ cup cooked rice, pasta, or cereal (all whole-grain products)
Sugar	≤ 5/week	1 tablespoon sugar, 1 tablespoon jelly or jam, ½ cup sorbet, 1 cup lemonade
Nuts, legumes, and seeds	≥ 4/week	⅓ cup or 1.5 oz nuts (avoid macadamia nuts and salted nuts), 2 tablespoons peanut butter, 2 tablespoons or ½ oz seeds, ½ cup cooked legumes (dry beans and peas)
Saturated fat	< 7% of total energy intake	Found in fried foods, fat on meat or chicken skin, packaged desserts, butter, cheese, sour cream, etc.
Cholesterol	< 150 mg/day	Found in animal meats, organ meats, eggs, etc.
Alcohol	≥ 1/day	4 oz wine, 12 oz beer, 1.5 oz of 80-proof alcohol, or 1 oz of 100-proof alcohol
Sodium	< 1,500 mg/day	
***Trans* fatty acids**	0	

2. Smoking Cessation
- Women should be advised not to smoke and to avoid environmental tobacco smoke. Provide counseling, nicotine replacement, and other pharmacotherapy as indicated in conjunction with a behavioral program or formal smoking cessation program.

3. Physical Activity
- Women should be advised to accumulate at least 150 minutes per week of moderate exercise, or 75 minutes per week of vigorous exercise, or an equivalent combination of moderate- and vigorous-intensity aerobic physical activity. Aerobic activity should be performed in episodes of at least 10 minutes, preferably spread throughout the week.
- For additional cardiovascular benefits, women should increase their aerobic activity to 5 hours (300 minutes) a week of moderate-intensity aerobic physical activity, or 2½ hours a week of vigorous-intensity physical activity, or an equivalent combination of both.
- Women should be advised to engage in muscle-strengthening activities that involve all major muscle groups performed on ≥ 2 days per week.
- Women who need to lose weight or sustain weight loss should be advised to accumulate a minimum of 60 to 90 minutes of at least moderate-intensity physical activity (e.g., brisk walking) on most, and preferably all, days of the week.

4. Weight Management
- Women should maintain or lose weight through an appropriate balance of physical activity, caloric intake, and formal behavioral programs when indicated to maintain or achieve a healthy body weight.

[a] The recommended serving amounts are based on a 2,000-calorie diet.

[b] Pregnant women should be counseled to avoid eating fish with the potential for the highest level of mercury contamination (e.g., shark, swordfish, king mackerel, or tile fish).

[c] 1.1 gram of fiber for every 10 grams of carbohydrates.

Source: Adapted with permission from L. Mosca and coauthors, "Effectiveness-Based Guidelines for the Prevention of Cardiovascular Disease in Women—2011 Update: A Guideline from the American Heart Association," *Circulation* 123 (2011): 1243–62. Copyright © 2011 Wolters Kluwer Health; for updated guidelines related to CHD risk reduction, go to *www.nhlbi.nih.gov*.

ENTREPRENEUR IN ACTION

Janelle L'Heureux, MS, RD, has been working in HIV care since 1995 at AIDS Project Los Angeles (APLA), a community-based HIV service organization established in 1983. From the beginning, Janelle was involved in the coordination and implementation of national HIV training programs for interns, dietitians, and other professionals. As early as 2003, she was involved in the discussions to develop HIV nutrition evidence-based guides. She was part of the Academy of Nutrition and Dietetics expert working group for the development of HIV/AIDS Evidence-Based Nutrition Practice Guidelines and Recommendations, published in 2010. In her current role as coordinator of nutrition education services at APLA, she and her dietetic interns and nutrition students provide nutrition education to more than 1,000 clients per year. Janelle develops, coordinates, and implements the nutrition education component via one-on-one consultations, classes, and food demonstrations. As a dietetic intern preceptor, it is important to her that those coming into the field receive firsthand experience about the issues surrounding people living with HIV. Her message is to: Take on challenges even if you do not feel qualified; realize that you are probably your own worst critic; and embrace your curiosity. Find out more about her work online at *www.cengagebrain.com.*

Care delivered according to a protocol has been linked with positive **outcomes** for the patient or client.[108] Examples of outcomes include measures of control (serum lipid profiles, glycolated hemoglobin), quality of life, dietary intake, and patient satisfaction. The Academy has developed a variety of client protocols that define the minimum number of office visits and activities required for successful nutrition intervention and the outcomes that can be expected from the nutrition and dietetics professional implementing the protocol. In addition, it has developed a series of evidence-based guides for practice.[109]

Nutrition protocols serve as frameworks to help practitioners in the assessment, development, and evaluation of nutrition interventions. Developing standardized protocols of care (practice guidelines) for nutrition intervention is considered a must for achieving payment for nutrition services and expanding current levels of third-party reimbursement.[110] Another step has been the development of the comprehensive strategy to implement the nutrition care process. See the Professional Focus feature in Chapter 5 for a detailed discussion of the nutrition care process. A comprehensive guide has been developed to implement the nutrition care process using standardized language for nutrition assessment, diagnosis, intervention, and monitoring and evaluation. Labels have been developed for (1) specific data used in nutrition assessment and reassessment, (2) specific nutrition problems, (3) types of nutrition interventions, and (4) types of data used to judge effectiveness of nutrition care.[111] The data are specific outcomes of nutrition intervention—clinical data, laboratory measures, anthropometric measures, and dietary intake data—that must be documented.

Outcome An end result of the health care process; a measurable change in the patient's state of health or functioning.

The contribution of nutrition to preventing disease, prolonging life, and promoting health is well recognized.[112] Accumulated evidence shows that when nutrition services are integrated into health care, diet and nutrition status change, with the following results:[113]

- The birthweight of infants born to high-risk mothers improves.
- The prevalence of iron-deficiency anemia is reduced.
- Serum cholesterol and the risk of heart attacks are reduced.
- Glucose tolerance in persons with diabetes improves.
- Blood pressure in hypertensive patients is lowered.

As demonstrated by the research highlighted on page 356, the benefits of providing nutrition services far outweigh the costs of providing those services.

Medical Nutrition Therapy and Medicare Reform

Since 1992, the legislative priority of the Academy of Nutrition and Dietetics has been the inclusion of **medical nutrition therapy** as a covered benefit in health care delivery.[114] The Academy's Health Care Reform Team is focused on securing a mechanism for nutrition reimbursement under existing federal insurance programs. Medicare was amended in 2000 to cover nutrition therapy as an outpatient benefit under Part B of the Medicare program.[115] Chapter 6 provides a discussion of the legislative process that led to Medicare's reimbursement of MNT for certain Medicare recipients.

An Academy-financed independent study projected the cost of extending coverage of medical nutrition therapy to all Medicare beneficiaries under Medicare Part B to be less than $370 million over seven years, when savings are considered. Savings would be greater than costs after the third year of enactment (**Figure 9-13**).[116] For example, if coverage had begun in 1998, in 2001 an additional cost to Medicare Part B of $389 million would have been offset by a reduction in cost to Part A of $401 million, resulting in a net savings of $11 million. The savings to the Medicare program would come from fewer hospital admissions and fewer complications requiring a physician's visit. The data used in the study were particularly significant for persons with diabetes and cardiovascular disease. Spending for diabetes and cardiovascular disease accounts for about 60% of annual Medicare spending.[117] In the long run, the program would save more in medical expenses than it costs to operate.

In summary, medical nutrition therapy is an integral component of cost-effective medical treatment. It can reduce health costs by improving patient outcomes and reducing recovery time. The Academy of Nutrition and Dietetics believes that the coverage of appropriate medical nutrition therapy, when medically necessary, should be included in any basic health care benefit package.

Medical nutrition therapy
The range of specific medical nutrition therapies for various conditions is determined following a complete assessment of the client's nutrition status. Medical nutrition therapy includes dietary modifications and nutrition counseling, as well as more complex methods of nutrition support using specialized nutrition therapies (e.g., nutritional supplements and enteral and parenteral feedings).

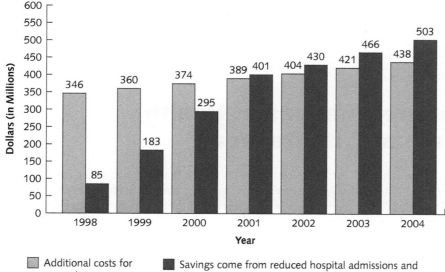

Additional costs for expanding coverage

Savings come from reduced hospital admissions and reduced complications requiring a doctor visit

FIGURE 9-13 Saving Medicare Millions
Go to *www.federalregister.gov* for the *Federal Register's* Final Rule for Medicare Part B Medical Nutrition Therapy Benefit.
Source: Lewin Group, 1997.

> ## Medical Nutrition Therapy Providing Return on Investment

Research demonstrates the cost-effectiveness of medical nutrition therapy.

- Oxford Health Plan[a] saved $10 for every $1 spent on nutrition counseling for at-risk older adult patients. Monthly costs for Medicare claims alone tumbled from $66,000 before the nutrition program to $45,000 afterward. As a result, the health plan continued use of nutrition screenings.
- The Lewin Group[b] documented an 8.6% reduction in hospital utilization and a 16.9% reduction in physician visits associated with medical nutrition therapy for patients with cardiovascular disease.
- The Lewin Group[b] additionally documented a 9.5% reduction in hospital utilization and a 23.5% reduction in physician visits when medical nutrition therapy was provided to persons with diabetes mellitus.
- The University of California Irvine[c] demonstrated that lipid drug eligibility was obviated in 34 of 67 subjects; the estimated annual cost savings from the avoidance of lipid medication was $60,652.
- Pfizer Corporation[d] projected $728,772 in annual savings from reduced employee cardiac claims because of an on-site nutrition/exercise intervention program.
- The U.S. Department of Defense[e] saved $3.1 million in the first year of a nutrition therapy program utilizing registered dietitians counseling 636,222 patients with cardiovascular disease, diabetes, and renal disease.
- Prenatal nutrition programs[f] that target high-risk pregnant women have been shown to improve long-term health outcomes in children, saving at least $8 for each dollar invested in the program.

[a] Oxford Health Plan's pilot nutrition screening program applied to the Medicare population in New York, between 1991 and 1993.

[b] Rachel Johnson, "The Lewin Group—What Does It Tell Us, and Why Does It Matter?" *Journal of the American Dietetic Association* (1999) 99: 426–27.

[c] G. Sikland et al., "Medical Nutrition Therapy Lowers Serum Cholesterol and Saves Medication Costs in Medicare Populations with Hypercholesterolemia," *Journal of the American Dietetic Association* 98 (1998): 889–94.

[d] Pfizer Corp., Lipid Intervention Program.

[e] "The Cost of Covering Medical Nutrition Therapy Services under TRICARE: Benefits Costs, Cost Avoidance and Savings," final report prepared by the Lewin Group, Inc., for the Department of Defense Health Affairs, 11/15/98.

[f] M. P. Duquette et al., "Validation of a Screening Tool to Identify the Nutritionally At-Risk Pregnancy," *Journal of Obstetrics and Gynaecology Canada* 30 (2008): 29–37.

Source: Adapted from American Dietetic Association, *Medical Nutrition Therapy Works* (April 2001).

Future Changes in Health Care and Its Delivery

The future of health care in the United States will be shaped by current trends in society at large and in the field of health care, as well as by the choices made for health care reform. The paradigm shift from sickness to wellness will undoubtedly be one of the strongest factors affecting health care.

For several decades, the dominant paradigm has been the medical model. During the 1970s, people were guided by the philosophy that the health care system would do everything possible in terms of curative and treatment services to make them well. In the 1990s, people began to view wellness as a function of prevention and accept responsibility for their own health. The focus on the pursuit of health, marked by an increased interest in nutrition, fitness, and health promotion, was reflected in the growth of corporate "wellness" programs and a widening choice of health care practitioners.

Our health care system still contains a number of barriers to focusing on prevention of poor health habits, however. The biomedical approach to illness underestimates and under-emphasizes behavioral and lifestyle influences on disease. Physicians think in terms of treating or correcting conditions rather than preventing them. To truly transform health care, medi-cal education will also undoubtedly need to change. Whereas most medical schools require some form of nutrition education, only 25% require a dedicated nutrition course and meet the minimum 25 required hours set by the National Academy of Sciences.[118]

The challenge for the next decade is to change the U.S. approach to health care from a system based on treatment of acute conditions to one based on disease prevention and health promotion. Physicians, public health workers, registered dietitians and other health practitioners, health educators, and community health organizations have joined ranks to emphasize health promotion and disease prevention as a more economical route to good health than the more costly procedures necessitated by sickness and disease.[119] According to physician Andrew Weil, "The medical facility of the future should look like a cross between a health spa and a hospital. Not only should it offer a smorgasbord of therapeutic options, its main focus should be on educating patients on how to stay well once they leave."[120]

The future offers much that is positive for the profession of nutrition and dietetics. The public's thinking about health and nutrition has matured, interest in positive health is growing steadily, and demand for health promotion products and services is increasing. Yet to be achieved, however, are the effective provision and allocation of resources such as nutrition services as part of preventive care. To accomplish this, political will, a coordinated strategy for health care, and active collaboration of health care professionals and consumers of health care services will be required. See Figure 6-10 on page 222 for a sample letter from a registered dietitian to his senator, supporting efforts to expand coverage and reimburse-ment of nutrition services—particularly for Medicare recipients with prediabetes.

As noted earlier, health care reform is a difficult undertaking. It involves more than cost containment and universal access. Community nutritionists need to educate the payers of health care about the inherent value of including nutrition services in their policies.[121] In arguing for reimbursable nutrition services, highlight its benefits:[122]

- Nutrition services are attractive, progressive health benefits that are relatively inexpen-sive compared with other types of benefits.
- Nutrition services benefits enhance the insurance product (the employee benefit package).
- Nutrition services have a preventive component (they help keep employees healthy).
- Nutrition services benefits attract healthy subscribers.
- Nutrition services are manageable—they can be easily documented.
- Nutrition services help patients become more self-reliant by helping them fight disease, avoid hospitalization, and reduce the use of other, more expensive medical therapies.
- Nutrition care speeds recovery.

Health care reform for the United States is certain, but the exact nature of the reform will continue to evolve. Undoubtedly, the changes required of the health care system will transform it slowly over time. Remember that change at the federal level begins with local advocacy and that the prescription for success is persistence.

❝ *To a greater extent than most of us are willing to accept, today's disorders of overweight, heart disease, cancer, blood pressure, and diabetes are by and large preventable. In this light, true health insurance is not what one carries on a plastic card but what one does for oneself.* ❞

—L. Power in G. Edlin and E. Golanty, Health and Wellness, *3rd ed.*

PROFESSIONAL **FOCUS**

Ethics and the Nutrition Professional

Life is full of paradoxes. For example, even though health promotion and disease prevention are paramount in halting the alarming escalation of the cost of health care in this country, the United States spends less than 5% of all dollars directed toward health care on public health and disease prevention.[1] Similarly, although one goal of nutrition is to apply scientific knowledge to feed all people adequately, every fifth child in the United States is vulnerable to hunger. The United States spends more on health care than other nations, but certain health disparities between racial and ethnic groups exist, particularly in pregnancy outcomes, infant mortality rate, nutrition status, life expectancy, and food insecurity. And finally, one issue that arises in connection with developing countries is whether it is fundamentally wrong that so much preventable sickness and death occur in the world.

As a community nutritionist, how do you address such issues? This feature reviews some of the ethical questions in the field of health promotion that are related specifically to community nutritionists. Its intent is not to arrive at a conclusion or present solutions to ethical dilemmas; rather, it seeks to present the issues for your consideration and stresses the need for moral sensitivity in the planning and implementation of community nutrition programs. As Aristotle said, "We are what we repeatedly do." Moral sensitivity and characteristics such as honesty, integrity, loyalty, and candor are developed through practice.[2]

What Is Ethics?

Philosophers throughout history have struggled with questions of how to live and work ethically. Ethics is a philosophical discipline that attempts to determine what is morally good and bad, right and wrong. Ethics helps decision makers seek criteria to evaluate different moral stances.[3]

As a community nutritionist, you may wonder what ethics has to do with your professional activities. Certainly, as a community nutritionist, you will not often confront such media issues as euthanasia, abortion, capital punishment, insider trading, maternal surrogacy, infanticide, the withdrawal of nutrition support for terminally ill patients, or the right to die. Nevertheless, situations arise in community settings that will force you to make ethical decisions.

Community nutritionists working with the media or food industry must consider the accuracy of product descriptions and claims, as well as words and images that can mislead the public.[4] As a manager, the community nutritionist may face ethical dilemmas in allocating resources. In setting priorities, she may have to make some decisions that necessitate ethical judgments. If she believes that all eligible clients have the right to receive optimal nutritional care, then how should she decide which clients will actually receive that care? (In this case, optimal nutritional care might mean a homebound older adult's receipt of home-delivered meals.) The community nutritionist involved in research exercises honesty, accuracy, and integrity in conducting studies and publishing the results. Consider the impact of using falsified data in determining nutrition policy for funding a new or existing nutrition program.

Codes of Ethics

Simple answers to ethical questions are elusive, but many health care organizations and professional associations have established codes of ethics to provide guidance in resolving ethical dilemmas.[5] Codes of ethics are written to guide decision making in areas of moral conflict; outline the obligations of the practitioner to self, client, society, and the profession; and "assist in protecting the nutritional health, safety, and welfare of the public."[6] The Academy of Nutrition and Dietetics published its first code of ethics in 1942.[7] The most recent code became effective in 2009 and applies to all Academy members and credentialed practitioners.

A code of ethics for nutritionists and other professionals working in international situations is likewise critical, as C. E. Taylor notes: "Needs are so obvious that the temptation is great to rush in with programs that seem reasonable; but international work is full of surprises. Each new activity needs to be carefully tested."[8] Consider the story of the monkey and the fish:

> After a dam burst, a flood raged through an African countryside. A monkey, standing in safety on the riverbank, watched a fish swim into its view. "I will save this poor fish from drowning," thought the monkey. And, swinging from a tree branch, he scooped up the fish and carried it, gasping, to land. "Throw me back," pleaded the fish. Reluctantly, the monkey agreed, scratching his head in bewilderment at the fish's lack of appreciation for the aid he had so selflessly offered.[9]

Code of Ethics for the Dietetics Profession
Preamble

The Academy of Nutrition and Dietetics and its credentialing agency, the Commission on Dietetic Registration (CDR), believe it is in the best interest of the profession and the public it serves to have a Code of Ethics in place that provides guidance to dietetics practitioners in their professional practice and conduct. Dietetics practitioners have voluntarily adopted this Code of Ethics to reflect the values and ethical principles guiding the dietetics profession and to set forth commitments and obligations of the dietetics practitioner to the *public, clients, the profession, colleagues, and other professionals.*

Application

The Code of Ethics applies to the following practitioners:

(a) In its entirety to members of the Academy of Nutrition and Dietetics who are Registered Dietitians (RDs) or Dietetic Technicians, Registered (DTRs);

(b) Except for sections dealing solely with the credential, to all members of the Academy of Nutrition and Dietetics who are not RDs or DTRs; and

(c) Except for aspects dealing solely with membership, to all RDs and DTRs who are not members of the Academy of Nutrition and Dietetics.

All individuals to whom the Code applies are referred to as "dietetics practitioners," and all such individuals who are RDs and DTRs shall be known as "credentialed practitioners." By accepting membership in the Academy of Nutrition and Dietetics and/or accepting and maintaining Commission on Dietetic Registration credentials, all members of the Academy of Nutrition and Dietetics and credentialed dietetics practitioners agree to abide by the Code.

Principles
Fundamental Principles

1. The dietetics practitioner conducts himself/herself with honesty, integrity, and fairness.

2. The dietetics practitioner supports and promotes high standards of professional practice. The dietetics practitioner accepts the obligation to protect clients, the public, and the profession by upholding the Code of Ethics for the Profession of Dietetics and by reporting perceived violations of the Code through the processes established by the Academy of Nutrition and Dietetics and its credentialing agency, the Commission on Dietetic Registration.

Responsibilities to the Public

3. The dietetics practitioner considers the health, safety, and welfare of the public at all times.

    The dietetics practitioner will report inappropriate behavior or treatment of a client by another dietetics practitioner or other professionals.

4. The dietetics practitioner complies with all laws and regulations applicable or related to the profession or to the practitioner's ethical obligations as described in this Code.

    a. The dietetics practitioner must not be convicted of a crime under the laws of the United States, whether a felony or a misdemeanor, an essential element of which is dishonesty;

    b. The dietetics practitioner must not be disciplined by a state for conduct that would violate one or more of these principles;

    c. The dietetics practitioner must not commit an act of misfeasance or malfeasance that is directly related to the practice of the profession as determined by a court of competent jurisdiction, a licensing board, or an agency of a governmental body.

5. The dietetics practitioner provides professional services with objectivity and with respect for the unique needs and values of individuals.

    a. The dietetics practitioner does not, in professional practice, discriminate against others on the basis of race, ethnicity, creed, religion, disability, gender, age, gender identity, sexual orientation, national origin, economic status or any other legally protected category;

    b. The dietetics practitioner provides services in a manner that is sensitive to cultural differences;

    c. The dietetics practitioner does not engage in sexual harassment in connection with professional practice.

6. The dietetics practitioner does not engage in false or misleading practices or communications.

    a. The dietetics practitioner does not engage in false or deceptive advertising of his/her services;

    b. The dietetics practitioner promotes or endorses specific goods or products only in a manner that is not false and misleading;

    c. The dietetics practitioner provides accurate and truthful information in communicating with the public.

7. The dietetics practitioner withdraws from professional practice when unable to fulfill his/her professional duties and responsibilities to clients and others.

    a. The dietetics practitioner withdraws from practice when he/she has engaged in abuse of a substance such that it could affect his/her practice;

    b. The dietetics practitioner ceases practice when he/she has been adjudged by a court to be mentally incompetent;

    c. The dietetics practitioner will not engage in practice when he/she has a condition that substantially impairs his/her ability to provide effective service to others.

Responsibilities to Clients

8. The dietetics practitioner recognizes and exercises professional judgment within the limits of his/her qualifications and collaborates with others, seeks counsel, or makes referrals as appropriate.

9. The dietetics practitioner treats clients and patients with respect and consideration.

    a. The dietetics practitioner provides sufficient information to enable clients and others to make their own informed decisions;

    b. The dietetics practitioner respects the client's right to make decisions regarding the recommended plan of care, including consent, modification, or refusal.

10. The dietetics practitioner protects confidential information and makes full disclosure about any limitations on his/her ability to guarantee full confidentiality.

11. The dietetics practitioner, in dealing with and providing services to clients and others, complies with the same principles set forth above in "Responsibilities to the Public" (Principles 3–7).

Responsibilities to the Profession

12. The dietetics practitioner practices dietetics based on evidence-based principles and current information.

13. The dietetics practitioner presents reliable and substantiated information and interprets controversial information without personal bias, recognizing that legitimate differences of opinion exist.

14. The dietetics practitioner assumes a lifelong responsibility and accountability for personal competence in practice, consistent with accepted professional standards, continually striving to increase professional knowledge and skills and to apply them in practice.

15. The dietetics practitioner is alert to the occurrence of a real or potential conflict of interest and takes appropriate action whenever a conflict arises.

    a. The dietetics practitioner makes full disclosure of any real or perceived conflict of interest;

    b. When a conflict of interest cannot be resolved by disclosure, the dietetics practitioner takes such other action as may be necessary to eliminate the conflict, including recusal from an office, position, or practice situation.

16. The dietetics practitioner permits the use of his/her name for the purpose of certifying that dietetics services have been rendered only if he/she has provided or supervised the provision of those services.

17. The dietetics practitioner accurately presents professional qualifications and credentials.

    a. The dietetics practitioner, in seeking, maintaining and using credentials provided by the Commission on Dietetic Registration, provides accurate information and complies with all requirements imposed by CDR. The dietetics practitioner uses CDR-awarded credentials ("RD/RDN" or "Registered Dietitian/Nutritionist"; "DTR" or "Dietetic Technician, Registered"; "CS" or "Certified Specialist"); only when the credential is current and authorized by CDR;

    b. The dietetics practitioner does not aid any other person in violating any Commission on Dietetic Registration requirements, or in representing himself/herself as Commission on Dietetic Registration credentialed when he/she is not.

18. The dietetics practitioner does not invite, accept or offer gifts, monetary incentives, or other considerations that affect or reasonably give an appearance of affecting his/her professional judgment.

Clarification of Principle:

    a. Whether a gift, incentive, or other item of consideration shall be viewed to affect, or give the appearance of affecting, a dietetics practitioner's professional judgment is dependent on all factors relating to the transaction, including the amount or value of the consideration, the likelihood that the practitioner's judgment will or is intended to be affected, the position held by the practitioner, and whether the consideration is offered or generally available to persons other than the practitioner.

    b. It shall not be a violation of this principle for a dietetics practitioner to accept compensation as a consultant or employee or as part of a research grant or corporate sponsorship program, provided the relationship is openly disclosed and the practitioner acts with integrity in performing the services or responsibilities.

c. This principle shall not preclude a dietetics practitioner from accepting gifts of nominal value, attendance at educational programs, meals in connection with educational exchanges of information, free samples of products, or similar items, as long as such items are not offered in exchange for or with the expectation of, and do not result in, conduct or services that are contrary to the practitioner's professional judgment.

d. The test for appearance of impropriety is whether the conduct would create in reasonable minds a perception that the dietetics practitioner's ability to carry out professional responsibilities with integrity, impartiality, and competence is impaired.

Responsibilities to Colleagues and Other Professionals

19. The dietetics practitioner demonstrates respect for the values, rights, knowledge, and skills of colleagues and other professionals.

a. The dietetics practitioner does not engage in dishonest, misleading, or inappropriate business practices that demonstrate a disregard for the rights or interests of others.

b. The dietetics practitioner provides objective evaluations of performance for employees and coworkers, candidates for employment, students, professional association memberships, awards, or scholarships, making all reasonable efforts to avoid bias in the professional evaluation of others.

Source: From the American Dietetic Association, *Code of Ethics for the Profession of Dietetics*.

Alignment of Values of the Academy of Nutrition and Dietetics to the Principles of the Code of Ethics for the Profession of Dietetics

Academy of Nutrition and Dietetics Values	Principles
Customer focus: Meets the needs and exceeds expectations of internal and external customers	#5, 9
Integrity: Acts ethically with accountability for lifelong learning and commitment to excellence	#1, 2, 4, 5, 6, 7, 10, 11, 12, 13, 17, 18
Innovation: Embraces change with creativity and strategic thinking	
Social Responsibility: Makes decisions with consideration for inclusivity as well as environmental, economic, and social implications	#3, 8, 9, 11, 13, 14, 15, 16, 17, 18, 19

Guiding Principles

Four basic principles are used in ethical decision making and in developing guidelines for professional practice:[10] (1) autonomy—respecting the individual's rights of self-determination, independence, and privacy; (2) beneficence—protecting clients from harm and maximizing possible benefits; (3) nonmaleficence—the obligation not to inflict harm intentionally; and (4) justice—striving for fairness in one's actions and equality in the allocation of resources.

To determine whether an issue in the community setting raises an ethical question, consider these ethical principles expressed as questions:[11]

1. Does the nutritional program, message, product, or service foster or deter the individual's ability to act freely?

2. Does the nutritional program, message, product, or service help people or harm them?

3. Does the nutritional program, message, product, or service unfairly or arbitrarily discriminate among persons or groups?

Consumers are eager to know about nutrition. The principle of beneficence moves us, as nutrition educators, to provide consumers with truthful and convincing information based on current scientific knowledge. In this way, we protect them from fraudulent misinformation and also motivate them to change their diet accordingly.[12] The principle of autonomy motivates us to provide consumers with factual information that includes both the weaknesses and the strengths of the scientific data supporting a given behavior, service, or product; with this information, individuals can exercise their right to make an informed choice or decision.

Health Promotion and Ethics

The purpose of health promotion is to motivate people to adopt and maintain healthful practices in order to prevent illness and functional impairment. Many hold that by investing in health promotion and disease prevention activities, we can avoid the much greater economic and social costs of disease and disability. The challenge today is to provide the public with the opportunity to benefit from appropriate nutrition knowledge and services. However, this challenge raises a hidden moral issue worthy of consideration. At what point is scientific knowledge sufficiently documented to warrant translating it into dietary messages to the public? What responsibilities and rights do we have to alter individual lifestyles in our effort to promote public health? As health promoters, we are sometimes criticized for taking a paternalistic approach with a "We know better than you" attitude. Moral sensitivity demands that we respect the dignity of persons—their right to make their own choices. For example, we may carefully and creatively design messages for older women at risk of osteoporosis, encouraging them to use dairy products in their daily diet, but our target audience has the right to resist our efforts and choose not to do so. An adequate calcium intake is a good thing, but life offers many other good things as well.

Health promotion for a number of issues (for example, cigarette smoking and drinking and driving) necessitates a paternalistic approach that both restricts private liberties and promotes group virtues such as beneficence and concern for the common good. Such paternalism is for the most part considered legitimate and reflects the view that the good of each of us is not the same thing as the good of all of us together.[13]

Community nutritionists, as health promoters, call attention to other health risks—a diet high in saturated fat or low in fiber, commercial advertising of empty-calorie foods to children, and nutrition fraud in the marketplace, among others. Should governments, therefore, move from taxing cigarettes and alcohol to taxing companies that manufacture high-fat confections or beverages high in sugar? Because obesity and a sedentary lifestyle are associated with a number of chronic diseases (for instance, hypertension, coronary artery disease, and diabetes) and with increased health care costs, should persons who eat or drink too many calories and those who fail to exercise regularly be taxed to discourage these lifestyles and raise revenues for health care? Should we fine pregnant women who smoke or drink? In other words, to what extent should society tolerate and bear the burden for the health risks that individuals choose to take? Such are the ethical dilemmas facing those who work in health promotion. The ethical conflict is how to achieve the goal of protecting and promoting public health while ensuring an individual's freedom of choice.

Ethical Decision Making

Analytical skills are necessary to resolve ethical dilemmas. One must objectively evaluate the individual circumstances of each situation, gather relevant data, consider possible alternatives, consult experts as necessary, and take appropriate actions to accomplish the greatest good for the greatest number. The particular action chosen must adhere to the general ethical principles of autonomy, beneficence, nonmaleficence, and justice.[14]

As community nutritionists, you are certain to face ethical dilemmas in both your professional and your personal lives. In closing this section, we leave you with a set of questions.[15] In the months to come, consider your responses to these questions in light of your moral sensitivity regarding these situations, your understanding of ethical principles, and your discussions with other professionals experienced in making ethical decisions.

- Do the United States, Canada, and other developed countries have a moral obligation toward less developed countries?

- When limited resources necessitate setting priorities in program planning, who should receive benefits? Infants? Children? Pregnant women? Working people? Older adults?

- What are the ethical limits to the promotional activities of multinational corporations? Is it acceptable to market infant formula or soft drinks in developing countries? Should we ban television advertising of empty-calorie foods to children?

- In setting program priorities, are there situations in which one ethnic group should be favored over another?

- Do we have the right to ask individuals to adjust and, in some cases, to abandon their ethnic and cultural customs, traditions, or cuisines in the interests of improved health?

> **THINK LIKE A COMMUNITY** NUTRITIONIST

The *Journal of the Academy of Nutrition and Dietetics* regularly publishes articles focused on ethics. Select one of the following articles to read, and make a list to indicate how the article could be applied.

- E. J. Ayers, The Impact of Social Media on Business and Ethical Practices in Dietetics, *Journal of the Academy of Nutrition and Dietetics*, 113 (2013): 1539–43.

- G. E. Gates, and L. Amaya, Registered Dietitian Nutritionists and Nutrition and Dietetics Technicians, Registered, Are Ethically Obligated to Maintain Personal Competence in Practice, *Journal of the Academy of Nutrition and Dietetics*, 115 (2015): 811–15.

- C. P. Fileti, Ethics Opinion: Eliminating Dietetics-Related Inequalities, *Journal of the American Dietetic Association*, 111 (2011): 307–9.

- J. O'Sullivan Maillet, D. B. Schwartz, and M. E. Posthauer, Position of the Academy of Nutrition and Dietetics: Ethical and Legal Issues in Feeding and Hydration, *Journal of the Academy of Nutrition and Dietetics*, 113 (2013): 828–33.

- R. San-Cristobal, F. I. Milagro, and J. A. Martinez, Future Challenges and Present Ethical Considerations in the Use of Personalized Nutrition Based on Genetic Advice, *Journal of the Academy of Nutrition and Dietetics*, 113 (2013): 1447–54.

case study

Insurance Access

by Alice Fornari, EdD, RD, Alessandra Sarcona, MS, RD, CSSD, and Alison Barkman, MS, RD, CDN

Scenario

You are a registered dietitian (RD) working in an ambulatory clinic that provides nutrition counseling to Medicaid clients. Nutrition services are not currently provided to Medicare clients because Medicare has historically not covered this service. An older adult client is referred to you for counseling regarding his elevated blood glucose levels, which remain high despite medications. Upon opening the client's record, you realize the client is on Medicare, not Medicaid. You ask the client to verify this information, and it is correct. You ask the client whether he can pay for your services. He cannot because of his fixed income from Social Security. You have on your bulletin board the memorandum from the clinic administrator reiterating the policy that no patients can be seen on clinic time if they are not able to pay for services and do not receive insurance reimbursement. You remember reading in the *Journal of the Academy of Nutrition and Dietetics*

(January 2002) about medical nutrition therapy (MNT) insurance coverage for Medicare clients diagnosed with diabetes mellitus. Although you want to investigate further this Medicare coverage of MNT, you cannot assume for this visit that the client will be covered for your services under Medicare. You decide to further investigate the specifications for Medicare coverage of MNT for diabetes by searching the Internet, which led you to this link: *www.medicare.gov/coverage/nutrition-therapy-services.html*.

Learning Outcomes

- Identify individuals who have access to health care/nutrition services through government and/or private insurance.
- Relate allocation of resources to health care issues, specifically considering the access to health care of clients with limited resources.

- Communicate to clients and colleagues policies and procedures for obtaining health care resources as an agency or individual provider.
- Integrate and monitor strategies that support MNT services and desired nutrition outcomes.

Foundation: Acquisition of Knowledge and Skills

1. Define terms specific to private and public insurance.
2. List comparative information about Medicare and Medicaid (refer to information on Medicare and Medicaid in this chapter).
3. Access and review the article "Becoming a Medicare Provider: Systems for Success," *Journal of the Academy of Nutrition and Dietetics* 101 (2001): 1412. As a member of the Academy of Nutrition and Dietetics, you can search the journal online at *www.eatright.org*.
4. List educational requirements of nutrition professionals receiving certification or licensure as applied to your state regulations, if applicable.

Step 1: *Identify Relevant Information and Uncertainties*

1. Explain the issue facing the nutritionist.
2. Identify a range of solutions focused on enabling the client to obtain nutrition counseling from a qualified nutrition professional.
3. Identify and analyze the information related to health care resources that would be useful to help resolve the issue.

Step 2: *Interpret Information*

1. Compare and contrast the arguments related to possible solutions on the basis of supporting evidence.
2. As you analyze the problem, how might you compensate for your own biases (e.g., your strong desire to provide nutrition counseling to this older client)?

Step 3: *Draw and Implement Conclusions*

Within the clinic structure, document in writing the steps you would need to pursue to ensure that the Medicare clients covered under the current MNT regulations are referred to you for nutrition services. Be sure to include the latest decision by CMS to cover intensive behavioral counseling for obesity, noting where this counseling must take place and by which health care practitioners in order for the service to be reimbursed.

Step 4: *Engage in Continuous Improvement*

To support your solution to the issue, develop an outcomes assessment plan to document that your intervention is cost-effective and beneficial to the client in terms of disease management and reducing risk for complications. Refer to the Evidence Analysis Library resources on diabetes mellitus on the Academy of Nutrition and Dietetics website at *www.andeal.org*. Refer to *www.eatright.org* and search for "diabetes resources" to identify criteria supporting the benefits of MNT specific to the management of diabetes mellitus.

CHAPTER **SUMMARY** . . . .

An Overview of the Health Care Industry

▶ In the United States, there are two general categories of health insurance: private and government/public health insurance.

- Private insurance can be in the form of traditional fee-for-service insurance or group contract insurance.

- A managed-care system is represented by health maintenance organizations (HMOs), preferred provider organizations (PPOs), point-of-service plans (POSs), and exclusive provider organizations (EPOs). The goal of managed care is improved quality of care with decreased costs.

- Government/public insurance: The two major public health insurance plans in the United States are Medicare and Medicaid (see Table 9-1).

Demographic Trends and Health Care

▶ The term "health care reform" refers to the efforts undertaken to ensure that everyone in the United States has access to affordable, high-quality health care.

▶ The level of health care activity is expected to grow due to various factors, including an aging population, technological advances requiring expensive equipment, increasing cost of and dependence on pharmaceutical products, increased demand (fostered in part by more consumer awareness of health issues), and continuing advances in medicine.

▶ Efforts to curb soaring health care costs include slowing hospital construction, modifying hospital and physician reimbursement mechanisms, reducing the length of hospital stays, increasing copayments and deductibles for insured employees and Medicare recipients, changing eligibility requirements for Medicaid, encouraging alternative delivery systems, emphasizing prevention, and using generic drugs.

Health Care Reform in the United States

▶ The Affordable Care Act (ACA) includes several measures that fundamentally change the health care system in the United States, including greater support for prevention, wellness, and public health activities.

▶ Practice guidelines or protocols enhance the quality, efficiency, and effectiveness of health care delivery. Nutrition protocols serve as frameworks to help practitioners in the assessment, development, and evaluation of nutrition interventions.

Future Changes in Health Care

▶ The challenge for the next decade is to change health care from a system based on treatment of acute conditions to one based on disease prevention.

▶ Medical nutrition therapy is an integral component of cost-effective medical treatment. Community nutritionists need to educate the payers of health care about the value of including nutrition services in their policies.

SUMMARY **QUESTIONS**

1. What medical nutrition therapy services are currently provided by Medicare and Medicaid?
2. If you were hired to design the nutrition component of a "new" national health care plan, what would it look like?
3. Compare and contrast traditional health care systems and managed-care systems. What are the benefits and drawbacks of each?
4. What strategies are consumers using to preserve resources spent on health care services?
5. What factors are affecting health care costs in the United States?

INTERNET **RESOURCES**

Agency for Healthcare Research and Quality
www.ahrq.gov

America's Health Insurance Plans
www.ahip.org

American Association of Retired Persons
www.aarp.org

Academy of Nutrition and Dietetics
www.eatright.org
Updates on medical nutrition therapy information and resources.

Centers for Medicare and Medicaid Services
www.cms.gov

CDC's Office of Minority Health and Health Disparities
www.cdc.gov/minorityhealth

Department of Health and Human Services
www.hhs.gov

Health Pages
www.thehealthpages.com
Issues report cards on major managed-care plans.

Healthfinder
http://healthfinder.gov
Find health information from federal and state agencies.

The Joint Commission
www.jointcommission.org
The primary accreditation organization for hospitals.

Medicare
www.medicare.gov

National Committee for Quality Assurance
www.ncqa.org

National Institutes of Health
www.nih.gov

Office of Minority Health
http://minorityhealth.hhs.gov

Social Security Administration
www.ssa.gov

Community Nutritionists in Action:
Delivering Programs

Serena M. sits on the edge of her bed and surveys the baby things spread around the room. A pearly white crib stands near the window on her left, and an old chest of drawers, newly painted yellow, fills the space on her right. On the floor next to her husband's crumpled jeans and T-shirt are a stuffed rabbit, a stack of disposable diapers, two rubber squeeze toys, a box of Q-tips, and an airplane mobile still in its box. She wonders whether she has everything she needs for the new baby—her first— due in just a few weeks.

Serena is excited about this change in her life and a little scared, too. Money is tight. She and her husband, Todd, live with his parents because they cannot afford their own apartment. They can't even afford a car, which is why Todd works at the auto body shop just four blocks over. She tries not to let her fear show, even though she frets daily about life with her in-laws and the prospect of being a mother. "I'm nearly 17," Serena says to herself. "My mother was about this age when she had my brother." As she gets up to take clothes out of the dryer, she wonders whether her mother ever felt scared, anxious, and alone.

Here is a young woman, in many respects a child herself, who is expecting her first baby. Does she know how to care for an infant? Is the family's income sufficient to cover the costs of providing for a child? Does this family need food assistance? Is there a way for this young woman to have her baby and continue in school? Is Serena eating properly during her pregnancy? Does she plan to breastfeed the baby? How can the health and nutritional outcome for this baby and its mother be improved?

This real-life scenario reflects the many activities undertaken by community nutritionists: identifying a nutritional problem in the community (a significant number of pregnant teenagers give birth to low-birthweight infants), selecting a target population (low-income pregnant teenagers), asking questions about why the problem developed (What do pregnant teenagers know about nutrition during pregnancy? Do pregnant teenagers use health services for prenatal counseling?), and figuring out how best to address the problem (programs that promote prenatal counseling and breastfeeding and enhance parenting skills among teenagers). The desired outcome is ultimately to reduce the number of low-birthweight babies born to teenagers and to improve infant health.

This section reviews the major food assistance and nutrition programs of the federal government and other noteworthy community-based programs. These programs help "protect" people like Serena and her family from environmental and social conditions that place them at risk for disease and poor health. They offer some security to people who have little money to spend on food, and they help control the problems associated with malnutrition. Following an overview chapter on domestic food security, the section is divided along life-cycle stages, with chapters on mothers and infants, children and adolescents, and adults. A chapter on global food insecurity is included because this area is increasingly important in a shrinking global community.

We encourage you to draw on the material you have already learned as you study the chapters that follow. By now, you can appreciate the complexities of community needs assessment, program planning, national nutrition monitoring, policymaking, and health care delivery systems. As you review the programs described in these chapters, consider how you would change the delivery of community-based nutrition programs and the policies that influence them.

CHAPTER 10

Food Insecurity and the Food Assistance Programs

LEARNING **OBJECTIVES**

After you have read and studied this chapter, you will be able to:

- Communicate the current status of food security in the United States.

- Link current trends in food insecurity and poverty to current food security and hunger policy initiatives.

- Describe the purpose, status, and current issues related to the U.S. food assistance programs.

- Describe actions that individuals might take to eliminate food insecurity.

- Interpret barriers to community food security and set priorities for action.

This chapter addresses such issues as interdisciplinary relationships in the community setting; aspects of the nutrition care process in community settings; the role of the environment, food, nutrition, and lifestyle choices in community health promotion and disease prevention; legislative issues related to community nutrition, including food and nutrition programs in the community, food availability and access, and local/state/national food security policy; food and nutrition laws/regulations/policies; and aspects of the food system, which have been designated by the Accreditation Council for Education in Nutrition and Dietetics (ACEND) as Foundation Knowledge and Learning Outcomes for dietetics education.

CHAPTER **OUTLINE**

Something to think about...

"Everyone has the right to a standard of living adequate for the health and well-being of himself [herself] and his [her] family, including food, clothing, housing, and medical care and necessary social services, and the right to security in the event of unemployment, sickness, disability, widowhood, old age, or other lack of livelihood in circumstances beyond his [her] control."

—*The United Nations General Assembly's Universal Declaration of Human Rights, Adopted More Than 50 Years Ago*

For a complete list of references, please access the MindTap Reader within your MindTap course.

Introduction

Although problems of overnutrition—obesity, heart disease, diabetes, cancer, and others—plague society, not everyone shares these problems. People in developing nations and people in the less privileged parts of developed nations instead suffer the effects of undernutrition. Characterized by chronic debilitating food insecurity and malnutrition, undernutrition has been a problem throughout history, and despite numerous development and assistance programs, food insecurity and malnutrition are not disappearing. They can be found among people of all ages and ethnic backgrounds. Even so, these problems hit some groups harder than others. Severe forms of undernutrition are not characteristic of the United States, but the problem of households not being able to consistently access food persists.

Everyone has known the uncomfortable feeling of hunger pangs, which pass with the eating of the next meal. But many people know hunger more intimately because often a meal does not follow to quiet the signal. For them, hunger is a constant companion, bringing ceaseless discomfort and weakness—the continuous lack of food and nutrients. People who live with chronic hunger pangs may have too little food to eat or may not receive an adequate intake of nutrients from the foods available to them; either way, malnutrition ensues.[1] The conceptual model found in **Figure 10-1** shows the large number of interrelated factors associated with food insecurity and its outcomes.

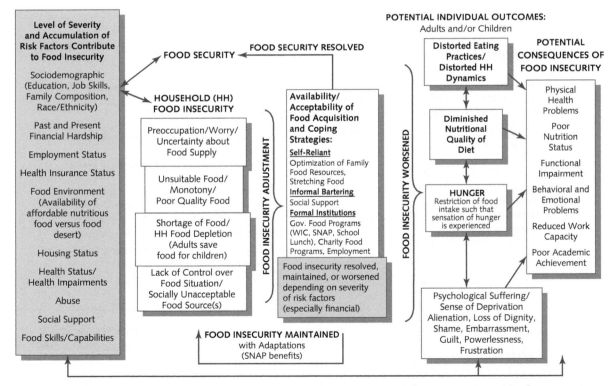

FIGURE 10-1 Conceptual Model of Factors Associated with Household (HH) Food Insecurity and Its Outcomes
The model describes the determinants and components of food insecurity, as well as the outcomes and consequences of food insecurity, which may be mediated by the availability and acceptability of various food-acquisition and coping strategies.
Source: Adapted from Katherine Alaimo, Ph.D., "Food Insecurity in the United States: An Overview," *Top. Clin. Nutr.* 20(4) (2005): 281–98.

Today this phenomenon is discussed in terms of **food security** or **food insecurity**.[2] Food security—access by all people at all times to enough food for an active, healthy life—is one of several conditions necessary for a population to be healthy and well nourished.[3] The concept of food security includes five components:[4]

- Quantity: Is there access to a sufficient quantity of food?
- Quality: Is food nutritionally adequate?
- Suitability: Is food culturally acceptable and the capacity for storage and preparation appropriate?
- Psychological: Do the type and quantity of food alleviate anxiety, lack of choice, and feelings of deprivation?
- Social: Are the methods of acquiring food socially acceptable?

A writer in Boston described food insecurity in more personal terms:[5]

> I've had no income and I've paid no rent for many months. My landlord let me stay. He felt sorry for me because I had no money. The Friday before Christmas he gave me $10. For days I have had nothing but water. I knew I needed food; I tried to go out but I was too weak to walk to the store. I felt as if I were dying. I saw the mailman and told him I thought I was starving. He brought me food and then he made some phone calls and that's when they began delivering these lunches. But I had already lost so much weight that five meals a week are not enough to keep me going.
>
> I just pray to God I can survive. I keep praying I have the will to save some of my food so I can divide it up and make it last. It's hard to save because I am so hungry that I want to eat it right away. On Friday, I held over two peas from the lunch. I ate one pea on Saturday morning. Then I got into bed with the taste of food in my mouth and I waited as long as I could. Later on in the day I ate the other pea.
>
> Today I saved the container that the mashed potatoes were in and tonight, before bed, I'll lick the sides of the container. When there are bones I keep them. I know this is going to be hard for you to believe and I am almost ashamed to tell you, but these days I boil the bones until they're soft and then I eat them. Today there were no bones.

The *Healthy People 2020* initiative set a goal of reducing food insecurity among U.S. households from 14.6% (2008) to 6% and, in so doing, reducing hunger by the end of the decade. This chapter examines the extent of food insecurity in the United States; Chapter 14 examines the incidence of food insecurity around the world. Both chapters offer suggestions for personal involvement with the issues presented. As you read, challenge yourself with the following question: What problems would you attack first in solving the problem of food insecurity? Although these issues are complex and often overwhelming from an individual's standpoint, the virtual elimination of food insecurity and the reduction of poverty are within our nation's reach.[6]

Counting the Food-Insecure in the United States

The United States is the world's biggest food exporter and one of the wealthiest nations on earth. Yet food insecurity persists, especially among the impoverished. In 2013, 14.5% of people in the United States (over 45.3 million people) lived in **poverty** (up from 12.5% in 2007); 20% of children under the age of 18 lived in poverty.[7] The poverty line was developed in 1963–1964 from the food budgets conceived by the U.S. Department of Agriculture for economically stressed families and considered the proportion of their

Food security Access by all people at all times to sufficient food for an active and healthy life. Food security includes at a minimum the ready availability of nutritionally adequate and safe foods and the ability to acquire them in socially acceptable ways (without resorting to emergency food sources, scavenging, stealing, or other coping strategies to meet basic food needs).

Food insecurity Limited or uncertain ability to acquire or consume an adequate quality or sufficient quantity of food in socially acceptable ways (e.g., not knowing where one's next meal is coming from constitutes food insecurity).

Poverty The state of having too little money to meet minimum needs for food, clothing, and shelter. As of 2015, the U.S. Department of Health and Human Services defined a poverty-level income as $24,250 annually for a family of four.

income spent on food.[8] This work became the basis for the current *poverty thresholds*—one of two slightly different versions of the federal poverty line—which are adjusted annually to reflect changes in the consumer price index for urban consumers. The poverty thresholds, which are the dollar amounts below which a family would be viewed as living in poverty, are used for calculating all official poverty population statistics (e.g., estimating the number of children and families in poverty each year). The food budget used in the poverty threshold calculation reflects a diet that is just barely adequate—one designed for short-term use when funds are extremely low.[9] Therefore, people with incomes below the poverty threshold undoubtedly have a difficult time buying nutritionally adequate foods even for a short-term, emergency diet.

The *poverty guidelines* are the other version of the federal poverty measure. The poverty guidelines are a simplified version of the poverty thresholds and are used for administrative purposes (e.g., determining eligibility for the Supplemental Nutrition Assistance Program [SNAP]). The Department of Health and Human Services issues the poverty guidelines each year based on the previous year's poverty thresholds.[10] The 2015 poverty guidelines are listed in **Table 10-1**. If you wanted to assess a person's income by comparing it with the "poverty line," you could use either the thresholds or the guidelines.

Despite their inadequacies, the official poverty guidelines define eligibility for many federal assistance programs; however, government aid programs do not have to use the official poverty measure as their eligibility criterion.[11] Individuals with incomes a certain amount above poverty are automatically ineligible for programs such as SNAP benefits or free and reduced-price school meals. Such criteria mean that some households are unable to participate in particular programs, which may prevent them from escaping poverty or improving food access (**Figure 10-2**).

Since 1995, the USDA has monitored food security through an annual survey of 50,000 to 60,000 households, conducted as a supplement to the U.S. Census Bureau's nationally representative Current Population Survey.[12] Households without children are asked

TABLE 10-1 Annual Poverty Guidelines, 2015[a]

HOUSEHOLD SIZE	POVERTY GUIDELINE[b] (100% POVERTY)[c]
1	$11,770
2	15,930
3	20,090
4	24,250
5	28,410
6	32,570
7	36,730
8	40,890

For each additional family member, add $4,160.

[a] The *poverty guidelines* are sometimes loosely referred to as the "federal poverty level" or "poverty line." Updates to the poverty guidelines can be found at *http://aspe.hhs.gov/poverty-guidelines*. The *poverty thresholds* are available on the Census Bureau website at *www.census.gov/hhes/www/poverty/data/threshld/index.html*.

[b] The poverty guideline for Alaska starts at $14,720 and rises by increments of $5,200, and that for Hawaii starts at $13,550 and rises by increments of $4,780.

[c] This table shows income levels equal to the poverty line (100% of the poverty line). Programs sometimes set program income eligibility at some point above the poverty line. For example, if a program sets income eligibility at 130% of the poverty guidelines, then the cutoff for a family of two living in the 48 contiguous states is $15,930 × 130% = $20,709.

Source: 2015 HHS Poverty Guidelines, *Federal Register*, 80 FR 3236, January 22, 2015, 3236–37. Available at *http://aspe.hhs.gov/2015-poverty-guidelines*.

Household Size	100% of Federal Poverty Guideline (Annual Income)	130% of Federal Poverty Guideline (Annual Income)	185% of Federal Poverty Guideline (Annual Income)
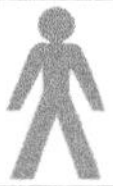 (1 person)	$11,770	$15,301	$21,775
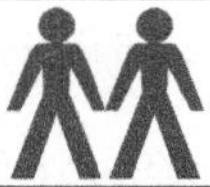 (2 people)	$15,930	$20,709	$29,471
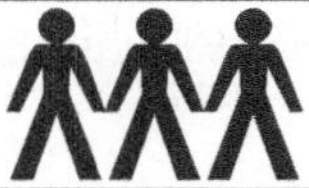 (3 people)	$20,090	$26,117	$37,167
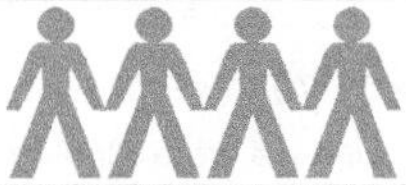 (4 people)	$24,250	$31,525	$44,863
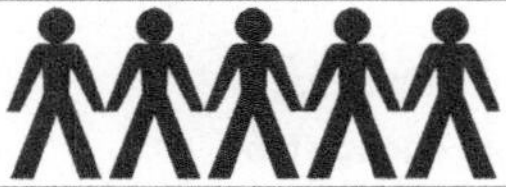 (5 people)	$28,410	$36,933	$52,559
For each additional family member add:	$4,160	$5,408	$7,696

* See Table 10-1 for poverty guidelines for Alaska and Hawaii.

FIGURE 10-2 Estimated Food Assistance Program Eligibility among Food-Insecure People
The majority of food-insecure households (57%) have incomes falling at or below 130% of the poverty guidelines, which is the federal income threshold for SNAP eligibility. An additional 17% of food-insecure households fall between 130 and 185% of the poverty guidelines. Although these households may not be eligible for SNAP, they may be eligible for WIC, The Emergency Food Assistance Program (TEFAP), or reduced-price meals through the National School Lunch Program (NSLP) and the School Breakfast Program (SBP). Twenty-six percent of food-insecure households report incomes greater than 185% of the poverty guideline, and thus are likely ineligible for any federal assistance, leaving the charitable sector as one of the few sources of food assistance that they receive.
Source: Adapted from Mapping the Meal Gap 2015: A Report on County and Congressional District Level Food Insecurity and County Food Cost in the United States in 2013 (Chicago: Feeding America, 2015), p. 16; and Income Eligibility Guidelines, *Federal Register* 80(61) (March 31, 2015).

a series of 10 questions; households with children are asked 18 questions (**Table 10-2**). The questions address such issues as:

- Fear and anxiety related to the insufficiency of the food budget to meet basic needs
- Experiencing food shortages without having the money to purchase more
- Perceived quality and quantity of food eaten by household members
- Atypical food usage (substituting fewer or cheaper foods)
- Episodes of reduced food intake, hunger, or weight loss by household members[13]

These questions reflect the different stages that households go through as food insecurity worsens—from worrying about running out of food to children missing meals for a whole day. A scale measuring the food security status of each household is calculated on the basis of the household's answers to the questions. This food security scale locates each household along a continuum extending from "high food security" at one end to "very low food

TABLE 10-2

Measuring Food Security: Questions from the Food Security Survey Module Used in the Current Population Survey and Other Surveys/Studies[a,b,d]

1. We worried whether our food would run out before we got money to buy more.

2. The food that we bought just didn't last, and we didn't have money to get more.

3. We couldn't afford to eat balanced meals.

4. In the last 12 months, did you or other adults in your household ever cut the size of your meals or skip meals because there wasn't enough money for food?

5. How often did this happen?[c]

6. In the last 12 months, did you ever eat less than you felt you should because there wasn't enough money for food?

7. In the last 12 months, were you ever hungry but didn't eat because there wasn't enough money for food?

8. In the last 12 months, did you lose weight because you didn't have enough money for food?

9. In the last 12 months, did you or other adults in your household ever not eat for a whole day because there wasn't enough money for food?

10. How often did this happen?[c]

(Questions 11–18 were asked only if the household included children age 0–17.)

11. We relied on only a few kinds of low-cost foods to feed our children because we were running out of money to buy food.

12. We couldn't feed our children a balanced meal because we couldn't afford that.

13. Our children were not eating enough because we just couldn't afford enough food.

14. In the last 12 months, did you ever cut the size of your children's meals because there wasn't enough money for food?

15. In the last 12 months, did any of the children ever skip meals because there wasn't enough money for food?

16. How often did this happen?[c]

17. In the last 12 months, were the children ever hungry but you just couldn't afford more food?

18. In the last 12 months, did any of the children ever not eat for a whole day because there wasn't enough money for food?

[a] The questionnaire for households with no children has 10 items (1–10).

[b] To score the questionnaire for a household with children, a "yes" response to 0 items is considered high food security; a "yes" response to any 1–2 items is marginal food security; 3–7 items, low food security; and 8–18 items, very low food security. For households with no children, a "yes" response to 0 items is considered high food security; 1–2 items, marginal food security; 3–5 items, low food security; and 6–10 items, very low food security.

[c] Counted as a "yes" if it occurred in three or more months during the previous year.

[d] USDA information should be accessed when formatting the food security questions for research or program evaluation.

Source: A. Coleman-Jensen, C. Gregory, and A. Singh, *Household Food Security in the United States in 2013* (ERR-173) (Alexandria, VA: U.S. Department of Agriculture, Economic Research Service, September 2014). For further information on measuring household food-security status, see G. Bickel and coauthors, *Guide to Measuring Household Food Security*, revised 2000 (Alexandria, VA: U.S. Department of Agriculture, Food and Nutrition Service, 2000).

security" at the other end, as shown in **Figure 10-3**. As defined in Figure 10-3, households with high or marginal food security are described as food-secure and those with low or very low food security are described as food-insecure.[14] **Figure 10-4** illustrates how households responded in 2013 to questions regarding food security.

If there are children in the household, the full set of 18 questions is used to identify food-insecure households, and a subset of the questions is used to identify those with food insecurity among children (see questions 11–18 in Table 10-2). Households with very low food security among children are those in which children's food intake has been reduced even further and children are hungry because of lack of financial resources.[15] In this case, adults' food intakes are typically also severely reduced.

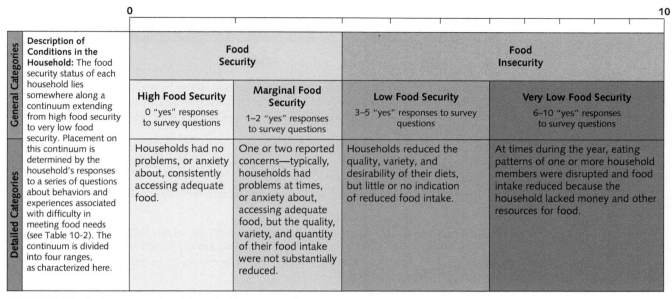

FIGURE 10-3 Household Food Security Measurement[a]

[a] To categorize a household with children, a "yes" response to 0 items is considered high food security; a "yes" to 1–2 items is considered marginal food security; a "yes" response to any 3–7 items is low food security; and 8–18 items, very low food security.

Source: Adapted from "Food Security in the United States: Definitions of Hunger and Food Security." *U.S. Department of Agriculture.* September 7, 2011; *www.ers.usda.gov/Briefing/FoodSecurity/labels.htm*.

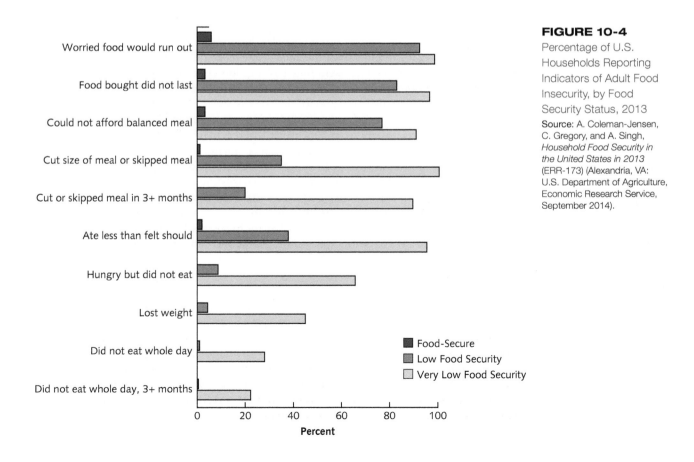

FIGURE 10-4

Percentage of U.S. Households Reporting Indicators of Adult Food Insecurity, by Food Security Status, 2013

Source: A. Coleman-Jensen, C. Gregory, and A. Singh, *Household Food Security in the United States in 2013* (ERR-173) (Alexandria, VA: U.S. Department of Agriculture, Economic Research Service, September 2014).

> ## A Glimpse at Mealtime in Households with Very Low Food Security
>
> U.S. households with very low food security reported:
>
> - 99% worried their food would run out before they got the money to buy more.
> - 98% reported that the food they purchased did not last and they had no money to get more.
> - 97% reported that an adult reduced the size of meals or skipped meals due to lack of money for food.
> - 94% could not afford to eat balanced meals.
> - 66% had been hungry but did not eat because they could not afford enough food.
> - 45% lost weight due to lack of money for food.
> - 29% reported an adult did not eat for a whole day because there was not enough money for food.
>
> Source: A. Coleman-Jensen, C. Gregory, and A. Singh, *Household Food Security in the United States in 2013* (ERR-173) (Alexandria, VA: U.S. Department of Agriculture, Economic Research Service, September 2014).

Who Are the Food-Insecure in the United States?

Over the past three decades, numerous studies on food security have been conducted throughout the United States, supporting the conclusion that food insecurity continues to be a serious and persistent problem that may lead to physical, social, and mental health problems, including overweight and obesity.[16] The number of people at risk of hunger increased by nearly 9.1 million since the 2008–2009 recession—from 36.2 million people in 2007 to 45.3 million people (including 14.7 million children) in 2013. This number represents 17.5 million households (approximately one in seven households) experiencing food insecurity—having difficulty providing enough food—because of lack of resources.[17] The increase in food insecurity mirrors the dramatic rise in unemployment, foreclosures, and economic distress present from 2007 to 2010 and evidenced in the increased demand for SNAP benefits and emergency food assistance during this period (**Figure 10-5**). For example, in 2009, **food pantry** use in suburban areas topped that in metropolitan areas for the first time since 2001.[18] **Figure 10-6** summarizes the trends in food insecurity in the United States from 1995 to 2013 and shows that food insecurity increased from 1999 to 2004 and then remained fairly steady until the recession, when it increased further. **Figure 10-7** shows the prevalence of food security measures in 2013. Poverty and food insecurity affect certain socioeconomic, geographical, and demographic groups more than others. As illustrated in **Figure 10-8**, the millions who experience food insecurity today in the United States include the following:

Food pantry Usually attached to existing nonprofit agencies, a food pantry distributes bags or boxes of groceries to people experiencing food emergencies. Distributed foods are prepared and consumed elsewhere. Pantries often require referrals or proof of need.

The Poor The most compelling single reason for this food insecurity is poverty. Between 40 and 50% of those who become poor live in a household where the head of the household, spouse, or other family member has lost his or her job.[19] Likewise, the majority of people leaving poverty do so because a family member gets a job or a pay raise. Over 40% of families with incomes below the federal poverty threshold were food-insecure in 2013. As noted in Figure 10-8, those living below the poverty threshold experienced food insecurity at nearly three times the national average of 14.3%. With an income of 130% and 185% of the poverty threshold—the income levels needed to qualify for several food

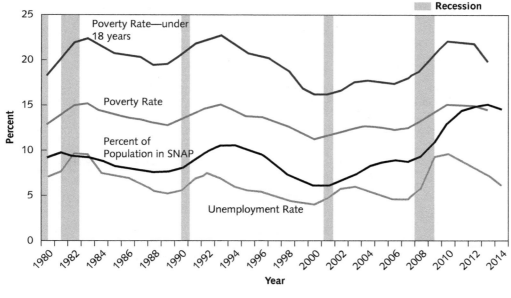

FIGURE 10-5
Percentage of
Population in SNAP
and Selected
Economic Indicators,
1980–2014

Note: Shaded bars indicate
recessions.

Source: V. Oliveira,
*The Food Assistance
Landscape: FY 2014
Annual Report* (EIB-137)
(U.S. Department of
Agriculture, Economic
Research Service, March
2015); data from USDA,
Food and Nutrition Service,
U.S. Department of Labor,
U.S. Bureau of Labor Sta-
tistics, U.S. Department
of Commerce, and U.S.
Census Bureau.

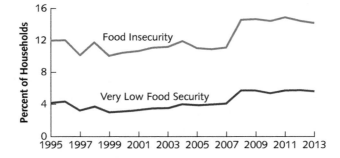

FIGURE 10-6 Trends
in Food Insecurity and
Very Low Food Security
in U.S. Households,
1995–2013
Food insecurity (including
low and very low food
security) in the United
States steadily increased
from 1999 to 2004,
declined in 2005, and rose
again in 2007.

Source: Prepared by ERS
(Economic Research Service)
using Current Population Sur-
vey Food Security Supplement
data; A. Coleman-Jensen,
C. Gregory, and A. Singh,
*Household Food Security in
the United States in 2013*
(ERR-173) (Alexandria, VA:
U.S. Department of Agricul-
ture, Economic Research
Service, September 2014).

assistance programs in the United States, the rate of food insecurity was still more than twice as high as the national average.

The Working Poor A job that pays the minimum wage does not lift a family above the federal poverty threshold, and many such jobs fail to provide fringe benefits to help meet rising health care costs. Many women live in poverty, struggling to provide childcare while working for the minimum wage. Of single-parent households, 35% headed by a single mother were food-insecure in 2013, as were 25% of those headed by a single father.[20] Additionally, the recent recession has contributed to significant declines in employer-sponsored health insurance coverage, as a high unemployment rate and increases in the number of individuals living below poverty have put employer-sponsored health care coverage out of reach for many individuals. States differ in the minimum wage they allow, but the federal minimum wage is $7.25 per hour.[21] Some states that require hourly rates greater than the federal minimum wage recognize that the minimum wage, even at 40 hours per week, is insufficient for a family's survival needs.[22] Consider the hypothetical budget scenario shown on page 379.

U.S. Households by Food Security Status, 2013

FIGURE 10-7

Prevalence of Food Security and Food Insecurity in U.S. Adult Households and in Households with Children, 2013

Source: A. Coleman-Jensen, C. Gregory, and A. Singh, *Household Food Security in the United States in 2013* (ERR-173) (Alexandria, VA: U.S. Department of Agriculture, Economic Research Service, September 2014).

U.S. Households by Food Security Status, 2013

Food-Secure Households—85.7%

Food-Insecure Households—14.3%
Households with Low Food Security—8.7%
Households with Very Low Food Security—5.6%

U.S. Households with Children by Food Security Status of Adults and Children, 2013

Food-Secure Households 80.5%

Food-Insecure Households—19.5%
Food Insecurity among Adults only in Households with Children—9.6%
Food-Insecure, Children and Adults—9.9%
Low Food Security among Children—9.0%
Very Low Food Security among Children—0.9%

FIGURE 10-8

Prevalence of Food-Insecurity Status by Selected Household Characteristics, Before and After the Great Recession

[a] Income below poverty threshold.

[b] Income < 130% of poverty threshold.

[c] Income < 185% of poverty threshold.

[d] Income ≥ 185% of poverty threshold.

Source: A. Coleman-Jensen, C. Gregory, and A. Singh, *Household Food Security in the United States in 2013* (ERR-173) (Alexandria, VA: U.S. Department of Agriculture, Economic Research Service, September 2014).

Category	Subcategories		2001–2007 Pre-Recession Average Food-Insecure	2008–2013 Post-Recession Average Food-Insecure
All Households	–	–	11.13	14.58
Household Composition	With children < 18 years	–	16.27	20.43
		With children < 6 years	17.39	21.72
		Married-couple families	10.57	13.78
		Female head, no spouse	31.43	35.92
		Male head, no spouse	19.23	25.40
		Other household with child	17.66	26.12
	With no children < 18 years	–	8.37	11.73
		More than one adult	6.50	9.63
		Women living alone	10.87	14.90
		Men living alone	11.27	14.72
	With older adult	–	6.11	8.23
		Older adult living alone	6.66	8.58
Race/Ethnicity of Household	White non-Hispanic	–	7.99	10.95
	Black non-Hispanic	–	22.21	25.25
	Hispanic	–	20.71	25.53
	Other	–	10.11	12.83
Household Income-to-Poverty Ratio	Under 1.00[a]	–	36.64	41.58
	Under 1.30[b]	–	33.29	38.50
	Under 1.85[c]	–	28.54	34.35
	1.85 and over[d]	–	5.19	7.20
	Income unknown	–	7.26	9.63
Area of Residence	Inside metropolitan area	–	10.97	14.55
		In principal cities	14.10	17.20
		Not in principal cities	8.83	12.75
	Outside metropolitan	–	11.93	14.85
Census Geographic Region	–	Northeast	9.33	12.53
		Midwest	10.27	13.75
		South	12.36	15.92
		West	11.60	14.90
			0 20 40 Average (%)	0 20 40 Average (%)

Of the 77.2 million hourly paid workers in the United States 16 years and older, 3 million workers earn at or below the minimum wage, with workers in service, sales, and office occupations leading the pack of those earning at or below the minimum wage.[23] Not surprisingly, 36% of emergency food recipient households (those served in soup kitchens, food pantries, and shelters) had at least one adult working in 2014.[24]

The Young Over 14.7 million children lived in food-insecure households in 2013; in fact, 20% of the households surveyed with children experienced food insecurity.[25] Not all persons living in food-insecure households experience food insecurity, however. In fact, children are typically protected by the adults in the households. As previously discussed, using a subset of the questions summarized in Table 10-2 (questions 11–18), the prevalence of households classified as "very low food security among children" can be measured.[26] In 2013, about 1% of children in the nation, or 765,000 children, lived in households with very low food security.[27] Research shows that children living in food-insecure households have poorer health, even after controlling for confounding factors such as poverty. A child's growth, cognitive development, academic achievement, and physical and emotional health are negatively affected by living in a family that does not have enough food to eat.[28] Additional forms of deprivation may accompany poverty, including poor housing, limited access to nutritious foods, and lack of adequate medical care.[29]

FOOD BUDGET EXERCISE[a]

Imagine that you are a single parent with three children. You take a job that pays $9 an hour (more than minimum wage), without benefits, in the fast-food industry. You work 40 hours per week for 52 weeks. Is your income above or below the poverty threshold (refer to Table 10-1)? After you subtract the monthly expenses shown here for rent, utilities, transportation, and childcare, how much money remains in your budget to feed yourself for one day?

1. Total number of household members ____**4**____
2. Monthly income $ ___**1,560**___ /month

Monthly expenses:
3. Rent (or mortgage) $ ____**725**____
4. Heat/electricity $ ____**150**____
5. Transportation $ ____**65**____
6. Phone $ ____**25**____
7. Childcare $ ____**475**____
8. TOTAL (add lines 3 through 8) $ ___**1,440**___

To calculate money for food for yourself for one day:
9. Monthly income   (line 2) $ _____
10. Total expenses   (minus line 8) $ _____
11. Money left over for food   (equals) $ _____
12. Divided by number of people in household   (divide by line 1) $ _____
13. Food money for one day   (divide by 30 days) $ _____

Money available for food for yourself, per day (line 13) $ _____

Calculations do not include emergencies, sick or vacation days, medical care, alimony, leisure, education, or other expenses, and it is assumed that the Earned Income Tax Credit would be approximately the same as the federal income tax, thus canceling out that cost.

[a] This exercise is meant to give you an idea of the difficulties of living on a low-wage budget.

Source: Hunger: A Picture of Washington, *www.childrensalliance.org*. Based on the Northwest Harvest website, *www.northwestharvest.org*.

Ethnic Minorities

Although the majority of the poor in the United States in 2013 were white, the median income of black and Hispanic households was lower than that of white households. The national data reveal marked disparity of hardship among racial and ethnic groups. Some demographic groups had greater food insecurity than the national average of 14.3% (see Figure 10-8). In 2013, the poverty rate was 10.6% for white individuals, 26.1% for black individuals, and 23.7% for Hispanic individuals (of any race).[30] Overall, non-Hispanic black and Mexican American children are more likely than non-Hispanic white children to be poor, food-insecure, and in poor health.[31]

Older Adults

Social Security and other programs have pulled many older people out of poverty, but large numbers of older people who cannot work and have no savings or families to turn to are facing rising bills for housing, utilities, food, and health care. In 2013, 9% of all Americans age 65 and over were poor; that is, they lived below the poverty threshold.[32] Although a lower proportion of households with older adults experience food insecurity than other groups, not all households with seniors are food-secure.[33] Low-income older adults often have health-related problems that necessitate special diets and costly drugs as part of their treatment, forcing many to choose between paying for rent, medication, and/or food. Food insecurity can prevent older adults from adhering to their recommended therapies, often with dire health consequences.[34]

Inner-City and Rural Dwellers

The prevalence of food insecurity in households in inner-city and rural areas exceeded that in suburbs and other metropolitan areas in 2013 (see Figure 10-8). A lack of adequate transportation and limited access to quality supermarkets can be problems for dwellers in low-income, inner-city communities, as well as for dwellers in remote rural areas. About 2.3 million households in the continental United States live more than a mile from a supermarket and do not have access to a vehicle.[35] Higher prices at small grocery stores and convenience stores compound the problem of limited access to healthy foods. Nutrition and consumer education may be one of the keys to improving household food-security status. One study showed that mothers from rural, low-income households using food and financial skills (including managing bills, making a budget, stretching groceries, and preparing meals) tended to have food-secure households, compared to mothers who used fewer of these types of skills.[36] Having a garden also appears to be positively related to the household food-security status of some rural families.[37]

Certain Southern and Western States

Percentages of food insecurity vary from state to state and, for 2011–2013, ranged from 8.7% in North Dakota to 21.2% in Arkansas. Very low food security also varied and ranged from 3.1% in North Dakota to 8.4% in Arkansas.[38] States in the Northeast, Midwest, and West had lower levels of food insecurity, whereas those in the South generally had higher-than-average rates (**Figure 10-9**).[39]

Many Farmers

Changes in the domestic economy have caused problems for producers as well as for consumers.[40] U.S. farmers today lack significant control over the products they produce, the prices they must pay for supplies, and the prices they receive for their commodities. While the costs for seed, fertilizer, equipment, and loans have steadily risen, crop prices have declined. Today, thousands of U.S. farmers are hungry, frustrated, and desperate about their debt. The number of hungry farm families is not known, but agencies that provide aid to the rural poor say the demand for food assistance is increasing.

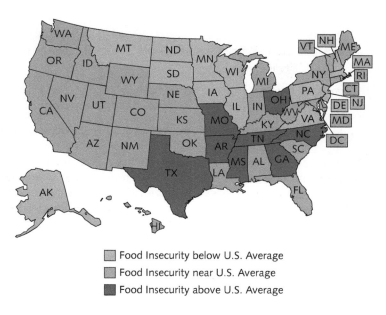

FIGURE 10-9

Prevalence of Food Insecurity and Hunger by State, Average 2011–2013

Source: A. Coleman-Jensen, C. Gregory, and A. Singh, *Household Food Security in the United States in 2013* (ERR-173) (Alexandria, VA: U.S. Department of Agriculture, Economic Research Service, September 2014).

☐ Food Insecurity below U.S. Average
☐ Food Insecurity near U.S. Average
■ Food Insecurity above U.S. Average

The Homeless The food-insecure are often faced with making choices between food and other necessities, including housing.[41] On any given night, almost 580,000 people were homeless in 2014.[42] About 110,000 people are chronically homeless—persons with severe disabilities and long homeless histories.[43] What characterizes the homeless?[44] A survey of 29 cities reported that about 26% of homeless adults were severely mentally ill, 16% were physically disabled, 15% were employed, 13% were victims of domestic violence, 13% were veterans, and 4% were HIV-positive. About 20% of homeless persons needing assistance did not receive it due to lack of resources. Among households with children, unemployment led the list of causes of homelessness. This was followed by lack of affordable housing and by poverty. Unemployment also led the list of causes of homelessness among individuals without children, followed by lack of affordable housing, mental illness and the lack of needed services, and substance abuse and the lack of needed services. Since 2008, the housing problems of Americans are making headlines across the country. With evictions and foreclosures on the rise, the housing wage—that is, the hourly wage that must be earned for a 40-hour work week in order to afford a two-bedroom housing unit (**Figure 10-10**)[45]—will undoubtedly continue to be a problem for many Americans. It is not surprising that lacking affordable housing and earning insufficient income are two of the factors cited most often as contributing to homelessness.

The majority of the survey cities have adopted policies or implemented programs aimed at preventing homelessness among households that have lost, or may lose, their homes to foreclosure. Several of the cities describe initiatives undertaken through the federal Homelessness Prevention and Rapid Re-Housing Program established under the American Recovery and Reinvestment Act in 2009. The top three actions needed to reduce homelessness, according to the city officials, were providing more mainstream assisted housing, more permanent supportive housing for people with disabilities, and an increase in higher-paying job opportunities.

Lack of food, inadequate diet, poor nutrition status, and nutrition-related health problems (stunted growth, failure to thrive, low-birthweight babies, infant mortality, anemia, and compromised immune systems) are problems among homeless persons.[46] Increasing numbers of people living with HIV are homeless because of the high costs of health care or lack of supportive housing.[47]

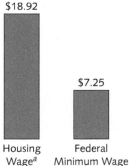

$18.92

$7.25

Housing Wage[a]   Federal Minimum Wage

FIGURE 10-10 The Gap between Affordable Housing and Low-Income Wages

[a] Hourly wage, at 40 hours per week, needed to afford U.S. median fair market rent (FMR) for a two-bedroom unit while spending no more than 30% of income on housing costs. Nationally, the average two-bedroom FMR for 2014 was $984.

Source: *Out of Reach, 2014* (Washington, D.C.: National Low Income Housing Coalition, 2014); available at *www.nlihc.org*.

Poverty Snapshots: A Look Inside the Everyday Lives of Five People Living in Poverty

It may appear to be one impossible choice after another—choosing between food and medicine, transportation to work, or paying the latest utility bill. However, for many, the government food assistance programs and charitable organizations help them move beyond poverty.

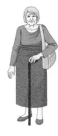

Rita, 82, lives outside a small town in a farming community. A widow for eight years, she loves her church and gardening in her vegetable patch. She and her husband were never able to save much, so she relies on Social Security for income. An unexpected bill—for health care, a new prescription, an unexpected home repair, or a high fuel bill—could be catastrophic for Rita. Rita is trying to manage her blood pressure and other health issues, but her health is failing. Medicare takes care of most of her health care expenses and prescription drugs, and is a vital support for her. Medicare, along with Social Security, helps keep millions of seniors from falling into poverty. Rita is less and less able to drive. Lack of transportation, especially in rural areas, can isolate seniors from support systems. Without services, they rely on a network of friends for everything from doctor visits to grocery shopping. Hunger is an issue for seniors. Rita is able to visit her church's food pantry, and it makes a big difference in her life—2.5 million households with seniors are food-insecure.

Estimated number of seniors in poverty: 4.2 million
Rita's annual income: $8,400
Single person over 65 poverty threshold: $11,354

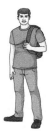

Carlos, 21, lives in the city with relatives, and has always dreamed of being a chef. After high school, he borrowed money for culinary school, but couldn't afford to finish. Today, Carlos is earning minimum wage at a fast-food restaurant, and is busy looking for a better-paying job to put him ahead of his student loan debt and other bills. Having his own car would give Carlos a greater capability to expand his search for work, but it's not in the cards right now. Public transportation is a vital lifeline for people in poverty. Payday loans for unexpected expenses are a short-term answer for many people in poverty. However, the costs and rates escalate quickly and become impossible to repay. New, fair options for micro-credit would help many people in poverty be able to repay their loans faster. A living wage will help many people work their way out of poverty. Today's federal minimum wage is $7.25, which yields $15,080 annually at 40 hours a week, but many low-wage workers like Carlos never reach this. Additionally, most low-wage work doesn't include vacation time or paid sick leave. The Supplemental Nutrition Assistance Program (SNAP) keeps millions of people out of poverty. More than one in seven people receive SNAP benefits. With these benefits, Carlos can save more of his income for housing and other expenses.

Carlos's annual income: $10,250
Single-person poverty threshold: $12,316

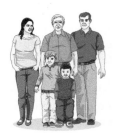

Marlene, 40, and her husband Rick live with their two sons and Marlene's dad in an apartment in a suburban Midwest community. Everybody helps, but Marlene and Rick have to work several part-time jobs to bring in a yearly income of $23,500. Marlene and Rick are typical of the "sandwich" generation; people with growing children and aging parents. Recently, Dad's diabetes has taken a turn for the worse and he can't help with supervision of the boys and homework as much as he did, not to mention his additional medical expenses. Marlene is wondering whether she will have to give up her day job so that she can take care of her father, which will drive them further into poverty. Both boys participate in the National School Lunch Program (NSLP), which ensures low-income children have access to at least one healthy meal daily, but the family struggles sometimes to put enough food on the table during the summer. Bryan and Rickie Jr. are smart kids, but they're at the age when they need attention and supervision. The family is starting to look ahead and wonder how they could possibly manage any college for the boys. Both Marlene and Rick have jobs. Rick works in a big-box store, and Marlene cleans hotel rooms during the day and office buildings at night. Many people under the poverty line do work. In 2014, 48 million people lived in low-income working families. Medical expenses for everyone in the family are a huge worry for Marlene and Rick. While Dad is eligible for Medicare, he still has out-of-pocket medical expenses, and Marlene and Rick are uninsured, a potentially catastrophic situation if either of the wage earners becomes too sick to work.

Marlene and Rick's annual income: $23,500
Family of five poverty threshold: $28,960

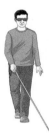

Jimmy, 35, has been legally blind since he was a boy. Like many people with disabilities, Jimmy is underemployed. He has a part-time job at the local service agency for the blind; however, they can only afford to give him a small stipend. He also receives government disability assistance. Jimmy has his own room at a house shared by three people with disabilities. Part of Jimmy's training at the agency involves daily living skills such as cooking and maintaining his own apartment that help him to live on his own. Jimmy is able to take public transportation to the agency for his daily work. However, the city is facing cutbacks, and schedules and routes will be affected. For many people with disabilities, transportation is one of the greatest challenges to employment. Adults with disabilities, whether physical or developmental, are chronically underemployed and live in poverty at twice the rate (28%) of adults without disabilities (12.5%). Many have more than one disability, which further hampers them from finding employment. Jimmy has received employment and skills training, and now uses a cane effectively to find his way around his work, apartment, and neighborhood. His goal is to be fully productive, without having to rely on assistance.

Jimmy's annual income: $5,000
Government assistance (SSDI): $6,500
Single-person poverty threshold: $12,316

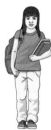

Mia is 10 years old and lives with her mom in the city. Her mom works as a cashier at the corner discount store, without benefits. During hard times, Mom's hours can be reduced, which can add up to hard choices for their little family. While Mia loves school, the real problem facing her mom is after-school daycare, which she can't afford, and how to take care of Mia in the summer when school is out. With the federal minimum wage at $7.25 an hour, Mia's mom can make about $15,080 a year working 40 hours a week. Unfortunately, that's still below the poverty threshold for a family of two. Today in the United States, more than 14.7 million (about 20%) of children live in poverty. Mia is on the waiting list to get into an after-school program that's expanding to a facility near her. The group offers homework help, activities, computer programs, mentoring, and health education. Without daycare, Mia has to get home to their apartment by herself, where she can do her homework and watch TV until Mom gets home. Mia is young for this. Generally the safe age for a so-called "latch-key kid" is considered to be 12. Mia's mom worries about her being alone, but can't afford the move to a safer neighborhood. There's a community garden down the street from Mia's apartment. The families in the area work together to grow fruits and vegetables (and some flowers, too). Sometimes Mia joins some friends from school and works in the garden, learning about fresh food. Every bit helps. According to the USDA, 8.6 million children live in food-insecure households. Federal food assistance—such as SNAP, the School Lunch Program, and Women, Infants, and Children (WIC)—help decrease the overall poverty rate and is one of the most effective antipoverty measures in the country.

Mia's mom's annual income: $15,080
Family of two poverty threshold: $16,317

Causes of Food Insecurity in the United States

Solving food insecurity and hunger in America is paramount.[48] Understanding the root causes of food insecurity, however, is necessary before a solution can be devised. Because poverty is the major cause of domestic food insecurity, reducing poverty in the United States is vital. Although a one-to-one relationship between poverty and food insecurity does not exist,[49] households with income below the poverty threshold have substantially higher rates of food insecurity than the national average.[50] Events that stress a household's budget, such as losing a job, gaining a household member, or losing SNAP benefits, often precipitate food insecurity.[51] Households must then make tough choices that compromise their ability to buy food, including having to choose between food and other necessities, such as utilities, heating fuel, rent or mortgage payment, and medicine or medical care.[52]

The U.S. Conference of Mayors–Sodexho Hunger and Homelessness Survey 2014, a 29-city survey on the need for emergency food assistance and homelessness in America's cities, revealed that the causes of hunger and food insecurity are many and interrelated.[53] The factor most frequently identified by the survey cities was unemployment, followed by poverty, low wages, and high housing and health care costs. Leading the list of actions recommended for reducing food insecurity was providing more affordable housing, followed by increasing SNAP benefits and providing more job-training programs.[54]

Considering the reports on food insecurity cited previously in this chapter, it appears that:

- Poverty is a chronic cause of food insecurity in the United States.
- The diets of households experiencing food insecurity are inadequate.
- Food insecurity can lead to physical, social, and mental health problems, including overweight and obesity (see the discussion on the next page about the paradox of hunger and obesity). Likewise, health problems, chronic disease, alcoholism, or substance abuse may precipitate an inability to purchase and prepare food, leading to food insecurity and hunger.
- Low-paying jobs result in incomes inadequate to meet the costs of housing, utilities, health care, and other fixed expenses; these items compete with and may take precedence over food, leading to food insecurity, which may be problematic among some ethnic minorities because they are overrepresented in the low-income population.
- Individuals stave off very low food security by using a variety of coping skills. Poor management of limited family resources may contribute to food insecurity. A lack of education and employment skills can make it difficult for individuals to exit poverty.
- Families and individuals rely on emergency food assistance facilities both in emergencies and as a steady source of food over long periods of time. However, insufficient community food resources are available to the hungry. Likewise, insufficient community transportation systems are linked to food insecurity.
- Individuals self-select to participate or not to participate in food assistance programs. The reluctance of some people, including older adults, to accept what they perceive as "welfare" or "charity" may delay their receiving SNAP benefits and other public/private assistance benefits, which may lead to hunger. Likewise, individuals and households may forgo seeking benefits because of intimidation, ineligibility, complicated paperwork, and other reasons.
- Private charity cannot solve the food insecurity problem. Voluntary activities may be limited in expertise, time, and resources.

Concern for food insecurity back in the 1930s and 1960s resulted in the creation of food assistance programs. Let us look first at how programs were developed to handle the problems of food insecurity and poverty in those times and then at how those programs are working now.

Historical Background of Food Assistance Programs

During the Great Depression of the 1930s, concern about the plight of farmers who were losing their farms and the widespread economic problems facing families in the United States led Congress to enact legislation giving the federal government the authority to buy and distribute excess food commodities. A few years later, Congress initiated an experimental Food Stamp Program to enable low-income people to buy food. Then, in

The Paradox of Food Insecurity and Obesity in America[1]

Hunger and food insecurity have been called America's "hidden crisis." At the same time, and apparently paradoxically, obesity has been declared an epidemic. Both obesity and food insecurity are serious public health problems, sometimes coexisting in the same families and the same individuals. Their coexistence sounds contradictory, but those with insufficient resources to purchase adequate food can still be overweight, for reasons that researchers now are beginning to understand.

The need to maximize caloric intake. Without adequate resources for food, families must make decisions to stretch their food money as far as possible and maximize the number of calories they can buy so that their members do not suffer from frequent hunger. Low-income families therefore may consume lower-cost foods with relatively higher levels of calories per dollar to stave off hunger when they lack the money or other resources (such as SNAP benefits) to purchase a more healthful balance of more nutritious foods.

The trade-off between food quantity and quality. Research on coping strategies among food-insecure households shows that, along the continuum of typical coping strategies, food quality is generally affected before the quantity of intake. Households reduce food spending by changing the quality or variety of food consumed before they reduce the quantity of food eaten.[2] As a result, although families may get enough food to avoid feeling hungry, they also may be poorly nourished because they cannot afford a consistently adequate diet that promotes health and averts obesity. In the short term, the stomach registers that it is full, not whether a meal was nutritious.

Overeating when food is available. In addition, obesity can be an adaptive response to periods when people are unable to get enough to eat. Research indicates that chronic ups and downs in food availability can cause people to eat more when food is available than they normally would.[3] When money or SNAP benefits are not available for food purchases during part of the month, for example, people may overeat on the days that food is available. Over time, this cycle can result in weight gain.[4] Research among food-insecure families also shows that low-income mothers first sacrifice their own nutrition by restricting their food intake during periods of food insufficiency in order to protect their children from hunger.[5] This practice may result in eating more than is desirable when food is available, thereby contributing to obesity among poor women.

Sources: 1. This discussion is adapted from *The Paradox of Hunger and Obesity in America*, developed by Center on Hunger and Poverty and Food Research and Action Center (*http://frac.org*). 2. K. L. Radimer and coauthors, "Understanding Hunger and Developing Indicators to Assess It in Women and Children," *Journal of Nutrition Education* 24 (1992): 36S–45S. 3. J. Polivy, "Psychological Consequences of Food Restriction," *Journal of the American Dietetic Association* 96 (1996): 589–92. 4. M. S. Townsend and coauthors, "Food Insecurity Is Positively Related to Overweight in Women," *Journal of Nutrition* 131 (2001): 1738–45.5. K. L. Radimer and coauthors, 1992.

1946, it passed the National School Lunch Act in response to testimony from the surgeon general that "70% of the boys who had poor nutrition 10 to 12 years ago were rejected by the draft." Despite these programs, in the 1960s large numbers of people were still going hungry in the United States, and some of them suffered seriously from malnutrition as a result.

As evidence accumulated during the 1960s and 1970s that hunger was prevalent in the United States, poverty and hunger became national priorities. Old programs were revised and new programs were developed in an attempt to prevent malnutrition in those people found to be at greatest risk. The Food Stamp Program was expanded to serve more people. School lunch and breakfast programs were enlarged to support children nutritionally while they learned. Feeding programs were started to reach senior citizens. To provide food and nutrition education during the years when nutrition has the most crucial impact on growth, development, and future health, a supplemental food and nutrition program (WIC) was established for low-income pregnant and breastfeeding women, infants, and children who were nutritionally at risk.

As a result of these efforts, hunger diminished as a serious problem for the United States. Several studies, including comparative observations made 10 years apart, documented the difference the food assistance programs had made.[55] In a baseline study in the late 1960s, a Field Foundation report stated,

> Wherever we went and wherever we looked we saw children in significant numbers who were hungry and sick, children for whom hunger is a daily fact of life, and sickness in many forms, an inevitability. The children we saw were . . . hungry, weak, apathetic . . . visibly and predictably losing their health, their energy, their spirits . . . suffering from hunger and disease, and . . . dying from them.

Ten years later, in 1977, the same group reported as follows:

> Our first and overwhelming impression is that there are far fewer grossly malnourished people in this country today than there were ten years ago. . . . This change does not appear to be due to an overall improvement in living standards or to a decrease in joblessness in those areas. . . . But in the area of food there is a difference. The Food Stamp Program, school lunch and breakfast programs, and the Women–Infant–Children programs have made the difference.

By 1973, the poverty rate in the United States had reached an all-time low of 11.1%. However, in the 1980s, federal spending for antipoverty programs was reduced in an attempt to reduce the national debt. Likewise, the Personal Responsibility and Work Opportunity Reconciliation Act of 1996 reduced federal spending on programs such as the Supplemental Nutrition Assistance Program that support needy families and children.[56] In 2013, the poverty rate was 14.5%, decreasing from 15.1% in 2010.[57] The national trends in poverty are shown in **Figure 10-11**.

Today, food insecurity affects all segments of the population without regard to age, marital status, previous employment or successes, family ties, or efforts to change the situation. Increasingly, national surveys show that food insecurity isn't just a problem for those who are homeless or unemployed. People who lack access to a variety of resources—not just food—are most at risk of food insecurity. Other causes cited in the surveys, in order of frequency, include unemployment, high housing costs, SNAP-benefit cuts, poverty or lack of income, economic downturn or weakening of the economy, utility costs, welfare reform, escalating health care costs, mental health problems, and the fact that available resources are failing to reach many groups.[58]

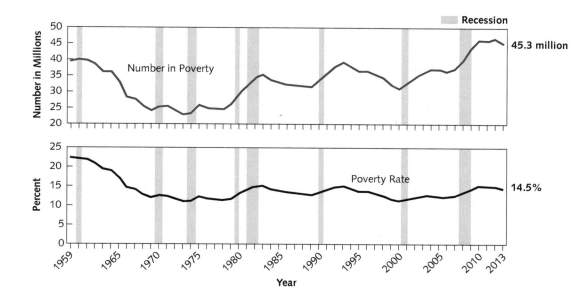

Welfare Reform: Issues in Moving from Welfare to Work

Welfare in the United States changed in the mid-1990s when the challenge to reform the welfare system resulted in the Personal Responsibility and Work Opportunity Reconciliation Act of 1996 (PRWORA).[59] **Table 10-3** summarizes key aspects of PRWORA. The challenge of the welfare reform legislation was to change the welfare system from an income-support-based system to a work-based system with a five-year time limit on benefits. This welfare reform law was intended to encourage self-sufficiency. It sought to promote personal responsibility by encouraging work, reducing nonmarital births, and strengthening and supporting marriage. It resulted in a decline in the numbers of those on welfare, a dramatic increase in employment of low-income mothers, increases in earnings by females heading low-income households, and a decline in child poverty.[60] The Department of Health and Human Services prepares an annual report to Congress on indicators and predictors of welfare dependence.[61]

As a result of the welfare reform law, the Temporary Assistance for Needy Families (TANF) Program replaced the former Aid to Families with Dependent Children (AFDC) Program. Under TANF, states determine the eligibility of needy families and the benefits and services those families will receive. The welfare reform law allows states greater flexibility in creating opportunities for job training and economic security for households with low incomes.[62] Single women with children are a major target group for job placement and training. Two critical issues for states to consider in their efforts to enhance the long-term successful placement of these women in jobs are transitional childcare assistance and the maintenance of health care benefits.[63]

Federal Domestic Nutrition Assistance Programs Today

The U.S. Department of Agriculture (USDA) has implemented an array of programs targeted at different populations with different nutritional needs to provide needy individuals with access to a more nutritious diet, to improve the eating habits of the nation's

FIGURE 10-11

Percentage of Total U.S. Population in Poverty

Note: Shaded bars indicate recessions.

Source: U.S. Census Bureau, Current Population Survey, 1960 to 2014 Annual Social and Economic Supplements.

TABLE 10-3 Key Provisions of the Personal Responsibility and Work Opportunity Reconciliation Act (PRWORA)

a A *block grant* is a grant from the federal government to states or local communities for broad purposes (e.g., community services or social services) as authorized by legislation.

Establishes Temporary Assistance for Needy Families (TANF) that:

• Replaces former entitlement programs with federal block grants*a*

• Shifts authority and responsibility for welfare programs from federal to state government

• Emphasizes moving from welfare to work through time limits and work requirements

Changes eligibility standards for Supplemental Security Income (SSI) child disability benefits:

• Denies benefits to certain formerly eligible children

• Changes eligibility rules for new applicants and eligibility redetermination

Requires states to enforce a strong child support program for collection of child support payments
Restricts aliens' eligibility for welfare and other public benefits:

• Denies illegal aliens most public benefits, except emergency medical services

• Restricts most legal aliens from receiving SNAP and SSI benefits until they become citizens or work for at least 10 years

• Allows states the option of providing federal cash assistance to legal aliens already in the country

• Restricts most new legal aliens from receiving federal cash assistance for five years

• Allows states the option of using state funds to provide cash assistance to nonqualifying aliens

Provides resources for foster care data systems and national child welfare study
Establishes a block grant to states to provide childcare for working parents
Alters eligibility criteria and benefits for child nutrition programs:

• Modifies reimbursement rates

• Makes families (including aliens) that are eligible for free public education also eligible for school meal benefits

Tightens national standards for Supplemental Nutrition Assistance Program (SNAP) benefits and commodity distribution:

• Institutes an across-the-board reduction in benefits

• Caps the standard deduction at fiscal year 1995 level

• Limits receipt of benefits to three months in every three years for childless, able-bodied adults aged 18–50 years unless working or in training

Source: Economic Research Service, U.S. Department of Agriculture, Food and Nutrition Assistance Programs: Welfare Reform and Food Assistance Briefing Room; *www.ers.usda.gov/briefing/foodnutritionassistance/gallery/keyprovisions.htm*.

children, and to help farmers in the United States by providing an outlet for the distribution of food purchased under farmer assistance authorities.[64] These programs, coupled with programs administered by other agencies, including the Departments of Health and Human Services and Homeland Security, are often referred to as a food or nutrition "safety net." Households with limited resources employ a variety of methods to help meet their food needs, including participating in one or more federal food assistance programs and/or obtaining food from emergency food providers in their community; in fact, about one in four Americans participate in a USDA food assistance program annually.[65] Current U.S. federal food assistance and nutrition education programs and initiatives are summarized in **Table 10-4**.

Food assistance programs are typically administered by federal agencies, and benefits are often delivered through state and local agencies such as welfare offices, schools, and public health clinics. The individual states determine most details regarding distribution of food benefits and eligibility of participants. In 2014, expenditures for the USDA Food

(Text discussion continued on page 394.)

TABLE 10-4 Federal Food and Nutrition Assistance and Nutrition Education-Related Programs and Initiatives

PROGRAM, YEAR STARTED, ADMINISTRATION,[a] AND PURPOSE(S)	TYPE OF ASSISTANCE PROVIDED	ELIGIBILITY REQUIREMENTS AND WEBSITE ADDRESS
SNAP and Related Education Program		
Supplemental Nutrition Assistance Program/ SNAP (formerly Food Stamp Program); 1961; USDA, Food and Nutrition Service (FNS) *Purpose(s):* Improve the diets of low-income households by increasing access to food/food-purchasing ability.	Direct payments in the form of electronic benefits transfer (EBT) redeemable at most retail food stores.	Household eligibility and allotments are based on household size, income, assets, housing costs, work requirements, and other factors. Online prescreening tool available on program website; *www.fns.usda.gov/snap*
SNAP Nutrition Education (SNAP-Ed, in some states called Family Nutrition Program); 1986; USDA, FNS *Purpose(s):* Increase the likelihood that those eligible for SNAP benefits will make healthful choices on a limited budget and choose active lifestyles consistent with the *Dietary Guidelines for Americans*.	Optional program, not offered in every state. States are reimbursed 50% by the USDA of the allowable administrative costs deemed necessary to operate the program. The National Institute of Food and Agriculture (NIFA) is the predominant sponsoring state agency, but state nutrition education networks, public health departments, welfare agencies, and other university academic centers are also sponsoring agencies.	Persons eligible to receive SNAP benefits; *https://snaped.fns.usda.gov*
Food Distribution Programs		
Commodity Supplemental Food Program (CSFP); 1969; USDA, FNS *Purpose(s):* Improve the health and nutrition status of low-income pregnant and breastfeeding women, other new mothers up to one year postpartum, infants, children up to age six, and older adults at least 60 years of age by supplementing their diets with nutritious USDA commodity foods.	Provides food and administrative funds to states.	Eligible persons must meet age and income requirements and must be determined to be at nutritional risk by a competent health professional at the local agency. (Eligible participants cannot participate in USDA's Special Supplemental Nutrition Program for Women, Infants, and Children [WIC] at the same time that they participate in CSFP); *www.fns.usda.gov/csfp/commodity-supplemental-food-program-csfp*
Food Distribution Program on Indian Reservations (FDPIR); 1976; USDA, FNS *Purpose(s):* Provide commodity foods and nutrition education to improve the dietary quality of low-income households, including older adults, living on Indian reservations, and of Native American families residing in designated areas near reservations.	Provides food and administrative funds to Indian tribal organizations and states.	Eligible households must have at least one person who is a member of a federally recognized tribe. Must meet income and resource criteria and be low-income American Indian or non-Indian households that reside on a reservation or in approved areas near a reservation or in Oklahoma. May not participate in the FDPIR and SNAP in the same month; *www.fns.usda.gov/fdpir/food-distribution-program-indian-reservations-fdpir*
The Emergency Food Assistance Program (TEFAP); 1981; USDA, FNS *Purpose(s):* Supplement the diets of low-income needy persons, including older adults, by providing them with emergency food and nutrition assistance.	Provides commodity foods to state distributing agencies, which are typically food banks, that then distribute foods to the public through soup kitchens and food pantries.	Needy individuals, usually including those who have low incomes, are unemployed, or receive welfare benefits; *www.fns.usda.gov/tefap/emergency-food-assistance-program-tefap*
Nutrition Services Incentive Program (NSIP); 1978; DHHS, Administration on Aging (AOA) (with financial support from USDA) *Purpose(s):* Provide incentives to states and tribes for the efficient delivery of nutritious meals to older adults.	Cash and/or commodities to agencies for meals served.	People 60 years of age or over and their spouses (or a younger age in tribes that define "older" adults differently). Disabled people under age 60 who live in older adult housing facilities where congregate meals are served; disabled persons who reside at home and accompany older adult participants to meals; and volunteers who assist in the meal service may also receive meals through NSIP; *www.fns.usda.gov/nsip/nutrition-services-incentive-program-home-page*

continued

TABLE 10-4 Federal Food and Nutrition Assistance and Nutrition Education-Related Programs and Initiatives—*continued*

PROGRAM, YEAR STARTED, ADMINISTRATION,[a] AND PURPOSE(S)	TYPE OF ASSISTANCE PROVIDED	ELIGIBILITY REQUIREMENTS AND WEBSITE ADDRESS
Commodity Foods; 1961; USDA, FNS *Purpose(s):* Support American agricultural producers by providing cash reimbursements for meals served in schools; provide nutritious, USDA-purchased food for the NSLP, CACFP, and SFSP.	Food commodities to eligible programs.	NSLP-participating schools or institutions participating in CACFP or SFSP are eligible to receive USDA-donated commodities; *www.fns.usda.gov/fdd/ frequently-asked-questionsfact-sheets*
Food Distribution Disaster Assistance (Food Assistance in Disaster Situations); 1977; USDA, FNS (Disaster Feeding Situations are administered by DHS's Federal Emergency Management Agency [FEMA].) *Purpose(s):* Supply food to disaster relief organizations such as the Red Cross and the Salvation Army for mass feeding or household distribution in a disaster situation, such as a storm, earthquake, civil disturbance, or flood.	Provides commodity foods for shelters and other mass feeding sites, distributes commodity food packages directly to households in need, and issues emergency SNAP benefits.	The USDA authorizes states to release commodity food stocks to disaster relief agencies for shelters and mass feeding sites; if the president declares a disaster, states can also, with USDA approval, distribute commodity foods directly to households (typically when normal commercial food supply channels have been disrupted, damaged, or destroyed or cannot function for some other reason); those who might not ordinarily qualify for SNAP may be eligible under the disaster food program if they have had disaster damage to their homes or expenses related to protecting their homes, if they have lost income as a result of the disaster, or if they have no access to bank accounts or other resources; those already participating in the regular SNAP may also be eligible for certain benefits under the disaster food program; each household's circumstances must be reviewed by the certification staff to determine eligibility; *www.fns.usda.gov/fd-disaster/ food-distribution-disaster-assistance*

Child Nutrition and Related Programs

National School Lunch Program (NSLP); 1946; USDA, FNS *Purpose(s):* Assist states in providing nutritious free or reduced-price lunches to eligible children.	Schools receive cash subsidies and USDA commodities for each meal served. (Meals must meet federal requirements.)	Public or nonprofit private schools of high school grade or under and public or nonprofit private residential childcare institutions may participate. Eligibility standards for children: All students attending schools where the program is provided may participate. Children from households with incomes at or below 130% of poverty guidelines are eligible for free meals. Children from households with incomes between 130 and 185% of the poverty guidelines are eligible for reduced-price meals. Children from households with incomes over 185% of the poverty guidelines pay full price, a price set by the school (foodservice operations must be nonprofit, however); *www.fns.usda.gov/ nslp/national-school-lunch-program-nslp*
Afterschool Snack Program in the NSLP; 1998; USDA, FNS *Purpose(s):* Assist school-based after-school educational or enrichment programs in providing healthful snacks to children through age 18; an expansion of the NSLP.	Available through NSLP. Schools receive cash subsidies for each snack served. Snacks must contain at least two different components of the following four: a serving of fluid milk; a serving of meat or meat alternative; a serving of vegetable(s) or fruit(s) or full-strength vegetable or fruit juice; a serving of whole-grain or enriched bread or cereal.	After-school snacks are provided to children on the same income eligibility basis as NSLP; however, programs that operate in areas where at least 50% of students are eligible for free or reduced-price meals serve all snacks free; *www.fns.usda.gov/school-meals/afterschool-snacks*

PROGRAM, YEAR STARTED, ADMINISTRATION,[a] AND PURPOSE(S)	TYPE OF ASSISTANCE PROVIDED	ELIGIBILITY REQUIREMENTS AND WEBSITE ADDRESS
School Breakfast Program; 1966; USDA, FNS *Purpose(s):* Assist states in providing nutritious breakfasts to children. Free and reduced-price meals must be offered to eligible children.	Schools and institutions receive cash subsidies for each meal served. (Meals must meet federal requirements.)	Public and nonprofit private schools and residential childcare institutions may participate. Operates in the same manner as NSLP; *www.fns.usda.gov/sbp/school-breakfast-program-sbp*
Special Milk Program; 1955; USDA, FNS *Purpose(s):* Encourage fluid milk consumption by children.	Schools receive reimbursement for milk served to children eligible for free milk and cash subsidies for each half-pint of milk sold. Pasteurized fluid types of unflavored or flavored fat-free or low-fat (1%) milk that meet state and local standards may be served. All milk should contain vitamins A and D at levels specified by the FDA.	Schools, childcare institutions, and eligible camps that do not participate in other federal meal service programs may participate; however, an institution may participate to provide milk to children in half-day prekindergarten and kindergarten programs where children do not have access to the school meal programs. Milk programs must be offered on a nonprofit basis. Any child from a family that meets income guidelines for NSLP free meals is eligible for free milk; *www.fns.usda.gov/smp/special-milk-program*
Summer Food Service Program (SFSP); 1968; USDA, FNS *Purpose(s):* Ensure that children in lower-income areas continue to receive nutritious meals during long school vacations, when they do not have access to school lunch or breakfast. All meals are served free to eligible children.	Approved sponsors receive reimbursement for serving meals that meet federal nutritional guidelines; payments are received through state agencies, based on the number of meals served and documented costs of running the program.	May be sponsored by organizations capable of managing a foodservice program: public or private nonprofit schools; units of local, municipal, county, tribal, or state government; private nonprofit organizations (including eligible emergency shelters); public or private nonprofit camps; and public or private nonprofit universities or colleges. Types of sites served include areas/programs with a majority of children eligible for free and reduced-price school meals, residential or day camps, migrant worker communities, and National Youth Sports Programs. All children 18 years of age or younger who come to an approved open site or to an eligible enrolled site may receive meals. At camps, only children who are eligible for free and reduced-price school meals may receive SFSP meals. People over age 18 who are enrolled in school programs for persons with disabilities may also receive meals; *www.fns.usda.gov/sfsp/summer-food-service-program-sfsp*
Child and Adult Care Food Program (CACFP); 1968; USDA, FNS *Purpose(s):* Improve the quality and affordability of daycare for low-income families by providing nutritious meals and snacks to children and to adults who receive care in nonresidential adult daycare centers, providing meals to children residing in homeless shelters, and providing snacks and suppers to youth participating in eligible after-school care programs.	Cash reimbursement for meals served that meet federal nutritional guidelines and reimbursement of associated administrative costs. (CACFP meal patterns vary by children's age and type of meal served.) Agricultural commodities or cash in lieu of commodities is also available.	Eligible institutions include public or private nonprofit childcare centers; outside-school-hours care centers; Head Start programs; some daycare homes; community-based programs that offer enrichment activities for at-risk children and teenagers after the regular school day ends; public or private nonprofit emergency shelters that provide residential and foodservices to homeless families; and public or private nonprofit adult daycare facilities that provide structured, comprehensive services to nonresidential adults who are functionally impaired or age 60 and older. Participant eligibility standards for free and reduced-price meals are the same as the NSLP; *www.fns.usda.gov/cacfp/child-and-adult-care-food-program*

continued

TABLE 10-4 Federal Food and Nutrition Assistance and Nutrition Education-Related Programs and Initiatives—*continued*

PROGRAM, YEAR STARTED, ADMINISTRATION,[a] AND PURPOSE(S)	TYPE OF ASSISTANCE PROVIDED	ELIGIBILITY REQUIREMENTS AND WEBSITE ADDRESS
Team Nutrition; 1995; USDA, FNS *Purpose(s):* Improve the health of children by having school meals reflect federal dietary guidelines.	Schools receive technical training and assistance to help school foodservice staff prepare healthful meals and provide nutrition education to help children understand the link between eating/physical activity and health.	Eligible schools include those who participate in school meal programs and other partners found in federal, state, and local programs, agencies, and organizations; *www.fns.usda.gov/tn/team-nutrition*
Fresh Fruit and Vegetable Program (FFVP); 2002; USDA, FNS *Purpose(s):* Introduce children to fresh fruits and vegetables. The Farm Security and Rural Investment Act of 2002 authorized the pilot program, and the Food, Conservation, and Energy Act of 2008 (Farm Bill) amended the Richard B. Russell National School Lunch Act by adding the Fresh Fruit and Vegetable Program, allowing for nationwide expansion of the program.	Provides fresh and dried fruits and fresh vegetables free to children nationwide in selected schools in 50 states, the District of Columbia, Guam, Puerto Rico, and the Virgin Islands.	Go to *www.fns.usda.gov/ffvp/ fresh-fruit-and-vegetable-program.*

Programs for Women and Young Children[b]

PROGRAM, YEAR STARTED, ADMINISTRATION,[a] AND PURPOSE(S)	TYPE OF ASSISTANCE PROVIDED	ELIGIBILITY REQUIREMENTS AND WEBSITE ADDRESS
Special Supplemental Nutrition Program for Women, Infants, and Children (WIC); 1972; USDA, FNS *Purpose(s):* Safeguard the health of low-income women, infants, and children up to age five who are at nutritional risk by providing nutritious foods to supplement diets, information on healthy eating, and referrals to health care.	Provides nutritious foods to supplement diets, nutrition education and counseling, and screening/referrals to other health, welfare, and social services.	Pregnant, breastfeeding, and postpartum women, infants up to one year of age, and children up to five years of age are eligible if they are individually determined by a qualified health professional to be in need of the special supplemental foods provided by the program because they are nutritionally at risk (having a medical-based or dietary-based condition), and if they meet an income standard (gross income at or below 185% of the poverty guidelines); *www.fns.usda.gov/wic*
WIC Farmers' Market Nutrition Program; 1992; USDA, FNS *Purpose(s):* Provide fresh, unprepared, locally grown fruits and vegetables to WIC recipients and expand the awareness, use of, and sales at farmers' markets.	FMNP coupons to purchase a variety of fresh, nutritious, unprepared, locally grown fruits, vegetables, and herbs. (Each state agency develops a list of the fresh fruits, vegetables, and herbs eligible for purchase.)	Eligibility is the same as WIC, but infants must be over four months of age (not operated in all states, territories, or tribal organizations); *www.fns.usda.gov/fmnp/ wic-farmers-market-nutrition-program-fmnp*
Head Start/Early Head Start (EHS); 1965/1994; DHHS, Administration for Children and Families *Purpose(s):* Increase the school readiness of young children in low-income households. Also, to promote healthy prenatal outcomes, enhance the development of infants and toddlers, and foster healthy family functioning.	Comprehensive, focused child development programs (including home-based programs) serve children from birth to age five, pregnant women, and their families. Health, education, nutrition, and social services are provided and are responsive and appropriate to each child's and family's heritage and experience; services encompass all aspects of a child's development and learning.	Eligible participants reside in households with incomes below the official poverty guidelines; *www.acf.hhs.gov/programs/ohs*

PROGRAM, YEAR STARTED, ADMINISTRATION,[a] AND PURPOSE(S)	TYPE OF ASSISTANCE PROVIDED	ELIGIBILITY REQUIREMENTS AND WEBSITE ADDRESS
Programs for Older Adults[b]		
Older Americans Nutrition Program, formerly known as the Elderly Nutrition Program (ENP); 1965; DHHS, AOA *Purpose(s):* Improve the dietary intakes and nutrition status of participating older adults and to offer them opportunities to form new friendships and create informal support networks.	Congregate and home-delivered meals and other nutrition services. Nutrition screening, assessment, education, and counseling to identify older adults' general and special nutritional needs; provided in a variety of settings, such as senior centers, schools, and individual homes. Meals served must provide at least one-third of recommended intakes established by the Food and Nutrition Board. Also provides an important link to other needed supportive in-home and community-based services (homemaker or home health aide services, transportation, fitness programs, and home repair and home modification programs).	Adults 60 years of age and older may participate. No means test for participation; however, services are targeted to older people with the greatest economic or social need, with special attention given to low-income minorities. Others who may receive services include a spouse of any age, disabled persons under age 60 who reside in housing facilities occupied primarily by older adults where congregate meals are served, disabled persons who reside at home and accompany older persons to meals, and nutrition service volunteers; *www.aoa.gov/AoA_Programs/HPW/Nutrition_Services/index.aspx*
Senior Farmers' Market Nutrition Program; 2001; USDA, FNS *Purpose(s):* Provide resources in the form of fresh, nutritious, unprepared, locally grown fruits, vegetables, and herbs from farmers' markets, roadside stands, and community-supported agriculture programs to low-income seniors; increase the domestic consumption of agricultural commodities by expanding or aiding in the expansion of these domestic agriculture programs; and develop or aid in the development of new and additional farmers' markets, roadside stands, and community-supported agriculture programs.	During the harvest season, coupons are provided that can be exchanged for eligible foods at farmers' markets, roadside stands, and community-supported agriculture programs. Fresh, nutritious, unprocessed fruits, vegetables, and fresh-cut herbs can be purchased; items not eligible for purchase include dried fruits and vegetables, potted fruit or vegetable plants, potted or dried herbs, wild rice, nuts of any kind, honey, maple syrup, cider, and molasses.	Older adults at least 60 years of age with incomes (generally) no more than 185% of the poverty guidelines; *www.fns.usda.gov/sfmnp/senior-farmers-market-nutrition-program-sfmnp*
Other Nutrition Education and Food/Nutrition-Related Programs		
The Expanded Food and Nutrition Education Program (EFNEP); 1968; USDA, National Institute of Food and Agriculture *Purpose(s):* Assist adults and youth with limited resources in acquiring the knowledge, skills, attitudes, and changed behavior necessary for nutritionally sound diets and to contribute to their personal development and the improvement of the total family diet and nutritional well-being.	Adults participate in a series of 10–12 or more lessons, often over several months, delivered by paraprofessionals and volunteers (trained by county extension educators), many of whom are indigenous to the target population, using a hands-on, learn-by-doing approach to imparting practical skills. Youth programs take various forms, including nutrition education at schools as an enrichment of the curriculum; in after-school care programs; and through 4-H EFNEP clubs, day camps, residential camps, community centers, neighborhood groups, and home gardening workshops. In addition to lessons on nutrition, food preparation, budgeting, and food safety, youth topics may also include fitness, avoidance of substance abuse, and other health-related topics.	Recruitment typically through referrals from neighborhood contacts and community agencies (such as SNAP and WIC); *http://nifa.usda.gov/program/expanded-food-and-nutrition-education-program-efnep*

[a] Programs are typically administered by federal agencies but often deliver benefits through state and local agencies such as welfare offices, schools, and public health clinics.

[b] SNAP and some food distribution and nutrition education–related programs/initiatives also serve women, infants, children, and older adults.

and Nutrition Service's food assistance programs were $103.6 billion—up from $33 billion in 1992 and $1.1 billion in 1969, the first year of the agency's operation (**Figure 10-12**).[66] Five programs—SNAP; the National School Lunch Program; the Special Supplemental Nutrition Program for Women, Infants, and Children (WIC); the School Breakfast Program; and the Child and Adult Care Food Program—together accounted for 96% of all federal expenditures for food assistance in 2014.[67]

Other food assistance programs and programs providing a nutrition component—the Nutrition Services Incentive Program, the Older Americans Nutrition Program, Head Start/Early Head Start—are administered by the Department of Health and Human Services (DHHS).[68] In addition, disaster feeding is administered by the Department

FIGURE 10-12 Food Program Costs, 1970–2013

About one in four Americans participates in at least one of the U.S. Department of Agriculture's (USDA) 15 domestic food and nutrition assistance programs at some point during the year. About three-quarters of USDA's annual budget goes to these programs, which vary by size, target population, and type of benefit provided. Together these programs form a nutritional safety net for millions of children and low-income adults.

[a] SNAP = Supplemental Nutrition Assistance Program.

[b] WIC = Special Supplemental Nutrition Program for Women, Infants, and Children.

Sources: V. Oliveira, *The Food Assistance Landscape: FY 2014 Annual Report* (EIB-137) (U.S. Department of Agriculture, Economic Research Service, March 2015); Fiscal 2016 Budget of the U.S. Government, as illustrated in "Policy Basics: Where Do Our Tax Dollars Go?," Center on Budget and Policy Priorities, 2015; *www.cbpp.org*.

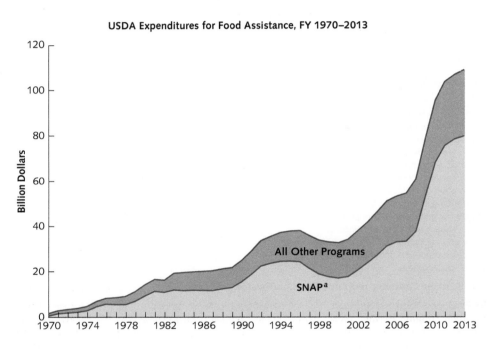

USDA Expenditures for Food Assistance, FY 1970–2013

Food and Nutrition Assistance Expenditures by Program, FY 2014

Expenditure for all food and nutrition assistance programs totaled $103.6 billion. SNAP[a] accounted for over two-thirds of food and nutrition assistance expenditures.

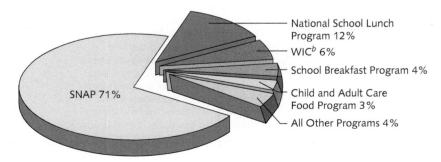

SNAP 71%

National School Lunch Program 12%

WIC[b] 6%

School Breakfast Program 4%

Child and Adult Care Food Program 3%

All Other Programs 4%

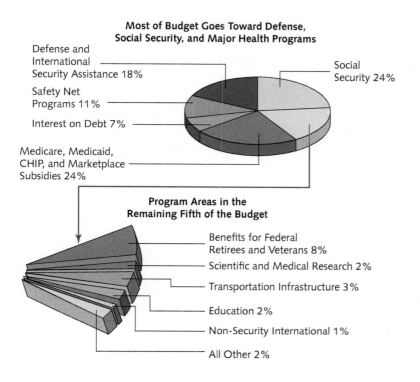

Most of Budget Goes Toward Defense, Social Security, and Major Health Programs

Defense and International Security Assistance 18%

Safety Net Programs 11%

Interest on Debt 7%

Medicare, Medicaid, CHIP, and Marketplace Subsidies 24%

Social Security 24%

Program Areas in the Remaining Fifth of the Budget

Benefits for Federal Retirees and Veterans 8%

Scientific and Medical Research 2%

Transportation Infrastructure 3%

Education 2%

Non-Security International 1%

All Other 2%

FIGURE 10-12

Food Program Costs, 1970–2013—*continued*

of Homeland Security (DHS). In addition to the information in Table 10-4, many food assistance programs are discussed in the sections that follow.

Supplemental Nutrition Assistance Program and Related Programs/Initiatives

Nutrition surveys in the United States have demonstrated consistently that the lower a family's income, the less adequate its nutrition status. Similarly, food insecurity negatively impacts the diet and health of individuals.[69] Improving food access and purchasing ability, as well as providing education to foster improved food choices within a limited budget, is one avenue to improving the diet and health of Americans.

Supplemental Nutrition Assistance Program (SNAP) The Food and Nutrition Act of 2008 established the Supplemental Nutrition Assistance Program (formerly the Food Stamp Program); however, the roots of this program date back to the food assistance programs of the Great Depression—a time when farmers were burdened with surplus crops they could not sell, while thousands stood in bread lines, waiting for something to eat.[70] To help both farmers and consumers, the government began distributing the surplus farm foods to hungry citizens. Milo Perkins, the first administrator of the program that preceded the current program by two decades, said, "We got a picture of a gorge, with farm surpluses on one cliff and under-nourished city folks with outstretched hands on the other. We set out to find a practical way to build a bridge across that chasm."[71] Today, SNAP enables recipients to buy approved food items at authorized food stores, with the goal of improving the diets of low-income households by increasing access to food and food-purchasing ability. The program

Feeding the hungry in the United States: then and now.

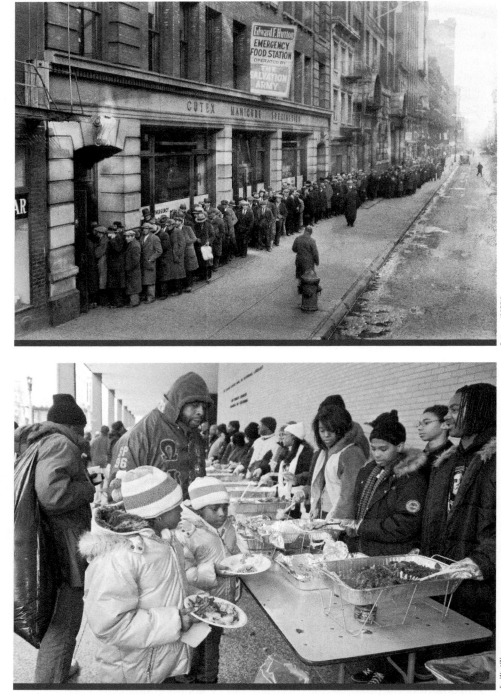

operates in the 50 states, the District of Columbia, some Indian tribe reservations, Guam, and the Virgin Islands.

During 2014, SNAP spending totaled $74 billion, 71% of all federal food assistance spending.[72] Average participation per month was 46.5 million people; one in seven Americans receives SNAP benefits. In 2015, monthly benefits averaged $134 per person per month.[73] Household characteristics give insight into the demographic and economic circumstances of households receiving SNAP:[74]

- 45% of all participants are children (18 or younger).
- 46% of all participants are adults (< age 60).
- 9% of all participants are older adults (age 60 or over).
- 75% of all benefits go to households that include a child, a disabled person, or an older adult.
- 33% of households with children are headed by a single parent, the overwhelming majority of which are headed by women.
- 40% of participants are white; 26% are African American, non-Hispanic; 10% are Hispanic; 2% are Asian; and 1% are Native American.

SNAP is an **entitlement program**, which means that anyone who meets eligibility standards is entitled to receive benefits. Eligibility and allotments are based on income, household size, assets, housing costs, work requirements, and other factors (see Table 10-4).[75] The program's website outlines eligibility standards, including current income guidelines.[76] In 2002, benefits were restored to adult legal immigrants—previously dropped from the program under welfare reform rules—who have been in the United States for at least five years and to all children of legal immigrants.[77] SNAP benefits are also available during disaster situations.[78]

Entitlement program
A government program that provides cash, commodities, or services to all qualifying low-income individuals or households.

In the past, state welfare or human services agencies gave households monthly allotments of coupons that were redeemable for food at authorized grocery stores. However, benefits are now issued in the form of electronic benefits on a debit card—known as the EBT card (electronic benefits transfer card). The EBT card acts in much the same way as a bank card to transfer funds from a SNAP recipient's account to a food retailer's account. With an EBT card, SNAP recipients purchase groceries without the use of paper coupons. EBT keeps an electronic record of all transactions and makes fraud easier to detect.

The amount of benefits that a household receives (called an *allotment*) varies according to its size and income (**Figure 10-13**).[79] Recipients may use the benefits to purchase food and seeds at stores authorized to accept them. They cannot buy food that will be eaten in the store, ready-to-eat hot foods, vitamins or medicines, pet foods, tobacco, cleaning items, alcohol, or nonfood items (except seeds and garden plants) with SNAP benefits.

Although the program potentially increases a household's ability to purchase nourishing foods, SNAP benefits may be used to buy most available human foods. Therefore, the effect of SNAP purchases on nutrient intakes of participants will vary depending on the nutritional composition of the foods they select. An optional program for states is SNAP-Ed, or Supplemental Nutrition Assistance Program Nutrition Education, which is intended to improve the likelihood that the program participants will make healthful choices within a limited budget and choose active lifestyles consistent with the *Dietary Guidelines for Americans*. Providers of SNAP-Ed vary by state, with the predominant agency providing

ENTREPRENEUR IN ACTION

As a community nutritionist, Shailja Mathur, MS, MEd, RDN, has provided leadership to nutrition education projects for New Jersey Supplemental Nutrition Assistance Program-Education (NJ SNAP-Ed) at the national, state, and county levels since 2001. Her typical day might include a morning session with elementary school students, presenting lessons on making healthy food choices; a stop at the Food Bank's Culinary School to talk about portion sizes; and an afternoon class at the Senior Center to introduce easy ways to incorporate physical activity into daily routines. She has been instrumental in expanding the NJ SNAP-Ed Support Network, a group of state agencies, private industries, and community-based, nonprofit, health, trade, and faith-based organizations that work cooperatively to ensure nutrition education for limited resource, at-risk families and individuals. Under her leadership, the Network has grown to over 200 partners across the state, allowing services to reach many more SNAP participants. As an enthusiastic educator, she hopes to continue to positively impact the lives of New Jersey residents. Find out what she has to say online at *www.cengagebrain.com*.

FIGURE 10-13 SNAP Allotments (2015)[a]

[a] The Supplemental Nutrition Assistance Program is currently authorized by the Food and Nutrition Act of 2008 (PL 110-246). Use the SNAP Map Machine to illustrate SNAP participation and benefit levels for a county, a state, or the nation. Go to *http://www.ers.usda.gov/ data-products/supplemental-nutrition-assistance-program-(snap)-data-system.aspx*.

[b] The SNAP Challenge gives nonparticipants a view of what life can be like for the millions of low-income Americans who live on about $4 per day worth of food—the average SNAP benefit. Take the Challenge at *http://frac.org/newsite/ wp-content/uploads/2009/09/ fsc_toolkit.pdf*.

[c] *Net income* is all the household's income that counts in figuring SNAP benefits minus the deductions for which the household is eligible. Most households may have up to $2,000 in countable resources (cash, bank accounts, stocks/ bonds, and so forth). House and property lot values are not included in this assets limit, and vehicles are in a special category. Households may have $3,000 if at least one person is age 60 years or older or is disabled.

[d] *Work requirements:* At the time of application and once every 12 months, all able-bodied household members between 18 and 60 years of age and 16- and 17-year-old heads of households who are not in school must register to work. Many adult recipients must participate in employment and training programs. Generally, able-bodied adults between 18 and 50 years of age who do not have any dependent children can get food stamps only for three months in a 36-month period if they do not work or participate in a workfare or employment and training program other than job search.

Source: U.S. Department of Agriculture, Office of Research and Analysis, Characteristics of SNAP Households, Center on Budget and Policy Priorities, 2015.

The amount of benefits the household gets is called an allotment. The net monthly income of the household is multiplied by 0.3, and the result is subtracted from the maximum allotment for the household size to find the household's allotment. This is because SNAP households are expected to spend about 30% of their resources on food.

People in Household	Maximum Monthly Allotment
1	$ 194
2	$ 357
3	$ 511
4	$ 649
5	$ 771
6	$ 925
7	$1,022
8	$1,169
Each additional person	$ 146

Benefit Computation[b]	Example
Multiply net income by 30%... (Round up)	$1,154 net monthly income x 0.3 = $346.20 (round up to $347)
Subtract 30% of net income[c] from the maximum allotment for the household size... (for example, a four-person household)[d]	$649 maximum allotment for 4 – $347 (30% of net income) = $302 **SNAP Allotment** for a full month

SNAP Benefits Are Modest

Average monthly SNAP benefit by demographic group

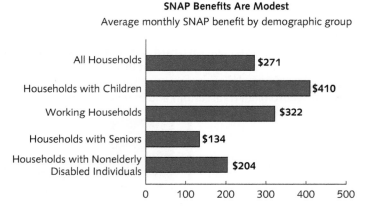

SNAP-Ed being the Cooperative Extension System (CES), supported by the National Institute of Food and Agriculture (NIFA).[80]

Two problems with SNAP are that benefit allotments are insufficient to meet needs and that environmental factors, including access to supermarkets and to high-quality, healthful foods, impact the dietary choices of participants.[81] Many households receiving SNAP benefits still need emergency food assistance by the end of the month because their benefits rarely last the entire month. In a study of 1,922 households, monthly food expenditures of SNAP participants—including cash, SNAP benefits, and WIC benefits—averaged just under 80% of the value of the food guide for low-income families known as the *Thrifty Food Plan*.[82] The Thrifty Food Plan (TFP) serves as a food guide for a nutritious diet at a minimal cost, is used as the basis for SNAP allotments, and is maintained by the USDA's Center for Nutrition Policy and Promotion. Results from national surveys have shown that only 12% of people purchasing food valued at 100% of the Thrifty Food Plan were eating nutritionally adequate diets, indicating that SNAP households spending only 80% of the value of the Thrifty Food Plan may be at nutritional risk.

Whereas SNAP participation tends to mirror economic conditions (see Figure 10-5), a second major problem is that many households who are eligible for SNAP and are in need do not participate. Approximately one in four people eligible for SNAP are not receiving benefits.[83] Potential reasons for nonparticipation include embarrassment about receiving assistance, complex rules and requirements, confusing paperwork, caseworker hostility, and lack of public information about eligibility requirements.

The USDA is trying to improve participation rates by those eligible through a number of outreach efforts targeted at low-participation groups, such as older adults and persons who are working poor, non-English-speaking, homeless, or living in rural areas. Outreach efforts include training community workers and volunteers to refer families to SNAP offices, community education and mass media campaigns, and individualized client assistance.

To improve SNAP's ability to meet the needs of low-income households, the following steps are recommended:[84]

- Improve and expand outreach about SNAP.
- Lower administrative barriers to participation in SNAP.
- Increase allotments so that families can afford to eat a nutritionally adequate diet throughout each month.
- Provide nutrition education materials to households that receive SNAP benefits.

Nutrition Assistance Program (NAP) in Puerto Rico, American Samoa, and the Commonwealth of the Northern Marianas Islands
Instead of SNAP, Puerto Rico, American Samoa, and the Commonwealth of the Northern Marianas Islands receive block grant funds that allow these United States territories to operate food assistance programs designed specifically for their low-income residents.* Through this program, eligible families receive benefits on an electronic benefits transfer (EBT) card to be used for the purchase of food. The Food Stamp Program in Puerto Rico was replaced in 1982 by the Nutrition Assistance Program. The same program was instituted in the Northern Marianas in 1982 and in American Samoa in 1994. Congress has begun to assess the feasibility and the potential impact of establishing SNAP (instead

▶ **THINK LIKE A COMMUNITY** NUTRITIONIST

The Supplemental Nutrition Assistance Program (SNAP) includes a component called SNAP-Education (or SNAP-Ed), which is focused on nutrition promotion and obesity prevention. This focus on both adult nutrition education as well as obesity prevention was established by the Healthy, Hunger-Free Kids Act of 2010 (Public Law 111-296), Section 241. Although program names and activities vary by state, a recent toolkit was developed by the USDA, Food and Nutrition Service (FNS), and National Collaborative on Childhood Obesity Research (NCCOR) to assist states in developing evidence-based policy, systems, and environmental approaches aimed at obesity prevention. Plans developed at the state level are intended to meet the particular needs of each state. The toolkit provides suggested strategies for intervening in a variety of settings, including childcare, school, communities, families, and social marketing/media, while indicating that comprehensive programs with multiple intervention mechanisms are more likely to be effective.

In this activity, you will review the toolkit (SNAP-Ed Strategies & Interventions: An Obesity Prevention Toolkit for States) and begin developing a plan for one suggested strategy.

1. Go to the toolkit available at *http://snap.nal.usda.gov/snap/SNAP-EdInterventionsToolkit.pdf*.
2. Select one of the five settings included in the toolkit.
3. Then select one nutrition strategy to intervene in your selected setting.
4. Imagine you are at the beginning stages of planning an intervention related to your chosen strategy. Address each of the following questions:

- Where would you start?
- What questions would you ask? To whom would you talk?
- With whom would you partner?
- What types of activities would you use?

To find out about SNAP-Ed activities in your state, visit *https://snap.nal.usda.gov/state-contacts*.

---

* A block grant is a grant from the federal government to states or local communities for broad purposes (e.g., maternal or child health or social services) as authorized by legislation. Recipients have great flexibility in distributing such funds as long as the basic purposes are fulfilled.

of providing funding through block grants) in Puerto Rico, including the administrative burden and costs to both the U.S. and Puerto Rican governments.[85]

Food Distribution Programs

Food distribution programs are another aspect of the U.S. national effort to improve access to food. Food distribution programs are intended to strengthen the nutrition safety net through commodity distribution and other nutrition assistance to low-income households, emergency feeding programs, Indian reservations, and older adults.[86]

Commodity Supplemental Food Program The Commodity Supplemental Food Program (CSFP) is a direct food distribution program. The CSFP was authorized by the Agriculture and Consumer Protection Act of 1973. It is intended to improve the health and nutrition status of low-income pregnant and breastfeeding women, other new mothers up to one-year postpartum, infants, children up to age six, and older adults at least 60 years of age by supplementing their diets with nutritious USDA commodity foods. Eligibility is reviewed in Table 10-4. Recipients may not participate in both WIC and CSFP. The commodities available vary from one year to another and are subject to market conditions. Food packages are designed to suit the nutritional needs of participants and may include a variety of foods, such as infant formula and cereal, nonfat dry and ultra-high-temperature fluid milk, juice, farina, oats, ready-to-eat cereal, rice, pasta, peanut butter, dried beans, canned meat or poultry or fish, and canned fruits and vegetables. Distribution sites make packages available on a monthly basis to participants, including more than 573,000 older adults and more than 19,000 women, infants, and children, with expenditures of $176.4 million in 2014.[87]

Food Distribution Program on Indian Reservations This program is intended to improve the dietary quality, through provision of commodity foods and nutrition education, of low-income households, including older adults, living on Indian reservations and of Native American families residing in designated areas near reservations or in Oklahoma. Currently, over 276 tribes are served through 100 Indian tribal organizations and five state agencies. Participants may select from a variety of products, including frozen ground beef, beef roast, canned meats, poultry, and fish; canned fruits, vegetables, beans, soups, and spaghetti sauce; pastas, cereals, rice, and other grains; cheese, egg mix, low-fat ultra-high-temperature milk, nonfat dry milk, and evaporated milk; flour, cornmeal, and crackers; dried beans and dehydrated potatoes; juices and dried fruit; and peanuts or peanut butter. On most reservations, participants can select fresh produce instead of canned fruits and vegetables. Nutrition counseling and classes, cooking classes, and tips for using and storing the commodities are among the nutrition education activities that can be provided as part of the program.[88] A Native American Nutrition Education Database is also available.[89]

Participants may choose from month to month whether they will participate in SNAP or the food distribution program. Many on Indian reservations prefer the food distribution program if they do not have easy access to grocery stores. Monthly participation in 2014 averaged more than 85,400 people, and expenditures were $104 million.[90]

The Emergency Food Assistance Program The Emergency Food Assistance Program (TEFAP) provides commodity foods to state distributing agencies, typically **food banks**, which then distribute foods to the public through **soup kitchens** and food pantries. This is not disaster relief. TEFAP reduces the level of government-held surplus commodities and supplements the diets of low-income needy persons, including older adults. Eligibility is summarized in Table 10-4. The types of foods vary with agricultural market

Food banks A nonprofit community organization that collects surplus commodities from the government and edible but often unmarketable foods from private industry for use by nonprofit charities, institutions, and feeding programs at nominal cost.

Soup kitchens A small feeding operation attached to an existing organization, such as a church, civic group, or nonprofit agency, that serves prepared meals that are consumed on-site. Soup kitchens generally do not require clients to prove need or show identification.

conditions. Foods typically available include canned and dried fruits, fruit juice, canned vegetables, meat, poultry, fish, rice, grits, cereal, dried egg mix, peanut butter, nonfat dried milk, and pasta products. In 2013, $311 million was appropriated for the program. In addition to these funds, TEFAP receives surplus commodities. In 2013, $229 million in such commodities was made available to the program.[91]

Nutrition Services Incentive Program (NSIP) The NSIP was established by the Older Americans Act in 1974 as the Nutrition Program for the Elderly in the United States Department of Agriculture. The NSIP was transferred to the Administration on Aging in 2003. NSIP provides grant funding to states, territories, and eligible tribal organizations that is used exclusively to purchase food and may not be used to pay for other nutrition-related services or for state or local administrative costs. States may choose to receive the grant as cash, USDA commodities, or a combination of cash and commodities. USDA also donates bonus foods to NSIP when feasible. This program provides incentives for efficient delivery of nutritious meals to older adults. NSIP costs were $180 million in 2013.[92]

Food Distribution Disaster Assistance This program provides food to state relief agencies and organizations (e.g., the Red Cross and the Salvation Army) in times of emergency such as civil disturbances, hurricanes, earthquakes, tornadoes, floods, and severe winter storms. FNS may provide commodity foods for distribution to shelters and mass feeding sites, distribute commodity food packages directly to persons in need, or approve issuance of emergency SNAP benefits. The program is administered by the Federal Emergency Management Agency (FEMA) in the Department of Homeland Security. Most disaster relief expenditures are provided through SNAP.[93]

Child Nutrition and Related Programs
Many federal programs address the special nutritional needs of children. The following sections describe the diversity of such programs. Table 10-4 highlights the programs below, as well as Team Nutrition and the Fresh Fruit and Vegetable Program. More about the Child Nutrition Programs appears in Chapter 12.

National School Lunch Program, School Breakfast Program The National School Lunch Program (NSLP) and the School Breakfast Program (SBP) assist schools in providing nutritious lunches and breakfasts, respectively, to children. The NSLP was authorized in 1946 by the National School Lunch Act (PL 79-396). The School Breakfast Program was authorized by the Child Nutrition Act of 1966 (PL 89-642). Participating schools get cash subsidies on the basis of the number of meals served and also receive food commodities through the NSLP. Program schools must serve meals that meet specified nutritional guidelines and must offer free or reduced-price meals to eligible students. These programs enable students in households with incomes at or below 130% of the poverty guidelines to receive meals at no cost and allow students from households with incomes between 130 and 185% of the poverty guidelines to receive a reduced-price meal. Children whose families participate in SNAP are automatically eligible for free school meals. Eligibility is summarized in Table 10-4. In 2012, more than 31.6 million children participated in the NSLP each school day (60% of all children attending a participating school or institution); 56% of these children received their meal free, and 10% received meals at a reduced price. Total cost of the NSLP was $11.6 billion in 2012. Approximately 12.9 million children participated in the School Breakfast Program each school day in 2012, at a total cost of $3.3 billion.[94]

Afterschool Snack Program School-based after-school programs can provide healthful snacks to children through age 18 via this expansion of the NSLP. Eligibility is summarized in Table 10-4. For 2012, the after-school snack program cost $169.7 million, up from $54 million in 2001.[95]

Special Milk Program The Special Milk Program (SMP) encourages fluid milk consumption by children by providing cash reimbursement for each half-pint of milk served to children in schools and childcare institutions that are not participating in the NSLP (see Table 10-4). Over 61 million half-pints of milk costing $12.3 million were served in 2012.[96] The SMP was incorporated into the Child Nutrition Act of 1966 (PL 89-642).

Summer Food Service Program for Children and Seamless Summer Option The Summer Food Service Program (SFSP) ensures that children in lower-income areas can continue to receive nutritious meals during long school vacations, when they do not have access to school lunch or breakfast. All meals are served free to eligible children. The SFSP was authorized in 1975 as an amendment to the National School Lunch Act (PL 94-105). The program operates in areas where half or more of the children are from households with incomes at or below 185% of the poverty guidelines or where half or more of the participants in a program are from households at that same income level. These are called "open" sites. "Migrant" sites primarily serve children of migrant workers, and "camp" sites offer foodservice as part of a residential or day camp. In the community, sponsors of the program include local schools or colleges, government units (e.g., parks and recreation departments), summer camps, community action agencies, and other non-profit organizations. The SFSP offers meals that meet the same nutritional standards as those provided by the NSLP at no cost to all children, up to age 18, who attend the program site (see Table 10-4). Over 2.3 million children participated in the SFSP in 2012 at 39,000 sites, with expenditures of $398 million.[97]

The Seamless Summer Option combines features of NSLP, SBP, and SFSP and eases the paperwork and administrative burden of schools in low-income areas in order to serve meals to children during traditional summer vacation periods and during long school vacation periods (year-round schools). Sites are similar to those of the SFSP.[98]

Child and Adult Care Food Program The Child and Adult Care Food Program (CACFP) is designed to help public and private nonresidential child and adult day-care programs provide nutritious meals for children up to age 12, older adults, and certain people with disabilities. The CACFP was permanently authorized in 1978 (PL 94-105). The 1987 amendments to the Older Americans Act authorized the Child Care Food Program to change its name and to expand its service to include older adults and persons with disabilities. Sponsors may also receive USDA commodity foods or cash in lieu of commodities. Eligibility guidelines are summarized in Table 10-4. Approximately 1.9 billion meals were served to 3.3 million children and 120,000 adults in 2013 at childcare centers, daycare homes, and adult care centers. Expenditures for this program totaled over $2.9 billion in 2013.[99]

Programs for Women and Young Children Many federal programs address the special nutritional needs of women and their young children. The following sections review some of these programs. Table 10-4 gives the highlights of the programs below, as well as those of Head Start and Early Head Start.

Special Supplemental Nutrition Program for Women, Infants, and Children (WIC) Congress created a pilot WIC project in 1972 (PL 92-433) and authorized WIC as a national program as part of the National School Lunch and Child Nutrition Act Amendments of 1975 (PL 94-105). WIC provides supplemental foods to infants, children up to age five, and pregnant, breastfeeding, and nonbreastfeeding post-partum women who qualify financially and are at nutritional risk. Financial eligibility is determined by income (at or below 185% of the poverty guidelines) or by participation in SNAP or Medicaid. Nutritional risks, determined by a health professional, may include one of three types: medically based risks (anemia, underweight, maternal age, history of high-risk pregnancies), diet-based risks (inadequate dietary pattern), or conditions that make the applicant predisposed to medically based or diet-based risks, such as alcoholism or drug addiction. Homelessness and migrancy are also considered nutritional risks for purposes of WIC.[100]

The WIC program serves both a remedial and a preventive role. Its services include:

- Checks or vouchers for supplemental foods rich in one or more of the following nutrients found to be lacking among WIC clients: protein, calcium, iron, vitamin A, and vitamin C (food packages or an electronic benefit card may be provided, rather than paper checks or vouchers; all WIC agencies are required to implement WIC electronic benefit transfer [EBT] statewide by October 1, 2020)[101]
- Nutrition education
- Referrals to health care services

In 2009, the WIC food packages changed to better meet participant nutritional needs by aligning with the *Dietary Guidelines for Americans* and infant feeding practice guidelines of the American Academy of Pediatrics. The foods in the packages are meant to supplement food intake and are intended to be consumed along with other wholesome foods needed for a balanced diet.[102]

Unlike most of the other food assistance programs, WIC is not an entitlement program. Of the 8.3 million people who received WIC benefits each month in 2014, approximately 4.32 million were children, 1.96 million were infants, and 1.97 million were women, with total expenditures of $6.2 billion. Women make up about 24% of participants, infants younger than one year make up 24%, and children one to four years make up 52%. The average monthly WIC food cost per person in 2014 was $43.65. Total expenditures for the program covered food benefits, nutrition services, and administrative funds, WIC Farmers' Market Nutrition Program, and other items in 2014.[103] More about WIC appears in Chapter 11.

WIC Farmers' Market Nutrition Program The WIC Farmers' Market Nutrition Program (FMNP) was created to accomplish two goals:

- Provide, from farmers' markets, fresh, nutritious, unprepared fruits and vegetables to low-income, at-risk women, infants, and children.
- Expand the awareness and use of farmers' markets and increase sales at such markets.

The FMNP was authorized in 1992 (PL 102-314) as a national program through an amendment to the Child Nutrition Act of 1966. In 2013, nearly 1.5 million WIC participants received benefits from this program at a cost of almost $20 million. In 2013, 46 state agencies offered the program, including Washington, D.C.; Guam; Puerto Rico; Indian tribal organizations; and many states. Eligible recipients are given coupons (not less than $10 but not more than $30 per year per participant) that can be used at authorized farmers' markets.[104] Coupons redeemed through the FMNP resulted in over $13.2 million in revenue to farmers in 2013.[105]

Programs for Older Adults Like people at other stages of the lifespan, older adults have unique needs. This section and Table 10-4 outline some of the programs designed to meet those needs.

Older Americans Nutrition Program The Congregate Meals Program and the Home-Delivered Meals Program were authorized by the Older Americans Act of 1965 (PL 89–73). The Older Americans Nutrition Program is intended to improve older people's nutrition status and enable them to avoid medical problems, continue living in communities of their choice, and stay out of institutions. Its specific goals are to provide:[106]

- Low-cost, nutritious meals
- Opportunities for social interaction
- Nutrition education and shopping assistance
- Counseling and referral to other social services
- Transportation services

One of the Title III efforts is the Congregate Meals Program. Administrators try to select sites for congregate meals that will attract as many eligible older adults as possible. Through the Home-Delivered Meals Program, meals are delivered to those who are homebound either permanently or temporarily. The home-delivery program ensures nutrition, but its recipients miss out on the social benefits of the congregate meal sites; every effort is made to persuade them to come to the shared meals if they can. The DHHS's Administration on Aging administers these programs.

All persons 60 years and older (and spouses of any age) are eligible to receive meals from these programs, regardless of their income level. Priority is given to those who are economically and socially needy. In 2010, total funding for the Title III congregate and home-delivered meal programs was almost $659 million (almost $218 million for home-delivered meal programs and over $441 million for congregate meal programs).[107] More about the Older Americans Nutrition Program appears in Chapter 13.

Senior Farmers' Market Nutrition Program (SFMNP) Under SFMNP, low-income older adults are provided with coupons (worth not less than $20 per year or more than $50 per year) that may be used to purchase fresh, unprepared, locally grown fruits, vegetables, and herbs at farmers' markets, roadside stands, and community-supported agriculture programs. Some programs may provide nutrition education or information to SFMNP participants through Cooperative Extension programs, local Area Agencies on Aging, local chefs, or other programs. In 2013, almost 835,795 older adults purchased products from over 20,617 farmers at 4,247 farmers' markets, as well as 3,083 roadside stands and more than 191 community-supported agriculture programs. In some areas, participants are provided with transportation to and from the markets by partnering with senior centers. Others have arranged to have local farmers transport their produce directly to senior housing locations. Table 10-4 lists eligibility guidelines. In 2013, $19.1 million was available to operate SFMNP in 52 state agencies, including many states, several Indian tribal organizations, Puerto Rico, and the District of Columbia.[108]

Filling In the Gaps to Strengthen the Food Resource Safety Net

Eight-year-old Jack dreams of becoming a doctor; Helen, a 69-year-old grandmother, dreams of seeing her first great-grandson turn 5; and Meg, a 26-year-old single mother, dreams of getting a college degree. These very different people have one thing in common. None of them ate dinner last night.

—Feeding America Annual Report

Despite all of the federal food assistance programs, emergency shelters and community food programs are straining to meet the rising requests for food. The public demand for emergency food assistance has increased in every region of the United States since 1980. The country has become a "soup kitchen society" to an extent unmatched since the breadlines of the Great Depression. The demand for emergency food assistance has increased steadily over the past three decades (**Figure 10-14**). One survey of 29 major cities indicated that in 2014, requests for emergency food assistance increased by an average of 7%, with 71% of the cities reporting an increase.[109] Much of the increased public demand for emergency food assistance is coming from the working poor and families with children, who report having to choose between food and other necessities, such as rent, utilities, or medicine.

The Rising Tide of Food Assistance Need

To help fill the gaps in the federal programs, concerned citizens are working through community programs and churches to provide meals to the hungry. **Feeding America**, the nation's largest supplier of surplus food, distributes over 4 billion pounds of food to 46,000 agencies operating some 58,000 food programs for direct distribution around the nation

Feeding America A national network hunger-relief organization to which the majority of food banks belong.

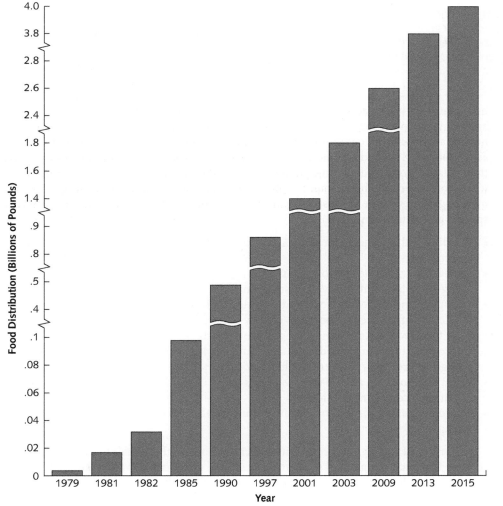

FIGURE 10-14

Demand for Emergency Food Assistance Donated foods distributed by the Feeding America network rose from 2.5 million pounds in 1979 to 100 million pounds in 1985 and to well over 860 million pounds in 1997. By 2015, Feeding America was collecting and distributing 4.0 billion pounds of food nationwide, reflecting the efforts of private organizations to cope with the public's demand for emergency food assistance.

Emergency foodservices:

• Soup kitchens

• Church charities

• Surplus food giveaways

• Food banks

• Food pantries

• Prepared and perishable food programs

Source: Adapted from Feeding America, *www.feedingamerica.org.*

Teri Underwood

**ENTREPRENEUR
IN ACTION**

As owner of Sustainable Diets, a nutrition counseling and education company, Teri Underwood, MS, RD, CD, counsels clients on a variety of nutrition issues. She also provides culinary services to restaurants and foodservice establishments, offers wellness programs, and teaches classes on nutrition, cooking, preventive health, gardening, and environmental nutrition. How did Teri incorporate environmental nutrition into her private practice? Says Teri: "Healthy Food, Healthy People, Healthy Planet, the tagline for the Sustainable Diets website, means that in order for us to be healthy—we must eat healthy food. To continue to grow healthy food—we need a healthy planet. It is all interconnected." Teri advanced her study of environmental health through years of volunteer work and leadership positions with local and regional environmental and nutrition organizations. She wrote and produced a weekly radio show called *The Environmental Update*. She is active in the Hunger and Environmental Nutrition (HEN) Dietetic Practice Group, which was the pivotal learning experience that launched her into work as an environmental nutritionist. Find out more about Teri at *www.cengagebrain.com*.

annually (**Figure 10-15**). An estimated 46.5 million people relied on food banks, soup kitchens, and other agencies for emergency food in 2013. Approximately 39% of those served are children and 8.4% are older adults.[110]

However, even the dramatic increases in the number of food banks, food pantries, soup kitchens, **prepared and perishable food programs (PPFPs)**, and other emergency food assistance programs cannot keep pace with the growing number of hungry people seeking food assistance.[111] It is estimated that on average, 27% of the requests for emergency food assistance go unmet.[112] Some facilities have had to decrease the number of bags of food provided and/or the number of times people can receive food. Moreover, each day's supply of meals lasts only for that day, leaving the problem of poverty unsolved.

Community Food Security: Enhancing Local Food Access

In an effort to reduce hunger, the USDA partnered with states, local municipalities, nonprofit groups, and the public sector to address **community food security**. The Professional Focus section of this chapter examines community food security, a relatively new concept with its roots in such disciplines as community nutrition, public health, nutrition education, sustainable agriculture, antihunger advocacy, and community development.[113] Community-based initiatives—such as farmers' markets and community gardens established on vacant city lots—can increase the availability of affordable, high-quality foods and serve to reconnect local farmers with urban consumers.[114] This chapter's Programs in Action feature describes a successful community garden venture in Wisconsin. The community food security initiatives focus on specific goals, including:[115]

Prepared and perishable food programs (PPFPs)
A nonprofit program that helps feed people in need by linking sources of unused, unserved cooked and fresh food—such as caterers, restaurants, hotel kitchens, and cafeterias—with social service agencies that serve meals to people who would otherwise go hungry.

Community food security
The development and enhancement of sustainable, community-based strategies to ensure that all persons in a community have access to culturally acceptable, nutritionally adequate food through local nonemergency sources at all times.

- Building and enhancing local infrastructures to reduce hunger and food insecurity in communities
- Increasing economic and job security for low-income people by helping people locate living-wage jobs and achieve self-sufficiency
- Strengthening the federal food and nutrition assistance safety net
- Bolstering supplemental food provided by nonprofit groups by assisting or developing local food recovery, gleaning, and donation efforts
- Improving community food production and marketing by aiding community projects that grow, process, and distribute food locally
- Boosting education and raising awareness about nutrition, food safety, and food security among community residents
- Improving research, monitoring, and evaluation efforts to help communities assess and strengthen food security

Examples of strategies and activities included under the label of community food security that fight hunger and strengthen local food systems are as follows:

- *Farmers' Markets.* Boost the income of small local farmers and increase consumers' access to fresh produce.

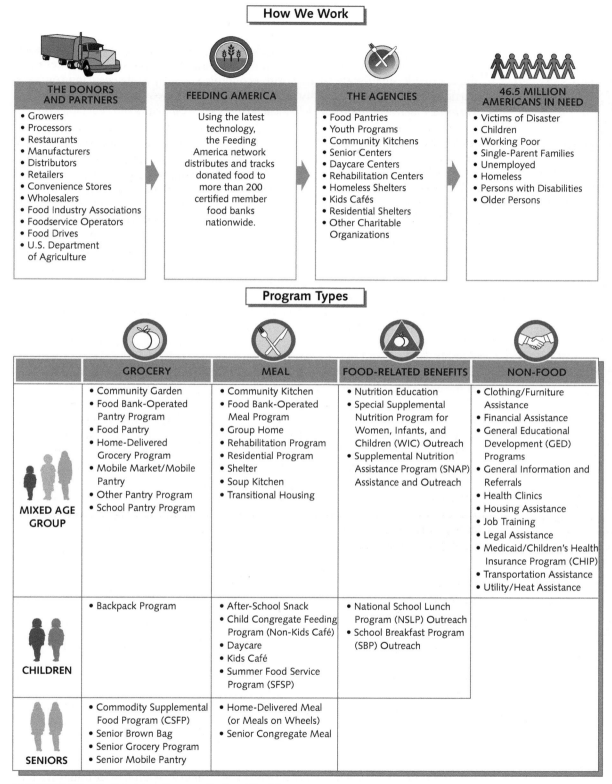

How We Work

THE DONORS AND PARTNERS	FEEDING AMERICA	THE AGENCIES	46.5 MILLION AMERICANS IN NEED
• Growers • Processors • Restaurants • Manufacturers • Distributors • Retailers • Convenience Stores • Wholesalers • Food Industry Associations • Foodservice Operators • Food Drives • U.S. Department of Agriculture	Using the latest technology, the Feeding America network distributes and tracks donated food to more than 200 certified member food banks nationwide.	• Food Pantries • Youth Programs • Community Kitchens • Senior Centers • Daycare Centers • Rehabilitation Centers • Homeless Shelters • Kids Cafés • Residential Shelters • Other Charitable Organizations	• Victims of Disaster • Children • Working Poor • Single-Parent Families • Unemployed • Homeless • Persons with Disabilities • Older Persons

Program Types

	GROCERY	MEAL	FOOD-RELATED BENEFITS	NON-FOOD
MIXED AGE GROUP	• Community Garden • Food Bank-Operated Pantry Program • Food Pantry • Home-Delivered Grocery Program • Mobile Market/Mobile Pantry • Other Pantry Program • School Pantry Program	• Community Kitchen • Food Bank-Operated Meal Program • Group Home • Rehabilitation Program • Residential Program • Shelter • Soup Kitchen • Transitional Housing	• Nutrition Education • Special Supplemental Nutrition Program for Women, Infants, and Children (WIC) Outreach • Supplemental Nutrition Assistance Program (SNAP) Assistance and Outreach	• Clothing/Furniture Assistance • Financial Assistance • General Educational Development (GED) Programs • General Information and Referrals • Health Clinics • Housing Assistance • Job Training • Legal Assistance • Medicaid/Children's Health Insurance Program (CHIP) • Transportation Assistance • Utility/Heat Assistance
CHILDREN	• Backpack Program	• After-School Snack • Child Congregate Feeding Program (Non-Kids Café) • Daycare • Kids Café • Summer Food Service Program (SFSP)	• National School Lunch Program (NSLP) Outreach • School Breakfast Program (SBP) Outreach	
SENIORS	• Commodity Supplemental Food Program (CSFP) • Senior Brown Bag • Senior Grocery Program • Senior Mobile Pantry	• Home-Delivered Meal (or Meals on Wheels) • Senior Congregate Meal		

FIGURE 10-15 What Is a Community Food Bank?

With extra groceries, hot meals, or daycare snacks, hundreds of thousands of individuals benefit from a food bank's partnerships with industry and the community.

Source: Adapted from *Hunger in America, 2014* (Chicago: Feeding America, 2014); *www.feedingamerica.org.*

- *Community-Supported Agriculture Programs.* Partnerships between local farmers and consumers who buy shares in the farm in exchange for weekly supplies of fresh produce. Provide small-scale farmers with economic stability, while ensuring consumer participants receive high-quality produce, usually at below-retail prices.
- *Farm-to-Cafeteria Initiatives.* Help local farmers sell fresh fruits and vegetables directly to school meals programs, hospitals, and worksites.
- *SNAP Outreach Programs.* Help increase the number of eligible households that participate in SNAP.
- *Community Gardens.* Connect local consumers to locally grown food; the food may be made available to members of the community or to local food banks and food pantries; improve access to fresh produce.
- *Food Recovery and Gleaning Programs.* The terms **food recovery** and **gleaning** refer to programs that collect excess wholesome food that would otherwise be thrown away and deliver it to nonprofit organizations for distribution to food-insecure individuals. Some 30% or more of America's food goes to waste each year, with an estimated 290 pounds of food waste per person ending up in landfills.[116] In 2013, USDA and the U.S. Environmental Protection Agency joined together to launch the U.S. Food Waste Challenge to provide information about the best practices to reduce, recover, and recycle food loss and waste. The USDA and the Food and Drug Administration worked together to produce a food recovery handbook, providing guidelines to restaurants, schools, airlines, and other groups for donating excess food, and providing technical assistance to community-based groups who seek to help. See the food recovery websites at the end of this chapter.
- *Food-Buying Cooperatives.* Help families save money by pooling resources (money, labor, purchasing, and distribution) to buy food in bulk quantities at reduced cost.
- *Directory of Supply and Demand for Community Food Surplus.* Creating a community directory can link farmers, retailers, and other sources of food surplus with local food pantries, soup kitchens, or other sites in need of emergency food.[117]

Food recovery Activities such as salvaging perishable produce from grocery stores; rescuing surplus prepared food from restaurants and caterers; and collecting nonperishable food from manufacturers, supermarkets, or people's homes. The items recovered are donated to hungry people.

Gleaning The harvesting of excess food from farms, orchards, and packing houses to feed the hungry.

PROGRAMS IN **ACTION**

Overcoming Barriers to Increasing Fruit and Vegetable Consumption

Even though messages abound telling us to eat a *minimum* of five servings of fruits and vegetables each day, the average American eats only three and a half servings.[1] People give many reasons for this, but most of the barriers they note are self-imposed.[2] Low-income families have cited difficulty of preparation, expense, and perishability as barriers to consuming more fruits and vegetables.[3]

Barriers to eating fruits and vegetables can be tackled in several ways. Programs such as WIC and the National School Lunch Program provide food or vouchers for free or reduced-price foods, including produce, to members of lower-income families, thereby alleviating the barriers related to

price and accessibility. Point-of-purchase education, such as a supermarket-based Fruits & Veggies—More Matters program, positively influences eating behaviors and can increase fruit and vegetable consumption.[4] Building self-efficacy—in this case, confidence in one's abilities to make healthful choices—is associated with increased intake of fruits and vegetables.[5] Demonstrating techniques for preparing fruits and vegetables and providing opportunities for hands-on practice may enhance self-efficacy and increase consumption. Encouraging family members to participate in intervention programs has also been shown to increase fruit and vegetable consumption.[6]

Community gardens can break down barriers to eating fruits and vegetables. They offer numerous other benefits to participants as well. "Community gardens are common ground for growing plants that feed, heal and give aesthetic pleasure. They are civic spaces where people work and recreate to nourish themselves, their families and friends. Most gardeners take satisfaction in having filled some part of their diet with food they have grown themselves."[7] The Kane Street Community Garden brought together educators, volunteers, and families to increase fruit and vegetable consumption among a low-income population in Wisconsin.

Inadequate fruit and vegetable consumption was common among low-income women participating in the WIC program in La Crosse County, Wisconsin. Barriers to consumption of fresh fruits and vegetables included the high cost of produce in a limited budget, lack of knowledge of preparation methods, unfamiliarity with numerous fresh fruits and vegetables, and family members' dislike of fruits and vegetables. Program initiatives were established to overcome these barriers.

Goals and Objectives

The Kane Street Community Garden was established to increase the consumption of fresh fruits and vegetables among low-income residents of La Crosse County. Program objectives were to establish a community garden on a vacant site, begin free distribution of community garden produce, and provide opportunities for learning to prepare fresh fruits and vegetables. The time frame for planting the garden, harvesting, hosting cooking classes, and evaluating the program ran from June to October.

Methodology

The Hunger Task Force of La Crosse County established a subcommittee to oversee the planting of a community garden in a low-income neighborhood. The City Planning Department donated a parcel of land for the garden. Volunteers prepared the garden for planting as part of a local community volunteer day. AmeriCorps volunteers were recruited to help the garden committee oversee garden maintenance and harvesting.

Produce was harvested and distributed to low-income families free of charge two nights a week throughout the harvest season; any remaining produce was donated to local food pantries and free meal sites. Cooperative extension staff members at the garden provided preparation tips, recipes, and fact sheets on harvest nights. Produce samples were offered to encourage families to take home unfamiliar fruits and vegetables. Local media aided in publicizing the garden and soliciting donations of money and materials. The garden was publicized through WIC sites, the Salvation Army, the local food pantry, community centers, and senior meal sites.

Results

The growing season ended with 5,006 pounds of produce grown and distributed. A total of 125 community residents volunteered to work or help in the garden, and 95 low-income families helped harvest. Six community organizations distributed surplus produce to needy families. Of the low-income families that responded to a survey, 71% stated that their fruit and vegetable consumption had increased.

Lessons Learned

As with many new projects, securing sufficient funding was and continues to be one of the biggest challenges. The subcommittee decided to expand the garden and sell a portion of the additional produce to raise additional funding for ongoing support. It also decided to hire a part-time coordinator to help protect the volunteers from burnout.

Source: From *Community Nutritionary* (White Plains, NY: Dannon Institute, Fall 2001). Used with permission. For more information about the Awards for Excellence in Community Nutrition, go to *www.dannon-institute.org.*

Beyond Public Assistance: What Can Individuals Do?

Solutions to the hunger problem depend on the willingness of people to take action and work together. Can we realistically hope to end hunger in the United States in the near future? Dr. J. Larry Brown, former director of the Center on Hunger and Poverty at Brandeis University, provides our response:

> The chief answer to those who question whether we can eliminate hunger lies in the fact that we virtually did so in our recent past. The programs created by the nation in the late 1960s and early 1970s worked. The evidence indicates that hunger significantly declined in the face of a national commitment expressed through the vehicles of school meals, food stamps, WIC, and elderly feeding programs. By fully utilizing these existing programs, we could again end hunger.

The larger question—the truly complicated one—is how to eliminate the cause of hunger: poverty. The United States pays a high price for poverty, and hunger is only one part of it. From a public health perspective it is the height of folly to permit such a significant risk factor for illness and premature mortality to persist. From a moral perspective the prevalence of poverty in one of the world's wealthiest nations is yet another matter.

Our nation has the ability to end hunger in a matter of months once we determine to do so. The larger issue is whether we will address poverty and, in doing so, not only eliminate hunger but prevent much untimely disease and death as well.[118]

Using Mapping Tools to Understand the Food Environment

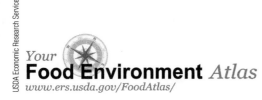

Your **Food Environment** *Atlas*
www.ers.usda.gov/FoodAtlas/

Food environment factors—such as store and restaurant proximity, food prices, food and nutrition assistance programs, and community characteristics—interact to influence food choices and diet quality. The USDA's *Food Environment Atlas* provides a spatial overview of a community's ability to access healthy food. County-level statistics can be viewed according to three broad categories of food environment factors:

- *Food Choices*—Indicators of access to and acquisition of healthy, affordable food, such as access and proximity to a grocery store, number of food stores and restaurants, expenditures on fast foods, food and nutrition assistance program participation, quantities of foods eaten, food prices, and availability of local foods
- *Health and Well-Being*—Indicators of success in maintaining healthy diets, such as food insecurity, diabetes and obesity rates, and physical activity levels
- *Community Characteristics*—Indicators of community characteristics that might influence the food environment, such as demographic composition, income and poverty, metro–nonmetro status, and recreation and fitness centers

What can users do with the *Atlas*?

- Create maps showing the variation in a single indicator across the United States; for example, variation in the prevalence of obesity or access to grocery stores across U.S. counties
- View all of the county-level indicators for a selected county
- Use the advanced tool to identify counties sharing the same degree of multiple indicators (e.g., counties with high poverty and high obesity rates)

More than 23 million Americans, including 6.5 million children, live in low-income urban and rural neighborhoods where the closest supermarket is more than one mile from their homes—making it difficult to access fresh, healthy, and affordable food. Part of the *Let's Move!* Initiative, the Healthy Food Financing Initiative (HFFI) will expand the availability of nutritious food to **food deserts**—low-income communities without ready access to healthy and affordable food—by developing and equipping grocery stores, small retailers, corner stores, and farmers' markets with fresh and healthy foods. To qualify as a low-income community, a census tract must have a poverty rate of 20% or higher. To qualify as a "low-access community," at least 500 people and/or at least 33% of the census tract's population must reside more than one mile from a supermarket or large

Food deserts A *low-income census* tract where a substantial number of residents has *low access* to a supermarket or large grocery store.

Regardless of the type and level of involvement a person chooses, each person can make a difference. The government programs described in this chapter need people's support in a number of ways. Individual people can:

- Document the hunger-related needs that exist in their own communities. The USDA's *Food Environment Atlas* provides a spatial overview of a community's ability to access healthy food. The *Food Access Research Atlas* maps and provides selected population characteristics of census tracts defined as food deserts (see the box below).[119]
- Help develop means of informing low-income people about food-related federal and local services and programs for which they are eligible—from SNAP, Medicaid, and

grocery store (for rural census tracts, the distance is more than 10 miles). The USDA *Food Access Research Atlas* (formerly, *The Food Desert Locator*) provides maps and selected population characteristics of census tracts defined as food deserts.

This map shows food desert census tracts in Atlanta, GA. The dark gray shaded census tracts meet the definition of food deserts. Users can view and download statistics on selected population characteristics of food desert census tracts—such as the number and percentage of children under age 18, seniors age 65 and older, people with low incomes, and housing units without a vehicle. The data for the highlighted food desert tract below indicate that 23% of households in the tract are over one mile from a supermarket and do not own a vehicle.

Food Access Research Atlas

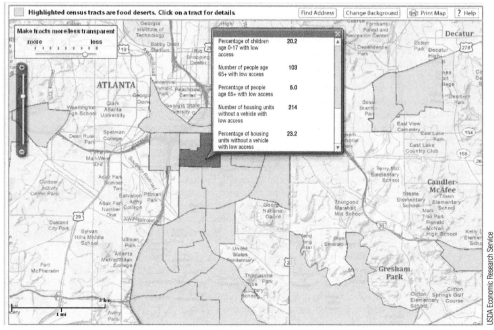

Source: Adapted from M. Ver Ploeg, D. Nulph, and R. Williams, "Mapping Food Deserts in the U.S.," *Amber Waves*, December 2011; *www.ers.usda.gov/AmberWaves/December11/DataFeature*.

WIC, to rent and utility assistance programs, to job-training programs that will help provide a living wage.[120]

- Help increase the accessibility of existing programs and services to those who need them.
- Assist in the food assistance programs as volunteers. Community nutritionists can educate providers about safe food-handling practices and healthful diets, identify the most effective means of providing the needed nutrients from limited resources, and teach participants how to shop for the most economical nutritious foods.[121]
- As a food and nutrition practitioner, monitor the household food security of the clients you serve.
- Support local food production such as farmers' markets, roadside stands, community gardens, and community-supported agriculture programs.[122]
- Join with others in the community who have similar interests. Use the "hunger-free" criteria listed in **Table 10-5** as guidelines for implementing comprehensive food assistance networks. The criteria are meant to provide a useful means of evaluating local antihunger networks.
- Conduct or participate in research to document the effectiveness of food assistance programs.[123]
- Represent nutrition issues at community health planning meetings.
- Document the impact of welfare reform on food security in local communities.
- Learn more about the problem of food insecurity and become familiar with organizations that advocate for sustainable solutions to the problems associated with food insecurity.
- Follow food security legislation; call and write legislators about food insecurity issues; lobby to draw political attention to employment and wages.

TABLE 10-5 Fourteen Ways to Reduce Food Insecurity in Communities

1. Establish a community-based emergency food delivery network.
2. Assess community food insecurity problems and evaluate community services. Create strategies for responding to unmet needs.
3. Establish a group of individuals, including low-income participants, to develop and implement policies and programs to combat hunger and the threat of food insecurity; monitor responsiveness of existing services; and address underlying causes of food insecurity.
4. Participate in federally assisted nutrition programs that are easily accessible to target populations.
5. Integrate public and private resources, including local businesses, to relieve food insecurity.
6. Establish an education program that addresses the food needs of the community and the need for increased local citizen participation in activities to alleviate food insecurity.
7. Provide information and referral services for accessing both public and private programs and services.
8. Support programs to provide transportation and assistance in food shopping, where needed.
9. Identify high-risk populations and target services to meet their needs.
10. Provide adequate transportation and distribution of food from all resources.
11. Coordinate foodservices with parks and recreation programs and other community-based outlets to which residents of the area have easy access.
12. Improve public transportation to human service agencies and food resources.
13. Establish nutrition education programs for low-income citizens to enhance their food purchasing and preparation skills and make them aware of the connections between diet and health.
14. Establish a program for collecting and distributing nutritious foods—either agricultural commodities in farmers' fields or prepared foods that would have been wasted.

Source: House Select Committee on Hunger, legislation introduced by Tony P. Hall, excerpted in *Seeds, Sprouts Edition*, January 1992, p. 3 with permission, © SEEDS Magazine, P.O. Box 6170 Waco, TX 76706.

Besides individual actions, all persons who are concerned about the problems of poverty and undernutrition in the United States can exercise their right to affect the political process. Anyone can decide what she or he thinks local, state, and national governments should do to help and can communicate these ideas to elected officials, urging them to support needed legislative changes. Individuals who volunteer their efforts and express their convictions to improve food assistance programs can also make a difference. Consider the following words, spoken over a hundred years ago:

I am only one,

But still I am one.

I cannot do everything,

But still I can do something;

And because I cannot do everything

I will not refuse to do the something that I can do.[124]

case study

Hunger in an At-Risk Population
by Alice Fornari, EdD, RD, Alessandra Sarcona, MS, RD, CSSD, and Alison Barkman, MS, RD, CDN

Scenario

As an AmeriCorps volunteer with an educational background in foods and nutrition, you are asked by the social service agency sponsoring you to help a current client budget for food within the allowance that she receives to feed herself and her children. This single African American mother with three children is renting a home in an urban environment; she has no access to a car and depends on public transportation. She currently is working 40 hours a week at a fast-food restaurant for minimum wage. Because the property she is renting is being sold, she has called the social service emergency housing program. No apartments are currently available, so she and her children must occupy a motel room subsidized by the county social service agency. There is a small refrigerator and a microwave oven. She received a $340 monthly SNAP allocation when she was renting a home. Since moving to the motel, she has depended on local restaurants and take-out food as her main supply of food for the family.

Learning Outcomes

- Identify food assistance programs and federal policies that are applicable to the family described in the case, including Internet sites providing this information; identify Internet sources of reliable statistics on hunger.
- Create a conceptual model (see the example on page 370) describing this client, considering household features (including nutritional needs of children), cultural food-related behaviors, food access, and economics.
- Identify variables that affect the food intake of the family, and characterize each of these variables as modifiable or not modifiable.
- Develop a plan for the family to incorporate adequate nutrition in their daily diet within the constraints of their socioeconomic status.

Foundation: Acquisition of Knowledge and Skills

1. Describe four food assistance programs and identify criteria for eligibility.

2. Access Internet sites supporting assistance for families that are hungry and homeless (refer to the Internet Resources listed at the end of this chapter).

Step 1: *Identify Relevant Information and Uncertainties*

1. Create a conceptual model (see the example on page 370) showing the interrelated factors associated with food insecurity and its outcomes for the family described in this case.
2. Identify information that the nutritionist does not have readily available and information that needs to be uncovered by the professional to help this family move forward.

Step 2: *Interpret Information*

1. Propose possible solutions for the family, supporting access to food and adequate nutrition; include federally funded food assistance programs that they are eligible for on the basis of their socioeconomic status. If applicable,

include community outreach programs supported by local agencies.
2. Prioritize issues and variables impacting solutions.

Step 3: *Draw and Implement Conclusions*

1. Describe the limitations of the proposed solution(s).
2. Design a memo to social service staff communicating possible solutions and suggestions applicable to the family; design a comparable communication for the head of the household in language that is "consumer-friendly."

Step 4: *Engage in Continuous Improvement*

1. Explain how conditions might change for the family in such a way as to impact the current proposed solutions (e.g., if this mother decides to relocate to a suburban community and has limited access to public transportation, or if she decides to move in with a family member).
2. Establish a plan for monitoring the implementation of the solution(s) over time.

PROFESSIONAL **FOCUS**

Moving Toward Community Food Security

Over the past decade, various entities within the United States, Canada, and Europe have applied a food systems approach to build community food security (CFS).[1] Using a food systems approach to build CFS requires understanding how communities interact with resources in their social and physical environments over extended periods of time. It also draws on strategies that address broad systemic issues affecting food availability, affordability, accessibility, and quality.[2] This Professional Focus discusses a three-stage continuum of evidence-based strategies and activities that applies a food systems approach to build community food security.

Community Food Security

CFS is an evolving concept that emphasizes long-term, systemic, and broad-based approaches to addressing food insecurity.[3] CFS can be defined as "a situation in which all community residents

obtain a safe, culturally acceptable, nutritionally adequate diet through a sustainable food system that maximizes self-reliance and social justice."[4] A combination of practical activities and policy development is required to achieve CFS.[5]

Food Systems, Sustainability, and Sustainable Community Food Systems

A *food system* is a set of interrelated functions that includes food production, processing, and distribution; food access and utilization by individuals, communities, and populations; and food recycling, composting, and disposal.[6] Food systems operate and interact at multiple levels, including community, municipal, regional, national, and global levels. Sustainability is defined as society's ability to shape its economic and social systems to maintain both natural resources and human life.[7] A sustainable community food system improves the health of the community, environment, and individuals over time, involving a collaborative effort in a particular setting to build locally based, self-reliant food systems and economies.[8]

Evidence-Based Strategies to Build Community Food Security

Examples of evidence-based strategies and activities that nutrition and dietetics professionals can use to build CFS are arranged on a continuum related to the time frame of the expected outcome (short to long term) (**Figure 10-16**). These strategies and activities fall into three progressive stages: initial food systems change, food systems in transition, and food systems redesign for sustainability.

In stage 1, participants create small but significant changes to existing food systems. In stage 2, food systems change is progressing, and efforts are directed toward facilitating and stabilizing that change. In stage 3, efforts are made to institutionalize

Stage 1: Initial Food Systems Change	Stage 2: Food Systems in Transition	Stage 3: Food Systems Redesign for Sustainability[a]
Strategies and Activities	**Strategies and Activities**	**Strategies and Activities**

• Counsel clients to maximize access to existing programs providing food and nutrition assistance, social services, and job training.
 	
 • Document the nutritional value of emergency foods.
 	
 • Identify food quality and price inequities in low-income neighborhoods.
 	
 • Educate consumers and institutions about the benefits of locally produced, seasonally available, and organically produced foods.
	• Connect emergency food programs with local urban agriculture projects.
	
	 • Create multisector partnerships and networks.
	
	 • Facilitate participatory decision making and policy development by serving on food policy councils and organizing community-mapping processes and multistakeholder workshops.
		• Advocate for minimum wage increase and more affordable housing.
		
		 • Advocate for food labeling standards about product history (e.g., place of origin, organic certified, Fair Trade certified[b]).
		
		 • Mobilize governments and communities to institutionalize:
		
		   1. land use policies that facilitate large-scale urban agriculture;
		
		   2. market promotion and subsidies;
		
		   3. tax incentives and financing mechanisms to attract local food businesses to low-income neighborhoods.

Time Frame: Short term	**Time Frame:** Short term	**Time Frame:** Long term

Evaluation
Data collection, monitoring, and evaluation are conducted at all stages of the CFS continuum.[c]

FIGURE 10-16 Evidence-Based Strategies and Activities Associated with a Three-Stage Community Food-Security Continuum

[a] Sustainability is defined as society's ability to shape its economic and social systems to maintain both natural resources and human life.

[b] Fair trade is an innovative, market-based approach to sustainable development. Fair trade helps family farmers in developing countries to gain direct access to international markets, as well as to develop the business capacity to compete in the global marketplace. In the United States, Fair Trade USA places the "Fair Trade Certified" label on coffee, tea, cocoa, bananas, and other fruits. For more information, see *www.fairtradeusa.org*.

[c] This three-stage CFS continuum was adapted from a framework that was originally developed by R. J. MacRae and coauthors, "Policies, Programs, and Regulations to Support Transition to Sustainable Agriculture in Canada," *American Journal of Alternative Agriculture* 5 (1990): 76–92.

Source: C. McCullum et al., "Evidence-Based Strategies to Build Community Food Security," *Journal of the American Dietetic Association* 105: 279. Copyright © 2005 by Elsevier. Reprinted with permission.

food systems change through advocacy and development of public policy. Data collection, monitoring, and evaluation are conducted at all stages. A detailed discussion of the strategies and activities outlined in the three-stage CFS continuum follows and is summarized in Figure 10-16.

Stage 1: Initial Food Systems Change

Stage 1 of the CFS continuum focuses on strategies and activities that create small but significant changes in existing food systems. An example of a strategy that food and nutrition practitioners can use to facilitate initial food systems change is client counseling to maximize access to existing programs that provide food and nutrition assistance, social services, and job training.[9] Furthermore, food and nutrition practitioners can collect data on the nutritional adequacy of foods served in emergency food programs because there is evidence that people who rely regularly on such sources may have inadequate nutritional intake.[10] There is also some evidence that people who live in low-income neighborhoods may not have easy access to food retail outlets that sell a variety of affordable and healthful foods.[11] Therefore, it is valuable to determine whether pricing and food quality inequities exist in food stores located in low-income neighborhoods.[12] Overall, this type of research and documentation is a useful early step to ensure that all community residents have access to nutritionally adequate and affordable foods.

Food and nutrition practitioners can also facilitate initial change in food systems by educating consumers and institutions about the benefits of purchasing locally produced, seasonally available, and organically grown food. When consumers purchase foods that have been produced locally, a greater proportion of the profits remain with local farmers, providing them with a livable income while supporting local economies.[13] Purchasing locally produced foods protects the environment by reducing the use of fossil fuel and packaging materials.[14] The benefits of organic farming systems extend to farmers, consumers, and the environment. The results of a Washington State study showed that organic apple production provided similar yields, better-tasting fruit, and higher profitability and that it was more environmentally sound and energy efficient than producing apples by conventional practices.[15]

Stage 2: Food Systems in Transition

Stage 2 of the CFS continuum focuses on strategies and activities that support food systems in transition toward initiatives that have not traditionally been utilized by the current food systems. In this stage, the social infrastructure needed to connect various food system processes is established or strengthened through capacity building and multisector partnerships and networks. Stage 2 involves connecting private food distribution activities (e.g., food banks) with public spaces (e.g., community gardens and community-supported agriculture [CSA] farms), and promoting economic renewal projects and job creation through farmers' markets and small-scale food businesses. Several types of transition strategies and activities are described below.

Connecting Emergency Food Programs with Urban Agriculture Projects

Urban agriculture involves producing food closer to where most consumers live; it is an increasingly important strategy for achieving food security in the twenty-first century because the world is becoming more urbanized.[16] Urban agriculture offers many potential benefits, such as reducing energy costs and pollution from food transportation and storage, absorbing greenhouse gas emissions, offering a viable use for urban waste as compost, and creating employment and economic development opportunities.[17]

An example of a successful effort to link urban agriculture projects with emergency food programs is the Michigan Food Bank Project, which administers 18 community gardens in the Lansing area. All garden participants receive supplies and training, which enable them to grow and preserve their own fresh vegetables. A second initiative of this project organizes volunteers to harvest surplus fruits and vegetables from local farms and distribute them to residents of low-income housing projects.[18]

Another successful example involves linking emergency food programs with CSA farms, an innovative strategy designed to connect local farmers with local consumers, develop a regional food supply and strengthen a local economy, maintain a sense of community, encourage land stewardship, and honor the knowledge and experience of local food producers.[19] CSA members pay a fee or volunteer their time in exchange for a share of the CSA farm's produce each week during the harvest season.[20]

Creating Multisector Partnerships and Networks

Food and nutrition practitioners can support food systems in transition by creating or joining multisector partnerships and networks that result in mutually beneficial programs and projects. For example, partnerships and networks are created by providing nutrition education at farmers' markets and conducting research on barriers to establishing, accessing, and participating in farmers' markets within low-income communities.[21] Farmers' markets improve consumers' access to fresh produce through reduced prices while stimulating the vitality and sustainability of the local economy.[22]

Research in Michigan revealed that the maximum positive impact on fruit and vegetable consumption was achieved among WIC Farmers' Market Nutrition Program (FMNP) participants when nutrition education accompanied the coupons that were distributed as incentives to improve affordability.[23] Evaluation of consumer participation in the Senior Farmers' Market Nutrition Program (SFMNP) in South Carolina suggested that participants receiving vouchers reported an intention to eat more fruits and vegetables year-round.[24] Food and nutrition practitioners can also create multisector partnerships that involve urban agriculture projects (e.g., CSA farms and community gardens) and farm-to-school programs. For example, one urban agricultural partnership in Colorado connected CSA farms with the WIC program to promote both fruit and vegetable consumption and physical activity for WIC participants.[25] Urban agricultural partnership projects such as community gardening exemplify an integrated approach to health promotion by increasing community networks, expanding green space, lowering crime rates in urban neighborhoods, and providing employment opportunities.[26] Farm-to-school partnerships provide local markets for farmers and integrate education about local food and farming issues with local foods served in school cafeterias. These partnerships may also lead to arranging special events with local farm organizations, creating nutrition curricula around school gardens, and providing opportunities for field trips to local farms. Farm-to-school programs have been shown to promote greater fruit and vegetable consumption.[27]

Facilitating Participatory Decision-Making Processes and Policy Development

Community residents must participate in decision-making processes and policy development in order to increase their access to resources.[28] Participatory decision making and policy development can promote social cohesion and reduce inequities by building connections between local food production and consumption.[29] Participatory CFS strategies and activities such as *food policy councils* (FPCs), *community-mapping processes*, and *multistakeholder workshops* offer a planning framework and tools to involve local residents in defining and analyzing their community's issues and in mobilizing community action around a range of food system problems.[30] Each of these strategies and activities is described in more detail below.

A food policy council (FPC) is an officially sanctioned body representing various segments of a state, city, or local food system. It is composed of diverse stakeholders representing a wide range of interests related to agriculture, food, nutrition, and health. The goal of an FPC is to foster a comprehensive and systematic examination of agriculture, food, nutrition, and health policies.[31]

The Toronto FPC has been instrumental in placing CFS and food policy development on the municipal agenda. Among its notable accomplishments, it has worked with the Economic Development Committee, the Board of Health, and Parks and Recreation to develop strategies for featuring farmers' markets at various civic centers. It has also chaired the School Garden and Compost Committee at the Toronto Board of Education, which entailed conducting 25 gardening workshops and developing a manual for school garden and compost projects.[32]

Food and nutrition practitioners can also facilitate participatory decision-making processes and policy development through organizing *community-mapping processes* and *multistakeholder workshops*. A community-mapping process involves analyzing the community environment, examining the causes and consequences of food insecurity, and implementing strategies for improving local CFS.[33] Diverse food system stakeholders—including urban planners, food producers and retailers, volunteers in food access projects, food-insecure individuals, and other concerned citizens—convene to engage in a process that examines how a local community food system can meet household and community needs by identifying available local food resources, food prices, transportation options, and employment opportunities. For example, the Portland–Multnomah County FPC has partnered with the regional government to create a geographical information system (GIS) map of grocery stores, farmers' markets, emergency food locations, and community gardens in the county.[34]

The purpose of a multistakeholder workshop is to provide a common vision and a platform for building consensus among diverse participants who may have divergent or competing interests.[35] One evaluation in upstate New York suggests that in their efforts to build CFS, practitioners may benefit from skills in facilitation, negotiation, and conflict resolution in order to transform conflict into greater capacity, equity, and justice.[36] See the Professional Focus feature in Chapter 12 for more about developing negotiation skills.

Stage 3: Food Systems Redesign for Sustainability

Stage 3 of the CFS continuum provides examples of strategies and activities in which citizens and government institutions play a larger role in building CFS. This stage involves advocacy and public policies that integrate different policy fields (such as education, labor, economic development, agriculture, food, social welfare, and health) in order to increase a community's food self-reliance and achieve nutritional goals (see Figure 10-16).[37] Integrated policies should ensure that all community members have the capacity to buy healthful foods rather than relying regularly on charitable food sources. It is also important that the proportion of the locally based food supply increase over time for the entire population, a goal that may be achieved through land-use policies, market promotion and subsidies, and tax incentives and financing mechanisms.

Norway is an example of a country that has used integrated policy instruments to redesign its food system. Norwegians aspired to increase their domestic food self-reliance from 39 to 52% of total calories and to achieve macronutrient intakes appropriate for a healthful diet using policy tools such as production and consumer subsidies, market promotion, consumer education, food labeling, and penalties for unhealthful foods.[38]

By 1988, Norway had reached 50% food self-reliance and had increased whole-grain consumption and the quality of locally produced grains and potatoes. Greater improvements were limited by the lack of human and financial resources.[39]

In summary, food and nutrition practitioners can use a three-stage continuum of evidence-based strategies and activities that applies a food systems approach to build community food security. Stage 1 creates small but significant changes in existing food systems through such strategies as identifying any inequities in food quality and pricing in low-income neighborhoods and educating consumers about the need and the possibilities for alternative food systems. Stage 2 stabilizes and augments change for food systems in transition by developing social infrastructure through multisector partnerships and networks and fostering participatory decision making and initial policy development. Based on these changes, Stage 3 involves advocacy and integrated policy instruments to redesign food systems for sustainability. Data collection, monitoring, and evaluation are key components of all stages of the CFS continuum.

Source: Adapted from C. McCullum, E. Desjardins, V. I. Kraak, P. Ladipo, and H. Costello, "Evidence-Based Strategies to Build Community Food Security," *Journal of the American Dietetic Association* 105 (2005): 278–83.

CHAPTER SUMMARY

Counting the Food-Insecure

▶ Food security is one of several conditions necessary for a population to be healthy and well nourished. The concept of food security includes five components: quantity, quality, suitability, psychological, and social.

▶ **Causes of Food Insecurity in the United States.** Poverty is the most compelling reason for food insecurity. Other causes include unemployment, high housing costs, SNAP-benefit cuts, economic downturn or weakening of the economy, utility costs, welfare reform, escalating health care costs, mental health problems, and the fact that available resources are failing to reach many groups.

Federal Nutrition Assistance Programs

▶ The nutrition safety net includes an array of 15 USDA nutrition assistance programs targeted at different populations with different nutritional needs to provide individuals with access to a more nutritious diet, to improve

the eating habits of the nation's children, and to help farmers in the United States by providing an outlet for the distribution of food purchased under farmer assistance authorities (see Table 10-4). Other programs are administered by the Department of Health and Human Services, and disaster feeding is administered by the Department of Homeland Security.

▶ The Supplemental Nutrition Assistance Program is an entitlement program with the goal of improving the diets of low-income households by increasing access to food and food-purchasing ability. Eligibility and allotments are based on income, household size, assets, housing costs, work requirements, and other factors.

  ● To improve SNAP's ability to meet the needs of low-income households, the following steps are recommended: improving and expanding outreach about SNAP, lowering administrative barriers to participation in SNAP, increasing allotments so that families can afford to eat a nutritionally adequate diet throughout each month, and providing nutrition education materials to participants.

▶ **Food Distribution Programs** are intended to strengthen the nutrition safety net through commodity distribution and other nutrition assistance to low-income households, emergency feeding programs, Indian reservations, and older adults.

▶ **Child Nutrition and Related Programs.** Many federal programs address the special nutritional needs of children. These programs include the National School Lunch Program and the School Breakfast Program, the Afterschool Snack Program, the Special Milk Program, the Summer Food Service Program for children, the Child and Adult Care Food Program, Team Nutrition, and the Fresh Fruit and Vegetable Program.

▶ **The Special Supplemental Nutrition Program for Women, Infants, and Children (WIC)** provides supplemental foods to infants; children up to age five; and pregnant, breastfeeding, and nonbreastfeeding postpartum women who qualify financially and are at nutritional risk. Its services include checks or vouchers for supplemental foods, nutrition education, and referrals to health care services.

▶ **The Older Americans Nutrition Program** is intended to improve older people's nutrition status and enable them to avoid medical problems and stay out of institutions. Its specific goals are to provide low-cost, nutritious meals (congregate meals or home-delivered meals); opportunities for social interaction; nutrition education and shopping assistance; and counseling and referral to other services.

Filling In the Gaps to Strengthen the Food Resource Safety Net

▶ Emergency shelters and community food programs are straining to meet the rising requests for food. Feeding America distributes food to food banks and other agencies for direct distribution around the nation.

▶ Community food security focuses on specific goals, including building and enhancing local infrastructures to reduce hunger and food insecurity in communities. Examples of strategies and activities are farmers' markets, community-supported agriculture programs, farm-to-cafeteria initiatives, SNAP outreach programs, and community gardens.

SUMMARY **QUESTIONS**

1. What households in the United States are prone to experiencing food insecurity?
2. What factors contribute to and what outcomes are associated with food insecurity in the United States?
3. You work with households composed of single women with children in a community characterized by food insecurity. What food assistance programs would you recommend to your clients, and what benefits would each program provide to the households?
4. Describe a community program that you could design as a community nutritionist to combat food insecurity.
5. Describe components of a needs assessment designed to evaluate the food security of a community where you are working as a community nutritionist.

INTERNET **RESOURCES**

See Table 10-4 for additional resources.

American Community Gardening Association
https://communitygarden.org

Bread for the World Institute
www.bread.org

Food Banks Canada
www.foodbankscanada.ca/

Community Supported Agriculture (CSA)
http://afsic.nal.usda.gov/
community-supported-agriculture-3

Congressional Hunger Center
www.hungercenter.org

National Institute of Food and Agriculture
http://nifa.usda.gov/program/
hunger-food-security-programs

Empty Bowls Project
www.emptybowls.net

Feeding America
www.feedingamerica.org

Food, Nutrition and Consumer Services (USDA)
www.fns.usda.gov/fncs

Food Assistance and Nutrition Research
www.ers.usda.gov/topics/food-nutrition-assistance/
food-nutrition-assistance-research.aspx

Food Access Research Atlas
www.ers.usda.gov/data-products/food-access-research-
atlas.aspx

Food Environment Atlas
www.ers.usda.gov/FoodAtlas

Food Research and Action Center
http://frac.org

Food Security in the United States
www.ers.usda.gov/topics/food-nutrition-assistance/
food-security-in-the-us.aspx

National Center for Children in Poverty
www.nccp.org

Rural Poverty and Well-Being
www.ers.usda.gov/topics/rural-economy-population/
rural-poverty-well-being.aspx

Share Our Strength
www.nokidhungry.org

USDA Food Recovery and Gleaning Toolkit
www.usda.gov/documents/usda_gleaning_toolkit.pdf

Food Recovery Guidelines
www.foodprotect.org/media/guide/food-recovery-
final2007.pdf

Think, Eat, Save Global Initiative
www.thinkeatsave.org

USDA and EPA Food Waste Challenge
www.usda.gov/oce/foodwaste

CHAPTER 11

Mothers and Infants: Nutrition Assessment, Services, and Programs

LEARNING OBJECTIVES

After you have read and studied this chapter, you will be able to:

- List the recommendations for maternal weight gain during pregnancy.
- Explain the relationship of maternal weight gain to infant birthweight.
- Identify nutritional factors and lifestyle practices that increase health risk during pregnancy.
- Describe the benefits of breastfeeding.
- Describe the purpose, eligibility requirements, and benefits of the federal nutrition programs available to assist low-income women and their children.

- Identify the common nutrition-related problems of infancy.
- Describe current recommendations for feeding during infancy.

This chapter addresses such issues as nutrient requirements across the lifespan, nutrition status assessment, use of information technologies, and program evaluation, which have been designated by the Accreditation Council for Education in Nutrition and Dietetics (ACEND) as Foundation Knowledge and Learning Outcomes for dietetics education.

CHAPTER OUTLINE

> *Something to think about...*
>
> All aspects of a society, whether it is relatively static or in a stage of dramatic upheaval, affect the health of every member of the family and of the community, and especially of its most physiologically and culturally vulnerable groups—mothers and young children.
>
> —*CICELY D. WILLIAMS*
> —*DERRICK B. JELLIFFE*

For a complete list of references, please access the MindTap Reader within your MindTap course.

TABLE 11-1

A Comparison of Infant Mortality Rates Worldwide, 2013

Finland	2.0
Iceland	2.0
Japan	2.0
Norway	2.0
Singapore	2.0
Sweden	2.0
Australia	3.0
Austria	3.0
Czech Republic	3.0
Denmark	3.0
Germany	3.0
Ireland	3.0
Israel	3.0
Italy	3.0
Netherlands	3.0
Portugal	3.0
Belgium	4.0
France	4.0
Greece	4.0
Spain	4.0
Switzerland	4.0
United Kingdom	4.0
Canada	5.0
Cuba	5.0
Hungary	5.0
New Zealand	5.0
Poland	5.0
United States	6.0

Source: Adapted from UNICEF, *The State of the World's Children 2013* (Oxford, UK: Oxford University Press, 2015).

Introduction

The effects of nutrition extend from one generation to the next, and this is particularly evident during pregnancy. Research has demonstrated that the poor nutrition of a woman during her early pregnancy can impair the health of her *grandchild*—and can do so even after that child has become an adult.[1] For example, if a mother's nutrient stores are inadequate early in pregnancy when the placenta is developing, the fetus will develop poorly, no matter how well the mother eats later. After getting such a poor start on life, the female child may grow up poorly equipped to support a normal pregnancy, and she, too, may bear a poorly developed infant.

Infants born of malnourished mothers are more likely than healthy women's infants to become ill, to have birth defects, and to have impaired mental or physical development.[2] Malnutrition in the prenatal and early postnatal periods also affects learning ability and behavior. Impaired intrauterine growth may also "program" the fetus for chronic diseases—such as coronary heart disease, hypertension, or type 2 diabetes—in adult life. According to the fetal origins hypothesis, if a woman's nutrient intake is under- or oversupplied—particularly at critical phases of fetal development—long-term alterations may occur in tissue function.[3] For example, if a woman's energy intake is low during the third trimester of pregnancy, pancreatic cell development in the fetus may be hindered, resulting in impaired glucose tolerance and an increased risk of developing diabetes later in life.[4] Clearly, it is critical to provide the best nutrition possible at the early stages of life. This chapter focuses on the nutrition and health recommendations for pregnancy, lactation, and infancy and examines the nutrition programs and services that target pregnant women and their infants.

Trends in Maternal and Infant Health

The health of a nation is often judged by the health status of its mothers and infants. One of the best indicators of a nation's health, according to epidemiologists, is the **infant mortality rate (IMR)**. Although the United States spends more money on health care than most other countries, its IMR of 6.0 infant deaths per 1,000 live births is considerably higher than that of several industrialized countries—for example, 2.0 for Norway, Sweden, and Japan (**Table 11-1**). Furthermore, important measures of increased risk of morbidity and death, such as incidence of low birthweight and fetal alcohol syndrome, have increased since 2000.[5] In addition, disparities in IMRs persist between ethnic groups and between poor and nonpoor infants, as shown in **Figure 11-1**. The IMR of 11.1 for black infants remains more than twice as high as the IMR of 5.1 for white infants. Although infant mortality rates among blacks and whites have been in steady decline throughout the last few decades, the discrepancy between the rates among blacks and rates among whites has remained largely unchanged. The failure to further improve the IMR in the United States has been attributed to the number of infants born with low birthweights. In 2013 the infant

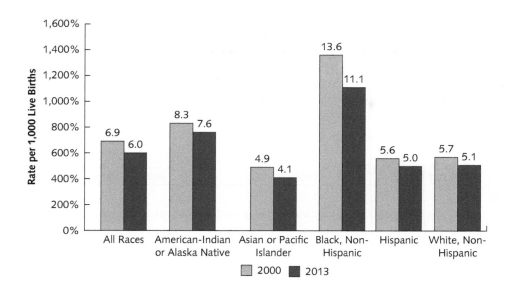

FIGURE 11-1 Total Infant Mortality Rates by Race and Ethnicity of Mother in the United States, 2000 and 2013

Source: National Vital Statistics System, National Center for Health Statistics, Centers for Disease Control and Prevention.

mortality rate ranged from a low of 4.2 in Massachusetts to a high of 9.6 in Mississippi.[6] The leading causes of death among infants are birth defects, preterm delivery and **low birthweight (LBW),** sudden infant death syndrome (SIDS), and maternal complications during pregnancy.

If a pregnant woman does not receive adequate nourishment and does not gain the recommended amount of weight, she may give birth to a baby of low birthweight. Not all small babies are unhealthy, but birthweight and length of gestation are the primary indicators of the infant's future health status. An LBW baby is more likely to experience complications during delivery than a normal-weight baby and has a statistically greater chance of having physical and mental birth defects, of contracting diseases, and of dying during the first year of life. Low birthweight in full-term infants is a major contributing factor to infant mortality. Clearly, a key to reducing infant mortality is reducing the incidence of LBW babies. Doing so requires that several factors be addressed: poverty, minority status, lack of access to health care, inability to pay for health care, poor nutrition, low level of educational achievement, and unhealthful habits such as smoking, drinking, and drug use. The percentage of LBW births ranges from a low of 6% in several states to a high of 12% in Mississippi.[7]

Improving the health and nutrition status of pregnant women and infants remains a national challenge. Although **maternal mortality rates** have decreased significantly from a high of 83.3 per 100,000 live births in the 1950s to 17.8 in 2011, considerable racial disparities in maternal mortality exist: 12.5 deaths per 100,000 live births for white women, 42.8 deaths per 100,000 live births for black women, and 17.3 deaths per 100,000 live births for women of other races.[8] Substantial improvements are needed to meet the *Healthy People 2020* objective for maternal mortality, which seeks a target of 11.4 maternal deaths per 100,000 live births.

Infant mortality rate (IMR) Infant deaths under one year of age, expressed as the number of such deaths per 1,000 live births.

Low birthweight (LBW) A birthweight of 5 pounds (2,500 grams) or less, used as a predictor of poor health in the newborn and as a probable indicator of poor nutrition status of the mother during and/or before pregnancy. *Very low birthweight* is defined as less than 1,500 grams, or 3 pounds, 4 ounces.

Maternal mortality rate Women's deaths assigned to causes related to pregnancy, expressed as the number of such deaths per 100,000 live births.

National Goals for Maternal and Infant Health: *Healthy People 2020*

Within the past decade, a number of research reports have established goals and recommendations designed to improve the nutrition and health status of mothers and infants.[9] *Healthy People 2020* takes a broad scope, encompassing maternal and infant health, as well as child health, birth defects, and developmental disabilities. It includes 72 objectives (some of these objectives are shown in **Table 11-2**). Objectives focusing on mortality include infant, fetal, and maternal deaths; perinatal deaths; and deaths of children, adolescents, and young adults. Objectives addressing risk factors include the areas of preterm births and infant sleep position. A focus on developmental disabilities is included, with objectives on the incidence of several specific conditions and folate intake among women of childbearing age.

TABLE 11-2 A Selection of *Healthy People 2020* Objectives from the Maternal, Infant, and Child Health (MICH) and Nutrition and Weight Status (NWS) Topic Areas[a]

OBJECTIVE NUMBER AND OBJECTIVE	BASELINE (YEAR)[b]	PROGRESS (YEAR)	*HEALTHY PEOPLE 2020* TARGET
Maternal, Infant, and Child Health			
MICH-1.3: Reduce the rate of all infant deaths within first year of life.	6.7 infant deaths per 1,000 live births (2006)	6.0 infant deaths per 1,000 live births (2012)	6.0 infant deaths per 1,000 live births
MICH-5: Reduce the rate of maternal mortality.	12.7 maternal deaths per 100,000 live births (2007)	–	11.4 maternal deaths per 100,000 live births[c]
MICH-8: Reduce low birthweight (LBW) and very low birthweight (VLBW).			
MICH-8.1 Low birthweight	8.2% of live births were low birthweight (2007)	8.0% of live births were low birthweight (2012)	7.8%[d]
MICH-8.2 Very low birthweight	1.5% of live births were very low birthweight (2007)	1.4% of live births were very low birthweight (2012)	1.4%[d]
MICH-10: Increase the proportion of pregnant women who receive early and adequate prenatal care.			
MICH-10.1 Prenatal care beginning in first trimester	70.8% (2007)	–	77.9%[c]
MICH-11: Increase abstinence from alcohol, cigarettes, and illicit drugs among pregnant women.			
MICH-11.1 Alcohol	89.4% of pregnant females reported abstaining from alcohol in the past 30 days (2007–2008)	90.6% of pregnant females reported abstaining from alcohol in the past 30 days (2012)	98.3%[c]
MICH-11.2 Binge drinking	95.0% of pregnant females reported abstaining from binge drinking during the past 30 days (2007–2008)	97.2% of pregnant females reported abstaining from binge drinking in the past 30 days (2012)	100%
MICH-11.3 Cigarette smoking	89.6% of females reported abstaining from smoking cigarettes during pregnancy (2007)	–	98.6%[c]
MICH-11.4 Illicit drugs	94.8% of pregnant females reported abstaining from illicit drugs in the past 30 days (2007–2008)	94.6% of pregnant females reported abstaining from illicit drugs in the past 30 days (2012)	100%
MICH-14: Increase the proportion of women of childbearing potential with intake of at least 400 μg of folic acid from fortified foods or dietary supplements.	23.8% (2003–2006)	22.8% (2007–2010)	26.2%[c]

OBJECTIVE NUMBER AND OBJECTIVE	BASELINE (YEAR)[b]	PROGRESS (YEAR)	*HEALTHY PEOPLE 2020* TARGET
Maternal, Infant, and Child Health—*continued*			
MICH-15: Reduce the proportion of women of childbearing potential who have low red blood cell folate concentrations.	24.5% (2003–2006)	24.9% (2007–2010)	22.1%[c]
MICH-16: Increase the proportion of women delivering a live birth who received preconception care services and practiced key recommended preconception health behaviors.			
MICH-16.2 Took multivitamins/folic acid prior to pregnancy	30.1% of females delivering a recent live birth took multivitamins/folic acid every day in the month prior to pregnancy (2007)	–	33.1%[c]
MICH-16.5 Had a healthy weight prior to pregnancy	48.5% of females delivering a recent live birth had a normal weight (i.e., a BMI of 18.5–24.9) prior to pregnancy (2007)	–	53.4%[c]
MICH-20: Increase the proportion of infants who are put to sleep on their backs.	69% (2007)	–	75.9%[c]
MICH-28: Reduce the occurrence of neural tube defects.			
MICH-28.1 Reduce the occurrence of spina bifida.	34.2 live births and/or fetal deaths with spina bifida per 100,000 live births were diagnosed (2005–2006)	30.5 live births and/or fetal deaths per 100,000 live births (2010)	30.8 live births and/or fetal deaths per 100,000 live births[c]
MICH-28.2 Reduce the occurrence of anencephaly.	24.6 live births and/or fetal deaths with anencephaly per 100,000 live births were diagnosed (2005–2006)	12.8 live births and/or fetal deaths per 100,000 live births (2010)	22.1 live births and/or fetal deaths per 100,000 live births[c]
Nutrition and Weight Status			
NWS-21: Reduce iron deficiency among young children and females of childbearing age.			
NWS-21.1 Children aged 1 to 2 years	15.9% (2005–2008)	–	14.3%[c]
NWS-21.2 Children aged 3 to 4 years	5.3% (2005–2008)	–	4.3%[c]
NWS-21.3 Females aged 12 to 49 years	10.5% (2005–2008)	–	9.4%[c]
NWS-22: Reduce iron deficiency among pregnant females.	16.1% (2003–2006)	–	14.5%[c]

[a] See Chapter 8 for objectives on obesity and weight status. See also Chapters 7, 12, and 13 for specific nutrition and weight status, child and adolescent, and adult-related *Healthy People 2020* objectives. See Figure 11-2 for objectives related to breastfeeding.

[b] Data sources include National Vital Statistics System (CDC), National Health and Nutrition Examination Survey (NHANES), National Survey on Drug Use and Health, National Health Interview Survey, Pregnancy Risk Assessment Monitoring System, and National Birth Defects Prevention Network.

[c] Target setting method: 10% improvement.

[d] Target setting method: 5% improvement.

In order for the United States to achieve further reductions in infant mortality and eliminate racial and ethnic differences in pregnancy outcomes, health care professionals must focus on changing the behaviors—both protective and risky—that affect pregnancy outcomes, as well as advocate for social and environmental changes to facilitate behavior change.[10] Health-related problems and behaviors such as smoking, substance abuse, poor nutrition, and limited access to prenatal care need to be addressed in preconception screening and counseling. Examples include daily folate consumption (a protective factor) and alcohol use (a risk factor). Presently, only 22.8% of women of childbearing age are consuming the recommended 400 micrograms of folate daily.[11] The proportion of pregnant women aged 15 to 44 years who had abstained from alcohol in the month preceding the survey was 90.6% in 2012, with little variance by race or ethnicity. The *Healthy People 2020* target is 98%.

Five new objectives relate to preconception care services and health behaviors prior to pregnancy: discussed preconception health with a health professional, took multivitamins/folic acid, did not smoke, did not drink, and had a healthy weight.[12] Two new objectives track postpartum health and behaviors: the relapse of smoking among women who quit smoking during pregnancy and the proportion of women giving birth who attend a postpartum care visit with a health care professional. Three new objectives target infant care: employers that have worksite lactation support programs, breastfed newborns not given formula within the first two days of life, and births in facilities that provide recommended care for lactating mothers and their babies.

The use of timely prenatal care can also help to mitigate risks by identifying women who are at high risk of high blood pressure or other maternal complications. Other actions, such as breastfeeding, newborn screening, and primary care in infancy, can significantly improve infants' health and chances of survival. For example, the incidence of SIDS, the leading cause of postneonatal mortality in the United States, decreased from 79 per 100,000 live births in 1996 to 55 per 100,000 in 2007. The *Healthy People 2020* objective seeks a 10% improvement and a target of 50 per 100,000 live births. This improvement reflects the success of the "Back to Sleep" education campaign that encourages parents to place healthy infants on their backs to sleep.[13] Approximately 69% of infants are now put to sleep as recommended, on their backs, compared to 36% in 1996. The *Healthy People 2020* target is 76%.

Uneven Progress for Maternal and Infant Health According to the final *Healthy People 2010* review, progress toward the *Healthy People 2010* maternal and infant objectives was uneven.[14] Improvement occurred in the following areas: (1) There has been a small decline in infant mortality rates for Hispanics, whites, and blacks. (2) The incidence (new cases) of spina bifida and other neural tube defects decreased from 60 per 100,000 live births in 1996 to 48 per 100,000 in 2007. The target was 30 per 100,000. The decrease was due in large part to increased consumption of folic acid from fortified foods or dietary supplements, as evidenced by the rise in the median red blood cell folate level in nonpregnant women aged 15 to 44 years. (3) There has been an increase in breastfeeding by women in all racial and ethnic groups. (4) Cigarette smoking during pregnancy continued to decline. In 2007, 11% of women smoked during pregnancy, compared to 20% of pregnant women in 1990.[15] However, either no progress or movement in the *wrong* direction occurred in the areas of maternal death for African American women, iron deficiency in women aged 12 to 49 years, and low birthweight.

The proportion of pregnant women who received prenatal care beginning in the first trimester showed little change in recent years. Long-standing racial and ethnic disparities among the recipients of prenatal care also remained much the same. An estimated 23% of minority women receive late or no prenatal care, compared to 11% of white women.

Many factors, including education, health care coverage, availability of health providers in neighborhoods, and language barriers, affect the use of prenatal care services.[16]

Improving the health of mothers and infants remains a national priority. As a follow-up to the *Healthy People 2010* initiative, and in order to continue to achieve gains in maternal and infant health in the current decade, an interagency workgroup, along with the surgeon general, has identified several key areas on which to focus attention:[17]

- Ensure the capacity for tracking the effects of welfare reform on the availability and utilization of prenatal care, particularly for immigrant populations.
- Seek to streamline eligibility requirements for maternal and infant programs so as to increase participation.
- Ensure that maternal and infant health care programs are culturally sensitive.
- Direct additional research toward determining the cause of black women's increased risk of dying from maternal complications.
- Increase research on genetic, environmental, and behavioral factors that have an influence on pregnancy outcomes for mother and child.
- Develop new interventions to reduce alcohol consumption during pregnancy, especially binge drinking.
- Increase dissemination of information to health care providers about the benefits of daily folate intake before, during, and after pregnancy.
- Help ensure that maternal and infant health care programs are tailored to the communities they serve by strengthening the nonmedical aspects of the programs, such as transportation and childcare.

Healthy Mothers

A number of factors contribute to maternal and infant health. Genetic, environmental, and behavioral factors affect risk and the outcome of pregnancy.[18] A woman's nutrition prior to and throughout pregnancy is crucial both to her health and to the growth, development, and health of the infant she conceives. Ideally, a woman starts pregnancy at a healthful weight, with filled nutrient stores and the firmly established habit of eating a balanced and varied diet (**Table 11-3**). In this section, we discuss maternal weight gain, adolescent pregnancy, and nutrition assessment in pregnancy.

Maternal Weight Gain

Normal weight gain and adequate nutrition support the health of the mother and the development of the fetus. The National Academy of Sciences recommendations for weight gain take into account a mother's prepregnancy weight-for-height or body mass index (BMI), as shown in **Table 11-4**. The committee recommends that a woman who begins pregnancy at a healthful weight should gain between 25 and 35 pounds. Women pregnant with twins need to gain 35 to 45 pounds; women pregnant with triplets need to gain 45 to 55 pounds. An underweight woman needs to gain between 28 and 40 pounds, an overweight woman between 15 and 25 pounds, and an obese woman between 11 and 20 pounds.

Approximately three-quarters of married women who deliver at full term gain the recommended weight during pregnancy. Two groups of women who continue to gain less than the recommended level of weight during pregnancy—pregnant teenagers and African American women—also are at particularly high risk for having LBW infants and other adverse pregnancy outcomes.[19]

Low weight gain in pregnancy is associated with increased risk of delivering an LBW infant; these infants have high mortality rates.[20] Excessive weight gain in pregnancy

---

POINTS TO CONSIDER FOR OPTIMAL WEIGHT GAIN IN PREGNANCY

If Weight Gain Is Slow or If Weight Loss Occurs:

- Is there a measurement or recording error?
- Is the overall pattern acceptable?
- Was there evidence of edema at the last visit, and is it resolved?
- Is nausea, vomiting, or diarrhea a problem?
- Is there a problem with access to food?
- Have psychosocial problems led to poor appetite?
- Does the woman resist weight gain? Does she understand the relationship between her weight gain and her infant's growth and health?
- Is she smoking? How much?
- Is she using alcohol or drugs?
- Does her energy expenditure exceed her energy intake?
- Does she have an infection or illness that requires treatment?

If Weight Gain Is Very Rapid:

- Is there a measurement or recording error?
- Is the overall pattern acceptable?
- Is there evidence of edema?
- Has the woman stopped smoking recently?
- Are twins a possibility?
- Are there signs of gestational diabetes?
- Has there been a dramatic decrease in physical activity?
- If serious overeating is occurring, explore why.

Source: Adapted from B. Worthington-Roberts and S. R. Williams, *Nutrition Throughout the Life Cycle*, 3rd ed. (St. Louis, MO: Times Mirror/Mosby, 1996).

TABLE 11-3 MyPlate Food Guide for Pregnant and Lactating Women

When you are pregnant or breastfeeding, you have special nutritional needs. Follow the plan below to help you and your baby stay healthy.

FOOD GROUP	1ST TRIMESTER	2ND AND 3RD TRIMESTERS	BREASTFEEDING ONLY	BREASTFEEDING PLUS FORMULA	WHAT COUNTS AS 1 CUP OR 1 OUNCE?	REMEMBER TO . . .
	EAT THIS AMOUNT FROM EACH GROUP DAILY[a]					
Fruits	2 cups	2 cups	2 cups	2 cups	1 cup fruit or juice ½ cup dried fruit	*Focus on fruits*—Eat a variety of fruits.
Vegetables	2½ cups	3 cups	3 cups	3 cups	1 cup raw or cooked vegetables or juice 2 cups raw leafy vegetables	*Vary your veggies*—Eat more dark-green and orange vegetables and cooked dry beans.
Grains	6 ounces	8 ounces	8 ounces	7 ounces	1 slice bread 1 ounce ready-to-eat cereal ½ cup cooked pasta, rice, or cereal	*Make half your grains whole*—Choose whole instead of refined grains.
Protein Foods	5½ ounces	6½ ounces	6½ ounces	6 ounces	1 ounce lean meat, poultry, or fish ¼ cup cooked dry beans ½ ounce nuts or 1 egg 1 tablespoon peanut butter	*Go lean with protein*—Choose low-fat or lean meats and poultry.
Dairy	3 cups	3 cups	3 cups	3 cups	1 cup milk 8 ounces yogurt 1½ ounces cheese 2 ounces processed cheese	*Get your calcium-rich foods*—Go low-fat or fat-free when you choose milk, yogurt, and cheese.

[a] Most pregnant and lactating women need a total of 2,200–2,900 calories per day; see "Pregnant & Breastfeeding Women" at *www.choosemyplate.gov/pregnancy-breastfeeding.html.*

Source: Adapted from USDA, Center for Nutrition Policy and Promotion.

increases the risk of complications during labor and delivery, and of postpartum obesity. Obese women also have an increased risk for complications during pregnancy, including hypertension and gestational diabetes.

Weight gain should be lowest during the first trimester—two to four pounds for the trimester—followed by a steady gain of about a pound per week thereafter. If a woman gains more than the recommended amount of weight early in pregnancy, she should not try to diet in the last weeks. Dieting during pregnancy is not recommended. A sudden large weight gain, however, may indicate the onset of pregnancy-induced hypertension, and a woman who experiences this type of weight gain should see her health care provider. Tips on counseling pregnant women regarding healthful weight gains are listed on the previous page.

TABLE 11-4

Recommended Weight Gain for Pregnant Women Based on Body Mass Index (BMI)

BMI	WEIGHT CATEGORY	RECOMMENDED GAIN (POUNDS)[a]
< 18.5	Underweight	28–40
18.5–24.9	Normal weight	25–35
25–29.9	Overweight	15–25
≥ 30	Obesity	11–20

[a] Teens should strive to gain the maximum pounds in their ranges; short women (less than 62 inches tall) should strive for the minimum. Weight gain varies widely, and these values are suggested only as guidelines for identifying individuals whose weights may be too high or low for health.

Source: Adapted from Institute of Medicine and National Research Council of the National Academies, *Weight Gain during Pregnancy: Reexamining the Guidelines* (Washington, D.C.: National Academies Press, 2009).

Adolescent Pregnancy

Approximately 273,000 babies were born to teenagers in the United States in 2013.[21] The complex social, emotional, and physical factors involved make teen pregnancy one of the most challenging situations for nutrition counseling. According to a paper from the Academy of Nutrition and Dietetics, pregnant adolescents are nutritionally at risk and require intervention early and throughout pregnancy.[22] Medical and nutritional risks are particularly high when the teenager is within two years of menarche (usually at 15 years of age or younger).[23] Risks include higher rates of pregnancy-related hypertension, iron-deficiency anemia, premature birth, stillbirths, LBW infants, and prolonged labor in pregnant teens than in older women. In addition, mothers under 15 years of age bear more babies who die within the first year than do any other age group.

The increased energy and nutrient demands of pregnancy place adolescent girls, who are already at risk for nutritional problems, at even greater risk. To support the needs of both mother and infant, adolescents are encouraged to strive for pregnancy weight gains at the upper end of the ranges recommended for pregnant women (see Table 11-4). Those who gain between 30 and 35 pounds during pregnancy have lower risks of delivering LBW infants. Adequate nutrition can substantially improve the course and outcome of adolescent pregnancy.[24]

Nutrition Assessment in Pregnancy

Nutrition assessment and monitoring during pregnancy can be divided into three categories: preconception care, the initial prenatal visit, and subsequent prenatal visits. Because a woman's nutrition status and lifestyle habits prior to pregnancy can influence the outcome of pregnancy, these are important factors to consider prior to pregnancy. Nutritional risk factors that may be present at the start of pregnancy are listed in **Table 11-5**. Preconception care should ideally be available to all women. It should include nutrition assessment, nutrition counseling, and appropriate supplementation and referral to correct nutritional problems existing prior to conception.

Assessment of pregnant teens follows the general pattern for assessment of older pregnant women. Assessment issues include acceptance of the pregnancy, food resources and food preparation facilities, body image, living situation, relationship with the father of the infant, peer relationships, nutrition status, prenatal care, nutrition attitudes and knowledge, preparation for infant feeding, financial resources, continuation of education, daycare, and knowledge of and attitudes toward different methods of feeding infants.[25] See **Table 11-6** for sample questions to include in a nutrition interview with a pregnant woman.

The nutrition status of all women should be assessed at their initial prenatal visit. This assessment should include:[26]

- *Dietary measures*. Diet history, including food habits, attitudes, and folklore; allergies; use of vitamin and mineral supplements; and lifestyles (e.g., substance abuse or existence of pica).

• Age 15 or under	• Iron-deficiency anemia early in pregnancy
• Unwanted pregnancy	• Cigarette smoking
• Many pregnancies close together (depletes nutrient stores)	• Alcohol or drug abuse
• History of poor pregnancy outcome	• Chronic disease requiring special diet (e.g., diabetes)
• Poverty	• Underweight or overweight
• Lack of access to health care	• Insufficient or excessive weight gain in pregnancy
• Low education level	• Carrying twins or triplets
• Inadequate diet (such as that due to food faddism or dieting)	

TABLE 11-5

Nutritional Risk Factors in Pregnancy

TABLE 11-6

Questions for a
Client-Focused
Nutrition Interview
in Pregnancy

What you eat and some of the lifestyle choices you make can affect your nutrition and health now and in the future. Your nutrition can also have an important effect on your baby's health. Please answer these questions by circling the answers that apply to you.

EATING BEHAVIOR

1. Are you frequently bothered by any of the following? Circle all that apply:

   Nausea   Vomiting   Heartburn   Constipation

2. Do you ever skip meals?	No	Yes
3. Do you try to limit the amount or kind of food you eat to control your weight?	No	Yes
4. Are you on a special diet now?	No	Yes
5. Do you avoid any foods now for health or religious reasons?	No	Yes

FOOD RESOURCES

6. Do you have a working stove?	No	Yes
Do you have a working refrigerator?	No	Yes
7. Do you sometimes run out of food before you are able to buy more?	No	Yes
8. Can you afford to eat the way you should?	No	Yes
9. Are you receiving any food assistance now?	No	Yes

   Circle all that apply:

   SNAP benefits   School breakfast   School lunch
   WIC   Donated food   Commodity foods

10. Do you feel you need help in obtaining food?	No	Yes

FOOD AND DRINK

11. Which of these did you drink yesterday? Circle all that apply:

   Soft drinks   Coffee   Tea   Fruit drink
   Orange juice   Grapefruit juice   Other juices   Milk
   Kool-Aid   Beer   Wine   Other alcoholic drinks
   Water   Other beverages (list)

12. Which of these foods did you eat yesterday? Circle all that apply:

   Cheese   Pizza   Macaroni and cheese
   Yogurt   Cereal with milk
   Other foods made with cheese (such as tacos, enchiladas, lasagna, cheeseburgers)
   Corn   Potatoes   Sweet potatoes   Green salad
   Carrots   Collard greens   Spinach   Turnip greens
   Broccoli   Green beans   Green peas   Other vegetables
   Apples   Bananas   Berries   Grapefruit
   Melon   Oranges   Peaches   Other fruit
   Meat   Fish   Chicken   Eggs
   Peanut butter   Nuts   Seeds   Dried beans
   Cold cuts   Hot dog   Bacon   Sausage
   Cake   Cookies   Doughnut   Pastry
   Chips   French fries
   Other deep-fried foods, such as fried chicken or egg rolls
   Bread   Rolls   Rice   Cereal
   Noodles   Spaghetti   Tortillas

Were any of these whole grain?	No	Yes
13. Is the way you ate yesterday the way you usually eat?	No	Yes

LIFESTYLE

14. Do you exercise for at least 30 minutes on a regular basis?	No	Yes
15. Do you ever smoke cigarettes?	No	Yes
16. Do you ever drink beer, wine, liquor, or other alcoholic beverages?	No	Yes

17. Which of these do you take? Circle all that apply:

   Prescribed drugs or medications
   Over-the-counter products (such as aspirin, antacids, or vitamins)
   Street drugs (such as marijuana, speed, downers, crack, or heroin)

INTENTIONS REGARDING INFANT FEEDING PRACTICES

18. Which of the following statements are true regarding your intentions? Circle all that apply:

    • I am planning to only formula feed my baby and do not plan to breastfeed at all.
    • I am planning to breastfeed my baby or at least try.
    • When my baby is one month old, I will be breastfeeding without using any formula or other milk.
    • When my baby is three months old, I will be breastfeeding my baby without using any formula or other milk.
    • When my baby is six months old, I will be breastfeeding my baby without using any formula or other milk.

19. What influences you to breastfeed or formula feed your infant?

20. Does your employer have a workplace lactation program or provide any workplace accommodations (such as reasonable breaks, an appropriate place to store milk, a place other than the bathroom to pump/express human milk)?

21. Have you received counseling on infant feeding and care and by whom?

22. What are your and your health care providers' views or beliefs regarding breastfeeding?

23. What recommendations have you received from your health care providers regarding breastfeeding?

Source: Adapted from National Academy of Sciences, *Nutrition during Pregnancy and Lactation: An Implementation Guide* (Washington, D.C.: National Academy Press) and L. May and coauthors, *WIC ITFPS-2 Infant Report: Intention to Breastfeed* (Rockville, MD: Westat), May 2015.

TABLE 11-6

Questions for a Client-Focused Nutrition Interview in Pregnancy—*continued*

• *Clinical measures.* Obstetric history, including outcome of previous pregnancies, interval between pregnancies, and history of problems during the course of previous pregnancies (pregnancy-induced hypertension [PIH], gestational diabetes, iron-deficiency anemia, or pattern of inadequate or excessive weight gain).

• *Anthropometric measures.* Measurement of weight-for-height or body mass index (BMI).

• *Laboratory values.* Screening for anemia by hematocrit and/or hemoglobin. A urine analysis for ketones, glucose, and protein spillage may be ordered for women with gestational diabetes or preeclampsia.

During each subsequent prenatal visit, weight gain should be monitored and the pattern of weight gain evaluated. Screening for anemia should be repeated on at least one other occasion during pregnancy. Routine assessment of dietary practices is recommended for all women so that their need for an improved diet or vitamin or mineral supplementation can be evaluated. The nutrition status of women in high-risk categories should be reevaluated at each visit.

Poor dietary practices should be improved by appropriate interventions. These may include general nutrition education, individualized diet counseling, and referral to food assistance programs (e.g., the Special Supplemental Nutrition Program for Women, Infants, and Children [WIC] and the Supplemental Nutrition Assistance Program [SNAP]) or to programs that promote improved food acquisition or preparation practices (such as the Expanded Food and Nutrition Education Program [EFNEP]).

Healthy Babies

The growth of infants directly reflects their nutritional well-being and is the major indicator of their nutrition status. A baby grows more rapidly during the first year of life than ever again; its birthweight doubles during the first four to six months and triples by the end of the first year. Adequate nutrition during infancy is critical to support this rapid rate of growth and development. Clearly, from the point of view of nutrition, the first year is the most important year of a person's life. This section provides a brief overview of nutrient requirements, current recommendations and health objectives for feeding healthy infants, and the relationship between infant feeding and selected pediatric nutrition issues.

Nutrient Needs and Growth Status in Infancy

The infant's rapid growth and metabolism demand an adequate supply of all essential nutrients. Because of their small size, infants need smaller total amounts of these nutrients than adults do, but relative to body weight, infants need over twice as much of many of the nutrients. After six months, energy needs increase less rapidly as the baby's growth rate begins to slow down, but some of the energy saved by slower growth is spent on increased activity.

Anthropometric Measures in Infancy Anthropometric measurements routinely obtained in the examination of infants include length, weight, and head circumference. These measures assess physical size and growth.

Infants should be weighed nude, using a table model beam scale that allows the infant to lie or sit. Length should be measured in the recumbent position on a measuring board that has a fixed headboard and a movable footboard attached at right angles to the surface.

Head circumference measures can confirm that growth is proceeding normally or help detect protein-energy malnutrition (PEM) and evaluate the extent of its impact on brain size. To measure head circumference, a nonstretchable tape is placed around the largest part of the infant's head: just above the eyebrow ridges, just above the point where the ears attach, and around the occipital prominence at the back of the head.[27] The head circumference percentile should be similar to the infant's weight and length percentiles.

In 2006, the World Health Organization (WHO) released new international growth standards for children for assessment of children of any ethnicity or socioeconomic status. There are growth standards for infants to one year, and for children up to five years. Similar to the 2000 CDC growth charts, these standards describe weight-for-age, length (or stature)-for-age, weight-for-length (or stature), and body mass index-for-age. CDC recommends that health care providers:

- Use the WHO Child Growth Standards to monitor growth for infants and children up to two years of age.
- Use the CDC growth charts for children age two years and older in the United States.

The CDC growth charts describe how the average child grows, but do not indicate how children should grow for the best health outcome.[28] The recommendation to use the 2006 WHO international growth charts recognizes that breastfeeding is the recommended standard for infant feeding. In the WHO charts, the healthy breastfed infant is intended to be the standard against which all other infants are compared; 100% of the reference population of infants for the WHO Child Growth Standards were breastfed for 12 months and were predominantly breastfed for at least four months. In contrast, approximately 50% of the infants in the CDC growth chart data set had ever been breastfed.[29]

Growth charts are used to analyze measures of growth status in infants. A single plotting is used to assess how an infant ranks in comparison with population data for that infant's specific age and sex. Excessive weight-for-length (above the 95th percentile) indicates obesity. An infant whose weight-for-length falls below the 5th percentile is classified as exhibiting **failure to thrive**, and those below the 10th percentile are suspect for failure to thrive. These infants require further evaluation and care. Under normal conditions, the growth rate usually varies within two percentiles. Greater variation indicates the possibility of inadequate nutrition and needs to be evaluated further. When using the WHO Child Growth Standards, health professionals should be aware that slower growth among breastfed infants during ages 3 to 18 months is normal, and gaining weight more rapidly than is indicated

Failure to thrive Inadequate weight gain of infants.

How to Measure Length and Height

To improve the accuracy of length and height measurements, keep the following in mind:

- Always measure—never ask! Self-reported heights are less accurate than measured heights. If height is not measured, document that the height is self-reported.
- Measure the length of infants and young children by using a measuring board with a fixed head-board and a movable footboard. It generally takes two people to measure length: one person gently holds the infant's head against the headboard, while the other straightens the infant's legs and moves the footboard to the bottom of the infant's feet. The measurement is taken while the infant is lying flat on its back, with chin and toes pointing upward and heels flat against the footboard.
- Measure height next to a wall on which a nonstretchable measuring tape or board has been fixed. Ask the person to stand erect without shoes and with heels together. The person's eyes and head should be facing forward, with heels, buttocks, and shoulder blades touching the wall. Place a ruler or other flat, stiff object on the top of the head at a right angle to the wall and carefully note the height measurement.
- Immediately record length and height measurements to the nearest ⅛ inch or 0.1 centimeter.
- For evaluating growth rate in young children, use the appropriate growth chart (Appendix A) when plotting results.

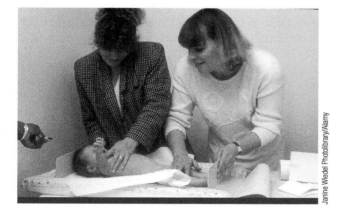

It generally takes two people to measure the length of an infant.

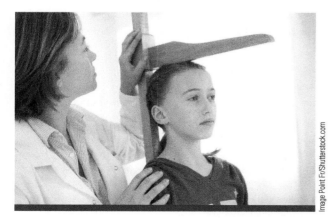

Standing erect allows for an accurate height measurement.

Source: E. Whitney, L. DeBruyne, K. Pinna, and S. Rolfes, *Nutrition for Health and Health Care*, 4th ed. (Belmont, CA: Wadsworth/Cengage Learning, 2011), 391.

on the WHO charts might serve as an early sign of overweight.[30] Appendix A provides an example of how to plot measures on a growth chart, and includes the WHO Child Growth Standards, which can be downloaded from *www.cdc.gov/growthcharts*.

Breastfeeding Recommendations

Breastfeeding offers both emotional and physical health advantages. Emotional bonding is facilitated by many events and behaviors of mother and infant during the early months and years; one of the first can be breastfeeding.

During the first two or three days of lactation, the breasts produce colostrum, a premilk substance containing antibodies and white cells from the mother's blood. Colostrum and breast milk both contain the bifidus factor that favors the growth of the "friendly" bacteria *Lactobacillus bifidus* in the infant's digestive tract so that other, harmful bacteria cannot grow there. Breast milk also contains the powerful antibacterial agent lactoferrin and other factors—including several enzymes, several hormones, and lipids—that help protect the infant against infection.

Breastfeeding provides other benefits as well (**Table 11-7**). It protects against allergy development during the vulnerable first few weeks, the act of suckling favors normal tooth and jaw alignment, and breastfed babies are less likely to be obese because they are less likely to be overfed. These attributes, along with the convenience and lower cost of breastfeeding, have led many organizations and medical experts to encourage breastfeeding for all normal full-term infants.[31] Breastfeeding in the United States declined after World War II to a low of about 25% of infants in 1970. Breastfeeding rates have increased since 1999, but continue to fall short of *Healthy People 2020* objectives regarding duration and exclusivity. Among children born in 2007, 74% initiated breastfeeding, whereas 43% were breastfeeding at six months and 22% at 12 months of age. Approximately 33% of infants born in 2007 were exclusively breastfed through three months of age, and 14%

TABLE 11-7 Benefits of Breastfeeding

For Infants:

• Provides appropriate balance of nutrients and supports healthy weight

• Improves cognitive development

• Protects against food allergies

• Reduces risk of sudden infant death syndrome (SIDS)

• May lower risk of chronic diseases such as asthma, atherosclerosis, diabetes, some cancers, childhood obesity, hypertension

• Protects against infections and illnesses such as ear infections, pneumonia, diarrhea, and vomiting

For Mothers:

• Contracts the uterus and delays the return of regular ovulation

• Conserves iron stores by prolonging amenorrhea

• May lead to a lower risk of type 2 diabetes, certain types of breast cancer, and ovarian cancer

For Society:

• **Breastfeeding saves lives.** Recent research shows that if 90% of families breastfed exclusively for six months, nearly 1,000 deaths among infants could be prevented.

• **Breastfeeding saves money.** Health care costs are lower for fully breastfed infants than never-breastfed infants. Breastfed infants usually need fewer sick care visits, prescriptions, and hospitalizations.

• **Breastfeeding helps make a more productive workforce.** Mothers who breastfeed miss less work to care for sick infants than mothers who feed their infants formula.

• **Breastfeeding is better for the environment.** Formula cans and bottle supplies create more trash and plastic waste.

Source: Adapted from U.S. Department of Health and Human Services' Office on Women's Health.

were exclusively breastfed for six months. The *Healthy People 2020* goal for breastfeeding is to increase the incidence of breastfeeding to 82% early postpartum, 60% at six months, and 34% at one year (**Figure 11-2**). Disparities in breastfeeding continue to exist, with non-Hispanic black and socioeconomically disadvantaged groups having lower breastfeeding

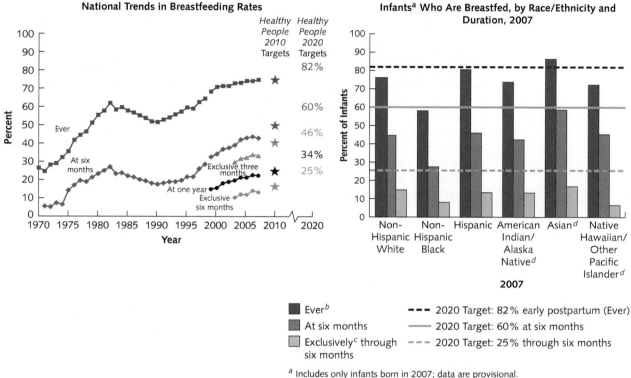

Health People 2020 Breastfeeding Objectives		Baseline (2006–2009) %	Progress (2011) %	2020 Target %
MICH-21: Increase the proportion of infants who are breastfed.				
MICH-21.1	Ever	74	79	82
MICH-21.2	At six months	43	49	60
MICH-21.3	At one year	23	27	34
MICH-21.4	Exclusively through three months	34	41	46
MICH-21.5	Exclusively through six months	14	19	25
MICH-22: Increase the proportion of employers that have worksite lactation support programs.		25	–	38
MICH-23: Reduce the proportion of breastfed newborns who receive formula supplementation within the first two days of life.		24	19	14
MICH-24: Increase the proportion of live births that occur in facilities that provide recommended care for lactating mothers and their babies.		3	–	8

FIGURE 11-2 Percentage of U.S. Children Who Were Breastfed, by Birth Year, with 2007 Breakdown by Race

Source: CDC National Immunization Survey, *Breastfeeding among U.S. Children Born 1999–2007* (Atlanta: Division of Nutrition, Physical Activity and Obesity, National Center for Chronic Disease Prevention and Health Promotion, 2011), CDC, Breastfeeding Report Card, 2014.

rates. In 2007, the highest percentages at each of the three stages were recorded for Asians and the lowest for blacks, with whites and Hispanics in between (see Figure 11-2). Breast-feeding rates continue to be the highest among women who are older, well educated, relatively affluent, and/or living in the western United States.[32]

Breastfeeding Promotion

Increasing a woman's knowledge about the benefits of breastfeeding is not enough to improve breastfeeding rates. Breastfeeding support after birth in the hospital and in the workplace, as well as positive social norms in families and communities, are important factors impacting breastfeeding rates. The *Surgeon General's Call to Action to Support Breastfeeding* identified a number of barriers to achieving the nation's health objective of increasing the incidence of breastfeeding. These include lack of experience or understanding among family members of how best to support mothers and babies, not enough opportunities to communicate with other breastfeeding mothers, lack of up-to-date instruction and information from health care professionals, hospital practices that make it hard to get started with successful breastfeeding, and lack of accommodation to breastfeed or express milk at the workplace.[33]

Health care professionals and hospitals can provide support by offering encouragement and supplying accurate information on breastfeeding. Duration of breastfeeding depends on the successful establishment of breastfeeding during the first days of a newborn's life. However, successful breastfeeding can be hampered by distribution of infant formula discharge packs at hospitals. Results from the Maternity Practices in Infant Nutrition and Care survey found the percentage of hospitals distributing infant formula discharge packets to breastfeeding mothers was 73% in 2007 and 32% in 2013. Based on these results, the authors concluded that "discontinuing the practice of distributing infant formula discharge packs is part of optimal, evidence-based maternity care to support mothers who want to breastfeed."[34] The U.S. Preventive Services Task Force concluded that multifaceted breastfeeding interventions are effective in increasing breastfeeding initiation, duration, and exclusivity.[35] **Table 11-8** lists 10 steps recommended by the World Health Organization that hospitals and health professionals can take to promote breastfeeding among women.[36]

Certain cultural beliefs and practices may also influence a woman's perception of normal feeding practices.[37] For example, the belief that larger babies are healthier is common among many racial and ethnic groups, and mothers may be encouraged by family and friends to supplement breastfeeding with formula or to inappropriately introduce solid foods if the infant is perceived as thin.[38] Another practice associated with cultural beliefs is the use of cereal in a bottle because of the false belief that it will help the infant sleep through the night.[39]

TABLE 11-8 Baby-Friendly Hospitals: Ten Steps to Successful Breastfeeding

To Promote Breastfeeding, Every Maternity Facility Should:

- Develop a written breastfeeding policy that is routinely communicated to all health care staff.
- Train all health care staff in the skills necessary to implement the breastfeeding policy.
- Inform all pregnant women about the benefits and management of breastfeeding.
- Help mothers initiate breastfeeding within a half hour of birth.
- Show mothers how to breastfeed and how to maintain lactation, even if they need to be separated from their infants.
- Give newborn infants no food or drink other than breast milk, unless medically indicated.
- Practice rooming-in, allowing mothers and infants to remain together 24 hours a day.
- Encourage breastfeeding on demand.
- Give no artificial nipples or pacifiers to breastfeeding infants.
- Foster the establishment of breastfeeding support groups and refer mothers to them at discharge from the facility.

Source: United Nations Children's Fund and World Health Organization, "Barriers and Solutions to the Global Ten Steps to Successful Breastfeeding."

Sustained breastfeeding requires adequate peer support and interventions that involve both prenatal and postnatal components. One study found that the strongest predictor of whether a woman would continue breastfeeding was whether or not she returned to work within six weeks of delivery. Establishing breastfeeding policies that are economically feasible (e.g., paid maternity leave) may be needed to ensure sustained breastfeeding, particularly among nonaffluent women.[40] An analysis of state laws and breastfeeding practices in the United States found that the most robust state laws associated with increased infant breastfeeding at six months were an enforcement provision for workplace pump laws and a jury duty exemption for breastfeeding mothers. In addition, having a private area in the workplace to express breast milk and having break time to breastfeed or pump breast milk were important provisions for infant breastfeeding at six months.[41]

One example of a successful approach to increasing breastfeeding rates in low-income, urban populations is the peer counseling method promoted by the La Leche League International.[42] The WIC program has initiated breastfeeding promotion projects among low-income women using the peer counselor method. With this approach, peer support counselors are trained to provide culturally appropriate interventions for initiating and maintaining breastfeeding in their communities. The peer counselor is paired with an expectant or new mother for individual assistance and informal discussions in their neighborhood. The peer counselor addresses any barriers to breastfeeding through breastfeeding education, support, and role modeling.[43] When a new mother has the support of someone from within her neighborhood with a similar cultural background, she has the opportunity to overcome her perceived barriers to breastfeeding. Results of similar grassroots approaches to breastfeeding promotion are encouraging; both the rate and the duration of breastfeeding among the women in the programs have shown significant increases (**Figure 11-3**).[44]

Focus groups can be useful in designing breastfeeding promotion projects. For example, the project Best Start: Breastfeeding for Healthy Mothers, Healthy Babies was organized by a coalition of nutrition and public health officials concerned about the rates of breastfeeding in the southeastern United States.[45] Focus groups were especially helpful in exploring topics related to breastfeeding among participants who were ambivalent or undecided. Research findings pointed to the need for a carefully coordinated campaign that utilized a combination of strategies (see the box of findings on page 439) to improve the image of breastfeeding and help women overcome the barriers they perceived to breastfeeding, including:[46]

- Lack of confidence in the ability to breastfeed or bad previous breastfeeding experience
- Competing demands on mother's time (work, school, social life)

FIGURE 11-3

Increased Breastfeeding Rates among WIC Participants
Breastfeeding is initiated in most parts of the country by an increasing percentage of WIC mothers. About 42% of WIC mothers nationwide initiated breastfeeding in 1998, whereas almost 59% of women initiated breastfeeding in 2008.
Source: National Academy of Sciences, Updating the USDA National Breastfeeding Campaign: Workshop Summary; data source: USDA/FNS, 2010.

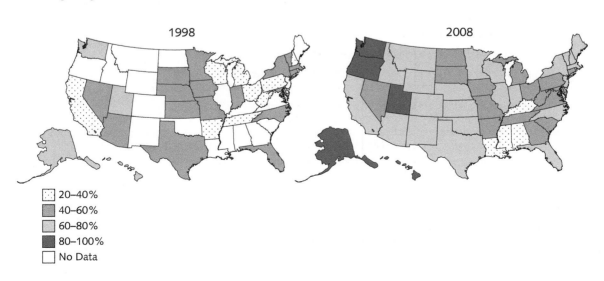

1998   2008

- [::] 20–40%
- [▨] 40–60%
- [▢] 60–80%
- [■] 80–100%
- [ ] No Data

- Need for social support and encouragement from baby's father and grandmother, family, and friends
- Hospital practices of offering free infant formula, separating mother and baby, or inadequately following-up about breastfeeding progress after discharge
- Lack of support in the workplace (limited leave, lack of breastfeeding/breast milk expression/childcare facilities)

On the basis of information derived from the focus group interviews, guidelines were formulated for program development (see the box on the next page).

Other Recommendations on Feeding Infants

Like the breastfeeding mother, the mother who offers formula to her baby has reasons for making her choice, and her feelings should be honored. Infant formulas are manufactured to approximate the nutrient composition of breast milk. The immunologic protection of breast milk, however, cannot be duplicated.

Many mothers breastfeed at first and then wean within the first one to six months. Whole cow's milk is not recommended during the first year of life, according to the American Academy of Pediatrics (AAP).[47] Therefore, when a woman chooses to wean her infant during the first six months of life, it is imperative that she shift to formula, not to plain milk of any kind. Only formula contains enough iron (to name but one of many factors) to support normal development in the baby's first months of life. National and international standards have been set for the nutrient content of infant formulas.

For infants with special problems, many variations of infant formulas exist. Special formulas based on soy protein are available for infants allergic to milk protein, and formulas with the lactose removed can be used for infants with lactose intolerance.

For most infants, breast milk and/or iron-fortified formula provide all the nutrients required for the first six months after birth. After that, breast milk and/or iron-fortified infant formula should remain an infant's primary beverage until the end of the first year of life, but solid foods should also be given to provide needed nutrients and to expose infants to a wide variety of flavors and textures, as well as to encourage the mastery of feeding skills. Introducing a variety of flavors and foods before age two may increase acceptance of a wider variety of flavors and foods in later childhood.[48] **Table 11-9** shows a suggested pattern for feeding infants.

TABLE 11-9 First Foods for the Infant

AGE (MONTHS)	FOOD ADDITIONS
4 to 6[a]	Iron-fortified rice cereal (mix with breast milk, formula, or water), followed by other cereals (baby can swallow nonliquid foods now);[b] pureed fruits and vegetables
6 to 8	Mashed vegetables and fruits, infant breads and crackers, unsweetened fruit juices[c]
8 to 10	Protein foods (soft cheeses, yogurt, tofu, mashed cooked beans, finely chopped meat, fish, chicken, egg yolk), toast, teething crackers (for emerging teeth), soft-cooked vegetables, fruit
10 to 12	Whole egg (allergies are less likely now), whole milk (at one year)

[a] The AAP supports exclusive breastfeeding for six months and continued breastfeeding for at least 12 months, but acknowledges that infants may be developmentally ready for certain foods between four and six months of age.

[b] Feeding skills: *0–3 months*: strong extrusion reflex. *3–6 months*: extrusion reflex diminishes, and the ability to swallow nonliquid foods develops; chewing action begins. *6–8 months*: able to feed self finger foods and begins to drink from cup. *8–10 months*: begins to hold own bottle; reaches for and grabs food and spoon. *10–12 months*: begins to master spoon.

[c] All baby juices are fortified with vitamin C. Orange juice may cause allergies; apple juice may be a better juice to feed first. Offer juices in a cup to prevent nursing bottle syndrome.

Source: Adapted from Committee on Nutrition, American Academy of Pediatrics, *Pediatric Nutrition Handbook*, 6th ed., ed. R. E. Kleinman (Elk Grove Village, IL: American Academy of Pediatrics, 2009); for more information, see also *Feeding Infants: A Guide for Use in Child Nutrition Programs*, FNS-258 (Washington, D.C.: Food and Nutrition Service, U.S. Department of Agriculture, 2002).

> ### Using Focus Group Findings

Using comments made by women participating in focus groups, planners of the Best Start breast-feeding promotion project formulated the following guidelines:[a]

- **Campaign tone.** The tone should be emotional to reflect the strong feelings women attach to their aspirations for their children and themselves as mothers.
- **Message design.** Educational messages should be succinct and easily understood to counter-act the mistaken belief that breastfeeding is complicated and requires major lifestyle changes. Promotional messages should emphasize confidence and the pride breastfeeding mothers gain from nursing.
- **Spokespersons.** Celebrities are not perceived as credible sources of advice on infant feeding. Also, most focus group respondents find it difficult to identify with the wealthy women featured on many of the pamphlets, posters, and other breastfeeding promotion materials used in health departments. Whenever possible, women featured in the materials should be of the same economic, ethnic, and age groups as those targeted or should not have a clear class affiliation. Visual images in print and broadcast materials should communicate modernity and confidence.
- **Educational approaches.** Educational strategies and materials need to be redesigned so that they no longer reinforce women's perceptions of breastfeeding as difficult. The emphasis on being healthy and relaxed and following special dietary guidelines needs to be replaced with reassurance that most women produce sufficient quantities of highly nutritious breast milk despite variations in diet, stress levels, and health status.
- **Professional training.** Motivational and training materials are needed to counter professionals' mistaken belief that their economically disadvantaged clients are not interested in breastfeeding and do not value health professionals' advice. Counseling strategies need to be redesigned to address the special needs of low-income women. Of special concern are recommendations for overcoming clients' lack of confidence and enabling them to realize their aspirations as women and mothers.
- **Program activities/components.** A variety of mutually reinforcing activities are needed to reach social network members who influence women's decisions about infant feeding and who create hospital, home, and community environments conducive to lactation.

[a] *Best Start*—the national breastfeeding promotion program for economically disadvantaged minorities and teenagers—was started in 1990.
Source: Adapted from C. Bryant and D. Bailey, "The Use of Focus Group Research in Program Development."

Primary Nutrition-Related Problems of Infancy

Iron deficiency and food allergies are two of the most significant nutrition-related problems of infants.

Iron Deficiency
Iron deficiency remains a prevalent nutritional problem in infancy, although it has declined in recent years largely because of increased use of iron-fortified formulas.[49] The use of cow's milk earlier than recommended in infancy can cause iron deficiency because of its poor iron content and its potential to cause gastrointestinal blood loss in susceptible infants.[50] Other factors contributing to iron deficiency during infancy include breastfeeding for more than six months without providing supplemental iron, feeding infant formula not fortified with iron, the infant's rapid rate of growth, low birth-weight, and low socioeconomic status. To prevent iron deficiency, the AAP recommends

> ▶ **THINK LIKE A COMMUNITY NUTRITIONIST**
>
> Using formative research to understand the needs and desires of the target audience can help improve effectiveness of breastfeeding promotion interventions. Review the box "Using Focus Group Findings" on this page. How would you apply these findings? What audience would be important to target? What strategies would you use to reach the audience?

exclusive breastfeeding for six months, followed by continued breastfeeding as complementary foods are introduced through the first year of life.[51]

Food Allergies

Genetics is probably the most significant factor affecting an infant's susceptibility to food allergies. Nevertheless, food allergies are much less prevalent in breastfed babies than in formula-fed infants. At-risk infants can be identified from elevated cord blood levels of immunoglobulin E (IgE) or by a family history. Breast milk is recommended for infants allergic to cow's milk protein and is preferable to soy or goat's milk formulas because infants are sometimes intolerant of these proteins as well. To reduce the risk of food sensitivity or allergic reactions to other foods, new foods should be introduced singly to facilitate prompt detection of allergies. For example, if a cereal causes irritability due to skin rash, digestive upset, or respiratory discomfort, discontinue its use before going on to the next food. At least two days should elapse between the introduction of one new food and that of another, to allow time for clinical symptoms to appear.[52] For infants with a strong family history of food allergies, solid foods should not be given before six months of age, and eggs, milk, wheat, soy, peanuts, tree nuts, shellfish, fish, and foods containing these major food allergens should not be given before one year of age.[53]

PROGRAMS IN **ACTION**

Using Peer Counselors to Change Culturally Based Behaviors

For many years, the Special Supplemental Nutrition Program for Women, Infants, and Children (WIC) clinics and organizations such as the La Leche League have used peer counselors to help women successfully breastfeed their infants. Incidence of breastfeeding among rural, low-income women in Iowa was far greater among women in a peer counseling group (82%) than among women in a control group (31%), and women in the peer counseling group also were more likely to continue breastfeeding.[1] Breastfeeding decisions among a group of low-income women in Georgia were influenced more by the women's social support networks than by the attitudes of health professionals.[2] These programs, along with the case that follows, demonstrate that a peer counselor who has breastfed a baby, has been trained in lactation support and counseling, and understands a pregnant woman's view on breastfeeding can be very influential in motivating women to initiate and continue breastfeeding.

Goals and Objectives

The goals of Best Beginnings of Forsyth County were to:

- Increase the number of women who breastfeed their newborn infants
- Increase the number of women who continue to breastfeed past the first few weeks of their baby's life

The program objectives were to develop the curriculum for the didactic and experiential components of the training and to add group discussions and breastfeeding classes.

Target Audience

The Best Beginnings breastfeeding education program was designed for pregnant women who applied for support under the WIC program in Forsyth County. Approximately one-third of those women were Hispanic.

Rationale for the Intervention

Best Beginnings of Forsyth County was initiated to increase breastfeeding and duration of breastfeeding among women in low-income settings. Prior to intervention, only about 10% of mothers in the target audience initiated breastfeeding, and almost no women continued breastfeeding past six weeks. The Forsyth County WIC Program decided to lay the groundwork for a peer counselor program to try to increase the rate of breastfeeding among WIC participants.

Methodology

The Forsyth County WIC program received a grant to begin a breastfeeding support program. Peer counselor training began with three women, all of whom had been enrolled in the WIC program and each of whom had breastfed a baby for more than six months. Peer counselor training included 20 hours of didactic instruction on lactation and counseling, a written test, and practical instruction on counseling. Course information included advantages of and myths about breastfeeding, breast physiology, mechanics of breastfeeding, common problems, and high-risk situations. On completion of the training course, peer counselors took a competency exam and completed a six-week internship.

Peer counselors encouraged breastfeeding among WIC participants through individual counseling, classes, and telephone support. They increased public awareness of breastfeeding by taking part in health fairs, baby fairs, and the county fair.

Results

The Best Beginnings program of breastfeeding education through peer counselors has been highly successful. Within six months after the start of the program, the breastfeeding initiation rate had increased from 10 to 26%. After one year, almost 50% of Forsyth County women enrolled in WIC had initiated breastfeeding, compared to 38% of WIC participants statewide. The percentage of participants who continued breastfeeding

for more than six weeks increased from virtually zero to over 27% in one year, compared to 19% of WIC participants statewide. Forsyth County was recognized for having the highest breastfeeding initiation rate among urban counties in North Carolina.

Lessons Learned

The enthusiasm of the peer counselors was important to the success of Forsyth County's breastfeeding support program. In addition, peer counselor programs can have a positive influence on the peer counselors themselves. Of the peer counselors who no longer work with Best Beginnings, a large percentage left to complete their education. Most now work full time and no longer depend on federally subsidized programs.[3]

Source: *Community Nutritionary* (White Plains, NY: Dannon Institute, Fall 2000). Used with permission. For more information about the Awards for Excellence in Community Nutrition, go to *www.dannon-institute.org*.

Domestic Maternal and Infant Nutrition Programs

As the first half of this chapter has indicated, nutrition plays a vital role in the outcome of pregnancy and in the growth and development of infants. A stable base of essential programs and services is required to meet maternal and infant health care needs. This section describes the nutrition programs and related services available to meet the demands of pregnancy and infancy, two of the most vulnerable periods of the life cycle (**Table 11-10**).

The WIC Program

In 1969, the White House Conference on Food, Nutrition, and Health recommended that special attention be given to the nutritional needs of pregnant and breastfeeding women, infants, and preschool children. As a result, the Special Supplemental Nutrition Program for Women, Infants, and Children (WIC) was authorized in 1972 by PL 92-433 as an amendment to the Child Nutrition Act of 1966. The legislation states that the WIC program is to "serve as an adjunct to good health care, during critical times of growth and development." To encourage earlier and more frequent utilization of health services, federal regulations mandate that local agencies may qualify as WIC sponsors only if they can make health care services available to WIC enrollees.[54]

The WIC program is based on two assumptions. One is that inadequate nutritional intakes and health behaviors of low-income women, infants, and children make them vulnerable to adverse health outcomes. The other is that nutrition intervention at critical periods of growth and development will prevent health problems and improve the health status of participants.

WIC is federally funded but is administered by the states. Cash grants are made to authorized agencies of each state and to officially recognized American Indian tribes or councils, which then provide WIC services through local service sites. Priority for the

TABLE 11-10 Federal Nutrition and Health Care Programs That Assist Mothers and Their Infants

PROGRAM[a]	PARTICIPANTS	BENEFITS
SNAP	Anyone with income < 130% of poverty guidelines[b]	Increased ability to purchase food
SNAP-Ed	Persons eligible for SNAP	Nutrition education
WIC	Pregnant women, postpartum and lactating women, infants, and children up to five years of age with incomes ≤ 185% of poverty guidelines	Checks or vouchers to purchase healthful foods or direct food supplements, nutrition education, and referral to health services
FMNP	Persons eligible for WIC	Increased fruit and vegetable consumption
Commodity Supplemental Foods	Pregnant and postpartum women, infants, and children < 6 years of age with incomes ≤ 185% of poverty guidelines	Monthly food package of fruits, vegetables, meats, infant formula, beans, and other available foods
EFNEP	Persons with incomes ≤ 125% of poverty guidelines who have children under 19 years of age	Nutrition education
Medicaid	Anyone with income < 133% of poverty guidelines	Complete health care
Healthy Start	Pregnant women with incomes < 185% of poverty guidelines; certain high-risk pregnancies	Prenatal and postpartum care
EPSDT	Infants, children, and adolescents up to 18 years of age	Health screening: dental checks, health education, hearing, vision

[a] SNAP, Supplemental Nutrition Assistance Program; WIC, Special Supplemental Nutrition Program for Women, Infants, and Children; FMNP, Farmers' Market Nutrition Program; EFNEP, Expanded Food and Nutrition Education Program; EPSDT, Early Periodic Screening, Diagnosis, and Treatment.

[b] See Table 10-1 in Chapter 10 for the 2015 Poverty Guidelines.

creation of local programs is given to areas whose populations need benefits most, judging on the basis of high rates of infant mortality, low birthweight, and low income. WIC began as a two-year pilot project for fiscal years 1973 and 1974. It provides supplemental foods to infants; children up to age five; and pregnant, breastfeeding, and nonbreastfeeding postpartum women who qualify financially and are considered by competent professionals to be at nutritional risk because of inadequate nutrition and inadequate income.[55] Competent professionals include physicians, nutritionists, nurses, and other health officials. Financial eligibility is determined by income (at or below 185% of the poverty guidelines) or by participation in SNAP or Medicaid. Nutritional risks, determined by a health professional, may include one of three types: medically based risks (anemia, underweight, obesity, maternal age, history of high-risk pregnancies, HIV infection); diet-based risks (inadequate dietary pattern, gastrointestinal disorders, renal or cardiorespiratory disorders); or conditions that make the applicant predisposed to medically based or diet-based risks, such as alcoholism or drug addiction (**Table 11-11**).

The WIC program plays both a remedial and a preventive role. Services provided include the following.

WIC foods WIC foods not only address specific nutritional deficiencies but also focus on "foods that promote the health of the population served, as indicated by relevant nutrition science, public health concerns, and cultural eating patterns."

- Checks or vouchers to purchase specific supplemental foods each month (food packages or an electronic benefit card may be provided, rather than paper checks or vouchers). **WIC foods** include iron-fortified infant formula and infant cereal, iron-fortified breakfast cereal, vitamin C–rich fruit or vegetable juice, eggs, milk, cheese, peanut

To be considered for the WIC program, an applicant must exhibit at least one of the nutritional risk factors listed below.

Women

Conditions complicating the prenatal and/or postpartum periods:

- Low hematocrit or hemoglobin
- Insufficient or excessive prenatal weight gain
- Insufficient or excessive pregravid or postpartum weight
- Excessive use of alcohol, drugs, or tobacco
- Inadequate dietary status (as assessed by WIC standards)

General obstetrical risks:

- Younger than age 18
- Multifetal gestation
- Closely spaced pregnancies
- High parity and young age

History of:

- Preterm delivery
- Low-birthweight infant
- Infant with congenital defect
- Miscarriage or stillbirth
- Neonatal death
- Gestational diabetes

Nutrition-related risk conditions:

- Eating disorders
- Gastrointestinal disorders
- Chronic or pregnancy-induced hypertension
- Thyroid disorders
- Diabetes
- Infectious diseases
- Depression
- Cancer
- Renal disease
- Homelessness
- Migrancy

Infants and Children

Low-birthweight or preterm infants

Abnormal pattern of growth: short stature, underweight, overweight

Failure to thrive

Inadequate growth

Low head circumference

Inadequate dietary status (as assessed by WIC standards)

Low hematocrit or hemoglobin (after six months of age)

Elevated blood lead levels

Food allergies/intolerances (as specified by WIC)

Fetal alcohol syndrome

Inborn errors of metabolism

TABLE 11-11

Nutritional Risk Criteria for the Special Supplemental Nutrition Program for Women, Infants, and Children

Source: USDA, "Nutrition Program Facts: WIC" (Washington, D.C.: USDA, December 2014) and *www.fns.usda.gov/wic*.

butter, dried beans and peas, canned fish, and fruits and vegetables. A review of the WIC food package was undertaken by a committee of the Institute of Medicine.[56] As a first step toward determining whether changes were needed to strengthen the nutritional quality of the WIC food packages, the committee evaluated the dietary intakes of the WIC-eligible population. In its final report, *WIC Food Packages: Time for a Change*, the committee recommended revisions to the WIC food packages. As a result, in December 2007, the USDA mandated that significant changes be made to the WIC program food package to make it more consistent with the *Dietary Guidelines for Americans* and more sensitive to cultural food preferences (**Table 11-12**).[57] The new changes to the WIC program also include incentives to promote breastfeeding among low-income women, who, according to the CDC, have lower rates of breastfeeding.[58] New foods added in

TABLE 11-12 WIC Foods

CRITERIA FOR WIC FOOD PACKAGES

- Reduce the prevalence of inadequate or excessive nutrient intakes
- Follow *Dietary Guidelines for Americans* and dietary recommendations for infants
- Support breastfeeding
- Are suitable for persons who may have limited transportation options, storage, and cooking facilities
- Are readily acceptable and available, and take into account cultural food preferences

SAMPLE WIC FOOD PACKAGE[a]

Pregnant and Partially Breastfeeding Women[b]

- 144 fluid oz vitamin C–rich juice
- 36 oz iron-fortified cereal
- 22 qt reduced-fat milk[c]
- 1 dozen eggs
- 1 lb whole-wheat bread[d]
- Legumes (1 lb dried or 64 oz canned)
- 18 oz peanut butter
- $10 cash value voucher for fruits and vegetables (fresh, frozen, canned)

---

[a] An enhanced food package is available for fully breastfeeding women whose infants do not receive formula from the WIC program (includes addition of cheese, canned fish, and larger quantities of milk and eggs).

[b] Maximum monthly allowance.

[c] Or yogurt, soy beverage, calcium-set tofu, cheese.

[d] Or brown rice, bulgur, oatmeal, whole-grain barley, whole-grain bread, whole-wheat macaroni products, soft corn or whole-wheat tortillas.

For more information about the WIC Food Packages, go to *http://wicworks.nal.usda.gov/food-packages*.

2009 include whole-grain tortillas; brown rice; soy beverages; tofu; a wider choice of fruits and vegetables for ethnic variety; canned salmon, mackerel, and sardines; and baby foods. WIC foods are intended to supplement participants' food intakes; each of the WIC foods is rich in one or more of the nutrients that tend to be low in the diets of the population that WIC serves (protein, calcium, iron, vitamin A, and vitamin C).

- Nutrition education and counseling, including individual nutrition counseling and breastfeeding counseling, and group nutrition classes.
- Screening and referral to health care services, including breastfeeding support, immunizations, prenatal care, family planning, and substance abuse treatment.

Providing nutritious supplemental foods to pregnant women is expected to improve the outcome of pregnancy. For infants and children, the food supplements are intended to reduce the incidence of anemia and to improve physical and mental development. Some states distribute food directly, but most provide vouchers, checks, or an electronic benefit transfer (EBT) card that participants can use at participating grocery stores. The food voucher lists the quantities of specific foods, including brand names that can be purchased. All WIC agencies will transition to using EBT by October 2020.

The combination of supplementary food, nutrition education, and preventive health care distinguishes WIC from other federal food assistance programs. Some of the potential impacts of program participation are summarized in **Figure 11-4**. Program benefits include improved dietary quality; more efficient food purchasing; better use of health services; and improved maternal, fetal, and child health and development.[59]

WIC Works WIC has been described as one of the most efficient programs undertaken by the federal government. Over the years, the program has expanded significantly; the 1.9 million women and children served in 1980 at a cost of $725 million had grown

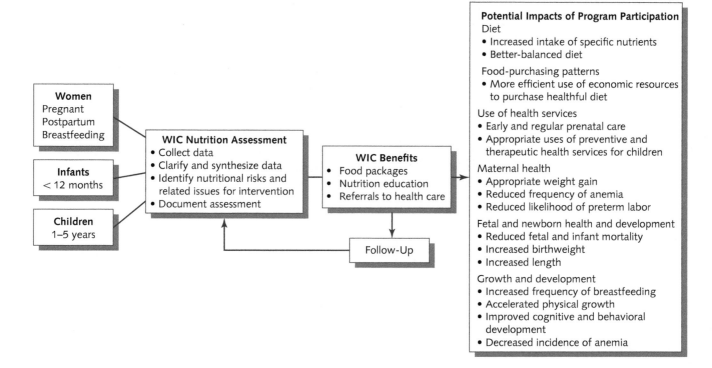

Potential Impacts of Program Participation

Diet
- Increased intake of specific nutrients
- Better-balanced diet

Food-purchasing patterns
- More efficient use of economic resources to purchase healthful diet

Use of health services
- Early and regular prenatal care
- Appropriate uses of preventive and therapeutic health services for children

Maternal health
- Appropriate weight gain
- Reduced frequency of anemia
- Reduced likelihood of preterm labor

Fetal and newborn health and development
- Reduced fetal and infant mortality
- Increased birthweight
- Increased length

Growth and development
- Increased frequency of breastfeeding
- Accelerated physical growth
- Improved cognitive and behavioral development
- Decreased incidence of anemia

Women
Pregnant
Postpartum
Breastfeeding

Infants
< 12 months

Children
1–5 years

WIC Nutrition Assessment
- Collect data
- Clarify and synthesize data
- Identify nutritional risks and related issues for intervention
- Document assessment

WIC Benefits
- Food packages
- Nutrition education
- Referrals to health care

Follow-Up

FIGURE 11-4 WIC Benefits and Potential Program Impacts

Source: Adapted from D. Rush, *The National WIC Evaluation* (Washington, D.C.: U.S. Department of Agriculture, 1987).

by 2014 to more than 8.3 million women, infants, and children served at a cost of nearly $6.9 billion. The dramatic growth of WIC since 1974 has prompted policymakers to focus attention on quantifying the program's benefits.[60] To date, the program's proven benefits include the following:

- A General Accounting Office review of previous WIC studies concluded that WIC reduces the incidence of low birthweight (< 2,500 grams) and very low birthweight (< 1,500 grams) by 25% and 44%, respectively.[61]
- A national WIC evaluation released by the USDA found that WIC has contributed to a reduction of 20–33% in fetal mortality and that the head size of infants whose mothers participated in the WIC program during pregnancy increased measurably.[62]
- Women who participate in WIC have longer pregnancies leading to fewer premature births. This not only benefits the infants but saves millions of dollars in Medicaid costs that would otherwise have been incurred for neonatal intensive care. It is estimated that every dollar spent on WIC for pregnant women can save as much as $4.21 in Medicaid costs.[63] (See the cost–benefit analysis of the WIC program provided in the box on page 447.)
- A study conducted in five states—Florida, North Carolina, Minnesota, Texas, and South Carolina—found that each dollar spent on WIC participants prenatally resulted in a $1.77 to $3.90 savings per participant in Medicaid costs.[64]
- A Yale University School of Medicine study found a remarkable decrease in the prevalence of anemia among low-income children in New Haven since the early 1970s. The researchers concluded, "The marked improvement can most probably be attributed to the nutritional supplementation with iron-fortified foods provided by the WIC program."[65]
- WIC also appears to lead to better mental performance. WIC children whose mothers participated in WIC during pregnancy had better scores than nonparticipants on vocabulary and memory tests.

- WIC participation can lead to improved breastfeeding rates.[66]
- WIC participation is associated with regular use of health care services; WIC children are more likely than not to receive some form of immunization against infectious diseases.
- Data show that the WIC program makes a significant contribution to reducing food insecurity among first-time program participants and suggest the need to consider food insecurity as a risk criterion for the WIC program.[67]
- The WIC program may contribute to the adequacy of iron intake among low-income infants and children.[68]

Unlike most of the other food assistance programs, WIC is not an entitlement program and therefore can serve only as many people as its annual appropriation from Congress permits (**Figure 11-5**).[69] Under federal regulations, once a local agency has reached its maximum caseload, vacancies must be filled in the following order of priority to ensure that program resources are allocated to those at greatest nutritional risk.

FIGURE 11-5

WIC Coverage Rate for All Participants by State, 2012

The percentage of the eligible population that receives WIC benefits is the program's *coverage rate*. In the average month of 2012, WIC served an estimated 63% of those eligible for WIC. For more than a decade, WIC's overall estimated coverage rate has fluctuated in a narrow range from 56–63%. State coverage rates range from 44% in New Hampshire to 82% in California.

Source: U.S. Department of Agriculture, Food and Nutrition Service, Office of Policy Support. *National and State-Level Estimates of Special Supplemental Nutrition Program for Women, Infants, and Children (WIC) Eligibles and Program Reach, 2012*, Alexandria, VA: January 2015.

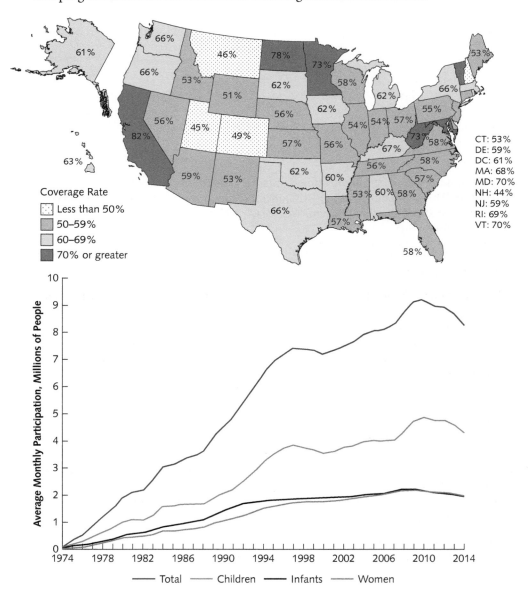

1. Pregnant women, breastfeeding women, and infants determined to be at nutritional risk by a blood test, anthropometric measures, or other documentation of a nutrition-related medical condition.
2. Infants up to six months of age whose mothers participated in WIC or could have participated and who had a medical problem.
3. Children at nutritional risk because of a nutrition-related medical condition.
4. Pregnant or breastfeeding women and infants at nutritional risk because of an inadequate dietary pattern.
5. Children at nutritional risk because of an inadequate dietary pattern.
6. Nonbreastfeeding, postpartum women at nutritional risk.
7. Persons certified for WIC solely because of homelessness or migrancy, and current participants who without WIC foods could continue to have medical and/or dietary problems.

ENTREPRENEUR IN ACTION

Celestine Onyango, RDN, LD, discovered her passion for community nutrition while working as a nutritionist with a local WIC agency in southwest Missouri. The most rewarding aspect of her work is in equipping individuals with the tools they need to live a healthy life. Says Celestine: "This is especially true when you are serving populations that would not have otherwise had access to the information you offer due to their socioeconomic status. At WIC, it is always exciting to work with pregnant women, especially if they come in very early in their pregnancy, because this is such a critical time to start nutrition education. Being able to continue passing on the appropriate information as their child grows is priceless. For community nutrition to grow and thrive, it needs passionate individuals who honestly care about the welfare of those they serve. Newcomers need vision and a hunger to make a big or small difference. They also need a sense of commitment to see it through—especially in this field, as results do not happen overnight. It is important to not let reality dampen your dream of making an impact." Find out more about Celestine online at *www.cengagebrain.com*.

Because of the caps placed on allocated federal funds, WIC currently reaches about 63% of eligible persons. Barriers to participation in WIC include limited government funding, lack of transportation, insufficient time or money to travel to the clinic, insufficient outreach to potential WIC recipients, the absence or expense of childcare, inconvenient clinic hours, and understaffing of WIC facilities.

Overall, research evaluating WIC's effectiveness finds positive outcomes for WIC participants compared to nonparticipants.[70] The following measures would help lower the barriers to program participation and improve the nutrition status and health care of women, infants, and children even further.

- Increase congressional funding for the program to enable more eligible women, infants, and children to receive WIC benefits.
- Improve the coordination between WIC and programs providing or financing maternal and child health care services.
- Implement outreach activities to increase access to WIC program benefits by all who are eligible.[71]

A Cost–Benefit Analysis of the WIC Program

A cost–benefit analysis helps managers gauge how well a program is meeting its clients' needs and provides data that can be used to influence policymakers. Let's consider an evaluation of prenatal participation in the Special Supplemental Nutrition Program for Women, Infants, and Children (WIC). This cost–benefit analysis involved the following steps:

1. **Identify the primary client.** The primary client was the Division of Maternal and Child Health of the Department of Environment, Health, and Natural Resources in Raleigh, North Carolina.

continued

A Cost–Benefit Analysis of the WIC Program —*continued*

2. **Specify the purpose of the evaluation.** The cost–benefit analysis was designed to assess the effect of participation in the prenatal WIC program on low birthweight and on Medicaid costs for the medical care of infants.

3. **Specify the objectives of the evaluation.** The objectives of the evaluation of WIC prenatal participation in North Carolina were to determine:

   - The birthweight of all infants born to WIC mothers
   - The birthweight of a random sample of infants born to non-WIC mothers
   - The cost per client of participating in the WIC program
   - The type and cost of hospital claims for newborn care paid by Medicaid

4. **Calculate a dollar value for each benefit of the program.** The direct benefits to participants in the WIC program included food and nutrition counseling. Indirect benefits included the birth of infants weighing more than 2,500 grams and reduced costs to Medicaid for the medical management of newborn care. (The dollar value assigned to these benefits was not reported in the published analysis.)

5. **Calculate the costs associated with the program.** Both personnel and material costs were considered. In this analysis, the direct costs included the total value of food vouchers redeemed through the WIC program; administrative costs, estimated at an average of $170 per woman; and the newborn medical care costs paid by Medicaid. Medicaid covered such costs for newborn care as physician services, medications, and inpatient or outpatient care. The direct costs are summarized in **Table 11-13**, which shows the Medicaid costs for infants whose mothers received WIC prenatal care, the Medicaid costs for infants whose mothers did not participate in WIC, and the estimated WIC program costs.

6. **Calculate the total cost per client.** The average cost of the program was $179 per white woman, $164 per black woman, and $170 overall (both groups taken together).

7. **Calculate the benefit-to-cost ratio and/or the net savings.** The benefit-to-cost ratio, also shown in Table 11-13, was calculated by subtracting the Medicaid costs for the WIC group (column 1) from the Medicaid costs for the non-WIC group (column 2) and dividing by the WIC costs (column 3). The net savings was the actual dollar difference between the total benefits and the total costs. The estimated net savings (column 1 subtracted from column 2) was $343 for whites and $615 for blacks.

The cost–benefit analysis revealed that the savings in Medicaid costs outweighed the costs of WIC services. The benefit-to-cost ratio was 1.92 for white women and 3.75 for black women, which means that for each dollar spent on WIC, Medicaid saved $1.92 on whites and $3.75 on blacks. In addition, women who received WIC prenatal care gave birth to fewer infants with low and very low birthweights than women who did not participate in WIC.

TABLE 11-13 Average Costs of Medicaid and Average Costs of WIC Services

	MEDICAID COSTS		WIC COSTS[a]	BENEFIT-TO-COST RATIO
	WIC	**NON-WIC**		
White	$1,778	$2,121	$179	1.92
Black	1,902	2,517	164	3.75
Total	1,856	2,350	170	2.91

[a] WIC costs include administrative and food costs.

Source: From the Journal of the American Dietetic Association 93 (1993): 16.

A cost–benefit analysis undertaken by another state with a different sample of women and infants would probably produce slightly different results in program costs and in the benefit-to-cost ratio. Even so, fiscal evaluations can be used to convince policymakers that money allocated for the WIC program is well spent and that cost savings can be achieved with nutrition intervention.

Source: The description of the cost–benefit analysis of the WIC program was adapted from P. A. Buescher and coauthors, "Prenatal WIC Participation Can Reduce Low Birthweight and Newborn Medical Costs: A Cost–Benefit Analysis of WIC Participation in North Carolina," *Journal of the American Dietetic Association* 93 (1993): 163–66. The procedure for conducting a cost–benefit analysis was adapted from the Ross Roundtable Report, *Benefits of Nutrition Services: A Costing and Marketing Approach* (Columbus, OH: Ross Laboratories, 1987), 24–29.

▶ **THINK LIKE A COMMUNITY NUTRITIONIST**

Read "A Cost–Benefit Analysis of the WIC Program" on pages 447–449. Imagine you are preparing to lobby for increased WIC funding. What would be your key messages? Make a list of talking points you would use in discussing the importance of WIC and convincing your legislator of the need for increased funding.

Other Nutrition Programs of the U.S. Department of Agriculture

Several programs of the U.S. Department of Agriculture (USDA) directly or indirectly provide nutrition support during pregnancy and infancy.

Supplemental Nutrition Assistance Program (SNAP)
SNAP is designed to improve the diets of people with low incomes by providing benefits to cover part or all of their household's food budget. Chapter 10 provided an overview of this program. As explained previously, program participants can use SNAP benefits to buy food in any retail store that has been approved by the Food and Nutrition Service to accept them. For many economically disadvantaged women, SNAP is the major means by which they are able to purchase adequate diets for their families. The Select Panel for the Promotion of Child Health reported that SNAP users purchase more nutritious foods per dollar spent on food than eligible households that do not participate in the program.[72]

WIC Farmers' Market Nutrition Program
The WIC Farmers' Market Nutrition Program (FMNP) was created to provide fresh, nutritious fruits and vegetables to WIC participants and to expand the awareness and use of farmers' markets by consumers. Eligible recipients receive FMNP coupons. A study reported by the Food Research and Action Center showed that women in the WIC program who received FMNP coupons increased both fruit and vegetable consumption by about 5% compared with WIC women who did not receive coupons. The FMNP participants also patronized farmers' markets more than nonrecipients, even after they were no longer eligible for WIC.[73]

Commodity Supplemental Food Program
The Commodity Supplemental Food Program (CSFP) is a direct food distribution program providing supplemental foods and nutrition education. The CSFP provides supplemental foods to infants and children and to pregnant, postpartum, and breastfeeding women with low incomes who are vulnerable to malnutrition and live in approved project areas. Recipients may not participate in both WIC and CSFP. The USDA purchases the foods for distribution through state agencies on a monthly basis.

Expanded Food and Nutrition Education Program (EFNEP)
The Expanded Food and Nutrition Education Program (EFNEP) is a federally funded program designed specifically for nutrition education. The EFNEP was authorized in 1968 and is administered by the USDA National Institute of Food and Agriculture. It is designed to assist limited-resource audiences in acquiring the knowledge, skills, attitudes, and changed

behavior necessary for nutritionally sound diets, and to contribute to their personal development and the improvement of the total family diet.[74] The program is implemented by trained paraprofessionals (peer educators) and volunteers from the local community under the supervision of county extension family and consumer science professionals. For more information about the Cooperative Extension System, go to *http://nifa.usda.gov/extension*.

Nutrition Programs of the U.S. Department of Health and Human Services

The U.S. Department of Health and Human Services (DHHS) also sponsors several programs that are concerned with health and nutrition status during pregnancy and infancy.

Title V Maternal and Child Health Program
Enacted in 1935, Title V of the Social Security Act is the only federal program concerned exclusively with the health of mothers, infants, and children. It provides federal support to the states to enhance their ability to "promote, improve, and deliver" maternal, infant, and child health (MCH) care and programs for children with special health care needs (CSHCN), especially in rural areas and regions experiencing severe economic stress. The aim of Congress in passing this legislation was to improve the health of mothers, infants, and children in areas where the need was greatest.

The states are allocated Title V MCH funds to be used for (1) services and programs to reduce infant mortality and improve child and maternal health and (2) services, programs, and facilities to locate, diagnose, and treat children who have special health care needs (e.g., chronic medical conditions) or who are at risk of physical or developmental disabilities.[75] The Title V MCH program provides for nutrition assessment, dietary counseling, nutrition education, and referral to food assistance programs for infants, preschool and school-age children, children with special health care needs, adolescents, and women of childbearing age. Title V helps create healthy communities by working with local groups to identify and address their local health needs, ranging from teen pregnancy to low immunization rates. It also supports training in nutrition for health and nutrition professionals who are involved in developing nutrition services (**Figure 11-6**).

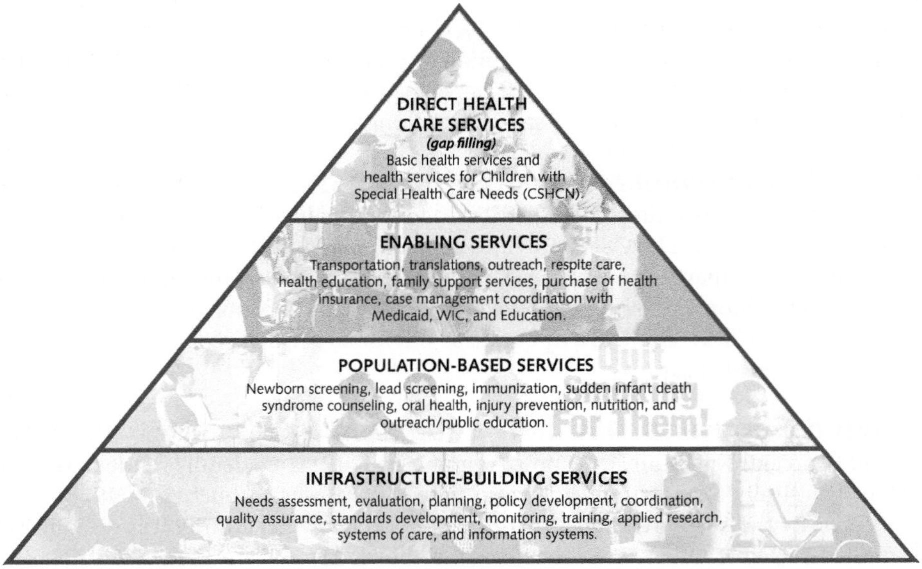

FIGURE 11-6

Maternal and Child Health Pyramid of Health Services

The conceptual framework for the services of the Title V Maternal and Child Health Bureau is envisioned as a pyramid with four tiers of services and levels of funding that provide comprehensive services for mothers and children.

Source: Reprinted from Understanding Title V of the Social Security Act, U.S. Department of Health and Human Services, Maternal and Child Health Bureau.

DIRECT HEALTH CARE SERVICES
(gap filling)
Basic health services and health services for Children with Special Health Care Needs (CSHCN).

ENABLING SERVICES
Transportation, translations, outreach, respite care, health education, family support services, purchase of health insurance, case management coordination with Medicaid, WIC, and Education.

POPULATION-BASED SERVICES
Newborn screening, lead screening, immunization, sudden infant death syndrome counseling, oral health, injury prevention, nutrition, and outreach/public education.

INFRASTRUCTURE-BUILDING SERVICES
Needs assessment, evaluation, planning, policy development, coordination, quality assurance, standards development, monitoring, training, applied research, systems of care, and information systems.

The Title V MCH program is administered federally by the Bureau of Maternal and Child Health in the Health Resources and Services Administration of the Public Health Service. Administration of the MCH program is the responsibility of the MCH unit within each state's health agency. Most of the CSHCN programs are also administered through state health agencies; some, however, are delivered through other state agencies, such as welfare departments, social service agencies, or state universities. Under the law, each state is required to operate a "program of projects" in each of five areas: (1) maternity and infant care, (2) intensive infant care, (3) family planning, (4) health care for children and youth, and (5) dental care for children.[76]

States have varying degrees of control over local use of Title V funds. Most state MCH funds are used to support well-child checkups, immunization programs, vision and hearing screenings, and school health services, as well as other programs. Funds for CSHCN programs are used to provide direct services to children with special health care needs through local clinics and/or fee-for-service arrangements with physicians in private practice. Regardless of the method of delivering CSHCN programs, a multidisciplinary approach to providing health care is used by nearly all states.[77]

The Select Panel for the Promotion of Child Health reported that Title V program efforts have resulted in significant improvements in maternal and child health. The program is believed to have contributed to the decline in infant and maternal mortality, to the reduction of disability in children with handicaps, and to a general improvement in the health status of children.[78]

Medicaid and EPSDT Congress created the Medicaid program in 1965 to ensure financial access to health care for the economically disadvantaged. It was enacted through Title XIX of the Social Security Act. The Medicaid program is a state-administered entitlement program built on the welfare model. It is constructed as a medical assistance program that reimburses providers for specific services delivered to eligible recipients. Under amendments enacted in 1967, the states are required to provide Early Periodic Screening, Diagnosis, and Treatment (EPSDT) as a mandatory Medicaid service. As outlined by Congress, the purpose of EPSDT is to improve the health status of children from low-income families by providing health services not typically found under the current Medicaid program. EPSDT requires an assessment of the nutrition status of eligible children and their referral for treatment.[79] Whereas Medicaid is mainly a provider payment program for medical services, EPSDT regulations stipulate that states must develop protocols for identifying eligible children; informing them of the EPSDT program; and ensuring that referral, preventive, and treatment services are made available to participants.

The federal administration of Medicaid is the responsibility of the Center for Medicare and Medicaid Services (CMS) within the DHHS. Medicaid and EPSDT have been credited with increasing the access of low-income women, infants, and children to health care services. EPSDT, by virtue of its aggressive preventive strategy, has been effective in improving child health.[80] However, strict eligibility requirements and federal statutory policies have limited the ability of these programs to reach their full potential.[81]

Health Center Program The Health Center Program was initiated by the Office of Economic Opportunity in 1966 and authorized by the Public Health Service Act. The health centers serve populations with limited access to health care, including low-income populations, the uninsured, those with limited English proficiency, migrant and seasonal farmworkers, individuals and families experiencing homelessness, and those living in public housing. The primary program focus is on comprehensive primary care services through federally funded community-based health centers.[82] Preventive services are also

TO REMEMBER THE ELEMENTS OF EPSDT, USE THE NAME OF THE PROGRAM:

Early — Identifying problems early, starting at birth;

Periodic — Checking children's health at periodic, age-appropriate intervals;

Screening — Doing physical, mental, developmental, dental, hearing, vision, and other screening tests to detect potential problems;

Diagnosis — Performing diagnostic tests to follow up when a risk is identified; and

Treatment — Treating the problems found.

Laura Sprauer

**ENTREPRENEUR
IN ACTION**

Laura Sprauer, MPH, RD, first gained an interest in nutrition while spending her summers in college working on community health initiatives in rural communities in Latin America. After her dietetic internship, Laura worked at a community health center as a dietitian with the WIC Program, serving a predominantly Hispanic population in an underserved Boston neighborhood. Working in a community health center gave Laura the ability to show her flexibility and become an asset to the organization. As an international board-certified lactation consultant (IBCLC) and certified childbirth educator, Laura can provide comprehensive and culturally appropriate education and support to the families in the community. Says Laura: "Community health centers are all about one-stop shopping, and clients should be able to have a wide variety of health concerns addressed in the same place. I was able to go from teaching diabetes classes as a certified diabetes educator to creating a childhood obesity program, to helping a mom breastfeed her newborn baby." Laura took advantage of her time spent in Latin America and used her Spanish language skills and knowledge of the Latino community to further connect with her clients. Find out more about her experiences online at *www.cengagebrain.com*.

offered through the health centers, including well-child care, nutrition assessment, and health education. The program is administered federally by the Health Resources and Services Administration of the Public Health Service.

The Healthy Start Program The fact that African Americans and other minorities continue to have increased rates of infant mortality and low birthweight constitutes a major public health problem. In 1991, the Health Resources and Services Administration (HRSA) of the U.S. Department of Health and Human Services funded 15 urban and rural sites in communities with infant mortality rates that were 1.5 to 2.5 times the national average.[83] The Healthy Start Program's goal is to identify and develop community-based approaches to reducing infant mortality and improving the health of low-income women, infants, children, and their families. Healthy Start projects address multiple issues, such as providing adequate prenatal care, promoting positive prenatal health behaviors, and reducing barriers to accessing health care services. Healthy Start specializes in outreach and home visits and focuses on getting women into prenatal care as early as possible. Improving the low-birthweight rate requires improvements in the practices and behavior of women while pregnant. Significant savings in health care costs can accrue from enabling mothers to add a few ounces to a baby's weight before birth. An increase of 250 grams (about 0.5 pound) in birthweight saves an average of $12,000 to $16,000 in first-year medical expenses. Prenatal interventions—such as the Healthy Start Program—that result in a normal-weight birth (over 2,500 grams, or 5.5 pounds) can save $59,700 in medical expenses in the infant's first year. In 2015, 105 Healthy Start projects were providing services in 39 states, the District of Columbia, and Puerto Rico. Over 90% of all Healthy Start families are African American, Hispanic, or Native American.

Looking Ahead: Improving the Health of Mothers and Infants

Many of the existing health care programs do not themselves offer nutrition counseling or education. These programs frequently refer their clients to the WIC program for nutrition services. The heavy caseloads in many WIC programs, however, limit the amount of personalized nutrition counseling they can provide. Clearly, more must be done to ensure that quality nutrition counseling is available and accessible for pregnant and lactating women and their infants. Some WIC agencies now provide qualifying WIC participants with the option of doing nutrition education online in place of coming to the WIC office. The nutrition education lessons typically take about 15 to 20 minutes to complete. Upon completion of the online lesson, the participants become eligible to receive their WIC checks either by mail or by coming into their WIC Center. Lesson topics available at *www.wichealth.org* include:[84]

- Offering regular meals and snacks
- Child feeding issues related to food demands and picky eating habits
- Creating good eating habits in your child
- Parent–child feeding issues related to trust
- Helping your child make good eating choices
- Support for breastfeeding
- Balancing physical activity with healthy eating
- Postpartum wellness
- Starting your infant on solid foods
- Teaching your baby how to drink from a cup
- Infusing concepts associated with "Choose MyPlate" into daily living
- How to give your child fun and healthy drinks
- Eating whole grains
- Making the most of your food dollars
- Following food safety guidelines
- Preparing for a healthy pregnancy
- Preparing meatless meals

Breastfeeding peer counselors can connect with WIC clients through a videoconferencing program following completion of the online breastfeeding or pregnancy-related lessons. Clients also gain access to *Health eKitchen*, a video library regarding shopping, preparing, cooking, and storing WIC food package items.[85]

A few states have been successful in providing reimbursable nutrition counseling services to maternal and child health programs. The South Carolina High Risk Channeling Project provides nutrition services, reimbursable by Medicaid, to all participants. The Kentucky Department for Health Services uses some of its MCH block grant funds to hire public health nutritionists specifically to provide nutrition counseling for high-risk clients in the local maternal and child health care programs.[86]

Some voluntary health organizations, such as local chapters of the La Leche League International and the March of Dimes Birth Defects Foundation, offer classes that are helpful to particular groups or can provide appropriate nutrition education materials and other resources to the community nutritionist working with mother–child populations (see the Internet Resources at the end of this chapter).

The increasing numbers of working women, including those who are planning families or have young infants, along with the growth in worksite health promotion programs, have implications for community nutritionists in providing nutrition education and related services to this population. Some worksites have included components designed for pregnant and lactating women (e.g., breastfeeding promotion and prenatal education programs) in their overall health promotion programs.[87]

Where adolescents are concerned, a variety of comprehensive community programs exist to help the pregnant teen with her educational, social, medical, and nutritional needs. Most of these programs include three components: (1) early and consistent prenatal care, (2) continuing education on a classroom basis, and (3) counseling on an individual or group basis.[88] The importance of these programs in improving maternal and child health is well recognized. Because teen pregnancy is usually unplanned, efforts should be made to improve the nutrition and health status of all adolescents through nutrition education and counseling in the classroom as well as in physicians' offices.

To ensure that all pregnant women have access to satisfactory prenatal services in the future, efforts must be made to convince policymakers of the importance of the following recommendations:[89]

- Food supplementation, nutrition education, and breastfeeding support should be available to all pregnant women with low incomes.
- Additional federal funds should be appropriated to make WIC available to all pregnant low-income women.
- Nutrition counseling and education should be provided to all pregnant women whose care is financed by Medicaid.
- State Medicaid programs should be required to include nutrition counseling and education as reimbursable services.
- Federal and state funds should be provided to health department clinics and community health centers to allow for employment of public health nutritionists to offer nutrition counseling to all pregnant women who use these facilities.
- Health insurance policies should include prenatal nutrition counseling as a reimbursable service for all pregnant women living in the United States.

case study

Promotion of Breastfeeding

by Alice Fornari, EdD, RD, Alessandra Sarcona, MS, RD, CSSD, and Alison Barkman, MS, RD, CDN

Scenario

As a lactation specialist (international board-certified lactation consultant) and registered dietitian, you have been doing consulting work for physicians specializing in obstetrics and gynecology. Most of your counseling has been geared to middle- and upper-class pregnant and lactating women. You have created nutrition education pamphlets outlining the benefits of breastfeeding, as well as lactation management to promote continued breastfeeding. Most of your visits were to patients' homes. You also held group sessions focusing on nutrition and lactation for pregnant mothers enrolled in birthing preparation classes.

The community hospital in your area has set up a Medicaid program called Healthy Start for pregnant women with incomes less than 185% of the poverty guidelines for prenatal and postpartum care and has requested your services in setting up a breastfeeding promotion program for program participants. The population is predominantly African American (70%), Hispanic (22%), and Caucasian (8%).

Learning Outcomes

- Describe the benefits of breastfeeding and identify the barriers to breastfeeding.
- Identify the tools for advocating breastfeeding using peer counselors to change culturally based behaviors.
- Distinguish cultural differences that affect delivery of nutrition education.

Foundation: Acquisition of Knowledge and Skills

1. Review the following Academy of Nutrition and Dietetics position paper titled "Promoting and Supporting Breastfeeding," which is available from the *Journal of the Academy of Nutrition and Dietetics.* (Visit *www.eatright.org* and go to Position Papers.) List the benefits of breastfeeding; choose one that you think is interesting and discuss. Then list the barriers to breastfeeding; choose one that you think is common and discuss.
2. Referring to your text, describe the rationale for using peer counselors to change culturally based behaviors.

Step 1: *Identify Relevant Information and Uncertainties*

1. In review of the breastfeeding trends in the United States, compare the Healthy Start population to the findings in the Academy of Nutrition and Dietetics position paper.
2. Identify the barriers to breastfeeding that may exist in the Healthy Start population.

Step 2: *Interpret Information*

1. Compare and contrast your experience with counseling pregnant women on lactation in a physician's referral practice to the present situation with Medicaid recipients in a Healthy Start program; take into account any bias you may have toward breastfeeding.
2. In order to make the breastfeeding peer counselor program a success, there are various strategies used to recruit women to become peer counselors. What tools do WIC and La Leche use to advocate a breastfeeding peer counselor program? Search these websites to find out more about the peer counseling program:

www.llli.org/llleaderweb/lv/lvaugsep99p92.html
www.llli.org/llleaderweb/lv/lvaugsep00p74.html
www.cdc.gov/breastfeeding/pdf/BF_guide_3.pdf

Search the following website to find out more on strategies used to advocate breastfeeding peer counseling:

www.cdph.ca.gov/programs/wicworks/Documents/BF/WIC-BF-PCHandbook.pdf

Step 3: *Draw and Implement Conclusions*

Judging on the basis of your interpretations in the questions posed in Step 2, what types of revisions would you make to your nutrition education materials, counseling, and group sessions in order to help minimize barriers to successful breastfeeding in the Healthy Start setting?

Step 4: *Engage in Continuous Improvement*

As you continue to work with breastfeeding promotion at Healthy Start, what steps would you take to encourage breastfeeding up to one year?

PROFESSIONAL **FOCUS**

Leading for Success

Supreme Court Justice Potter Stewart once said about obscenity, "I cannot define it for you, but I know it when I see it."[1] The same might be said about leadership, although the wealth of research in this area has helped define the behaviors and attitudes of good leaders.

Leading is not the same as managing. The difference between the two has been described by Warren Bennis, an internationally recognized consultant, writer, and researcher on leadership: "Leaders are people who do the right thing; managers are people who do things right. Both roles are crucial, but they differ profoundly."[2] In general, managers crunch numbers; orchestrate activities; and control supplies, projects, and data. Leaders fertilize and catalyze. They enhance people, allowing them to stretch and grow. Where managers push and direct, leaders pull and expect.[3]

What exactly is leadership? Leadership is "the process whereby one person influences others to work toward a goal."[4] Leaders understand how an organization works (or doesn't work, as the case may be) and how people work—that is, what motivates them to be top performers. Leaders have the power to project onto other people their vision, their inspiration, and their ideas.[5]

The traits of successful leaders number more than 100, according to recent studies, though not all experts agree on the importance of every trait.[6] Some of the attributes commonly ascribed to leaders are intelligence, credibility, energy, sociability, discipline, courage, and generosity. Integrity is essential. Integrity has been described as "the most important leadership principle that you will demonstrate to your leadership team and your followers."[7] Integrity means adhering to a high standard of honesty. Leaders with integrity strive to present their values and character honestly in their dealings with other people.

Accountability is also important. Accountability means doing what you say you are going to do. Whether the issue is large or small, leaders follow through on their promises and commitments. They know that *not* following through on a promise or commitment reduces their credibility and diminishes the trust other people have placed in them.[8] Leaders hold themselves accountable.

Leaders are forward-thinking. They see the big picture and have a vision about where they are going—and where they want their teams to go. Leaders can describe what a team, department, or organization will look and feel like in six months, one year, or five years. Make no mistake, though, leaders are not ones to complain about the way things are or dwell on the way things might have been. They are optimistic about the future, seeing many possibilities and positive outcomes. Their enthusiasm is contagious. Leaders come in all shapes, sizes, and temperaments. They are found in the executive suite and on the factory floor, among support staff and across middle management. In their seminar programs on leadership, James Kouzes and Barry Posner used to say, "Leaders go places. The difference between managing and leading is the difference between what you can do with your hands and what you can do with your feet. . . . You can't lead from behind a desk. You can't lead from a seated position. The only way you can go anyplace is to get up from behind the desk and use your feet."[9] Then they received a letter from the president of a computer software services company who indicated that although about one-third of his employees had disabilities and several were in wheelchairs, they led quite effectively. Kouzes and Posner reformulated their example to reflect the diversity of leaders. You can have a disability and be a leader; you can be a manager and be a leader; you can be a newly minted community nutritionist in your first job and be a leader.

Warren Bennis believes that leaders all have a guiding vision, passion, integrity, curiosity, and daring.[10] They are self-confident and instill self-confidence in others. They are willing to take risks and responsibility.[11] Following is a description of the principles of leadership outlined by General H. Norman Schwarzkopf, who guided U.S. troops to victory in the Gulf War.*

- **You must have clear goals.** Having specific goals and articulating them clearly makes it easy for everyone involved to understand the mission.
- **Give yourself a clear agenda.** First thing in the morning, write down the five most important things you need to accomplish that day. Whatever else you do, get those five things done first.

- **Let people know where they stand.** You do a great disservice to an employee or student when you give high marks for mediocre work. The grades you give the people who report to you must reflect reality.
- **What's broken, fix now.** If it's a problem, fix it now. Problems that aren't dealt with lead to other problems, and in the meantime, something else breaks down and needs fixing.
- **No repainting the flagpole.** Make sure that all the work your people are doing is essential to the organization.
- **Set high standards.** Too often we don't ask enough of people. People generally won't perform above your expectations, so it is important to expect a lot.
- **Lead and then get out of the way.** Yes, you must put the right people in the right place to get the job done, but then step back. Allow them to own their work.
- **People come to work to succeed.** Nobody comes to work to fail. Why do so many organizations operate on the principle that if people aren't watched and supervised, they'll bungle the job?
- **Never lie. Ever.** Lying undermines your credibility. Be straightforward in your thinking and actions.
- **When in charge, take command.** Leaders are often called upon to make decisions without adequate information. It is usually a mistake to put off making a decision until all the data are in. The best policy is to decide, monitor the results, and change course if necessary.
- **Do what's right.** "The truth of the matter," said Schwarzkopf, "is that you *always* know the right thing to do. The hard part is doing it."

* From *Inc.* magazine, Goldhirsh Group, Inc., 38 Commercial Wharf, Boston, MA 02110 (*www.inc.com*). "Schwarzkopf on Leadership," *Inc.* 14 (January 1992): 11.

CHAPTER **SUMMARY** ....

Trends in Maternal and Infant Health

▶ One of the best indicators of a nation's health, according to epidemiologists, is the infant mortality rate (IMR). In order to achieve further reductions in infant mortality and eliminate racial and ethnic differences in pregnancy outcomes, health care professionals must focus on changing the behaviors—both protective and risky—that affect pregnancy outcomes.

▶ The use of timely prenatal care can help to mitigate risks by identifying women who are at high risk of high blood pressure or other maternal complications. Other actions, such as breastfeeding, newborn screening, and primary care in infancy, can significantly improve infants' health and chances of survival.

▶ *Healthy People 2020* takes a broad scope, encompassing maternal and infant health, birth defects, and developmental disabilities (see Table 11-2).

Healthy Mothers

▶ Genetic, environmental, and behavioral factors affect risk and the outcome of pregnancy.

▶ Normal weight gain and adequate nutrition support the health of the mother and the development of the fetus.

▶ Nutrition assessment and monitoring during pregnancy can be divided into three categories: preconception care, the initial prenatal visit, and subsequent prenatal visits. The nutrition status of all women should be assessed at their initial prenatal visit.

Healthy Babies

▶ The growth of infants directly reflects their nutritional well-being and is the major indicator of their nutrition status. The WHO Child Growth Standards are used to analyze measures of growth status in infants.

▶ Breastfeeding offers both emotional and physical health advantages.

▶ Barriers to achieving the nation's health objective of increasing the incidence of breastfeeding include lack of knowledge, an absence of work policies and facilities that support lactating women, and the lack of breastfeeding support for low-income women (see Table 11-8).

▶ Iron deficiency and food allergies are two of the most significant nutrition-related problems of infants.

Domestic Maternal and Infant Nutrition Programs

▶ WIC provides supplemental foods to infants; children up to age five; and pregnant, breastfeeding, and nonbreastfeeding postpartum women who qualify financially and are considered to be at nutritional risk because of inadequate nutrition and inadequate income (see Table 11-11). The WIC program plays both a remedial and a preventive role. Services provided include the following: food packages or checks or vouchers to purchase specific foods each month, nutrition education, and referral to health care services.

- Program benefits include improved dietary quality; more efficient food purchasing; better use of health services; and improved maternal, fetal, and child health and development.

- WIC is not an entitlement program and therefore can serve only as many people as its annual appropriation from Congress permits.

▶ Other USDA programs that directly or indirectly provide nutrition support during pregnancy and infancy include SNAP, WIC Farmers' Market Nutrition Program, Commodity Supplemental Food Program, and the Expanded Food and Nutrition Education Program.

▶ The U.S. Department of Health and Human Services also sponsors programs for women, infants, and children.

- The Title V Maternal and Child Health Program provides federal support to the states for (1) services and programs to reduce infant mortality and improve child and maternal health and (2) services, programs, and facilities to locate, diagnose, and treat children who have special health care needs or who are at risk of physical or developmental disabilities.
- Congress created the Medicaid program to ensure financial access to health care for the economically disadvantaged. States are required to provide Early Periodic Screening, Diagnosis, and Treatment (EPSDT) as a mandatory Medicaid service.
- The Health Centers Program is designed to provide health services and related training in medically underserved areas.
- The Healthy Start Program's goal is to identify and develop community-based approaches to reducing infant mortality and improving the health of low-income women, infants, and children and their families.

Looking Ahead: Improving the Health of Mothers and Infants

▶ To ensure that all pregnant women have access to satisfactory prenatal services in the future, the following recommendations are made: Food supplementation and nutrition education should be available to all pregnant women with low incomes. Additional federal funds should be appropriated to make WIC available to all pregnant low-income women. Nutrition counseling and education should be provided to all pregnant women whose care is financed by Medicaid. Health insurance policies should include prenatal nutrition counseling as a reimbursable service for all pregnant women living in the United States.

SUMMARY **QUESTIONS**

1. Discuss the progress made or not made in meeting the *Healthy People 2010* objectives in regard to maternal and infant nutrition. What efforts are needed to make the *Healthy People 2020* objectives a reality?
2. Explain the relationship of maternal weight gain to infant birthweight.
3. Discuss the benefits of breastfeeding and provide an example of a successful approach to increasing breastfeeding rates in the United States.
4. Describe the purpose, eligibility requirements, and benefits of the federal food and nutrition assistance programs available to assist low-income women and their children.
5. What improvements would you recommend to enhance the effectiveness of the WIC program in meeting the needs of those who are eligible to participate?

INTERNET **RESOURCES**

American Academy of Pediatrics
www.aap.org

Bright Futures
http://brightfutures.org

Center for Food Safety and Applied Nutrition
www.fda.gov/Food/default.htm

Expanded Food and Nutrition Education Program (EFNEP)
http://nifa.usda.gov/program/expanded-food-and-nutrition-education-program-efnep

Feeding Infants: A Guide for Use in the Child Nutrition Programs
www.fns.usda.gov/tn/Resources/feeding_infants.pdf

Healthy Start Program
www.nationalhealthystart.org

La Leche League International
www.llli.org

March of Dimes
www.marchofdimes.org

Maternal and Child Health Bureau
www.mchb.hrsa.gov

Mayo Clinic Healthy Living Centers
www.mayoclinic.org

National WIC Breastfeeding Promotion Project
www.fns.usda.gov/wic/breastfeeding-promotion-and-support-wic

National Center for Education in Maternal and Child Health
http://ncemch.org

National Women's Health Information Center (DHHS)
www.womenshealth.gov

Nutrition for Limited Resource Groups
http://extension.psu.edu/health/nutrition-links

WIC Breastfeeding Promotion
http://wicworks.nal.usda.gov/breastfeeding

WIC Program
www.fns.usda.gov/wic/women-infants-and-children-wic

WIC Assessment Tools/Growth Charts
https://wicworks.fns.usda.gov/assessment-tools

WIC Studies
www.fns.usda.gov/ops/wic-studies

WIC Works Educational Materials Database
https://wicworks.fns.usda.gov/nutrition-education

WISEWOMAN
www.cdc.gov/wisewoman

CHAPTER 12

Children and Adolescents: Nutrition Issues, Services, and Programs

LEARNING **OBJECTIVES**

After you have read and studied this chapter, you will be able to:

- Describe three nutritional problems currently experienced by U.S. children and adolescents.

- Specify four *Healthy People 2020* nutrition objectives for children and adolescents.

- Discuss four nutrition assistance programs aimed at improving the health and nutrition status of children, including their purposes and types of assistance offered.

- Describe factors that increase the likelihood of obesity in children.

This chapter addresses such issues as the influence of age, growth, and normal development on nutrition requirements; availability of food and nutrition programs in the community; and current information technologies, which have been designated by the Accreditation Council for Education in Nutrition and Dietetics (ACEND) as Foundation Knowledge and Learning Outcomes for dietetics education.

CHAPTER **OUTLINE**

For a complete list of references, please access the MindTap Reader within your MindTap course.

Introduction

Good health is fundamental to the growth, development, and well-being of all children and adolescents and ultimately helps to protect them from chronic diseases as adults. Widespread immunization, improved sanitation, public education on nutrition and health, and the discovery of antibiotics have dramatically reduced the rates of child morbidity and mortality due to infectious diseases. Unfortunately, the status of this group today is far from satisfactory, and new perils have arisen in the past few decades: motor vehicle accidents; violence due to suicide, homicide, and abuse; increased incidence of bullying; sexually transmitted diseases; substance abuse; exposure to environmental pollutants; and the increased prevalence of overweight and obese children and adolescents.[1] Despite advances in clinical and preventive medicine, children and adolescents in the United States have significant health and nutritional concerns that deserve attention.

This chapter reviews the eating patterns of children and adolescents, the factors that influence these patterns, and current nutrition-related problems of children and adolescents. It also examines the nutrition programs that target children and teenagers and the challenges of operating and improving the child nutrition programs. These programs all have the objective of improving child and adolescent nutrition and, ultimately, enhancing health. For our purposes, children are generally categorized as ages 1–11 years and adolescents as ages 12–19 years. Other age categories appear in this chapter, however, because the literature is not entirely consistent on the ages that constitute childhood and adolescence.

Healthy People 2020 National Nutrition Objectives

In 2010, the U.S. Department of Health and Human Services (DHHS) outlined a set of health and nutrition objectives for children and adolescents in its publication *Healthy People 2020*.[2] The priority health-related areas for children and adolescents include physical activity and fitness, nutrition, and dental health.

Healthy People 2020 includes separate targets for fruits, vegetables, and whole grains in order to be consistent with the current set of *Dietary Guidelines for Americans*. Objectives are included for foods eaten at school and for nutrition education in schools. **Table 12-1** shows several of the major *Healthy People 2020* objectives for children and adolescents.

Healthy People 2010 Final Review

The final review for the *Healthy People 2010* initiative shows an overall trend for the worse in the data on the weight status of children.[3] The prevalence of overweight among

TABLE 12-1 A Selection of *Healthy People 2020* Objectives from the Nutrition and Weight Status, Physical Activity, and Adolescent Health Topic Areas[a]

OBJECTIVE NUMBER AND OBJECTIVE	BASELINE (YEAR)[b]	HEALTHY PEOPLE 2020 TARGET
Nutrition and Weight Status		
NWS-1: Increase the number of states with nutrition standards for foods and beverages provided to preschool-age children in childcare.	24 states (2006)	34 states
NWS-2: Increase the proportion of schools that offer nutritious foods and beverages outside of school meals.		
NWS-2.1 Increase the proportion of schools that do not sell or offer calorically sweetened beverages to students.	9.3% (2006)	21.3%
NWS-2.2 Increase the proportion of school districts that require schools to make fruits or vegetables available whenever other food is offered or sold.	6.6% (2006)	18.6%
NWS-10: Reduce the proportion of children and adolescents who are considered obese.		
NWS-10.1 Children ages 2–5 years	10.4% (2005–2008)	9.4%[c]
NWS-10.2 Children ages 6–11 years	17.4% (2005–2008)	15.7%[c]
NWS-10.3 Adolescents ages 12–19 years	17.9% (2005–2008)	16.1%[c]
NWS-12: Eliminate very low food security among children.	1.3% (2008)	0.2%
Physical Activity		
PA-3: Increase the proportion of adolescents who meet current federal physical activity guidelines for aerobic physical activity and for muscle-strengthening activity.		
PA-3.1 Aerobic physical activity	28.7% (2011)	31.6%[c]
PA-3.2 (Developmental) Muscle-strengthening activity	TBD[d]	TBD
PA-4: Increase the proportion of the nation's public and private schools that require daily physical education for all students.		
PA-4.1 Elementary schools	3.8% (2006)	4.2%[c]
PA-4.2 Middle and junior high schools	7.8% (2006)	8.6%[c]
PA-4.3 Senior high schools	2.1% (2006)	2.3%[c]
PA-5: Increase the proportion of adolescents who participate in daily school physical education.	33.3% (2009)	36.6%[c]
PA-8.2: Increase the proportion of children and adolescents age 2 years through 12th grade who view television or play video games for no more than two hours a day.		
PA-8.2.1 Children ages 2–5 years	75.6% (2005–2008)	83.2%
PA-8.2.2 Children and adolescents ages 6–14 years	78.9% (2007)	86.8%[c]
PA-8.2.3 Adolescents in grades 9–12	67.2% (2007)	73.9%[c]
Adolescent Health		
AH-6: Increase the proportion of schools with a school breakfast program.	68.6% of schools had a school breakfast program (2006)	75.5%[c]

[a] See Chapter 8 for objectives for obesity and weight status. See also Chapter 7 for other nutrition and weight status *Healthy People 2020* objectives.

[b] Data sources include School Health Policies and Programs Study, National Resource Center for Health and Safety in Child Care and Early Education, National Vital Statistics System (CDC), National Health and Nutrition Examination Survey (NHANES), Youth Risk Behavior Surveillance System.

[c] Target setting method: 10% improvement.

[d] Potential data source: Youth Risk Behavior Surveillance System (YRBSS), CDC/NCHHSTP.

Source: National Center for Health Statistics, Department of Health and Human Services, *Healthy People 2020* and *Healthy People 2010 Final Review* (Hyattsville, MD: Public Health Service, 2011); available at *www.healthypeople.gov*.

children and adolescents of all ethnic groups increased substantially.[4] The proportion of children and adolescents ages 6–19 years who are overweight increased from 11% in the late 1980s to 18% in 2010.

Progress was made in moving toward some of the objectives for the year 2010. The prevalence of growth retardation among low-income children, for example, decreased for all races combined and for some Hispanics and Asian/Pacific Islanders. The percentage of elementary and secondary schools offering low-fat choices for breakfast and lunch increased considerably, although only about one in five schools offered lunches that met goals for total fat and saturated fat content.[5]

The proportion of students in grades 9–12 who participated in daily physical education increased slightly. Both the incidence and the prevalence of diabetes increased for the population as a whole and among the special population groups for whom there are data, including American Indians, Alaska Natives, Mexican Americans, and African Americans. No progress was made in reducing the prevalence of iron deficiency among young children overall, although the prevalence did decline for low-income children.

The three objectives for fruit, vegetable, and grain consumption showed little or no progress. The average number of daily servings of fruit consumed by people two years of age and older changed little, going from 1.6 in 1994–1996 to 1.5 in 2008. Two to four servings are recommended. Vegetable intake also showed little change: an average of 3.4 daily servings in 1994–1996, compared with 3.3 in 2008. Three to five servings are recommended, with at least one-third being dark green or orange vegetables. In 2007–2008, only 8% of vegetable servings consumed by children aged 2–19 years were dark green or orange, whereas fried potatoes constituted about one-half.[6]

Significant efforts should be made to achieve the *Healthy People 2020* objectives that promote healthful weights and food choices in children and adolescents. The following steps are recommended.[7]

- Because most postpubertal children regain any lost weight within a year, promote the initiation of behavioral therapy for overweight children before the onset of puberty. Such therapy should include the teaching of social skills to counter taunting and to maintain and develop friendships.
- Educate children and their families about the health benefits of being physically active and the possible added benefit of thereby attaining modest weight reduction.
- Encourage schools to find ways to offset potential revenues lost from removal of competitive foods that do not meet USDA Food and Nutrition Service nutrition standards. Recommendations include offering healthier competitive food choices and substituting sales of nonfood items in fundraising activities.[8]
- Promote partnerships among schools, families, and community members to increase resources that support a health-promoting environment.[9]
- Demonstrate to schools that setting aside regularly scheduled periods for physical education during the school day can boost students' academic achievement.
- Develop and implement strategies to increase physical activity among children with disabilities. This step should include the use of media that feature disabled adults who can serve as role models of physical fitness for youth who have disabilities.
- Advocate for public health policies that address not only individual behaviors but also the environmental context and conditions in which people live and make choices.[10]
- Implement strategies to make healthful food choices available, identifiable, and affordable to people of all races and income levels and in all types of geographic locations (e.g., urban, suburban, rural).[11]

What Are Children and Adolescents Eating?

Since the early 1990s, government agencies, nonprofit groups, and the medical community have given considerable attention to identifying nutritional problems in children's diets and developing initiatives to help improve what children eat. Studies from a number of organizations have shown that children are failing to meet the recommended nutrition guidelines by not consuming enough fruits, vegetables, and whole grains and by eating too many foods high in saturated fat, added sugars, and sodium.

Children's eating habits have changed over the past two decades. Dietary data, collected in large nationwide surveys to determine trends in nutrient intakes, have shown that most children and adolescents have either a poor diet or one that needs improvement. The USDA's Center for Nutrition Policy and Promotion uses the **Healthy Eating Index (HEI)** as an indicator of diet quality.[12] It provides an overall picture of the types of foods people choose to eat and of their adherence to the *Dietary Guidelines for Americans*. The HEI consists of 12 dietary components, including nine for which adequacy of consumption is measured and three for which moderation of intake is measured. The total score is a measure of overall diet quality.

As shown in **Table 12-2**, the dietary quality of most children and adolescents ages 2–17 is less than optimal. The average scores for all of the categories were below recommendations. Consumption of dairy products and protein foods were closest to the standards;

Healthy Eating Index (HEI) A summary measure of the quality of one's diet. The HEI provides an overall picture of how well one's diet conforms to the *Dietary Guidelines for Americans*. The index factors in such dietary practices as consumption of whole fruits, dark green and orange vegetables, whole grains, milk, meat and beans, oils, saturated fat, sodium, and the calories from solid fats and added sugars in the diet.

DIETARY COMPONENT (MAXIMUM SCORE)	2003–2004[a] SCORE (%)	2005–2006[a] SCORE (%)	2007–2008[a] SCORE (%)
Adequacy (higher score indicates higher consumption)			
Total fruit (5)	3.3 (66)	3.4 (68)	4.0 (80)*
Whole fruit (5)	2.9 (58)	3.4 (68)	4.6 (92)*
Total vegetables (5)	2.3 (46)	2.3 (46)	2.3 (46)
Greens and beans (5)	0.7 (14)	0.8 (16)	0.9 (18)
Whole grains (10)	1.6 (16)	1.7 (17)	1.8 (18)
Dairy (10)	8.6 (86)	8.4 (84)	8.3 (83)
Total protein foods (5)	4.0 (80)	4.1 (82)	4.2 (84)
Seafood and plant protein (5)	2.4 (48)	2.4 (48)	2.1 (42)
Fatty acids (10)	3.1 (31)	2.9 (29)	3.0 (30)
Moderation (higher score indicates lower consumption)			
Refined grains (10)	4.5 (45)	4.3 (43)	4.6 (46)
Sodium (10)	5.5 (55)	5.1 (51)	5.0 (50)
Empty calories[b] (20)	8.0 (40)	8.3 (42)	9.0 (45)**
Total Score (100)	46.9 (47)	47.1 (47)	49.8 (50)

[a] Excludes children under two years of age and breast- and formula-fed infants.

[b] *Empty calories* refers to calories from solid fats (i.e., sources of saturated fats and *trans* fats) and added sugars (i.e., sugars not naturally occurring), plus calories from alcohol beyond a moderate level.

* Significantly different from 2003–2004 and 2005–2006 ($p < 0.05$).

** Significantly different from 2003–2004 ($p < 0.05$).

Source: USDA Nutrition Insight 52, July 2013.

TABLE 12-2

The Quality of American Children's Diets, as Measured by the Healthy Eating Index, 2010 The Healthy Eating Index is a dietary assessment tool consisting of 12 components: Nine components address nutrient adequacy. The remaining three components assess refined grains, sodium, and empty calories. For adequacy components, a score of zero is assigned for no intake, and the scores increase proportionately as intakes increase up to the standard. For moderation components, a reverse scoring is applied; that is, levels of intakes meeting dietary recommendations get the maximum score, with scores decreasing as intakes increase. For all components, a higher percentage indicates a higher quality diet.

intake of dark green vegetables and beans were farthest from recommendations. More-over, children who live in low-income families, compared to those who do not live in poverty, are more likely to have a diet rated as poor or needing improvement. Dietary quality continues to decline from childhood to adolescence, especially with the decreased consumption of fruits and the increased intake of sodium and empty calories from solid fats and added sugars.[13]

By not following the current nutrition recommendations, children are missing impor-tant daily nutrients, as shown in the results of national surveys. Children of all ages, races, and ethnic groups were shown to be at risk of inadequate intakes of folate, calcium, mag-nesium, and vitamins A, C, D, and E; iron is underconsumed by adolescent females.[14] The diet quality scores of children would be improved by replacing refined grains with whole grains; increasing the intake of vegetables, especially dark greens and beans; and by decreasing the intake of sodium and empty calories from solid fats and added sugars.[15]

Survey data showed that beverage choices for all ages changed from whole milk to lower-fat milk, soft drinks, and fruit and fruit-flavored drinks. On any given day, approxi-mately one-half of the population ages two and older consumes sugar drinks. Adolescents ages 12–19 show the highest percentage of total calories from these beverages.[16] **Figure 12-1** shows the mean calorie intake from sugar drinks for ages two and over. Additional sources of energy for children and teenagers are grain desserts such as cakes and cookies and dough-based dishes such as pizza.[17] These foods not only are high in calories but are often high in saturated fat and sodium and low in fiber.

Over the past 20 years, the portion sizes of commonly consumed foods, such as soft drinks and hamburgers, have increased. Large food portions that provide more calories than smaller portions may be contributing to the increasing prevalence of overweight in children and teens. For example, children three to five years of age consumed 25% more of an entrée when they were presented with portions that were double an age-appropriate standard size.[18]

Influences on Child and Adolescent Eating Patterns and Behaviors

Despite the importance of healthful eating habits during the growing years, children and youth are not meeting the current nutrition recommendations for health. As children grow into teens, unhealthful eating patterns become more pronounced. The reasons for this decline in good eating habits can be correlated with growing independence from parents, eating away from home, concern with physical appearance and body weight, the need for peer acceptance, and busy schedules.

FIGURE 12-1 Mean Kilocalories from Sugar Drinks for Ages Two and Over: United States, 2005–2008

* Significantly different from males.

Source: Adapted from C. L. Ogden and coauthors, *Consumption of Sugar Drinks in the United States, 2005–2008*, NCHS Data Brief No 71, 2011.

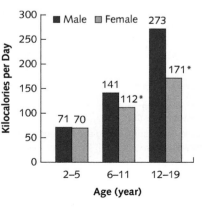

Social Influences Eating family meals is associated with improved diet quality in children, a benefit that may continue into young adulthood.[19] Over the past several years, the traditional pattern of the family gathered around the kitchen table has changed, and fewer families are eating meals together. The increasing popularity of fast food, dining out, and take-out meals, and the increasing demand for convenience and prepared foods, are related to shifts in family structure and work schedules. As the number of single parents and the number of women in the workforce increase, it is likely that dining out will continue to increase. Nearly half of family food expenditures are spent on food and beverages outside the home, and more than one-third of the dollars spent on food away from home are spent on fast foods.[20]

Individual Influences When dining in environments other than home, the majority of adolescents do not make food choices primarily in terms of health and nutrition. Instead, taste, appearance of the food, hunger, and price are the primary factors influencing food selections.[21] Dining out is more prevalent among older teens, who have the greatest freedom, mobility, and income. More than 52% of "dining out" takes place at schools, followed by quick-serve restaurants, vending machines, convenience stores, and worksites.[22]

Physical Environment Influences Quick-serve restaurants provide almost one-third of the meals adolescents eat away from home. An average teen visits a quick-serve restaurant at least twice a week and spends more than $5 a visit, for a nationwide total of over $13 billion annually.[23] These restaurants typically offer foods high in saturated fat and sodium, and low in fiber, iron, and calcium. Adolescents also spend $5.2 billion each year on after-school snacks in convenience stores.[24] Quick-serve outlets and convenience stores are often located near school buildings, making them easily accessible food sources. Furthermore, because many quick-serve restaurants and convenience stores employ adolescents, these worksites influence dietary habits through food discounts and free meals that are often provided as part of employee benefits.

Lifestyle Adolescent lifestyles show that convenience and peer pressure strongly influence food choices. As we have noted, adolescents frequently turn to vending machines, quick-serve restaurants, and convenience stores for foods that can be prepared and served quickly. They also want to sleep longer in the morning instead of taking time to eat breakfast. Breakfast is the most commonly missed meal, and studies show that 20% of 9- to 13-year-old children and 36% of 14- to 18-year-old adolescents skip breakfast.[25] Adolescents also spend a substantial amount of time socializing with friends while eating. Friends help to define acceptable behavior for the peer group, including eating patterns and habits.

Media and Advertising Persons under age 18 make up 24% of the U.S. population, which represents a considerable share of the retail market.[26] In a media-saturated world, children and adolescents are the target of intense and specialized marketing efforts.[27] They often influence their parents' decisions on where the family dines, what types of foods are eaten at home, and what brands are purchased. Approximately 70% of the food marketing directed toward children under age 12 falls into three categories: breakfast cereal, snack foods, and restaurant foods. The industry targets adolescents ages 12–17 with the promotion of carbonated beverages, noncarbonated beverages, and restaurant foods.[28]

In 2012, the fast-food restaurant industry spent $4.6 billion in advertising, including television, magazines, and Internet.[29] Current research acknowledges some improvements in child-targeted advertising trends. From 2009 to 2012 there was a 10% decline in total fast-food television advertising to children ages 6–11 and three child-targeted websites were discontinued. Some progress was also made in fast-food marketing to teens. The percent

▶ **THINK LIKE A COMMUNITY** NUTRITIONIST

Food marketing to children has been a controversial policy topic in recent years. To learn more about the debate, visit the websites below.

- Public Health Law Center: *http://publichealthlawcenter.org/topics/healthy-eating/food-marketing-kids*
- Prevention Institute: *www.preventioninstitute.org/focus-areas/supporting-healthy-food-a-activity/supporting-healthy-food-and-activity-environments-advocacy/get-involved-were-not-buying-it/735-were-not-buying-it-the-facts-on-junk-food-marketing-and-kids.html*
- HBO Weight of the Nation: *http://theweightofthenation.hbo.com/themes/marketing-food-to-children*

These sites all argue against food marketing to children. What arguments do you think are used *for* food marketing to kids (i.e., against policies to restrict food marketing to children)? After you have considered both sides of the debate, develop your own stance.

- What key messages would you use to back up your stance?
- Consider how the food and beverage industry could use food advertisements in a way that would have a positive influence on children's and adolescents' food choices.

of calories from sugar and saturated fat declined in the foods advertised and the number of display ads placed on teen websites also declined.[30]

Despite this progress, there continues to be cause for concern. During this same period, television advertising to very young children (ages two to five) did not change, 19 of the top 25 advertisers increased advertising to preschoolers, and 14 increased advertising to older children.[31] Several restaurants continued to target teens with marketing strategies promoting unhealthy products. Marketing through media that is popular with teens, such as branded apps for mobile devices with interactive features such as ordering and discount offers and postings to social media (e.g., Facebook, Twitter) increased.

The IOM expert committee report *Food Marketing to Children and Youth: Threat or Opportunity?* provides a comprehensive review of the influence of food marketing on the dietary patterns and health of children and youth. The committee found that the child-targeted marketing strategies did have an influence on children's food and beverage preferences, diets, and health. Unfortunately, the majority of the branded products marketed to children were not supportive of a healthy diet. According to the report, "Creating an environment in which U.S. children and youth can grow up healthy should be a high priority for the nation. Yet the prevailing pattern of food and beverage marketing to children and youth in America represents, at best, a missed opportunity, and at worst, a direct threat to the health prospects of the next generation. . . . Ensuring that environments are supportive of good health is a fundamental responsibility, requiring leadership and action from all sectors."[32] The report concluded with recommendations to guide industry stakeholders to use a variety of integrated communications to promote a healthy diet for children and adolescents. A subsequent progress report noted that moderate progress was made by the food and beverage companies in promoting a healthy diet and limited progress was shown by restaurants and industry trade associations.[33]

Weighing In on the Problem of Childhood Obesity

Eating practices influence a child's physical growth, cognitive development, and overall health. The lack of good nutrition habits, coupled with physical inactivity, has led to an epidemic of overweight children and adolescents during the past two decades.[34] During this period, the percentage of overweight children has nearly doubled, and the percentage of overweight adolescents has almost tripled. The same conditions associated with overweight adults, such as type 2 diabetes, high blood lipids, and hypertension, are now appearing in young children and teens with greater frequency. See Chapter 8 for more about factors contributing to, and proposed solutions to, the epidemic of child obesity.

Unlike BMI values for adults, BMI values for children and adolescents are gender- and age-specific and can be calculated using growth charts for children and adolescents from 2 to

20 years old. For children, obesity is defined as a BMI at or above the CDC growth chart criterion of 95th percentile based on gender and age standards. Overweight reflects a BMI above the CDC growth chart criterion of 85th percentile but lower than the 95th percentile based on gender and age standards. For a fourth-grade child (nine years of age), overweight is approximately 10 pounds over the maximum ideal weight, whereas for an eighth-grade child (13 years of age), overweight is approximately 20 pounds over maximum ideal weight. BMI changes with age and gender, so as children and adolescents increase in age, BMI also increases.

The CDC Growth Charts are available at *www.cdc.gov/GrowthCharts/*. Refer to Appendix A for information on assessing children's BMI and growth status.

- Underweight = BMI-for-age < 5th percentile
- Healthy Weight = BMI-for-age ≥ 5th percentile to < 85th percentile
- Overweight = BMI-for-age ≥ 85th percentile to < 95th percentile
- Obese = BMI-for-age ≥ 95th percentile

Dietary intake and nutrition status affect the maturation rate of children and youth. Early maturation, characterized in adolescents by a skeletal age greater than three months in advance of chronological age, is associated with increased fatness in adulthood and an increase in abdominal fat.[35] Overweight children tend to be taller, to have advanced bone ages, and to mature earlier than children who are not overweight.[36]

Childhood Obesity and the Early Development of Chronic Diseases
Childhood obesity is associated with hyperinsulinemia, hypertriglyceridemia, and reduced HDL-cholesterol concentrations. Overweight children are at risk for cardiovascular disease, insulin resistance and type 2 diabetes, sleep apnea, gallbladder disease, psychosocial dysfunction, and other serious health problems. A variety of orthopedic complications in overweight children can affect the feet, legs, and hips because the tensile strength of bone and cartilage has not fully developed to carry substantial quantities of excess weight. The economic impact of childhood obesity on health care costs has been documented. Studies have shown that children diagnosed with overweight or obesity had higher annual health care costs than children with a normal BMI.[37] Moreover, overweight children and adolescents are more likely to become overweight and obese adults.[38]

The health consequences related to excess weight can begin early in life, especially with respect to cardiovascular disease. Nearly 60% of overweight children have been shown to have at least one cardiovascular risk factor, compared to 10% of those with a BMI less than the 85th percentile.[39] Furthermore, 25% of overweight children had two or more risk factors. Hypertension occurs with low frequency in children. However, in a study of nearly 7,000 children, persistent elevated blood pressure occurred nine times more frequently in those who were overweight.[40]

Diabetes mellitus, the seventh deadliest disease in the United States, is the third most chronic disease of childhood.[41] The prevalence of both type 1 and type 2 diabetes in individuals younger than 20 years has increased rapidly, with approximately 0.25% in this age category diagnosed with diabetes.[42] Children diagnosed with type 2 diabetes are generally overweight, have a strong family history of the disease, are older than 10 years of age, and tend to be members of certain racial and ethnic groups (e.g., African American, Hispanic, and Native American). Researchers have also examined the possible association of childhood obesity with the development of type 1 diabetes.[43] The complications of diabetes include heart disease, stroke, vision loss and blindness, amputation, and kidney disease.

Social stigmatization and low self-esteem are other childhood consequences of excess weight. Overweight children often become targets of early discrimination. For example, children ages 6–10 associate obesity with negative characteristics, such as laziness and sloppiness.[44] Research examining friendship networks has shown that overweight and obese children have less friends than normal-weight children.[45] Overweight children may choose younger friends, who are less inclined to discriminate and be judgmental about the older child's weight. Furthermore, overweight children and youth often experience psychological stress from teasing by peers that can lead to poor body image and low self-esteem. A negative self-image in adolescence often persists into adulthood and may have a long-term impact on achievement and income-earning potential.[46]

Genetic susceptibility to obesity, lifestyle, family eating patterns, and lack of access to neighborhood environments that support physical activity all contribute to overweight and obesity in this population. Three major behavioral components have also been identified: dietary intake of energy-dense foods with poor nutritional quality, physical inactivity, and sleep deprivation.[47] The data on the morbidity and mortality associated with overweight and obesity demonstrate the importance of the prevention of weight gain in maintaining and improving health and quality of life. Although a number of programs and interventions have been developed to address this problem, progress in obesity prevention has been slow. The Institute of Medicine's (IOM) Committee on Accelerating Progress in Obesity Prevention was formed to address this challenge. The committee was charged with developing a set of recommendations and measures of progress for accelerating obesity prevention over the next decade. The committee identified five interrelated environments for change along with implementation strategies, actions, and outcome indicators (see Table 8-5 on page 297).[48] The committee envisioned the five goals would work synergistically to influence the success of each goal.

A significant and widespread governmental social marketing campaign for prevention of childhood obesity is *Let's Move!*, championed by First Lady Michelle Obama. President Obama appointed a White House Task Force on Childhood Obesity to guide the campaign. The program has since grown to include several new initiatives, including *Let's Move Cities and Towns*, *Let's Move Salad Bars to Schools*, *Let's Move Outside*, and *Let's Move Child Care*, as well as a new focus on faith-based communities. Recommendations for *Let's Move!* focus on five pillars: (1) creating a healthy start for children; (2) empowering parents and caregivers; (3) providing healthy foods in schools; (4) improving access to healthy, affordable foods; and (5) increasing physical activity.[49] *Let's Move!* is dedicated to solving the problem of obesity within a generation and urges everyone to play a role in reducing childhood obesity, including parents and caregivers, elected officials, schools, health care professionals, faith-based and community-based organizations, and private industry.

Other Nutrition-Related Problems of Children and Adolescents

The physical, developmental, and social changes that occur during childhood and the teen years can markedly affect eating behaviors and may have long-term health implications. Childhood is a critical time in human development. Children typically grow taller by 2–3 inches and heavier by five or more pounds each year between the age of one and adolescence.[50] They master fine motor skills (including those related to eating and drinking), become increasingly independent, and learn to express themselves appropriately. Adolescence is a time of change. Between the ages of about 10 and 18 years in girls and about 12 and 20 years in boys, there are marked changes in physical, intellectual, and emotional growth and development. Many aspects of the maturation process are influenced by dietary intake and nutrition status. Failure to meet nutrition needs during the early years can potentially affect growth, delay sexual maturation, and lead to chronic illnesses as an adult.[51]

In general, the nutritional health of U.S. children is better today than ever before.[52] Overt nutrient deficiencies, with the exception of iron deficiency, are not the public health problems they once were, although low calcium intakes during the peak bone-building years increase the risk of osteoporosis in later life, especially among females. Specific nutrition-related problems among children and adolescents include undernutrition, iron-deficiency anemia, high blood cholesterol levels, dental caries, eating disorders, and overweight and obesity.

Undernutrition

Undernutrition is a problem for some children in the United States, especially those from low-income and migrant families or certain ethnic and racial minority groups (e.g., African Americans and Asians).[53] Some groups of adolescents are at risk for reduced energy and food intakes. Adolescents from low-income families and those who have run away from home or who abuse alcohol or drugs are at risk nutritionally. African American and Hispanic teenagers are nearly twice as likely as white teenagers to live in poverty.

In 2012, approximately 49 million people in the United States were food-insecure, meaning that at some time during the year, these households were unable to acquire enough food for all household members because of insufficient resources.[54] Nearly 16 million children lived in food-insecure households in 2012. The prevalence of hunger in children was six times higher in single-mother families; three times more prevalent among racial and ethnic minorities, particularly African Americans and Hispanics; and 10 times more prevalent in households with incomes below 185% of the poverty threshold.[55]

The widespread practice of dieting among adolescents, especially girls, makes them at risk for undernutrition.[56] In a survey of 7- to 13-year-old children, almost half were concerned about their weight, more than one-third had dieted, and almost one-tenth demonstrated signs of anorexia nervosa. As girls increase in age, concerns about weight also increase. About 13% of the 17,354 females in grades 7–12 who were interviewed in the Minnesota Adolescent Survey reported being chronic dieters, which is defined as always being on a diet or having been on a diet for 10 of the previous 12 months.[57] The results of the 2013 National Youth Risk Behavior Survey found that 47% of high school students were trying to lose weight. The prevalence of engaging in extreme weight-loss behaviors, such as vomiting, using laxatives, or taking diet pills, powders, or liquids, was higher among female than male students.[58]

Iron Deficiency and Iron-Deficiency Anemia

Iron deficiency is one of the most common nutritional deficiencies, not only in the United States but throughout the world. Iron-deficiency anemia results from depletion of total body iron and impaired hemoglobin production. It is associated with diminished cognitive function, behavior changes, delayed growth and development, and impaired immune function in children.[59]

The *Healthy People 2020* target is to reduce iron deficiency by 10% for children ages one to two years.[60] Current prevalence estimates of impaired iron status indicate that nearly 16% of children ages one to two years are iron deficient. Roughly 5% of children ages three to four years are iron deficient. The target for the year 2020 is 4%.

The incidence of iron-deficiency anemia has decreased in recent years, thanks to iron fortification of infant formula and cereal and increased emphasis on breastfeeding.[61] However, the prevalence of iron deficiency is higher among children living at or below the poverty threshold than among other children.[62] The problem still exists in 10% of minority children one to three years of age.[63] Mexican American and non-Hispanic black children are more likely to be iron deficient than children of other ethnic groups.[64]

Adolescents have special iron needs. In boys, the requirements for absorbed iron increase from about 1.0 to 2.5 milligrams/day.[65] This increase reflects the expanding blood volume and rise in hemoglobin concentration that accompany sexual maturation. The total daily iron loss of menstruating women is about 1.4 milligrams.[66] Whereas most males have an adequate iron intake during adolescence, many females do not. Data from the NHANES indicate that females between 12 and 19 years of age have iron intakes below what is recommended.

Blood Lead Level

Concern about the link between high blood lead levels and lowered intelligence (IQ) in children led to a large-scale public health effort and legislation to eliminate or reduce lead in gasoline, food cans, drinking water, and house paint over the last four decades. Recent findings suggest that adverse effects of children's exposure to lead extends beyond deficits in IQ to additional concerns such as attention-deficit disorder and cardiovascular, immunological, and endocrine complications. Today, small children are most likely to be exposed to lead if they live in houses built before 1978 when the use of lead-based paints was restricted. Additional sources are drinking water coming through lead pipes, some imported items including clay pots, and certain home remedies.

Until recently, children were identified as having a "blood lead level of concern" if the result was 10 micrograms per deciliter (μg/dL) or greater. The current value used is based on the U.S. population of children ages one to five years who are in the top 2.5% of children when tested for lead, currently > 5 micrograms per deciliter (μg / dL).[67] In a recent report, the CDC's Advisory Committee on Childhood Lead Poisoning Prevention notes that "because no measurable level of blood lead is known to be without deleterious effects, and because once engendered, the effects appear to be irreversible in the absence of other interventions, public health, environmental and housing policies should encourage prevention of all exposures to lead."[68]

Although there has been an overall decline in the prevalence of lead levels, data indicates that poverty, age, and being non-Hispanic black are major risk factors for higher blood lead levels. Certain vitamins and minerals such as calcium, iron, and vitamin C function in minimizing lead absorption; therefore, children with inadequate intake of these nutrients may also be at increased risk.[69] Continued efforts are needed to minimize disparities in childhood blood lead levels and prevent all exposure of children to lead.

Dental Caries

Although dental caries are largely preventable, this remains the most common chronic disease of children ages 5–17 years.[70] By age five, 60% of all children have had tooth decay, and more than 90% of 18-year-olds have experienced decay.[71] Children in low-income households, and especially those who are American Indian, African American, or Hispanic, have three times the risk of tooth decay because they lack access to or encounter barriers to accessing dental services.[72]

School-based sealant programs are an excellent means of reaching low-income children with preventive dental care. At no cost to children 6–14 years of age, some schools offer oral hygiene instruction, fluoride rinses, and dental sealants for permanent molars.[73] There is typically a 60% decrease in tooth decay on teeth after sealant application.[74]

Fortunately, the incidence of dental caries in children has decreased by as much as 30–50% over the last two decades, owing in part to fluoridation of public drinking water, improved dental hygiene, and the use of fluoride in toothpastes and mouthwashes.[75] Children living in communities with water fluoridation experienced 30–50% fewer cavities than those who lived where there was no fluoridated water.[76] In the United States, about 100 million people are still not receiving the benefits of community water fluoridation.[77] Community coalitions are essential in educating citizens about the benefits of water fluoridation.

High Blood Cholesterol

Multiple risk factors have been associated with the early development of lipid disorders and atherosclerosis in children and adolescents. The increased prevalence of childhood obesity has contributed to the incidence of elevated triglycerides, reduced high-density lipoprotein cholesterol (HDL-C), insulin resistance, and elevated blood pressure—what is referred to as metabolic syndrome in adults. Additional behavioral risk factors include physical inactivity, tobacco use, and a diet high in saturated and *trans* fat.[78] Identifying and controlling dyslipidemia early on in childhood is critical to reduce the risk of cardiovascular disease (CVD) in adulthood.

Because total cholesterol and low-density lipoprotein cholesterol (LDL-C) can fall from 10 to 20% or more during puberty, it is recommended the initial routine screening be completed between the ages of 9 and 11 years with an additional screening completed once between 17 and 21 years. Children with risk factors such as a strong family history of CVD or certain medical conditions should have their initial screening at a younger age. The Expert Panel on Integrated Guidelines for Cardiovascular Health and Risk Reduction in Children and Adolescents classifies a total blood cholesterol level of $\geq$ 200 mg/dL, an LDL-cholesterol level of $\geq$ 130 mg/dL, and a triglyceride level of $>$ 100 (zero to nine years) or $>$ 130 (10–19 years) as high, and a high-density lipoprotein cholesterol (HDL-C) level of $<$ 40mg/dL as low.[79] The panel recommends that children with high blood cholesterol be evaluated further and receive medical nutrition therapy if appropriate. Drug therapy is recommended only for children over 10 years of age whose blood cholesterol level has not responded to an adequate trial of medical nutrition therapy and who have undergone detailed risk factor assessment.[80]

The development and progress of atherosclerosis in childhood has a direct influence on developing CVD later in life. In addition, several of the risk factors associated with childhood atherosclerosis track from childhood into adult life. Interventions to lower the risk will have a lasting benefit across the lifespan.

Eating Disorders Eating disorders have become serious health problems in recent years. The most common eating disorders are anorexia nervosa and bulimia nervosa. A constellation of individual, familial, sociocultural, and biological factors contribute to these disorders, which threaten physical health and psychological well-being. Some individuals are more predisposed to develop an eating disorder than others. For example, about 90% of people with eating disorders are female. Caucasians are more likely than African Americans and other minority groups to develop an eating disorder.[81] African American females have greater acceptance of increased body weight and are less preoccupied with social consequences of obesity.[82] Finally, most individuals who develop eating disorders are adolescents or young adults who typically begin experiencing food-related and self-image problems between the ages of 14 and 30 years. Because these syndromes are surrounded by secrecy, their prevalence is not known with certainty, although it has increased dramatically within the past three decades. These types of eating disorders are often seen in adolescent athletes, many of whom compete in sports such as gymnastics, wrestling, distance running, diving, figure skating, and swimming that demand a rigid control of body weight.[83] See Programs in Action: Combating Disordered Nutrition in Young Female Athletes that follows.

PROGRAMS IN **ACTION**

Combating Disordered Nutrition in Young Female Athletes

A serious commitment to sport and exercise may predispose some female athletes to the development of eating disorders, particularly for those participating in sports where a low body weight is desired, such as skating, gymnastics, and ballet. The energy restriction and low calcium intake often associated with eating disorders may increase risk of injury. Low body weight and its often accompanied amenorrhea are significant predictors of osteoporosis. The development of osteoporosis among women with eating disorders has been confirmed by several researchers.[1, 2] Adequate calcium and vitamin D intake, along with balanced nutrition, are recommended as part of the preventive guidelines against osteoporosis. The program Osteoporosis Prevention for Female Athletes in High Risk Sports targeted potentially at-risk female athletes directly and through their coaches in an attempt to change eating behavior early enough to boost bone health.

Osteoporosis Prevention for Female Athletes in High-Risk Sports

The Female Athlete Triad is characterized by amenorrhea, osteoporosis, and eating disorders, and is most common in sports that are appearance-related (gymnastics, ballet, and ice skating) or require repetitive movement (basketball, soccer, tennis, track/field, and cross-country running). The target population for this project was female athletes between the ages of 12 and 22, who participated in sports that placed them at high risk for the Female Athlete Triad. This target age group was selected because preadolescence, the teen years, and early adulthood offer the opportunity to build bone density through nutrition and lifestyle changes. Program goals were to increase awareness of the Female Athlete Triad and osteoporosis among preadolescent, adolescent, and college-age female athletes in high-risk sports; to increase educational efforts to modify their nutrition behaviors; and to increase awareness among coaches of female athletes of osteoporosis and its prevention.

Innovation/Creativity

The professor in charge of the project, with assistance from a college senior majoring in health promotion, developed two lesson plans, as well as slide masters, handouts, and a brochure on osteoporosis geared toward the target market. PowerPoint slide sets were developed on two topics: Preventing Osteoporosis in Female Athletes and Female Athletes, Nutrition, and Eating Disorders. The project staff also created a website titled Osteoporosis and the Female Athlete. The college senior was trained to use the lesson kits to conduct educational sessions for high school and college athletes participating in women's soccer, track, cross country, cheerleading, tennis, and volleyball. Each participating athlete received a folder, key articles, and the project's brochure Preventing Osteoporosis in Female Athletes. Project staff conducted educational sessions with 12 coaches in "high-risk" sports and provided them with the materials distributed to athletes, as well as the lesson kit with PowerPoint slides and background articles. Additional materials were developed. A press release was published in two area newspapers. The university newspaper printed the program's public service announcement. A bulletin board on the Female Athlete Triad was designed and placed in a university hall. Staff conducted two television interviews.

Replicability

The materials developed for this project could easily be used by "peer mentor" athletes, middle and high school health teachers, coaches, or other interested persons. All materials are available for replication through the project coordinator.

Theory Base/Rationale

Among this study group, 33.4% reported menstrual irregularities, 23% had calcium intakes below recommended levels, and 8.6% reported a previous or present eating disorder as measured by information obtained from their completion of paper-and-pencil surveys. The program was framed around four social–cognitive theory constructs. Observational Learning was met through the use of a "peer" female athlete to conduct the educational sessions; the peer athlete also served as a role model whose image and, more importantly, message were respected by the participants. Behavioral Capability was addressed by providing the athletes with exposure to a knowledge base of proper nutrition and training to improve bone strength, and teaching them skills for changing their behavior based on this new knowledge. Self-Control of Performance was met through personal goal setting for future bone health and personal satisfaction from attaining those goals. Management of Emotional Arousal was met by designing sessions that had a positive tone and were not overly emotional, negative, or overbearing. A positive environment can boost self-efficacy, a participant's belief that she can achieve success.

Outcomes/Evaluation Data

A total of 309 female athletes were reached through educational sessions. A pre- and post-test evaluated nutrition knowledge and changes in attitudes and beliefs regarding calcium consumption and osteoporosis prevention. Attitudes and beliefs improved significantly ($p < 0.05$) regarding naming risk factors for osteoporosis, needing calcium from foods and supplements, and naming and increasing foods high in calcium.

Lessons Learned

This project made us aware of the paucity of research and materials related to early risk of osteoporosis in female athletes. Education and intervention can help prevent this.

Source: Adapted from *Community Nutritionary* (White Plains, NY: Dannon Institute, Spring 2000). Used with permission. For more information about the Awards for Excellence in Community Nutrition, go to *www.dannon-institute.org*.

Children with Special Health Care Needs

Children with special needs from infancy through adolescence are served by public school systems and early-intervention services. Several terms and classifications have been used in describing the population with special needs, including developmental disabilities, developmental social needs, handicapping conditions, chronic disorders, and chronic illnesses.[84]

An estimated 14–19% of U.S. children age 18 years or younger experience some form of disability that limits their participation in school, play, and social activities.[85] A person with a disability is any person who has a physical, developmental, behavioral, or emotional impairment that substantially limits one or more major life activities, has a record of such impairment, or is regarded as having such impairment.[86] Children with special health care needs include those with birth defects, chromosomal abnormalities, asthma, autism, cerebral palsy, epilepsy, metabolic disorders, insulin-dependent diabetes, cancer, fetal alcohol syndrome, mental retardation, and other chronic health conditions.[87] Children with special health care needs are at increased nutritional risk because of feeding problems, metabolic aberrations, drug–nutrient interactions, decreased mobility, and alterations in growth patterns. In addition to experiencing a range of health problems, such as loss of hearing and vision and poor fitness, 70–90% of children with special health care needs also have unique nutritional requirements.[88] An interdisciplinary approach to managing children with special health care needs is recommended. The interdisciplinary team may include a physician; a nurse; a psychologist; a dentist; a dietitian; a school administrator; a food-service director; special education staff; and occupational, physical, and speech therapists. The child and his or her parents or caregivers are important team members whose insights and observations help the team determine which foods and feeding strategies work.[89]

The interdisciplinary team evaluation of the health and nutrition status of children with special needs includes the dietary history, medical history, anthropometric measurements, clinical assessment, and feeding assessment.[90] The nutritional assessment forms the basis for the development of a nutrition plan for the toddler or school-age child and his or her family. The nutrition plan describes the child's food preferences, the family's beliefs and values about foods, and the child's mealtime behavior, nutritional needs, and ability to feed him- or herself. It includes feeding goals for the child—for example, "David will learn to chew solid food" or "Karen will learn to hold a spoon in her right hand"—and provides detailed information about the child's special diet and any equipment required during feeding. The primary feeding goal is to help the child learn to feed her- or himself.

Fortunately, nutrition care for these children has improved because of legislation, increased involvement of various agencies, improved delivery of community-based programs, and better home health care. In 1986, Congress passed the Education of the Handicapped Act Amendments (PL 99-457), which mandate the provision of comprehensive nutrition services to children with special needs who are three to five years of age, using a community-based approach that focuses on the family. The legislation also recognizes nutritionists as the health professionals qualified to provide developmental services to children with special health care needs.

Hallie Halsey

ENTREPRENEUR IN ACTION

As a registered dietitian with a foodservice management company, Hallie Halsey, RD, SNS, has created and implemented nutrition curriculum materials for students in kindergarten through 12th grade. She designs and analyzes school lunch menus, supervises operational activities of the school meal programs, and implements the company's Food Allergy Management Plan. Developing special substitute meals for the various allergies and disabilities that exist in schools can be challenging, but she affirms her company's philosophy: "Healthy Meals Grow Healthy Kids." Says Hallie: "It is rewarding to accommodate the students with disabilities with safe menu choices and even more gratifying to see them enjoy this special school experience of eating lunch with their friends. Small steps lead to bigger results. The smallest changes that one can make can have the biggest impact on a child's life." Learn more about her experiences online at *www.cengagebrain.com*.

In recent years, there has also been increased emphasis on ensuring that children with special health care needs who participate in school feeding programs are able to receive substitutions for food items because of their disabilities. This is mandated by the U.S. Department of Agriculture's nondiscrimination regulations and the National School Lunch and Breakfast policies. The regulations require that a physician's statement be provided, listing the disability—such as diabetes, PKU, or lactose intolerance—along with the reason for meal modification and the specific substitution that is required. Additionally, nutrition goals should be included in the child's or adolescent's individualized education plan (IEP), a written statement that contains the program of special education and related services to be provided to a child with a disability.[91]

One program that gives children and youth with special needs an opportunity for year-round training and competition is Special Olympics. The nutrition section of Special Olympics offers locally based, ongoing health-promotion programs with the goal of making good nutrition and physical fitness routine for athletes with special needs. *Healthy People 2020* lists goals for individuals with special health care needs to accomplish, such as increasing employment opportunities; improving social support; and improving access to health care and clinical preventive services.[92]

PROGRAMS IN **ACTION**

Nutrition Education Strategies for Preadolescent Girls

Studies have documented the high prevalence of unhealthful dieting behaviors among adolescent girls.[1,2] These behaviors may have a negative impact on nutritional intake and psychological well-being. Of even greater concern are the increasing rates of unhealthful dieting behaviors and body dissatisfaction among girls of elementary school age. Television shows, commercials, magazines, and movies filled with images of thin models fuel body image problems.

Despite the high prevalence of unhealthful dieting behaviors, disordered eating, and body dissatisfaction among youth, few primary prevention programs—programs that prevent a problem from occurring at all—have been both implemented and evaluated. Several have been school based, with the school serving as a catalyst for community outreach interventions that are directed toward groups of individuals,[3,4] namely preadolescent and adolescent girls. It has been suggested that children and adolescents can learn at school about the dangers of unsafe weight-loss methods and about safe ways to maintain a healthful weight.[5] Other possible avenues for reaching preadolescent and adolescent girls include religious institutions, community centers, and clubs such as the Boys and Girls Club and the YMCA and YWCA. These institutions are well established and trusted, so they may be better able to reach the target population and attract participants.

The Free to Be Me program directed its attention toward social and environmental factors (the media and the family), personal factors (body image), and behavioral factors (dieting behaviors). It also worked within the framework of an established, widely accepted community program, the Girl Scouts, as a catalyst for connecting with the target population and creating trust in the program.

Free to Be Me was a Girl Scout badge program that helped young girls feel good about their bodies. It was designed to decrease unhealthful weight control behaviors in preadolescent girls. Its primary emphasis was on improving body image by taking an in-depth look at what young girls see in the media and on helping fifth- and sixth-grade Girl Scouts accept a wide variety of body shapes and sizes.

Goals and Objectives

A research study was undertaken to assess the feasibility and short-term impact of Free to Be Me, a program aimed at preventing unhealthful dieting and promoting a healthful body image among preadolescent girls. Objectives for participants upon completion of the six-session intervention study were to decrease incidence of unhealthful weight control behaviors, to increase knowledge of media influences on body image and food choices, to increase the interest in healthful eating and body image, to improve participants' ability to critically evaluate media messages, and to improve overall body image.

Methodology

Free to Be Me included six 90-minute sessions that were presented during consecutive biweekly Girl Scout meetings. The girls completed activities on body development, the media's impact on body image and self-esteem, and combating negative images. For example, they critically analyzed media messages and looked for alternative positive messages. After analyzing media messages, the girls were encouraged to write letters to the media about positive body image. Following completion of the program, they were awarded a "Free to Be Me" badge designed specifically for the program.

A three-hour training session taught troop leaders to teach the program. Each troop leader received a detailed handbook, along with materials and supplies. A registered dietitian served as project coordinator and worked closely with troop leaders. Parental involvement included receiving weekly mailings, assisting with take-home activities, preparing healthful snacks, and viewing end-of-session skits.

Results

A group-randomized, controlled study was designed to evaluate program effectiveness using 12 troops that participated in Free to Be Me and 13 nonparticipating troops as controls. The evaluation focused on program feasibility and short-term effectiveness, to be assessed on the basis of changes exhibited upon program completion and at a three-month follow-up. The program was found to have had a significant influence on media-related attitudes and behaviors, including internalization of sociocultural ideals, self-efficacy to affect weight-related social norms, and print media habits. A modest program impact on body-related knowledge and attitudes (i.e., on acceptance of body size, knowledge about puberty, and perceived weight status) was apparent immediately after the intervention, but not at follow-up. No significant changes were noted for dieting behaviors. Nevertheless, satisfaction with the program was high among girls, parents, and leaders.

Lessons Learned

Community nutrition programs may be successfully implemented within Girl Scout troops. Intervention programs for young adolescent girls have the potential to promote a positive body image and prevent unhealthful dieting behaviors.

Source: Adapted from *Community Nutritionary* (White Plains, NY: Dannon Institute, Spring 2000). Used with permission. For more information about the Awards for Excellence in Community Nutrition, go to *www.dannon-institute.org*.

The History of Child Nutrition Programs in Schools

Federal programs addressing the nutritional needs of children and adolescents have existed for more than 150 years. The Children's Bureau, at one time part of the U.S. Department of Labor, issued dietary advice to parents and teachers and conducted nutrition surveys of low-income children. School feeding programs, augmented by the financial support of local school districts, philanthropic organizations, and private donors, began in the early 1900s. Federal involvement in school food programs increased during the 1930s with the passage of an amendment to the Agricultural Act of 1933, which established a fund to purchase surplus agricultural commodities for donation to needy families and child nutrition programs, including school lunch programs.

As a result of testimony from the surgeon general that "70% of the boys who had poor nutrition 10 to 12 years ago were rejected by the draft," legislation was introduced to give the school lunch program permanent status and to authorize the appropriations necessary to keep it running in the future.[93] In 1946, President Harry Truman signed into law the National School Lunch Act (as amended, P.L. 79-396) with the following policy objectives:

> It is hereby declared to be the policy of Congress, as a measure of national security, to safeguard the health and well-being of the Nation's children and to encourage the domestic consumption of nutritious agricultural commodities and other food, by assisting the states, through grants-in-aid and other means, in providing an adequate supply of foods and other facilities for the establishment, maintenance, operation, and expansion of non-profit school lunch programs.[94]

To receive cash and commodity assistance under the statute, states had to operate school lunch programs on a nonprofit basis, serve free or reduced-price lunches for needy children, and provide lunches that met certain federal standards. Twenty years later, in 1966, the Child Nutrition Act was passed. It expanded federal efforts to improve child nutrition by establishing numerous programs of year-round food assistance to children of all ages. Many of the programs and policies developed during the 1960s and 1970s still exist today, although most have been modified over the years. This section describes the major domestic nutrition programs for children and adolescents.

Nutrition Programs of the U.S. Department of Agriculture

The Food and Nutrition Service was established in 1969 to administer the food assistance programs of the U.S. Department of Agriculture (USDA). The primary aim of this agency is to make food assistance available to people who need it. Other goals include improving the eating habits of U.S. children and stabilizing farm prices through the distribution of surplus foods. In this section, we examine five of the agency's largest food assistance programs for children: the National School Lunch Program, the School Breakfast Program, the Summer Food Service Program, the Afterschool Snack Program, and the Commodity Distribution Program. **Table 12-3** gives a brief description of the programs designed

TABLE 12-3 USDA Food Assistance Programs Specifically for Children

PROGRAM PURPOSE(S)		TYPE OF ASSISTANCE	ELIGIBILITY REQUIREMENTS OF PROGRAM PARTICIPANTS
National School Lunch Program	Assists states in making the school lunch program available to students and encourages the domestic consumption of nutritious agricultural commodities. Public and nonprofit private schools of high school grade and under, public and private nonprofit residential childcare institutions (except Job Corps Centers), residential summer camps that participate in the Summer Food Service Program for Children, and private foster homes are eligible to participate.	Formula grants[a]	1. All students attending schools where the lunch program is operating may participate. 2. Lunch is served free to students who are determined by local school authorities to live in households with incomes at or below 130% of the federal poverty guidelines. 3. Lunch is served at a reduced price to students who live in households with incomes between 130% and 185% of the poverty guidelines. 4. Students from families with incomes over 185% of the poverty guidelines pay full price for lunch.
School Breakfast Program	Assists states in providing a nutritious, nonprofit breakfast for school students. Eligible schools and residential childcare facilities are the same as for the National School Lunch Program.	Formula grants	Eligibility requirements are the same as for the National School Lunch Program.
Afterschool Snack Program	Assists school-based after-school programs in providing healthful snacks to children.	Available through NSLP	Sites can qualify to serve all children free of charge based on the percentage of children receiving free and reduced-price meals at the school.
Special Milk Program for Children	Provides subsidies to schools and institutions to encourage the consumption of fluid milk by children. Any public or private nonprofit school or childcare institution (e.g., nursery school, childcare center) of high school grade or under (except Job Corps Centers) may participate on request if it does not participate in a meal service program authorized under the National School Lunch Act or the Child Nutrition Act of 1966.	Formula grants	All students attending schools and institutions in which the program is operating may participate.
Summer Food Service Program for Children	Assists states in conducting nonprofit foodservice programs for low-income children during the summer months and at other approved times, when area schools are closed for vacation.	Formula grants	Homeless children and children attending public or private nonprofit schools and residential camps or participating in the National Youth Sports Program can receive free meals.

[a] Formula grants are a type of funding mechanism in which the funding agency distributes funds to states on the basis of a "formula" that takes into account a variety of factors, such as the number of breakfasts or lunches served to eligible children, the number of breakfasts or lunches served free or at a reduced price, and the national average payment for the program.

Source: Catalog of Federal Domestic Assistance Programs, 2012; available at *www.cfda.gov.*

TABLE 12-4 Other USDA Food Assistance Programs That Benefit Children[a]

PROGRAM	PURPOSE(S)
Child and Adult Care Food Program	Assists states in initiating, maintaining, and expanding nonprofit foodservice programs for children and older adults or impaired adults in nonresidential daycare facilities. After-school programs operated by community groups may also serve snacks to teenagers age 12–18 in low-income areas.
Commodity Supplemental Food Program	Improves the health and nutrition status of low-income pregnant, postpartum, and breastfeeding women; infants and children up to six years of age; and older adults through the donation of supplemental foods.
Emergency Food Assistance Program	Makes food commodities available to states for distribution to needy persons such as the unemployed, welfare recipients, and low-income individuals.
Food Distribution Program	Improves the diets of preschool- and school-age children and other groups and increases the market for domestically produced foods acquired under surplus removal or price support operations.
Food Distribution Program on Indian Reservations	Improves the diets of needy persons in households on or near Indian reservations and increases the market for domestically produced foods acquired under surplus removal or price support operations.
Supplemental Nutrition Assistance Program (SNAP)	Improves the diets of low-income households by increasing their ability to purchase foods.
Special Supplemental Nutrition Program for Women, Infants, and Children (WIC)	Provides, at no cost, supplemental nutritious foods, nutrition education, and referrals to health care to low-income pregnant, breastfeeding, and postpartum women; infants; and children to age five who are determined to be at nutritional risk.
WIC Farmers' Market Nutrition Program	Provides fresh, nutritious unprepared foods such as fruits and vegetables from farmers' markets to low-income women, infants, and children; expands the awareness and use of farmers' markets; and increases sales at farmers' markets.

[a] Refer to Table 10-4 on pages 389–393 for a complete description of the programs shown in this table.

Source: *Catalog of Federal Domestic Assistance Programs*, 2012.

specifically for children, and **Table 12-4** outlines programs that benefit children by assisting their families. These programs are also described in Chapter 10.

The National School Lunch Program

The National School Lunch Program (NSLP) operates in more than 100,000 public and nonprofit private schools and residential childcare institutions. In 2012, it provided nutritionally balanced, low-cost, or free lunches to more than 31 million school children each school day, at a cost of $11.6 billion.[95] Public school districts and independent private, nonprofit schools that participate in the NSLP are entitled to receive reimbursement dollars and donated commodities for each meal served. In return, they must offer free or reduced-price lunches to eligible children and meet specific nutrition guidelines. As a result of the Healthy, Hunger-Free Kids Act, the USDA is making the first major changes in school meals in 15 years.[96] **Table 12-5** compares the new meal standards and dietary specifications with the former standards. A sample lunch menu with a before and after comparison is shown in the box on page 486.

In accordance with the *Dietary Guidelines for Americans*, schools must increase the availability of fruits, vegetables, whole grains, and fat-free and low-fat milk in school meals, and reduce the levels of sodium and saturated fat in meals. Regulations also require that lunches provide one-third of the DRI for calories, protein, calcium, iron, vitamin A, and vitamin C for the applicable age or grade groups. Even though school lunches must meet federal nutrition requirements, local school food authorities make decisions about what specific foods to serve and how they are prepared.

Any child at a participating school may purchase a meal through the NSLP. Children from families with incomes at or below 130% of the poverty guidelines are eligible for free meals. Those with incomes between 130 and 185% of the poverty guidelines are eligible for reduced-price meals, where students can be charged no more than $0.40. Children

TABLE 12-5 New Meal Patterns and Dietary Specifications for National School Lunch Program

	NATIONAL SCHOOL LUNCH PROGRAM MEAL PATTERN		SAMPLE MEAL PATTERN GRADES 9–12	
FOOD GROUP	**PREVIOUS REQUIREMENTS K–12**	**NEW REQUIREMENTS K–12**	**LUNCH MEAL PATTERN**	**AMOUNT OF FOOD PER WEEK (MINIMUM PER DAY)**
Fruit and Vegetables	½–¾ cup of fruit and vegetables combined per day	¾–1 cup of vegetables plus ½–1 cup of fruit per day	**Fruits**[a] (cups) **Vegetables**[a] (cups)	5 c (1 c) 5 c (1 c)
Vegetables	No specifications as to type of vegetable subgroup	Weekly requirement for: • dark green • red/orange • beans/peas (legumes) • starchy • other	**Dark green**[b] **Red/orange**[b] **Legumes**[b] **Starchy**[b] **Other**[b] **Additional vegetable to meet total**	½ c 1¼ c ½ c ½ c ¾ c 1½ c
Meat/Meat Alternate (M/MA)	1½–2 oz eq. (daily minimum)	Daily minimum and weekly ranges: Grades K–5: 1 oz equivalent minimum daily (8–10 oz weekly) Grades 6–8: 1 oz equivalent minimum daily (9–10 oz weekly) Grades 9–12: 2 oz equivalent minimum daily (10–12 oz weekly)	**Meats/meat alternates** (oz eq.)	10–12 oz equivalent (2 oz/day)
Grains	8 servings per week (minimum of 1 serving per day)	Daily minimum and weekly ranges: Grades K–5: 1 oz equivalent minimum daily (8–9 oz weekly) Grades 6–8: 1 oz equivalent minimum daily (8–10 oz weekly) Grades 9–12: 2 oz equivalent minimum daily (10–12 oz weekly)	**Grains**[c] (oz eq.)	10–12 oz equivalent (2 oz/day)
Whole Grains[c]	Encouraged	All grains must be whole grain–rich.		
Milk	1 cup (variety of fat contents allowed; flavor not restricted)	1 cup; must be fat-free (unflavored/flavored) or 1% low-fat (unflavored)	**Fluid milk** (cups)	5 c (1 c)

OTHER NEW SPECIFICATIONS: DAILY AMOUNT BASED ON THE AVERAGE FOR A 5-DAY WEEK, GRADES 9–12

Minimum to maximum calories:[d]	750–850
Saturated fat (% of total calories):	< 10
Sodium (mg):[e]	< 740

Trans fat: Nutrition label or manufacturer specifications must indicate zero grams of *trans* fat per serving.

[a] One quarter-cup of dried fruit counts as ½ cup of fruit; 1 cup of leafy greens counts as ½ cup of vegetables. No more than half of the fruit or vegetable offerings may be in the form of juice. All juice must be 100% full-strength under new standards.

[b] Larger amounts of these vegetables may be served.

[c] All grains must be whole grain–rich by July 1, 2014.

[d] The average daily amount of calories for a five-day school week must be within the range (at least the minimum and no more than the maximum values). Discretionary sources of calories (solid fats and added sugars) may be added to the meal pattern if within the specifications for calories, saturated fat, *trans* fat, and sodium. Foods of minimal nutritional value and fluid milk with fat content greater than 1% milk fat are not allowed.

[e] Final sodium specifications are to be reached by July 1, 2022. Intermediate sodium specifications are established for SY 2014–2015 and 2017–2018.

Source: United States Department of Agriculture, Food and Nutrition Service, "Nutrition Standards in the National School Lunch and School Breakfast Programs," *Federal Register* 77 (January 26, 2012), 4088–167. Information related to the new meal requirements are available on a special webpage on the FNS website: *www.fns.usda.gov/cnd/Governance/Legislation/nutritionstandards.htm.*

HOUSEHOLD SIZE	FEDERAL POVERTY GUIDELINES 100% OF POVERTY*a*	FREE MEALS 130% OF POVERTY	REDUCED-PRICE MEALS 185% OF POVERTY
1	$11,670	$15,171	$21,590
2	15,730	20,449	29,101
3	19,790	25,727	36,612
4	23,850	31,005	44,123
5	27,910	36,283	51,634
6	31,970	41,561	59,145
7	36,030	46,839	66,656
8	40,090	52,117	74,167
Each additional person	$4,060	$5,278	$7,511

TABLE 12-6 Annual Income Eligibility Guidelines for the Federal Child Nutrition Programs, 2014–2015

a Guidelines are adjusted annually. Income guidelines are higher in Alaska and Hawaii.

Source: *Federal Register* 79, No. 43 (2014): 12467–69.

from families with incomes greater than 185% of the poverty guidelines pay full price, although their meals are still federally subsidized by a small amount. **Table 12-6** lists the income eligibility guidelines for the Child Nutrition Programs. Local districts set their own prices for paid meals but must still operate as a nonprofit program. In addition to cash reimbursements listed in **Table 12-7**, schools are entitled to receive commodity foods for each lunch meal served.[97]

There has been a strong effort by the School Nutrition Association and other education organizations to seek legislation that would eliminate the reduced-price category by raising "free" eligibility to the "reduced" limit of 185% of the poverty guidelines, thereby allowing these children a free meal. Children classified as eligible only for reduced-price meals are often from the "working poor"—households that are ineligible for free meals but do not have enough money to pay for reduced-priced meals.

A recent study explored the impact of the updated USDA national school meal standards on students' food choices and consumption rates.[98] Data was collected on the eating habits of elementary and middle-school children at four schools in a low-income district in Massachusetts before and after the implementation of the new standards. The researchers found that after implementation of the new standards, the proportion of entrées consumed increased 15.6% and the proportion of students selecting fruit increased 23%. While the percentage of students selecting vegetables did not change, portion consumption increased by 16.2%, which resulted in significantly more cups of vegetables consumed. The authors concluded that, overall the new standards have led to improvements in students' diets.

NATIONAL SCHOOL LUNCH PROGRAM	REIMBURSEMENT RATE PER MEAL
Paid lunches	$0.28
Reduced-price lunches	$2.58
Free lunches	$2.98
SCHOOL BREAKFAST PROGRAM	
Paid breakfasts	$0.28
Reduced-price breakfasts	$1.32
Free breakfasts	$1.62

TABLE 12-7 2014–2015 Reimbursement Rates for Sponsors of the National School Lunch and School Breakfast Programs*a*

a Payment rates are higher in Alaska and Hawaii to reflect the higher cost of providing meals in those states.

Source: *Federal Register* 79, No. 136 (2014): 41405–630.

The School Breakfast Program The 1966 Child Nutrition Act established funding for a pilot breakfast program, which was made permanent in 1975. By 2014, the program had grown annually to 13.5 million children participating at a federal cost of $3.7 billion.[99] Even though a school may offer the NSLP, it does not have to offer the breakfast program. This program, operated in the same manner as the School Lunch Program, provides a nutritious breakfast to all students attending a school where the program is offered (**Table 12-8**).

Breakfast is served free, or at a reduced price of no more than $0.30, to students from households with incomes at or below the income eligibility guidelines. Breakfasts served to students paying full price are also subsidized. To receive federal reimbursement, participating schools must follow standard meal patterns in which breakfasts provide one-fourth of the DRI values for protein, calcium, iron, vitamin A, vitamin C, and calories.

Although student participation in the school breakfast program has grown over the years, the number of children who participate, including those who qualify for a free or reduced-price meal, is far below the number of children who participate in the school lunch program. State agencies and local school boards are exploring alternative ideas to encourage more children to take advantage of this important program. Maryland's Meals for Achievement (MMFA) is a classroom breakfast project that started in 1998 in six Maryland elementary schools. Under state law, any school that has at least 40% of its enrollment approved for free or reduced-price meals can apply for state funding to cover the cost of providing free breakfast for all students. Participating schools offer in-class breakfast at no cost to students, regardless of family income. This innovative program removes common barriers such as transportation issues, getting to school late, or fear of being stigmatized that prevent students from participating in traditional cafeteria-based school breakfasts that are served before the school day starts. As of the 2014–2015 school year, 473 schools throughout Maryland are participating in the Meals for Achievement

TABLE 12-8 Foods Required for Breakfasts Provided under the School Breakfast Program

FOOD GROUP	OLD REQUIREMENTS, K–12	NEW REQUIREMENTS, K–12
Milk	• ½ pt of fluid milk as a beverage, on cereal, or both—one serving; AND	• 1 c must be fat-free (unflavored/flavored) or 1% low-fat (unflavored); AND
Fruit	• ½ c serving fruit OR ½ c full-strength fruit or vegetable juice—one serving; AND	• 1 c per day (vegetable substitution allowed); AND
Grains	• Bread or bread alternate (one slice whole-grain or enriched bread, or an equivalent serving of cornbread, biscuits, rolls, muffins, etc.; or ¾ c or 1 oz serving of cereal)—two servings; OR	• Daily minimum and weekly ranges for grains:[a,b] • Grades K–5: 1 oz equivalent minimum daily (7–10 oz weekly) • Grades 6–8: 1 oz equivalent minimum daily (8–10 oz weekly) • Grades 9–12: 1 oz equivalent minimum daily (9–10 oz weekly)
Meat/Meat Alternate[b]	• Meat or meat alternate (one serving of protein-rich foods such as an egg; or a 1 oz serving of meat, poultry, fish, or cheese; or 2 tbsp of peanut butter)—two servings; OR • One bread AND one meat	

[a] By July 1, 2014, all grains must be whole grain–rich.

[b] There is no separate meat/meat alternate component in the new standards for the SBP. Schools may substitute 1 oz equivalent of meat/meat alternate for 1 oz equivalent of grains after the minimum daily grains requirement is met.

Source: United States Department of Agriculture, Food and Nutrition Service, "Nutrition Standards in the National School Lunch and School Breakfast Programs," *Federal Register* 77 (January 26, 2012), 4088–167. Information related to the new meal requirements are available on a special webpage on the FNS website: *www.fns.usda.gov/cnd/Governance/Legislation/nutritionstandards.htm.*

program.[100] Researchers have examined the program's impact on students' behavior and academic achievement and found that both student tardiness and suspensions declined and the scores for the state's standardized achievement test improved significantly more in MMFA schools.[101] The success of this program has prompted other states to adopt similar efforts. Some 14 states provide financial incentives to school districts that offer a breakfast program, and 22 states mandate that districts offer school breakfast. Recognizing the important effect that breakfast has on a child's ability to learn in the classroom, school foodservice operators are using a number of approaches to increase participation, such as serving in the classroom, providing "grab 'n go" breakfasts, or offering breakfast after the first class. Some districts are offering breakfast free of charge to *all* students, regardless of whether the child's eligibility status is "free," "reduced-price," or "paid," and without additional state and federal funding.

The Afterschool Snack Program In 1998, Congress expanded the National School Lunch Program to include reimbursement for snacks served to children through the age of 18 in after-school educational and enrichment programs.[102] After-school snacks are provided to children on the same income eligibility basis as school lunches and must meet federal nutrition standards to qualify for reimbursement. However, programs that operate in schools where 50% or more of the enrolled students are eligible for free and reduced-priced meals, called "area-eligible" sites, may receive the "free" rate of reimbursement for all snacks served to children.

The Summer Food Service Program for Children The Summer Food Service Program (SFSP) is an entitlement program created by Congress in 1968 to ensure that children will have access to nutritious meals when school is not in session during summer vacation. During the 2014 Summer Food Service Program, close to 45,170 sites served 160 million meals to children, for a federal expenditure of $464.9 million.[103]

For the program to operate in a community, it must have a local sponsor that either contracts for foodservices or prepares its own food. Many school districts act as both the sponsor and the provider. For example, a district may provide food not only in its own locations but also to other school districts and to local parks and recreation programs. Programs operate as either open or enrolled sites:

- *"Open sites"* are located in areas where 50% or more of the children come from families whose household income is below 185% of the federal poverty guidelines. Any child or teen who lives in the area of an open site, even if she or he is not enrolled in the site's program, may participate free of charge in the SFSP. Sponsors of open-site programs may be reimbursed for all meals served, regardless of the income of each individual child, provided that the meals meet specified nutrition requirements.
- *"Enrolled sites"* are those where 50% of the children attending the program come from families whose income is greater than 185% of the federal poverty guidelines. Sponsors of enrolled sites, unlike those of open sites, must document the incomes of participating children in order to claim reimbursement.

The SFSP has faced a lack of sponsors, often because of the labor-intensive accounting and application procedures required by the program, as well as insufficient funding. To increase the number of sponsors, the Seamless Summer Feeding Waiver, begun in 2002, gives school districts the option of claiming meals under the National School Lunch Program instead of the SFSP. Another initiative to increase participation was launched as a result of the 2002 Farm Bill. Fourteen states were eligible to participate in a pilot study where the cost of meals served by sponsors was reimbursed at the maximum allowable rate, which reduced the amount of administrative record keeping.

In 2007, Congress simplified the summer foodservice program and extended it to include all states. Simplifying the program eliminated complex accounting requirements, reduced paperwork, and ensures that all sponsors receive the maximum federal reimbursement.[104]

Over 24 million children live in working-poor families.[105] The SFSP provides a critical safety net for their parents by providing nutritious meals at sites that offer educational enrichment and physical and recreational activities, keep children safe and out of trouble, and provide vital childcare. Currently, only one in six of the low-income children who rely on the school lunch program during the school year participates in the SFSP.[106] It is essential that national, state, and local stakeholders support efforts to provide funding and grow participation in this program to support the health and well-being of this population.

The Food Distribution Program The food distribution division of the USDA's Food and Nutrition Service coordinates the distribution of commodities to public and private nonprofit schools that provide meals to students. This program purchases food only of U.S. origin with funds provided through direct appropriations from Congress and price supports.

School districts are given an entitlement dollar value, based on the number of lunches served during the previous year, which is used to determine the amount of commodity food items that will be allocated to the district. Schools received 22.75 cents' worth of commodity foods per meal for the 2013 school year, but the entitlement is adjusted annually to reflect changes in the Price Index of Foods Used in Schools and Institutions.[107] The amount of entitlement commodities provided (such as fruits, vegetables, meats, dairy, grains, and ready-to-eat cereal) is based on the number of lunches served multiplied by the annual per-meal commodity rate.

Nutrition Programs of the U.S. Department of Health and Human Services

Recall from Chapter 11 that several DHHS programs include a childcare component: the Title V Maternal and Child Health Program; Medicaid and the Early and Periodic Screening, Diagnosis, and Treatment (EPSDT) program; and the primary-care programs of community-based health centers. Another DHHS program that benefits children is the Head Start Program.

Initiated in 1965 by the Office of Economic Opportunity, Head Start was authorized by the Economic Opportunity and Community Partnership Act of 1967 (P.L. 93-644, as amended in 1974). The program is coordinated by the Administration for Children and Families within the DHHS. It is one of the most successful federal government programs for child development. Head Start provides children from low-income families with comprehensive social, education, health, and nutrition services. Eligible children range in age from birth to the age at which they begin to attend school. Parental involvement in the program planning and operation is emphasized. Head Start projects provide meals and snacks as well as nutrition assessment and education for children and their parents. The nutrition services are meant to complement the health and education components of the program. Head Start programs served over 1 million children from birth to age five years and pregnant women throughout the 2013–2014 program year. The Select Panel for the Promotion of Child Health reported that Head Start has been shown to improve children's health. Children participating in Head Start have a lower incidence of anemia, receive more immunizations, and have better nutrition and improved overall health than children who do not participate.[108] Initiated in 1995, the Early Head Start Program expands the benefits of Head Start's early childhood development and family support services to low-income families with children under age three and to pregnant women.[109]

Improving Nutrition in the Childcare Setting

Over the past two decades there has been an increase in the number of households with two parents working outside the home, which makes childcare an important part of life for U.S. families. Almost two-thirds of preschool-age children were in some form of regular childcare arrangement in 2011. Nearly one-quarter were cared for in organized facilities, with daycare being the most common.[110] The American Academy of Pediatrics Policy Statement *Quality Early Education and Child Care from Birth to Kindergarten* maintains that early education includes all of a child's experiences at home, in childcare, and in other preschool settings. When those experiences are of high quality, it improves the child's health and promotes their development and learning.[111] The amount of time that children spend in childcare centers has increased over time and as a result, preschool-age children can be consuming many of their meals outside the home. Children's early experiences with food can influence both their food preferences and consumption. Studies have shown that early exposure to a variety of foods can increase children's acceptance and intake of these foods, thus improving the overall quality of their diet. In addition, these preferences have been shown to track from early age until early adulthood.[112] The foods and beverages served at childcare centers present an opportunity to affect children's healthy food intake patterns.

The Child and Adult Care Food Program (CACFP) is a federally funded nutrition program through the U.S. Department of Agriculture. The program's purpose is to ensure that nutritious meals and snacks are served to low-income children in qualifying daycare facilities by providing reimbursement for foods served. Individual state agencies are responsible for administering the program. The CACFP has recently proposed changes to its meal pattern requirements to better align them with the *Dietary Guidelines for Americans* as required by the Healthy, Hunger-Free Kids Act (HHFKA) of 2010. In addition, the amendments made by the HHFKA require the USDA, through its CACFP, to promote health and wellness in childcare settings through guidance and technical assistance that focuses on physical activity and limiting electronic media use.[113]

Under the proposed rule, the infant meal pattern would allow only breast milk and/or infant formula for infants up through five months of age, allow the introduction

ENTREPRENEUR IN ACTION

Kristine Smith, MS, RD, is Director of Nutrition Services at Neighborhood House Association (NHA) in San Diego, CA. Kristine leads a team of 14 at the central kitchen where more than 6,000 meals are produced daily for preschool-age children in Head Start and child development programs throughout the county. The foodservice operation is primarily funded by the USDA's Child and Adult Care Food Program. Nine years ago, Kristine hired a chef and completely redesigned the menu and overhauled the entire foodservice operation with a goal of reducing childhood obesity. NHA's preschool menu uses the Harvest of the Month program to feature a new and seasonal fruit or vegetable every month. NHA's Head Start program implemented Farm to Preschool in an effort to teach children and families where their food comes from, how to grow it, and how to cook with the different fruits and vegetables. NHA was awarded the inaugural First Lady's 2012 *Let's Move! Child Care* Recognition Award, of which the healthy menu was a focal point. Kristine finds it very rewarding for young children to thoroughly enjoy the nutritious food her team prepares every day. Even more impactful to her is that she believes foodservice can be more than just providing healthy meals; she is making a difference in young children's lives by helping them develop healthy eating habits that can last a lifetime. Learn more about Kristine online at *www.cengagebrain.com.*

of additional foods at six months of age (as developmentally appropriate), prohibit the service of fruit juice to infants through 11 months, and require a fruit or vegetable in the snack. Child meal patterns would require that:

- The currently combined fruit/vegetable component be divided into two separate components
- At least one serving per day, across all eating occasions, of grains be whole grain–rich
- Breakfast cereals conform to requirements as outlined by WIC
- Grain-based desserts be excluded from being used to meet the grain component
- A meat or meat alternate be allowed as a substitute for up to one-half of the required grains at breakfast meals
- Tofu be allowed as a meat alternative
- Unflavored whole milk be served to children 12–23 months and 1% or fat-free milk be served to children age two and older
- Flavored milk served is fat-free only
- Frying is disallowed as an on-site preparation method for daycare institutions[114]

Participation in the CACFP depends on the low-income status of children attending a childcare center, so not all childcare centers are required to comply with the meal standard requirements. In some states, childcare centers are required to meet that state's menu and dietary regulations. In 2011, First Lady Michelle Obama introduced *Let's Move Child Care*, an effort to promote children's health by encouraging physical activity and healthy nutrition practices for children in childcare settings within five goal areas: physical activity, reducing screen time, improving food choices, providing healthy beverages, and supporting infant feeding.[115] At the time of the launch of this program, data from the National Resource Center for Health and Safety in Child Care and Early Education showed that most states' childcare licensing regulations addressed the *Let's Move Child Care* goal to provide opportunities for daily outdoor play when the weather permits, make drinking water freely available throughout the day, and make provisions regarding breastfeeding to children in care. However, less than half of the states had requirements regarding screen time and few states specified the duration of physical activity, prohibited soft drinks and other sugary drinks, limited servings of fruit juice, or required that children age two and older be served low-fat or nonfat milk.[116]

Impact of Child Nutrition Programs on Children's Diets

Child Nutrition Program foodservice directors use federal dietary guidelines to plan menus for the National School Lunch and Breakfast Programs. Because of these standards, school meal programs have promoted healthful eating habits and contributed to the quality of children's overall diets. However, despite progress that has enhanced the nutrition quality of school meals, results of research conducted in the 1990s indicated that school meals were failing to meet certain key nutritional goals.[117]

The USDA's Continuing Survey of Food Intakes by Individuals (CSFII) assessed dietary intake in more than 5,000 children aged 6–18. One objective was to examine relationships between their participation in school meal programs and their dietary intake. Researchers reported that children who ate both breakfast and lunch at school on any given day received over 50% of their daily food energy from these meals.[118] Participation was also associated with higher intakes of total fat, saturated fat, and sodium, and with lower intakes of added sugars, than the intakes of those who did not participate. Students who participated in both

FIGURE 12-2 Consumption of Low-Nutrient, Energy-Dense Items at School, by NSLP[a] Participation Status

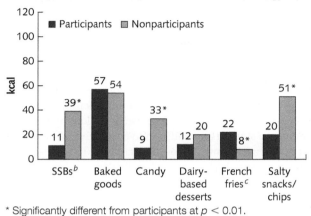

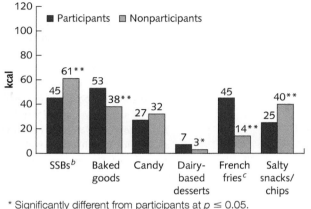

* Significantly different from participants at $p < 0.01$.

* Significantly different from participants at $p \leq 0.05$.
** Significantly different from participants at $p \leq 0.01$.

A. Elementary Schools
Mean energy intake from specific categories of low-nutrient, energy-dense items at elementary schools. On average, NSLP participants consumed significantly more energy from french fries and similar potato products in elementary school and significantly less from sugar-sweetened beverages, candy, and chips/salty snacks compared with nonparticipants.

B. Secondary Schools
Mean energy intake from specific categories of low-nutrient, energy-dense items at secondary schools. On average, NSLP participants consumed significantly more energy from french fries/similar potato products, baked goods, and dairy-based desserts in secondary school and significantly less from sugar-sweetened beverages and salty snacks compared with nonparticipants.

[a] NSLP, National School Lunch Program.
[b] SSBs, sugar-sweetened beverages.
[c] Includes similar potato products.

Source: R. R. Briefel, A. Wilson, and P. M. Gleason, "Consumption of Low-Nutrient, Energy-Dense Foods and Beverages at School, Home, and Other Locations among School Lunch Participants and Nonparticipants," *Journal of the American Dietetic Association* 109 (2009): S79–S90.

the school breakfast and lunch programs came much closer to meeting the recommended goals for fruits and vegetables, consumed more grains, and drank more milk, while eating fewer sweet and salty snacks and drinking fewer sweetened beverages, compared to those students not participating in the school meal programs (**Figure 12-2**). Participation in only the NSLP was associated with higher intakes of nutrients, such as the B vitamins, calcium, magnesium, and zinc, than the intakes of those who did not eat a school lunch.[119] Children who ate a school lunch got 15% of their lunch calories from saturated fat and 13% from added sugars. Those who did not participate received only 11% of their lunch calories from fat but got 23% from added sugars, possibly from soda consumption. School lunch participants drank about three times as much milk, but only half as much soda, as children who did not participate in the program. School breakfast participants had higher intakes of many vitamins and minerals, and had no increase in saturated fat and added sugars, compared to those who skipped breakfast at school and at home.

Even though school meal programs appeared to have a positive effect on children's consumption of milk, fruits, vegetables, and some vitamins and minerals, there was evidence that school meals contributed too much fat in menu items such as pizza, chicken sandwiches, french fries, and baked goods. In light of these findings, the USDA launched a reform of the NSLP in 1994, starting with public hearings and a proposed rule. In 1995, a final rule was adopted that directed schools to upgrade the nutritional value of their meals. Several elements of this reform are collectively referred to as the *School Meals Initiative for Healthy Children*, or SMI.[120] The USDA requires that states perform an SMI compliance review of school programs to determine whether menus are adhering to the *Dietary Guidelines for Americans* and meeting specified energy and nutrient standards for calories, total fat, saturated fat, protein, carbohydrate, calcium, iron, and vitamins A and C.

By 2000, nearly two-thirds of all school districts said they had "fully implemented" their menu upgrades.[121] To meet the nutrition standards, menus included more fruits, vegetables, whole grains, and low-fat and reduced-fat foods. These items, often served as larger portions to meet calorie requirements for specific ages, did not contribute to increasing fat percentages. More vegetarian and vegan options are now being offered, as well as salad bars and a variety of prepared salads. The creative use of packaging for food items helped to market healthful choices to students. In addition to complying with federal regulations, school foodservice directors throughout the country have also implemented a number of creative concepts to improve the quality and nutritional value of school meals.

> ## The New 2012 Nutrition Standards for Healthy School Meals

A Sample Elementary School Lunch Menu Before and After the Healthy, Hunger-Free Kids Act of 2010
The sample lunch menu below compares former NSLP elementary school meals to those offered under the new standards for school meals.

The USDA published a final rule in January 2012 to update nutrition standards for meals served through the National School Lunch and School Breakfast Programs as part of the Healthy, Hunger-Free Kids Act of 2010, which was signed into law by President Obama. The rule revises the meal patterns and nutrition requirements for the NSLP and SBP to align them with the *Dietary Guidelines for Americans*. The rule requires schools to increase the availability of fruits, vegetables, whole grains, and fat-free and low-fat fluid milk in school meals; reduce the levels of sodium and saturated fat in meals; and help meet the nutritional needs of school children within their calorie requirements. The new standards will ensure that school-age children are offered fruits and vegetables on every school day, given increased offerings of whole grain–rich foods, and offered only fat-free or low-fat milk varieties (see Tables 12-5 and 12-8). The new standards also address proper portion sizes for children.

Monday	Tuesday	Wednesday	Thursday	Friday
BEFORE	BEFORE	BEFORE	BEFORE	BEFORE
Bean and Cheese Burrito (5.3 oz) with Mozzarella Cheese (1 oz) Applesauce (1/4 cup) Orange Juice (4 oz) 2% Milk (8 oz)	Hot Dog on Bun (3 oz) with Ketchup (4 T) Canned Pears (1/4 cup) Raw Celery and Carrots (1/8 cup each) with Ranch Dressing (1.75 T) Low-fat (1%) Chocolate Milk (8 oz)	Pizza Sticks (3.8 oz) with Marinara Sauce (1/4 cup) Banana Raisins (1 oz) Whole Milk (8 oz)	Breaded Beef Patty (4 oz) with Ketchup (2 T) Wheat Roll (2 oz) Frozen Fruit Juice Bar (2.4 oz) 2% Milk (8 oz)	Cheese Pizza (4.8 oz) Canned Pineapple (1/4 cup) Tater Tots (1/2 cup) with Ketchup (2 T) Low-fat (1%) Chocolate Milk (8 oz)
AFTER	AFTER	AFTER	AFTER	AFTER
Submarine Sandwich (1 oz turkey, .5 oz low-fat cheese) on Whole Wheat Roll Refried Beans (1/2 cup) Jicama (1/4 cup) Green Pepper Strips (1/4 cup) Cantaloupe Wedges, Raw (1/2 cup) Skim Milk (8 oz) Mustard (9 g) Reduced-fat Mayonnoise (1 oz) Low-fat Ranch Dip (1 oz)	Whole Wheat Spaghetti with Meat Sauce (1/2 cup) and Whole Wheat Roll Green Beans, Cooked (1/2 cup) Broccoli (1/2 cup) Cauliflower (1/2 cup) Kiwi Halves, Raw (1/2 cup) Low-fat (1%) Milk (8 oz) Low-fat Ranch Dip (1 oz) Soft Margarine (5 g)	Chef Salad (1 cup romaine, .5 oz low-fat mozzarella, 1.5 oz grilled chicken) with Whole Wheat Soft Pretzel (2.5 oz) Corn, Cooked (1/2 cup) Baby Carrots, Raw (1/4 cup) Banana Skim Chocolate Milk (8 oz) Low-fat Ranch Dressing (1.5 oz) Low-fat Italian Dressing (1.5 oz)	Oven-Baked Fish Nuggets (2 oz) with Whole Wheat Roll Mashed Potatoes (1/2 cup) Steamed Broccoli (1/2 cup) Peaches (canned, packed in juice - 1/2 cup) Skim Milk (8 oz) Tartar Sauce (1.5 oz) Soft Margarine (5 g)	Whole Wheat Cheese Pizza (1 slice) Baked Sweet Potato Fries (1/2 cup) Grape Tomatoes, Raw (1/4 cup) Applesauce (1/2 cup) Low-fat (1%) Milk (8 oz) Low-fat Ranch Dip (1 oz)

Source: USDA Economic Research Service.

To recognize schools that are actively engaged in fostering healthy school environments, the USDA is implementing the HealthierUS School Challenge, which is a voluntary program that provides monetary incentives and certifications to schools that are promoting healthy food and physical activity.[122]

Improving child nutrition is the focal point of the Healthy, Hunger-Free Kids Act of 2010, which authorizes funding and sets new policy for the USDA child nutrition programs. The Healthy, Hunger-Free Kids Act allows the USDA to reform the nutrition standards of the school lunch and breakfast programs. These improvements to the school meal programs—largely based on recommendations from the 2009 IOM report *School Meals: Building Blocks for Healthy Children*—aim to enhance the diet and health of school children and reduce childhood obesity (see the box that follows).[123]

The meals provided through the USDA's school nutrition programs provide most of the food and beverages for children at school. Most schools also sell "competitive foods" such as á la carte sales in the cafeteria, vending machines, school stores, or snack bars. Until recently, competitive foods have been required to meet minimal nutrition standards. Starting with the 2014–2015 school year, competitive foods sold to children during the school day must meet specific standards (the Smart Snack Rule) regarding nutrient content and amount of sodium, sugar, fats, and calories. For many schools, the sale of competitive foods represents additional income. School foodservices, especially those where competitive food revenues make up a large portion of their overall revenue, have expressed concern that the change in standards would impact sales. However, evidence from schools that had initiated strong nutrition standards for competitive foods prior to the mandatory school year suggests they can remain financially stable and have increased school meal participation.[124] **Figure 12-3** shows a comparison of snack foods offered before and after implementation of the Smart Snack Rule standards.

Building Healthful School Environments

The surgeon general's call to action to prevent and decrease overweight and obesity outlines the following actions for creating healthful school environments:[125]

- Provide age-appropriate nutrition and health education to help students develop lifelong healthy lifestyle habits.
- Ensure that meals offered through school breakfast and lunch programs meet healthy standards.
- Adopt policies that require all foods and beverages available on school campuses and at school events to contribute toward eating patterns that are consistent with the *Dietary Guidelines for Americans*.
- Provide food options that are low in solid fat, calories, and added sugars.
- Ensure that healthy snacks and foods are provided in vending machines, school stores, and other venues.
- Prohibit access to vending machines that compete with healthy school meals in elementary schools; restrict access in middle, junior, and high schools.
- Provide adequate time for students to eat school meals, and schedule lunch periods at reasonable hours around midday.

In response to the epidemic of overweight children that has resulted from unhealthy eating behavior and a lack of physical activity, the Local School Wellness Policy was established through the Child Nutrition and WIC Reauthorization Act of 2004 and further strengthened through the Healthy, Hunger-Free Kids Act of 2010. This law requires every school district that participates in the NSLP and/or SBP to adopt policies that support a

FIGURE 12-3 Smart Snacks in School

Source: U.S. Department of Agriculture, Food and Nutrition Service. See *www.fns.usda .gov/healthierschoolday/ tools-schools-focusing-smart-snacks*.

United States Department of Agriculture

SMART SNACKS IN SCHOOL

The Healthy, Hunger-Free Kids Act of 2010 requires USDA to establish nutrition standards for all foods sold in schools — beyond the federally-supported meals programs. This new rule carefully balances science-based nutrition guidelines with practical and flexible solutions to promote healthier eating on campus. The rule draws on recommendations from the Institute of Medicine, existing voluntary standards already implemented by thousands of schools around the country, and healthy food and beverage offerings already available in the marketplace.

● Equals 1 calorie   ○ Shows empty calories*

Before the New Standards

286 TOTAL CALORIES	**249** TOTAL CALORIES	**242** TOTAL CALORIES	**235** TOTAL CALORIES	**136** TOTAL CALORIES
Chocolate Sandwich Cookies (6 medium)	**Fruit Flavored Candies** (2.2 oz. pkg.)	**Donut** (1 large)	**Chocolate Bar** (1 bar-1.6 oz.)	**Regular Cola** (12 fl. oz.)
182 Empty Calories	**177** Empty Calories	**147** Empty Calories	**112** Empty Calories	**126** Empty Calories

After the New Standards

170 TOTAL CALORIES	**161** TOTAL CALORIES	**118** TOTAL CALORIES	**95** TOTAL CALORIES	**68** TOTAL CALORIES	**0** TOTAL CALORIES
Peanuts (1 oz.)	**Light Popcorn** (Snack bag)	**Low-Fat Tortilla Chips** (1 oz.)	**Granola Bar (oats, fruit, nuts)** (1 bar-.8 oz.)	**Fruit Cup (w/100% Juice)** (Snack cup 4 oz.)	**No-Calorie flavored Water** (12 fl. oz.)
0 Empty Calories	**17** Empty Calories	**0** Empty Calories	**32** Empty Calories	**0** Empty Calories	**0** Empty Calories

*Calories from food components such as added sugars and solid fats that provide little nutritional value. Empty calories are part of total calories.

the School Day Just got Healthier
United States Department of Agriculture

school environment that provides nutrition education, physical activity, and other school-based activities designed to promote student wellness. Schools must also comply with federal nutrition standards for all foods that are available on each school campus during the school day. The law also requires school districts to establish wellness policy leadership that includes parents, students, school board members, school administrators, members of the public, and school foodservice staff members, and to designate one or more district and/or school officials responsible for ensuring compliance with the policies. Annual progress reports that summarize the school's events and activities and the progress in meeting the wellness policy goals are to be submitted and triennial assessment on school compliance and alignment with the model wellness policies are required.

An analysis from the first five years following the required implementation date for wellness policies showed areas of strength and opportunities for improvement in the development and implementation of school wellness polices.[126] As of the beginning of the school year 2010–2011, nearly all (99%) of students nationwide were enrolled in a school district with a wellness policy. However, less than half (46%) of students were in a district that included all of the required elements: nutrition education, school meals, physical activity, implementation and evaluation, and competitive food guidelines. The degree of progress varied by element. Most students were in a district with a policy that had goals for nutrition education (95%), guidelines for school meals (91%), and physical activity (90%). Areas for improvement in adopting/implementing policy goals were implementation and evaluation plans (83%) and competitive food guidelines (61%). (Note this data was collected prior to the required implementation date for the Smart Snacks Rule for competitive foods and beverages [2014–2015]. Subsequent analysis of this element should show improvement.) Nutrition education was the most comprehensively addressed and most likely to be required component of the wellness policies. Although physical education was not a required element, 95% of all students were in a district with a wellness policy that addressed physical education.

Nutrition Education Programs

Nutrition education strategies aimed at children or their caregivers are found in both the public and private sectors. Their goal is to improve eating patterns among children. Numerous government and commercial sites on the Internet provide databases of educational materials and resources and, in some cases, offer interactive games and puzzles for children. Refer to the Internet Resources at the end of the chapter for a list of government and commercial websites related to children and adolescents. Public-sector and private-sector nutrition education initiatives are described in this section.

Nutrition Education in the Public and Private Sectors

Schools can play a key role in reversing the trend of obesity and lack of physical activity by offering comprehensive nutrition education programs. Schools are an ideal setting for nutrition education for the following reasons:

- More than 95% of all children and adolescents are enrolled in school.
- More than 50% eat at least one of three meals at school.
- Professionally prepared teachers and staff can provide nutrition education that teaches students to resist social pressures for unhealthful eating.

Action for Healthy Kids

Action for Healthy Kids (AFHK) is an integrated national–state initiative that addresses childhood obesity by focusing on changes in the school environment. AFHK includes a partnership of 40 national organizations, industry groups, and government agencies representing education, physical activity, and health and nutrition—such as the Association for Supervision and Curriculum Development, the National Association of State Boards of Education, the National Association for Sport and Physical Education, the Academy of Nutrition and Dietetics, the American Academy of Pediatrics, the United States Department of Agriculture, and the United States Department of Education.

In the short term, AFHK is working to increase the number of health-promoting schools that support sound nutrition and physical activity in order to slow the rate of increasing obesity among American children. In the long term, AFHK aims to play a key role in preventing childhood obesity nationwide. To achieve these goals, AFHK has three main objectives:

- Improving school children's eating habits by increasing access to nutritious food and beverages on school grounds, while decreasing access to high-calorie, low-nutrient options, as well as by integrating nutrition education into the curriculum for all school children.
- Increasing school children's physical activity through physical education courses, recess, the integration of physical activity into academic classes, and after-school and co-curricular fitness programs.
- Educating administrators, educators, students, and parents about the role of sound nutrition and physical activity in academic achievement.

Fifty-one *Action for Healthy Kids* state teams are implementing a variety of creative interventions at the grassroots level to promote sound nutrition and physical activity throughout the school environment. Each team has developed an action plan that is appropriate for its own state's educational system, culture, and resources. For instance:

- The Alabama team conducted a school vending machine survey with 1,400 school principals. The team used the results to develop a "Guide to Healthy Vending," which it distributed to all principals in the state.
- The Delaware team is working to provide staff training on how to test students' physical fitness in order to ensure that 50% of students show an improvement on physical fitness tests.
- The Indiana team is providing all superintendents with a position paper summarizing the relationship between recess and academic performance, and a resource kit of selected before-school and after-school activities and nutrition programs.
- The Texas team is working to ensure that the majority of its school districts have a school health advisory council responsible for making recommendations and monitoring nutrition and physical activity programs within the district.
- The Massachusetts team has developed nutrition guidelines for foods and beverages sold à la carte in all school districts, positively impacting nearly 1 million students by improving choices of healthful foods and beverages on campus and by increasing physical activity during and after school.

Check out the *www.actionforhealthykids.org* website for the latest information, resources, and success stories for improving nutrition and physical activity in schools. The AFHK website provides a one-stop source for information on its national and state team initiatives, statistics on nutrition and physical activity in schools, and a variety of resources for school-based change. Additionally, AFHK has collaborated with the CDC and other agencies to develop a wellness policy tool that is available as a resource for schools.

Source: Action for Healthy Kids; *www.actionforhealthykids.org*.

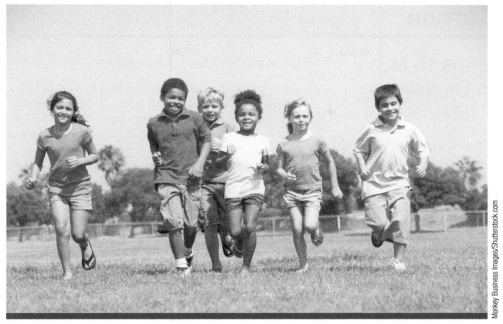

Successful nutrition education activities help children and teenagers focus on their interests and on the relationship of good eating and physical activity to health.

Severe drops in funding from year to year have decreased the capacity of the USDA, state agencies, and local sponsors to deliver effective nutrition education to children. Even though the number of students participating in child nutrition programs has continued to grow, these same programs have received limited funding for nutrition education.

Despite the lack of significant and consistent federal funding for national nutrition education initiatives, successful nutrition projects have been implemented. The Fresh Fruit and Vegetable Program is a program designed to increase fruit and vegetable availability to schools and improve fruit and vegetable consumption of children. The 2002 Farm Bill appropriated $6 million for schools in Iowa, Indiana, Michigan, Ohio, and the Zuni Indian Tribal Organization in New Mexico to purchase fresh and dried fruit and fresh vegetables to be available free of charge to children throughout the school day in the Fresh Fruit and Vegetable Program.[127] The Fresh Fruit and Vegetable Program showed several positive benefits. Students reported enjoying the healthful snack option and being involved in preparing the fruits and vegetables for distribution. School administrators commented that the USDA offered flexibility: Each school was allowed to implement the program with the approach that best met the needs of the school. Foodservice staff reported that not only did lunch participation increase, but so did the consumption of fruits and vegetables at mealtime. The pilot program showed that, if given the resources, schools can create an environment where healthful snack options can be a reality.

The 2004 Child Nutrition Reauthorization made the pilot Fresh Fruit and Vegetable Program a permanent program, increased funding to $9 million, and added four more states (Mississippi, Washington, Pennsylvania, and North Carolina) and two tribal organizations in Arizona and South Dakota. Federal dollars are used by schools to purchase fresh fruits and vegetables for snacks. As a result of the 2008 Farm Bill, this program was expanded to all states.[128] Research has shown that children who report a high preference for fruits and vegetables are less likely to be overweight or obese than those who report a very low preference for fruits and vegetables.[129]

PROGRAMS IN **ACTION**

Empowering Teens to Make Better Nutrition Decisions

Unhealthful eating and lack of physical activity are major contributors to adult morbidity and mortality in the United States.[1] These habits are also prevalent among youth. By the time children graduate from high school, more than 70% do not eat enough fruits and vegetables, 84% eat too much fat, and nearly one-third do not engage in regular vigorous physical activity.[2] Fast food is increasingly common in high schools,[3] and fast-food advertising is widespread.[4] These elements contribute to the fact that more than 17% of young people are considered overweight or obese. The incidence of obesity has significant public health implications today and for years to come.

The Food on the Run project recognized the importance of empowering teens to make better decisions about their diet, activity, and health. It was born out of collaboration among 10 California communities that recognized the lack of nutrition education materials and programs for high school students.

Participating communities worked with California Project LEAN, a program of the Public Health Institute and the California Department of Health Services, to develop the framework for Food on the Run.

Goals and Objectives

Food on the Run sought to improve the health of high school students through the promotion of accurate nutrition information in the classroom and increased availability of healthful food options on campus. Its primary objectives were:

- To create a high school youth advocacy model that motivates students to advocate for more healthful food and physical activity options in their communities.
- To advance locally identified policy and environmental changes that increase the number and promotion of healthful food items and physical activity options on participating school campuses.
- To motivate students to make more healthful food choices and to become physically active.

Target Audience

Program participants were low-income students in high schools where at least 40% of the students were eligible for free and reduced-price meals. During the year of implementation, the 28 Food on the Run schools reached 11% of California's low-income high school students.

Rationale for the Intervention

In general, high school students need to improve their eating habits and level of physical activity. It is believed that these students will be more motivated to change if they play an integral role in the formulation of health program strategies and messages.

Food on the Run uses the spectrum of prevention as a basis for its intervention.[5] This framework states that the following components are necessary to impact change at the individual and community levels:

- Strengthening individual knowledge and skills
- Promoting community education
- Educating providers
- Fostering coalitions and networks
- Changing organizational practices
- Influencing policy and legislation

Methodology

Each Food on the Run school, in conjunction with students, set its own nutrition and physical activity policy agenda. During the school year, each school worked with a coalition of local organizers, health providers, and private industry to build its program. Components included the recruitment and training of 10–20 high school student advocates, the implementation of at least seven school-based activities, and at least two activities to increase parent awareness and involvement. Specific activities included taste tests of low-fat foods, presentations to school boards, setting up of a sports equipment checkout table at lunch, initiation of a cafeteria salad bar, and a change from reduced-fat (2%) to low-fat (1%) milk in school cafeterias.

California Project LEAN supported Food on the Run communities with training, resources, media tools, research, and development of food and physical activity messages.

Results

Program success was evaluated with student surveys and an assessment of the school environment. The environment assessment described the eating and physical activity environment at participating high schools using pre- and post-test measures. During the school year, statistically significant increases ($p = 0.05$) were observed for physical activity knowledge (6%) and attitude (4%); nutrition knowledge (5%), attitude (5%), and behavior (9%); healthy eating options (5.7 out of a possible 11 points); healthy eating promotional efforts on school campuses (2.3 out of a possible 5 points); and physical activity options available to students at the schools (3.3 out of a possible 6 points).

Lessons Learned

Contrary to popular belief, high school students want opportunities to "eat healthy" and be more physically active. Student involvement is the key to offering healthful foods that sell and

physical activity classes that are full. When high school students are involved in the formulation of nutrition and physical activity messages and policy strategies, behavior change can occur.

Source: Adapted from *Community Nutritionary* (White Plains, NY: Dannon Institute, Spring 2001). Used with permission. For more information about the Awards for Excellence in Community Nutrition, go to *www.dannon-institute.org*. The California Project LEAN program is available at *www.californiaprojectlean.org*.

Two other successful USDA nutrition education programs, the Expanded Food and Nutrition Education Program (EFNEP) and Team Nutrition, target the improvement of children's health. EFNEP, a cooperative extension program, began in 1968 to assist low-income youth and families in acquiring knowledge, skills, and attitudes that contribute to their nutritional well-being and to the improvement of the total family's diet. Team Nutrition, begun in 1995, focuses attention on the role of school meals, nutrition education, and a healthful school environment in teaching students the importance of good dietary habits and physical activity.[130] The Team Nutrition logo is shown in **Figure 12-4**. Team Nutrition has three behavior-focused strategies:

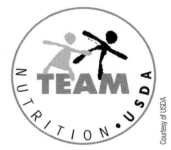

FIGURE 12-4
The Team Nutrition Logo

1. Provide training to school foodservice professionals that enables them to prepare and serve nutritious meals.
2. Promote nutrition education in schools that teaches and encourages students to make healthful lifestyle choices.
3. Build school and community support for healthful school environments that promote positive nutrition messages throughout.

There are many government and nonprofit organizations at the national, state, and local levels that are also implementing initiatives that aim to reduce overweight and increase physical activity among youth. An excellent example of a coordinated school health program that addresses both nutrition and physical activity is the Coordinated Approach to Child Health, or CATCH, program described in the Programs in Action feature in Chapter 8. Another such program is the Centers for Disease Control and Prevention's Coordinated School Health Program (CSHP), which combines health education and promotion, disease prevention, and access to health and social services in an integrated, comprehensive manner. To reach beyond the classroom and cafeteria, CSHP also provides opportunities for parental and community involvement in promoting healthful behaviors to students.

The following are some examples of programs that effectively promote healthful eating to children using a variety of methods.

Eat Smart. Play Hard.   This national FNS nutrition education and promotion campaign is designed to convey motivational messages about healthful eating and physical activity. The campaign uses a mascot, Power Panther, as the primary communication vehicle for delivering messages about nutrition and physical activity to children and their caregivers. The target audience for this campaign is children ages 2–18 years who are participating, or are eligible to participate, in FNS nutrition assistance programs. Campaign messages are based on the *Dietary Guidelines for Americans* and focus on four basic themes: eating breakfast, healthful snacking, achieving balance, and physical activity.

Farm-to-School Programs

Through farm-to-school programs, students gain access to healthy, local foods and experiential learning opportunities. Implementation of the program typically includes one or more of the following: (1) Procurement: local foods are purchased and served in the cafeteria, frequently as part of a social marketing campaign in the schools; (2) Education: includes activities such as school gardens, cooking classes, and field trips to local farms; (3) School gardens: students engage in hands-on learning through gardening. Currently 44% of schools and 23.5 million students participate in some form of farm-to-school program in the United States.[131]

Fruits & Veggies—More Matters

This is a large public/private nutrition partnership to promote the increased consumption of fruits and vegetables by adults and children. The campaign includes many resources, including a program for elementary schools, There's a Rainbow on My Plate, that promotes a colorful diet of fruits and vegetables. It includes curriculum guides for teachers and techniques to promote healthful eating in the school foodservice program. The campaign also targets the produce sections of supermarkets.

Best Bones Forever

This is a national bone health campaign that partners the National Osteoporosis Foundation with the Centers for Disease Control and Prevention and the Department of Health and Human Services.[132] It is a multiyear campaign to promote optimal bone health in girls 9–12 years of age and thus to reduce their risk of osteoporosis later in life. The goal is to encourage calcium consumption and physical activity for building and maintaining strong bones. The campaign also targets adults who influence "tweens," including parents, teachers, and health care professionals.

Fuel Up to Play 60

Launched in 2009, this is a nationwide movement focused on fighting childhood obesity by empowering children to take control of their own health. The in-school program encourages the availability and consumption of nutrient-rich foods and at least 60 minutes of daily physical activity. The program was founded by the National Dairy Council and the National Football League in collaboration with the USDA. The program—now in more than 70,000 schools—helps schools create a healthier environment for students. Fuel Up to Play 60 provides a free "playbook" of tools, resources, rewards, and activities to empower youth to make healthy choices. Some member schools have started walking clubs, while others have conducted "taste tests" of foods such as whole grains, fruit, and reduced-fat cheese. Students then vote on which ones they would like to see in the school cafeteria.[133]

Kids Café Program

Kids Café is a program of Feeding America—the nation's leading domestic hunger-relief charity. Since the program's inception in 1993, Kids Cafés have become one of the nation's largest free meal service programs for children.[134] The primary goal of the Kids Café Program is to provide free prepared food and nutrition education to hungry children. Kids Cafés across the country achieve this goal by utilizing existing community resources, such as Boys and Girls Clubs, community recreation centers, or schools—places where children already congregate naturally. In 2014 Kids Cafés served 14.5 million meals to 155,000 children. In addition to providing hot meals to hungry kids, some Kids Café programs also offer a safe and welcoming place where, under the supervision of caring staff, a child can get involved in educational, recreational, and social activities that draw on existing community programs and often include family members.

Keeping Children and Adolescents Healthy

Programs and services designed to keep children and adolescents healthy can have a lasting effect on the nation's public health. Healthy children and adolescents mean healthy communities. Children and youth who learn good eating habits, exercise regularly, refrain from smoking, learn to manage stress, and develop a strong sense of self are less likely to turn to drugs and alcohol to solve problems and more likely to know how to live constructively.

Successful, effective programs or services for children and youth recognize the stresses of life in the early twenty-first century and the mixed messages in the media about products and values. Programs and services founded on basic health promotion principles must consider the urgent health issues facing today's young people: suicide, child abuse, teen pregnancy, sexually transmitted diseases, eating disorders, obesity, substance abuse, and others. Positive nutrition messages support and expand on other health promotion concepts.

What types of programs work? Health educators have found that programming for children and adolescents succeeds when it is fun and informative. Programs work best when they are geared to a specific health or nutritional objective, such as weight loss, improved eating patterns, or increased activity levels. For instance, Girls on the Run is a positive physical activity–based youth development program for girls in grades 3–8 that uses an experience-based curriculum that integrates running. The goal of the program is to "unleash confidence through accomplishment while establishing a lifetime appreciation of health and fitness." A 2002 pilot study on Girls on the Run found that pre- to post-test improvements were significant ($p < 0.05$) for the program participants' self-esteem, eating attitudes and behaviors, and body size satisfaction.[135] Involving children and adolescents in the planning and implementation of a program increases its effectiveness, as does using peer support to help the participants make decisions about their health. Effective programs also employ trained staff who work well with these populations. The youth development approach offers a strategy for linking young people meaningfully with their communities and involving them in designing and implementing programs and services.[136]

In the final analysis, developing programs and services that meet the needs of our nation's children and youth means recognizing that as today's children grow, they have to perform increasingly complex tasks in a world of constant technological and environmental change. Improving the health of today's young people will enhance the quality of their lives in the immediate future and enlarge their potential for contributing to our nation's future as adults. In promoting the health and well-being of children and youth, we are recognizing "that children matter for themselves, that childhood has its own intrinsic value, and that society has an obligation to enhance the lives of children today."[137]

case study

The Child Nutrition Program

by Alice Fornari, EdD, RD, Alessandra Sarcona, MS, RD, CSSD, and Alison Barkman, MS, RD, CDN

Scenario

A school district in a suburban community has offered you the position of director of the Child Nutrition Program.

The school district consists of one high school, two middle schools, and four elementary schools. You have accepted the position, seeing it as an exciting challenge after your 15 years of experience directing hospital foodservice. The district has expressed interest in developing a nutrition and health intervention program for the students as part of the Child Nutrition Program.

After a month of "settling in" to the job, you begin to look at the goal of developing a nutrition and health intervention program for the students. You have done a nutrient analysis of the school lunch menu that revealed that 40% of the calories in the average lunch are derived from fat. Twenty percent of the student body receives free and reduced-price lunches. Government commodities are provided but are not fully utilized. A large percentage of the sales of the lunch program—and therefore a large percentage of its revenues—comes from snack items. Recently, the school nurse has released statistics on the weight status of the students. She outlined the percentage of students with a BMI greater than the 85th percentile to determine overweight trends: 12% of the high school students, 20% of the middle school students, and 14% of the elementary school students fell in this category. Another relevant issue is that the middle school physical education curriculum has been reduced from daily to two days per week because of budget constraints and the need for more classroom time in order to meet rigorous academic requirements.

Learning Outcomes

- Identify the *Healthy People 2020* objectives for children and adolescents.
- Identify USDA nutrition guidelines for Child Nutrition Program meals. Outline the latest updates by the USDA to all school lunch programs as part of the Healthy, Hunger-Free Kids Act of 2010.
- Outline the process for implementing a school-based nutrition/health intervention program.

Foundation: Acquisition of Knowledge and Skills

1. Acquire from the text the *Healthy People 2020* objectives for children and adolescents.

2. Go to the USDA website, *www.usda.gov*, and search for food and nutrition and child nutrition programs. Review the guidelines for menu planning for the national school lunch program for healthful school meals.
3. From the USDA website, go to *www.fns.usda.gov/tn/about.html*, "About Team Nutrition," and outline the objectives of Team Nutrition.

Step 1: *Identify Relevant Information and Uncertainties*

1. To set up a pilot program for a specific target group, sort the pieces of information presented in the case to determine which school in the district has the most risk factors.
2. Identify conditions in the school and aspects of the lunch menu that are affecting the population determined to be at greatest risk; list a range of possible ways to address these issues.

Step 2: *Interpret Information*

1. Identify the strengths and weaknesses of incorporating Team Nutrition for your target school; on the Team Nutrition website, review some projects/activities other schools have implemented that might be feasible for your school.
2. Devise a plan to develop a task force from appropriate groups within the school to support the implementation of Team Nutrition; include a written letter.

Step 3: *Draw and Implement Conclusions*

Outline a timeline for implementing Team Nutrition.

Step 4: *Engage in Continuous Improvement*

1. Outline the variables that would need to be monitored in the first phase to evaluate a desired outcome for your intervention program.
2. From the Team Nutrition website, investigate the availability of grants. Develop a fact sheet for the task force that would support applying for a grant.

The Art of Negotiating

Whether we like it or not, we are all negotiators. Every day, we negotiate with family, friends, and coworkers to get something we want. Although each of us negotiates every day, most of us don't negotiate particularly well. Our negotiations tend to leave us feeling frustrated, taken advantage of, dissatisfied, or just plain worn out. This is unfortunate because negotiation is the heart of all business deals.

The reason that people sometimes emerge from negotiations feeling this way is that they tend to see only two ways to negotiate: hard or soft.[1] Hard negotiators view the other participants as adversaries. Their goal is victory—their side wins and the other side loses. Hard negotiators tend to distrust the other party and to make threats. They perceive the negotiation process as a contest of wills. Soft negotiators, on the other hand, think of the participants as friends. Their goal is agreement among the parties. They tend to be trusting, avoid a battle of wills, change positions easily, and make concessions to maintain the relationship. Many of us use soft negotiation tactics in our dealings with our parents, siblings, friends, or other people who are important to us.

Are these the only ways of negotiating? There is a better way to negotiate than either the soft or the hard approach, according to Roger Fisher and William Ury of the Harvard Negotiation Project. The method they developed is called *principled negotiation*. Its main precept is that a decision about an issue should be based on its merits, not on what each side says it will or will not do. The method can be boiled down to four basic elements:

- People—Separate the people from the problem.
- Interests—Focus on interests, not positions.
- Options—Generate a variety of possibilities before deciding what to do.
- Criteria—Insist that the result be based on some objective standard.

Separate the People from the Problem

When people sit down at the bargaining table, they bring with them certain perceptions about the relationships among the participants and about the problem itself. Whether these perceptions are accurate or false, they pervade the proceedings. There is a tendency to confuse the participants' relationships with the "issue" or "problem." One of the first steps to take in negotiating is to separate the problem from the people and to deal with relationship goals and problem goals separately. This means

thinking about how to get good results from the negotiation and what kind of relationship is likely to produce those results.

Another challenge in negotiating is having to deal with a problem when emotions are running high. People sometimes come to the bargaining table with strong feelings. They may be angry or frightened, may feel threatened or misunderstood, or may be worried about the outcome. A good way to handle the emotional aspects of the negotiation process is to recognize such emotions and give them legitimacy. The bottom line, write Fisher and Brown, is to "do only those things that are both good for the relationship and good for us."[2]

Focus on Interests, Not Positions

The purpose of negotiating is to serve our interests. Interests motivate people to reach certain decisions. The primary problem in most negotiations is not the difference in positions but the conflicts between the two sides' needs, fears, desires, and concerns—in other words, their interests. In addition, most of us tend to think that the other party's interests are similar to our own. This is almost never the case. When negotiating, begin by defining, as precisely as possible, your own interests, and then allow the other participants to define theirs. Work through the discussion until mutual interests are identified.[3]

Consider a Variety of Options

We sometimes approach a negotiating session with only one outcome in mind. We operate with blinders on and fail to see other dimensions to the problem that may be a source of possible solutions. To get around this barrier, bring the participants together to brainstorm about potential solutions and options. In a good brainstorming session, judgments about possible solutions are suspended, and everyone involved in the negotiation is allowed to contribute ideas. At the end of the session, the parties discuss the various options, picking several that offer the most promise. The parties give themselves time to evaluate each of these "best and brightest" ideas and consider which of them, if any, would best suit their purpose. Once again, when exploring options, consider the interests of both parties.

Use Objective Criteria

Suppose your roommate wants to buy your car, but you cannot agree on a price. She thinks that your asking price is too high; you think her offer is too low. Where do you go from here? One option is to consult the *Blue Book* price for your car's make and model. Another is to examine the newspaper listings of used cars for sale to determine the asking price for cars like yours. These options are the criteria or standards that help you reach an agreement. The type of criteria you use will depend on the nature of the issue being negotiated. In this case, the criterion was the fair market value of your car. In other situations, a court decision, tradition, precedent, scientific judgment, cost, or moral standard might serve as the criterion. The important thing is to choose an objective standard that all parties are comfortable with.

Build Good Relationships

The negotiating process is much like a tango—a little give and a little take on both sides. Regardless of the issue, a "good" negotiation is fueled by a good relationship. When next you enter into a negotiation, take a few minutes to evaluate your relationship with the other person or party. The questions below will help you determine how good your working relationship is and where improvements can be made.[4] With practice, you can help build good working relationships.

Do we want to work together? In a good relationship, people want to work together. They respect each other and actively pursue strategies for sorting out differences. They work to keep problems to a minimum.

Are we reliable? Good relationships are built on trust and constancy. All parties have confidence that verbal and written commitments will be kept. The parties work to allay any concerns about trustworthiness.

Do we understand each other? Even in the best of working relationships, there will be differences of opinion, values, perceptions, and motives. In good relationships, the parties strive to accept each other and work toward understanding their differences.

Do we use our powers of persuasion effectively? In good relationships, persuasion is used to influence and inform the other party about an issue or proposed action. The parties refrain from using coercive tactics and rely instead on rational, logical discussions of the merits of a particular position or action.

Do we communicate well? Good communication is based on sound and compassionate reasoning. In good relationships, sensitive issues can be discussed in a supportive environment where candor is valued. The parties in a good relationship communicate often, consult each other before making decisions, and practice "active listening," where the parties work to hear each other with an open, flexible mind.

Work Toward Success

Good negotiating means that all parties leave the bargaining table feeling they have won. A successful negotiation is one in which the outcome advances both parties' interests. It is seen as fair. The solution was arrived at with an efficient use of everyone's time. Neither party feels that he or she is at a disadvantage. And the solution will be implemented according to plan. A successful negotiation leaves the parties feeling respect for their counterparts and a desire to work together again.[5]

CHAPTER **SUMMARY** . . . .

Healthy People 2020 National Nutrition Objectives

▶ In 2010, the U.S. Department of Health and Human Services outlined a set of health and nutrition objectives for children and adolescents in its publication *Healthy People 2020* (see Table 12-1).

▶ Significant efforts are needed to achieve the *Healthy People 2020* objectives that promote healthful weights and food choices in children and adolescents. Suggested actions include advocating for public health policies that address not only individual behaviors but also the environmental conditions in which people live; and implementing strategies to make healthy food choices available, identifiable, and affordable to people of all races and income levels and in all types of geographic locations.

What Are Children and Adolescents Eating?

▶ Nationwide surveys show that most children and adolescents have either a poor diet or one that needs improvement. Children are failing to meet the recommended nutrition guidelines by not consuming enough fruits, vegetables, and whole grains and by eating too many foods high in saturated fat, added sugars, and sodium.

▶ Influences on child and adolescent eating patterns and behaviors include growing independence from parents, convenience, eating away from home, concern with physical appearance and body weight, the need for peer acceptance, busy schedules, and food marketing.

▶ The lack of good nutrition habits, coupled with physical inactivity, has led to an epidemic of overweight children and adolescents of all ethnic groups. Genetic susceptibility to obesity, lifestyle, family eating patterns, lack of positive role models, and inactivity all contribute to overweight and obesity in this population.

▶ A significant and widespread governmental social marketing campaign for prevention of childhood obesity is *Let's Move!*, which focuses on creating a healthy start for children; empowering parents and caregivers; providing healthy foods in schools; improving access to healthy, affordable foods; and increasing physical activity.

▶ Other nutrition-related problems among children and adolescents include undernutrition, iron-deficiency anemia, high blood cholesterol levels, dental caries, and eating disorders.

▶ Children with special needs from infancy through adolescence are served by public school systems and early-intervention services. Children with special health care needs are at increased nutritional risk because of feeding problems, metabolic aberrations, drug–nutrient interactions, decreased mobility, and alterations in growth patterns.

The History of Child Nutrition Programs in Schools

▶ The Food and Nutrition Service was established to administer the 15 food and nutrition assistance programs of the USDA. The aim of this agency is to make food assistance available to people who need it, improve the eating habits of children, and stabilize farm prices through the distribution of surplus foods. Five programs for children include the National School Lunch Program, the School Breakfast Program, the Summer Food Service Program, the Afterschool Snack Program, and the Commodity Distribution Program (see Table 12-3).

▶ Several DHHS programs include a childcare component: the Title V Maternal and Child Health Program; Medicaid and the Early and Periodic Screening, Diagnosis, and Treatment (EPSDT) program; Head Start and Early Head Start programs; and the primary-care programs of community-based health centers.

Impact of Child Nutrition Programs on Children's Diets

▶ To recognize schools that are actively engaged in fostering healthy school environments, the USDA is implementing the HealthierUS School Challenge, a voluntary program that provides monetary incentives and certifications to schools that are promoting healthy food and physical activity.

▶ Improving child nutrition is the focal point of the Healthy, Hunger-Free Kids Act of 2010, which authorizes funding and allows the USDA to reform the nutrition standards of the school lunch and breakfast programs in order to enhance the diet and health of school children and reduce childhood obesity.

▶ The new nutrition standards for meals served through the National School Lunch and School Breakfast Programs align school meals with the *Dietary Guidelines for Americans*. Schools must increase the availability of fruits, vegetables, whole grains, and fat-free and low-fat fluid milk in school meals; reduce the levels of sodium and saturated fat in meals; and help meet the nutritional needs of school children within their calorie requirements (see Tables 12-5 and 12-8).

▶ Factors that have been shown to influence children's weight status include consumption of sugar-sweetened beverages; consumption of low-nutrient, energy-dense foods; and presence or absence of fruits and vegetables.

▶ Many school districts have developed wellness policies that support a school environment that provides nutrition education, physical activity, and other school-based activities designed to promote student wellness.

Nutrition Education Programs

▶ Nutrition education strategies aimed at children or their caregivers are found in both the public and private sectors. Their goal is to improve eating patterns among children.

▶ Schools can play a key role in reversing the trend of obesity and lack of physical activity by offering comprehensive nutrition education programs. Successful programs include the Fresh Fruit and Vegetable Program, the Expanded Food and Nutrition Education Program, and Team Nutrition.

▶ Many other government and nonprofit organizations at the national, state, and local levels are implementing initiatives that aim to reduce overweight and increase physical activity among youth.

SUMMARY **QUESTIONS**

1. Discuss some of the influences on current food consumption patterns and behaviors of children and adolescents.
2. Discuss factors that increase the likelihood of obesity in children and adolescents.
3. Describe four of the common nutrition-related problems among U.S. children and adolescents and provide a rationale for why each of the problems is prevalent.
4. Describe the impact of the school food environment and practices on children's nutrition and health status.

5. Discuss four nutrition assistance programs aimed at improving the health and nutrition status of children, including:
   a. Purpose of the program
   b. Types of assistance offered to clients
   c. Eligibility requirements
   d. Improvements you would recommend to enhance the program

INTERNET **RESOURCES**

Government and University Websites

CDC Growth Charts
www.cdc.gov/growthcharts/

Administration for Children and Families
www.acf.hhs.gov

Let's Move!
www.letsmove.gov

Child Nutrition Education Resources
http://fnic.nal.usda.gov/professional-and-career-resources/nutrition-education/sources-nutrition-education-materials

Food and Nutrition Information Center/Lifecycle Nutrition
http://fnic.nal.usda.gov/lifecycle-nutrition

Food and Nutrition Assistance Programs
www.fns.usda.gov

Office of Head Start
www.acf.hhs.gov/programs/ohs/

Lead Program at CDC
www.cdc.gov/nceh/lead

National Center for Education in Maternal and Child Health
http://ncemch.org

National Clearinghouse on Families and Youth
http://ncfy.acf.hhs.gov

National Institute of Child Health and Human Development
www.nichd.nih.gov

President's Council on Fitness, Sports, and Nutrition
www.fitness.gov

School Nutrition Dietary Assessment Study II
www.fns.usda.gov/school-nutrition-dietary-assessment-study-ii

School Nutrition Program (Nutrient Analysis Protocols)
www.fns.usda.gov/tn/resources/nutrientanalysis.html

MyPlate for Preschoolers
www.choosemyplate.gov/preschoolers.html

MyPlate Information for Children
www.choosemyplate.gov/children

Team Nutrition's Local Wellness Policy Webpage
www.fns.usda.gov/tn/local-school-wellness-policy

Action for Healthy Kids (AFHK)
www.actionforhealthykids.org

U.S. Department of Housing and Urban Development Office of Healthy Homes and Lead Hazard Control
www.hud.gov/offices/lead

U.S. Government Health Information Site
http://healthfinder.gov

Websites Related to Disabilities

Nutrition Interventions for Children with Special Health Care Needs
http://here.doh.wa.gov/materials/nutrition-interventions

Cornucopia of Disability Information (CODI)
http://codi.tamucc.edu

National Council on Disability
www.ncd.gov

Other Websites

Academy for Eating Disorders
www.aedweb.org

American Academy of Pediatrics
www.aap.org

School Nutrition Association
https://schoolnutrition.org

Canadian Paediatric Society
www.cps.ca/en

Childhood Obesity Prevention Partnership
www.kidnetic.com

Farm to School Network
www.farmtoschool.org

Feeding America's Child Hunger Programs
http://feedingamerica.org

Food Research and Action Center
http://frac.org

International Life Sciences Institute's Take10!™ Program
http://take10.net

Fuel Up to Play 60
www.fueluptoplay60.com

Kids Eat Right
www.eatright.org/resources/for-kids

Kids Count
www.aecf.org/work/kids-count/

KidsHealth
http://kidshealth.org

Produce for Better Health Foundation
www.fruitsandveggiesmorematters.org

Children's Nutrition Research Center at Baylor College of Medicine
www.bcm.edu/cnrc

Best Bones Forever
www.bestbonesforever.org

Dairy Council of California
www.healthyeating.org

TeensHealth
http://kidshealth.org/teen

CHAPTER 13

Healthy Aging: Nutrition Assessment, Services, and Programs

LEARNING **OBJECTIVES**

After you have read and studied this chapter, you will be able to:

- Describe the demographic trends in aging in America and the potential impact on health care services.

- List national objectives for health promotion for adults.

- Identify factors influencing the nutrition status of older adults.

- List and define essential components of a nutrition assessment for older adults.

- Describe community nutrition programs that are intended to provide nutrition services to older adults.

This chapter addresses such issues as the influence of age on nutrient requirements, screening individuals for nutritional risk, collecting pertinent information for nutrition assessments, availability of food and nutrition programs in the community, and current information technologies, which have been designated by the Accreditation Council for Education in Nutrition and Dietetics (ACEND) as Foundation Knowledge and Learning Outcomes for dietetics education.

CHAPTER **OUTLINE**

Something to think about...

"How far you go in life depends on your being tender with the young, compassionate with the aged, sympathetic with the striving, and tolerant of the weak and the strong. Because someday in life you will have been all of these."

—*GEORGE WASHINGTON CARVER*
(1864–1943, American botanist)

For a complete list of references, please access the MindTap Reader within your MindTap course.

Introduction

Americans are living longer than ever before, and the *average* age at death (life expectancy) has changed dramatically. A child born in 2013 can expect to live 78.8 years, about 30 years longer than a child born in 1900. Among women, life expectancy from birth is 81.4 years for white females and 78.4 years for black females (**Figure 13-1**).[1] For men, life expectancy from birth is 76.7 years for white males and 72.3 years for black males. On the other hand, the *maximum* age at which people die—that is, the *maximum lifespan*—has changed less dramatically. It seems that the aging phenomenon cuts off life at a rather fixed point in time.

To what extent is aging inevitable? Apparently, aging is an inevitable, natural process programmed into our genes at conception. Nevertheless, we can adopt lifestyle habits—such as consuming a healthful diet, exercising, and paying attention to our work and recreational environments—that will slow the process within the natural limits set by heredity. Life expectancy has also risen as a result of better prenatal and postnatal care and improved means of combating disease in older adults. For example, the death rate from heart disease began to decline in the 1960s and continues to fall today. Over half of the drop is attributed to a decline in smoking and in the numbers of people with high blood pressure or high blood cholesterol. Clearly, good nutrition can retard and ease the aging process in many significant ways.

One approach to the prevention of aging has been to study other cultures in the hope of finding an extremely long-lived people and then learning their secrets of long life. Older adults in Okinawa, Japan, have among the lowest mortality rates in the world from a multitude of chronic diseases of aging. The Okinawa Centenarian Study seeks to uncover the genetic and lifestyle factors responsible for this successful aging phenomenon (see the "Eating Pattern for Longevity" box). The views of the experts can best be summed up by saying that disease can *shorten* people's lives and that poor nutrition practices make diseases more likely to occur, but poor health is not an inevitable consequence of aging. Thus, by postponing and slowing disease processes, optimal nutrition can help to prolong life up to the maximum lifespan—but cannot extend it further.[2] This chapter focuses on the diseases that seem to arise with age, their risk factors, and the nutrition assessment of older adults; it also examines the programs and services that target older adults for health

FIGURE 13-1 Life Expectancy in the United States, 1970–2013

Source: *National Vital Statistics Reports* 63, no. 7 (Hyattsville, MD: National Center for Health Statistics, 2014).

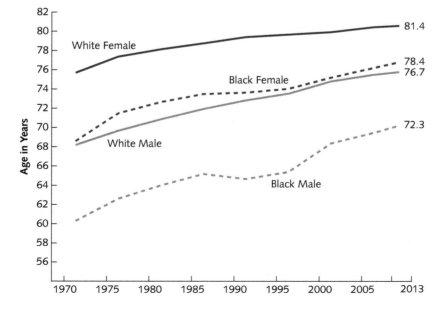

promotion and disease prevention. We begin with a look at the demographic trends characteristic of this segment of the population and the national nutrition and health goals for improving the quality of life of Americans as they age.

Eating Pattern for Longevity[3]

Do you need proof that good dietary choices can have a profound effect on health and longevity? Look no further than the Okinawans. These people dwell on a group of islands—known collectively as Okinawa—that lie southwest of mainland Japan. Okinawans enjoy one of the longest lifespans of anyone on earth, and they do so while maintaining a very high quality of life. This fact has sparked much interest in Okinawan culture and resulted in the 25-year Okinawa Centenarian Study that began in 1976 to investigate what makes these people so healthy.[4] Researchers studied more than 600 Okinawan centenarians and numerous others in their 70s, 80s, and 90s.

When the study began, researchers were surprised to find that many centenarians were still very active, free of health problems, and looked years younger than their chronological age. Upon further investigation, they also discovered that Okinawan elders have low levels of cancer-causing free radicals, low cardiovascular risks, extremely healthy bone densities, and a lower prevalence of dementia than those of the same age in other countries. Indeed, they have among the lowest mortality rates in the world from many chronic diseases, including cancer, stroke, osteoporosis, and heart disease. Although there is no magic bullet that results in the Okinawans' longevity and health, Okinawan centenarians have a number of variables in common.

Enough Is Enough. Okinawan elders have an average body mass index (BMI) that ranges from 18 to 22. The Okinawans stay lean by eating a low-calorie diet and practicing calorie control in a cultural habit known as *hara hachi bu* (only eating until they are 80% full) and keeping physically active every day. In contrast, middle-aged Okinawans,

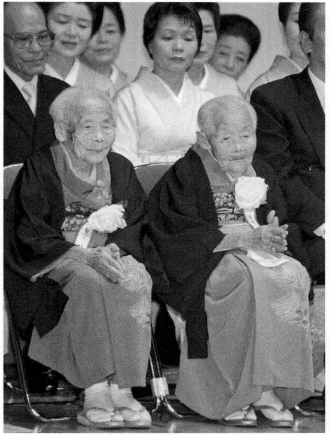

Okinawan twin sisters—Gin Kanie and Kin Narita at age 106— celebrate with family and friends. Okinawan centenarians maintain optimistic attitudes and strong social bonds throughout their lives.

Yoshida-Fujitotos/The Image Works

who have a less traditional lifestyle, have a BMI of 26, the highest in Japan and similar to Americans. A BMI of 25 and greater is considered overweight and places a person at greater risk for chronic diseases, especially heart disease and stroke.

Moderation and a Healthy Lifestyle Are Key Cultural Values. Okinawan elders never smoke. They consume a diet that is 80% plant-based and naturally high in unrefined whole grains, soy, vegetables, and fruits—all of which are rich in antioxidants and phytochemicals. They consume higher intakes of good fats from omega 3–rich fish and monounsaturated fats, and they have rather low amounts of saturated and *trans* fat in their diet. They keep active every day throughout their lives in a variety of activities such as gardening, traditional dance, and martial arts. In fact, many of those studied still participated in competitive games and karate past the age of 100!

Psychological and Spiritual Health Matters. Okinawans put family first. They keep socially engaged, maintaining strong bonds with friends and family. They have an easygoing approach to life. Centenarians score high on optimistic attitudes and adaptability. They possess a strong sense of purpose, which translates roughly to "that which makes one's life worth living."

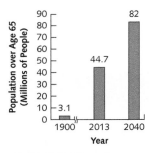

FIGURE 13-2 The Aging of the Population[a]

In 1900, 4% of the U.S. population (3.1 million people) were more than 65 years of age; in 2013, 14.1% (44.7 million people) were more than age 65; and by 2040, 21.7% (about 82 million people) will have reached age 65.

[a] Researchers and marketing analysts have struggled to find a useful way to segment—and, therefore, target—the older adult market. One frequently used segmentation divides older adults into the "mature," age 55–64; the "young-old," age 65–74; and the "old-old," over age 74.

Source: Data from *A Profile of Older Americans, 2014*; available at *www.aoa.gov*.

Demographic Trends and Aging

The number of older adults (aged 65 years and older) in the United States will nearly double by 2040 to more than 82.3 million people. In 2013, people aged 65 and over accounted for 14.1% of the population, but are expected to grow to be 21.7% of the population by 2040. The 85+ population is projected to grow from 6 million in 2013 to 14.6 million in 2040.[5] The increased growth in the older adult population in the United States is illustrated in **Figure 13-2**.

The baby boom that took place between 1946 and 1964 and improved life expectancy are important contributors to the growing older adult population in the United States. Baby boomers increased the numbers of the older middle-aged (ages 46–63) until 2011, when they began to swell the ranks of the retired population. The growth rate of the older population is expected to slow after 2030, when the last baby boomers turn 65 years old. By 2030, minority groups will represent 26.4% of the population of older adults (up from 17.2% in 2002), with the largest increases in Hispanics and Asians (**Figure 13-3**).

Policymakers and others concerned with meeting the health needs of older adults are alert to the implications of these demographic changes because older adults tend to consume a large amount of total health care and long-term care resources. Consider that persons aged 65 years and older represented just over 12% of the total population in 2008, yet they accounted for more than 30% of the country's health care costs—utilizing more hospital services and consuming more than 40% of all prescription drugs.[6] With the "graying of America," these health care demands can only increase. As Joseph A. Califano, a former secretary of health and human services, testified before the Committee on a National Research Agenda on Aging,

> The aging of America will challenge all our political, retirement, and social service systems. As never before, it will test our commitment to decent human values. Nowhere is the aging of America freighted with more risk and opportunity than in the area of health care.[7]

FIGURE 13-3

Population Age 65 and Over, by Race and Hispanic Origin, 2008 and Projected 2050

This graph shows the strong projected growth of the minority older population, which will reach 41% of the 65-and-over population in 2050. Black older adults are projected to grow to 12% in 2050, and Hispanic older adults are projected to grow to 20%.

Source: Federal Interagency Forum on Aging-Related Statistics, *Older Americans 2012: Key Indicators of Well-Being* (Washington, D.C.: U.S. Government Printing Office, 2012).

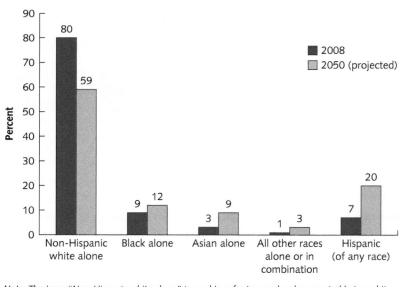

Note: The term "Non-Hispanic white alone" is used to refer to people who reported being white and no other race and who are not Hispanic. The term "Black alone" is used to refer to people who reported being black or African American and no other race, and the term "Asian alone" is used to refer to people who reported only Asian as their race. The race group "All other races alone or in combination" includes American Indian and Alaska Native alone; Native Hawaiian and other Pacific Islander alone; and all people who reported two or more races.

Healthy Adults

The most important goal of health promotion and disease prevention for adults as they age is maintaining health and functional independence. Many of the health problems associated with the later years are preventable or can be controlled. An individual's current health profile is substantially determined by behavioral risk factors. As shown in **Table 13-1**, the leading causes of death for adults of various ages include heart disease, cancer, chronic lung disease, stroke, diabetes, injuries, and liver disease; all have been associated with behavioral risk factors. Thus, many adults today would benefit from changes in their lifestyle behaviors. For example, changing certain risk behaviors into healthful ones can improve the quality of life for older persons and lessen their risk of disability. Improvements in diet and nutrition status and weight management can enhance the health of older adults and help control risk factors for disease in middle-aged and younger adults.

For the past four decades, health professionals have provided the public with health-related messages to lower risk of chronic diseases such as cardiovascular disease, cancer, diabetes, osteoporosis, and obesity.[8] These messages have encouraged such things as avoidance or cessation of cigarette smoking; maintenance of a healthy body weight; reduced intake of saturated fats, *trans* fat, and sodium; regular physical activity; regular health screenings for blood pressure and cholesterol; cancer-related screenings; and consumption of a diet rich in whole grains, fruits, vegetables, and fiber.

National Goals for Health Promotion

Primary *Healthy People 2020* topic areas for adults include reducing the prevalence of and the overall number of people who suffer from diseases such as arthritis, osteoporosis, cancer, heart disease, diabetes, and kidney disease. Other age-specific goals include increasing the number of older persons receiving pneumonia and influenza vaccinations and colorectal cancer screenings, along with increasing daily physical activity and cardiovascular health.[9] **Table 13-2** lists selected *Healthy People 2020* objectives for adults and older adults and includes the data achieved during the *Healthy People 2010* initiative.

TABLE 13-1 The Leading Causes and Numbers of Deaths among Adults, Aged 25–44, 45–64, and 65+; All Races, Both Sexes, 2012

	AGE GROUPS		
RANK	**25–44**	**45–64**	**65+**
1.	Unintentional injury: 28,149	Cancer: 159,379	Heart disease: 477,840
2.	Cancer: 15,389	Heart disease: 103,812	Cancer: 403,497
3.	Heart disease: 13,447	Unintentional injury: 32,667	Chronic low respiratory disease: 122,375
4.	Suicide: 12,119	Chronic low respiratory disease: 18,616	Cerebrovascular: 109,127
5.	Homicide: 6,674	Liver disease: 18,348	Alzheimer's disease: 82,690
6.	Liver disease: 2,900	Diabetes mellitus: 17,224	Diabetes mellitus: 52,881
7.	HIV: 2,638	Cerebrovascular: 16,565	Unintentional injury: 44,698
8.	Cerebrovascular: 2,396	Suicide: 14,912	Influenza and pneumonia: 43,355
9.	Diabetes mellitus: 2,365	Nephritis: 7,306	Nephritis: 37,740
10.	Influenza and pneumonia: 1,146	Septicemia: 6,957	Septicemia: 27,022

Sources: Office of Statistics and Programming, National Center for Injury Prevention and Control, CDC; *National Center for Health Statistics (NCHS) Vital Statistics Report* 64 (August 2015).

TABLE 13-2 *Healthy People 2020* Selected Topic Areas and Objectives Relevant to Adults and Older Adults with Final Data from *Healthy People 2010*

TOPIC AREA	OBJECTIVE NUMBER AND OBJECTIVE	BASELINE (YEAR)[a]	PROGRESS (YEAR)	*HEALTHY PEOPLE 2020* TARGET
Arthritis, Osteoporosis, and Chronic Back Conditions	**AOCBC-10:** Reduce the proportion of adults with osteoporosis.	5.9% of adults aged 50 years and older had osteoporosis (2005–2008)		5.3%[b]
Arthritis, Osteoporosis, and Chronic Back Conditions	**AOCBC-11:** Reduce hip fractures among females aged 65 and older.	824 hospitalizations for hip fractures per 100,000 females (2007)	778 (2010)	741 hospitalizations per 100,000 females[b]
Cancer	**C-16:** Increase the proportion of adults who receive a colorectal cancer screening.	52% of adults aged 50 to 75 years received a colorectal cancer screening (2008)	58.2% (2013)	70.5%
Heart Disease	**HDS-7:** Reduce the proportion of adults with high total blood cholesterol levels.	15.0% of adults had total blood cholesterol levels of 240 mg/dL or greater (2008)	12.9% (2009–2012)	13.5%[b]
Heart Disease	**HDS-8:** Reduce the mean total blood cholesterol levels among adults.	198 mg/dL was the mean total blood cholesterol level for adults (2008)		177.9 mg/dL (mean)[b]
Immunizations and Infectious Diseases	**IID-12.7:** Increase the percentage of adults aged 65 and older who are vaccinated annually against seasonal influenza.	67% (2008)		90%[c]
Nutrition and Weight Status	**NWS-6.1:** Increase the proportion of physician office visits made by patients with a diagnosis of heart disease, diabetes, or hyperlipidemia that include counseling or education related to diet and nutrition.	20.8% (2007)	19.1% (2010)	22.9%[b]
Nutrition and Weight Status	**NWS-7:** (Developmental) Increase the proportion of worksites that offer nutrition or weight-management classes or counseling.	TBD		TBD
Nutrition and Weight Status	**NWS-8:** Increase the proportion of adults who are at a healthy weight.	30.8% of persons 20 years and older (2005–2008)	29.5% (2009–2012)	33.9%[b]
Nutrition and Weight Status	**NWS-4:** Increase the proportion of Americans who have access to a food retail outlet that sells a variety of foods that are encouraged by the *Dietary Guidelines for Americans*.	TBD		TBD
Nutrition and Weight Status	**NWS-13:** Reduce household food insecurity and in so doing reduce hunger.	14.6% of households were food-insecure (2008)	14.5% (2012)	6%[c]

TABLE 13-2 *Healthy People 2020* Selected Topic Areas and Objectives Relevant to Adults and Older Adults with Final Data from *Healthy People 2010—continued*

TOPIC AREA	OBJECTIVE NUMBER AND OBJECTIVE	BASELINE (YEAR)[a]	PROGRESS (YEAR)	*HEALTHY PEOPLE 2020* TARGET
Older Adults	**OA-11:** Reduce the rate of emergency department (ED) visits due to falls among older adults.	5,235 ED visits per 100,000 (2007)	6,894 ED visits (2011)	4,712 ED visits per 100,000[b]
Older Adults	**OA-7.6:** Increase the proportion of registered dietitians with geriatric certification.	0.30% of registered dietitians had geriatric certification (2009)	0.56% (2012)	0.33%[b]
Physical Activity	**PA-1:** Reduce the proportion of adults who engage in no leisure-time physical activity.	36.2% of adults engaged in no leisure-time physical activity (2008)	29.6% (2012)	32.6%[b]
Physical Activity	**PA-2.4:** Increase the proportion of adults who meet the objectives for aerobic physical activity and for muscle-strengthening activity.	18.2% of adults (2008)	20.8% (2014)	20.1%

[a] Baseline data derived from *Healthy People 2010 Final Review*; sources of data include: National Health and Nutrition Examination Survey, National Ambulatory Medical Care Survey, follow-up survey to the 2004 National Worksite Health Promotion Survey, National Hospital Discharge Survey, Commission on Dietetic Registration, National Health Interview Survey; TBD, Developmental objective; data to be determined.

[b] Target setting method: 10% improvement.

[c] Retention of *Healthy People 2010* target.

Source: Adapted from U.S. Department of Health and Human Services, *Healthy People 2020* at *http://healthypeople.gov/2020*. See Table 7-6 in Chapter 7 for the current status of the U.S. adult population on various "healthy lifestyle" habits. *Healthy People 2020* presents the key national health objectives for the year 2020, which focus on improving the health of adults as they age. See also *www.healthypeople.gov*.

Overall, a review of data on the *Healthy People 2020* objectives for the weight status of adults reflect a trend for the worse.[10] The proportion of adults aged 20 years and older who are at a healthy weight—that is, who have a body mass index (BMI) in the range of 18.5 to 24.9—decreased from 42% in 1988–1994 to 29.5% in 2012. The age-adjusted proportion of adults aged 20 years and older who are obese (with a BMI of 30 or more) increased from 23% in the survey period 1988–1994 to 35% in 2009–2012.

As illustrated in **Figure 13-4**, the four objectives for fruit, vegetable, grain, and sodium consumption show little or no progress. Eating fruits and vegetables adds key nutrients to our diets; reduces the risk for chronic diseases such as heart disease, stroke, and certain cancers; and can help manage body weight when consumed in place of more energy-dense foods.[11] Adults are advised to consume 1.5–2.0 cup equivalents of fruit and 2.5–3 cups of vegetables daily. However, during 2007–2010, half of the total U.S. population consumed < 1 cup of fruit and < 1.5 cups of vegetables daily; 76% did not meet fruit intake recommendations, and 87% did not meet vegetable intake recommendations. Figure 13-4 shows the average daily intakes of fruits and vegetables by adults.[12] In 2013, only 13.1% of respondents to the Behavioral Risk Factor Surveillance System (BRFSS) met fruit intake recommendations, ranging from 7.5% in Tennessee to 17.7% in California, and 8.9% met vegetable recommendations, ranging from 5.5% in Mississippi to 13.0% in California.[13] Since the variations may be due to factors such as differences in population demographics and access, and availability and affordability of produce, the Centers for Disease Control and Prevention urges new public health efforts to increase consumer intakes of fruits and vegetables through competitive pricing, placement, and promotion in childcare, schools, grocery stores, communities, and worksites.[14]

FIGURE 13-4 *Healthy People* Review: Fruits, Vegetables, Whole Grains, and Sodium

[a] 2,300 mg/day is the Tolerable Upper Intake Level (UL) for sodium intake in adults; UL for children are listed on the inside front cover of this book. The average intake for men is 4,240 mg/day, and for adult women, the average is 2,980 mg/day.

[b] 1,500 mg/day is the Adequate Intake (AI) for individuals ages nine years and older.

Source: *Healthy People 2010 Final Review: Nutrition and Overweight,* December 2010; L. V. Moore and F. E. Thompson, Adults Meeting Fruit and Vegetable Intake Recommendations, United States, 2013, *Morbidity and Mortality Weekly Report* 64 (2015): 709-13; *2015–2020 Dietary Guidelines for Americans,* 8th ed. (Washington, D.C.: U.S. Government Printing Office, 2015).

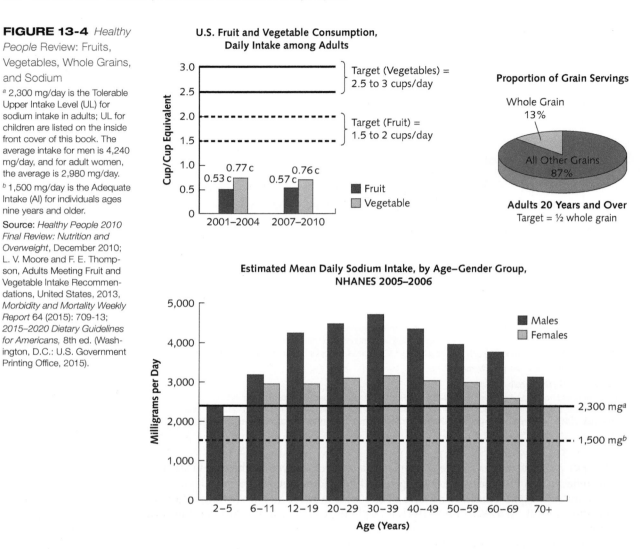

The proportion of all grain products consumed that were whole grain was 13% for adults. The target is that one-half be whole grain. Sodium intakes were significantly higher than the target amount of 2,300 milligrams per day (see Figure 13-4).

There has also been little or no change since the past decade in the status of most objectives for physical activity and fitness. Since the *Healthy People 2010* initiative, modest improvements are noted: (1) A slightly smaller proportion of the adult population (aged 18 years and older) reported pursuing no leisure-time physical activity, and (2) a larger proportion of adults perform physical activities that enhance muscular strength. In 2008, 36% of adults engaged in no leisure-time physical activity, compared with 40% in 1997. The 2010 target for all population groups was 20%. Among five racial and ethnic groups, Hispanics had the highest rate of being sedentary during leisure time; whites had the lowest. **Figure 13-5** shows that as age increased, the percentage of adults who met the 2008 federal physical activity guidelines for aerobic activity decreased. The annual percentage of adults aged 18 and over who met the 2008 federal physical activity guidelines for both aerobic and muscle-strengthening activities increased from 16.0% in 2006 to 20.8% in 2014.[15]

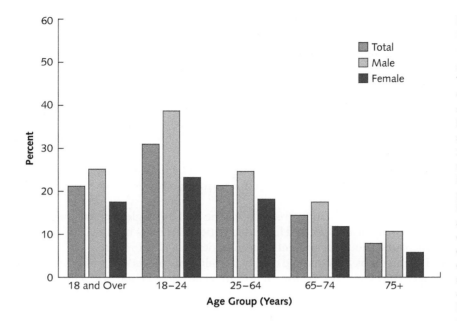

FIGURE 13-5 Adults Engaging in Adequate Physical Activity by Age and Gender, 2014

The 2008 Physical Activity Guidelines for Americans state that for substantial health benefits, adults should engage in at least 2½ hours per week of moderate intensity (e.g., brisk walking) or 1¼ hours per week of vigorous-intensity aerobic physical activity (e.g., jogging or kick-boxing), or an equivalent combination of both, plus muscle-strengthening activities on at least two days per week. For both sexes combined, as age increased, the percentage of adults who met the 2008 federal physical activity guidelines for aerobic activity (based on leisure-time activity) decreased. The percentage of adults who met the 2008 federal physical activity guidelines for both aerobic and muscle-strengthening activities increased from 16.0% in 2006 to 20.8% in 2014.

Source: Data from the 2014 National Health Interview Survey, National Center for Health Statistics, June 2015. Available at *http://www.cdc.gov/nchs/nhis.htm.*

Health professionals from a number of government agencies and organizations suggest steps listed below for achieving the *Healthy People 2020* objectives that promote healthy weights and food choices.[16]

- Improve communications with the public to convey the message that there are recommended actions that can be effective in weight management (see Chapter 8).
- Educate the public about the health benefits of being physically active at any size and the possible added benefit of thereby attaining modest weight reduction. For example, the Go4Life physical activity campaign from the National Institute on Aging is designed to help adults fit physical activity into their daily life.
- Promote partnerships with community planners to design neighborhoods that encourage and support increased opportunities for physical activity in appropriate and safe locations.
- Educate the public on how to use the Nutrition Facts Panel on food products and on how to select appropriate portion sizes for healthful diets.
- Explore the use of tax incentives for worksites to provide safe, convenient, and affordable venues for employees to engage in physical activity.
- Also recommended as effective were "point-of-decision" prompts, such as motivational signs that encourage people to use the stairs instead of elevators.
- Educate older adults on nutrition and food safety to promote health, reduce risk, and manage diseases in order to improve and maintain health, independence, and quality of life.[17]
- Use adequately funded federal food and nutrition assistance programs to promote successful aging and increase access to and availability of fruits, vegetables, and whole grains to older adults.[18]

Understanding Baby Boomers

Baby boomers, or the approximately 76 million individuals who were born between 1946 and 1964, represent almost one-fourth of the U.S. population. By virtue of their large numbers, baby boomers are a driving force for current and future trends. An understanding of their preferences, character, lifestyle, and location is and will continue to be critical to health promotion programs and services. In 1991 the first of this generation turned 45, and in 2030 the last of the baby boomers will turn 65.

Although there are several subsets of baby boomers, some general characteristics can be noted:[19]

- Boomers have the power to change the marketplace. Because of their numbers and affluence, they are able to drive trends, especially as they age. Of importance to community nutritionists, these consumers are generally concerned about what is healthful and convenient.
- Boomers make decisions based on personal beliefs and want to be empowered. They prefer health programs that offer information and options in a learner-involved format, such as a supermarket tour.
- Boomers are constantly pressed for time as they juggle careers, childcare, elder care, home responsibilities, and leisure activities. Programs need to be practical and convenient and should be presented in an understandable format.
- Boomers look for value and quality in their investments and are becoming thriftier with age. They seek information on how to relate market choices to value.
- Boomers will not age gracefully. Programs must be upbeat and dynamic for these on-the-go consumers. Community nutritionists can ease baby boomers' transition into retirement by providing accurate and practical nutrition information in settings such as supermarkets, health fairs, farmers' markets, and community centers.
- Boomers like nostalgia. Nostalgia can be used to reinforce nutrition messages—for example, modifying traditional family recipes and holiday menus to reflect current nutritional advice.

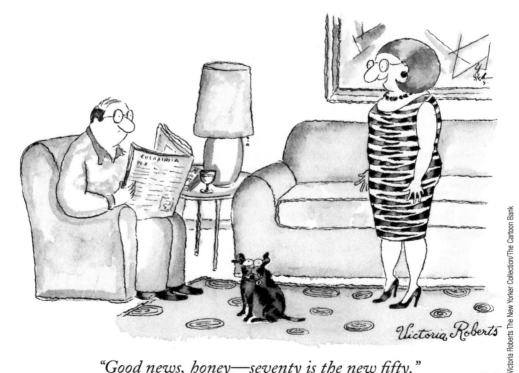

"Good news, honey—seventy is the new fifty."

Victoria Roberts The New Yorker Collection/The Cartoon Bank

Nutrition Education Programs

Nutrition education strategies aimed at adults are found in both the public and private sectors. They strive to increase knowledge and skills about nutrition and physical activity to improve eating and physical activity patterns among adults of all ages. Chapter 16 offers strategies for designing nutrition education programs for adult learners.

Nutrition education for health promotion is generally based on the *Dietary Guidelines for Americans* and other food guidance systems. The nutritional goals of these educational tools are to help consumers select diets that provide an appropriate amount of energy to maintain a healthy weight; meet the recommended intakes for all nutrients; are low in solid fat and *trans* fat, added sugars, sodium, and alcohol; and are adequate in whole grains and fiber. In *What's on Your Plate?: Smart Food Choices for Healthy Aging*, the National Institute on Aging introduces consumers to the basic facts for making healthy food choices and for adjusting those choices as they grow older. *What's on Your Plate?* is based on the nutrition recommendations for adults in the *Dietary Guidelines for Americans*.[20] At *ChooseMyPlate.gov*, individuals can create customized eating patterns for consuming age- and gender-appropriate daily portions and calorie levels. The USDA *SuperTracker* tool provides users with free diet and physical activity planning and assessment tools.

Public nutrition education programs include the Expanded Food and Nutrition Education Program, described in Chapter 11, and the Food and Drug Administration (FDA) and U.S. Department of Agriculture (USDA) public education campaigns on topics such as food labels and food safety in cooperation with other federal, state, and local agencies. The Family Nutrition Program (FNP) is part of a national nutrition education effort (SNAP-Ed) funded through the U.S. Department of Agriculture's Supplemental Nutrition Assistance Program (SNAP). FNP provides nutrition education programs and activities that help limited-resource families eligible for SNAP to establish healthy eating habits and physically active lifestyles.[21]

A primary challenge facing nutrition educators is to improve strategies to reduce the major risk factors for coronary heart disease and cancer, the leading causes of death among adults. The National Heart, Lung, and Blood Institute (NHLBI) conducts educational activities, including the development of the Dietary Approaches to Stop Hypertension (DASH) diet. DASH emphasizes that a healthy eating plan can reduce the risk for developing high blood pressure and can lower elevated blood pressure. The Centers for Disease Control and Prevention and its partners designed the Fruits & Veggies—More Matters program to increase per capita fruit and vegetable consumption. The program promotes a simple nutrition message that physicians, nurses, community nutritionists, and other health care professionals can reinforce to their clients: *Eat more servings of fruits and vegetables every day for better health.*[22]

A number of trade and professional organizations are likewise directing some of their nutrition education strategies to help adults understand the role of nutrition and physical activity in health promotion and disease prevention. The Academy of Nutrition and Dietetics, the American Association for Retired Persons, the National Dairy Council, and the Produce Marketing Association, among others, offer brochures, booklets, newsletters, videos, and interactive websites that offer simple ways to reduce dietary intake of solid fats, added sugars, refined grains, and sodium; interpret nutrition labels; implement the *Dietary Guidelines for Americans*; or improve shopping skills. For example, the International Food Information Council's *Weight Loss: Finding a Weight Loss Program that Works for You* is a booklet that helps consumers choose safe and effective weight-loss methods. Likewise, their *Foods for Health: Living Well, Living Longer* video provides food safety, nutrition, and healthful eating and physical activity tips to help adults make healthy food choices, prepare foods safely, and maintain a healthy weight.[23]

There are also numerous free and commercial apps with nutrition and health-related information available for iPhone, iPod Touch, Android, and other handheld smart devices. An example is Calorie Counter, a free downloadable nutrition app that tracks food, exercise, weight, and all the nutrients listed on a Nutrition Facts label.[24] Go to *www.eatright.org* for reviews regarding which apps are helpful and based on fact, not fad. The Food4Bones app by the National Osteoporosis Foundation is designed to help individuals understand and manage their nutritional requirements, especially related to bone health or other dietary concerns.

In many communities, food retailers and foodservice establishments provide point-of-purchase information and literature to their customers. Other communities offer grocery store tours to help consumers understand food labels and healthy food choices.

Health Promotion Programs

Evidence continues to indicate that adults of all ages need to modify their current eating patterns and other behaviors to reduce the risk of chronic diseases. However, changes in behavior can be very difficult to make. Chapter 3 discussed evidence-based theories and models of behavior change and strategies for incorporating these theories in community nutrition interventions. An important characteristic of community nutrition interventions is that they can reach people in many different contexts of their daily lives. Supportive social environments can help individuals change their behavior.[25] For this reason, community- and employer-based programs for health promotion are expanding and are facilitating lifestyle changes. For example, many employers now provide worksite health promotion programs offering classes and activities for smoking cessation, weight management, and stress reduction. These programs vary widely—some are simple and inexpensive (distribution of online newsletters or health information brochures), whereas others are more complex (comprehensive risk factor screening and intensive follow-up counseling). In general, worksite health promotion efforts can be classified under four main areas:[26]

- *Policies.* Smoking and alcohol and other drugs.
- *Screenings.* Health risk/health status, cancer, high blood pressure, glucose, and cholesterol.
- *Information or activities.* Individual counseling, group classes, workshops, lectures, special events, and resource materials such as posters, brochures, pamphlets, videos, podcasts, pedometers, and interactive online tools. Topics typically covered include cancer, high blood pressure, cholesterol, smoking, physical activity and fitness, nutrition, weight management, and stress reduction.
- *Facilities or services.* Nutrition, physical fitness, alcohol and other drugs, and stress reduction.

Two new *Healthy People 2020* objectives address the need for community-based programs designed to prevent disease and injury, improve health, and enhance quality of life: (1) Increase the proportion of worksites that offer an employee health promotion program to their employees, and (2) increase the proportion of employees who participate in employer-sponsored health promotion activities.[27] The Centers for Disease Control and Prevention's Healthier Worksite Initiative (HWI) has worked on a number of demonstration projects, policies, and environmental changes that affect the

> ## Worksite Health Promotion Programs

As the evidence mounts that worksite health promotion (WHP) cuts costs and produces a healthier workforce, more employers are giving WHP programs greater attention. Much of this newfound respect is probably due to the impressive savings reported by 12 companies in *Fortune* magazine. Here are some of the highlights:

- *Aetna:* Five state-of-the-art centers kept exercisers' health care costs nearly $300 lower than those of nonexercisers.
- *L.L. Bean:* Thanks to a healthy workforce, annual insurance premiums were half the national average.
- *Dow Corporation:* On-the-job injury strains dropped 90%.
- *Johnson & Johnson:* Health screening saved $13 million a year in absenteeism and health care costs.
- *Quaker Oats:* Because of an integrated health management approach, health insurance premiums were nearly a third less than the national average.
- *Steelcase:* Personal health counselors motivated high-risk employees to reduce major risk factors, generating an estimated $20 million in savings over 10 years.
- *Union Pacific:* Reduced hypertension and smoking saves more than $3 million a year.

Source: Adapted from D. H. Chenoweth, *Worksite Health Promotion*, 3rd ed. (Champaign, IL: Human Kinetics, 2011), 10–11. © D. H. Chenoweth.

---

entire CDC workforce. HWI has worked on improving the stairs and the cafeteria at headquarters, developed a walking trail, conducted walkability audits at almost every CDC campus, and implemented a discount fitness center membership program for employees.[28] The CDC's LEAN *Works!*—Leading Employees to Activity and Nutrition— is a free web-based resource that offers interactive tools and resources to help program planners design effective worksite obesity prevention and control programs. The Kaiser Permanente HealthWorks Program offers a comprehensive health promotion program to employers.[29] Successful nutrition promotion programs range from introducing heart-healthy menus into company cafeterias to reducing blood cholesterol levels through screening and intervention. The nutrition theme can be carried through group weight-loss and fitness classes, online videos and webinars, cooking demonstrations and taste tests, lunch-and-learn programs, individualized health coaching sessions, and nutrition counseling.

While individuals need to be held accountable for the lifestyle choices they make, employers can promote wellness and provide employees with incentives, knowledge, and opportunities that promote individual behavior change. One innovative approach to preventing obesity is the Texas Farm to Work Initiative, a program established through a partnership between the Sustainable Food Center (an Austin-based nonprofit organization) and the Texas Department of State Health Services (see the discussion that follows).[30]

Current efforts to help younger adults identify their familial risk factors for chronic disease conditions and programs that tout the benefits of lifelong healthful eating and regular physical activity should enable the older adults of tomorrow to enjoy *successful aging*[31]—a healthy, productive, and satisfying life well into advanced age.

PROGRAMS IN **ACTION**

The Farm to Work Initiative: An Innovative Approach to Obesity Prevention

According to the Centers for Disease Control and Prevention (CDC), 35.7% of adults (aged 20 years and older) were obese in 2009–2010, compared with 22.9% in 1988–1994.[1] The estimated prevalence of obesity was higher in the South and Midwest and lower in the Northeast and West. According to CDC data, in 2010, none of the 50 states nor the District of Columbia had achieved the *Healthy People 2010* target for obesity prevalence among adults.[2]

In their new book, *The Fattening of America: How the Economy Makes Us Fat, If It Matters, and What to Do About It*, health economist Eric Finkelstein, PhD, MHA, and coauthor Laurie Zuckerman argue that the economy is the main driver of behaviors that lead to high rates of overweight and obesity. These authors conclude that successful obesity prevention strategies need to make it cheaper and easier to maintain a healthful weight.[3,4] Such strategies need to address identified barriers to solving the problem of adult obesity, including a lack of funding for health promotion and disease prevention; environmental factors (such as limited sidewalks and green space, urban sprawl, and reliance on cars); workplace settings not conducive to healthful eating and physical activity; lack of political leadership; and limited access to nutritious foods (e.g., fruits and vegetables) due to high prices or limited availability.[5] Approaches to encourage more healthful eating were highlighted in a meeting of representatives from 25 community programs that was held at the CDC in July 2008. Examples of strategies included increasing access to healthful foods through community gardens, farmers' markets, and local grocery stores.[6]

According to Susan Combs, Texas comptroller of public accounts, "The phrase, 'Everything is bigger in Texas,' rings true when we consider the current state of Texans' health."[7] Nearly two-thirds (65.8%) of the state's population is overweight or obese.[8] Being overweight or obese increases one's risk of developing chronic illnesses or comorbidities, such as coronary heart disease, hypertension, stroke, congestive heart failure, high cholesterol, and diabetes.[9] These diseases cost employers—either directly in higher health care costs, or indirectly through lost productivity when employees are sick, disabled, or not functioning up to the standard.[10]

Projecting the costs of obesity to 2025, it is estimated that obesity and obesity-related illnesses could cost Texas businesses $15.8 billion per year.[11] In a separate report, it was estimated that if Texas were to invest $10 per person per year in proven community-based programs that improve nutrition, increase physical activity, and prevent smoking and tobacco use, Texas could save $1 billion annually within five years through reductions in health care spending. This is a return of $4.70 for every $1.00.[12] Combs believes that "we must become a society focused on preventing obesity, rather than treating the diseases it causes."[13]

The Farm to Work Program

The Farm to Work Initiative is a worksite wellness program that provides employees with the opportunity to purchase a basket of fresh local produce that is delivered to individual worksites every week. The program was created to change the worksite environment in order to make eating fruits and vegetables an easy choice for employees. The goals of the program are to (1) increase fruit and vegetable consumption to levels that increase health through worksite-based approaches, (2) provide a supportive work environment to promote employee wellness and health, and (3) improve quality of life among employees and their families through chronic disease prevention and improved health. The program's logic model is highlighted in **Figure 1**.[14]

In November 2007, the Farm to Work program began as a pilot project at two locations, the Texas Department of State Health Services (DSHS) main campus and Austin State Hospital. Since then, the program has grown substantially. The Farm to Work program has delivered approximately 85,000 pounds of local, farm-fresh produce to over 1,600 Austin-area employees at six worksites, and participating farmers have grossed nearly $140,000 in sales. The program also delivers to a handful of recreation centers and to the program offices of the Special Supplemental Nutrition Program for Women, Infants, and Children (WIC).[15] The program is a win–win situation for everyone involved: employees, worksites, and the local farmers participating in the program.[16] Currently, the Farm to Work program has more business than it can handle. The waiting list for the program included 17 businesses and city and state agencies.[17]

The local produce provided in the weekly baskets—which consists of 10 to 12 different fruits and vegetables—is comparatively priced, or in some cases a bit cheaper than grocery store prices. For example, one cost comparison found that items in the first weekly Farm to Work basket cost 13% less than the same items found in a local grocery store.[18] According to Andrew Smiley, Farm Direct projects director at the Sustainable Food Center, "I think one reason we have succeeded is that it's an easy and convenient choice, and people appreciate the simplicity of going online to order."[19] Unlike traditional farm subscription delivery services, Farm to Work requires no long-term commitment to participate. Instead, the program operates on a weekly cycle so participants can order produce baskets as frequently as they prefer. The program operates on a year-long basis with two possible exceptions depending on the weather—a three- to four-week break in August/September and another three- to four-week break in January/February.[20] Sonny Naegelin, owner of Naegelin Farm—a family farm that has been farming in Lytle, Texas, for five generations—supplies produce for the Farm to Work programs at the DSHS main campus, DSHS Austin State Hospital, Asuragen Inc. (a small private business), and the city of Austin. Kevin and Becky Ottmers, owners of Ottmers Family Farm, supply produce to Convio Inc. (an Austin technology company), and Gundermann Farm supplies produce for the DSHS Howard Lane worksite. While the produce is not certified as organic, participating

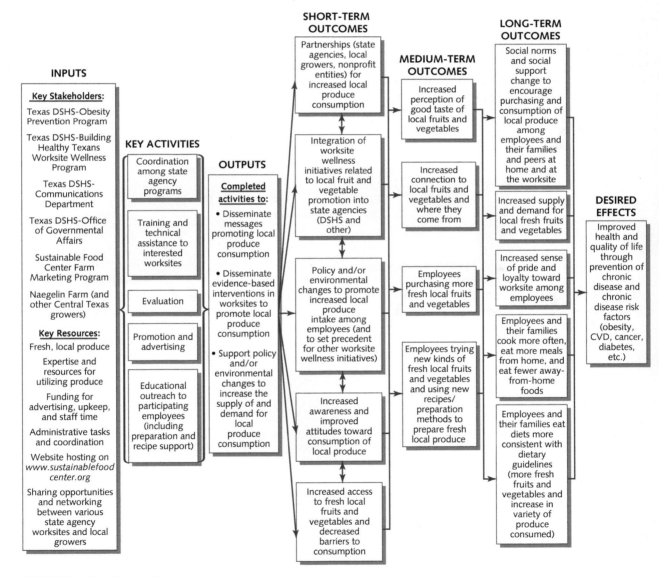

FIGURE 1 The Farm to Work Logic Model

farmers provide worksite employees with produce that is sustainably grown—that is, the farms use natural methods to build healthy soils and avoid use of synthetic pesticides and fertilizers.[21]

Each week, employees at participating worksites have the option to place an online order for a basket, which costs $25. **Figure 2** outlines the process by which employees receive their Farm to Work produce baskets each week. The Farm to Work ordering website, hosted at *www.sustainablefoodcenter.org*, lists available seasonal produce. Employees often welcome the surprises they receive, but there is a trade box available at the pick-up site where they can exchange produce with other employees. Recipes, food preparation tips, and storage information are available to help employees learn to use the produce they receive. Unclaimed produce is donated to a charitable organization. In the case of DSHS, unclaimed vegetables are brought to Austin State Hospital's Child and Adolescent Psychiatric Services, where an activity-therapy program helps patients learn cooking skills and participate in an event called Stir-Fry Thursdays. The children's enthusiasm for these vegetables has spawned a new project for the children—raised in-ground gardens on campus.

Where to Find More Information

Those interested in starting a similar worksite wellness program can find more information in the *Farm to Work Toolkit* and *Farm to Work Toolkit Supplement*. The *Farm to Work Toolkit* includes a summary of key program components, tips for obtaining legal clearance and other legal concerns, a worksite feasibility checklist, a timeline for implementation, information on produce distribution and staffing produce distribution, evaluation tools (including a farmer survey and online pre/post employee surveys), and website content. The *Farm to Work Toolkit Supplement* includes sample memos, internal communications, and marketing artwork used to implement the program. Both resources are available online at *www.dshs.state.tx.us/CWWObesityF2W*.

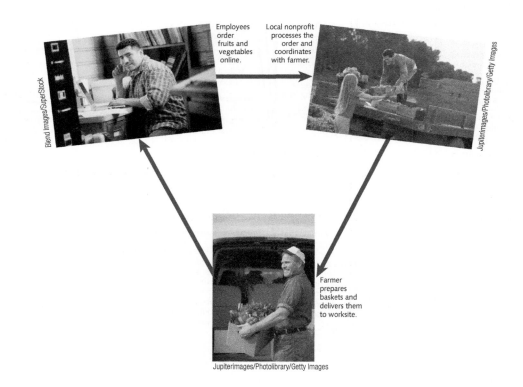

FIGURE 2   How the Farm to Work Program Operates Each Week

Source: C. McCullum-Gómez, PhD, RD, LD, food and nutrition consultant, and Lindsay Rodgers, MA, RD, LD, obesity prevention specialist, Nutrition, Physical Activity, and Obesity Prevention Program, Texas Department of State Health Services, "The Farm to Work Initiative: An Innovative Approach to Obesity Prevention," *Hunger and Environmental Nutrition Dietetic Practice Group Newsletter* (Fall 2008).

Aging and Nutrition Status

Although older adults in our society do experience chronic illness and associated disabilities, this population is very heterogeneous: Older people vary greatly in their social, economic, and lifestyle situations; functional capacity; and physical condition. Each person ages at a different rate, sometimes making chronological age different from biological age. Most older persons live at home, are fully independent, and have lives of good quality. Only 3.4% of the 65+ population live in nursing homes. However, the percentage increases with age, ranging from about 1% for persons 65–74 years to 3% for persons 75–84 years and 10% for persons 85 and older.[32]

Primary Nutrition-Related Problems of Aging

Although aging is not completely understood, we know that it involves progressive changes in every body tissue and organ: the brain, heart, lungs, digestive tract, and bones (**Table 13-3**). After age 35, functional capacity declines in almost every organ system. Such changes affect nutrition status. Some, including oral problems, interfere with nutrient intake; others affect absorption, storage, and utilization of nutrients; and still others increase the excretion of, and need for, specific nutrients. Examples of various conditions associated with aging that can affect nutrition status include sensory impairments; altered endocrine, gastrointestinal, and cardiovascular functions; and changes in the renal and musculoskeletal systems. Both genetic and environmental factors contribute to these declines. Many of the changes are inevitable, but a healthful lifestyle that combines physical activity with optimal intakes of all essential nutrients can forestall degeneration and improve quality of life into the later years.

TABLE 13-3 The Effects of Aging on Biological Function

ORGAN SYSTEM	AGING EFFECT
Skin	Dryness, wrinkling, mottled pigmentation, loss of elasticity, dilation of capillaries
Head and neck	Macular degeneration, hearing loss
Cardiovascular	Thickening heart wall and valves, decreased cardiac output, increased collagen rigidity, decreased elasticity of blood vessels with calcification
Pulmonary	Stiffening of tissue, decreased vital capacity, decreased maximum oxygen consumption, decreased breathing capacity
Renal	Decreased size, decreased GFR,[a] decreased renal blood flow, decreased renal concentrating ability
Endocrine	Altered circulating hormone levels and actions
Gastrointestinal (GI) tract	Altered perception of taste and smell, altered GI motility, decreased muscle strength, decreased digestive secretions, decreased absorption (calcium, iron, vitamin B_{12}, vitamin D)
Nervous	Decreased sensory perception, decreased muscle response to stimuli, decreased cognition and memory, loss of brain cells
Musculoskeletal	Progressive loss of skeletal muscle, degeneration of joints, decalcification of bone

[a] GFR, Glomerular filtration rate.

Source: Adapted from G. L. Jensen, M. McGee, and J. Binkley, "Nutrition in the Elderly," *Gastroenterology Clinics of North America* 30 (2001): 314; American Dietetic Association, *Nutrition Care of the Older Adult*, 2nd ed. (Chicago: American Dietetic Association, 2004), 65.

Older adults face the challenge of choosing a nutrient-dense diet. Although caloric needs may decrease with age, the need for certain nutrients such as calcium, vitamin D, and vitamin B_{12} may actually increase with the effects of aging.[33] For example, as many as 30% of persons older than 50 years may experience reduced stomach acidity, which can interfere with their ability to absorb vitamin B_{12}, calcium, and iron effectively from foods. In addition, there may be increased needs for vitamin D in older adults who have low intakes of fortified dairy products and have less ability to make the vitamin when their skin is exposed to sunlight. General nutrition guidelines for older adults are given in **Figure 13-6**.

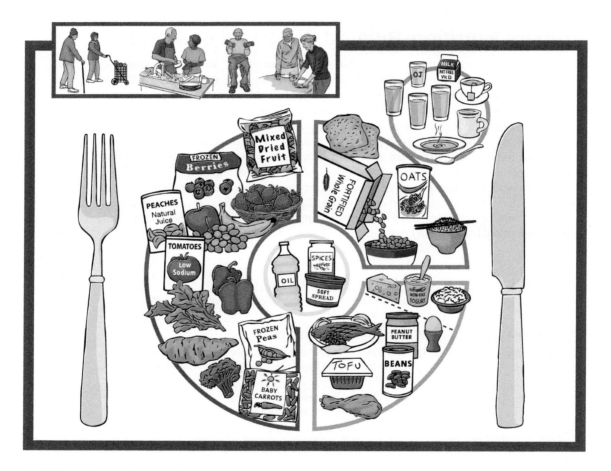

FIGURE 13-6 MyPlate for Older Adults

This food guide highlights the nutritional and physical activity requirements for older adults. Half of the plate has icons for a variety of fruits and vegetables in a range of colors that include representations of frozen, pre-peeled fresh, dried, and low-sodium, low-sugar canned options as they are affordable and convenient. The other half provides examples of whole, enriched, and fortified grains that are good sources of fiber and lean protein sources such as beans, tofu, fish, lean meat, and low-fat and fat-free dairy products. Water, tea, coffee, and soup are represented to emphasize the importance of adequate fluid intake because decline in thirst is a common issue with the older population. MyPlate for Older Adults has icons showing common daily activities such as running errands and housework as a reminder that there are a variety of options available for regular physical activity. Because overall calorie requirements decline with age due to a slowing of metabolism and physical activity, it is important to consume a variety of foods that are good sources of vitamins and minerals but low in *trans* and saturated fats and added sugars to meet nutritional and calorie needs.

Source: 2011© Tufts University.

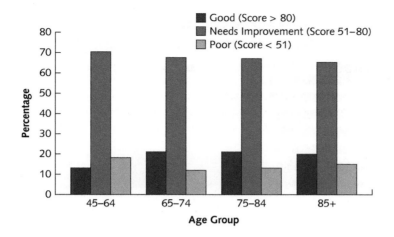
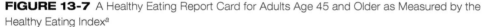

FIGURE 13-7 A Healthy Eating Report Card for Adults Age 45 and Older as Measured by the Healthy Eating Index[a]

The diet quality standards were met or exceeded by all age groups for total grains and protein foods. Average intakes of saturated fat, sodium, and calories from solid fats, alcoholic beverages, and added sugars were too high and failed to meet the recommended standards. To improve their diet quality, adults need to increase their intakes of whole grains, dark green and orange vegetables, legumes, and nonfat or low-fat dairy foods; choose more nutrient-dense forms of foods, that is, foods low in solid fats and free of added sugars; and lower their intake of sodium and saturated fat. These changes, if made, would provide substantial health benefits.

[a] The Healthy Eating Index gives a summary measure of people's overall diet quality and physical activity status. The interactive tool measures the degree to which a person's diet conforms to the serving recommendations from the USDA food guide's five major food groups: Grains, Vegetables, Fruits, Dairy, and Protein Foods. A high score for these components is reached by maximizing consumption of recommended amounts. The tool also measures compliance of intakes of sodium, saturated fat, and calories from solid fats and added sugars according to the *Dietary Guidelines for Americans*. A high score is reached by consuming at or below recommended amounts.

Source: Center for Nutrition Policy and Promotion, U.S. Department of Agriculture, *Nutrition Insights*.

Assessing the diet quality of older adults is important for identifying issues relevant to their health and nutrition status. According to the Healthy Eating Index, a composite measure of overall dietary quality based on the *Dietary Guidelines for Americans*, the majority of the population age 45+ does not consume a "good" diet.[34] Only 13% of the population age 45–64 years consumes a "good" diet, with the dairy, whole grains, fruit, and dark green and orange vegetable groups needing the most improvement. **Figure 13-7** summarizes the overall dietary quality of adults age 45 and older.

As a person gets older, the chances of suffering a chronic illness or functional impairment are greater, thereby increasing nutritional risk. In the United States, some type of **disability** (difficulty in hearing, vision, cognition, ambulation, self-care, or independent living) was reported by 36% of all persons 65 years of age and older in 2013.[35] A majority of older persons have at least one chronic condition and many have multiple conditions. Among the most frequently occurring chronic conditions in older persons are hypertension (71%), diagnosed arthritis (49%), all types of heart disease (31%), any cancer (25%), and diabetes (21%). Other chronic conditions contributing to disability include strokes and disorders of vision and hearing (**Figure 13-8**). Dementia (especially Alzheimer's disease) is a major contributor to disability and placement in nursing homes for those over age 75.[36] Malnutrition can occur secondary to these conditions, as noted in **Table 13-4**. Many of these conditions require special diets that can further compromise nutrition status in the older adult. Also, there are differences in disease prevalence among racial and ethnic groups. For this reason, nutrition interventions designed to reduce disease

Disability Any restriction on or impairment in performing an activity in the manner or within the range considered normal for a human being.

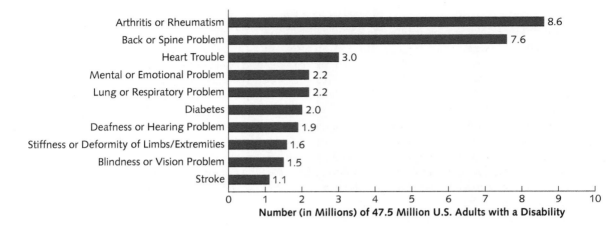

FIGURE 13-8 Common Causes of Disability in Older Persons

The number of people reporting a disability increases with age, and women have a higher prevalence of disability than men at all ages. The prevalence of disability doubles in successive age groups (18–44 years, 11.0%; 45–64 years, 23.9%; ≥ 65 years, 51.8%). Given the size of the baby-boom generation, the number of adults with a disability is likely to increase along with the need for appropriate medical and public health services, as the baby boomers enter into higher-risk age groups over the next 20 years. Increasing physical activity and reducing or preventing obesity and tobacco use can eliminate some of the underlying causes of disability for some people and prevent secondary conditions in those already affected.

Source: Centers for Disease Control and Prevention, Prevalence and Most Common Causes of Disability among Adults, United States, *Morbidity and Mortality Weekly Report* 58 (2009): 421–26.

TABLE 13-4 Malnutrition That Is Secondary to Disease, Physiologic State, or Medication Use

DISEASE OR CONDITION	EFFECTS ON NUTRITION STATUS
Atherosclerosis	May increase difficulties in regulating fluid balances if caused by congestive heart failure.
Cancer	Weight loss, lack of appetite, and secondary malnutrition are common.
Dental and oral disease	May alter the ability to chew and thus reduce dietary intake. Increased likelihood of choking and aspiration.
Depression and dementia	Increased or decreased food intakes are common. A person with dementia may have decreased ability to get food, or the appetite may be very small or very great. Judgment and balance in meal planning are generally absent.
Diabetes mellitus	Increased risk of other diet-related diseases such as hyperlipidemia; weight loss is needed if obesity is present.
Emphysema and chronic obstructive pulmonary diseases (COPD)	May be difficult to eat due to breathing problems.
End-stage kidney disease	Alters fluid and electrolyte needs; uremia may alter appetite and increase risk of malnutrition.
Gastrointestinal disorders	Increased risk of malabsorption of nutrients and consequent undernutrition.
High blood pressure	Weight gain may exacerbate high blood pressure.
Osteoarthritis	Makes motion difficult, including those activities related to meal preparation. Predisposes people to a sedentary lifestyle and may give rise to obesity.
Osteoporosis	Limits the ability to purchase and prepare food if mobility is affected. If severe scoliosis is present, the appetite may be altered.
Stroke	May alter abilities in the cognitive and motor realms related to food and eating.

Source: Adapted from Institute of Medicine, *The Second Fifty Years: Promoting Health and Preventing Disability* (Washington, D.C.: National Academy Press, 1992), 168–69.

risks must be sensitive to ethnic, cultural, and linguistic differences and preferences. Minority-group older adults are more likely to have malnutrition secondary to chronic diseases such as heart disease, renal disease, diabetes mellitus, obesity, and certain cancers. Low socioeconomic status can further increase risk of malnutrition. Many times, low-income older adults have less access to health care and food assistance programs, limited access to healthful foods in poorer neighborhoods, and decreased quality of life and increased mortality.[37]

Polypharmacy, or the use of multiple drugs, is problematic for many older adults. The average older person fills more than 30 prescriptions a year and often takes three or more drugs at a time.[38] Cardiac drugs are most widely used by older adults, followed by drugs to treat arthritis, mental disorders, and respiratory and gastrointestinal conditions. Many older adults also use over-the-counter medications such as antacids, as well as nutritional herbal remedies and supplements.[39] Long-term use of a variety of medications and supplements increases the risk of drug–nutrient and drug–drug interactions. Individuals with impaired nutrition status and poor dietary intakes are at the highest risk.

Polypharmacy The taking of three or more medications regularly; occurs in one-third of those over 65 years of age.

Nutrition Policy Recommendations for Health Promotion for Older Adults

As we noted in Chapter 1, efforts at health promotion and disease prevention are conducted at several levels and are designed to help adults of all ages change their eating patterns and other behaviors to reduce the risk of chronic disease. Optimal nutrition contributes to healthy aging. As primary prevention, nutrition helps promote health and affects the quality of life in older adults. As secondary prevention, nutrition can lessen risks from chronic diseases. As tertiary prevention, medical nutrition therapy slows disease progression and reduces symptoms.[40] The Academy of Nutrition and Dietetics has designated life-cycle nutrition as a priority area for its current public policy advocacy program and supports efforts to help older adults better manage their health. Several policy recommendations for promoting the health of older adults are related to the value of nutrition services:[41]

- Good nutrition is essential to the health, independence, and quality of life of older adults and one of the major determinants of successful aging.
- Nutrition services are needed in the wide variety of settings in which older adults live, dine, and receive health care. These include rehabilitation, community health, congregant feeding, home care, adult daycare, assisted-living, and nursing facilities.
- More than a quarter of all Americans and two out of every three older Americans have multiple chronic conditions (e.g., cardiovascular disease, diabetes mellitus, kidney disease, hypertension, obesity, and osteoporosis) that can benefit from nutrition intervention by food and nutrition practitioners.[42]
- The majority of homebound older adults rely on informal caregivers, most of whom are untrained and unprepared for care management.
- A broad array of culturally appropriate food and nutrition services as well as physical activities and supportive care are vital for maintaining the health of this growing segment of the U.S. population.
- Enjoyment of food, along with its social and nurturing aspects, contributes to quality of life for older adults.
- Evidence shows that services that improve nutrition among older adults produce positive health outcomes and reduce their health care costs.
- Adults with poor nutrition status, especially those consuming inadequate food and fluids, are more likely to have serious complications, require institutional or home-based care, and have greater reliance on prescription drugs.

- Many long-term care residents are at risk for malnutrition and dehydration.
- Government, academia, the health care community, civic and religious institutions, and individuals all have roles to play in ensuring that older adults' nutritional needs are met. Support and coordination of activities and partnerships are vital if improvements are to be made and sustained.

To promote healthful aging, improve care, and broaden access to food and nutrition programs and services for older adults, the Academy of Nutrition and Dietetics supports the following strategies:[43]

- Expansion and funding of federal and state nutrition services in home- and community-based programs, such as the Older Americans Nutrition Program. Funding for nutrition services, such as home care, risk reduction and management, nutrition education, health promotion, and caregiver training can yield substantial savings in health care costs. Reimbursement for medical nutrition therapy for unintended weight loss, dehydration, and wounds would mean more older adults could obtain services.
- Applied nutrition and aging research is needed to determine the nutritional needs and optimal diets in nursing homes and home care and for the very old.
- Recruitment and retention in allied health professions is needed to meet future projected health care demands.

The Academy of Nutrition and Dietetics recommends that nutrition services (including nutrition assessment, diagnosis, intervention, and monitoring) and nutrition counseling and education be included throughout the continuum of health care services for older adults.[44] A discussion of the guidelines and tools for nutrition screening and assessment of older adults follows in the next section.

Evaluation of Nutrition Status

Up to one-quarter of all older adults and one-half of all hospitalized older adults may be suffering from malnutrition.[45] About 4.2 million older adults (9.5%) had incomes below the poverty threshold in 2013; another 2.5 million were classified as "near poor," with incomes up to 125% of the poverty threshold. In addition, a national survey found that about 28% of all noninstitutionalized people over the age of 65 lived alone in 2014 (8.8 million women and 3.8 million men) and 46% of older women age 75+ live alone. People identified as living in poverty are at risk of having inadequate resources for food, housing, health care, and other needs.[46] Older persons living alone were much more likely to be poor than were older persons living with families. The highest poverty rates were experienced among Hispanic women who lived alone and older black women who lived alone. Additionally, 45% of all noninstitutionalized older adults take multiple prescription drugs that can interfere with appetite and nutrient absorption, 45% have difficulty in performing one or more **activities of daily living (ADLs)**, and an additional 15% have difficulties with **instrumental activities of daily living** (e.g., preparing meals and taking medications)—all factors that place older persons at nutritional risk. Older persons who have problems with the activities of daily living depend on others to perform these essential activities and are more likely to be at risk for malnutrition.[47] Identifying older adults at nutritional risk is an important first step in maintaining quality of life and functional status.

Activities of daily living (ADLs) Bathing, dressing, grooming, transferring from bed or chair, going to the bathroom (toileting), and feeding oneself.

Instrumental activities of daily living (IADLs) Food preparation, use of telephone, housekeeping, laundry, use of transportation, responsibility for medication, managing money, and shopping.

Nutrition Screening The Academy of Nutrition and Dietetics, the American Academy of Family Physicians, and the National Council on Aging promote nutrition screening and early intervention as part of routine health care, particularly among older

RISK FACTORS	MAJOR INDICATORS	MINOR INDICATORS

• Inappropriate food intake
• Poverty
• Social isolation
• Dependence/disability
• Acute/chronic diseases or conditions
• Chronic medication use
• Advanced age (80+)
	• Weight loss of 10 lb or more
	• Under-/overweight
	• Serum albumin below 3.5 g/dL
	• Change in functional status
	• Inappropriate food intake
	• Mid-arm muscle circumference < 10th percentile
	• Triceps skin fold < 10th percentile or > 95th percentile
	• Obesity
	• Nutrition-related disorders
	   Osteoporosis
	   Osteomalacia
	   Folate deficiency
	   B_{12} deficiency
		• Alcoholism
		• Cognitive impairment
		• Chronic renal insufficiency
		• Multiple concurrent medications
		• Malabsorption syndromes
		• Anorexia, nausea, dysphagia
		• Change in bowel habits
		• Fatigue, apathy, memory loss
		• Poor oral/dental status
		• Dehydration
		• Poorly healing wounds
		• Loss of subcutaneous fat or muscle mass
		• Fluid retention
		• Reduced iron, ascorbic acid, zinc

TABLE 13-5 Risk Factors and Indicators of Poor Nutrition Status in Older Adults

Source: Adapted from Nutrition Screening Initiative, *Incorporating Nutrition Screening and Interventions into Medical Practice* (1994): 28.

adults, believing that nutrition status is a "vital sign"—as vital to health assessment as blood pressure and pulse rate.[48] **Table 13-5** identifies a number of specific risk factors and indicators of poor nutrition status in older adults. Some of the risk factors shown in the marginal box increase the risks for dietary inadequacy, excess, or imbalance and involve social, economic, and psychological factors rather than physical health problems. Others indicate risks of malnutrition secondary to disease rather than those caused primarily by lack of food.[49]

Several simplified assessment tools are available to screen and assess nutritional risk and maintain health in older adults.[50] The *Mini Nutritional Assessment (MNA)* shown in **Figure 13-9** is a validated screening tool for assessing early malnutrition in older adults and can be completed relatively quickly.[51] The MNA addresses functional ability, diet and lifestyle, anthropometric indicators, and self-perception of health status. The Nutrition Screening Initiative developed a 10-question self-assessment "checklist" that addresses disease, eating status, tooth loss or mouth pain, economic hardship, reduced social contact, multiple medications, involuntary weight loss or gain, and need for assistance with self-care (**Table 13-6**), but the tool has not yet been validated.[52]

Health professionals should follow up with people identified as being at risk, performing more in-depth screening and assessment of nutrition status. A good assessment examines four major areas: physical health, functional ability, psychological health, and socioenvironmental factors. In-depth screening tools focus on the components of nutrition assessment, including anthropometric indicators (e.g., weight, height, and body composition); clinical indicators (e.g., oral health and general physical exam); biochemical indicators (e.g., serum albumin, serum cholesterol, hemoglobin, and blood glucose); dietary indicators (including dietary history); chronic medication use and the living environment of the individual (assistance, facilities, support systems, safety); and cognitive, emotional, and functional status.[53]

Nutrition Assessment Periodic nutrition assessment is useful for identifying and tracking older adults at nutritional risk. The components of nutrition assessment for older adults include the elements discussed in the list that follows:[54]

- *Anthropometric measures.* Height, weight, and skin fold measures are affected by aging. Height decreases over time because of changes in the integrity of the skeletal system as a result of bone loss. Measurements of height are sometimes difficult to obtain as a

Risk Factors Influencing Nutrition Status

PHYSIOLOGICAL
- Dietary intake
- Lack of appetite
- Inactivity/immobility
- Poor taste and smell
- Alcohol or drug abuse
- Chronic disease
- Polypharmacy
- Physical disability
- Oral health problems

PSYCHOLOGICAL
- Dementia
- Cognitive impairment
- Depression
- Loss of spouse
- Social isolation

ENVIRONMENTAL
- Inadequate housing
- Inadequate cooking facilities
- Lack of transportation

SOCIOECONOMIC
- Cultural beliefs
- Poverty
- Limited education
- Literacy level
- Limited access to health care
- Institutionalization

Mini Nutritional Assessment
MNA®

Nestlé Nutrition INSTITUTE

Last name:	First name:	Sex:	Date:

Age:	Weight, kg:	Height, cm:	I.D. Number:

Complete the screen by filling in the boxes with the appropriate numbers.
Add the numbers for the screen. If the score is 11 or less, continue with the assessment to gain a Malnutrition Indicator Score.

Screening

A Has food intake declined over the past 3 months due to loss of appetite, digestive problems, chewing or swallowing difficulties?
0 = severe loss of appetite
1 = moderate loss of appetite
2 = no loss of appetite

B Weight loss during the last 3 months
0 = weight loss greater than 3 kg (6.6 lbs)
1 = does not know
2 = weight loss between 1 and 3 kg (2.2 and 6.6 lbs)
3 = no weight loss

C Mobility
0 = bed or chair bound
1 = able to get out of bed/chair but does not go out
2 = goes out

D Has suffered psychological stress or acute disease in the past 3 months
0 = yes   2 = no

E Neuropsychological problems
0 = severe dementia or depression
1 = mild dementia
2 = no psychological problems

F Body Mass Index (BMI) (weight in kg) / (height in m²)
0 = BMI less than 19
1 = BMI 19 to less than 21
2 = BMI 21 to less than 23
3 = BMI 23 or greater

Screening score (subtotal max. 14 points)
12 points or greater   Normal – not at risk – no need to complete assessment
11 points or below   Possible malnutrition – continue assessment

Assessment

G Lives independently (not in a nursing home or hospital)
0 = no   1 = yes

H Takes more than 3 prescription drugs per day
0 = yes   1 = no

I Pressure sores or skin ulcers
0 = yes   1 = no

Ref. Vellas B, Villars H, Abellan G, et al. Overview of the MNA® - Its History and Challenges. J Nut Health Aging 2006;10:456-465.
Rubenstein LZ, Harker JO, Salva A, Guigoz Y, Vellas B. Screening for Undernutrition in Geriatric Practice: Developing the Short-Form Mini Nutritional Assessment (MNA-SF). J. Geront 2001;56A: M366-377.
Guigoz Y. The Mini-Nutritional Assessment (MNA®) Review of the Literature - What does it tell us? J Nutr Health Aging 2006; 10:466-487.

© Nestlé, 1994, Revision 2006. N67200 12/99 10M
For more information : www.mna-elderly.com

J How many full meals does the patient eat daily?
0 = 1 meal
1 = 2 meals
2 = 3 meals

K Selected consumption markers for protein intake
• At least one serving of dairy products (milk, cheese, yogurt) per day   yes ☐   no ☐
• Two or more servings of legumes or eggs per week   yes ☐   no ☐
• Meat, fish or poultry every day   yes ☐   no ☐
0.0 = if 0 or 1 yes
0.5 = if 2 yes
1.0 = if 3 yes

L Consumes two or more servings of fruits or vegetables per day?
0 = no   1 = yes

M How much fluid (water, juice, coffee, tea, milk…) is consumed per day?
0.0 = less than 3 cups
0.5 = 3 to 5 cups
1.0 = more than 5 cups

N Mode of feeding
0 = unable to eat without assistance
1 = self-fed with some difficulty
2 = self-fed without any problem

O Self view of nutritional status
0 = views self as being malnourished
1 = is uncertain of nutritional state
2 = views self as having no nutritional problem

P In comparison with other people of the same age, how does the patient consider his/her health status?
0.0 = not as good
0.5 = does not know
1.0 = as good
2.0 = better

Q Mid-arm circumference (MAC) in cm
0.0 = MAC less than 21
0.5 = MAC 21 to 22
1.0 = MAC 22 or greater

R Calf circumference (CC) in cm
0 = CC less than 31   1 = CC 31 or greater

Assessment (max. 16 points)

Screening score

Total Assessment (max. 30 points)

Malnutrition Indicator Score
17 to 23.5 points   At risk of malnutrition
Less than 17 points   Malnourished

FIGURE 13-9 Mini Nutritional Assessment (MNA)
®Société des Produits Nestlé S.A., Vevey, Switzerland, Trademark Owners. An interactive version of the Mini Nutritional Assessment (MNA) tool is available at *www.mna-elderly.com/mnaregforms_interactive.php.*
Source: Nestle Nutrition Services, USA, 2005.

The word *DETERMINE* is used as a mnemonic device with the checklist. Each letter in the word stands for a risk factor:

DETERMINE the Warning Signs of Poor Nutrition:

Disease
Eating poorly
Tooth loss or mouth pain
Economic hardship
Reduced social contact
Many medicines
Involuntary weight loss or gain
Needs assistance in self-care
Elder years above age 80

TABLE 13-6

Nutritional Health Checklist

STATEMENT	YES
I have an illness or condition that made me change the kind or amount of food I eat.	2
I eat fewer than two meals per day.	3
I eat few fruits, vegetables, or milk products.	2
I have three or more drinks of beer, liquor, or wine almost every day.	2
I have tooth or mouth problems that make it hard for me to eat.	2
I don't always have enough money to buy the food I need.	4
I eat alone most of the time.	1
I take three or more different prescription or over-the-counter drugs per day.	1
Without wanting to, I have lost or gained 10 lb in the past six months.	2
I am not always physically able to shop, cook, or feed myself.	2

Note: The Nutritional Health Checklist was developed for the Nutrition Screening Initiative. Read the statements above and circle the number in the "yes" column for each statement that applies to you. Add up the circled numbers to get your nutritional score.

SCORING

0 to 2 = You have good nutrition. Recheck your nutritional score in six months.
3 to 5 = You are at moderate nutritional risk, and you should see what you can do to improve your eating habits and lifestyle. Recheck your nutritional score in three months.
6 or more = You are at high nutritional risk, and you should bring this checklist with you the next time you see your physician, dietitian, or other qualified health care professional. Talk with any of these professionals about the problems you may have. Ask for help to improve your nutrition status.

Source: B. Elsawy and K. E. Higgins, "The Geriatric Assessment," *American Family Physician* 83 (2011): 48–56. Adapted with permission from *The Clinical and Cost-Effectiveness of Medical Nutrition Therapies: Evidence and Estimates of Potential Medical Savings from the Use of Selected Nutritional Intervention* (June 1996). Summary report prepared for the Nutrition Screening Initiative, a project of the American Academy of Family Physicians, the American Dietetic Association, and the National Council on the Aging, Inc.

consequence of poor posture or the inability to stand erect unassisted. In such cases, a recumbent anthropometric measure such as knee-to-heel height can be used instead.[55]
- *Clinical assessment.* The clinical assessment should evaluate the condition of hair, skin, nails, musculature, eyes, mucosa, and other physical attributes. An oral examination is useful for determining the condition of the mouth and teeth, the need for dentures or the condition of existing dentures, and oral lesions.[56] An assessment of the client's ability to chew, swallow, and self-feed is recommended.
- *Biochemical assessment.* Biochemical parameters are affected by the aging process, as well as by polypharmacy, chronic disease, and hydration status. However, serial measures of blood parameters can be useful in evaluating nutritional risk. Serum albumin is generally used to assess visceral protein status. Low serum albumin levels are associated

with increased morbidity and mortality in older adults. Measurements of serum cholesterol, hemoglobin, blood glucose, and antigen-recall skin tests are also included.

- *Dietary assessment.* A detailed record of current food consumption and a history of changes in eating habits over time are needed to assess diet adequacy. The evaluation should detect persons who avoid certain food groups, adhere to unusual dietary practices, or consume excessive or insufficient amounts of essential nutrients. The adequacy of fluid intake should be assessed as well.
- *Functional assessment.* A functional assessment measures changes in the basic functions necessary to maintain independent living. Activities of daily living (ADLs) are self-care activities (e.g., bathing, dressing, and feeding). Instrumental ADLs, or IADLs, which require a higher level of functioning, include activities such as meal preparation, financial management, and housekeeping. Many of these activities (e.g., shopping, cooking, and self-feeding) are closely related to adequate nutrition status.
- *Medication assessment.* Note the types and doses of various prescription and over-the-counter drugs. Evaluate the individual's drug intake for possible nutrient–drug interactions that could affect the absorption and metabolism of, and requirements for, specific nutrients. Also identify any drugs that may depress the appetite or alter the perception of taste.
- *Social assessment.* Financial resources, living arrangements, and social support network, including availability of caregivers, should be evaluated as part of the nutrition assessment because these factors can directly affect a person's nutrition status. Poverty (annual income of less than $11,770 per person in 2015) and social isolation particularly impair the nutrition status of many older adults, as noted perceptively by a professor of psychiatry:

> It is not what the older person eats but with whom that will be the deciding factor in proper care for him. The oft-repeated complaint of the older patient that he has little incentive to prepare food for only himself is not merely a statement of fact but also a rebuke to the questioner for failing to perceive his isolation and aloneness and to realize that food . . . for one's self lacks the condiment of another's presence which can transform the simplest fare to the ceremonial act with all its shared meaning.[57]

Home- and Community-Based Programs and Services

Until the early 1970s, nutrition services for older adults, with the exception of food stamps, were found primarily in hospitals and long-term care facilities. Efforts were then made to expand services from the hospitals to include communities and homes.

In response to the socioeconomic problems that trouble many older adults and may lead to malnutrition—low income, inadequate facilities for preparing food, lack of transportation, and inability to afford dental care, among others—federal, state, and local agencies have mandated nutrition programs for older adults.[58] An individual's need for nutrition services depends on his or her level of independence, which can be depicted as a continuum (**Figure 13-10**). Currently, home- and community-based nutrition programs support the functional independence of older individuals in ambulatory care centers, adult daycare centers, hospices, and home settings. Community nutritionists need to be familiar with organizations and programs providing nutrition and other health-related services to older adults. A summary of the nutrition programs for older adults is provided

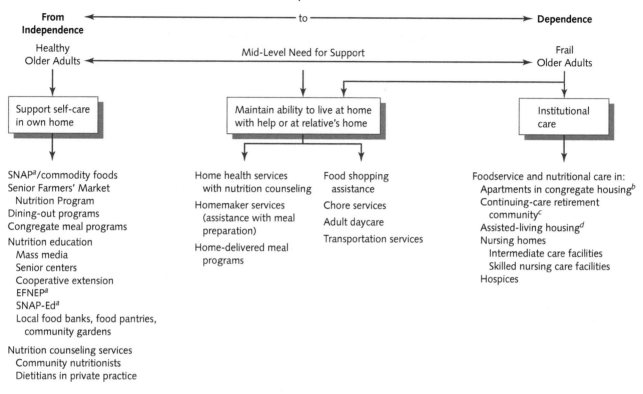

Semidependence

From Independence ← to → **Dependence**

Healthy Older Adults ← Mid-Level Need for Support → Frail Older Adults

Support self-care in own home

Maintain ability to live at home with help or at relative's home

Institutional care

SNAP[a]/commodity foods
Senior Farmers' Market
  Nutrition Program
Dining-out programs
Congregate meal programs
Nutrition education
  Mass media
  Senior centers
  Cooperative extension
  EFNEP[a]
  SNAP-Ed[a]
  Local food banks, food pantries,
    community gardens
Nutrition counseling services
  Community nutritionists
  Dietitians in private practice

Home health services
  with nutrition counseling
Homemaker services
  (assistance with meal
  preparation)
Home-delivered meal
  programs

Food shopping
  assistance
Chore services
Adult daycare
Transportation services

Foodservice and nutritional care in:
  Apartments in congregate housing[b]
  Continuing-care retirement
    community[c]
  Assisted-living housing[d]
  Nursing homes
    Intermediate care facilities
    Skilled nursing care facilities
  Hospices

[a] SNAP = Supplemental Nutrition Assistance Program; EFNEP = Expanded Food and Nutrition Education Program; SNAP-Ed = Supplemental Nutrition
  Assistance Program-Education.
[b] *Apartments in congregate housing*: allows older persons to maintain a private apartment but makes supportive services easily available
  (transportation, common dining room, other personal services).
[c] *Continuing-care retirement community*: offers full spectrum of services as needed—from meal service only to assisted-living services to
  skilled nursing care.
[d] *Assisted-living housing*: offers older adults more supportive services and supervision than congregate housing (for example, help
  with ADLs, meals provided in common dining room, emergency assistance available 24-hours/day).

FIGURE 13-10 Overview of Community Nutrition Programs for Older Adults
Community-based services can be located by contacting the Eldercare Locator at 800-677-1116 or *www.eldercare.gov*. The National
Council on Aging has created *www.benefitscheckup.org* to help older adults quickly identify federal and state assistance programs that
may improve the quality of their lives.
Source: Adapted from H. T. Phillips and S. H. Gaylord, eds., *Aging and Public Health* (New York: Springer, 1985). Copyright Springer Publishing Company,
Inc., New York 10012. Used by permission.

in **Table 13-7.** Check out the resources available online from the organizations listed at the
end of the chapter.

General Assistance Programs

The Supplemental Security Income (SSI) Program improves the financial plight of the very
poor directly by increasing a person's or family's income to the defined poverty threshold.
This sometimes helps older people retain their independence.

Another system of financial support to older Americans is the third-party reimbursement system, which was discussed in Chapter 9. Third-party payers (e.g., Medicare,

TABLE 13-7 Nutrition Programs for Older Adults

PROGRAM	TYPE OF INTERVENTION	FUNDING SOURCE[a]	ELIGIBLE/AVAILABLE SERVICES
Older Americans Nutrition Program	Congregate and home-delivered meals, special diets	DHHS AoA	Meals; transportation; shopping assistance; limited nutrition education, information, referral, and attention to needs of homebound older adults.
SNAP[a]	Income subsidy	USDA	Electronic benefits transfer (EBT) for food purchases.
SNAP Nutrition Education	Nutrition education	USDA NIFA	Provide information about making healthful food choices.
Adult Day Care Food Program	Meal program, supervised daycare	USDA	Meals and snacks to participating daycare programs.
Senior Farmers' Market Nutrition Program	Income subsidy	USDA	Provide low-income seniors with coupons that can be exchanged for eligible foods at farmers' markets, roadside stands, and community-supported agriculture programs.
Medicare/Medicaid	Third-party payment system	DHHS CMS SSA	Covers medical and related services provided by participating hospitals, HMOs, private medical practices, ambulatory centers, rehabilitation and skilled nursing facilities, home health agencies, and hospice programs. Eligible nutrition services vary depending on the setting of care and the deemed medical necessity.

[a] AoA, Administration on Aging; DHHS, U.S. Department of Health and Human Services; SNAP, Supplemental Nutrition Assistance Program; NIFA, National Institute of Food and Agriculture; CMS, Centers for Medicare and Medicaid Services; SSA, Social Security Administration; USDA, U.S. Department of Agriculture.

Source: Food and Nutrition Service, *Food Program Facts* (Washington, D.C.: U.S. Department of Agriculture, 2014). See Table 10-4 on page 389 for more information about federal nutrition assistance and nutrition education programs for older adults.

Medicaid, and Blue Cross/Blue Shield) sometimes reimburse the costs of health-related services, including such nutrition services as nutrition screening, assessment, and counseling and enteral or parenteral nutrition support. Generally, the nutrition service must be deemed "medically necessary." Whether a service is reimbursable and the extent of reimbursement vary from state to state and from case to case.

Social work agencies can provide older adults with information about appropriate nutrition resources in the community, such as congregate meal sites and home-delivered meal programs. On physician referral, Home Health Services, offered through local private and public organizations, provide home health aides to assist older people with shopping, housekeeping, and food preparation.[59]

Nutrition Programs of the U.S. Department of Agriculture

The Supplemental Nutrition Assistance Program (SNAP) (formerly the Food Stamp Program) was not designed specifically for older people, but it can nevertheless help older adults in need of financial assistance. SNAP, which is administered by the USDA, enables qualifying people to obtain an Electronic Benefits Transfer (EBT) debit-type card that they can use to buy food at authorized grocery stores or at Senior Farmers' Markets.

Currently, about 9% of participants in SNAP are older adults (aged 60 or over), and only 42% of eligible older adults participate in the program.[60] Reasons for nonparticipation by older adults include the "stigma" of receiving assistance, confusing paperwork, and a lack of public information about eligibility requirements.

The USDA also sponsors meal and snack programs for the Adult Day Care Centers operating in many communities through its Child and Adult Day Care Program. Adult daycare facilities care for seniors while their care providers are away from the home. The USDA's Commodity Supplemental Food Program is also available in a limited number of states and can provide monthly food packages to persons 60 years of age and older.

Nutrition Programs of the U.S. Department of Health and Human Services

The Administration on Aging (AoA) in the Department of Health and Human Services (DHHS) administers the Older Americans Nutrition Program, which includes (1) the Congregate Nutrition Services Program, (2) the Home-Delivered Nutrition Services Program, and (3) the Nutrition Services Incentive Program (NSIP). All persons over 60 years of age and their spouses (regardless of age) are eligible to receive meals from these programs, regardless of their income level. However, for the Congregate and Home-Delivered Programs, services must be targeted at persons with the greatest social and economic need, with particular attention to low-income older persons, including low-income minority older persons, older persons with limited English proficiency, older persons residing in rural areas, and those at risk for institutionalization.[61] The Older Americans Act (OAA) of 1965, which authorizes and funds the Administration on Aging and all of its programs, was amended in 1972 (PL 92-258) to establish and fund the federal Older Americans Nutrition Program (formerly called the Elderly Nutrition Program). The Older Americans Nutrition Program is authorized to provide grants to promote the delivery of nutrition services in local communities: (1) Under Title III, Grants for State and Community Programs on Aging, grants are made to the 655 Area Agencies on Aging, and (2) under Title VI (added in 1978), Grants for Native Americans, grants are made to 233 tribal organizations representing American Indians, Alaska Natives, and Native Hawaiians. These grants are used to fund local congregate and home-delivered meal programs. The following section provides an overview of the congregate and home-delivered meal programs.

The Older Americans Nutrition Program

With the graying of America, increased attention is being given to delivering cost-effective nutrition and health-related services to older persons in the community. The Older Americans Nutrition Program is intended to improve older people's nutrition status and enable them to avoid medical problems, continue living in communities of their own choice, and stay out of institutions. Its specific goals are to:[62]

- Reduce hunger and food insecurity by providing low-cost, nutritious meals
- Provide opportunities for social interaction among older individuals
- Promote the health and well-being of older individuals and delay adverse health conditions through access to nutrition and other disease prevention and health promotion services, including:

  - Nutrition screening and assessment
  - Nutrition education and shopping assistance
  - Counseling and referral to other social and rehabilitation services
  - Transportation services

The current Older Americans Nutrition Program legislation makes meals available at least five days a week, supplying about a third of the dietary reference intakes (DRI) for one meal, two-thirds of the DRI for two meals, and 100% of the DRI when three meals are served (**Table 13-8**). States must also ensure that meals comply with the *Dietary Guidelines for Americans* and take into account local cultural preferences. Menu planning is done with the advice of a registered dietitian or someone with comparable experience.[63] Meals can be breakfast, lunch, or dinner, depending on the needs of participants. There is no cost for meals, but participants sometimes make voluntary contributions.

One aspect of the Older Americans Nutrition Program is the Congregate Meals Program. Administrators try to select sites for congregate meals that will be accessible to as many of the eligible older adults as possible. The congregate meal sites are often community centers, senior centers, faith-based facilities, schools, adult daycare facilities, or older adult housing complexes. Through the Home-Delivered Meals Program, meals are delivered to those who are homebound either permanently or temporarily. The home-delivery program—often referred to as "Meals on Wheels"—ensures nutrition, but its recipients miss out on the social benefits of coming to congregate meal sites; every effort is made to persuade them to come to the shared meals if they can. The home-delivered meals can be hot, cold, frozen, dried, or canned. Breakfast, lunch, dinner, or some combination of meals may be provided five to seven days per week, where feasible. The DHHS's Administration on Aging administers these feeding programs, whereas the states, usually in conjunction with local county and city agencies, have responsibility for their daily operation and administration.

Because American Indians, Alaska Natives, and Native Hawaiians tend to have lower life expectancies and higher rates of illness at younger ages, Title VI allows tribal organizations to set the age at which older people can participate in the program. Since 1972, these programs have grown significantly, accounting for annual federal funding of about $818 million in 2012. In total, the Older Americans Nutrition Program provides 86.3 million meals to about 1.6 million congregate meal participants and 137.4 million meals to about 841,000 home-delivered meal participants (**Figure 13-11**). Characteristics of current participants in the Congregate and Home-Delivered Nutrition Programs are shown in **Figure 13-12**.[64] For every federal dollar spent, the program collects more than $2 from state, local, and private donations. Funding assists with food purchasing and preparation, facilities, and transportation for persons otherwise unable to participate. Current evaluations of home-delivered meal programs assess whether the most needy older adults are going unserved and who should be given priority for receiving food assistance—those who lack access to food because of social or economic disabilities, or those with medical disabilities.[65] Criteria of nutritional risk are needed in order to assign priority

TABLE 13-8

Sample Title III Meal Pattern

FOOD TYPE	RECOMMENDED PORTION SIZE
Protein foods	3 oz, cooked portion
Vegetables and fruits	Two ½ c portions[a]
Enriched white or whole-grain bread or alternative	1 serving (one slice bread or equivalent)
Butter or margarine	1 tsp
Dairy	8 oz fat-free or low-fat milk or calcium equivalent
Dessert	One ½ c serving (fruit, pudding, gelatin, ice cream, sherbet, etc.)

[a] A vitamin C–rich fruit or vegetable is to be served each day; a vitamin A–rich fruit or vegetable is to be served at least three times per week.

Source: U.S. Department of Health and Human Services.

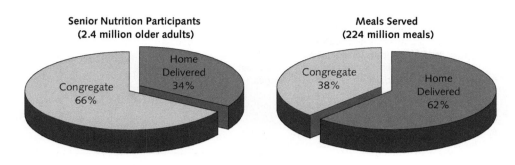

Senior Nutrition Participants
(2.4 million older adults)

Home Delivered 34%

Congregate 66%

Meals Served
(224 million meals)

Congregate 38%

Home Delivered 62%

FIGURE 13-11

Proportion of Participants and Meals Served for the Congregate and Home-Delivered Nutrition Programs, 2013[a]

[a] Congregate meal participants represent a larger proportion of all meal participants but a smaller proportion of total meals served. On the other hand, home-delivered meal participants are relatively fewer but likely to receive more meals. Many home-delivered meal participants receive more than one meal delivered during a week. Congregate meal settings are designed to serve many participants but may serve meals less frequently. In addition, congregate meal participants may partake in meals on a less frequent basis, compared to home-delivered meal participants.

Source: Administration for Community Living (2013). State Program Report Data from *www.agid.acl.gov/*.

status among older adults experiencing food insecurity. One such assessment tool was designed in Great Britain so that social workers would be able to identify nutritional risk factors related to poverty, frailty, and loss of coping skills among homebound older adults (**Table 13-9**). In the United States, eligibility criteria for home-delivered meals vary according to whether the program is a federally, state-, or locally operated program.

In an effort to reduce the cost of providing home-delivered meals, some states have initiated "luncheon clubs." These clubs have permitted several older adults living in close proximity to one another and receiving home-delivered meals to congregate in neighbors' homes. Only one meal delivery stop is therefore required, and the participants benefit from the social interaction.

A two-year congressionally mandated evaluation of the programs for congregate and home-delivered meals generally shows that the programs improve the dietary intake and nutrition status of their clients (**Figure 13-13**).[66] Participants generally have greater diversity in their diets and higher intakes of essential nutrients, and they are less likely than

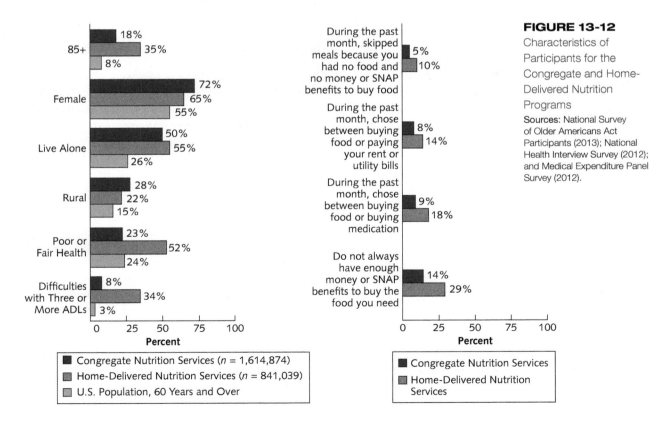

FIGURE 13-12

Characteristics of Participants for the Congregate and Home-Delivered Nutrition Programs

Sources: National Survey of Older Americans Act Participants (2013); National Health Interview Survey (2012); and Medical Expenditure Panel Survey (2012).

TABLE 13-9 Ten Nutritional Risk Factors Diagnostic for the Need for Assistance among Older Adults

1. Consumption of fewer than eight main meals (hot or cold) per week
2. Drinking of very little milk or milk alternate (less than half a pint per day)
3. Little or no intake of fruits or vegetables
4. Wastage of food, even if supplied hot and ready to eat
5. Long periods of the day without food or beverages
6. Depression or loneliness
7. Unexpected weight change (gain or loss)
8. Shopping difficulties
9. Low income
10. Presence of disabilities (including alcoholism)

Source: L. Davies, "Nutrition and the Elderly: Identifying Those at Risk," *Proceedings of the Nutrition Society* 43 (1984): 299. ©1984, reprinted with the permission of Cambridge University Press.

FIGURE 13-13

Intakes of Selected Nutrients by Participants and Nonparticipants in the Congregate Meal and Home-Delivered Meal Programs

Meal participants have a higher calorie intake and reach a higher percentage of the recommended intakes for most nutrients than nonparticipants similar in age and socioeconomic status. Homebound older adults have lower nutrient intakes than older adults who can leave their home.

Source: Data from M. Ponza, J. Ohls, and B. Millen, *Serving Elders at Risk: The Older Americans Act Nutrition Programs: National Evaluation of the Elderly Nutrition Program 1993–1995, Vol. I, Title III Evaluation Findings* (Princeton, NJ: Mathematica Policy Research, 1996).

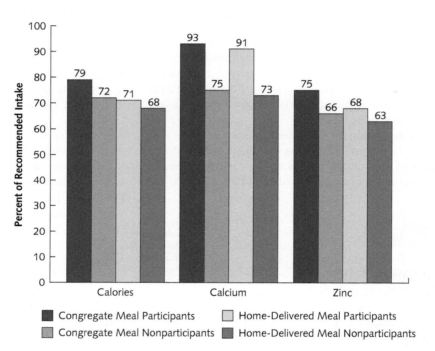

nonparticipants to report food insecurity.[67] Other benefits come as a result of screening and the referrals generated by such programs. Additional benefits are derived from the activities associated with the congregate meals services: nutrition counseling, physical activity programs, adult education, and other classes and activities. Participants benefit, too, from the opportunity for increased socializing.

However, despite these positive outcomes, deficiencies in the meal programs are noted in the lack of regular provision of weekend or evening meals to those who cannot get food or cannot cook. In addition, 41% of Title III Older Americans Nutrition Program providers have waiting lists for home-delivered meals, suggesting a significant unmet need for these meals.[68]

The special needs of homebound older adults need to be given greater priority.[69] The dietary intake of homebound older adults might improve if more than one meal per day were provided, if the meal furnished to the client were prepared with greater percentages of the DRI, and if meals were provided seven days a week rather than five.[70]

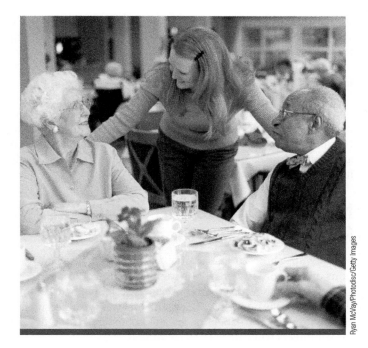

The social atmosphere at congregate meal sites can be as valuable as the foods served.

Ryan McVay/Photodisc/Getty Images

Although Title III nutrition programs are required to provide nutrition education to their clients at least twice a year, these efforts are usually limited to the congregate meal sites. With the exception of a limited amount of printed material, virtually no education is provided to the staff who purchase and prepare these meals. Greater emphasis on nutrition education for both the helper and the client receiving home-delivered meals is warranted. One such effort—the Senior Nutrition Awareness Project of Rhode Island—in partnership with the Meals-on-Wheels program, provides home-delivered meal participants with easy-to-read nutrition tips and information via a brief monthly newsletter called *Nutrition to Go*.[71] The newsletter is delivered to participants by the meal drivers each month and includes low-cost recipe ideas, self-assessment quizzes, and nutrition information on a monthly topic. As effective as it has been, the Older Americans Nutrition Program faces certain challenges on the horizon:[72]

- Changing demographics are likely to increase the demand for program services—particularly for home-delivered meals. The number of persons 85 years and older is expected to double by 2030; because of disabling conditions, this group is less likely to live independently.[73]
- Changes in the present health care system will affect the Older Americans Nutrition Program as more people are discharged early and in need of home- and community-based health services.
- Depending on changes in public policy and funding, the Older Americans Nutrition Program may be challenged to meet increased demand at a time of decreasing federal funding.

Private-Sector Nutrition Assistance Programs

In some communities, food banks enable older people on limited incomes to buy good food for less money. A food bank project buys industry "irregulars"—products that have been mislabeled, underweighted, redesigned, or mispackaged and would therefore ordinarily be thrown away. Nothing is wrong with this food; the industry can claim it, for tax purposes, as a donation, and the buyer (often a food-preparing site) can obtain the food for a small handling fee and make it available at a greatly reduced price.

The Meals On Wheels Association of America (MOWAA) provides leadership and professional training to those who provide congregate and home-delivered meals, develops partnerships, and offers grant opportunities to its members (e.g., volunteer coordinators or nutrition directors at congregate meal and home-delivered meal programs).[74] MOWAA helps to reach older adults in communities not fully serviced by the Older Americans Nutrition Program. In some communities, MOWAA member programs provide weekend and holiday meals in addition to the Older Americans Nutrition Program's typical five luncheon meals.

Nutrition Education and Health Promotion Programs for Older Adults

Nationwide, about 20% of all older adults live in rural areas—communities with populations of 2,500 or less.[75] Few nutrition education efforts for these individuals are available, although some new programs have been designed to target this large audience. In Florida, the Area Agency on Aging of Central Florida has teamed with Florida Cooperative Extension to provide food-labeling educational materials for older adults and training programs for volunteers working with older adults.

Focus group interviews show that older adults are interested in changing their eating behavior.[76] Including practical activities in programs can help motivate these changes. For example, monthly cooking classes at Chicago's White Crane Wellness Center, a combination health care and wellness center founded by older adults, provide an opportunity to modify and taste new recipes, try new foods, and practice healthy eating habits.

The supermarket can serve as a forum to promote healthful diets to older persons. At some supermarkets, dietitians interact with older consumers through store tours for people on special diets and in-store cooking classes showing how to prepare meals with foods that help lower the risks for chronic diseases. Retailers now recognize the value of providing customers with point-of-purchase information about nutrition and health. Supermarket programs for older adults can increase product sales, attract new customers, and contribute to customer loyalty. Many quality nutrition programs exist that can be implemented with a minimum of cost and effort, such as the interactive Share Our Strength *Shopping Matters* grocery store tours. The Food Marketing Institute's website describes several in-store nutrition and labeling programs, such as the Guiding Stars program, that offer tools and ideas for promoting healthful eating and activity habits for shoppers.[77]

Whatever the setting, nutrition programs for adults can be designed for cost-effectiveness by considering the following elements that have been found to contribute to the cost-effectiveness of past interventions involving adults.[78]

- Begin nutrition programs with a personalized approach, such as a self-assessment of nutrition status or behaviors and subsequent comparison with recommendations.
- Use a behavioral approach that combines self-assessment with self-management techniques (e.g., goal setting or social support).
- Allow for active participation in the program (e.g., hands-on cooking classes and small-group discussions).
- Pay attention to motivators and reinforcements (e.g., ease of food preparation and opportunities for social interaction).
- Empower participants by enhancing personal choice and self-control of health-related behaviors.

- Target specific subgroups of older adults. Needs and interests differ by age, income, and health status.
- Be sensitive to age-related physical changes. For example, consider the visual and hearing capabilities of the audience.

Finally, remember to plan for the evaluation of the program. Clarify and document program outcomes in order to measure the impact of the intervention. Who benefits? How does the impact vary by type of person served? Is the program cost-effective? Chapter 5 provides steps for evaluating program elements and effectiveness.

The USDA Food and Nutrition Service released Eat Smart, Live Strong—a program designed to improve fruit and vegetable consumption and physical activity among older adults eligible for federal food and nutrition assistance programs. The program's activity kit includes a leader's guide and four sessions designed to reinforce these behaviors.[79] The intervention is designed to help nutrition educators working in communities deliver science-based nutrition education to low-income older adults.

The National Institute on Aging's national outreach campaign for promoting physical activity for older adults—the Go4Life Campaign—is designed to increase the number of older adults who are active and healthy.[80] The campaign encourages people to make healthier lifestyle choices that can keep them healthy, active, and independent as they age. Go4Life offers exercises, motivational tips, and free resources to help adults start and maintain a physically active lifestyle. Go4Life uses a partnership approach to mobilize communities to create public awareness strategies and make programs available to older adults.

> ▶ **THINK LIKE A COMMUNITY NUTRITIONIST**
>
> Review the bulleted list on the previous page. Then list nutrition education topics that link with the needs and desires of this audience. Next to each topic, indicate the need or desire that it addresses.

PROGRAMS IN **ACTION**

Bringing Food and Nutrition Services to Homebound Seniors

Mobile health services have been successful in improving the well-being of individuals who are physically isolated from traditional health settings. For example, one Virginia organization created a mobile health unit to reach rural residents who could not obtain conventional health services because of illness, transportation problems, or financial factors.[1] Participants reached by the mobile health unit demonstrated increased participation in cancer screenings and increased immunization rates.

The Mobile Market Program offers a creative solution for reaching homebound older adults whose major limitation to food access is transportation. By bringing a traveling market to their clients, volunteers in the Mobile Market Program empower older adults and the homebound to overcome their isolation and take more responsibility for their own health and well-being.

Goals and Objectives

Mobile Meals of Toledo, Ohio, devised the Mobile Market, a grocery store on wheels, to improve the independence and quality of life for older adults and those who are convalescing, chronically ill, disabled, or homebound by giving them an easy way to shop for their groceries. Ongoing objectives include providing shopping opportunities to those who lack them and encouraging clients to progress from receiving home-delivered meals to using the Mobile Market Program.

Target Audience

The Mobile Market serves seniors, the physically and mentally challenged, the homebound, and residents of center-city neighborhoods with limited availability of supermarkets. The Market visits residents of 46 housing facilities for seniors and the disabled on a weekly basis.

Rationale for the Intervention

Mobile Meals of Toledo's existing Home-Delivered Meal Program had a waiting list in some parts of the city. The organization realized that some clients needed assistance only in obtaining groceries rather than in meal preparation and delivery. These clients were able to prepare their own meals but lacked shopping options and transportation. Thus, moving clients from Mobile Meals to the Mobile Market Program would reduce the waiting time for those who needed the full meal program. With the services of the Mobile Market available, agency caseworkers could better serve their neediest clients.

Methodology

The Mobile Market is a grocery store on wheels that visits 46 housing facilities for seniors and the disabled on a weekly basis to provide residents with the opportunity to shop for their groceries. The Market carries more than 1,200 grocery items, including meats; fresh produce; frozen items; dairy products; baked goods; and other nonfood items typically carried by grocery stores, such as greeting cards, cleaning supplies, and reading materials. The Market is small—37 feet long—to enable shoppers to focus easily and not become overwhelmed. Shoppers who are unable to visit the Mobile Market during its regularly scheduled stop can phone in orders for delivery. A voucher program allows the clients of mental health agencies to purchase groceries without using cash. The Mobile Market helps promote health screenings and other community health programs to its clients and arranges for flu and pneumonia vaccinations.

The Mobile Market has several partners in the community. The program is partially funded by United Way of Greater Toledo and the Area Office on Aging of Northwestern Ohio. The Market also receives a Community Development Block Grant. A local grocery store provides technical advice and sells the Market merchandise at cost to provide significant savings to its customers, who are frequently those most in need yet least able to pay for services.

Results

Approximately 7,500 clients now use the services of the Market each year, with over 150 clients purchasing groceries from the Mobile Market on a weekly basis. Caseworkers report that they made fewer home visits because they knew many of their clients' dietary needs were being met. Site managers acknowledged the positive effect of the opportunity to socialize offered by the Mobile Market; it was the only social outlet of the week for many homebound residents.

Lessons Learned

The Mobile Market Program is particularly beneficial to rural areas and inner-city neighborhoods that have limited options for grocery shopping. It also has led to fewer people on waiting lists for meal programs.

Source: Adapted from *Community Nutritionary* (White Plains, NY: Dannon Institute, Fall 2000). Used with permission.

ENTREPRENEUR IN ACTION

Alberta Scruggs, RDN, LDN, DTR, is owner of Nutritional Concerns, Inc, a consulting company. Initially, Alberta worked seven years as a clinical DTR in a long-term care facility, where she became aware of the urgent need to focus on disease prevention. Alberta has since designed and implemented nutrition components in programs of many organizations, including the YMCA of Greater Dayton, a diabetes prevention program, and a Diabetes and Obesity Wellness Opportunity Program. Alberta expanded her sphere of influence to faith-based organizations by initiating a program that challenged parishioners to increase fruit, vegetable, and water intake. She is also an older adult fitness instructor and a certified group fitness instructor who works with people who require modifications to regular exercise programs. As an entrepreneur, Alberta believes that autonomy, tenacity, innovation, vision, a plan B for when plan A fails, out-of-the-box thinking, and focus are essential for success. Read her sage advice for students online at *www.cengagebrain.com*.

The Eat Better & Move More program encourages older adults to take simple steps for better health.[81] A multisite study enrolled approximately 750 ethnically diverse participants aged 60 and over in the Eat Better & Move More program of the Older Americans Nutrition Program. The subjects were participants at congregate meal centers, churches, neighborhood recreation centers, and housing complexes in urban inner-city, suburban, and rural sites. Eat Better & Move More is designed to fit the interests and needs of older adults who want to maintain their quality of life and independence and live longer and better lives. The programs follow the *Steps to Healthy Aging Guidebook*, a 12-week program consisting of mini-lectures on nutrition and walking. The mini-lecture topics emphasize the benefits of eating more fruits and vegetables, the relationship of dairy foods with bone health, the importance of dietary fiber, sensible portion sizes, and the benefits of physical activity. Step counters are used to encourage older adults to take more steps each day.

For adults over age 50, health promotion efforts seek to preserve independence, productivity, and personal fulfillment.[82] The premise of health promotion is that individuals can enjoy benefits from healthful behaviors at any age. To this end, most states now offer community wellness centers for older adults that include services at all levels of prevention. Resource people for these efforts at the local level include public health nutritionists employed by county health departments, registered dietitians working with local nursing homes and community hospitals as consultants, and county cooperative extension educators. In addition, some community groups and churches offer support and self-help groups.

Looking Ahead: Successful Aging

As a nation, we tend to value the future more than the present, putting off enjoying today so that we will have money, prestige, or time to have fun tomorrow. Older adults feel this loss of future. The present is their time for leisure and enjoyment, but often they have no experience in using leisure time.

The solution is to begin to prepare for old age early in life, both psychologically and nutritionally (**Figure 13-14**). Preparation for this period should, of course, include financial planning, but other lifelong habits should be developed as well. Each adult needs to learn to reach out to others to forestall the loneliness that will otherwise ensue. Adults need to develop some skills or activities—volunteer work with organizations, reading, games, hobbies, or intellectual pursuits—that they can continue into their later years and that will give meaning to their lives. Each adult needs to develop the habit of adjusting to change,

FIGURE 13-14

The Aging Well Pyramid
The time to prepare for the later years is early in life. Practice the items found at the base of the pyramid to achieve an optimal sense of well-being. Use the inner four compartments of the pyramid to create a balance among all aspects of your life: nutrition, physical activity, social health, and emotional well-being. Use the tip of the pyramid to manage everyday stresses such as traffic gridlock, exams, and work deadlines.

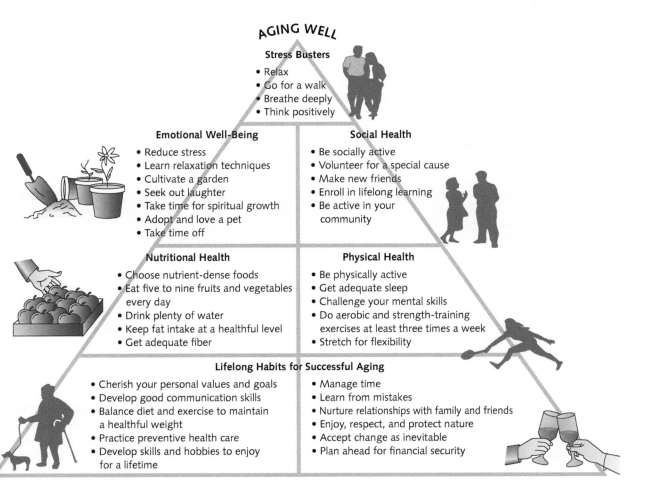

AGING WELL

Stress Busters
- Relax
- Go for a walk
- Breathe deeply
- Think positively

Emotional Well-Being
- Reduce stress
- Learn relaxation techniques
- Cultivate a garden
- Seek out laughter
- Take time for spiritual growth
- Adopt and love a pet
- Take time off

Social Health
- Be socially active
- Volunteer for a special cause
- Make new friends
- Enroll in lifelong learning
- Be active in your community

Nutritional Health
- Choose nutrient-dense foods
- Eat five to nine fruits and vegetables every day
- Drink plenty of water
- Keep fat intake at a healthful level
- Get adequate fiber

Physical Health
- Be physically active
- Get adequate sleep
- Challenge your mental skills
- Do aerobic and strength-training exercises at least three times a week
- Stretch for flexibility

Lifelong Habits for Successful Aging
- Cherish your personal values and goals
- Develop good communication skills
- Balance diet and exercise to maintain a healthful weight
- Practice preventive health care
- Develop skills and hobbies to enjoy for a lifetime
- Manage time
- Learn from mistakes
- Nurture relationships with family and friends
- Enjoy, respect, and protect nature
- Accept change as inevitable
- Plan ahead for financial security

especially when it comes without consent, so that it will not be seen as a loss of control over one's life. The goal is to arrive at maturity with as healthy a mind and body as possible; this means cultivating good nutrition status and maintaining a program of daily exercise.

In general, the ability of older adults to function well varies from person to person and depends on several factors. The "life advantages" listed below seem to contribute to good physical and mental health in later years.[83]

- Genetic potential for extended longevity. Some people seem to have inherited a reduced susceptibility to degenerative diseases.
- A continued desire for new knowledge and new experiences. Some studies suggest that "active" minds, ever involved in learning new things, may be more resistant to decline.
- Socialization, intimacy, and family integrity. Older persons thrive in situations where love, understanding, shared responsibility, and mutual respect are nurtured.
- Adherence to a nutritious diet, combined with avoidance of excesses of food energy, solid fat, added sugars, cholesterol, and sodium. A balanced diet with adequate intakes of all essential nutrients has a positive impact on health and weight management.
- Avoidance of substance abuse.
- Acceptable living arrangements.
- Financial independence.
- Access to health care, including a family physician, health clinic, public health nursing service providing home health care, dentist, podiatrist, physical therapist, pharmacist, and community nutritionist.

Everyone knows older people who have maintained many contacts—through relatives, church, synagogue, or fraternal orders—and have not allowed themselves to drift into isolation. Upon analysis, you will find that their favorable environment came about through a lifetime of effort. These people spent their entire lives reaching out to others and practicing the art of weaving others into their own lives. Likewise, a lifetime of effort is required for good nutrition status in the later years. A person who has eaten a wide variety of foods, maintained a healthy weight, and remained physically active will be best able to age successfully.

case study

Postmenopausal Nutrition and Disease Prevention Program

by Alice Fornari, EdD, RD, Alessandra Sarcona, MS, RD, CSSD, and Alison Barkman, MS, RD, CDN

Scenario

A physician (gynecological specialist) wants to create a nutrition program for the patients in his private practice who are postmenopausal or are at a target age of approximately 50–65 years old. The physician is leaving you, the consulting RD, responsible for identifying the nutrition topics that would best meet the needs of this population. The physician states that many of his patients have been asking him about soy, calcium, heart-healthy eating, and weight management. The target group consists of middle-income to upper-middle-income females, predominantly Caucasian. The physician's office has a conference room that could be utilized for nutrition lectures.

Learning Outcomes

- Identify the national goals for health promotion and disease prevention for adults.
- Recognize the leading nutrition-related diseases and causes of death of women.
- Select appropriate nutrition strategies for disease prevention among postmenopausal women.

Foundation: Acquisition of Knowledge and Skills

1. Review the *Healthy People 2020* objectives for adults presented in Chapter 7 and this chapter.
2. From the Centers for Disease Control and Prevention (CDC) website, *www.cdc.gov*, list the top killers/conditions of women. Alternatively, go to *www.nhlbi.nih.gov/whi/whywhi.htm* and list the diseases that were the focus of the Women's Health Initiative; give an explanation for why these conditions were studied.

Step 1: *Identify Relevant Information and Uncertainties*

1. Research the Women's Health Initiative (WHI), *www.nhlbi .nih.gov/whi/factsht.htm*, and extract from this initiative the nutrition information that could be useful for your program.
2. Besides reading the physician's report, how would you go about determining what nutrition issues take precedence among the women in the physician's private practice and among those in your target group, aged 50–65?

Step 2: *Interpret Information*

On the basis of the nutrition issues identified, what resources would you use to determine the legitimacy of nutrition topics relative to health issues and disease prevention? For example, how would you explore the impact of soy on the chronic diseases affecting women?

Step 3: *Draw and Implement Conclusions*

Based on the information gathered from the CDC and WHI and on the target group's nutrition issues and resources used, prioritize a list of nutrition topics that would be appropriate to discuss in a program with five 90-minute sessions. From your list, create an outline of a program proposal to present to the physician that includes a rationale for having a nutrition program, a list of the program's nutrition topics, and information and activities that will be utilized to assist the participants in learning about these topics.

Step 4: *Engage in Continuous Improvement*

Identify variables that could be used to monitor the impact of the program on women's health.

PROFESSIONAL **FOCUS**

Lighten Up—Be Willing to Make Mistakes and Risk Failure

If you knew that you had only a few months to live, would you live differently than you do right now? Would you find time to take dancing lessons, learn inline skating, snorkel off the Great Barrier Reef, study the stock market, get a pilot's license, or try your hand at papier-mâché? Would you take more chances and worry less about your image?

Most of us would probably answer that last question in the affirmative. We would choose to live differently if we knew that only a few grains of sand were left in the hourglass. Nadine Stair, at the age of 85, said the same thing: "If I had my life to live over again, I'd try to make more mistakes next time.

I would relax. I would limber up. I would be sillier than I have been this trip. I know of a very few things I would take seriously. I would take more trips. I would climb more mountains, swim more rivers and watch more sunsets. I would do more walking and looking. I would eat more ice cream and fewer beans. . . . If I had it to do over again, I would go places, do things and travel lighter than I have. . . . I'd pick more daisies."[1]

Notice that the first thing Nadine Stair said she would do differently "next time" was to try to make more mistakes. Most people work hard to *avoid* making mistakes, and few of us are willing to undertake a venture so risky that mistakes are almost guaranteed and the probability of failure looms large. In our culture, these activities are to be avoided at all costs.

Virtually every successful entrepreneur, adventurer, and risk taker has made mistakes and has failed at some point in his or her struggle to reach a personal or professional goal. In an essay in *Science*, Harold T. Shapiro, president of Princeton University, remarked that "the world too often calls it failure if we do not immediately reach our goals; true failure lies, rather, in giving up on our goals."[2] What would our world be like if the following individuals had given up on their goals?

- In 1842, at a time when most young British women of position were concerned mainly with parties and pending marriages, Florence Nightingale felt a call to perform some lifework. Although she sensed that her destiny "lay among the miserable of the world," the precise nature of this vocation eluded her for many years. Not until she was in her early thirties did she begin to pursue a career in nursing despite the persistent objections of her mother and sister, a cultural bias against nursing care, and the resistance of the traditional medical establishment. Over a lifetime of hard work, her determination and vision radically altered the practice and professionalism of nursing. Nightingale was among the first to document and describe hospital conditions, and she became an expert on sanitation. She reformed the health administration of the British army in response to the brutal mortality of the Crimean War and thereby influenced medical practice for years to come. Her reports on proper hospital construction, the training of nurses, and patient care led to the establishment of sanitary commissions and eventually to the public health service.[3]

- Thomas Alva Edison, born in 1847, has been described as "one of the outstanding geniuses in the history of technology."[4] He received very little formal schooling, having been expelled by a schoolmaster as "addled," and was taught history, science, and philosophy primarily by his mother. His fascination with the wireless telegraph as a young boy led to a lifelong enjoyment of experimentation and research. At his death in 1931, he held 1,093 patents on such devices as the incandescent electric lamp, the phonograph, the carbon telephone transmitter, and the motion picture projector.

  At one point in his career, Edison struggled to develop a storage battery. "I don't think Nature would be so unkind as to withhold the secret of a *good* storage battery if a real earnest hunt for it is made," he said. "I'm going to hunt."[5] This was no mean feat. He knew what was required of a good battery—it must last for years, should not lose capacity when recharged, and needed to be nearly indestructible. He began by testing one chemical after another in a series of experiments that spanned a decade. When 10,000 experiments failed to give the desired results, Edison remarked, "I have not failed. I've just found 10,000 ways that won't work."[6] He eventually succeeded.

- When he was a 20-year-old student at Yale University, Fred Smith wrote a term paper that analyzed freight services existing at the time. He concluded that there was a market for a company that moved "high-priority, time-sensitive" goods such as medicines and electronic components. He believed the existing system was cumbersome and failed to respond quickly to consumers' needs. In his paper, he proposed an overnight delivery service based on a "hub-and-spokes" air freight system. His professor was unimpressed with Smith's proposal, citing a restrictive regulatory environment and competition from airlines as major barriers to implementing such a service. The paper earned a grade of C.

  Smith did not give up on his idea, although he could not do anything about it for several years. Eventually, at the age of 29, he founded a company, Federal Express, designed to deliver packages "absolutely, positively overnight." In March 1973, his first planes flew over the eastern United States, carrying a total of six packages. One month later, the volume had increased to 186 packages. In its first years, the company nearly folded from a lack of capital, concerns about Smith's leadership, and a formal charge of fraud against him. The company—with Smith at its helm—survived this difficult period. By 1983, its earnings were more than $1 billion. Today, with annual revenues of $39 billion, FedEx delivers 8.5 million shipments to 220 countries every day and has altered American business practices substantially.[7]

The Secret of Success

Risk takers make mistakes and sometimes fail. If they all share one feature, however, it is their willingness and determination to persevere, sometimes against great odds. In our professional lives, it is impossible to avoid risk and the chance of failure. The trick is to learn how to minimize risk and capitalize on your mistakes. Here are a few points to keep in mind when you are next faced with undertaking a risky venture:

1. *Do your homework.* There are risks and there are calculated risks. The difference between the two is substantial. To prepare for a calculated risk, talk with people who have undertaken similar ventures. Find out about the unexpected problems they experienced and how they handled them.

2. *Write down your options and the potential outcome of each.* This activity will help you focus on the option that may stand the best chance for success. Then write down the worst possible thing that could happen if you proceeded with that option. Is it something you can live with? If not, how can the option be changed to protect you or your employees?

3. *Learn from your mistakes or failures.* We all make them, but we don't all learn from them. In the business world, bankruptcy is often viewed as the ultimate failure. One entrepreneur commented that "if you hadn't been bankrupt at least once, you hadn't really learned much about business."[8] Although it is certainly painful, business failure

can be an opportunity to learn new lessons both personally and professionally. The successful entrepreneur and risk taker has the ability to learn from his or her experiences and regain control of his or her destiny.

4. *Be committed to your goal.* A high level of commitment to the work at hand is one element that distinguishes the successful entrepreneur from the also-rans.[9]

Words to Work By

In his book of wildlife portraits, artist Robert Bateman remarked, "A great master teacher once said, 'In order to learn how to draw you have to make two thousand mistakes. Get busy and start making them.'"[10] These are apt words to keep in mind as you begin traveling your career path.

CHAPTER SUMMARY

Demographic Trends and Aging

▶ The number of older adults (age 65 years and older) in the United States will nearly double by 2040.

▶ The baby boom that took place between 1946 and 1964 and improving life expectancy are important contributors to the growing older adult population in the United States.

▶ By 2030, minority groups will represent 26.4% of the population of older adults, with the largest increases in Hispanics and Asians.

Healthy Adults

▶ The most important goal of health promotion and disease prevention for adults as they age is maintaining health and functional independence. Many of the health problems associated with the later years are preventable or can be controlled.

▶ Health professionals suggest steps for achieving the *Healthy People 2020* objectives that promote healthy weights and food choices, such as using the federal nutrition assistance programs to increase access to and availability of fruits, vegetables, and whole grains to low-income families.

▶ Baby boomers are a driving force for current and future trends. An understanding of their preferences, character, lifestyle, and location is and will continue to be critical to health promotion programs and services.

▶ An important characteristic of community nutrition interventions is that they can reach people in many different contexts of their daily lives. Supportive social environments can help individuals change their behavior.

▶ Community- and worksite-based programs for health promotion are expanding and are facilitating lifestyle changes. Worksite health promotion efforts can be classified under four main areas: policies, screenings, information or activities, and facilities or services.

Aging and Nutrition Status

▶ Older people vary greatly in their social, economic, and lifestyle situations; functional capacity; and physical condition.

▶ Older adults face the challenge of choosing a nutrient-dense diet. Although caloric needs may decrease with age, the need for certain nutrients may actually increase with the effects of aging.

▶ Individually or in combination, the social, economic, psychological, cultural, and environmental factors associated with aging may interact with physiological changes and further affect nutrition status in older adults.

Nutrition Policy Recommendations for Health Promotion for Older Adults

▶ Good nutrition is essential to the health, independence, and quality of life of older adults and is one of the major determinants of successful aging. A broad array of culturally appropriate food and nutrition services as well as physical activities and supportive care are vital for maintaining the health of older adults.

▶ Identifying older adults at nutritional risk is an important first step in maintaining quality of life and functional status.

● In-depth screening tools focus on the components of nutrition assessment, including anthropometric indicators; clinical indicators; biochemical indicators; dietary indicators; chronic medication use and the living environment of the individual; and cognitive, emotional, and functional status.

Home- and Community-Based Programs and Services

▶ An individual's need for nutrition services depends on his or her level of independence, which can be depicted as a continuum (see Figure 13-10).

▶ The Administration on Aging administers the Older Americans Nutrition Program, which includes (1) the Congregate Nutrition Services Program, (2) the Home-Delivered Nutrition Services Program, and (3) the Nutrition Services Incentive Program (NSIP).

▶ Nutrition programs for adults can be designed for cost-effectiveness by incorporating the following elements: Use a behavioral approach that combines self-assessment with self-management techniques, allow for active participation in the program, and plan for program evaluation.

Looking Ahead: Successful Aging

▶ The ability of older adults to function well varies from person to person and depends on factors such as genetic potential for extended longevity, a continued desire for new knowledge and new experiences, socialization, adherence to a nutritious diet, regular physical activity, financial independence, and access to health services.

SUMMARY QUESTIONS

1. Identify some of the characteristics of baby boomers and describe how they could be incorporated into a worksite wellness program that addresses some of the *Healthy People* nutrition-related objectives for adults.
2. Describe the physiological, environmental, socioeconomic, and psychological factors that influence the nutrition status of older adults.
3. Discuss the various components of a thorough nutrition assessment for older adults.
4. Describe community nutrition programs that are intended to provide nutrition assistance to older adults.
5. What improvements would you recommend to enhance the ability of the Older Americans Nutrition Program to meet the needs of those who are eligible to receive its benefits?

INTERNET RESOURCES

Government Sites

Administration on Aging
www.aoa.gov

Alzheimer's Disease Education and Referral Center
www.nia.nih.gov/alzheimers

CDC's Health Data Interactive
www.cdc.gov/nchs/hdi.htm

Eldercare Locator
www.eldercare.gov

Federal Interagency Forum on Aging
www.agingstats.gov

Food Safety for Older Adults
www.fda.gov/Food/FoodborneIllnessContaminants/
PeopleAtRisk/ucm312705.htm

Go4Life
https://go4life.nia.nih.gov

Healthier Worksite Initiative
www.cdc.gov/nccdphp/dnpao/hwi/index.htm

Information on Men's Health
www.cdc.gov/men

Medicare Program
www.medicare.gov

National Center for Health Statistics
www.cdc.gov/nchs

National Heart, Lung, and Blood Institute
www.nhlbi.nih.gov

National Institute on Aging
www.nia.nih.gov

National Women's Health Information Center
www.womenshealth.gov

NIH Senior Health
http://nihseniorhealth.gov

Office of Minority Health
http://minorityhealth.hhs.gov

Seniors at Nutrition.gov
www.nutrition.gov/life-stages/seniors

United States Senate Special Committee on Aging
http://aging.senate.gov

USDA Food and Nutrition Service
www.fns.usda.gov/fns/

Weight-Control Information Network
http://win.niddk.nih.gov/index.htm

Women's Health Initiative
www.nhlbi.nih.gov/whi/

Organizations

American Association of Retired Persons
http://healthtools.aarp.org/health-encyclopedia

American Diabetes Association
www.diabetes.org

American Federation of Aging Research
www.afar.org

American Geriatrics Society
www.americangeriatrics.org

American Heart Association
www.heart.org/HEARTORG

American Institute for Cancer Research
www.aicr.org

Gerontological Society of America
www.geron.org

Home- and Community-Based Services
www.nasuad.org/hcbs

Leadership Council of Aging Organizations
www.lcao.org

Meals On Wheels Association of America
www.mealsonwheelsamerica.org

National Association of Area Agencies on Aging
www.n4a.org

National Association of Child and Adult Care Food Programs
www.cacfp.org

National Association of Nutrition and Aging Services Programs
www.nanasp.org

National Association of States United for Aging and Disabilities
www.nasuad.org

National Council on Aging
www.ncoa.org

National Council on Aging's BenefitsCheckUp
www.benefitscheckup.org

National Osteoporosis Foundation
http://nof.org

North American Menopause Society
www.menopause.org

Universities

Florida International University's National Resource Center on Nutrition, Physical Activity and Aging
http://nutritionandaging.fiu.edu

Tufts University Human Nutrition Research Center on Aging
http://hnrca.tufts.edu

University of Michigan's Health and Retirement Study (HRS)
http://hrsonline.isr.umich.edu

Commercial

ElderNet
www.eldernet.com

CHAPTER 14

Global Food and Nutrition Security: Challenges and Opportunities

LEARNING OBJECTIVES

After you have read and studied this chapter, you will be able to:

- Describe the current status of global hunger and food insecurity.

- List causes of global food insecurity.

- Give reasons that women and children are particularly at risk with regard to hunger.

- Describe the purpose and goals of recent international food policy initiatives.

- Describe the global public health issues related to malnutrition and food insecurity that will continue

to challenge policymakers and program designers in the next decade.

- List actions that individuals might take to eliminate global hunger and food insecurity.

This chapter addresses such issues as the influence of socioeconomic and cultural factors on food behavior; food availability and access for the individual, family, and community; and using current information technologies, which have been designated by the Accreditation Council for Education in Nutrition and Dietetics (ACEND) as Foundation Knowledge and Learning Outcomes for dietetics education.

CHAPTER OUTLINE

For a complete list of references, please access the MindTap Reader within your MindTap course.

Nutrition security Requires that all people have access to a variety of nutritious foods and potable drinking water; knowledge, resources, and skills for healthy living; prevention, treatment, and care for diseases affecting nutrition status; and safety-net systems during crisis situations such as natural disasters or deleterious social and political systems.

Introduction

All people need food. Food security consists of access by all people at all times to sufficient, safe, and nutritious food for an active and healthy life. Food security has two aspects: ensuring that adequate food supplies are available and ensuring that households whose members suffer from undernutrition have the ability to acquire food, either by producing it themselves or by being able to purchase it. **Nutrition security** requires that all people have access to a variety of nutritious foods and potable drinking water; knowledge, resources, and skills for healthy living; prevention, treatment, and care for diseases affecting nutrition status; and safety-net systems during crisis situations such as natural disasters or deleterious social and political systems.[1]

Regardless of race, religion, sex, or nationality, our bodies experience similarly the effects of hunger and its companion, malnutrition—listlessness, weakness, failure to thrive, stunted growth, mental retardation, muscle wastage, scurvy, anemia, rickets, osteoporosis, goiter, tooth decay, blindness, and a host of other effects, including death.[2] Apathy and shortened attention span are two of a number of behavioral symptoms that are often mistaken for laziness, lack of intelligence, or mental illness in undernourished people.[3] Malnutrition is the biggest risk factor for illness worldwide. Some 2 billion people, mostly women and children, are deficient in one or more of four essential micronutrients: iron, zinc, iodine, and vitamin A.[4] For the year 2050, the projected United Nations figure for total world population is approximately 9 billion—up from 7.3 billion in 2015, thus further stretching the world's food resources.[5]

Mapping Poverty and Undernutrition

World Bank A group of international financial institutions owned by the governments of more than 150 nations. The bank provides loans for economic development.

Food insecurity was once viewed as a problem of overpopulation and inadequate food production, but now many people recognize it as a problem of poverty. Food is available but not accessible to the poor who have neither land nor money. In 1978, Robert McNamara, then president of the **World Bank**, gave what stands as the classic description of absolute poverty: "A condition of life so limited by malnutrition, illiteracy, disease, squalid surroundings, high infant mortality, and low life expectancy as to be beneath any reasonable definition of human decency" (**Table 14-1**).[6]

The Food and Agriculture Organization of the United Nations (FAO) estimates that of the more than 7.3 billion people in the world, at least 795 million people suffer from

REGION	GNI[a]	INFANT MORTALITY RATE (IMR)	LIFE EXPECTANCY	LITERACY RATE	SAFE WATER SUPPLY (%)	UNDER-5 MORTALITY RATE (U5MR)
General Differences[b]						
Least developed countries	$2,046	55	62	53	67	80
World	$14,012	34	71	81	89	46

	GNI	IMR	Children (Under Five Years of Age with Moderate or Severe Stunting) (%)	U5MR
Regional Differences				
Sub-Saharan Africa	$1,665	61	37	92
South Asia	$1,478	45	38	57
Middle East and North Africa	$6,254	24	18	31
East Asia and Pacific	$6,343	16	12	19
Latin America and Caribbean	$9,445	15	11	18

TABLE 14-1 The Gap between Developed and Developing Countries

[a] GNI, Gross national income.

[b] Notice that the poorer nations have higher infant and under-5 mortality rates, shorter life expectancies, and lower literacy rates than richer nations. In short, poverty negatively affects quality of life.

Source: Data from UNICEF, *The State of the World's Children 2015* (New York: UNICEF, 2015).

chronic undernutrition, consuming too little food each day to meet even minimum energy requirements (**Figure 14-1**).[7] To qualify as chronically and severely undernourished by FAO standards, a person must consume fewer than the calories required to perform the basic physiological functions and light physical activity. This minimum is usually in the range of 1,700 to 2,100 calories/day. Approximately 1 billion people live in extreme poverty, or on less than $1.25 per day. Living standards declined during the past two decades, partly because of accelerated rates of population growth, global warming, and environmental decline, but also as a result of lower export earnings, rising global food prices, and the recent worldwide economic crisis.[8] In other words, the poor earned less and paid more. According to the FAO, widespread chronic hunger is most likely to be found in developing countries that can neither produce enough food to feed their populations fully nor earn enough foreign exchange to import food to cover their food deficits.[9]

Those who live with chronic poverty often face unsafe drinking water, intestinal parasites, insufficient food, a low-protein diet, stunted growth, low birthweights, illiteracy, disease, shortened lifespans, and death. In *Quiet Violence: View from a Bangladesh Village*, Hartman and Boyce provide a good introduction to life in the villages of the developing world. The lives of these villagers are more difficult than anything we have ever known, and yet their hopes and dreams are not unlike our own. They exhibit resourcefulness, hard work, and dignity in the midst of circumstances that require a persistence and personal strength that most of us will never need to call upon in our lifetimes. Hari, one of the landless laborers in the village, reflects on his life just days before his death: "Between the mortar and the pestle, the chili cannot last. We poor are like chilies—each year we are ground down, and soon there will be nothing left."[10]

Poverty is much more than an economic condition. It exists for many reasons, including overpopulation; greed; unemployment; and the lack of productive resources such as land, tools, and credit.[11] Consequently, if we are to provide adequate nutrition for all the earth's hungry people, we must transform the economic, political, and social structures that both limit food production, distribution, and consumption and create a gap between rich and poor.[12]

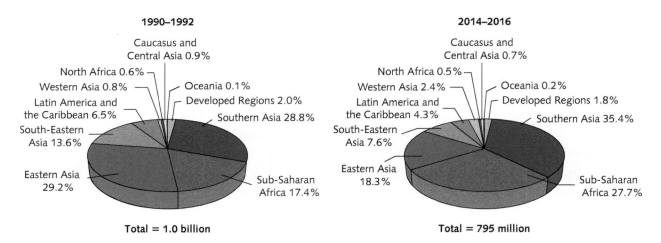

1990–1992

Caucasus and Central Asia 0.9%
North Africa 0.6%
Western Asia 0.8%
Latin America and the Caribbean 6.5%
South-Eastern Asia 13.6%
Eastern Asia 29.2%
Oceania 0.1%
Developed Regions 2.0%
Southern Asia 28.8%
Sub-Saharan Africa 17.4%

Total = 1.0 billion

2014–2016

Caucasus and Central Asia 0.7%
North Africa 0.5%
Western Asia 2.4%
Latin America and the Caribbean 4.3%
South-Eastern Asia 7.6%
Eastern Asia 18.3%
Oceania 0.2%
Developed Regions 1.8%
Southern Asia 35.4%
Sub-Saharan Africa 27.7%

Total = 795 million

FIGURE 14-1 Hunger Hotspots: Changing Distribution of the Proportion of the World's Chronically Undernourished Populations (Millions), 1990–1992 and 2014–2016

At present, there are around 795 million undernourished people worldwide.[a] They are of all ages, from babies whose mothers cannot produce enough milk to older adults with no relatives to care for them. They are the unemployed inhabitants of urban slums; the landless farmers tilling other people's fields; the orphans of AIDS; and the sick, who need special or increased food intake to survive. The percentage of hungry people is highest in east, central, and southern Africa. Around three-quarters of undernourished people live in low-income rural areas of developing countries, principally in higher-risk farming areas. However, the share of the hungry in urban areas is rising. Of the total number of chronically hungry people, over half are in Asia and the Pacific and over a quarter are in sub-Saharan Africa. Today, one in nearly nine people do not get enough food to be healthy and lead an active life.

[a] *Undernourished* is used to describe the status of people whose food intake does not include enough calories to meet minimum physiological needs for an active life.

Source: Food and Agriculture Organization (FAO) of the United Nations, *The State of Food Insecurity in the World 2015*, 10.

A Snapshot of Global Hunger and Food Insecurity: Facts and Figures Provide Perspective

Global Hunger and Nutrition Security

- The leading health risk in the world is hunger—killing more people every year than AIDS, malaria, and tuberculosis combined. About 25,000 people (adults and children) die every day from hunger and related causes.
- There is enough food in the world for everyone to have the nourishment needed for a healthy and productive life. Yet one in nine people—some 795 million people in the world—are chronically malnourished and do not have enough food to lead a healthy life.
- One-third of all food produced (1.3 billion tons) is never consumed. This food wastage represents a missed opportunity to improve global food security in a world where one in nine is hungry.
- The majority of the world's hungry people live in developing countries. Asia is the continent with the most hungry people. Sub-Saharan Africa is the region with the highest *prevalence* (percentage of population) of hunger—where one in four people are undernourished. See the World Food Program's interactive hunger map for presentations on hunger hot spots and poverty around the world. Go to *www.wfp.org/hunger* and click on Hunger Map. Where is hunger the worst?

  - Asia: 525.6 million
  - Sub-Saharan Africa: 214 million
  - Latin America and the Caribbean: 37 million

- About 663 million people still use unimproved drinking water sources and some 2.4 billion people lack adequate sanitation. Millions of people in developing countries, most of them children, die every year from diseases associated with lack of access to safe drinking water, inadequate sanitation, poor hygiene, and overcrowding.
- According to the World Health Organization (WHO), deficiencies of iron, vitamin A, and zinc rank among the top 10 leading causes of death through disease in developing countries. Iron deficiency is the most prevalent form of malnutrition worldwide. Vitamin A deficiency produces blindness in about 500,000 children and claims the lives of almost 670,000 children age five years and younger. Approximately one-third of the world's population lives in areas of high-risk for zinc deficiency.
- More than 60% of chronically hungry people are women. Every day, approximately 1,000 women die from preventable causes related to pregnancy and childbirth. In developing countries, more than one in four newborns and their mothers do not receive skilled care during and immediately after birth.
- Empowering women is essential to global food security. Almost half of the world's farmers are women, but they lack the same tools—land rights, financing, training—that their male counterparts have, and their farms are less productive as a result.
- HIV/AIDS directly affects people's ability to provide enough food to feed themselves or their families, compromising their household's food security. By 2020, the AIDS epidemic will have claimed one-fifth or more of the agricultural labor force in most southern African countries. The World Food Programme and UNAIDS estimate that it costs an average of 66 cents per day to provide nutritional support to an AIDS patient and his or her family.
- The cost of undernutrition to national economic development is estimated at U.S.$20–30 billion per year.
- Hunger can be eliminated in our lifetimes. The *Zero Hunger Challenge*, launched by the UN Secretary General Ban ki-Moon, seeks global action around this very objective. Learn more at *www.un.org/en/zerohunger*.

Child Hunger

- Nearly 6 million children under the age of five die every year. Poor nutrition causes nearly half (45%) of deaths in children under five each year. Over two-thirds of child deaths are due to conditions that could be prevented or treated with access to simple, affordable interventions. Within countries, child mortality is higher in rural areas and among poorer and less educated families.
- In the developing world, one child in four is stunted, meaning that their physical and mental growth is impaired because of inadequate nutrition.
- The first 1,000 days of a child's life, from pregnancy through age two, are critical. Appropriate infant feeding practices in this period can protect children from the mental and physical stunting that can result from malnutrition.
- On average, about 44% of infants are exclusively breastfed. It is estimated that 1.5 million children under age five die each year because they were not breastfed, particularly not exclusively breastfed through six months of age. In general, babies who do not breastfeed are 14 times more likely to die from diarrhea or respiratory infections than babies who are exclusively breastfed in the first six months.

Sources: Food and Agriculture Organization (FAO) of the United Nations, *The State of Food Insecurity in the World*, 2015; World Health Organization, World Health Statistics 2011; United Nations World Food Programme, Hunger Stats, 2015; UN Standing Committee on Nutrition, 6th Report on the World Nutrition Situation: Progress in Nutrition, 2010; FAO News Release, 2010; World Health Organization, Fact Sheet on Children: Reducing Mortality, February 2012; Fact Sheet on HIV/AIDS, November 2011; Rehydration Project, Facts about Hunger; *The Lancet's* Series on Maternal and Child Undernutrition, 2008, *www.globalnutritionseries.org*; The International Micronutrient Malnutrition Prevention and Control (IMMPaCt) Program, Micronutrient Facts, 2012; *www.cdc.gov/immpact/micronutrients/index.html*; R. E. Black et al., Maternal and Child Nutrition: Building Momentum for Impact, *The Lancet's* Series on Maternal and Child Nutrition, 2013, *The Lancet* 382 (2013): 372–75; *UN Inter-agency Group for Child Mortality Estimation, Levels and Trends in Child Mortality Report 2011.*

Protein-energy malnutrition (PEM) PEM is the world's most widespread malnutrition problem; characterized by a depletion of both energy stores and tissue proteins; usually accompanied by micronutrient deficiencies.

Kwashiorkor Severe malnutrition caused by inadequate protein and calories leading to apathy, anemia, loss of body proteins, and poor growth.

Marasmus Severe emaciation from energy deficiency with chronic wasting of fat, muscle, and other tissues; starvation.

Malnutrition and Health Worldwide

Nearly 23% of the world's population experiences some form of malnutrition.[13] Almost 6 million children under the age of five years die each year from the parasitic and infectious diseases associated with poverty.[14] At least 75% of all child deaths are caused by neonatal disorders and a few treatable infectious diseases, such as diarrhea, pneumonia, malaria, and measles (**Figure 14-2**). These diseases interact with poor nutrition to form a vicious cycle in which the outcome for many is death, as shown in **Figure 14-3**.

More than 146 million children—one out of four children—in developing countries suffer from malnutrition (**Figure 14-4**). Protein deficiency and energy deficiency very often go hand in hand and are called **protein-energy malnutrition (PEM)**, which is the most widespread form of malnutrition in the world today. Children who are thin for their height may be suffering from acute PEM (recent severe food restriction), whereas children who are short for their age may be suffering from chronic PEM (long-term food deprivation). PEM involves a depletion of both the body's energy stores and tissue proteins, and is usually accompanied by multiple vitamin and mineral deficiencies as well. Historically, severe child malnutrition was characterized as either protein deficiency called **kwashiorkor**—the disease of the weaned child, or **marasmus**—the emaciation caused by energy deficiency. Today, child malnutrition is described in terms of chronic malnutrition—evidenced by stunting from long-term undernutrition, and

FIGURE 14-2 Top Child Killers: Causes of Child Mortality (Percentages) Globally, malnutrition contributes to a third or more of child deaths.
Source: World Health Organization, 2013.

FIGURE 14-3 The Vicious Circle of Malnutrition Malnutrition is a deadly cycle. Malnourished children are more likely to suffer from diarrhea and disease, and the more they experience diarrhea (or disease), the more likely they are to be malnourished. Inadequate nutrient intake, poor digestion, and poor absorption of nutrients leads to weight loss, a weakened immune system, and loss of appetite, which extend the disease cycle further.
Source: UNICEF.

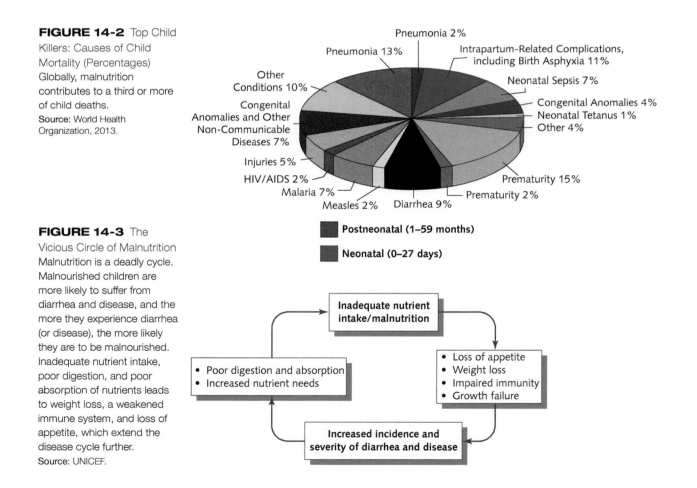

Pneumonia 2%

Pneumonia 13%

Intrapartum-Related Complications, including Birth Asphyxia 11%

Other Conditions 10%

Neonatal Sepsis 7%

Congenital Anomalies and Other Non-Communicable Diseases 7%

Congenital Anomalies 4%
Neonatal Tetanus 1%
Other 4%

Injuries 5%

HIV/AIDS 2%

Malaria 7%

Measles 2%

Diarrhea 9%

Prematurity 2%

Prematurity 15%

■ **Postneonatal (1–59 months)**

■ **Neonatal (0–27 days)**

Inadequate nutrient intake/malnutrition

• Poor digestion and absorption
• Increased nutrient needs

• Loss of appetite
• Weight loss
• Impaired immunity
• Growth failure

Increased incidence and severity of diarrhea and disease

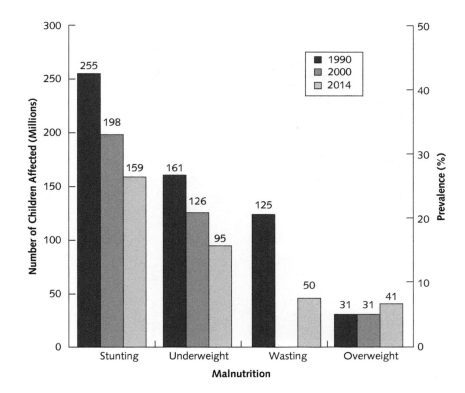

FIGURE 14-4 Trends in Percentage and Number of Children (Under Five Years of Age) with Malnutrition (1990–2014)
In developing countries, progress is being made, but millions of children are still malnourished. Between 1990 and 2014, the prevalence of stunting, underweight, wasting, and severe wasting fell, while overweight increased. Indicators of child malnutrition include:
Stunting (short-for-age): Children aged 0–59 months with a low *height-for-age* measure[a,b] (measure of linear growth); a measure of chronic malnutrition.
Underweight: Children aged 0–59 months with a low *weight-for-age*[c] (a synthesis of height-for-age and weight-for-height); reflects both stunting and wasting.
Wasting (thin-for-height): Children aged 0–59 months with a low *weight-for-height* measure[d]; a measure of acute malnutrition.
Overweight: Children aged 0–59 months whose weight-for-height is above two standard deviations (overweight) or above three standard deviations (obese) from the median of the WHO Child Growth Standards.
[a] Children who are below minus two standard deviations (−2 z-score) from median height-for-age of the WHO Child Growth Standards (see Appendix A and *www.who.int/childgrowth/en*).
[b] A z-score is the number of standard deviations (SDs) below or above the reference median value.
[c] Children who are below minus two standard deviations from median weight-for-age of the WHO Child Growth Standards.
[d] Children who are below minus two standard deviations from median weight-for-height of the WHO Child Growth Standards.
Source: The United Nations Children's Fund, the World Health Organization, and the World Bank, Levels & Trends in Child Malnutrition: UNICEF–WHO–The World Bank Joint Child Malnutrition Estimates, 2014; World Health Organization, *WHO Child Growth Standards: Length/Height-for-Age, Weight-for-Age, Weight-for-Length, Weight-for-Height and Body Mass Index-for-Age: Methods and Development* (Geneva, World Health Organization, 2006).

severe acute malnutrition—characterized by rapid weight loss, nutritional edema, and wasting from recent or sudden food deprivation or illness (diarrhea, infection).[15]

Apathy is one of the earliest signs of PEM. As PEM progresses, all growth ceases, and the child is no larger at age four than at age two. As the protein and energy deficits worsen, new hair grows without the protein pigment that gives hair its color. The skin also loses its color, and open sores fail to heal. Digestive enzymes are in short supply, the digestive tract lining deteriorates, and absorption fails. The child can't assimilate what little food is eaten. Proteins and hormones that previously kept the fluids correctly distributed among the compartments of the body now are diminished, so that fluid leaks out of the blood

This child has the characteristic edema and swollen belly often seen with kwashiorkor.

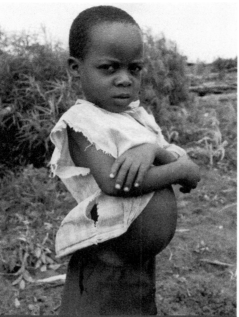

Stephen Dorey ABIPP/Alamy

This child is suffering from the extreme emaciation of marasmus.

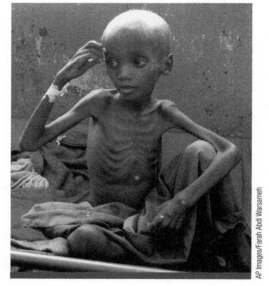

AP Images/Farah Abdi Warsameh

Severe acute malnutrition (SAM) SAM is characterized by very low weight-for-height (below −3 z-scores, or −3 standard deviations [SDs], of the median of the WHO Child Growth Standards), by visible severe wasting, and/or by the presence of nutritional edema associated with recent severe food deprivation. *Moderate acute malnutrition* in children is defined as weight-for-height between −3 and −2 z-scores of the median of the WHO Child Growth Standards without edema. *Note*: A z-score is the number of standard deviations (SDs) below or above the reference median value.

(edema) and accumulates in the belly and legs. Blood proteins, including hemoglobin, are not synthesized, so the child becomes anemic, which increases the child's weakness and apathy. Antibodies to fight off invading bacteria are degraded to provide amino acids for other uses; hence, the child becomes an easy target for any infection. The child is often sick because his or her resistance to disease is low. Measles, which might make a healthy child sick for a week or two, can kill the malnourished child within two or three days.

Worldwide, four micronutrient deficiencies are of particular concern: vitamin A deficiency, the world's most common cause of preventable child blindness and vision impairment; iron-deficiency anemia; iodine deficiency, which causes high levels of goiter and mental retardation; and zinc deficiency.[16]

- *Vitamin A deficiency.* More than 140 million preschool children are affected by vitamin A deficiency (VAD). Of these, an estimated 500,000 children become partially or totally blind as a result of insufficient vitamin A in the diet. Vitamin A deficiency compromises the immune systems of approximately 40% of the developing world's under-5s and leads to the early deaths of an estimated 1 million young children each year. This chapter's Programs in Action highlights the international activities that target vitamin A deficiency.

  - *Progress report:* More than 40 developing countries are now reaching 70% or more of their young children with at least one vitamin A supplement capsule every year. Coverage providing two doses is significantly lower, but the effort to date is estimated to be saving the lives of more than 300,000 young children a year and preventing many hundreds of thousands of cases of irreversible blindness.

- *Iron deficiency.* Iron-deficiency anemia is estimated to affect some 1.6 billion people. Iron deficiency in infancy and early childhood is associated with decreased cognitive abilities and resistance to disease. Iron deficiency in the 6- to 24-month age group impairs the mental development of 40–60% of the developing world's children. Severe iron-deficiency anemia causes the deaths of an estimated 50,000 young women a year in pregnancy and childbirth. Iron deficiency in adults is so widespread that it lowers the productivity of workforces—with estimated losses of up to 2% of GDP in the worst affected countries.

  - *Progress report:* An international movement to fortify all wheat flour with iron and folic acid is beginning to gain momentum. Indonesia, Jordan, Nigeria, and South Africa have recently acted, bringing to 49 the total number of countries adding iron to flour. Many more developing countries have begun the process of fortifying other staple foods and condiments—from salt, sugar, and margarine to noodles, cooking oil, and soy sauce—with essential vitamins and minerals.

- *Iodine deficiency.* Iodine deficiency, the major preventable cause of mental retardation worldwide, is risk factor for both physical and mental retardation in about 780 million people. About 700 million people worldwide—especially in mountainous regions—are estimated to have goiter, and more than 16 million suffer from overt cretinism. Iodine deficiency in pregnancy causes as many as 20 million babies a year to be born mentally impaired.

  - *Progress report:* The global prevalence of iodine deficiency has been halved from 30% to 15%. This has been brought about by a sustained effort to add iodine to the world's household salt. UNICEF supports salt iodization efforts around the world, including programs like the Smart Salt campaign led by the Ghana Health Service. The Ghana program achieved success educating the community (especially parents) using a radio campaign and other activities in schools and clinics to raise awareness regarding the benefits of iodine. Salt traders were given iodine kits to test salt sold by the many small-scale salt producers and refused to purchase non-iodized salt. As a result, salt producers had a commercial incentive to comply. The number of community households with adequate levels of iodized salt increased from 24% to 63% in a two-year period.[17]

- *Zinc deficiency.* Zinc deficiency contributes to growth failure and weakened immunity in young children; it results in some 800,000 child deaths per year from extreme diarrhea, pneumonia, and malaria.[18] Zinc deficiency is typically the result of inadequate dietary intake, as children in the developing world have mainly plant-based diets, which are often low in zinc.

  - *Progress report:* Research demonstrates the usefulness of zinc supplements in treating diarrhea and reducing diarrheal mortality by 50%. The World Health Organization issued a joint statement with UNICEF recommending use of zinc for 10–14 days for all episodes of diarrhea among children under age five. However, the recommendation has not yet been widely adopted.[19]

The malnutrition that comes from living with food insecurity is one of the major factors influencing life expectancy. According to the *2015 State of the World's Children Report*, life expectancy at birth is 79 years in the United States and about 81 years in Canada.[20] Worldwide, life expectancy averages about 71 years, but in sub-Saharan Africa it is approximately 57 years. In countries heavily affected by HIV/AIDS, life expectancy ranges from 48 years in Botswana, to the lowest of all—only 46 years—in Sierra Leone.

Hunger and malnutrition can be found in people of all ages, sexes, and nationalities. Even so, these problems hit some groups harder than others.

" The global community should be outraged by the millions of children that either die or are disabled each year because of malnutrition. We know how to prevent and treat it. The missing link is the political will to place nutrition squarely on the development agenda and to commit the necessary resources to implement programs, particularly food fortification, that we know can deliver sustainable improvements not only to the current generation of people at risk but to the lives of generations to come. "

—Marc Van Ameringen, Executive Director, Global Alliance for Improved Nutrition (GAIN)

Effects of Malnutrition on Those Most Vulnerable

When nutrient needs are high (as in times of rapid growth), the risk of undernutrition increases. If family food is limited, pregnant and lactating women, infants, and children are the first to show the signs of undernutrition. The effects of food insecurity can be devastating to these segments of the population.

What is a life worth? Infants and young children can be the first to show the signs of undernutrition due to their high nutrient needs. More than 6 million children less than five years of age died in 2015—some 16,000 every day (11 every minute). Malnutrition is an underlying cause of a third or more of children's deaths—over 2 million every year. More than half of these children die during the first month of life, usually at home and without access to essential health services and basic commodities that might save their lives.

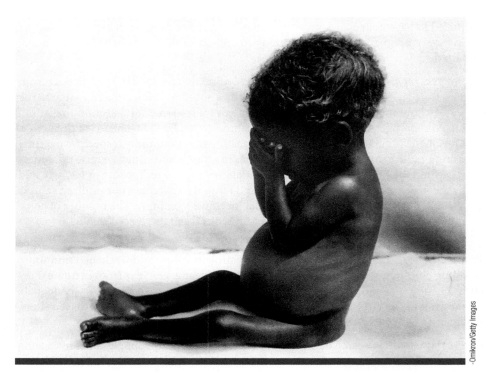

Omikron/Getty Images

As we noted in Chapter 11, women must gain adequate weight during pregnancy to support normal fetal growth and development. Healthy women in developed countries gain an average of about 27 pounds. Studies among poor women reveal that they have an average weight gain of only 11–15 pounds. In some areas, women may have caloric deficits of up to 42% and do not gain any weight at all during pregnancy.[21] As a consequence, they give birth to babies with low birthweights.

Birthweight is a potent indicator of an infant's future health status. A low-birthweight baby (less than 5.5 pounds, or 2,500 grams) is more likely to experience complications during delivery than a baby of normal weight and has a statistically greater-than-normal chance of exhibiting stunted physical and cognitive growth during childhood, contracting diseases, and dying early in life. More than 14% of infants born between 2009 and 2013 in developing countries had low birthweights [22] Low birthweight contributes to more than half of the deaths of children under five years of age.

Almost one-third of all children in developing countries are stunted—suffering from chronic undernutrition. If stunting occurs during the first five years of life, the physical and cognitive impairments are usually irreversible.[23] Mortality statistics reflect the hazards to those most vulnerable. The **infant mortality rate** ranges from about 8 (Costa Rica) to 107 (Sierra Leone) in the poorest of the developing countries. The death rate for children from one to five years of age is no more favorable; it ranges from 10 to 30 times higher in developing countries than in developed countries.[24] Maternal mortality rates depicted in **Figure 14-5** are equally shocking.

UNICEF regards the **under-5 mortality rate (U5MR)** as the single best indicator of children's overall health and well-being (**Figure 14-6**).[25] UNICEF argues that this rate reflects the overall resources a country directs at children:

> The U5MR reflects the nutritional health and the health knowledge of mothers; the level of immunization and ORT (oral rehydration therapy) use; the availability of maternal and health services (including prenatal care); income and food availability in the family; the availability of safe drinking water and basic sanitation; and the overall safety of the child's environment.[26]

The Economic Burden of Malnutrition and Hunger

The "grim tally of human lives cut short or scarred by disability leaves no doubt that hunger is morally unacceptable," states the FAO in *The State of Food Insecurity in the World.*[27] However, calculating the economic costs of hunger shows that it is also unaffordable—not only to those affected by hunger but also to the future development of the countries in which they live.

The burden of hunger includes both direct and indirect costs. The most obvious are the direct health-related expenses associated with maternal complications in pregnancy and with the poor health of low-birthweight babies and malnourished children, who are at increased risk of conditions such as diarrhea, measles, malaria, and pneumonia, as well as chronic diseases. A very rough estimate indicates that these direct costs add up to about $30 billion per year.[28]

The indirect costs of hunger include lost productivity and income caused by problems associated with chronic hunger: premature death, disability, absenteeism in the workplace, and reduced educational and occupational opportunities.[29] The FAO estimates these indirect costs to be hundreds of billions of dollars. Studies that measure the impact of malnutrition on physical and mental development have established correlations with reduced productivity and earnings. Every child whose physical and mental development is stunted by hunger and malnutrition stands to lose 5–10% or more in lifetime earnings.

Every year that hunger persists at current levels will cost developing countries future productivity of $500 billion from lives lost to disease or disability.[30] On the other hand, UNICEF estimates that most child malnutrition in the developing world could be eliminated with the expenditure of an additional $24 billion a year.[31] This amount would cover the cost of the

Infant mortality rate (IMR) Infant deaths under one year of age, expressed as a rate per 1,000 live births.

UNICEF The United Nations International Children's Emergency Fund, now referred to as the United Nations Children's Fund.

Under-5 mortality rate (U5MR) The number of children who die before the age of five for every 1,000 live births.

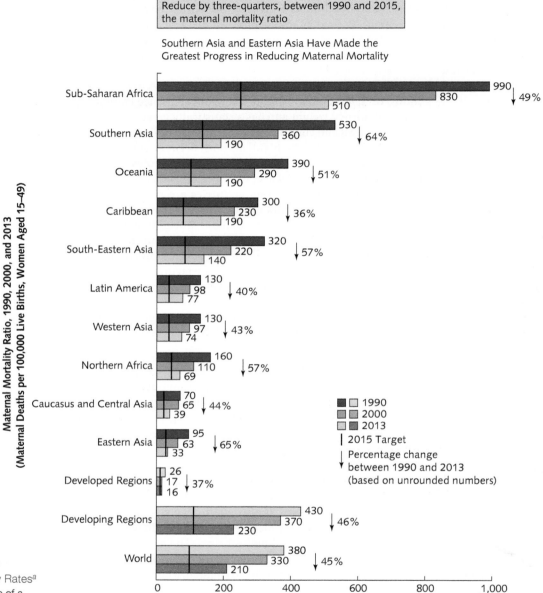

FIGURE 14-5

Maternal Mortality Rates[a]
The lifetime chance of a woman dying in pregnancy or childbirth in a least-developed country is almost 300 times greater than for a woman in an industrialized country.

[a] Annual number of maternal deaths from pregnancy-related causes per 100,000 live births.

Source: L. Jensen, editor, *The Millennium Development Goals Report 2015* (New York: United Nations, 2015).

resources needed to control the major childhood diseases, halve the rate of child malnutrition, bring clean water and safe sanitation to all communities, make family planning services universally available, and provide almost every child with at least a basic education.[32]

The World Bank estimates that the total cost of tackling malnutrition in the 36 countries that account for 90% of child malnutrition would be approximately $10–12 billion a year.[33]*

---

* The 36 countries that carry 90% of the burden of malnutrition: Afghanistan, Angola, Bangladesh, Burkina Faso, Burundi, Cambodia, Cameroon, Côte d'Ivoire, Democratic Republic of Congo, Egypt, Ethiopia, Ghana, Guatemala, India, Indonesia, Iraq, Kenya, Madagascar, Malawi, Mali, Mozambique, Myanmar, Nepal, Niger, Nigeria, Pakistan, Peru, Philippines, South Africa, Sudan, Tanzania, Turkey, Uganda, Vietnam, Republic of Yemen, and Zambia.

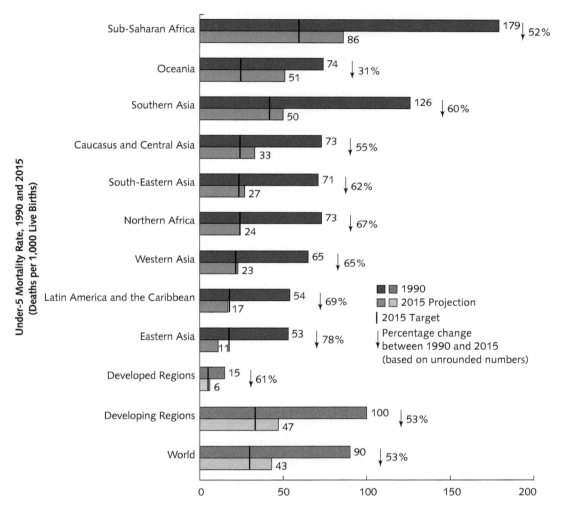

This amount would cover the cost of scaling up a minimal package of 13 cost-effective nutrition interventions from current coverage levels to full coverage of the target populations in the 36 countries (**Table 14-2**). These measures include improved maternal nutrition, improved breastfeeding practices, micronutrient and deworming interventions, and complementary and therapeutic feeding interventions.[34] Adding another 32 smaller countries with levels of stunting and/or underweight exceeding 20% would increase this cost estimate by only 6%.**

** Additional 32 countries with underweight or stunting rates > 20%: Albania, Bhutan, Bolivia, Botswana, Central African Republic, Comoros, Republic of Congo, Ecuador, Equatorial Guinea, Eritrea, Djibouti, Gambia, Guinea, Guinea-Bissau, Haiti, Honduras, Lesotho, Liberia, Maldives, Mauritania, Mongolia, Namibia, Rwanda, São Tomé and Príncipe, Sierra Leone, Somalia, Sri Lanka, Swaziland, Tajikistan, Timor-Leste, Togo, and Zimbabwe.

FIGURE 14-6

Under-5 Mortality Rate, 1990 and 2015 Achieving the goal for child survival hinges on action to address the leading causes of death.
Source: L. Jensen, editor, *The Millennium Development Goals Report 2015* (New York: United Nations, 2015).

TABLE 14-2 Examples of Thirteen Cost-Effective Interventions to Reduce Malnutrition

TYPE OF INTERVENTION	EXAMPLE OF INTERVENTION OR PRACTICE	TARGET POPULATION	METHOD OF DELIVERY
Behavior Change Interventions			
1. **Breastfeeding promotion and support**	• Early initiation of breastfeeding • Exclusive breastfeeding for six months and continued breastfeeding until two years of age	Pregnant women and parents of infants under six months of age	Community nutrition programs; health system; social marketing
2. **Promotion of complementary feeding**	Delivery of educational messages	Pregnant women and parents of infants and young children under two years of age	Community nutrition programs; health system; social marketing
3. **Safe hygiene behaviors, including handwashing with soap**	Delivery of educational messages	Entire population	Social marketing
Micronutrient Supplementation and Deworming Interventions			
4. **Vitamin A supplementation**	Semi-annual doses for children	Children six months to five years of age	Vitamin A outreach campaigns; health system
5. **Therapeutic zinc supplements**	As part of diarrhea management	Children six months to five years of age	Community nutrition programs; health system; social marketing; market system
6. **Supplements for pregnant women**	• Iron–folic acid supplements • Calcium supplements	Pregnant women	Community nutrition programs; outreach programs; health system
7. **Deworming (to reduce loss of micronutrients)**	Treat with deworming drugs (one or two rounds per year)	Children six months to five years of age	Community nutrition programs; outreach programs; health system
Home and Community Food Fortification Interventions			
8. **Home and community food fortification**	• Multiple micronutrient powders (sachets or "Sprinkles")[a] for in-home fortification of complementary foods • Ready-to-use supplementary[b] feeding (RUSF) (e.g., Plumpy'Doz®); intended to be an adjunct to the diet; provides energy with the full daily requirement of micronutrients	Children age 6–24 months and pregnant women; or may provide the complete recommended nutrient intake for children age six months to five years of age	Community nutrition programs; health system; market systems

Ready-to-use supplementary foods (RUSF) such as Plumpy'Doz™ are intended to compensate for deficiencies of the traditional diet of infants and young children—6 to 36 months of age—who are at risk of acute malnutrition. Plumpy'Doz™ contains micronutrients, proteins, and essential fatty acids and can help reduce the incidence of acute malnutrition in high food insecurity regions. Plumpy'Doz™ is designed to be eaten in small quantities, as a supplement to the regular diet.

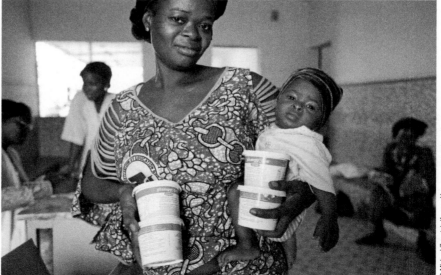

© Michael Zimstein/Agence Vu

TABLE 14-2 Examples of Thirteen Cost-Effective Interventions to Reduce Malnutrition—*continued*

TYPE OF INTERVENTION	EXAMPLE OF INTERVENTION OR PRACTICE	TARGET POPULATION	METHOD OF DELIVERY
Mass or Universal Fortification[c] Interventions			
9. **Iron fortification of staples**	Iron fortification of staples (e.g., flour, rice, oil, condiments)	Entire population	Market systems; social marketing
10. **Salt iodization**	Salt iodization	Entire population	Market systems
11. **Iodine supplements**	Iodized oil capsules	Pregnant women in highly endemic areas if iodized salt is not available	Community nutrition programs; outreach programs; health system
Complementary and Therapeutic Feeding Interventions			
12. **Prevention or treatment of moderate malnutrition (underweight)**	• Screening to determine circumstances in which food supplementation is needed • Provision of complementary foods	Populations with high prevalence of children 6–24 months with low weight-for-age measures	Community nutrition programs; health system; market system (coupons)
13. **Treatment of severe acute malnutrition (severe wasting)**	• Screening to identify cases of severe acute malnutrition • Therapeutic feeding with high-energy, fortified, ready-to-use therapeutic foods (RUTF)[d] (e.g., Plumpy'Nut®)	Children six months to five years of age with very low weight-for-height measures	Community nutrition programs; health system

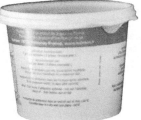

© Michael Zumstein/Agence Vu

[a] Large-scale distribution has been limited to a small number of countries thus far, but the number of sachets bought and supplied by UNICEF and the World Food Programme (WFP) increased from just over 50 million in 2008 to around 350 million in 2010.

[b] Home fortification is recommended where children have low dietary diversity or when a child has infectious diseases or worm infestation.

[c] Biofortification is the development of staple crops that are rich in micronutrients through traditional or conventional agricultural breeding practices or through modern biotechnology. Biofortification is an area in need of further research, including whether farmers would accept the new technology and whether consumers would buy and eat biofortified foods. An example is the large-scale introduction in Mozambique of the orange-flesh sweet potato, which is rich in vitamin A. Other commercial or market-driven fortification involves food companies voluntarily fortifying products, such as cereals or porridge for infants and young children, within regulatory limits set by the national government.

[d] Plumpy–Nut® is a ready-to-use therapeutic spread packaged in individual sachets of 500 calories each. It is a paste of groundnut composed of vegetable fat, peanut butter, skimmed milk powder, sugar, minerals, and vitamins.

Sources: Adapted from United Nations Standing Committee on Nutrition, *Scaling Up Nutrition: A Framework for Action* (Geneva: United Nations Standing Committee on Nutrition, 2010); S. Horton, M. Shekar, C. McDonald, A. Mahal, and J. K. Brooks, *Scaling Up Nutrition: What Will It Cost?* (Washington, D.C.: The International Bank for Reconstruction and Development, 2010); Save the Children, *A Life Free from Hunger: Tackling Child Malnutrition* (Westport, CT: The Save the Children Fund, 2012).

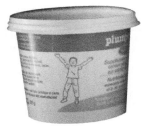

© Michael Zumstein/Agence Vu

Ready-to-use supplementary feedings (RUSF) are energy- and nutrient-dense with essential fats and recommended micronutrients. One example is Plumpy'Doz®, which has about 245 calories per recommended dose and comes in tubs containing a weekly ration. It contains peanut paste, vegetable fat, skimmed milk powder, whey, maltodextrins, and sugar.

Food Insecurity in Developing Countries

FIGURE 14-7 Causes of Global Food Insecurity and Malnutrition

Source: Adapted from *The State of the World's Children* 1990 (Oxford, UK: Oxford University Press, 1990); M. Ruel, "Addressing the Underlying Determinants of Undernutrition: Examples of Successful Integration of Nutrition in Poverty-Reduction and Agriculture Strategies," *SCN News* 36 (2008): 21–29; Save the Children, *A Life Free from Hunger: Tackling Child Malnutrition* (Westport, CT: The Save the Children Fund, 2012).

Global food insecurity is more extreme than domestic food insecurity. In fact, most people would find it hard to imagine the severity of poverty in the developing world:

> Many hundreds of millions of people in the poorest countries are preoccupied solely with survival and elementary needs. For them, work is frequently not available or pay is low, and conditions barely tolerable. Homes are constructed of impermanent materials and have neither piped water nor sanitation. Electricity is a luxury. Health services are thinly spread, and in rural areas only rarely within walking distance. Permanent insecurity is the condition of the poor. . . . In the wealthy countries, ordinary men and women face genuine economic problems. . . . But they rarely face anything resembling the total deprivation found in the poor countries.[35]

Figure 14-7 shows some of the many causes of global food insecurity and malnutrition. Global food insecurity is a problem of supply and demand, inappropriate technology, environmental abuse, demographic distribution, unequal access to resources, extremes

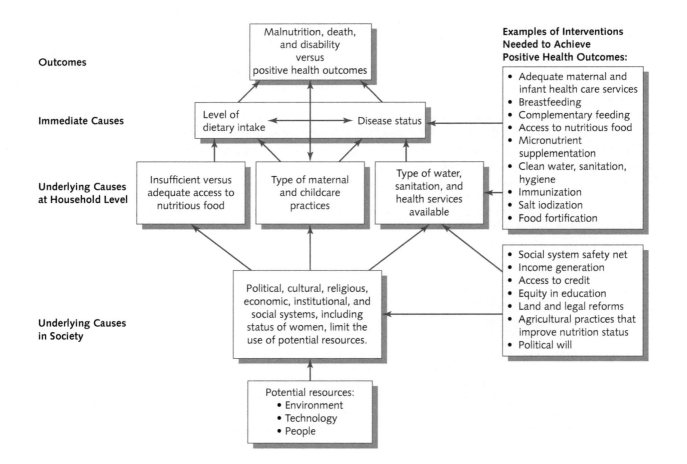

in dietary patterns, and unjust economic systems. Two generalizations and an important question are suggested by Figure 14-7:

- The underlying causes of global food insecurity and poverty are complex and interrelated.
- Food insecurity is a product of poverty resulting from the ways in which governments and businesses manage national and international economies.
- The question, then, is "Why are people poor?"

Poverty contributes to hunger and food insecurity in many important ways. Often, people who are poor are powerless to change their situation because they have little access to vital resources such as education, training, food, health services, and other vehicles of change. The roots of hunger and poverty, like those of many other current problems, can be found in numerous historical and natural developments, including colonialism, economic institutions, corporate systems, population pressure, resource distribution, and agricultural technology.

The Role of Colonialism

The colonial era led to hunger and malnutrition for millions of people in developing countries. Although no longer called colonialism, much of this same activity still continues today. The African experience provides a good example of the colonial process. Britain, the Netherlands, Germany, France, and other nations originally colonized the African continent largely to gain a source of raw materials for industrial use. Accordingly, the colonial powers created a governing infrastructure designed merely to move Africa's minerals, metals, cash crops, and wealth to Europe. They provided few opportunities for education, disrupted traditional family structures and community organization, and greatly diminished the ability of the African people to produce their own food.

Before the Europeans arrived, small landowners throughout much of Africa had cleared forests to grow beans, grains, or vegetables for their own use. With colonialism, wealthy Africans and foreign investors took over the fertile farmland and forced the rural poor onto marginal lands that could produce adequate food only with irrigation and fertilizer, which were beyond the means of the poor. The fertile lands were used to grow cotton, sesame, sugar, cocoa, coffee, tea, tobacco, and livestock for export. As more raw materials were exported, more food and manufactured products had to be imported. Imported goods cost money—also beyond the reach of the poor.

Per capita production of grains for food use has declined for the last 30 years in Africa, while sugar cane production has doubled and tea production has quadrupled. The country of Chad recently harvested a record cotton crop in the same year that it experienced an epidemic of famine. Sixty percent of the gross national product of Ghana, Sudan, Somalia, Ethiopia, Zambia, and Malawi is derived from cash crops that finance both luxury imported goods for the minority and international debts. Huge amounts of soybeans and grains are fed to livestock to produce protein foods that the poor cannot afford to purchase.

International Trade and Debt

Over the years, developing countries have seen the prices of imported fuels and manufactured items rise much faster than the prices they receive for their export goods—such as bananas, coffee, and various raw materials—on the international market. The combination of high import costs and low export profits often pushes a developing country into accelerating international debt that sometimes leads to bankruptcy.

Debt and trade are closely related to the progress a country can make toward achieving adequate diets for its people. As import prices increase relative to export prices, a country's money "moves abroad" to pay for the imports. With more and more of its money abroad, the country is forced to borrow money, usually at high interest rates, to continue functioning at home. Many of its financial resources must then go to pay the interest on the borrowed money, thus draining the economy further. Creditor nations may not demand much, or any, capital back, but they do require that interest be paid each year, and the interest can consume most of a country's gross national product. Large and growing debts can slow or halt a nation's attempt to deal effectively with its problems of local food insecurity. As more and more of its financial resources are used to pay interest on the country's trade debts, less and less money is available to deal with food insecurity at home.[36] Each year, the debt crisis worsens and leads to further problems with hunger.

Since 2000, 27 countries have benefited from some debt relief under the Heavily Indebted Poor Countries (HIPC) Initiative—a collaborative effort between the World Bank and other financial institutions.[37] This initiative has identified one of the key steps in solving debtor countries' hunger problems. Once the tremendous financial drain caused by their international debt is eliminated, the countries can choose to allocate more financial resources for the tasks of developing the infrastructure, agriculture, and other types of development that would lead to less hunger, such as investments in education, health, nutrition, water supply, and sanitation. Enhancing market access to help countries diversify and expand trade is also necessary.[38]

The Role of Multinational Corporations

Multinational corporations Transnational companies (TNC) with direct investments and/or operative facilities in more than one country. U.S. oil and food companies are examples.

National economic policies in the developing countries based on the export of cash crops, such as coffee, often have a negative effect on household food security. The competition between cash crops and food crops for farmland provides a classic example of the plight of the poor. Typically, the fertile farmlands are controlled by large landowners and **multinational corporations** that hire indigenous people for below-subsistence wages to grow crops to be exported for profit, leaving little fertile land for the local farmers to grow food. The local people work hard cultivating cash crops for others, not food crops for themselves. The money they earn is not even enough to buy the products they help produce. As a result, imported foods—bananas, beef, cocoa, coconuts, coffee, pineapples, sugar, tea, winter tomatoes, and the like—fill the grocery stores of developed countries, while the poor who labored to grow these foods have less food and fewer resources than when they farmed the land for their own use. Additional cropland is diverted for nonfood cash crops such as tobacco, rubber, and cotton. These practices have also had an adverse effect on many U.S. farmers. The foreign cash crops often undersell the same U.S.-grown produce. The U.S. farmers cannot compete with these lower-priced imported foods, so they may be forced out of business.

Export-oriented agriculture thus consumes the labor, land, capital, and technology that is needed to help local families produce their own food. For example, the resources used to produce bananas for export could be reallocated to provide food for the local people. Some have suggested that the developed countries could help alleviate the world food problem not by *giving* more food aid to the poor countries, but by *taking* less food away from them.[39]

Countless examples can be cited to illustrate how natural resources are diverted from producing food for domestic consumption to producing luxury crops for those who can afford them:

- Africa is a net *exporter* of barley, beans, peanuts, fresh vegetables, and cattle (not to mention luxury crops such as coffee and cocoa), yet 40% of Africans cannot obtain sufficient food on a day-to-day basis, and Africa has a high incidence of protein-energy malnutrition among young children.[40]

- Over half of the U.S. supply of several winter and early spring vegetables comes from Mexico, where infant deaths associated with poor nutrition are common.
- Half of the agricultural land in Central America produces food for export, while in several Central American countries, the poorest 50% of the population eat only half the protein they need.[41]

Besides diverting acreage from the traditional staples of the local diet, some multinational corporations also contribute to hunger through their marketing techniques. Their advertisements lead many consumers with limited incomes to associate products such as cola beverages, cigarettes, infant formulas, and snack foods with Western culture and prosperity. A poor family's nutrition status suffers when its tight budget is pinched further by the purchase of such goods.

The Role of Overpopulation

The current world population is approximately 7.3 billion, and the United Nations projects that it will reach 9 billion by the year 2050. Earth may not be able to support this many people adequately.[42] The world's present population is certainly of concern, as is the projected increase in that population. Nevertheless, population is only one aspect of the world food problem. Poverty seems to be at the root of both problems—food insecurity and overpopulation.

Three major factors affect population growth: birth rates, death rates, and standards of living. The transition of population growth rates from a slow-growth stage (high birth rates and high death rates) through a rapid-growth stage (high birth rates and low death rates) to a low-growth stage (low birth rates and low death rates) is known as the demographic transition. Low-income countries have high birth rates, high death rates, and low standards of living. When people's standard of living rises, giving them better access to health care, family planning, and education, the death rate falls. In time, the birth rate also falls. As the standard of living continues to improve, the family earns sufficient income to risk having smaller numbers of children. A family depends on its children to cultivate the land, secure food and water, and provide for the adults in their old age. Under conditions of ongoing poverty, parents will choose to have many children to ensure that some will survive to adulthood. Children represent the "social security" of the poor. Improvements in economic status help relieve the need for this "insurance" and so help reduce the birth rate. The relationships between the infant mortality rate and the population growth rate reveal that hunger and poverty reflect both the level of national development and the people's sense of security.[43]

In many countries where economic growth has occurred and all groups share resources relatively equally, the rate of population growth has decreased. Examples include Costa Rica, Sri Lanka, Taiwan, and Malaysia. In countries where economic growth has occurred but the resources are unevenly distributed, population growth has remained high. Examples include Mexico, the Philippines, and Thailand, where a large family continues to be a major economic asset for the poor.[44]

As the world's population continues to grow, it threatens the world's capacity to produce adequate food in the future. The activity of billions of human beings on Earth's limited surface is seriously and adversely affecting our planet: wiping out many varieties of plant life, using up our freshwater supplies, and destroying the protective ozone layer that shields life from the sun's damaging rays—in short, overtaxing Earth's ability to support life.[45] Population control is one of the most pressing needs of this time in history. Until the nations of the world resolve the population problem, they must all deal with its effects and make efforts to support the life of the populations that currently exist.

Distribution of Resources

Land reform—giving people a meaningful opportunity to produce food for local consumption, for example—can combine with population control to increase everyone's assets. However, in much of the developing world, control over land and other assets is highly inequitable. Resources are distributed unequally not only between the rich and the poor within nations, but also between rich and poor nations.

Developing nations must be allowed to increase their agricultural productivity. Much is involved, but to put it simply, poor nations must gain greater access to five things simultaneously: land, capital, water, technology, and knowledge.[46] Increasing people's access to assets, including credit, is also essential to ending hunger (**Figure 14-8**). A number of microcredit initiatives, such as the Grameen Bank in Bangladesh, offer small loans to help very poor women generate income through small-scale projects such as basket weaving and chicken raising. As the microenterprise income raises the women out of poverty, nutritional benefits can be seen. For example, their children have increased arm circumferences and their daughters are more likely to be enrolled in school.[47] Equally important, each nation must make improving the condition of all its people a political priority. International food aid may be required temporarily during the development period, but eventually this aid will be less and less necessary.

FIGURE 14-8

Breaking Out of the Cycle of Despair

Source: Adapted from Bread for the World Institute, *Hunger 1996: Causes of Hunger* (Silver Spring, MD: Bread for the World Institute, 1995), 91.

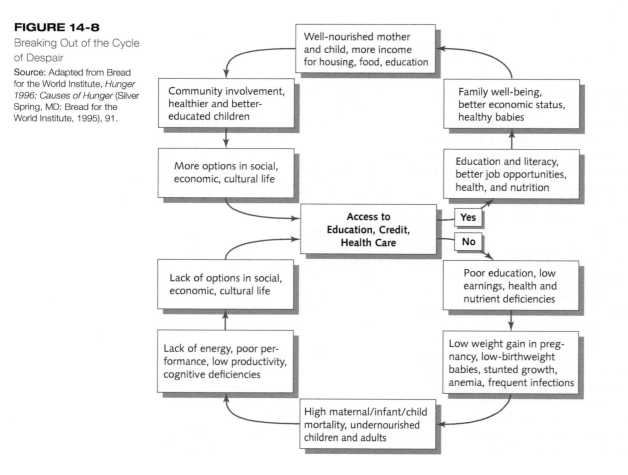

Agricultural Technology

Governments can learn from recent history the importance of developing local agricultural technology. A major effort made in the 1960s and 1970s—the **green revolution**—demonstrated both the potential for increased grain production in Asia and the necessity of considering local conditions. The industrial world made an effort to bring its agricultural technology to the developing countries, but the high-yielding strains of wheat and rice that were selected required irrigation, chemical fertilizers, and pesticides—all costly and beyond the economic means of many of the farmers in the developing world.

International research centers need to examine the conditions of developing countries and orient their research toward **appropriate technology**—labor-intensive rather than energy-intensive agricultural methods. Instead of transplanting industrial technology to the developing countries, small, efficient farms and local structures for marketing, credit, transportation, food storage, and agricultural education should be developed.

For example, labor-intensive technology, such as the use of manual grinders for grains, is appropriate in some places because it makes the best use of human, financial, and natural resources. A manual grinder can process 20 pounds of grain per hour, replacing the mortar and pestle, which can grind a maximum of only 3 pounds in the same time.[48] The specific technology that is appropriate for use varies from situation to situation.

Biotechnology and Genetically Modified Food

Biotechnology may result in the development of drought-tolerant crop varieties with increased yield and resistance to pests, herbicides, and plant diseases. Some researchers believe that a form of plant biotechnology known as **genetic engineering** may also help mitigate problems of malnutrition by enhancing the nutritional content of staple foods, such as rice high in beta-carotene and iron.[49] However, more research is needed to determine the long-term environmental and health effects of the large-scale utilization of genetically modified (GM) crops.

GM crops grown by U.S. farmers include corn, cotton, soybeans, alfalfa, canola, squash, sugar beet, and papaya. In the United States, 94% of soybean acreage, 93% of cotton, 86% of corn, and 95% of sugar beet are planted with GM varieties.[50] The five developing countries with the most acreage in GM crops are China (cotton, papaya, poplar, tomato, sweet pepper), India (cotton), Brazil (soybeans, corn, cotton), Argentina (soybeans, corn, cotton), and South Africa (corn, soybeans, cotton).[51] In Europe, no genetically modified fruits or vegetables are approved for commercial use.

The introduction of GM food has been controversial. Some people are concerned about the potential impact of an organism that would not have evolved under normal conditions. We cannot know the long-term environmental consequences as these GM plants multiply and mutate. Some people believe that naturally occurring cross-pollination between GM plants with nearby weeds may spread traits from plants to weeds. Potentially, this so-called "superweed" would be resistant to insects and herbicides.

People with food allergies express concern that new varieties of food produced by transgenetics may introduce allergens not found in the food before it was altered. Indeed, researchers have shown that allergens can be transferred through bioengineering, as in one case where an allergenic protein showed up in soybeans that had been genetically altered with proteins from Brazil nuts.[52]

Another widely debated issue surrounding genetic engineering involves labeling. Many consumer groups have called for across-the-board labels on GM foods. But according to the FDA, with some exceptions, the food must carry distinct consequences to consumers who eat it before it requires special labeling. When genes from peanuts

Green revolution
The development and widespread adoption of high-yielding strains of wheat and rice in developing countries. The term *green revolution* is also used to describe almost any package of modern agricultural technology delivered to developing countries.

Appropriate technology
A technology that utilizes locally abundant resources in preference to locally scarce resources. Developing countries usually have a large labor force and little capital; the appropriate technology would therefore be labor-intensive.

Biotechnology The use of biological systems or living organisms to make or modify products. Includes traditional methods used in making products such as wine, beer, yogurt, and cheese; cross-breeding to enhance crop production; and modification of living plants, animals, and fish through the manipulation of genes (the latter is called genetic engineering).

Genetic engineering
A form of biotechnology in which a plant's genes are altered in an effort to create a new plant with different traits; in some cases, a plant's gene(s) may be deleted or altered, or a gene(s) may be introduced from different organisms or species. The foods or crops produced are called genetically modified (GM) or genetically engineered (GE).

and other foods known to be common causes of allergies are put into a food, the label must indicate that the food contains an allergen, unless the manufacturer can prove that the item's potential to cause allergies has not been transferred via the gene. In addition, a food that has been genetically engineered to significantly change, say, its fiber content or nutrient composition, must bear a label that states the nature of the change.[53] A number of petitions currently calling for labeling of foods with GM ingredients may lead to FDA approval of required labeling for these foods in the future.[54] The accompanying box highlights some of the potential benefits and risks associated with genetically altered crops.[55]

Risks versus Benefits: The Debate over Genetically Modified (GM) Foods and Crops

Potential Benefits of GM Foods and Crops

- **Increased nutritional value of staple foods:** Genes can be inserted into rice to make it produce beta-carotene, which the body converts into vitamin A. This transgenic "golden rice" has the potential to reduce vitamin A deficiency, a leading cause of blindness and a significant factor in many child deaths.
- **Reduced environmental impact:** Scientists are developing trees with modified cell lignin content. When used to make pulp and paper, the modified wood requires less processing with harsh chemicals.
- **Increased fish yield:** Researchers have modified the gene that governs growth hormones in tilapia, a farmed fish, offering the prospect of increased yield and greater availability of fish protein in local diets.
- **Increased nutrient absorption by livestock:** Animal feed under development will improve animals' absorption of phosphorus. This reduces the phosphorus in animal waste, which pollutes groundwater.
- **Tolerance of poor environmental conditions:** Scientists are working to produce transgenic crops that are drought-resistant or salt-tolerant, allowing the crops to be grown on marginal land.

Potential Risks of GM Foods and Crops

- **Inadequate controls:** Although safety regimens are being improved, control over GM crop releases is not completely effective. In 2000, for example, a maize variety cleared only for animal consumption was found in food products.
- **Transfer of allergens:** Allergens can be transferred inadvertently from an existing to a target organism, and new allergens can be created. For example, when a Brazil nut gene was transferred to soybean, tests found that a known allergen had also been transferred. However, the danger was detected in testing, and the soybean was not released.
- **Unpredictability:** GM crops may have unforeseen effects on farming systems—for example, by taking more resources from the soil or using more water than normal crops.
- **Undesired gene movement:** Genes brought into a species artificially may cross accidentally to an unintended species. For example, resistance to herbicide could spread from a GM crop into weeds, which could then become herbicide resistant themselves.
- **Environmental hazards:** GM fish might alter the composition of natural fish populations if they escape into the wild. For example, fish that have been genetically modified to eat more in order to grow faster might invade new territories and displace native fish populations.

Examples of GM Crops

GMO*ᵃ* SPECIES	GENETIC MODIFICATION	SOURCE OF GENE	PURPOSE OF GENETIC MODIFICATION
Corn	Insect resistance	*Bacillus thuringiensis*	Reduced insect damage
Soybean, Cotton, Corn	Herbicide tolerance	*Streptomyces spp.*	Greater weed control
Cotton	Insect resistance	*Bacillus thuringiensis*	Reduced insect damage
Rice	Produce beta-carotene	*Erwinia* daffodil	Increase vitamin A supply

ᵃ GMO, Genetically modified organism; full biotechnology glossary available at *www.fao.org/biotech/biotech-glossary/en*.

For more information:
- Get a "pro" biotechnology perspective from the Council for Biotechnology Information: *www.sourcewatch.org/index.php/Council_for_Biotechnology_Information*.
- Get a "con" biotechnology perspective from the Union of Concerned Scientists: *www.ucsusa.org*.

Source: Adapted from "World Food Summit Fact Sheet: Biotechnology and Food Security" (Rome, Italy: The Food and Agriculture Organization of the United Nations, WFS FS 01-E).

A Need for Sustainable Development

Environmental concerns must be taken more seriously as well. The amount of land available for crop production is as important as the condition of the soil and the availability of water. Soil erosion is now accelerating on every continent at a rate that threatens the world's ability to continue feeding itself. Erosion of soil has always occurred; it is a natural process. But in the past, processes that build up the soil—such as the growth of trees—have compensated for erosion.

Where forests have already been converted to farmland and there are no trees, farmers can practice crop rotation, thus alternating soil-devouring crops with soil-building crops. An acre of soil planted one year in corn, the next in wheat, and the next in clover loses 2.7 tons of topsoil each year, but if it is planted only in corn three years in a row, it loses 19.7 tons a year. When farmers must choose whether to make three times as much money planting corn year after year or to rotate crops and earn less money, many choose the short-term profits. Ruin may not follow immediately, but it will inevitably follow.[56]

There is a growing recognition that governments need to encourage and support efforts at sustainable development. **Sustainable development** is defined as the successful management of agricultural resources to satisfy changing human needs while maintaining or enhancing the natural resource base and avoiding environmental degradation. In other words, sustainable development "meets the needs of the present without compromising the ability of future generations to meet their own needs."[57]

Consider that:

> Poverty drives ecological deterioration when desperate people overexploit their resource space, sacrificing the future to salvage the present. The cruel logic of short-term needs forces landless families to raise plots in the rain forest, plow steep slopes, and shorten fallow periods. Ecological decline, in turn, perpetuates poverty as degraded ecosystems offer diminishing yields to their poor inhabitants. A self-defeating spiral of economic deprivation and ecological degradation takes hold.[58]

Sustainable development entails the reduction of poverty and food insecurity in environmentally friendly ways. It includes the following four interrelated objectives:[59]

1. Expand economic opportunities for low-income people, to increase their income and productivity in ways that are economically, environmentally, and socially viable in the long term.

Sustainable development Development that meets the needs of the present without compromising the ability of future generations to meet their own needs.

2. Meet basic human needs for food, clean water, shelter, health care services, and education.
3. Protect and enhance the natural environment by managing natural resources in a way that respects the needs of present and future generations.
4. Promote democratic participation by all people in economic and political decisions that affect their lives.

People-Centered Development

We have used the word *developing* in this chapter to classify certain countries, but what is development? According to Oxfam America, a nonprofit international agency that funds self-help development and disaster relief projects worldwide, development enables people to meet their essential needs, extends beyond food aid and emergency relief, reverses the process of impoverishment, enhances democracy, and makes possible a balance between populations and resources. It also improves the well-being and status of women; respects local cultures; sustains the natural environment; measures progress in human (not just monetary) terms; and involves change, not just charity. Finally, development requires the empowerment of the poor and promotes the interests of the majority of people world-wide, in the global *North* as well as the *South*.[60] (The more developed countries, with the exceptions of New Zealand and Australia, are located geographically to the *north* of most of the developing countries.)

Development cannot be measured by gross national product or the quantity of the community harvest. Instead, development should serve the people and requires ongoing community involvement and participation in project development and implementation. In Tanzania, the Iringa Nutrition Program involves community members in the assessment and analysis of problems and decisions about appropriate actions.[61] The program is designed to increase people's awareness of malnutrition and thus improve their capacity to take action. Fundamental to the program are the United Nations' child survival activities; these include the regular quarterly weighing of children under five years of age in the villages, with discussion of the results by the village health committees. From this analysis, a set of appropriate interventions for solving problems can be identified. Recent evaluations indicate that this process has contributed to significant decreases in infant and child malnutrition and mortality.[62]

The cornerstone of true development was best expressed decades ago by Mahatma Gandhi: "Whenever you are in doubt . . . apply the following test. Recall the face of the poorest and the weakest man whom you may have seen, and ask yourself if the step you contemplate is going to be of any use to him. Will he gain anything by it? Will it restore him to a control over his own life and destiny?"[63]

Nutrition and Development

The United Nations views a healthful, nutritious diet as a basic human right—one that the FAO and WHO are pledged to secure. However, achieving improved nutritional well-being worldwide requires broad action on many issues, including the following:[64]

- Ensuring that the poor and malnourished have adequate access to food
- Preventing and controlling infectious diseases by providing clean water, basic sanitation, and effective health care
- Promoting healthful diets and lifestyles
- Protecting consumers through improved food quality and safety

- Preventing micronutrient deficiencies
- Assessing, analyzing, and monitoring the nutrition status of populations at risk around the world
- Incorporating nutrition objectives into development policies and programs

Nutrition and health are now seen as instruments or tools of economic development as well as goals in themselves. The inclusion of nutrition objectives in growth and development policies holds the promise of increasing the productivity and earning power of people worldwide. Well-nourished people are more productive, are sick less often, and earn higher incomes.[65]

The world's political leaders met at the 2000 Millennium Summit of the United Nations to set goals that called for a dramatic reduction in poverty and marked improvements in the lives of the world's poor by the year 2015.[66] The Millennium Development Goals set targets for progress in eight areas: poverty and hunger, primary education, women's equality, child mortality, maternal health, disease, environment, and a global partnership for development (**Table 14-3**). The summit leaders concluded that although sustainable

TABLE 14-3 Progress in Efforts to Meet the Millennium Development Goals (MDGs)

FACTOR	GOAL	TARGETS, 2015	PROGRESS, 1990–2015
Poverty	Eradicate extreme poverty and hunger	Reduce by half the proportion of people living on less than $1.25 a day.	**Mixed.** The number of people in developing countries living on less than $1.25 a day fell from 1.9 billion in 1990 to 836 million in 2015. Most sub-Saharan African countries missed the target.
		Reduce by half the proportion of people who suffer from hunger.	The proportion of people in the developing world who went hungry declined from 23.3% in 1990–1992 to 12.9% in 2014–2016.
Primary education	Achieve universal primary education	Ensure that all boys and girls complete a full course of primary schooling.	**Mixed.** The primary school net enrollment rate in the developing regions reached 91% in 2015, up from 83% in 2000. Shortfalls appear across sub-Saharan Africa. Being female, being poor, and living in a country affected by conflict are three factors keeping children out of school.
Gender equality	Promote gender equality and empower women	Eliminate gender disparity in education by 2015.	**Insufficient.** Many more girls are now in school compared to 15 years ago. Despite significant progress toward gender parity in primary schools, shortfalls still exist at the secondary and tertiary levels.
Child survival	Reduce child mortality	Reduce by two-thirds the mortality rate among children under five.	**Off track.** The fourth MDG is commonly regarded as the furthest from being achieved. The global under-5 mortality rate has declined by more than half, dropping from 90 to 43 deaths per 1,000 live births between 1990 and 2015 (from 12.6 million deaths in 1990 to 6 million in 2015). However, 16,000 children under five continue to die every day, mostly from preventable causes. The rate of decline in under-5 mortality is insufficient to reach the MDG goal, particularly in sub-Saharan Africa and South Asia.
Families and women	Improve maternal health	Reduce by three-quarters the maternal mortality ratio.	**Off track.** The maternal mortality ratio dropped by 45% worldwide between 1990 and 2013, from 380 maternal deaths per 100,000 live births to 210. More than one in four babies and their mothers are without access to crucial medical care during childbirth.

continued

TABLE 14-3   Progress in Efforts to Meet the Millennium Development Goals (MDGs)—*continued*

FACTOR	GOAL	TARGETS, 2015	PROGRESS, 1990–2015
Health	Combat HIV/AIDS, malaria, and other diseases	Halt and begin to reverse the spread of HIV/AIDS. Halt and begin to reverse the incidence of malaria, tuberculosis, and other major diseases.	**Mixed.** Between 2001 and 2015, the HIV incidence rate declined steadily, by nearly 40% worldwide, falling from an estimated 3.5 million new infections to 2.1 million. Only 33% of young men and 20% of young women in developing regions have a comprehensive and correct knowledge of HIV. Major progress has been made in the fight against malaria, particularly in the increased production and use of insecticide-treated nets in endemic regions. Since 2000, the incidence of tuberculosis has fallen by about 1.5% a year.
Water and sanitation	Ensure environmental sustainability	Reduce by half the proportion of people without sustainable access to safe drinking water and basic sanitation.	**Mixed.** Of the 2.6 billion people who gained access to improved drinking water since 1990, 1.9 billion gained access to piped drinking water on premises. However, about 663 million people still use unimproved drinking water sources, including unprotected wells and springs and surface water. Nearly half of all people using unimproved sources live in sub-Saharan Africa, while one-fifth live in South Asia. Sanitation remains an even greater challenge: Since 1990, the proportion of the global population using an improved sanitation facility increased from 54% to 68%, but over 2.4 billion people still lack flush toilets and other forms of improved sanitation.
Policy changes in developed countries regarding development aid, trade, and debt	Develop a global partnership for development	Deal comprehensively with the debt problems of developing countries. Develop further an open, nondiscriminatory trading and financial system.	**Mixed.** Some countries have benefited from debt relief under the Heavily Indebted Poor Countries (HIPC) Initiative, but much more needs to be done. Lower trade barriers are needed to improve market access by developing countries.

Sources: UNICEF, *The State of the World's Children*, 2005, 2008, 2009; United Nations, *The Millennium Development Goals Report, 2015* (New York: United Nations, 2015); United Nations Children's Fund, *Progress for Children: Achieving the MDGs with Equity* (New York, NY: UNICEF, September 2010); Food and Agriculture Organization of the United Nations (FAO), the International Fund for Agricultural Development, World Food Programme, *The State of Food Insecurity in the World 2015. Meeting the 2015 International Hunger Targets*: *Taking Stock of Uneven Progress* (Rome, FAO, 2015).

development to overcome chronic undernutrition is difficult both economically and politically, the payoff is high: more people contributing to the economic, social, and cultural life of their communities, their nations, and the world. **Figure 14-9** shows the progress made on meeting the Millennium Development Goals.

The final MDG Report demonstrated that with a 15-year focused effort by national governments and the private sector, much success is possible as noted in Table 14-3. For example, since 1990, the number of people living in extreme poverty has declined by more than half; the proportion of undernourished people has fallen by almost half; the primary school enrollment rate in the developing regions has reached 91%; and the under-5 mortality rate has declined by more than half. However, the work is unfinished. To that end, world leaders at the United Nations 2015 Sustainable Development Summit, adopted a challenging Agenda for Sustainable Development to achieve by 2030.[67] The plan includes a set of 17 Sustainable Development Goals (SDGs) that serve to guide policy and funding efforts moving forward (see the box on page 574). United Nations

| Goals and Targets | Africa | | Asia | | | | Oceania | Latin America and the Caribbean | Caucasus and Central Asia |
	Northern	Sub-Saharan	Eastern	South-Eastern	Southern	Western			
GOAL 1 | Eradicate extreme poverty and hunger.									
Reduce extreme poverty by half	low poverty	very high poverty	low poverty	moderate poverty	high poverty	low poverty	—	low poverty	low poverty
Reduce hunger by half	low hunger	high hunger	moderate hunger	moderate hunger	high hunger	moderate hunger	moderate hunger	moderate hunger	moderate hunger
GOAL 2 | Achieve universal primary education.									
Universal primary schooling	high enrollment	moderate enrollment	high enrollment	high enrollment	high enrollment	high enrollment	high enrollment	high enrollment	high enrollment
GOAL 3 | Promote gender equality and empower women.									
Equal girls' enrollment in primary school	close to parity	close to parity	parity	parity	parity	close to parity	close to parity	parity	parity
Women's share of paid employment	low share	medium share	high share	medium share	low share	low share	medium share	high share	high share
GOAL 4 | Reduce child mortality.									
Reduce mortality of under-five-year-olds by two-thirds	low mortality	high mortality	low mortality	low mortality	moderate mortality	low mortality	moderate mortality	low mortality	low mortality
GOAL 5 | Improve maternal health.									
Reduce maternal mortality by three-quarters	low mortality	high mortality	low mortality	moderate mortality	moderate mortality	low mortality	moderate mortality	low mortality	low mortality
Access to reproductive health	moderate access	low access	high access	moderate access	moderate access	moderate access	low access	high access	moderate access
GOAL 6 | Combat HIV/AIDS, malaria, and other diseases.									
Halt and begin to reverse the spread of HIV/AIDS	low incidence	high incidence	low incidence	low incidence	low incidence	low incidence	low incidence	low incidence	low incidence
Halt and reverse the spread of tuberculosis	low mortality	high mortality	low mortality	moderate mortality	moderate mortality	low mortality	moderate mortality	low mortality	moderate mortality
GOAL 7 | Ensure environmental sustainability.									
Halve proportion of population without improved drinking water	high coverage	low coverage	high coverage	high coverage	high coverage	high coverage	low coverage	high coverage	moderate coverage
Halve proportion of population without sanitation	moderate coverage	very low coverage	moderate coverage	low coverage	very low coverage	high coverage	very low coverage	moderate coverage	high coverage
GOAL 8 | Develop a global partnership for development.									
Internet users	moderate usage	low usage	high usage	moderate usage	low usage	high usage	low usage	high usage	high usage

The progress chart operates on two levels. The text in each box indicates the present level of development. The colors show progress made toward the target according to the legend below:

■ Target met or excellent progress
■ Good progress
  Fair progress

▨ Poor progress or deterioration
▨ Missing or insufficient data

For the regional groupings and country data, see *mdgs.un.org*.

FIGURE 14-9 Progress on Meeting the Millennium Development Goals (MDGs)

Source: United Nations, based on data and estimates provided by: Food and Agriculture Organization of the United Nations; Inter-Parliamentary Union; International Labour Organization; International Telecommunication Union; UNAIDS; UNESCO; UN-Habitat; UNICEF; UN Population Division; World Bank; World Health Organization—based on statistics available as of June 2015. Compiled by the Statistics Division, Department of Economic and Social Affairs, United Nations.

Development Program Administrator Helen Clark noted:[68] "This agreement marks an important milestone in putting our world on an inclusive and sustainable course. If we all work together, we have a chance of meeting citizens' aspirations for peace, prosperity, and well-being, and to preserve our planet."

The Sustainable Development Goals (SDGs)

At the United Nations 2015 Sustainable Development Summit, world leaders adopted the Agenda for Sustainable Development, which includes a set of 17 Sustainable Development Goals (SDGs) to achieve by 2030.

SDG 1: End poverty in all its forms everywhere. This involves targeting those living in vulnerable situations, increasing access to basic resources and services, and supporting communities affected by conflict and climate-related disasters.

SDG 2: Zero Hunger: End hunger, achieve food security and improved nutrition, and promote sustainable agriculture. End all forms of hunger and malnutrition, making sure all people have access to sufficient and nutritious food all year round. This involves promoting sustainable agricultural practices: improving the livelihoods and capacities of small-scale farmers, allowing equal access to land, technology, and markets. It also requires international cooperation to ensure investment in infrastructure and technology to improve agricultural productivity.

SDG 3: Ensure healthy lives and promote well-being for all. End the epidemics of AIDS, tuberculosis, malaria, and other communicable diseases by 2030. Achieve universal health coverage, and provide access to safe and effective medicines and vaccines for all.

SDG 4: Ensure inclusive and equitable quality education and promote lifelong learning opportunities for all. This goal reaffirms the belief that education is one of the most powerful and proven vehicles for sustainable development. This goal ensures that all girls and boys complete free primary and secondary schooling by 2030, and have increased access to affordable vocational training, and higher education.

SDG 5: Achieve gender equality and empower all women and girls. Ending all forms of discrimination against women and girls is not only a basic human right, but it also has a multiplier effect across all other development areas.

SDG 6: Ensure access to water and sanitation for all. Ensuring universal access to safe and affordable drinking water by 2030 requires we invest in adequate infrastructure, provide sanitation facilities, and encourage hygiene at every level. Protecting and restoring water-related ecosystems such as forests, mountains, wetlands, and rivers is essential if we are to mitigate water scarcity.

SDG 7: Ensure access to affordable, reliable, sustainable, and modern energy for all. Ensuring universal access to affordable electricity by 2030 means investing in clean energy sources such as solar, wind, and thermal.

SDG 8: Promote inclusive and sustainable economic growth, employment, and decent work for all. Encourage sustained economic growth by achieving higher levels of productivity and through technological innovation. Promoting policies that encourage entrepreneurship and job creation are key to this, as are effective measures to eradicate forced labor, slavery, and human trafficking.

SDG 9: Build resilient infrastructure, promote sustainable industrialization, and foster innovation. With over half the world population now living in cities, mass transportation and renewable energy are becoming ever more important, as are the growth of new industries and information and communication technologies.

SDG 10: Reduce inequality within and among countries. Adopt sound policies to empower the bottom percentile of income earners and promote economic inclusion of all regardless of sex, race, or ethnicity.

SDG 11: Make cities inclusive, safe, resilient, and sustainable. Making cities safe and sustainable means ensuring access to safe and affordable housing, and upgrading slum settlements. It also involves investment in public transportation, creating green public spaces, and improving urban planning and management in a way that is both participatory and inclusive.

SDG 12: Ensure sustainable consumption and production patterns. Achieving economic growth and sustainable development requires that we urgently reduce our ecological footprint by changing the way we produce and consume goods and resources. The efficient management of our shared natural resources, and the way we dispose of toxic waste and pollutants, are important targets to achieve this goal. Encouraging industries, businesses, and consumers to recycle and reduce waste is equally important (see the box "How to Reduce Your Ecological Footprint" on page 588).

SDG 13: Take urgent action to combat climate change and its impacts. The goal aims to mobilize $100 billion annually by 2020 to address the needs of developing countries and help mitigate climate-related disasters.

SDG 14: Conserve and sustainably use the oceans, seas, and marine resources. Create a framework to sustainably manage and protect marine and coastal ecosystems from land-based pollution, as well as address the impacts of ocean acidification.

SDG 15: Protect, restore, and promote sustainable use of terrestrial ecosystems, sustainably manage forests, combat desertification, halt and reverse land degradation, and halt biodiversity loss. Promote the sustainable management of forests and reduce the loss of natural habitats and biodiversity.

SDG 16: Promote peaceful and inclusive societies for sustainable development, provide access to justice for all, and build effective, accountable, and inclusive institutions at all levels. Reduce all forms of violence, and work with governments and communities to find lasting solutions to conflict and insecurity.

SDG 17: Revitalize the global partnership for sustainable development. Improving access to technology and knowledge is an important way to share ideas and foster innovation. Coordinating policies to help developing countries manage their debt, as well as promoting investment for the least developed, is vital to achieve sustainable growth and development.

Sources: Adapted from United Nations, *The Millennium Development Goals Report 2015* (New York: United Nations, 2015); United Nations, Resolution adopted by the General Assembly on 25 September 2015, *Transforming Our World: The 2030 Agenda for Sustainable Development*, October 2015; and United Nations Development Program, *www.undp.org/content/undp/en/home/mdgoverview/post-2015-development-agenda.*

Scaling Up Nutrition

In January 2008, *The Lancet* medical journal published a five-part series providing systematic evidence regarding the impact of undernutrition on infant and child morbidity and mortality.[69] The series highlighted a set of 13 cost-effective interventions that could address undernutrition and save millions of lives (shown previously in Table 14-2). *The Lancet* series sparked widespread agreement among diverse groups on the need to scale up actions to improve global nutrition—and led to the creation of the Scaling Up Nutrition (SUN) movement in 2010.[70]

SUN unites more than 100 key stakeholders, including the United Nations, various governments, development agencies, foundations, researchers, developing countries, and other organizations. The main elements of the SUN framework for action are as follows:[71]

- Individual country nutrition strategies and programs, while drawing on international evidence of good practice, must be country owned and built on the country's specific needs and capacities.
- Sharply scale up evidence-based interventions to prevent and treat undernutrition, especially during the critical 1,000-day period (from conception until a child's second birthday).
- Use a multisectoral approach that integrates nutrition interventions into related sectors, such as health (breastfeeding promotion), agriculture (small-scale farming and home

gardens), education (nutrition and hygiene in school curricula), and social protection (food assistance for those in poverty and during natural disasters).

- Provide substantially scaled-up domestic and external aid for country-owned nutrition programs.

Since 2010, 56 countries have joined the SUN movement.[72] Countries that join commit to increasing coverage of specific interventions to improve nutrition, such as support for exclusive breastfeeding, optimal micronutrient intake, safe and adequate complementary feeding practices, and food fortification interventions.

Agenda for Action

Although the problem of global food insecurity may seem overwhelming, it can be broken down into many small, local problems. Significant strides can then be made toward solving them at the local level. Even if the problem of poverty itself is not immediately or fully solved, progress is possible. Lessons can be learned from the countries that met the Millennium Development Goal of cutting extreme poverty rates in half by 2015.[73] Several of these countries applied a twin-track approach: strengthening social safety nets while at the same time addressing the underlying causes of food insecurity with new initiatives to stimulate agricultural production, increase education and employment opportunities, and reduce poverty.[74] The twin-track approach is illustrated in **Figure 14-10**. Brazil's Zero Hunger Program demonstrates the success of the twin-track approach: By buying food for school lunch and other food assistance programs directly from local farmers, it improves dietary intakes of children, increases food availability for families, increases the income of farmers, and contributes to national food security.[75]

Although good progress was made in achieving the Millennium Development Goals, more accelerated action is needed to resolve the problem of malnutrition. The World Health Assembly recently endorsed a comprehensive plan for improving maternal, infant, and young child health.[76] The plan specifies an ambitious set of six global nutrition targets to reach by 2025 (**Table 14-4**). The World Health Organization has produced a series of policy briefs, linked to each of the global nutrition targets to guide policymakers regarding strategies necessary to achieve the nutrition targets.

Making the World Fit for Children

The first World Summit for Children in history was convened by UNICEF in September 1990, bringing together representatives of 159 nations for the purpose of making a renewed commitment to improving the plight of the world's children. Significantly, *nutrition* was mentioned for the first time in world history as an internationally recognized human right.[77] The overall goal of ending child deaths and malnutrition was broken down into specific targets in a plan of action agreed upon by the countries in attendance. An immediate result of this summit was an increase in the number of governments actively adopting the child survival strategies of UNICEF and WHO. UNICEF's goals for nutrition and food security included the following:

- A 50% reduction in the levels of moderate to severe malnutrition among children under five years old
- A 50% reduction in the levels of low-birthweight infants
- The virtual elimination of blindness and other consequences of vitamin A deficiency

Strategies devised to achieve these goals included universal immunization, oral rehydration therapy, a massive effort to promote breastfeeding as the ideal food for at least the

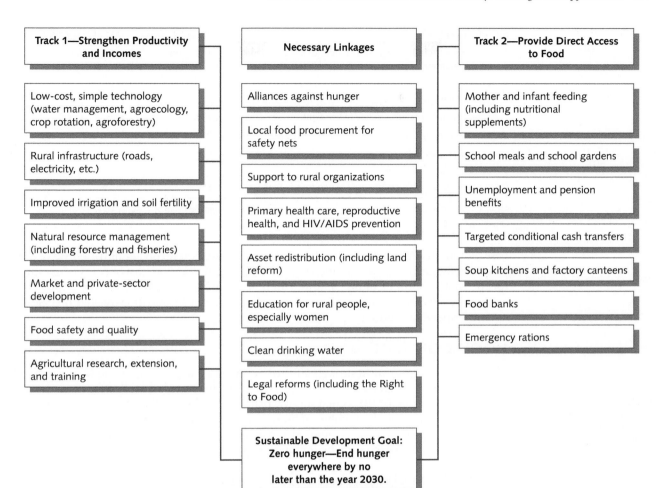

Track 1—Strengthen Productivity and Incomes	Necessary Linkages	Track 2—Provide Direct Access to Food
Low-cost, simple technology (water management, agroecology, crop rotation, agroforestry)	Alliances against hunger	Mother and infant feeding (including nutritional supplements)
Rural infrastructure (roads, electricity, etc.)	Local food procurement for safety nets	School meals and school gardens
Improved irrigation and soil fertility	Support to rural organizations	Unemployment and pension benefits
Natural resource management (including forestry and fisheries)	Primary health care, reproductive health, and HIV/AIDS prevention	Targeted conditional cash transfers
Market and private-sector development	Asset redistribution (including land reform)	Soup kitchens and factory canteens
Food safety and quality	Education for rural people, especially women	Food banks
Agricultural research, extension, and training	Clean drinking water	Emergency rations
	Legal reforms (including the Right to Food)	

Sustainable Development Goal: Zero hunger—End hunger everywhere by no later than the year 2030.

FIGURE 14-10 A Twin-Track Strategy to Escape Poverty and Eliminate Hunger

The Food and Agriculture Organization (FAO) believes that the Sustainable Development goal of "Zero Hunger—Ending all forms of hunger and malnutrition everywhere by no later than 2030" is both attainable and affordable. The FAO recommends a twin-track strategy that addresses both the *causes* and the *consequences* of poverty and hunger. Track 1 includes interventions for improving personal income and food availability for the poor by strengthening income-generating opportunities (e.g., by improving the productivity of small farmers). Track 2 supplies a safety net to provide direct assistance to the most vulnerable groups, including pregnant and lactating women, infants and small children, school children, unemployed urban youth, older adults, disabled persons, and the sick, including people living with HIV/AIDS.

Source: Adapted from FAO, *The State of Food Insecurity in the World 2004*, 32.

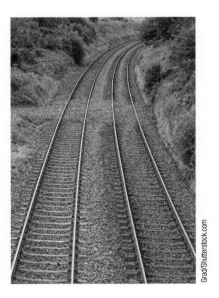

Grad/Shutterstock.com

TABLE 14-4 Global Nutrition Targets 2025

NUTRITION TARGET	BASELINE (2012)	TARGET FOR 2025
1. Achieve a 40% reduction in the number of children under five who are stunted.	162 million	~100 million
2. Achieve a 50% reduction of anemia in women of reproductive age.	29%	15%
3. Achieve a 30% reduction in low birthweight.	15%	10%
4. Ensure that there is no increase in childhood overweight.	7%	≤ 7%
5. Increase the rate of exclusive breastfeeding in the first six months up to at least 50%.	38%	≥ 50%
6. Reduce and maintain childhood wasting to less than 5%.	8%	< 5%

Source: WHO, Global Nutrition Targets 2025: Policy Brief Series (WHO/NMH/NHD/14.2) (Geneva: World Health Organization, 2014).

first six months of an infant's life, an attack on malnutrition involving nutrition surveillance that focuses on growth monitoring and weighing of infants at least once every month for the first 18 months of life, and nutrition and literacy education that will empower women in developing countries and lead to a reduction in nutrition-related diseases among vulnerable children.[78]

Focus on Children

Children are the group most strongly affected by poverty, malnutrition, and food insecurity and its related effects on the environment.[79] However, there is hopeful news for children in developing countries. **GOBI**, a child survival plan set forth by UNICEF, has made outstanding progress in cutting the number of hunger-related child deaths. GOBI is an acronym formed from four simple but profoundly important elements of UNICEF's Child Survival campaign: growth charts, oral rehydration therapy, breast milk, and immunization.

GOBI An acronym formed from the elements of UNICEF's Child Survival campaign—growth charts, oral rehydration therapy, breast milk, and immunization.

Growth Monitoring
The use of growth monitoring to determine the adequacy of child feeding requires a worldwide education campaign. A mother can learn to weigh her child every month and chart the child's growth on specially designed paper. She can learn to detect the early stages of hidden malnutrition that can leave a child irreparably impaired in mind and body. Then at least she will know she needs to take steps to remedy the malnutrition—if she can.

Oral Rehydration Therapy
Most children who die of malnutrition do not starve to death—they die because their health has been compromised by dehydration from infections causing diarrhea. Until recently, there was no easy way of stopping the infection–diarrhea cycle and saving their lives; now, the spread of **oral rehydration therapy (ORT)** is preventing an estimated 1 million dehydration deaths each year.[80] ORT involves the administration of a simple solution that mothers can make themselves, using locally available ingredients; the solution increases a body's ability to absorb fluids 25-fold.[81] International development groups also provide mothers with packets of premeasured salt and sugar to be mixed with boiled water in rural and urban areas. A safe, sanitary supply of drinking water is a prerequisite for the success of the ORT program. Contaminated water perpetuates the infection–diarrhea cycle.

Oral rehydration therapy (ORT) The treatment of dehydration (usually due to diarrhea caused by infectious disease) with an oral solution; as developed by UNICEF, ORT is intended to enable a mother to mix a simple solution for her child from substances that she has at home.

Promotion of Breastfeeding
Until the middle of the twentieth century, in most developing countries, babies were breastfed for their first year of life—with supplements of other milk and cereal gruel added to their diets after the first several months.[82] Despite

improved overall rates of breastfeeding during the last two decades, only 35% of all infants are now being exclusively breastfed for up to six months of age. A number of factors contributed to this unfortunate decline, including the aggressive promotion and sale of infant formula to new mothers; the encouragement of bottle-feeding by health care practitioners, who send mothers home from the hospital with free samples of formula after delivery of the newborn; and the global pattern of urbanization and accompanying loss of cultural ties supporting breastfeeding, combined with more women working outside the home.[83] The global recommendation now is for exclusive breastfeeding for the first six months of life, joined thereafter by timely complementary foods along with continued breastfeeding up to two years of age (**Figure 14-11**).[84] Overall, the World Health Organization estimates that improved breastfeeding practices could save the lives of more than 1.5 million children each year.[85]

Breastfeeding versus Formula Feeding Replacing breast milk with infant formula in environments and economic circumstances that make it impossible to feed formula safely may lead to infant undernutrition. Breast milk, the recommended food for infants, is sterile and contains antibodies that enhance an infant's resistance to disease. In the absence of sterilization and refrigeration, formula in bottles is an ideal breeding ground for bacteria. In countries where poor sanitation is prevalent, breastfeeding should take priority over feeding formula. Studies indicate that a bottle-fed infant living in poverty is up to 14 times as likely to die from diarrhea-related causes and 4 times more likely to die of pneumonia than an exclusively breastfed baby.[86]

The promotion of breastfeeding among mothers in developing countries has many benefits. Breast milk is hygienic, readily available, and nutritionally sound, and it provides infants with immunologic protection specific to their environment. In the developing world, its advantages over formula feeding can mean the difference between life and death.

The finding that HIV can be transmitted through breast milk has complicated infant feeding recommendations. New guidelines released by the Joint United Nations Programme on HIV/AIDS, WHO, and UNICEF call for urgent action to educate, counsel, and

FIGURE 14-11 Key Proven Practices, Services, and Policy Interventions for the Prevention and Treatment of Stunting and Other Forms of Undernutrition throughout the Life Cycle Stunting and other forms of malnutrition can be reduced by improving maternal nutrition, especially before, during, and immediately after pregnancy; early and exclusive breastfeeding; and timely introduction of safe, appropriate, and high-quality complementary food for infants, accompanied by appropriate micronutrient interventions.

Source: Policy and guideline recommendations based on UNICEF, WHO, and other United Nations agencies; Z. A. Bhutta et al., Maternal and Child Undernutrition 3: What Works? Interventions for Maternal and Child Undernutrition and Survival, *The Lancet* 371 (2008): 417–40.

During Adolescence and Pregnancy	Birth	0–6 Months	6–23 Months
• Improved use of locally available foods • Food fortification, including salt iodization • Micronutrient supplementation and deworming • Fortified food supplements for undernourished mothers • Prenatal care, including HIV testing	• Early initiation of breastfeeding within one hour of delivery (including colostrum) • Appropriate infant feeding practices for HIV-exposed infants, and antiretroviral drug therapy (ARV)	• Exclusive breastfeeding • Appropriate infant feeding practices for HIV-exposed infants, and ARV • Vitamin A supplementation in first eight weeks after delivery • Multi-micronutrient supplementation • Improved use of locally available foods, fortified foods, micronutrient supplementation/home fortification for undernourished women	• Timely introduction of adequate, safe, and appropriate complementary feeding • Continued breastfeeding • Appropriate infant feeding practices for HIV-exposed infants, and ARV • Micronutrient supplementation, including vitamin A, multi-micronutrients; zinc treatment for diarrhea; deworming • Community-based management of severe acute malnutrition; management of moderate acute malnutrition • Food fortification, including salt iodization • Prevention and treatment of infectious disease; hand washing with soap and improved water and sanitation practices • Improved use of locally available foods, fortified foods, micronutrient supplementation/home fortification for undernourished women

Note: Blue refers to interventions for women of reproductive age and mothers.
Black refers to interventions for infants and young children.

support HIV-positive women regarding safe infant feeding practices. Evidence shows that giving antiretroviral drugs (ARVs) to either the HIV-infected mother or the HIV-exposed infant can significantly reduce the risk of transmission of HIV through breastfeeding. According to the World Health Organization guidelines on infant feeding:[87]

- Where ARVs are available, mothers known to be HIV-infected should exclusively breastfeed their infants for the first six months of life, introducing appropriate complementary foods thereafter, and should continue breastfeeding for the first 12 months of life. Even when ARVs are not available, mothers should be counseled to exclusively breastfeed in the first six months of life and continue breastfeeding thereafter *unless* environmental and social circumstances are safe for, and supportive of, replacement feeding.

Recent reports indicate that transmission of HIV may be lower among exclusively breastfed three-month-old infants of HIV-positive women than among such infants who were only partially breastfed. However, confirmation of any protective effect of exclusive breastfeeding on the risk of mother-to-infant transmission of HIV is urgently needed.[88]

Baby-Friendly Initiatives In 1981, the World Health Assembly—comprising the health ministers of nearly all countries—adopted the International Code of Marketing of Breastmilk Substitutes. The code stipulates that health facilities must never be involved in the promotion of infant formula and that free samples should not be provided to new mothers. In 1992, WHO and UNICEF began the Baby-Friendly Hospital Initiative to help transform hospitals into centers that promote and support good infant feeding practices. The Baby-Friendly Hospital Initiative has fostered an increased awareness of the importance of breastfeeding worldwide and of exclusive breastfeeding in the early months of life; as a consequence, both breastfeeding rates and the average duration of breastfeeding are increasing globally.[89] Table 11-8 on page 436 provides a list of 10 steps to successful breastfeeding from the WHO Baby-Friendly Hospital Initiative. Today, there are Baby-Friendly Hospitals in 152 countries.[90] Nearly 80 developing countries have now banned the free or subsidized distribution of infant formula to new mothers in hospitals and clinics.[91]

Timely and Appropriate Complementary Feeding Breastfeeding permits infants in many developing countries to achieve weight and height gains equal to those of children in developed countries until about six months of age, but then the majority of these children fall behind in growth and development because inadequate complementary foods are added to their diets. The **weaning period** is one of the most dangerous times for children in developing countries for a number of reasons. For one thing, newly weaned infants often receive nutrient-poor diluted cereals or starchy root crops. For another, infants' foods are often prepared with contaminated water, making infection almost inevitable. Attitudes toward food may also affect nutrition. In some areas of India, for example, a child may be forbidden to eat curds and fruit because they are "cold" or bananas because they "cause convulsions."[92]

An important contributor to children's malnutrition in developing countries is the high bulk and low energy content of the available foods. The diet may be based on staple grains, such as wheat, rice, millet, sorghum, and corn, as well as starchy root crops, such as cassava and sweet potato. These may be supplemented with legumes (peas or beans), but rarely with animal proteins. Infants have small stomachs, and most cannot eat enough of these staples (grains or root crops) to meet their daily energy and protein requirements. They need to be fed more nutrient-dense foods during the weaning period. The most promising weaning foods are usually concentrated mixtures of grain and locally available

Weaning period The time during which an infant's diet is changed from breast milk to other nourishment.

pulses—that is, peas or beans—which are both nourishing and inexpensive. Mothers are advised to continue breastfeeding their children up to two years of age or beyond while they introduce safe, appropriate, and adequate complementary foods (**Table 14-5**).[93]

Pulses A term used for legumes, especially those that serve as staples in the diets of developing countries.

TABLE 14-5

Guiding Principles for Complementary Feeding of the Breastfed Child

---

1. Practice exclusive breastfeeding from birth to six months of age, and introduce complementary foods at six months of age while continuing to breastfeed.
2. Continue frequent, on-demand breastfeeding until two years of age or beyond.
3. Practice responsive feeding: Feed slowly and patiently, and encourage children to eat. If children refuse foods, experiment with different food combinations, tastes, textures, and methods of encouragement. Minimize distractions during meals.
4. Practice good hygiene and proper food handling.
5. Start at six months of age with small amounts of food and increase the quantity as the child gets older, while maintaining frequent breastfeeding.
6. Gradually increase food consistency and variety as the infant grows older, adapting to the infant's requirements and abilities.

How to feed infants 6–11 months
- Continue breastfeeding.
- Give adequate servings of:

  - Thick porridge made out of maize, cassava, or millet; add milk, soy, ground nuts, or sugar.
  - Mixtures of pureed foods made out of matoke (green cooking bananas), potatoes, cassava, maize, millet, or rice mixed with fish, beans, or pounded groundnuts; add green vegetables.
  - Give nutritious snacks: egg, banana, bread, papaya, avocado, mango, other fruits, yogurt, milk, and puddings made with milk, biscuits or crackers, bread or chapati with butter, margarine, groundnut paste, bean cakes, and/or cooked potatoes.

How to feed children 12–23 months
- Continue breastfeeding.
- Give adequate servings of:

  - Mixtures of mashed or finely cut family foods made out of matoke, potatoes, cassava, posho (maize or millet), or rice; mix with fish or beans or pounded groundnuts; add green vegetables.
  - Thick porridge made out of maize, cassava, or millet; add milk, soy, ground nuts, or sugar.
  - Give nutritious snacks: egg, banana, bread, papaya, avocado, mango, other fruits, yogurt, milk, and puddings made with milk, biscuits or crackers, bread or chapati with butter, margarine, groundnut paste, bean cakes, and/or cooked potatoes.

7. Increase the number of times that the child is fed complementary foods as the child gets older.
8. Feed a variety of nutrient-rich foods to ensure that all nutrient needs are met.

Appropriate foods for complementary feeding
- The basic ingredient of complementary foods is usually the local staple that consists mainly of carbohydrate and provides energy. Examples: cereals (rice, wheat, maize, millet, and quinoa), roots (cassava, yam, and potatoes), and starchy fruits (plantain and breadfruit). A variety of other foods should be added to the staple every day to provide other nutrients. These include:

  - Protein foods from animals or fish as good sources of protein, heme iron, and zinc.
  - Dairy products, such as milk, cheese, and yogurt are useful sources of calcium, protein, energy, and B vitamins.
  - Pulses—peas, beans, lentils, peanuts, and soybeans—are good sources of protein and some iron. Eating sources of vitamin C at the same time helps iron absorption.
  - Orange-colored fruits and vegetables such as carrot, pumpkin, mango, and papaya, and dark-green leaves such as spinach, are rich in beta-carotene.
  - Fats and oils are concentrated sources of energy, and of certain essential fats.
  - Nuts and seeds provide energy. Examples: groundnut paste or other nut pastes, and soaked or germinated seeds such as pumpkin, sunflower, melon, and sesame.

9. Use fortified complementary foods or vitamin–mineral supplements for the infant, as needed.
10. Increase fluid intake during illness, including more frequent breastfeeding, and encourage the child to eat soft, favorite foods. After illness, give food more often than usual and encourage the child to eat more.

Source: Adapted from World Health Organization, *Infant and Young Child Feeding: Model Chapter for Textbooks for Medical Students and Allied Health Professionals* (Geneva: World Health Organization, 2009).

> ► **THINK LIKE A COMMUNITY** NUTRITIONIST

Develop an outline of a community campaign advocating for either exclusive breastfeeding or appropriate complementary feeding in the global context. Research indicates that good communication to address these practices should be motivational rather than informational, and should be administered via mass media and interpersonal routes (rather than primarily through posters and brochures). In your outline, include motivational messages and how they will be delivered. Then develop a formative evaluation plan for testing messages prior to rolling out the campaign.

Immunizations As for immunizations (the *I* of GOBI), they could prevent most of the 2 million deaths each year from measles, diphtheria, tetanus, whooping cough, poliomyelitis, and tuberculosis. However, adequate protein nutrition is necessary for vaccinations to be effective; otherwise, the body may use the vaccine itself as a source of protein. It used to be difficult to keep vaccines stable in their long journeys from laboratory to remote villages. Now, however, the discovery of a new measles vaccine that does not require refrigeration has made universal measles immunization for young children possible, and many countries are reporting coverage rates of 80–90%. The immunization achievements of the last 20 years are credited with preventing approximately 3 million deaths a year and with protecting many millions more from disease, malnutrition, blindness, deafness, and polio.[94] Still, more than 30 million children in the world are unimmunized because vaccines are unavailable, because health services are poorly provided or inaccessible, or because families are uninformed or misinformed about when and why to bring their children for immunization.[95]

Focus on Women

Women make up 50% of the world's population. With their children, they represent the majority of those living in poverty. Thus, any solution to the problems of poverty and hunger is incomplete—indeed, is hopeless—if it fails to address the role of women in developing countries.[96]

Development projects are often large in scale and highly technological, but they frequently overlook women's needs. Typically, only men have access to education and training programs. Yet women play a vital role in the well-being of their nation's people, and are often extensively involved in food production as well. Their nutrition during pregnancy and lactation determines the future health of their children. The poor nutrition of some women results both from their family's lack of access to food and from unequal distribution of food within the family itself. If women are weakened by malnutrition themselves or ignorant about how to feed their families, the consequences ripple outward to affect many other individuals. The importance of women in these countries is increasingly being appreciated, and many countries now offer development programs with women in mind.

Seven basic strategies are at the heart of women's programs:

• Removing barriers to financial credit so that women can obtain loans for raw materials and equipment to enhance their role in food production
• Providing access to time-saving technologies—seed grinders, for example
• Providing appropriate training to make women self-reliant
• Teaching management and marketing skills to help women avoid exploitation
• Making health and daycare services available to provide a healthful environment for the women's children
• Forming women's support groups to foster strength through cooperative efforts
• Providing information and technology to promote planned pregnancies

The recognition of women's needs by some development organizations is an encouraging trend in the efforts to contend with the world hunger crisis. The following examples from Sierra Leone and Ghana illustrate how women's development programs work.[97]

Balu Kamara is a farmer in Sierra Leone in West Africa, where farming is difficult, particularly for women. There women have little money and must take out loans to buy seed rice and to pay for the use of oxen. The price of rice is so low, though, that at the end of the growing season the women do not earn enough money to repay their loans. Yet, as the economy worsens, it is up to the women to carry the burdens; it is up to the women to stretch what resources are available to feed their families regardless of hardships.

Balu is the leader of the Farm Women's Club, a basket cooperative the women formed to make and sell baskets so they could pay their debts and continue farming. Finding time to weave baskets is difficult. Yet the women and their cooperative are succeeding. On the value of the Farm Women's Club, Balu says, "We have access to credit and a cash income. We have the opportunity to learn improved methods of agriculture and marketing and to increase our belief in ourselves and ease our families through the hungry season."

Gari (processed cassava) is becoming increasingly popular in Ghana because of the shortage of many other food items and because, once prepared, it is easy to cook. But it is very time-consuming to prepare gari—peeling and grating the fresh cassava, fermenting it over several days, squeezing the water from the fermented cassava, and finally roasting it over a wood fire.

To help village women in the Volta Region increase their income through gari processing, an improved technology was introduced with the help of the National Council on Women and Development. The process involves a special mechanical grater, a pressing machine to squeeze the water from the grated cassava, and a large enamel pan for roasting. This pan holds 10 times the volume of the traditional cassava pot. The system was developed locally, with advice from the women themselves contributing to the success of the project. Before, the women produced 50 bags of gari every week. Now they are able to produce 5,000–6,000 bags a week. However, this increased output of gari can be maintained only with a higher yield of cassava in the area. Therefore, a male cassava growers' association has been formed to step up cassava production, and a tractor has been acquired by the women's cooperative to put more land under cassava cultivation.

International Nutrition Programs

Nutrition programs in developing countries vary considerably. A sample job description for a nutrition specialist working with the FAO is shown in **Figure 14-12**. International nutrition programs include both large-scale and small-scale operations, may be supported with private or public funds, and may focus on emergency relief or long-term development.[98] In developing countries, emphasis has generally been placed on four types of nutrition interventions:

1. Breastfeeding promotion programs with guidance on preparing appropriate weaning foods
2. Nutrition education programs typically focusing either on infant and child feeding guidelines and practices and child survival activities or on the incorporation of nutrition education into primary school curricula and teacher training programs
3. Food fortification and/or the distribution of nutrient supplements (e.g., vitamin A capsules) and the identification of local food sources of nutrients in short supply
4. Special feeding programs designed to provide particularly vulnerable groups with nutritious supplemental foods[99]

FIGURE 14-12

Sample Job Description for a Nutrition Specialist with the Food and Agriculture Organization

Source: Adapted from Vacancy Announcement (No. 130-ESN) of the Food and Agriculture Organization of the United Nations. Used with permission.

International Public Health Nutrition Employment Opportunities can be found in such places as:

- National and international health agencies and non-governmental organizations
- Humanitarian organizations
- Government health prevention and treatment programs
- International reproductive health programs
- Programs serving the HIV-infected population
- Health advocacy organizations
- Non-governmental organizations such as:
  - Catholic Relief Services
  - UNICEF
  - United Nations World Food Programme
  - World Bank
  - World Health Organization
  - World Vision International

See also the many organizations listed in the Internet Resources at the end of this chapter. For more information on careers, see the Association of Professional Schools of International Affairs at *www.apsia.org/career-guide.*

Position Title: Nutrition Officer (Nutrition Information)
Responsible To: Senior Officer (Nutrition Assessment)
Level Grade: P–4

Responsibilities:
Under the general direction of the Chief of the Nutrition Planning, Assessment and Evaluation Service, Food Policy and Nutrition Division, and the supervision of the Senior Officer (Nutrition Assessment), this specialist is responsible for the development of activities aimed at improving information necessary for assessing and analyzing nutrition status of populations at global, national, and local levels, especially in the drought-prone African countries.

Job Duties:
In accordance with departmental policies and procedures, this specialist carries out the following duties and responsibilities:

- Assists member countries in the design and implementation of data collection and analysis activities to meet the needs of policymakers and planners concerned with food and nutrition issues.
- In cooperation with other organization units, strengthens the skills and technical capacity of member countries, particularly within the agricultural sector, to assess, analyze, and monitor the food and nutrition situation of their own population.
- Provides data and background information for Expert Committees and Councils.
- Provides consultations on energy and nutrient requirements, dietary assessment methodology, and foodways.
- Prepares relevant reports for the organization and its committees.
- Performs other related duties.

Qualifications and Experience—Essential
The specialist should have the following educational qualifications and experience:

- A university degree in Nutrition or Biological Science with postgraduate qualification in Nutrition.
- Seven years of progressively responsible professional experience, including the planning and implementation of nutrition data collection, processing, and analysis.
- Experience in the management and analysis of nutrition-related data using advanced statistical applications software.

Qualifications and Experience—Desirable

- Experience in international work and research.
- Relevant work experience in Africa.
- Experience in the organization of seminars, training courses, or conferences.

Skills

- Working knowledge of English and French (level C).
- Demonstrated ability to write related technical reports. Familiarity with project design techniques.
- Courtesy, tact, and ability to establish and maintain effective work relationships with people of different national and cultural backgrounds.
- Experience using word-processing equipment and software.

In many countries, there is mounting evidence of grassroots progress in improving agricultural, water, education, and health services, especially for children.[100] Experiences in Sierra Leone, Nepal, and Bangladesh are encouraging examples.

- In Sierra Leone, a food product was developed from rice, sesame (benniseed), and peanuts that were hand pounded and cooked to make a flour meal. The local children not only found it tasty, but whereas they had been malnourished before, they thrived when this product supplemented their diets. The village women formed a cooperative to reduce the drudgery of preparing the food and rotated the work on a weekly or monthly basis.[101] The government also established a manufacturing plan to produce and market the mixture at subsidized prices. The success of the venture can be directly attributed to the involvement of the local people in identifying the problem and devising a solution that met their needs.

- A similar success story unfolded in Nepal. A supplementary food made from soybeans, corn, and wheat, mixed in a ratio of 2 to 1, yielded a concentrated "superflour" of high biological value suitable for young children. A nutrition rehabilitation center tested this superflour by giving undernourished children and their mothers two cereal-based meals a day and giving the children three additional small meals of superflour porridge daily. Within 10 days, the undernourished children had gained weight, lost their edema, and recovered their appetites and social alertness. The mothers, who saw the remarkable recoveries of their children, were motivated to learn how to make the tasty supplementary food and incorporate it into their local foodstuffs and customs.

These examples offer hope, but the real issue of poverty remains to be addressed. One-shot intervention programs offering nutrition education, food distribution, food fortification, and the like are not enough. It is difficult to describe the misery a mother feels when she has received education about nutrition but cannot grow or purchase the foods her family needs. She now knows *why* her child is sick and dying but is unable to *apply* her new knowledge.

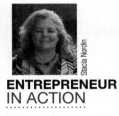

ENTREPRENEUR IN ACTION

Stacia Nordin, RD, has lived in Malawi, Africa, since 1997, and her home has become a demonstration venue for sustainable living at *www.NeverEndingFood.org*. Her career path as a registered dietitian began in Jamaica with the Peace Corps—as a nutrition officer at a local health department. After working with senior care in Wisconsin and marrying a fellow Peace Corps Jamaica volunteer, she and her husband were invited to join the Peace Corps program in Malawi, Africa. They worked primarily with local health and agriculture staff on issues of nutrition and HIV education, prevention, and care for the communities they served. Eventually, the Peace Corps hired Stacia as a staff member to manage their HIV and Food Security program in Malawi. Stacia is a strong advocate for sustainable living and developed a manual on food and nutrition security with the World Food Programme. She has worked with the Ministry of Education to develop and pilot a National School Health and Nutrition Program, which is now gaining momentum. She also works with the Ministry of Agriculture on improving nutrition policies and programs. Says Stacia: "A person with knowledge of food and nutrition security issues can really help to guide society toward what is healthy for people and the environment, often simultaneously. We all need to start thinking more about the sustainability of our Earth." Find out more about Stacia online at *www.cengagebrain.com*.

Grow Your Own: Tackling Poor Nutrition in Bangladesh[a]

One program that has been highly successful in improving child nutrition is *Jibon o Jibika* (Life and Livelihoods) in Bangladesh. Over five years, the program enrolled more than 400,000 children under two years of age. During these five years, in the three districts where the program operated, rates of malnutrition among young children came down against stunting and wasting indicators, and exclusive breastfeeding rates rose dramatically.

The program consisted of four components:

1. Setting up and supporting homestead gardens, where local communities grow different varieties of micronutrient-rich vegetables and fruits throughout the year.
2. Improving access to key services such as basic health care, safe water, and sanitation facilities, and ensuring mothers are given nutritional advice.
3. Giving women a route to market, by setting up a system where a local farmer purchases the surplus vegetables produced by women in their home gardens and then sells them at market. This enabled women to generate income despite limited mobility and lack of access to markets.
4. Supporting women's home food production by enlisting a local farmer to provide information on year-round gardening techniques, new nutrient-rich vegetable varieties, rearing poultry, and preserving seeds.

continued

> ## Grow Your Own: Tackling Poor Nutrition in Bangladesh[a]—*continued*
>
> The final evaluation found that stunting levels among children under two years of age were reduced in villages where homestead gardens had been established, as opposed to where they had not. It suggests that increasing the amount of food households produce contributed to reductions in chronic malnutrition. However, a greater improvement in nutrition was seen when homestead gardens were implemented alongside the second component of the program—improved access to maternal and child health and nutrition services, and to clean water and sanitation programs. The evaluation also found that the income women earned from selling surplus vegetables they had grown was used to pay for children's education and other household needs. Women also reported that this income gave them more status in their household.
>
> [a] The USAID-funded *Jibon o Jibika* program was led by Save the Children, working in partnership with Helen Keller International and local non-government agencies.
>
> Source: Save the Children, *A Life Free from Hunger: Tackling Child Malnutrition* (Westport, CT: The Save the Children Fund, 2012), 55.

Looking Ahead: The Global Challenges

In the developing world, the health care crisis revolves around the daily struggle for survival and the growing disparity between the haves and the have-nots. For the poor, the struggle for safe water, adequate nutrition, and access to basic health care leaves no energy or resources for other concerns—and most have little hope of winning the battle. For most of us living in the developed world, health care reform means we are assured of meeting our own and our family's ongoing health care needs, including access to the latest miracle drug or the availability of a bone marrow transplant. But as one physician from the hospital ship *M/V Anastasis* remarked on visiting Ghana in West Africa, "We are foolhardy to believe that we can be a healthy society when the world around us is languishing with diseases and poverty that we could alleviate."[102]

In addition, we face many new challenges if we are to meet the World Health Organization's main social target of "health for all in the twenty-first century." Consider the following list of issues that we must deal with, among others:

- *The pandemic of HIV/AIDS.* By the end of 2014, an estimated 36.9 million people in the world were living with HIV/AIDS. More than 95% of them are living in developing countries, and approximately 2.6 million are children less than 15 years of age.[103] The majority of these children were born to mothers with HIV, acquiring the virus during pregnancy, at birth, or during breastfeeding. More than 13 million children worldwide have lost one or both parents to AIDS.[104] Children orphaned by the rampant HIV/AIDS pandemic are more likely than other children to be malnourished and unschooled. Poverty itself increases the risk of infection because AIDS education is hampered by less access to health services and mass media, and by lower levels of literacy, among the poor in many countries.[105] Additionally, the loss of adult lives to AIDS deprives families and communities of healthy workers. Not only do these lost workers make up the most economically productive age group, but they also are the very same household members who previously had the responsibility to care for their elders.

- *The trend toward urbanization.*[106] According to FAO estimates, most of the increase in the world's population between 2000 and 2030 will occur in urban areas.[107] Urbanization has been a factor in the worldwide decline in breastfeeding; the increased consumption of fats, sugars, meat, and wheat; and the outbreak of cholera in several countries due to contamination of the urban water supply. As nations continue the rural-to-urban transition, the incidence of chronic diarrhea from polluted water and foodborne contamination remains a major public health problem in urban slums.
- *Rapid population growth.* The earth's population will increase from 7.3 to 9 billion by 2050—most of these people will be born into poor families in developing countries. Agricultural production will need to increase to feed these people. The number of nonagricultural jobs must also increase to support those not working in agriculture.
- *Destruction of the global environment.* The earth's capacity to sustain life is being impaired by many complex interrelated developments, including overconsumption, industrial pollution, overgrazing, and deforestation. This destruction of natural resources threatens the health and well-being of today's people and future generations.
- *The challenges of global aging.* The number of people age 65 or older is projected to grow from an estimated 524 million in 2010 to nearly 1.5 billion in 2050, with most of the increase in developing countries.[108] As both the proportion of older people and the length of life increase throughout the world, health and policy analysts are asking key questions:[109] Will population aging be accompanied by a longer period of good health and productivity, or will it be associated with more illness, disability, and dependency? How will aging affect health care costs? Global efforts to understand and find cures or ways to prevent such age-related diseases as Alzheimer's disease and frailty are needed, as well as efforts to prevent heart disease, stroke, diabetes, and cancer.[110] Some researchers suggest that nutrition status during pregnancy and infancy has a direct bearing on the development of risk factors for adult diseases—especially cardiovascular disease. Many people in developing countries may be at greater risk of health problems in older age as a result of poor nutrition in their early years. Data are needed to understand the health risks faced by older people in developing countries and to target appropriate prevention and intervention programs. Smaller family size, increasing urbanization, and fewer extended family households introduce challenges for families caring for older relatives.[111] The WHO Study on Global Aging and Adult Health (SAGE) involves nationally representative cohorts of respondents age 50 and over in six countries (China, Ghana, India, Mexico, Russia, and South Africa), who will be followed as they age.[112] This longitudinal study aims to generate data, raise awareness of the health issues of older people, and inform public policies regarding healthy aging.

Personal Action: Opportunity Knocks

The problems addressed in this chapter may appear to be so great that they can be approached only through worldwide political decisions. Indeed, the members of the International Conference on Nutrition stressed that intensive worldwide efforts were needed to overcome hunger and malnutrition and to foster self-reliant development. To this end, many individuals and groups are working to improve the future well-being of the world and its people through a number of national and international organizations. Check out the resources available online from the organizations listed in the Internet Resources section at the end of this chapter.

Consider working with others who have similar interests, raising awareness of world food security issues, following current hunger-related legislation, and calling for change by writing and telephoning local and national political representatives and expressing concern about foreign aid, trade, and other domestic policy issues relevant to world food security. Encourage your church or synagogue or mosque to support both overseas work and domestic outreach efforts to address food insecurity; support these efforts with monetary contributions.[113]

Individuals can help change the world through their personal choices.[114] Our choices have an impact on the way the rest of the world's people live and die. The world food problem derives in part from the demands we in the developed world place on the world's finite natural resources. In a sense, we contribute to the world food problem. People in affluent nations have the freedom and means to choose their lifestyles; people in poor nations do not. We can find ways to reduce our consumption of the world's resources by using only what we need (see the box that follows). Choosing a diet at the level of necessity, rather than excess, would reduce the resource demands made by our industrial agriculture. In fact, those who study the future are convinced that the hope of the world lies in "the widespread simplification of life that is vital to the well-being of the entire human family."[115] Personal lifestyles do matter, for a society is nothing more than the sum of its individuals. As we go, so goes our world.

How to Reduce Your Ecological Footprint

Electricity

1. Turn all lighting, appliances, and electronics off when not in use.

2. Unplug things when not in use and when traveling.

3. Keep the heat at or below 68 degrees in the winter and keep the air conditioner at or above 75 degrees in the summer. Don't open windows when the heat or A/C is on!

4. Use the clothes dryer as seldom as possible and wash clothes in cold water.

5. Use compact fluorescent light bulbs.

Food and Water

1. Eat local. Type in your zip code at Local Harvest (*www.localharvest.org*) to see a list of all the sustainably farmed foods in your area.

2. Eat in season. It reduces the amount of energy (and associated CO_2 emissions) needed to grow and transport the food we eat. To find out which foods, go to *www.eattheseasons.com*.

3. Grow it yourself, shop farmer's markets, and/or join a CSA.

4. Make it yourself. Enjoy cooking and baking (or at least learning to).

5. Eat lower on the food chain. The single greatest thing you can do to help stop climate change is to eat less meat or none at all.

6. Take shorter showers. Limit yourself to five minutes.

7. Turn off the water while brushing your teeth and while washing dishes. Use it only for rinsing.

Transportation

1. Keep your car clean and tuned up. Check your tire pressure and air filter regularly.

2. Drive efficiently (don't speed; avoid idling).

3. Carpool or use public transportation; fly less often.

4. Walk, jog, bike, skateboard, roller blade...

5. Plan ahead. Try to consolidate all your weekly errands into one outing to reduce the number of trips you take.

Goods (Reduce, Reuse, Recycle)

1. **REDUCE.** There's a reason it comes first. The less we use in the first place, the fewer resources are required and the less space we take up in landfills.

    a. Cancel any catalog and magazine subscriptions you can live without.

    b. Use both sides of sheets of paper.

    c. When shopping, take a list in order to avoid impulse purchases.

    d. Forgo convenience-oriented products such as individually packaged snack foods and single-use cleaning wipes.

2. **REUSE.** There's a reason it comes second.

    a. Take cloth bags to the store; carry a reusable coffee mug and water bottle, set of utensils, and food container.

    b. Opt for real dishes and utensils and cloth towels and napkins that you can launder instead of paper and plastic goods.

3. **RECYCLE.** There's a reason it comes last. Recycling should only happen once a product is absolutely not usable by anyone any longer.

Always

1. Think hard about whether you really need it or not, what went into it, and where it came from.

2. Read labels! Check out *www.greenerchoices.org/eco-labels*.

Source: *How to Reduce Your Ecological Footprint On (and Off) Campus*; more tips available at *http://www.smcm.edu/sustainability/*.

George McGovern, former U.S. senator and U.S. ambassador to the UN Agencies on Food and Agriculture in Rome, calls us all to action with the following words—excerpted from his book *The Third Freedom: Ending Hunger in Our Time:*

> Hunger is a political condition. The earth has enough knowledge and resources to eradicate this ancient scourge. Hunger has plagued the world for thousands of years. But ending it is a greater moral imperative now than ever before, because for the first time humanity has the instruments in hand to defeat this cruel enemy at a very reasonable cost.
>
> What will it cost if we don't end the hunger that now afflicts so many of our fellow humans? The World Bank has concluded that each year malnutrition causes the loss of 46 million years of productive life, at a cost of $16 billion annually, several times the cost of ending hunger and turning this loss into productive gain.
>
> Of course it is impossible to evaluate with dollars the real cost of hunger. What is the value of a human life? The twentieth century was the most violent in human history—with nearly 150 million people killed by war. But in just the last half of that century nearly three times as many died of malnutrition or related causes. How does one put a dollar figure on this terrible toll silently collected by the Grim Reaper? What is the cost of 800 million hungry people dragging through shortened and miserable lives, unable to study, work, play, or otherwise function normally because of the ever-present drain of hunger and malnutrition on body, mind, and spirit? What is the cost of millions of young mothers breaking under the despair of watching their children waste away and die from malnutrition? This is a problem we can resolve at a fraction of the cost of ignoring it. We need to be about that task now. I give you my word that anyone who looks honestly at world hunger and measures the cost of ending it for all time will conclude that this is a bargain well worth seizing. More often than not, those who look at the problem and the cost of its solution will wonder why humanity didn't resolve it long ago.[116]

ENDING HUNGER IS POSSIBLE.

#RethinkWorldHunger

THE HUNGER PROJECT

Anna Zhu for The Hunger Project

PROGRAMS IN **ACTION**

Vitamin A Field Support Projects

At least 140 million children under the age of five suffer from vitamin A deficiency (VAD) worldwide.[1] Millions more children consume inadequate amounts of vitamin A–rich foods and are thus at risk for VAD. Manifestations of VAD range from mild xerophthalmia (night blindness and/or Bitot's spots) to dryness of the conjunctiva and cornea and, in severe cases, to melting of the cornea and blindness. An estimated 250,000 to 500,000 vitamin A–deficient children become blind every year, half of them dying soon after losing their sight. Epidemiologic research has identified a relationship between marginal VAD, documented by reduced levels of circulating serum retinol, and higher mortality and morbidity rates from infectious diseases in children.[2] Researchers have confirmed that even mild VAD significantly increases the death rate among children age six months to six years. In particular, VAD significantly increases the severity of and risk for diarrheal disease, measles, and pneumonia—three of the main health threats facing children in the developing world.[3] Evidence from Africa suggests that vitamin A supplements can substantially reduce mortality and complications among children with measles, presumably by protecting epithelial tissue and ensuring the proper maintenance and functioning of the immune system.[4]

The most common factor contributing to the magnitude of VAD worldwide is the chronic inadequate dietary intake of vitamin A. Other contributors include poor nutrition status of mothers during pregnancy and lactation, low prevalence of breastfeeding, delayed or inappropriate introduction of complementary foods, high incidence of infection (such as diarrhea, acute respiratory infection, and measles), low levels of maternal education, drought, civil strife, poverty, and ecological deprivation in some regions resulting in limited availability of vitamin A–rich foods.[5] For example, the production and consumption of vitamin A–rich foods in Africa (dark green, leafy vegetables; orange-colored fruits and tubers; and red palm oil) are influenced strongly by seasonal trends and cultural practices.[6]

The U.S. Agency for International Development (USAID) developed a comprehensive global initiative for micronutrient programs—the Micronutrient Operational Strategies and Technologies (MOST) project.[7] MOST worked within 11 countries: Ghana, Madagascar, Uganda, and Zambia in Africa; Bangladesh, India, Morocco, Nepal, and the Philippines in Asia and the near East; and El Salvador and Nicaragua in Latin America.

MOST was a $45 million program administered by USAID for the promotion of activities designed to improve the micronutrient status of at-risk populations throughout the world, especially for vitamin A. Like other programs designed to eradicate and prevent VAD in developing countries, MOST sought an appropriate balance among dietary diversification, food fortification, and supplementation to deliver micronutrients to at-risk populations in an effective yet affordable way.

Dietary Diversification

MOST strategies included stimulating the production and consumption of vitamin A–rich foods through agricultural production, home gardening, food preservation, nutrition education, and social marketing. For example, MOST promoted the consumption of papayas, an excellent source of vitamin A, by pregnant women in the South Pacific. In some regions, foods containing vitamin A—especially vegetables and fruits—are readily available but are underutilized by vulnerable groups, particularly weaning-age children and pregnant and lactating women, because of traditional customs and beliefs. Consequently, dietary diversification programs in these areas focus on intensive nutrition education and social marketing campaigns to foster necessary community understanding, motivation, and participation.

Home gardens play a critical role in alleviating VAD in many communities. They provide a regular and secure supply of household food.

USAID also sponsors several VAD projects aimed at increasing vitamin A consumption by improving food processing techniques. Solar drying has been introduced as the appropriate technology for the preservation of mangoes, papayas, sweet potatoes, pumpkins, green leaves, and other vitamin A–rich foods in several countries. When solar-dried, these foods retain both flavor and carotene content and can alleviate seasonal variation in the availability of food. For example, the MANGOCOM Project in Senegal attempts to improve the vitamin A intake of weaning-age children by promoting dried mangoes, produced by women's cottage industries, as finger foods and fruit purees for toddlers.[8]

Food Fortification

Fortifying food is generally a large-scale undertaking and will be effective only if the target groups can buy and will consume the fortified product. In several developed countries, commonly consumed foods (such as margarine and milk) have been successfully fortified with vitamin A. Sugar is fortified with the vitamin in several regions of Central America, notably through VAD projects in Guatemala, El Salvador, and Honduras.[9] Pilot trials with vitamin A–fortified rice are under way in Brazil. A pilot program in the Philippines is currently testing vitamin A–fortified margarine as an alternative means of improving the vitamin A status of children.

Distribution of Vitamin A Supplements

Most commonly, VAD intervention programs periodically distribute vitamin A supplements in the form of high-dose capsules or oral dispensers. UNICEF typically donates the vitamin A capsules and helps organize the distribution efforts.* Often, supplements are delivered in conjunction with ongoing local health services, primary health care programs (e.g., maternal–child health projects), or national vaccination campaigns. UNICEF estimates that as many as 330,000 child deaths are prevented each year by vitamin A supplementation.

Vitamin A supplementation programs to date have reported a number of operational obstacles: low priority given to distribution of the supplements by primary health care workers, a lack of community demand for vitamin A, and a lack of awareness among policymakers of the critical nature of vitamin A nutrition status. However, similar obstacles have been overcome by immunization programs, which now reach 80% of targeted children worldwide.[10] For this reason, WHO and UNICEF have encouraged that vitamin A supplementation be integrated into existing immunization programs: "The provision of vitamin A supplementation through immunization services could dramatically expand the coverage of children in late infancy, giving a boost to vitamin A status before the critical period of weaning."[11]

Since immunization programs primarily target infants under 12 months of age, similar coverage would need to be provided by other means to children from one to six years old.

Supplementation is considered a temporary measure for the control and prevention of VAD. More lasting solutions include cultivating vitamin A–rich foods, fortifying foods with vitamin A, promoting improved food habits, eliminating poverty, and improving sanitation worldwide (**Table 14-6**).[12] Therefore, countries pursuing the high coverage achieved by integrating vitamin A supplement distribution into immunization programs are encouraged to allocate resources to these alternative efforts, as well.

Fortunately, the problem of VAD is not insurmountable. The numerous VAD projects worldwide have demonstrated three principles critical to successful VAD intervention efforts. First, successful interventions include preliminary formative research (such as focus group interviews), target audience segmentation, pretesting, and evaluation in program planning. Second, support by policymakers and participation by local community members is critical to sustaining the program. Finally, multiple channels of communication are recommended (mass media, traditional forms of media, and personal communications).

In the final analysis, individual countries will need to choose the most practical and cost-effective mix of VAD interventions given local customs, resources, and needs. Numerous international agencies—including WHO, UNICEF, the FAO, the World Bank, and USAID—continue their commitment to support country efforts to meet the World Summit for Children's goal of virtually eliminating VAD.

INTERVENTION	EXAMPLES	
Food-/menu-based	Modification in quantity and/or quality and diversity of menus Improved bioavailability through modified preservation/preparation procedures Household food-to-food fortification	**TABLE 14-6** Examples of Cost-Effective Interventions to Reduce Micronutrient Malnutrition
Fortification	Sugar, salt, and other condiments Oils and margarine Cereals and flours	
Supplementation	Periodic high doses Frequent low doses	
Public health measures	Breastfeeding promotion Immunizations Parasite control Sanitation/safe water	
Social and economic developmental measures	Female literacy Family spacing Income generation	

Source: Adapted from B. A. Underwood, "Micronutrient Malnutrition," *Nutrition Today* 33 (1998): 125; B. A. Underwood, "From Research to Global Reality: The Micronutrient Story," *Journal of Nutrition* 128 (1998): 145–51.

* The recommended dosing schedule for a vitamin A capsule distribution program is 200,000 IU given twice a year. The dose for children less than one year of age and for those who are significantly underweight is 100,000 IU twice a year. (A. Gadomski and C. Kjolhede, *Vitamin A Deficiency and Childhood Morbidity and Mortality* [Baltimore: Johns Hopkins University Publications, 1988].)

case study

UNICEF's Child Survival Campaign

By Alice Fornari, EdD, RD, Alessandra Sarcona, MS, RD, CSSD, and Alison Barkman, MS, RD, CDN

Scenario

You and seven other dietetic interns are embarking on a journey to Guatemala for a four-week community rotation. Each semester for the past three years, students from your university have been visiting the same village through Friends World and have done constructive projects, such as building a small schoolhouse and a church and cultivating a garden. This is the first year the dietetic interns will participate, with a focus on nutrition. The dietetic internship director will also attend to supervise; she is fluent in Spanish (the primary language of Guatemala), as are four of the eight interns. In the village there is a high incidence of dehydration from diarrhea and undernutrition. Most infants are formula-fed because there is little support for breastfeeding and a lack of knowledge about this practice. The goal of this rotation is to provide nutrition education on UNICEF's Child Survival campaign called GOBI (an acronym for the following elements of the UNICEF campaign: *growth charts, oral rehydration therapy, breast milk,* and *immunization*). UNICEF has initiated this program in many developing countries and will be setting up GOBI within the year in the Guatemalan village you will be visiting. Another goal of your rotation is to identify data that could be useful for a nutritional assessment and monitoring tool for the children of this village.

Learning Outcomes

- Describe the current status of malnutrition and health worldwide.
- Identify the components of UNICEF's Child Survival campaign.
- Recognize barriers to meeting nutrition and health goals in developing countries.
- Practice the nutrition care process specific to the GOBI program.

Foundation: Acquisition of Knowledge and Skills

1. Identify at least three organizations working toward the goal of ending world hunger.
2. Describe the current status of malnutrition and health worldwide.

3. Access the Millennium Development Goals (MDGs) and Sustainable Development Goals (SDGs).
4. Describe the basic principles of UNICEF's GOBI program from your text and at *www.rehydrate.org/index.html*. Also review the three "Fs"—female education, family spacing, and food supplements—which are the focus of the GOBI–FFF Program, at *http://rehydrate.org/facts/gobi-fff.htm*.

Step 1: *Identify Relevant Information and Uncertainties*

1. Which goals from the MDG and SDG are related to the GOBI program?
2. Note studies that support zinc supplementation as part of the oral rehydration component of GOBI for reducing severity of diarrhea at *www.rehydrate.org*.
3. List some major contributors to children's malnutrition in developing countries.

Step 2: *Interpret Information*

1. Create a list of data that will be useful to include in a nutritional assessment of the children in this village.
2. Describe some barriers that you and your group may encounter in delivering your nutrition messages relative to the GOBI program to the local population.

Step 3: *Draw and Implement Conclusions*

1. Select an element of GOBI (growth charts, oral rehydration therapy, breast milk, or immunization) that you and your fellow interns would view as a priority during your four weeks in the Guatemalan village and create a nutrition diagnosis using a PES statement. Include your rationale for choosing this element.
2. Describe intervention strategies that you might utilize with the Guatemalan community for the element of GOBI that you selected.

Step 4: *Engage in Continuous Improvement*

Establish a plan for monitoring and evaluating the outcomes of the GOBI element you selected that coincides with your nutrition diagnosis.

CHAPTER **SUMMARY**

Mapping Poverty and Undernutrition

▶ The underlying causes of global food insecurity and poverty are complex and interrelated. An estimated 795 million people suffer from chronic undernutrition, consuming too little food each day to meet even minimum energy requirements.

▶ Four micronutrient deficiencies are of particular concern: vitamin A deficiency, the world's most common cause of preventable child blindness and vision impairment; iron-deficiency anemia; iodine deficiency, which causes high levels of goiter and mental retardation; and zinc deficiency.

Food Insecurity in Developing Countries

▶ The current world population is approximately 7.3 billion, and the United Nations projects 9 billion by the year 2050. Three major factors affect population growth: birth rates, death rates, and standards of living.

▶ Developing nations must be allowed to increase their agricultural productivity by gaining greater access to five things simultaneously: land, capital, water, technology, and knowledge. Increasing people's access to assets, including credit, is also essential to ending hunger.

▶ Biotechnology may result in the development of drought-tolerant crop varieties with increased yield and resistance to pests, herbicides, and plant diseases. More research is needed to determine the long-term environmental and health effects of GM crops.

▶ Sustainable development meets the needs of the present without compromising the ability of future generations to meet their own needs.

People-Centered Development

▶ The Scaling Up Nutrition (SUN) movement seeks to scale up evidence-based interventions to prevent and treat undernutrition, especially during the critical 1,000-day period (see Table 14-2).

▶ The Millennium Development Goals set targets for progress in eight areas: poverty and hunger, primary education, women's equality, child mortality, maternal health, disease, environment, and a global partnership for development (see Table 14-3).

▶ GOBI is an acronym formed from four simple but profoundly important elements of UNICEF's Child Survival campaign: growth charts, oral rehydration therapy, breast milk, and immunization.

▶ In developing countries, emphasis is placed on four types of interventions: (1) breastfeeding promotion programs with guidance on preparing appropriate weaning foods, (2) nutrition education programs, (3) food fortification and/or the distribution of nutrient supplements and the identification of local food sources of nutrients in short supply, and (4) special feeding programs designed to provide vulnerable groups with nutritious supplemental foods.

Looking Ahead: The Global Challenges

▶ We face many new challenges if we are to meet the World Health Organization's main social target of "health for all in the twenty-first century": the pandemic of HIV/AIDS, the trend toward urbanization, rapid population growth, the destruction of the global environment, and the challenges of global aging.

SUMMARY **QUESTIONS**

1. List four causes of world food insecurity.
2. Describe the components of the GOBI intervention.
3. Describe two types of nutrition interventions that are commonly used in international nutrition programs and provide an example of each.
4. Describe the global public health issues related to global food insecurity that continue to challenge policymakers and program designers.
5. Identify the possibilities for personal action that can be taken to help solve the problem of world hunger.

INTERNET **RESOURCES** . . . .

Bread for the World Institute
www.bread.org

CARE
www.care.org

Catholic Charities USA
www.catholiccharitiesusa.org

Church World Service
http://cwsglobal.org

Development in Gardening (DIG)
www.reaplifedig.org

Eldis Information Resources
www.who.int/pmnch/topics/maternal/eldis/en

Food and Agriculture Organization
www.fao.org

Food First: Institute for Food and Development Policy
http://foodfirst.org

Freedom from Hunger
www.freedomfromhunger.org

Global Alliance for Improved Nutrition
www.gainhealth.org

Global Health Affairs, U.S. Department of Health and Human Services
www.globalhealth.gov

Global Health Council
http://globalhealth.org

Heifer International
www.heifer.org

Helen Keller International (HKI)
www.hki.org

The Hunger Project and Sustainable Development
www.thp.org

International Micronutrient Malnutrition Prevention Program
www.cdc.gov/immpact/index.html

International Food Policy Research Institute
www.ifpri.org

International Fund for Agricultural Development
www.ifad.org

International Institute for Sustainable Development
www.iisd.org/sd

Micronutrient Initiative
http://micronutrient.org

Oxfam America
www.oxfamamerica.org

Pan American Health Organization
www.paho.org

Partners in Information Access for the Public Health Workforce
http://phpartners.org/nutrition.html

Rehydration Project
www.rehydrate.org

RESULTS
www.results.org

Save the Children Fund
www.savethechildren.net

UNAIDS
www.unaids.org

UNICEF
www.unicef.org

UNICEF Maternal and Child Information
http://data.unicef.org

United Nations Development Programme (UNDP)
www.undp.org

UN System Standing Committee on Nutrition
www.unscn.org

U.S. Agency for International Development
www.usaid.gov

U.S. National Committee for World Food Day
www.worldfooddayusa.org

The World Bank
www.worldbank.org

World Food Programme
www.wfp.org

World Health Organization
www.who.int/en

WHO Nutrition Publications and Databases
www.who.int/nutrition/en/

Worldwatch Institute
www.worldwatch.org

Community Nutritionists in Action:
Planning Nutrition Interventions

Leon T. can't decide what to do next. "I could go downstairs and finish the pull-toy for young Kevin," he muses. Leon remembers leaving a pile of sawdust and wood chips scattered about the floor down there. "Or I could read the new *Reader's Digest*, just arrived today." Leon pats his shirt pocket for his glasses. Even with the magazine's large print, he can't read it very well without his glasses. Nope, they aren't in his shirt pocket, and they aren't in his pants pocket either, or on the end table. "I can't keep track of anything these days." He stands and starts a search of the easy chair and sofa. No luck.

He moves to the dining table, where he picks among the dirty dishes, magazine flyers, newspapers, and mail. His frustration mounts quickly when he realizes he can't remember what he's looking for. "Ah, look what I found—my pills!" Momentarily satisfied, he goes to the kitchen to take his medications. He's being treated for high blood pressure, underactive thyroid, and angina. He's suddenly confused, though, knowing there was something he was aiming to do. What was it?

Things just haven't been the same for Leon since his oldest, dearest friend Bill moved to Memphis a year ago to be close to his only daughter. Leon and Bill played golf regularly and met for dinner several nights a week. Now Leon doesn't seem to have the energy for much of anything, and he no longer enjoys puttering around his woodworking shop or reading.

At 76, Leon lives alone and likes it that way. But how much longer can he live independently? Does he need assistance with meals, medications, and doctor's visits? Are some of his symptoms due to depression or some other medical condition? Does he have family living nearby and, if so, what is the nature of his relationship with them?

These are the types of questions the community nutritionist asks when assessing Leon's needs. The community nutritionist aims to determine whether existing nutrition services and programs can improve his quality of life and help him continue to live independently.

This section illustrates several additional aspects of designing interventions and describes strategies to consider when designing a nutrition intervention program that targets lifestyle change related to eating patterns and physical activity. You will learn strategies to influence—and eventually change—the behavior of a target population. In this section you will learn how to work with culturally diverse groups, choose nutrition messages, market your program, evaluate its impact, and locate funding to cover program costs. As in Section One, the thread running through these discussions is entrepreneurship and how its essential principles—creativity and innovation—help community nutritionists "do more with less." The ultimate goal of community nutrition is to design programs that improve people's health and nutrition status.

CHAPTER 15

Gaining Cultural Competence in Community Nutrition

Kathleen D. Bauer, PhD, RD

LEARNING OBJECTIVES

After you have read and studied this chapter, you will be able to:

- Define cultural competence as exhibited by community nutrition practitioners.
- Identify and explain two cultural competence models.
- Describe the influence of culture on beliefs, values, and behaviors.
- Explain the importance of recognizing one's own cultural values and biases.
- Describe the basics of developing cross-cultural communication skills.

- Explain strategies for providing culturally competent nutrition interventions.

This chapter addresses such topics as sociocultural and ethnic food consumption patterns and the influence of cultural factors on food behavior, interpersonal communication skills, health behaviors and educational needs of diverse populations, and diversity issues, which have been designated by the Accreditation Council for Education in Nutrition and Dietetics (ACEND) as Foundation Knowledge and Learning Outcomes for dietetics education.

CHAPTER OUTLINE

Father and Mother, and Me
Sister and Auntie say
All the people like us are We,
And every one else is They
And They live over the sea,
While We live over the way,
But—would you believe it?
—They look upon We
As only a sort of They!
We eat pork and beef
With cow-horn-handled knives.
They who gobble Their rice off a leaf,
Are horrified out of Their lives;
And They who live up a tree,
Feast on grubs and clay,
(Isn't it scandalous?) look upon We
As a simply disgusting They!

—*RUDYARD KIPLING,*
"We and They"

For a complete list of references, please access the MindTap Reader within your MindTap course.

Introduction

How receptive would you be to a community education program featuring heart-healthy ways to prepare dog meat? How would you respond to a mandate that lobster could no longer be consumed because such practices are morally repugnant to the majority population? How would you like to be treated in a hospital where most of the décor was black and everyone wore black? If you were told to eat insects to improve the quality of your bones, would you readily change your eating habits? Does imagining such situations evoke feelings of confusion, shock, and anger? These examples may help you imagine how Hindus, who regard cows as sacred animals, may feel about community programs educating people on healthful ways to prepare beef; how Hmong may have felt about laws restricting healing ceremonies that include animal sacrifices; and how recent Asian immigrants may feel about going to a health center where everyone wears white, the color of mourning.

These scenarios highlight gaps in understanding food practices among various ethnic groups; however, differences between cultures occur on many levels—communication, sense of time, family practices, beliefs about the cause of illness, and healing beliefs, to name a few. Because North American society is composed of a large variety of groups, community health professionals and organizations need to have strategies to bridge cultural gaps. These strategies can be learned through gaining cultural competence.

Gaining Cultural Competence

Attitude A collection of beliefs that includes an evaluative aspect.

Gaining cultural competence in community health care is a developmental process and means developing **attitudes**, skills, knowledge, and levels of awareness that enable one to provide culturally appropriate, respectful, and relevant interventions. The foundation of cultural competence is development of an awareness of one's own cultural matrix and an understanding that cultural beliefs influence our behavior and our conscious and unconscious thoughts. There also needs to be an understanding that culture strongly influences food behavior, and interventions need to be culturally appropriate as well as nutritionally sound for clients. A food and nutrition practitioner needs to approach cross-cultural interactions with a nonjudgmental attitude and a willingness to explore and understand different values, beliefs, and behaviors. To work successfully with individuals from substantially different cultures or to develop cross-cultural programming, culturally sensitive communication, negotiation, and education skills are required. Consideration must also be given to the overall organizational cultural competence that community service agencies need in order to provide appropriate services and to support individual community health professionals to work effectively. In addition, health professionals need to recognize the importance of including clients as integral parts of planning and implementation of interventions.

Terms Related to Cultural Competence

An understanding of the relevant concepts and terminology is an important first step toward gaining cultural competence.

Culture Culture is shared history, consisting of "the integrated pattern of thoughts, communications, actions, customs, beliefs, values, and institutions associated, wholly or partially, with racial, ethnic, or linguistic groups, as well as with religious, spiritual, biological, geographical, or sociological characteristics."[1] The societal groups can include gender, age, sexual orientation, physical or mental ability, health, occupation, and socioeconomic status. We develop cultural characteristics and beliefs, including health beliefs, through life experiences and education. Culture directly and indirectly influences how we view the world and interact with others. Because each of us is a member of a number of societal groups interacting with each other and we have unique life experiences, no two people acquire exactly the same cultural attributes. In addition, culture is fluid. We tend to migrate to and away from various cultures throughout our lives. For example, an individual may change religious membership, residence, career, or recreational pursuits, resulting in the loss or acquisition of cultural attributes.

Cultural Values Munoz and Luckman[2] describe cultural **values** as "principles or standards that members of a cultural group share in common." Because cultural values are the grounding forces that provide meaning, structure, and organization in our lives, we hold on to them in the face of numerous obstacles. There are many examples in history of people practicing an outlawed religion in secrecy, despite the certainty of severe consequences if they were caught. See **Table 15-1** for a list of functions of cultural values.

Value Any belief or quality that is important, desirable, or prized.

• Provide a set of rules by which to govern lives.
• Serve as a basis for attitudes, beliefs, and behaviors.
• Guide actions and decisions.
• Give direction to lives and help solve common problems.
• Influence how to perceive and react to others.
• Help determine basic attitudes regarding personal, social, and philosophical issues.
• Reflect a person's identity and provide a basis for self-evaluation.

TABLE 15-1

Functions of Cultural Values

Source: Adapted from J. Luckmann, *Transcultural Communication in Health Care* (Albany, NY: Delmar/Thomson Learning, 2000), 23.

Diversity In the cultural context, diversity consists of differences among groups of people. Some forms of diversity are visible, such as physical differences, abilities and disabilities, and language differences. Other forms of diversity that may not be visible or obvious include sexual orientation, gender identification, socioeconomic status, and age.

Cross-Cultural The term *cross-cultural* denotes interaction between or among individuals who represent distinctly different cultures. Because individuals develop behavior patterns and views of the world on the basis of unique life experiences and membership in several cultural groups, no two people exhibit identical behavior patterns. Therefore, all encounters between two people can be viewed as linking cultures. However, encounters between individuals or groups are not labeled as cross-cultural unless the attributes of the cultures they represent are substantially different.

Ethnocentric People tend to be ethnocentric—that is, to consider the beliefs, values, customs, and viewpoints of their own group superior to those of every other group. Every culture teaches its members to regard its beliefs and views of reality as the best, and some cultures even teach that their beliefs are the only acceptable ones.

Need for Cultural Competence

There is a compelling need for health professionals to communicate with clients, families, communities, and fellow professionals in a culturally competent manner. The reasons include demographic diversity and projected population shifts, disparities in health status, increased utilization of traditional therapies, and legislative, regulatory, and accreditation mandates.

Demographics—Population Trends The United States has always had a rich mix of ethnic, racial, and societal groups, but the challenge of meeting the needs of a **multicultural** and dynamic population seems greater than ever (**Figure 15-1**). Since the 1970s, the United States has been moving toward a cultural plurality, where no single ethnic or racial group is a majority. Census data indicate that diverse racial and ethnic groups in the United States have increased from approximately one-fourth to one-third of the population, with those reporting belonging to two or more racial groups as the fastest-growing segment.[3] This trend is expected to continue, with minority groups climbing to 56% of the total population by the year 2060, as compared with 38% in 2014 (**Figure 15-2**).[4] Hispanics, Asians, and Pacific Islanders have been increasing more rapidly than the rest of the U.S. population. In 2010, Hispanics accounted for nearly 16% of the U.S. population,

Multicultural In this chapter, a property of groups wherein several cultures are represented.

FIGURE 15-1 Percent Distribution of the U.S. Population by Race/Ethnicity, 2014 Hispanic origin is considered an ethnicity, not a race. Hispanics may be of any race. The sum of the five racial groups adds to more than 100% because individuals may report more than one race.

Source: S. L. Colby and J. M. Ortman, *Projections of the Size and Composition of the U.S. Population: 2014 to 2060*, Current Population Reports, P25–1143, U.S. Census Bureau, Washington, D.C., 2014.

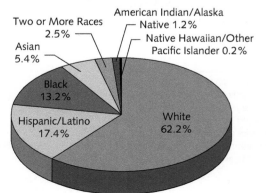

Total Population = 318,857,056

Two or More Races 2.5%
Asian 5.4%
Black 13.2%
Hispanic/Latino 17.4%
White 62.2%
American Indian/Alaska Native 1.2%
Native Hawaiian/Other Pacific Islander 0.2%

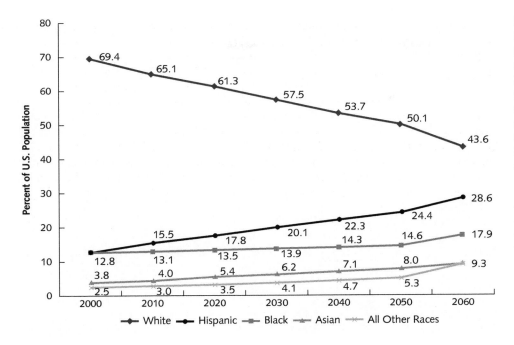

FIGURE 15-2

Projected U.S. Population by Race and Hispanic Origin from 2000 to 2060 Percentages for 2000 and 2010 are actual. Hispanic can be any race. Totals do not equal 100% for this reason. "All Other Races" includes American Indian and Alaska Native alone, Native Hawaiian and Other Pacific Islander alone, and two or more races.

Source: S. L. Colby and J. M. Ortman, *Projections of the Size and Composition of the U.S. Population: 2014 to 2060*, Current Population Reports, P25–1143, U.S. Census Bureau, Washington, D.C., 2014.

exceeding African Americans as the largest minority group, who accounted for 13% of the population.[5] These changes have been brought about by alterations in immigration laws (the foreign-born population has more than doubled in the past 20 years), by corporate expansions into the global market, and by the tendency for minorities and **immigrants** to have higher birth rates. In addition, the population mosaic is shifting in response to internal migration and the greater percentage of older adults.[6]

Linguistic diversity accompanies population shifts. Over 300 languages are spoken in the United States, and during the last decade the number of people who cannot speak English has increased substantially. Census results reveal that approximately 21% of the U.S. population spoke a language other than English at home. In some states the percentages were substantially higher than the national average, such as New Mexico (36%) and California (43%).[7]

Along with changes in ethnic and racial diversity, there are also dramatic changes in the number of people who make up the older segment of the American population. For example, the percentage of people 65 years of age and older was 14% in 2014, but is expected to increase to 24% by 2060.[8] An older population increases the need for health professionals to have expertise in dealing with chronic diseases and the ability to communicate with those who have disabilities, such as limitations in sight and hearing.

Immigrants Individuals who move to a new country seeking permanent residence.

Increased Utilization of Traditional Therapies

Community health professionals cannot ignore the substantial increase in the utilization of complementary, alternative, and traditional therapies, such as meditation, acupuncture, and herbal medicine, which are often culture based. The Centers for Disease Control and Prevention reported in 2007 that almost 4 out of 10 adults (38.3%) had used some type of **complementary and alternative medicine**, including diet-based therapies, in the past 12 months.[9] The Academy of Nutrition and Dietetics has set standards of practice and standards of professional performance for registered dietitians in integrative and functional medical nutrition therapy (IFMNT).[10] IFMNT uses both conventional and complementary therapies as well

Complementary and alternative medicine (CAM) Complementary medicine is used together with conventional treatments (e.g., using acupuncture to help with side effects of cancer treatment), whereas alternative medicine is used instead of conventional medicine. See Appendix B.

The United States has always had a rich mix of ethnic, racial, and societal groups; the challenge for community nutritionists is in meeting the needs of this diverse and dynamic audience.

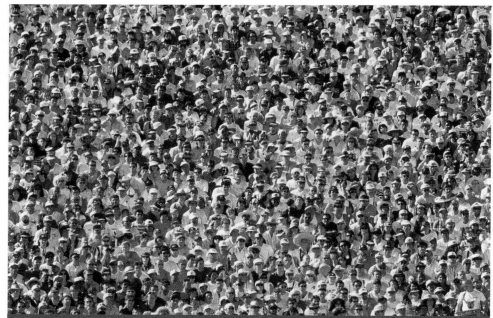

Bob Thomas/Stone/Getty Images

as traditional products and practices that are not part of standard care, such as massage or homeopathy. Diana Dyer, popular lecturer and author of *A Dietitian's Cancer Story: Information and Inspiration for Recovery and Healing from a Three-Time Cancer Survivor*, has been an advocate of learning about and combining conventional and complementary approaches to healing. She made many changes in her lifestyle to enhance healing but states in her book that "although I am a nutritionist to the core, learning to meditate, and doing it faithfully, has been the most important change I have made."[11] Kanjana also found a positive effect of using complementary therapies in her study of adolescent girls.[12] She found an improvement in various nutritional parameters after the girls participated in 80 minutes of yoga exercises each morning for six months. Developing an understanding and an appreciation of traditional health practices of various cultures can help health practitioners plan and implement meaningful interventions.

Health disparities Health disparities exist when a segment of the population bears a disproportionate incidence of a health condition or illness.

Race Refers to a category of population based on physical characteristics and shared ancestry.

Ethnicity A property of a group that consists of its sharing cultural traditions, having a common linguistic heritage, and originating from the same land. Ethnicity refers to membership in a national or tribal group.

Health Disparities

Not all cultural groups have the same health status. There are substantial **health disparities** (also called health inequalities) in segments of the population—disparities based on gender, age, **race** or **ethnicity**, education, income, religion, disability, geographic location, sexual orientation, or other characteristics historically linked to discrimination or exclusion. Disparities can exist in regard to access to health care; delivery of quality, competent health care services; and health outcomes. The incidence of chronic disease, disability, and death is higher among American Indian or Alaska Native, Asian American, black or African American, Hispanic or Latino, and Native Hawaiian or Other Pacific Islander.[13] (See **Table 15-2** for specific examples of health disparities among these groups.) Women and minorities were often excluded from research until a federal mandate in 1993 required inclusion. Studies indicate that adults with physical disabilities are four times more likely to report being in fair or poor health as compared to those without disabilities (40.3% vs 9.9%).[14] Rural Americans have higher rates of chronic illness and poorer overall health than those living in urban areas.[15] Lesbians are more likely than women of other sexual orientations to be overweight and obese. In addition, lesbian, gay, bisexual, and transgender (LGBT) individuals are more likely than

TABLE 15-2 Specific Examples of Health Disparities

African Americans	In 2010, the life expectancy at birth of whites was 79 years but only 75 for blacks. Infant mortality rate for blacks is more than double that of white Americans, and African American infants are four times as likely to die from issues related to low birthweight than white infants. In 2010, African Americans had a 30% higher chance of dying from heart disease and were twice as likely to die from a stroke than white individuals. They have the highest cancer-related mortality rate of any racial or ethnic group in America, as the death rate for all cancers is 30% higher. African American women are almost 40% more likely to die of breast cancer than white women. As of 2012, African Americans were 20% more likely to have asthma and three times more likely to die from asthma than whites. African Americans are also 70% more likely to be diagnosed with diabetes and 2.2 times more likely to die from diabetes than whites. African American women are 80% more likely to be obese compared to white women.
Hispanics	Obesity is an issue for Hispanic Americans, as adults are 1.2 times as likely to be obese and children are 1.6 times as likely to be overweight compared to white counterparts. Hispanics are also twice as likely to have diabetes as whites. Although overall cancer rates are lower for Hispanic Americans than non-Hispanic white populations, Hispanic Americans are twice as likely to have and die from liver cancer, and Hispanic women are 2.2 times more likely to have stomach cancer and 1.4 times more likely to die from cervical cancer than white women. Hispanic Americans account for a disproportionately high 20% of HIV infection. Hispanic men were three times more likely to have HIV/AIDS and women were four times as likely to have AIDS than white counterparts in 2011.
Native Hawaiians/ Pacific Islanders	Native Hawaiian/Pacific Islanders are 30% more likely to be obese, have high blood pressure, or be diagnosed with cancer as compared to white adults. Compared with white populations, Native Hawaiian/Pacific Islanders are three times more likely to develop coronary heart disease. They are also four times as likely to die from stroke than white adults. In Hawaii, Native Hawaiians are twice as likely as whites to be diagnosed with diabetes.
Asian Americans	In 2012, tuberculosis was 24 times more common among Asians. In 2010, Asian Americans were 5.5 times more likely to have chronic hepatitis B than whites. While the overall prevalence of AIDS in America has been declining within the white population over the past five years, it has increased among Asian Americans. Different subsets of the Asian American population have unique health concerns; for example, Filipino adults are 70% more likely to be obese than other Asian Americans, and Chinese Americans have higher asthma rates than white Americans.
American Indians/ Alaska Natives	American Indians/Alaska Natives are 1.3 times as likely to have high blood pressure, 60% more likely to be obese, and twice as likely to have a stroke as white populations. Overall, American Indians/Alaska Natives have a 50% higher AIDS rate, while American Indian/Alaska Native women were three times as likely as white women to be diagnosed with HIV. Adults in this population were two times as likely as white adults to be diagnosed with and die from diabetes. Cirrhosis deaths were 2.6 times that of non-Hispanic whites. Pima American Indians have the highest incidence of diabetes in the world.

Sources: E. Arias, United States Life Tables, 2010, National Vital Statistics Reports 63, no. 7 (2014). Hyattsville, MD: National Center for Health Statistics, Office of Minority Health, *Minority Populations*. Available at *http://minorityhealth.hhs.gov/omh/browse.aspx?lvl=2&lvlID=26*.

heterosexuals to rate their health as poor, have more chronic conditions, and have higher prevalence and earlier onset of disabilities than heterosexuals.[16]

Besides ethical, physical, and emotional turmoil for individuals who are the recipients of inadequate health care, there is a national cost to the health care system. Between 2003 and 2006, the combined costs of health inequalities and premature death in the United States were $1.24 trillion.[17]

Causes of Health Disparities
A number of interrelated factors are thought to contribute to health disparities:

Minorities Individuals designated by the 2010 U.S. Census Bureau as American Indians and Alaska Natives, Asian Americans, Native Hawaiians and Other Pacific Islanders, blacks or African Americans, or Hispanics or Latinos.

- **Socioeconomic status. Minorities** often have lower levels of income and education, reside in poorer housing, live in unsafe neighborhoods, and have fewer opportunities to engage in health-promoting behaviors. They are more likely to live in food deserts, where nutritious food may be expensive or unavailable.[18]
- **Culture.** Some beliefs and health practices of minorities may contribute to health risks. In a study of African American health attitudes, beliefs, and behaviors, only about 50% of respondents identified health as a high priority in their lives.[19] Mistrust and racism, two primary concerns within the African American community, have been negatively correlated to patient satisfaction and lead to a decreased desire to seek health care.[20] An evaluation of Hispanic health beliefs and practices indicates a greater emphasis on the power of God and less on preventive health care.[21] Degree of **acculturation** among immigrants and length of time in the United States have been shown to negatively influence food practices and health, especially among men.[22] Many immigrants are in better health than their counterparts who were born in the United States. The health advantages decrease the longer the immigrants live in the United States. For example, generational analyses of Asian Americans show significant increases in BMI in succeeding generations as compared to first-generation residents of the United States.[23] In addition, African immigrants who reported greater acculturation to American eating habits such as high fast-food intake and low intake of fruits and vegetables were more likely to have poor self-rated health scores.[24]

Acculturation Process of adopting the beliefs, values, and behaviors of another culture.

- **Access to and utilization of quality health care services.** Research has shown that many minority populations are less likely to receive routine medical checkups, obtain immunizations, undergo examinations for cancer, and receive treatment for hypertension.[25] Factors found to limit utilization of available services include inconvenient location, unawareness of services, feelings of discomfort with providers, health provider attitudes, lack of translators, and waiting in long lines.[26] Rural communities suffer from a lack of physicians and dentists.
- **Discrimination/racism/stereotyping.** Individuals who perceive that they have been treated in a racist manner are more likely to exhibit psychological distress, depressive symptoms, substance use, and physical health problems.[27] The majority of health care professionals find prejudice morally repugnant, but several studies indicate that even well-meaning health care professionals often demonstrate unconscious negative racial attitudes and make decisions based on **bias**, prejudice, and **stereotypes**, contributing to disparities in health care outcomes.[28]

Bias "A mental slant or leaning to one side; a highly personal and unreasoned distortion of judgment."[30]

Stereotypes Assumptions that information about a cultural group applies to all individuals who appear to represent that group.

- **Environment.** Minorities and the poor are more likely to live in polluted environments and to work in hazardous occupations that increase the likelihood of exposure to toxins.[29]
- **Insurance issues.** Lack of insurance has frequently been identified as a cause of health disparities. One of the major goals of the Affordable Health Care Act is to bring an end to this national problem. Hopefully, this will no longer be a component cause of health disparities in the future.

Underrepresentation of Health Care Providers from Culturally and Linguistically Diverse Groups
Community nutrition practitioners are frequently challenged to provide services for cultural groups they have never encountered. At the present time, health professionals represent limited ethnic and linguistic diversity. For example, the majority of registered dietitians (82%) are non-Hispanic whites.[31] Whites make up the majority of the U.S. health workforce (77.6%) compared with blacks or African Americans (13.6%), Asians (6%), and individuals reporting multiple races or

other race (2%).[32] Diversity in the composition of the health care workforce is important because it affects outcomes, quality, safety, and satisfaction. According to the 2013 National Healthcare Disparities Report, "A more ethnically and linguistically diverse population of health care providers could help break down cultural barriers to health care access."[33] In addition, minority health care professionals are more likely to work in medically underserved communities.

The health care workforce is expected to diversify along with the rest of the country due to increasing opportunities and the efforts of government and health professional organizations, including the Academy of Nutrition and Dietetics, to encourage minorities to train for health professional careers. Census Bureau predictions for the 2005–2050 time period indicate that in general, a more diverse population will be available in the future to fill openings in the health care field. Baby boomers (Americans born between 1946 and 1964) will steadily exit the labor force, and the numbers of minorities will considerably increase.[34] The challenge of serving a diverse and rapidly changing public underscores the need for diversity in the health professions and also highlights the importance of universal cultural competence skills because the mix of professionals will never be identical to the population it serves.

Legislative, Regulatory, and Accreditation Mandates
Recognizing the need to develop cultural competence skills, professional and government organizations mandate culturally appropriate standards.[35,36] **Title VI of the Civil Rights Act** of 1964 reads, in part, "No person in the United States shall, on ground of race, color or national origin, be excluded from participation in, be denied the benefits of, or be subjected to discrimination under any program or activity receiving federal financial assistance." Guidance issued by the Office of Civil Rights further clarifies Title VI as it relates to persons with limited English proficiency, stating that providers should include "reasonable steps to provide services and information in appropriate languages other than English to ensure that persons with limited English proficiency are effectively informed and can effectively benefit."[37] With a specific focus on the health care system, a congressionally mandated report, *Unequal Treatment: Confronting Racial and Ethnic Disparities in Health Care*, included the contribution of health care practitioners to health disparities.[38] In order to address this problem and provide guidance to health care providers, the United States Department of Health and Human Services (DHHS) created national standards for culturally and linguistically appropriate services in health care.[39] (See the section on organizational cultural competence later in this chapter as well as Table 15-15.)

The most recent government initiative dealing with health care disparities is the Patient Protection and Affordable Care Act of 2010. This act has a number of provisions to improve the health of underserved populations including insurance reform, improved access to health care, quality improvement, cost containment, and public health initiatives.[40,41] Title V of this act specifically addressed the need for a culturally competent health care workforce, as it specifies that funding, loan repayment, and scholarships for medical professionals will favor programs with cultural competency curriculum and individuals with a background of cultural competence.[42] The Act also specifies support for the development and implementation of programs that aim to reduce health disparities, improve prevention techniques, and focus on health care for disabled individuals.[43]

An overarching objective of *Healthy People 2020* is to improve the linguistic and cultural competency of public health professionals.[44] The Academy of Nutrition and Dietetics and the Accreditation Council for Education in Nutrition and Dietetics (ACEND) has integrated diversity requirements into numerous components of the organization, including curriculum requirements, a diversity philosophy statement, code of ethics, strategic planning, and member resources.[45]

Title VI of the Civil Rights Act The provision that a recipient of federal money may not discriminate on the basis of race, color, or national origin.

A culturally competent health care system may not completely eradicate health dispari-ties, but it does provide the means to "respond to the needs of individuals, families, and communities in an acceptable, meaningful, and equitable manner."[46] In order to help guide food and nutrition practitioners to develop interventions to eliminate health disparities, the Academy of Nutrition and Dietetics developed discipline-specific recommendations (**Figure 15-3**).[47] Particularly salient strategies for community nutrition practitioners are addressed throughout this chapter.

FIGURE 15-3 Ways in Which Food and Nutrition Practitioners Can Influence the Elimination of Racial and Ethnic Health Disparities

Source: "Practice Paper of the American Dietetic Association: Addressing Racial and Ethnic Health Disparities," *Journal of the American Dietetic Association* 111 (2011): 446–456 (p. 450).

Cultural Competence Models

Learning to communicate across cultures is an evolutionary process and requires practice, time, and effort. In order to work effectively, food and nutrition practitioners need to con-tinually assess their own cultural competence as well as the organization/system in which they work and the environment as a whole. The National Center for Cultural Competence website and the Office of Minority Health have a number of tools and processes to conduct self and organization assessments.[48,49] To provide a framework for the process, a number of models have been developed. Two of them have particular significance for community nutrition practitioners: the cultural competence continuum and the Campinha-Bacote cultural competence model.

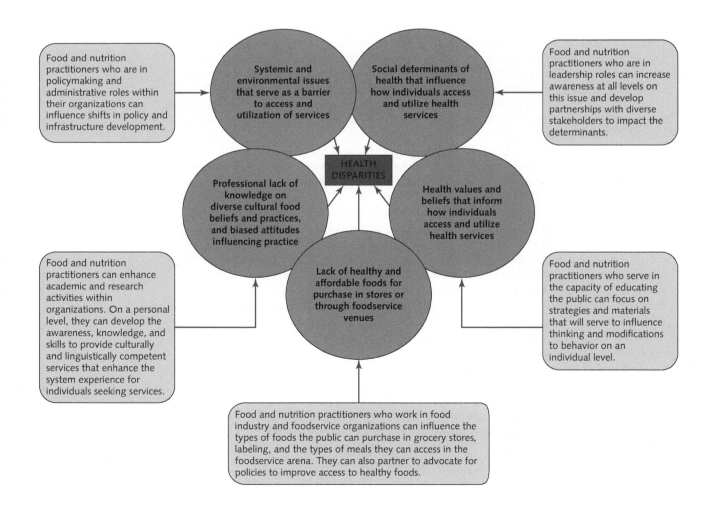

Cultural Competence Continuum Model In the cultural competence continuum model, the process of gaining cultural competence is envisioned as a succession of stages (**Table 15-3**). The continuum provides a visual guide for assessing individual or agency progress. However, movement through the stages cannot be expected to occur in lockstep for all cultural groups. For example, a person could be at a high level of proficiency for interacting with individuals who have disabilities but be at a lower stage for working with lesbians and gays.

The Campinha-Bacote Cultural Competence Model A dynamic conceptual model of cultural competence developed by Campinha-Bacote[50] for health care professionals views cultural competence as a process rather than an end result: "the process in which the health care provider continuously strives to achieve the ability and availability to effectively work within the cultural context of a client (individual, family, or community)." This model views cultural awareness, cultural skill, cultural knowledge, cultural encounters, and cultural desire as five interdependent constructs of cultural competence (**Table 15-4**). Although health care professionals can work on any one of the constructs to improve balance of the others, cultural encounters play a critical role by having the greatest impact.

STAGE	DESCRIPTION
Cultural destructiveness	Attitudes, practices, and policies are destructive to other cultures.
Cultural incapacity	Paternalistic attitude toward the "unfortunates." No capacity to help.
Cultural blindness	Belief that culture makes no difference. Everyone is treated the same. Approaches of the dominant culture are applicable for everyone.
Cultural precompetence	Weaknesses in serving culturally diverse populations are realized, and there are some attempts to make accommodations.
Cultural competence	Differences are accepted and respected, self-evaluations are continuous, cultural skills are acquired, and a variety of adaptations are made to better serve culturally diverse populations. Situations can be evaluated from multiple frames of reference.
Cultural proficiency	Engages in activities that add to the knowledge base, conducts research, develops new approaches, publishes, encourages organizational cultural competence, and works in society to improve cultural relations.

TABLE 15-3 Cultural Competence Continuum

Source: Adapted from T. Cross, B. Bazron, K. Dennis, and M. Isaac, *Toward a Culturally Competent System of Care*, Volume I (Washington, D.C.: Georgetown University Child Development Center, 1989).

CULTURAL CONSTRUCT[a]	DESCRIPTION
Awareness	Health care providers become appreciative of the influence of culture on the development of values, beliefs, lifeways, practices, and problem-solving strategies. A basic requirement for cultural awareness is an in-depth exploration of one's own cultural background, including biases and prejudices toward other cultural groups.
Skill	Health care providers learn to perform culturally sensitive assessments and interventions.
Knowledge	Health care professionals develop a sound educational foundation concerning various worldviews in order to understand behaviors, including food practices, health customs, and attitudes toward seeking help from health care providers. They also acquire knowledge of physical needs, such as common health problems and nutrition issues of different cultures.
Encounters	Providers seek and engage in cross-cultural encounters and reflect on experiences allowing integration of cultural competence constructs.
Desire	To appear **genuine** and to be effective cross-culturally, the health care provider must have a true inner feeling of wanting to engage in the process of becoming culturally competent.

TABLE 15-4 Constructs of the Campinha-Bacote Model of Cultural Competency

Genuine Behavior and words are congruent, appear open and spontaneous; opposite is phony.

[a] The mnemonic ASKED can assist health care professionals in assessing their level of cultural competence.

Source: Adapted for community nutrition practitioners from J. Campinha-Bacote, *The Process of Cultural Competence in the Delivery of Healthcare Services: The Journey Continues*, 5th ed. (Cincinnati, OH: Transcultural C.A.R.E. Associates, 2007).

Public markets often provide a venue for engaging in cross-cultural encounters. Many of the nation's public markets maintain a public space that builds upon the economic, social, and cultural assets within the surrounding communities. The markets provide an opportunity to sample the foods, crafts, and other aspects of diverse cultural groups.

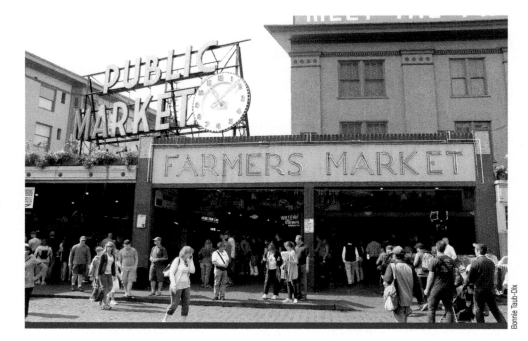

Bonnie Taub-Dix

Worldview Perception of the world including opinions, judgments, and beliefs biased by culture, values, and experience.

Cultural Awareness

The foundation of cultural competence is an awareness of your own beliefs, values, and attitudes and an understanding that these attributes reflect your own biases and are really just one point of view among many. Without cultural self-awareness, there is a tendency to be ethnocentric, devalue alternative cultural practices, blindly impose your own cultural procedures, and miss seeing opportunities for successful interventions.

Developing cultural self-awareness takes a concerted effort because our views are part of our essence and feel so natural. They are the basic components of how we believe the world should function. Because most of our life experiences occur within the same cultural context, our **worldviews** are repeatedly reinforced. We experience culture shock when we realize that our view of the world is not universally accepted. For example, nutritionists and other health care providers belong to the culture of biomedicine—health care based on the principles of natural sciences—and may be surprised to find that a client believes that illness is a spiritual matter and in fact may be due to a transgression of an ancestor.

An awareness of the high degree of importance you place on your own particular beliefs, values, and cultural practices can help you appreciate individuals from a culture different from yours holding dear specific beliefs, values, and cultural practices. Also, you can then empathize with individuals from non-Western cultures who are experiencing confusion and problems as they try to participate in the North American health care system.

A method of becoming aware of your beliefs, values, and biases is to compare some of them to those of cultures different from your own. **Table 15-5** provides a comparison of majority American values to those of various other cultures. One of the best ways to become aware of differences is to immerse yourself in the perceptual world or culture of others, as can be done by traveling or working in other countries.

Cultural Skill

Community health practitioners need a variety of skills to provide culturally meaningful interventions. Guidelines for cross-cultural communication, recommendations for working with interpreters, and a review of selected culturally appropriate intervention strategies are covered later in this chapter.

MAJORITY AMERICAN CULTURE	OTHER CULTURES
Mastery over nature	Harmony with nature
Individuality/control over the environment	Fate
Action, task oriented	Being
Time dominates, punctual	Personal interaction dominates
Human equality	Hierarchy/rank/status/authority
Individualism/privacy	Group welfare
Youth/thin/fit	Elders
Self-help/earned	Birthright/inheritance
Competition/free enterprise	Cooperation
Future orientation	Past or present orientation
Informality	Formality
Directness/openness/honesty	Indirectness/ritual/"face"
Practicality/efficiency	Idealism
Materialism	Spiritualism/detachment
Mind, body, and soul separate	Mind, body, and soul integrated
Disease is preventable	Humans cannot control disease
Confidentiality	Family decision making
Provider–client partnership	Provider-directed health care

TABLE 15-5

Comparison of Common Values and Beliefs

Sources: Adapted from readings of two authorities: P. G. Kittler, K. P. Sucher, and M. Nahikian-Nelms, *Food and Culture*, 6th ed. (Belmont, CA: Wadsworth/Cengage, 2012); Debra P. Keenan, "In the Face of Diversity: Modifying Nutrition Education Delivery to Meet the Needs of an Increasingly Multicultural Consumer Base," *Journal of Nutrition Education* 28 (1996): 86–91.

Cultural Knowledge When possible, community nutrition practitioners should invest time in learning about unfamiliar cultures that they are likely to encounter. There are a variety of strategies that health care professionals can employ to learn about other cultures. Eat at ethnic restaurants, explore stories about other cultures in the media, establish focus groups to gain insight into a target population's culture, read about cultural customs and etiquette, read local newspapers, travel, take language lessons, familiarize yourself with diverse neighborhoods, and attend professional development and training classes. Understanding various cultures provides a vehicle for developing attitudes congruent with cultural competence and discourages reliance on stereotypes. (**Table 15-6** lists values and attitudes congruent with cultural competence.) Cultural knowledge also provides the tools needed to develop culturally effective and relevant programs.

By exploring various cultures, you learn about new ways of interpreting reality and can develop alternative lenses through which to view your interactions with those who appear different from you. Keep in mind that it will be natural to experience some discomfort during your investigations as you learn about values and beliefs that conflict with yours. However, the process helps you develop attitudes congruent with cultural competence, such as appreciation, respect, and understanding of people who have cultural beliefs and behaviors different from your own.

An understanding of the generalities of cultural groups enables community nutrition practitioners to develop relevant programming that builds on strengths and respects cultural differences. Without cultural understanding, there is a risk that the program you develop could conflict with common beliefs, values, and customs of the group. (See **Table 15-7** for specific examples.)

TABLE 15-6 Values and Attitudes Congruent with Cultural Competence

For you to behave in a culturally competent manner, your attitudes need to convey an understanding and acceptance of diverse values and behaviors such as the following:

- Family is defined differently by different cultures (e.g., extended family members, fictive kin, godparents).
- Individuals from culturally diverse backgrounds may desire varying degrees of acculturation into the dominant culture.
- Male–female roles in families may vary significantly among different cultures (e.g., who makes major decisions for the family as well as play and social interactions expected of male and female children).
- Age and life-cycle factors must be considered in interactions with individuals and families (e.g., high value placed on the decisions of elders or the role of the eldest male or female in families).
- Meaning or value of medical treatment, health education, and wellness may vary greatly among cultures.
- Religion and other beliefs may influence how individuals and families respond to illnesses, disease, and death.
- Folk and religious beliefs may influence a family's reaction and approach to a child born with a disability or later diagnosed with a disability or special health care needs.
- Customs and beliefs about food, its value, its preparation, and its use differ from culture to culture.

Source: Adapted from material developed by T. D. Goode, National Center for Cultural Competence, Georgetown University Child Development Center.

TABLE 15-7 Specific Examples of Value Conflicts That May Arise in Program Planning

- Messages that stress eating certain foods to prevent specific diseases may not have much of an effect if ill health is viewed as "God's will."
- Prevention may be looked at as a useless attempt to control fate. Doing good deeds and requesting forgiveness from a spiritual leader may appear to be the best courses of action for those who believe that illness is a curse for sins.
- Food programs that require that only particular family members eat donated foods may not be well received in cultures where the welfare of the group is placed before that of the individual.

Source: B. Schilling and E. Brannon, *Cross-Cultural Counseling: A Guide for Nutrition and Health Counselors* (Washington, D.C.: U.S. Government Printing Office, 1990).

Learning useful generalizations about a cultural group is only the starting point for developing relevant community interventions. Your programs need to be community based and must address the specific needs of the people you serve. As you assess a particular person or group, you must keep general characteristics in mind but make no assumptions. For example, even though you know that many Hindus are vegetarians, you would want to explore that behavior with the individuals involved, rather than just assuming that any particular Hindu is following a vegetarian diet.

There are many areas of cultural food practices that can be explored, including commonly eaten foods and how food is obtained (purchased or grown), stored, and served. Food behaviors are an integral component of cultural identity and can be observed among descendants of immigrants even after many generations have passed. People of various cultures consume foods for religious, nutritional, and health reasons, as well as for self-indulgent reasons. See **Table 15-8** for examples of common cultural foods of various ethnic groups; see **Table 15-9** for examples of traditional food practices used to influence health.

Cultural encounters may lead to learning about alternative health care beliefs, customs, and traditions that favor a non-Western view of the cause of illness. For example, belief in a supernatural, spiritual, or religious cause is common, and healers may look for chi imbalance or a broken taboo. This contrasts with the value European Americans place on scientific reasoning, where bacteria, viruses, or environmental toxins are likely to be blamed for illness, and technology is expected to cure poor health. In a number of cultures, spirituality is viewed as a vital element in health and healing. For example, Hispanics may bring a broad definition of health to a clinical setting, viewing health as a

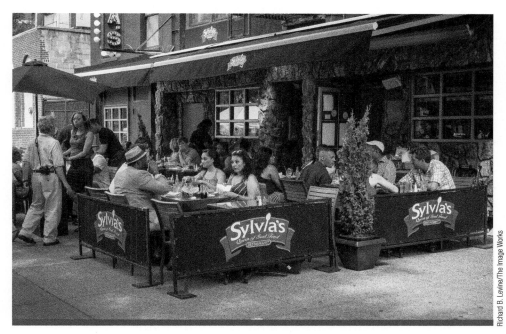

At many American-style restaurants, you can experience other cultures by sampling from the various ethnic cuisines represented on the menu.

Richard B. Levine/The Image Works

TABLE 15-8

Common Cultural Foods of Various Ethnic Groups

	COMMONLY CONSUMED FOODS	DIETARY CONCERNS/ISSUES
European Americans	Beef, chicken, pork, pasta, rice, bread, dairy foods, potatoes, bananas, apples, citrus juices, lettuce	High intake of fat, salt, sugar, and fast foods
Southern African Americans	Pork, organ meats, corn bread, rice, black-eyed peas, okra, greens, lard, hot sauce	Lactose intolerance is common; fried foods; low intake of fresh fruit and whole grains; pica common in rural South; breastfeeding rates are low
Asian/Pacific Island Americans	Pork, chicken, eggs, rice, wheat, bok choy, Chinese eggplant, mushrooms, water chestnuts, ginger root, soymilk, soy sauce	High salt intake; lactose intolerance is common; milk use is rare
Mexican Americans	Chicken, eggs, beans, flour or corn tortillas, rice, tomatoes, squash, lard, chili peppers, onions, tropical fruits, pine nuts	High intake of carbonated beverages; limited dental care among migrant workers
American Indians	Game, fish, berries, roots, wild greens, commodity foods, fried bread	Broad differences exist among the subgroups; lack of refrigeration; high intake of refined sugar, cholesterol, fat, and energy; lactose intolerance and obesity are common
Puerto Rican	Beans, various meats, rice, cornmeal, yams, sweet potatoes, onions, green peppers, tomatoes, lard, pineapple, bananas, sugar	Overweight and obesity are common; breastfeeding is not common; low intake of green, leafy vegetables; dairy intake is low
Middle Eastern Americans	Fermented dairy products, feta cheese, lamb, legumes, pita bread, rice, olive oil, figs, dates, pomegranates, lemons, eggplants, phyllo pastries, honey	High incidence of lactose intolerance

Sources: Adapted from readings of two authorities: P. G. Kittler, K. P. Sucher, and M. Nahikian-Nelms, *Food and Culture,* 6th ed. (Belmont, CA: Wadsworth/Cengage, 2012); Association for the Advancement of Health Education, *Cultural Awareness and Sensitivity: Guidelines for Health Educators* (Reston, VA: Association for the Advancement of Health Education, 1994).

TABLE 15-9

Traditional Health Beliefs
Related to Food of
Various Ethnic Groups

	TRADITIONAL BELIEFS[a]
Chinese	The body is kept in harmony through a balance of yin and yang. Yin foods include those that are raw or cooked at low temperatures and are white or light in color. Yang foods usually are high-calorie foods, are cooked at high temperatures, and have red-orange-yellow colors. Some foods, such as rice, are considered neutral. Ginseng is used as a general health-promoting tonic and is thought to help cure a variety of ailments. Sometimes the "like cures like" concept is used to treat specific illnesses, such as attempting to cure impotence by eating male genital organs from sea otters.
Italian	Foods may be categorized as heavy or light, wet or dry, and acid or nonacid. Light foods (gelatin and soups) are thought to be easy to digest and are fed to those who are ill. Wet meals may be served once a week to cleanse the system. They include escarole, spinach, and cabbage cooked in fluid. Citrus foods, tomatoes, and peaches are considered acid foods and are believed to aggravate skin conditions. Too many dairy products are thought to cause kidney stones.
Korean	A balance of yin and yang maintains health. Eating too much or too little food can disrupt the balance. Too much food, even of good quality, can block ki (energy), resulting in cold hands and feet, cold sweats, or fainting.
Mexican	A balance of strengthening hot foods and weakness-promoting cold foods are needed to maintain health. If someone has a "hot" condition such as menstruation or pregnancy, then hot foods are avoided. Examples of hot foods include alcohol, beef, pork, chilies, cornhusks, oils, and onions; cold foods include citrus fruits, dairy products, most fresh vegetables, and goat.

[a] Note that many factors affect food intake and health practices. These are examples of traditional beliefs and behaviors that may or may not be practiced by individuals who represent the specific cultural group.

Source: P. G. Kittler, K. P. Sucher, and M. Nahikian-Nelms, *Food and Culture*, 6th ed. (Belmont, CA: Wadsworth/Cengage, 2012).

► **THINK LIKE A COMMUNITY NUTRITIONIST**

Review the stages of the Cultural Continuum in Table 15-3. Select an ethnic group (e.g., Italians), religious group (e.g., Greek Orthodox), disability group (e.g., blind), gender group (e.g., males), and age group (e.g., over 65). Identify your stage on the continuum for each group. Answer the following questions.

- Do the stages differ according to the group you selected?
- What do you believe influenced your cultural competence ability for each group?
- Describe your reaction to this experience.

continuum of body, mind, and espíritu (spirit).[51] Some consumers may seek traditional healers and have more confidence in their services than in those offered by Western biomedicine. Others may mistrust organizations that represent authority because they have experienced severe oppression or were victims of atrocities in their homelands. Positive experiences over time can help build trust and respect. In many cultures, religion and health are not separate. (See **Table 15-10** for examples of common dietary practices of selected religious groups.)

Cultural Encounters Although the Campinha-Baccote Model posits that working on any of the five constructs of the model influences all the others, cultural encounters is believed to have the greatest impact on the other constructs. Valuing diversity and viewing the world through multiple cultural lenses are at the heart of cultural competence. Direct (face-to-face) and indirect (e.g., reading) experiences with individuals from diverse backgrounds provide a catalyst for revising existing beliefs and reduce the likelihood of stereotyping. During interactions, be alert to economic, communication, religious, and familial factors (including eating rituals). Pay special attention to socioeconomic issues and environmental risks because they can affect health and treatment. For example, lead is a common contaminant of inner-city environments because of the lead-based paint found on the interiors and exteriors of older buildings. Children who are chronically exposed to lead and who eat a high-fat diet that is also low in calcium and iron absorb more lead than those who eat a more nutritious diet.

Cultural Desire Motivation to engage in cross-cultural encounters stimulates the process of becoming culturally competent. Many studies have produced helpful suggestions for developing and instituting culturally sensitive interventions on an individual and organizational level, but without a sincere desire to make cultural competency a goal, changing standard practices is not likely to happen.

DIETARY PRACTICES[a]		**TABLE 15-10** Dietary Practices of Selected Religious Groups
Buddhists	Dietary customs vary depending on sect. Many are lacto-ovo vegetarians because there are restrictions on taking a life. Some eat fish, and some eat no beef. Monks fast at certain times of the month and avoid eating solid food after the noon hour.	
Hindus	All foods thought to interfere with physical and spiritual development are avoided. Many Hindus are lacto vegetarians and/or avoid alcohol. The cow is considered sacred—an animal dear to the Lord Krishna. Beef is never consumed, and often pork is avoided.	
Jewish	Kashrut is the body of Jewish law dealing with foods. The purpose of following the complex dietary laws is to conform to the Divine Will as expressed in the Torah. The term *kosher* denotes all foods that are permitted for consumption. (Many Jews also eat nonkosher foods.) To "keep kosher" means that the dietary laws are followed in the home. There is a lengthy list of prohibited foods, called *treyf*, which include pork and shellfish. The laws define how birds and mammals must be slaughtered, how foods must be prepared, and when they may be consumed. For example, dairy foods and meat products cannot be eaten at the same meal. During Passover, special laws are observed, such as the elimination of any foods that can be leavened.	
Mormons	Alcoholic drinks and hot drinks (coffee and tea) are avoided. Many also avoid beverages containing caffeine. Mormons are encouraged to limit meat intake and to emphasize grains in the diet. Many store a year's supply of food and clothing for each member of the household.	
Muslim	Overeating is discouraged, and consuming only two-thirds of capacity is suggested. Dietary laws are called *halal*. Prohibited foods are called *haram*, and they include pork and birds of prey. Laws define how animals must be slaughtered. Alcoholic drinks are not allowed. Fasting is required from sunup to sundown during the month of Ramadan.	
Roman Catholics	Meat is not consumed on Fridays during Lent (40 days before Easter). No food or beverages (except water) are to be consumed one hour before taking communion.	
Seventh-Day Adventists	Most are lacto-ovo vegetarians. If meat is consumed, pork is avoided. Tea, coffee, and alcoholic beverages are not allowed. Water is not consumed with meals but is drunk before and after meals. Followers refrain from using seasonings and condiments. Overeating and snacking are discouraged.	

[a] Many of the religious guidelines regarding food have practical applications for the society. For example, the Hindu prohibition against killing cattle respects the need of Indian farmers to use cattle for power and their dung for fuel. Cows also supply milk to make dairy products, and the skin of dead cows is used to make leather goods.

Cross-Cultural Communication

Cultural orientation has a major impact on the process of communication. When individuals share a common culture, or at least are familiar with each other's cultural background, it is much more likely that differences in perceptions will be minimal and communication will flow smoothly. Each society has a conscious and an unconscious set of expected reciprocal responses. For example, an Iranian woman may politely refuse an offer of coffee or tea and expect a second request, accompanied by insistence that she have something to drink. When such an expected interchange does not happen, a feeling of discomfort ensues that can set the stage for a breakdown in communication.

Communication Styles

Table 15-11 provides a summary of key differences in communication styles among cultures. While reviewing this list, keep in mind that considerable variation exists within any particular cultural group. Community nutrition practitioners are increasingly required to provide services for those who have communication styles that are unfamiliar. Professionals need to learn about these styles and find ways to communicate so that clients can be confident that their voices have been heard and that their values, beliefs, and behaviors are respected. The next section reviews some common cultural barriers to communication and offers practical suggestions for communicating in cross-cultural encounters.

TABLE 15-11 Communication Styles of Various Cultural Groups

CATEGORY	COMMUNICATION STYLE
Emotional expressiveness	The dynamic and expressive body language of African Americans may be considered excessive and too intense to European Americans. Vigorous handshaking can be considered a sign of aggression for Native Americans but a gesture of good will for European Americans. Some Asian American cultures value stoicism and may use a smile or laugh to mask other emotions.
Volume of speech	Asian Americans tend to speak quietly, whereas African and European Americans generally speak loudly.
Touching	Friendly behavior for Hispanics often involves touching that Native Americans and Asians may find uncomfortable. Asian Americans and Hispanics are not likely to appreciate a slap on the back. Many Asians totally avoid physical contact with strangers, even in transactions such as giving change.
Vocal style	Latinos often use expressive language and engage in lengthy pleasant talk before getting down to business. European Americans prefer a quiet, controlled style that other groups may consider manipulative and cold.
Verbal following	Asians and Native Americans are more likely to use indirect and subtle forms of communication by avoiding direct questions and answers. The direct styles of African and European Americans are considered too confrontational. Native Americans find direct personal questions particularly offensive.
Eye contact	For European Americans making eye contact is a sign of respect, but among Hispanics, Native Americans, and Asian Americans avoidance of eye contact is often considered proper behavior. Hispanics and Filipinos use sustained eye contact to challenge authority. Many African Americans use more eye contact during talking than when listening, whereas the opposite is true of most European Americans.
Physical space	Conversational space in Arab and Middle Eastern cultures is commonly 6 to 12 inches, whereas among European Americans a comfortable distance is ordinarily "arm's length." Hispanics prefer closer proximity, and Asian Americans a greater distance, than European Americans.
Silence	Duration of silence considered acceptable differs among cultures. Native Americans may take 90 seconds to formulate a response to a question, but that amount of silence can seem intolerable to others. European Americans are particularly uncomfortable with silence and will quickly fill the void with small talk. Some European Americans feel it is appropriate to start speaking before the other person has finished.
Question authority	Questioning authority comes naturally to Native and African Americans, but Asian Americans are not likely to disagree with an elder or a person in a position of authority. Some clients will appear to agree by giving answers they believe are desired and then disregard information that does not make sense to them.
Aggression	Some cultural groups may have learned that aggressive behavior or bribery is required to get what they want from bureaucracy.
Gender roles	Different cultures prescribe who will talk during interviews. Even during female dietary and medical assessments, a husband may answer all questions, no matter how personal.

Sources: Adapted from readings of three authorities: P. G. Kittler, K. P. Sucher, and M. Nahikian-Nelms, *Food and Culture*, 6th ed. (Belmont, CA: Wadsworth/Cengage, 2012); A. E. Ivey, N. Gluckstern, and M. B. Ivey, *Basic Attending Skills*, 3rd ed. (North Amherst, MA: Microtraining Associates, 1997); C. Elliott, R. J. Adams, and S. Sockalingam, *Multicultural Toolkit (Toolkit for Cross-Cultural Collaboration)* (Portland, OR: Evaluation and Development Institute, 1999), *www.awesomelibrary.org*.

Barriers to Cross-Cultural Communication In your career as a community nutrition practitioner, you may work with clients who do not speak your language. Even similar words that the two cultures share may not have the same meaning. Two individuals who speak the same language but are from different countries or even different areas of the same country may not give the same meaning to a specific word. For example, the word *bad* generally means something negative, but among some subgroups the word actually means something good.

Nonverbal behavior may not be interpreted correctly either. Very few gestures can be universally translated across all cultural groups.[52] More than 7,000 different gestures have been identified, so there are many opportunities for misunderstanding. For example, the same hand gesture that means "come here" in Nigeria signals "hello" in the United States. Nonverbal cues need to be interpreted very cautiously because meanings vary from one culture to the next. Your interpretation may be quite different from the speaker's intent.

Stereotyping means assuming that individuals will behave a certain way because they are from a particular culture. Kittler et al.[53] report that only about one-third of the individuals in a particular group of people actually behave in ways considered typical of that group.

Practical Guidelines for Cross-Cultural Communication Learning culturally sensitive communication skills facilitates more favorable community intervention outcomes and increases the likelihood of more rewarding interpersonal experiences for health care providers. The following suggestions can enhance cross-cultural communication.[54,55]

1. Smile, show warmth, and be friendly.
2. Attempt to learn and use key words, especially greetings and titles of respect, in languages spoken by populations serviced by your organization.
3. Thank clients for trying to communicate in English.
4. Suggest that clients choose their own seat (to make comfortable personal space and eye contact possible).
5. Articulate clearly; speak in a normal tone. Often people mistakenly raise the volume of their voice when they feel someone is having difficulty understanding them.
6. Paying attention to children appeals to women of most cultures; however, some believe that accepting a compliment about a child is not appropriate, especially in front of the child.
7. When interacting with individuals who have limited English proficiency, always keep in mind that limitations in English proficiency do not reflect their level of intellectual functioning. Limited ability to speak the language of the dominant culture has no bearing on ability to communicate effectively in their language of origin. Clientele may or may not be literate in their language of origin or in English.
8. Explain to clients that you have some questions to ask and that there is no intention to offend. Request that they let you know if they prefer not to answer any of the questions.
9. If you are not sure how to interpret a particular behavior, Magnus[56] suggests that you should ask for clarification. For example, you could ask, "I notice that you are mostly looking down. Would you tell me what that means for you?"
10. Follow your intuition if you believe something you are doing is causing a problem. Magnus[57] suggests that you ask, "There seems to be a problem. Is something I am doing offending you?" Once informed of a difficulty, immediately apologize and admit, "I am sorry. I didn't mean to offend you."

Suggestions for Communicating Information

1. Consider using a less direct approach than is common among Americans. Gardenswartz and Rowe[58] suggest some communication approaches that may lower the risk of misunderstanding and hurt feelings:

   - Make observations rather than judgments about behaviors. For example, do not say, "Your fruit intake is low." Instead, say, "Your food record indicates no servings of fruit each day, and the authorities tell us to eat two."
   - Refrain from using "you." For example, say, "People who have a low intake of calcium are at an increased risk for osteoporosis" rather than "You are at an increased risk for osteoporosis."
   - Be positive, saying what you want rather than what you do not want. For example, say, "Use a pencil to fill out the form" rather than "Don't use a pen to complete the form."

2. Use visual aids, food models, gestures, and physical prompts during interactions with those who have limited English proficiency.
3. If answers are unclear, ask the same question a different way.
4. Consider using alternatives to written communications because word of mouth may be a preferred method of receiving information.
5. Write numbers down, just as they would appear in recipes, because spoken numbers are easily confused by those with limited skills in a language.
6. Written communication should be made available in the major languages spoken in the area.

Ways in Which Discussions about Food Can Open Dialogue

1. Most people are pleased to educate others about their food ways, but some may feel that questions are probing. If you believe there is resistance, explain that you are asking questions to gain understanding of the client's experience and beliefs about food in order to develop a workable food plan that also incorporates evidence-based guidelines.
2. Ask about foods used for celebrations and special occasions.
3. Ask about favorite foods and discuss how they can be incorporated into a diet plan.
4. Tell your own food stories. Letting clients know that you do not always make the best food choices can help them feel more comfortable being truthful about their behavior patterns.

Working with Interpreters

Translator A person who works in converting written words into another language.

Interpreter A person who works in converting spoken words into another language.

As of 2011, about 21% of American households speak a language other than English at home and approximately half the individuals in those homes claim they speak English less than "very well."[59] As a result, community nutritionists are likely to need the services of professional interpreters or translators to provide effective services. A **translator** works with written information, and an **interpreter** explains spoken words.

Community nutritionists should insist on using professional interpreters who have expertise in the language and are familiar with the culture of their clients. Too often, health care providers resort to using nonprofessional interpreters, such as friends or relatives of clients or housekeeping staff. This has been shown to present numerous problems.[60] Sometimes clients are reluctant or embarrassed to discuss certain problems in front of close relations, or the nonprofessional interpreter may decide that certain information is irrelevant or unnecessary and may therefore not do a complete interpretation. Other nonprofessional interpreters may be unfamiliar with medical terminology and unknowingly make mistakes. All of these problems are compounded when a child is used as an interpreter. One study of well-trained professional interpreters made one-third the amount of translation errors as compared to untrained interpreters such as confusion between "teaspoon" and "tablespoon" when discussing medication dosage.[61] The difficulty of communication across cultures is illustrated in the story of a Hmong child experiencing severe epileptic seizures who was moved from a community hospital to a children's hospital with an intensive care unit. With the help of an interpreter, the situation was explained to Lia's non-English-speaking parents. Later investigation revealed that the parents thought their child had to go to another hospital because the doctors at the community hospital were going on vacation.[62]

In clinical settings, interpreters should be available to represent the major languages spoken in the area. Interpreter services by phone can be used to accommodate clients who speak languages not encountered frequently in the setting. There are several phone-based interpreter services available, such as *in WHAT LANGUAGE, CyraCom*, and *LanguageLine Solutions*, each providing 24-hour service in over 100 languages. In addition, smart medical translation apps are available for smartphones and tablets. Phone interpreters and mobile tools are useful for emergencies but cannot take the place of in-person professionals; some clients may have difficulty communicating personal issues with a faceless voice. Guidelines for using an interpreter are given in **Table 15-12**.

ENTREPRENEUR IN ACTION

It was during her internship at the Yavapai County Health Department in Arizona that Tracy Gregg, RD, LD, CLC, realized how important a role the community nutritionist can have in nurturing the health of a community. Now, as coordinator of the WIC Program for the Maniilaq Association in Kotzebue, Alaska, she travels to all the villages at least once a year. This gives her the opportunity to meet with her clients and observe some of the challenges confronting them. She assists families with incorporating traditional foods (such as seals, shee fish, moose, and caribou) with the fortified WIC foods. Tracy is a member of the Healthy Kotzebue Steering Committee. The Steering Committee includes members of local organizations and community experts donating time and knowledge to develop an action plan for strategies contributing to the prevention and control of diabetes, heart disease, and stroke and their associated risk factors. Those strategies include increasing the use of traditional and healthy foods and beverages, increasing opportunities for breastfeeding, improving opportunities for physical activity, and increasing knowledge about health. Find out what she has to say about entrepreneurship online at *www.cengagebrain.com*.

TABLE 15-12

Guidelines for Using an Interpreter

- Request an interpreter of the same gender and similar age. (Be sensitive and flexible in your selections, as interpreters who are considerably older than a client may receive greater respect.)
- Decide before the meeting what questions will be asked.
- If possible, go over the questions with the interpreter before the meeting. A professional interpreter should be able to assist you in formulating new questions if certain ones are deemed offensive.
- Try to learn a few phrases of the client's language to use at the beginning and/or the end of the interview.
- Remember that sessions will take extra time. Schedule adequate time.
- Look at and speak directly to the client, not the interpreter.
- Speak clearly in short units of speech. Do not ask more than one question at a time.
- Avoid using slang, similes, metaphors, and idiomatic expressions. For example, do not say, "Do you have your ups and downs?"
- Listen carefully and watch body language for any changes in expression.
- Do not just follow prepared questions, but ask clients to expand upon new issues.
- To avoid misunderstandings, begin some of your sentences with "Did I understand you correctly that . . . ?" or "Tell me about . . ."
- To check on the client's understanding and the accuracy of the interpretation, ask the client to back-translate important dietary instructions or guidelines. This technique may also encourage the client to ask questions.
- Be aware that interpreters come to sessions with their own cultural biases and may not completely convey everything that has been said.
- If your client appears tired, you and the interpreter may need to schedule another session.

Sources: Adapted from C. Munoz and J. Luckmann, *Transcultural Communication in Nursing*, 2nd ed. (Belmont, CA: Delmar Cengage Learning, 2004); K. Bauer and D. Liou, *Nutrition Counseling and Education Skill Development*, 3rd ed. (Belmont, CA: Wadsworth/Cengage Learning, 2016).

Culturally Appropriate Intervention Strategies

Learning about the food habits, health beliefs, and behaviors of specific cultural groups can be extremely valuable. Deep exploration of target populations helps community nutrition practitioners identify resources and find ways to build on community strengths to find solutions to problems related to health and nutrition. However, given the time constraints of busy health professionals and the great variety of cultures, community health professionals cannot be expected to have intimate knowledge of all cultural groups they encounter. Therefore, community nutrition practitioners need universal skills in cultural competence that can be utilized with clients from any cultural group. Fundamentally, what providers must have in order to use intervention strategies effectively is an inherent caring, appreciation, and respect for their clients and the ability to display warmth, empathy, and genuineness.

Explanatory Models

Medical anthropologists have developed explanatory models as a culturally sensitive tool for opening conversation to learn a client's viewpoint regarding the origin, treatment, and impact of an illness on daily life. Health care practitioners are encouraged to be open to understanding alternative frames of reference and put aside their own biases. There are six steps to using this approach:[63]

- **Step 1: Ethnic identity.** Ask clients to identify their ethnicity and inquire as to the importance their ethnicity plays in self-identity. The specific terms used to identify an individual's ethnicity can be a touchy issue. For example, Asian, Oriental, Chinese, and Chinese American have been used to describe individuals of a similar background, but not all of these terms are acceptable to all individuals. To avoid alienation, a counselor could directly inquire about heritage with questions such as "How do you describe your ethnicity?" and "Do you feel this is an important part of your life?"
- **Step 2: What is at stake?** By questioning clients regarding the impact of an illness, practitioners are better able to understand their perceptions of the effect on the quality of clients' lives. Evaluation responses are likely to vary and include such areas as relationships, commitments, resources, and even life itself.
- **Step 3: The illness narrative.** **Table 15-13** lists examples of open-ended questions that can be a guide for using the explanatory model. In this client-centered respondent-driven approach, food and nutrition practitioners ask simple, open-ended questions to initiate conversations, prompt clients for a better understanding when necessary, but for the most part exert little control over responses. By showing an unbiased and sincere desire to understand and accept traditional views and practices, you increase the likelihood that your clients will not fear criticism or ridicule, but will feel comfortable telling their stories, feel a sense of control over their condition, and be open to accepting suggestions for treatment.

    The questions in Table 15-13 and in Table 4-9 on page 129 aid in understanding illness and food issues from a client's perspective. However, not every question is appropriate for every cross-cultural encounter, so health care professionals must use their judgment to select suitable ones. If you are going to use a lot of the questions, consider

Questions to understand view and treatment of health problems:

- What do you call this problem you are having? (*Note:* Use this term instead of it in the following questions.)
- What do you think caused your problem?
- When did it start and why did it start when it did?
- What does your sickness do to your body?
- Will you get better soon, or will it take a long time, in your opinion?
- What do you fear about your sickness?
- What problems has your sickness caused for you personally? For your family? At work?
- What kind of treatment will work for your sickness? What results do you expect from treatment?
- What home remedies are common for this sickness? Have you used them?
- Are there benefits to having this illness?
- Is there anyone else in your family that I should talk to?

Question to understand about traditional healers:

- How would a healer treat your sickness? Are you using that treatment?

Questions to understand food habits:

- Can what you eat help cure your sickness or make it worse?
- Do you eat certain foods to keep healthy? To make you strong?
- Do you balance eating some foods with other foods?
- Are there foods you will not eat? Why?

TABLE 15-13

Culturally Sensitive Respondent-Driven Interview Questions

Sources: Modified from P. G. Kittler, K. P. Sucher, and M. Nahikian-Nelms, *Food and Culture*, 6th ed. (Belmont, CA: Wadsworth/Cengage, 2012); A. Kleinman and P. Benson, "Anthropology in the Clinic: The Problem of Cultural Competency and How to Fix It," *PLoS Med* 3, no. 10 (2006): e294. DOI: 10.1371, available at *www.plosmedicine.org/article/info:doi/10.1371/journal.pmed.0030294*, accessed May 26, 2015.

changing some of them into statements. A series of questions can feel like an interrogation, and in some cultures questions may evoke defensiveness. Variety can be accomplished by starting sentences with "Tell me . . ." or "Please describe . . ."

- **Step 4: Psychosocial stress.** The ability of clients to fulfill treatment plans can be hampered by lack of social supports or resources. For example, if getting a child to a clinic appointment requires loss of work and pay, there are added stresses that need to be addressed. By knowing the context of the psychosocial issues a client faces, health practitioners can help the client to search for options.
- **Step 5: Influence of culture on clinical relationships.** In this step, health practitioners are encouraged to reflect on the culture of biomedicine and the formative effect on "bias, inappropriate and excessive use of advanced technology interventions, and, of course, stereotyping."
- **Step 6: The problems of a cultural competency approach.** This step acknowledges that there can be cases where an overemphasis on the cultural context of a health concern can be viewed as intrusive or lead to misguidance when determining the root cause. Also, one should not assume that by understanding cultural factors of a complex case, easy solutions will be found.

LEARN Intervention Guidelines

Explanatory models are useful for assessment, and the LEARN guidelines given in **Table 15-14** provide a framework for negotiating a culturally sensitive treatment plan to address a given illness episode.

TABLE 15-14 LEARN
Communication
Guidelines for Health
Practitioners

L		Listen with sympathy and understanding to a client's perception of a problem.
E		Explain your perceptions of the problem.
A		Acknowledge and discuss differences and similarities.
R		Recommend treatment that is relevant, concise, and practical.
N		Negotiate agreement.

Source: Adapted from E. A. Berlin and W. C. Fowkes, "A Teaching Framework for Cross-Cultural Health Care," *Western Journal of Medicine* 139 (1983): 934–38.

1. **Listen.** Active listening is the foundation of successful cross-cultural communication. Your demeanor should come across as curious and nonjudgmental, and clients should be recognized as experts regarding information about their experiences. Not only are you learning, but you are demonstrating that what your client has to say is very important to you—a key relationship-building skill. Make sure you come to a common understanding of the issues and problems. Request clarification when necessary by saying, "I didn't quite understand. . . ." Probe to understand who does the food preparation and shopping, and determine whether there are others in the extended family who are responsible for decision making.

2. **Explain.** Make sure that you have understood correctly by explaining back to the client your perception of what was related. For example: "You feel that diarrhea is a hot ailment, and your baby should not be given a hot food like infant formula but should drink barley water, a cool food. Did I understand you correctly?" Your explanation creates an opportunity to clarify any misunderstandings.

3. **Acknowledge.** Acknowledge the similarities and differences in your perspectives regarding the cause and/or treatment of the problem. For example: "Both you and your doctor feel that what your baby drinks will help her feel better. You feel your baby needs a cool food like barley water, and the health care providers at this clinic feel that your baby needs a drink with minerals to get better."

4. **Recommend.** The client should be given several options that are culturally relevant, concise, and practical. For example, an Indian woman who is a vegetarian and wishes to lose weight might be given the following recommendations: "You could start a walking program, reduce the amount of ghee used when making rice or bean dishes, use skim milk to make yogurt, or eat smaller portions of fried bread."

5. **Negotiate.** After reviewing the options, negotiate a culturally sensitive plan of action with your client and any significant family members who are part of the decision-making process. Begin by asking, "Which of these options do you think would be a good place to start?" If there appears to be a conflict between the biomedical approach to healing and the client's cultural practices, then look for ways to "neutralize" the biomedical treatment. Ask, "You feel that to drink water with minerals is a 'hot' remedy and inappropriate for a hot ailment. Is there a way to use this treatment but reduce the hot effect?" Possibly the client will make a suggestion, such as combining treatments, or administering the treatment with a spiritual blessing, or giving the treatment at a certain time of day. If the condition is life-threatening and the cultural differences are great, such as resistance to having a blood transfusion, consider including a respected member of the community in the negotiations. If the counselor appreciates the powerful influence of the client's culture and the equally powerful culture of biomedicine, then the need for compromise and mediation becomes obvious.[64]

> ## Community-Based Intervention Strategies

In 2002, the Centers for Disease Control and Prevention established Racial and Ethnic Approaches to Community Health across the United States (REACH U.S.), a national program to eliminate racial and ethnic health disparities. Evaluation of the initial 28 community programs selected to participate demonstrated that well-designed community intervention programs can successfully improve health-related behaviors and reduce health disparities. As of 2014, 104 programs were funded through REACH, including community-based organizations, universities, tribes, and health departments. REACH places special focus on funding projects and creating partnerships using evidence-based strategies capable of reaching people who are particularly affected by chronic disease. Some of the REACH community successes included an increase in cholesterol screenings in African American and Hispanic communities, an increase in the number of American Indians and Hispanics taking medication for high blood pressure, improved intake of fruits and vegetables among African American and Hispanic adults, and a decrease in the prevalence of cigarette smoking among Asian American men and African American and Hispanic populations.

Keys to REACH U.S. Community Intervention Success:

- **Trust.** Building a culture of collaboration with communities that is based on trust.
- **Empowerment.** Giving individuals and communities the knowledge and tools needed to create change by seeking and demanding better health and building on local resources.
- **Culture and History.** Designing health initiatives that acknowledge and are based in the unique historical and cultural context of racial and ethnic minority communities in the United States.
- **Focus on Causes.** Assessing and focusing on the underlying causes of poor community health and implementing solutions designed to stay embedded in the community infrastructure.
- **Community Investment and Expertise.** Recognizing and investing in local community expertise and working to motivate communities to mobilize and organize existing resources.
- **Trusted Organizations.** Embracing and enlisting organizations within the community valued by community members, including groups with a primary mission unrelated to health.
- **Community Leaders.** Helping community leaders and key organizations to act as catalysts for change in the community, including forging unique partnerships.
- **Ownership.** Developing a collective outlook to promote shared interest in a healthy future through widespread community engagement and leadership.
- **Sustainability.** Making changes to organizations, community environments, and policies to help ensure that health improvements are long-lasting and community activities and programs are self-sustaining.

Source: Centers for Disease Control and Prevention, "Investments in Community Health: Racial and Ethnic Approaches to Community Health (REACH)," available at *www.cdc.gov/nccdphp/dch/programs/reach/pdf/2-reach_factsheet-for-web.pdf*, accessed May 26, 2015.

Practical Considerations for Community Interventions

When working with people of various cultures, be sure that the items available in the agency (e.g., pictures, food guides, magazines, media resources, snack foods, and toys) reflect sensitivity to cultural backgrounds, literacy levels, and linguistic preferences. In order to respond to the needs and preferences of a particular community, encourage community members to participate at all levels of intervention—program development, implementation, and evaluation. Here are some suggestions to consider:

- Include questions related to culture in community assessments.
- Conduct focus groups to obtain opinions and suggestions.
- Have a representative of the population groups you are targeting review any publications you intend to use to ensure that they are meaningful and do not contain offensive material.
- Seek assistance from community representatives in identifying places that your target audience frequents so that you can take your literature and programs to high-traffic areas.
- Ask volunteers to make the initial contacts with community organizations for outreach presentations.
- Recruit volunteers to distribute program literature to hair salons, barbershops, laundromats, dry cleaners, libraries, restaurants, and the like.
- Report outcomes to any individuals or groups that provided assistance. This will make them feel vested in the projects, and the likelihood of participation in the future will be greater.
- Show appreciation to volunteers—distribute certificates, provide appreciation lunches, list their names in publications.

Take time to learn about the community being served before designing a program. Identify and enlist the support of principal people in the community (examples include clergy, funeral planners, politicians, marriage brokers, and healers) and enlist their support. Individuals in these roles can incorporate your message into their work, play, or prayer. It is also a good idea to utilize the local media outlets, such as minority radio or cable television programs. Radio and television stations are often required to provide airtime for community messages, which can publicize local programs that are teaming up with the American Diabetes Association or the American Heart Association.

When working with an immigrant population,[65] create a resource list of grocery stores and specialty markets and offer a chart that demonstrates lower-cost substitutions for high-cost familiar foods. On this chart, give the English words equivalent to a list of foreign words for traditional foods and spices. Keep on hand up-to-date public transportation schedules that will facilitate traveling to and from the markets.

PROGRAMS IN **ACTION**

Encouraging Breastfeeding among African American Women

Both the rate and the duration of breastfeeding are low in the United States, despite efforts to communicate its numerous health benefits. In 2007, only 43% of all mothers were breastfeeding six months after delivery, and the rates among African American women were significantly lower.[1] A few of the factors associated with choosing bottle-feeding over breastfeeding in African American populations are that breastfeeding is too complicated, that it is not supported by family members, and that it takes too much time.[2,3] In contrast, a significant predictor is having a friend or relative who breastfed her infant, a correlation that emphasizes the importance of role models and peer support.[4] The Northside Breastfeeding Media Campaign is a grassroots, community-based breastfeeding promotion project.

Goals and Objectives

The goals of the campaign were to raise awareness and increase knowledge of breastfeeding in an African American population and to create a supportive environment for breastfeeding through culturally specific images, messages, and materials.

Target Audience

The target audience was African American women in the Near North Community of Minneapolis. The campaign aimed to reach 30% of African American women in the community.

Rationale for the Intervention

In November 2000, the U.S. Department of Health and Human Services released the "Blueprint for Action on Breastfeeding," a comprehensive plan outlining the critical need to promote breastfeeding in minority communities as a way to reduce health disparities.[5] This campaign recognized the importance of community norms in influencing breastfeeding practices and involved extensive research to ensure that the right messages would reach the target audience.

Methodology

The campaign developed culturally specific materials and tested them prior to publication and distribution. Community advisors and African American women who had breastfed were integrally involved in every step of the design and testing. A media advisory committee was formed to provide guidance to the media specialists and graphic designers to identify appropriate media channels, messages, and images. Media promotion materials from other campaigns, along with a survey of infant feeding practices, were used to develop message concepts. The concepts were pretested with the target audience.

Media strategies included bus stop posters, newspaper articles, public service announcements, radio and television newsrooms, and pamphlets to distribute to media audiences. The target audience was reached directly through pamphlets and promotional gifts that displayed the campaign themes— "Healthier Babies," "Faster and Easier," and "Get Back in Shape." The campaign educational and media materials were featured on the government's WIC site at *https://wicworks.fns.usda.gov* and are available at *http://ncemch.org/knowledge-base.php*.

The League of Catholic Women sponsored the campaign, with evaluation funding provided by a grant from the Allina Foundation. Participants in the overall Northside Breastfeeding Campaign included members of the community, along with representatives from WIC, two hospitals, several health clinics, and a Way to Grow program.

Results

Through interviews, researchers collected quantitative and qualitative data on the effectiveness of campaign intervention strategies in reaching the target audience. Some 31% of females and 15% of males who were surveyed reported that they had seen or heard the campaign messages. Bus stop posters, newspaper articles, and posters in health clinics were most effective. Acceptance of breastfeeding increased with age in both males and females, with females being more accepting.

Lessons Learned

The Northside Breastfeeding Campaign demonstrated the positive impact of involving community members and organizations in the development of nutrition materials and messages. Social marketing campaigns such as this can potentially increase the rate of breastfeeding initiation and the duration of breastfeeding in African American communities.

Source: From *Community Nutritionary* (White Plains, NY: Dannon Institute, Fall 2001). Used with permission. For more information about the Awards for Excellence in Community Nutrition, go to *www.dannon-institute.org*.

Essential Organizational Elements of Cultural Competence

Health care delivery organizations have a responsibility to provide appropriate care that is sensitive to cultural norms, values, and beliefs of individuals; linguistically accessible; and physically available. Incentives to address these needs include state and federal guidelines, *Healthy People 2020* goals, and a desire to attract a growing share of business among racial and ethnic minorities. To be effective, health care agencies must scrutinize and periodically review all aspects of their organizational structure to infuse cultural competence at every level. These levels include:

- Culturally sensitive mission statements
- Evaluation of policies, structures, and services that both support and act as barriers to providing culturally competent services
- Structures to ensure consumer and community participation (e.g., the involvement of traditional healers) in the planning, delivery, and evaluation of services
- Policies and procedures for the recruitment, hiring, and retention of a diverse and culturally competent workforce
- Policies and resources for staff development in cultural competence
- Adequate fiscal resources to support translation and interpretation services
- Assessment of environmental resources for obtaining affordable and accessible food
- Evaluation of the social and political landscape that influences health disparities

To provide guidance for instituting the above elements of organizational cultural competence, the Office of Minority Health of the USDHHS has issued National Standards for Culturally and Linguistically Appropriate Services (CLAS) in Health Care (**Table 15-15**). To assist in the implementation of these services, this office also sponsored the development of *A Blueprint for Advancing and Sustaining CLAS Policy and Practice*, which discusses implementation strategies for each Standard.[66]

Both increasing globalization around the world and diversity in the United States require health professionals to acquire skills to work with varied cultural groups. Because of their intimate knowledge of community resources and needs and nutrition expertise, community nutrition practitioners are in a unique position to provide culturally relevant interventions. For example, Heather Greenlee, ND, PhD, and colleagues successfully increased fruit and vegetable intake and decreased fat intake among Hispanic breast cancer survivors by creating a partnership with a nonprofit organization to develop *¡Cocinar Para Su Salud!* (Cook for Your Health!).[67]

TABLE 15-15 National Standards for Culturally and Linguistically Appropriate Services (CLAS) in Health Care	**PRINCIPAL STANDARD**	
	Standard 1	Health care organizations should provide effective, equitable, understandable, and respectful quality care and services that are responsive to diverse cultural health beliefs and practices, preferred languages, health literacy, and other communication needs.
	Governance, Leadership, and Workforce	
	Standard 2	Health care organizations should advance and sustain organizational governance and leadership that promotes CLAS and health equity through policy, practices, and allocated resources.
	Standard 3	Health care organizations should recruit, promote, and support a culturally and linguistically diverse governance, leadership, and workforce that are responsive to the population in the service area.
	Standard 4	Health care organizations must educate and train governance, leadership, and workforce in culturally and linguistically appropriate policies and practices on an ongoing basis.
	Communication and Language Assistance	
	Standard 5	Health care organizations must offer language assistance to individuals who have limited English proficiency and/or other communication needs, at no cost to them, to facilitate timely access to all health care and services.
	Standard 6	Health care organizations must inform all individuals of the availability of language assistance services clearly and in their preferred language, verbally and in writing.

Standard 7 Health care organizations must ensure the competence of individuals providing language assistance, recognizing that the use of untrained individuals and/or minors as interpreters should be avoided.

Standard 8 Health care organizations should provide easy-to-understand print and multimedia materials and signage in the languages commonly used by the populations in the service area.

Engagement, Continuous Improvement, and Accountability

Standard 9 Health care organizations should establish culturally and linguistically appropriate goals, policies, and management accountability, and infuse them throughout the organization's planning and operations.

Standard 10 Health care organizations should conduct ongoing assessments of the organization's CLAS-related activities and integrate CLAS-related measures into measurement and continuous quality improvement activities.

Standard 11 Health care organizations should collect and maintain accurate and reliable demographic data to monitor and evaluate the impact of CLAS on health equity and outcomes and to inform service delivery.

Standard 12 Health care organizations should conduct regular assessments of community health assets and needs and use the results to plan and implement services that respond to the cultural and linguistic diversity of populations in the service area.

Standard 13 Health care organizations should partner with the community to design, implement, and evaluate policies, practices, and services to ensure cultural and linguistic appropriateness.

Standard 14 Health care organizations should create conflict and grievance resolution processes that are culturally and linguistically appropriate to identify, prevent, and resolve conflicts or complaints.

Standard 15 Health care organizations should communicate the organization's progress in implementing and sustaining CLAS to all stakeholders, constituents, and the general public.

TABLE 15-15

National Standards for Culturally and Linguistically Appropriate Services (CLAS) in Health Care—*continued*

Source: USDHHS, Office of Minority Health, *National Standards for Culturally and Linguistically Appropriate Services in Health Care* (Washington, D.C.: U.S. Department of Health and Human Services, 2010).

case study

Gaining Cultural Competence in a Muslim Community

by Alice Fornari, EdD, RD, Alessandra Sarcona, MS, RD, CSSD, and Alison Barkman, MS, RD, CDN

Scenario

An Indian physician has contacted you for a nutrition intervention with a community group where he is also a participant. This group consists of Indian Muslims who have emigrated to the United States. The group meets one evening per week as a social support event and shares a meal. The physician, as a member of the group, has noted a growing interest in nutrition among members but cannot field many of the questions that are directed to him. He has invited you to come to share the meal with them and hold an informal question-and-answer discussion twice a month, as well as to set up nutrition counseling sessions with individuals who have health risks. He says that they are particularly interested in nutrition and in prevention of cardiovascular disease. You have done a lot of consulting for this physician and would enjoy the challenge of working with this Indian Muslim community; however, you do not know anything about their culture or their dietary habits. You decide you need to research the Muslim culture before you can provide any nutrition intervention with this group. You find information about the Islamic dietary laws, including foods considered haram and halal. You speak with an Indian colleague who informs you that traditional women dress conservatively and cover their hair with a scarf, that men and women tend to avoid mixed groups, and that many Muslims avoid contact between sexes, such as shaking hands and hugging. The Indian physician states that his group is traditional and consists mostly of married couples.

Learning Outcomes

- Identify the National Standards for Culturally and Linguistically Appropriate Services and understand how these standards are related to health care.
- Cite various ways to explore unfamiliar cultures in an effort to become culturally competent.
- Interpret generalizations about the tastes and values of a particular cultural group in order to provide culturally competent nutrition interventions.

Foundation: Acquisition of Knowledge and Skills

1. Review the National Standards for Culturally and Linguistically Appropriate Services in Health Care from the chapter text (see Table 15-15) or on the Web.
2. Access the website *www.ifanca.org* (go to What is Halal?) or any website on Muslim/Islamic dietary laws. Outline the basic principles of Muslim/Islamic dietary laws; identify foods considered haram and halal.

Step 1: *Identify Relevant Information and Uncertainties*

1. Identify and discuss cultural food practices and any other components that may be relevant to Muslims.
2. Outline cultural beliefs, attitudes, or practices that you discovered in your research on the Muslim way of life that would be different from those of your ethnicity. How might this affect your interaction with the Muslim immigrants when you hold a group session, share a meal, and conduct individual counseling sessions?

Step 2: *Interpret Information*

1. Indicate what questions you may need to ask the physician before coming to a meeting and what questions you may need to ask the group when you meet with them, to gain a greater understanding of Muslim food habits and behaviors.
2. Review the chapter text for any practical considerations for interventions when dealing with people from various cultures. What strategies will help you to provide culturally sensitive interventions for your target group?

Step 3: *Draw and Implement Conclusions*

1. On the basis of your research on Muslim dietary practices, create a Muslim pictorial food guide. For ideas on international pictorial food guides, locate the *Journal of the Academy of Nutrition and Dietetics* in your library, or go to the Academy of Nutrition and Dietetics website, *www.eatright.org*, to search for the article in the April 2002 issue titled "Comparison of International Food Guide Pictorial Representations." This can be accessed with your Academy of Nutrition and Dietetics member number; then go to the journal. You may also visit the USDA's Food and Nutrition Information Center website at *https://fnic.nal.usda.gov/*; go to Dietary Guidance → MyPlate and Historical Food Pyramid Resources → Past Food Pyramid Materials → Ethnic/Cultural Food Pyramids to access various international food guides.
2. Describe how you would use this pictorial food guide with your target group.

Step 4: *Engage in Continuous Improvement*

Develop additional interventions (resources, community participation, activities, shopping, food preparation, and the like) for presenting information about nutrition and prevention of heart disease as you become more familiar with the Muslim population.

PROFESSIONAL **FOCUS**

Cross-Cultural Nutrition Counseling

Community nutrition practitioners are often involved in counseling clients who come from cultures substantially different from their own. A cross-cultural nutrition counseling algorithm[1] provides a visual representation of a counseling session and illustrates how to incorporate basic cross-cultural communication tools, as covered in this chapter, into an intervention. See **Figure 15-4**. This cross-cultural nutrition counseling algorithm highlights relationship-building skills and the four phases of a counseling session: involving, exploration–education, resolving, and closing. The following paragraphs offer an overview of each of these components. For a more in-depth analysis of them, refer to *Nutrition Counseling and Education Skill Development*.[2]

FIGURE 15-4 Cross-Cultural Nutrition Counseling Algorithm

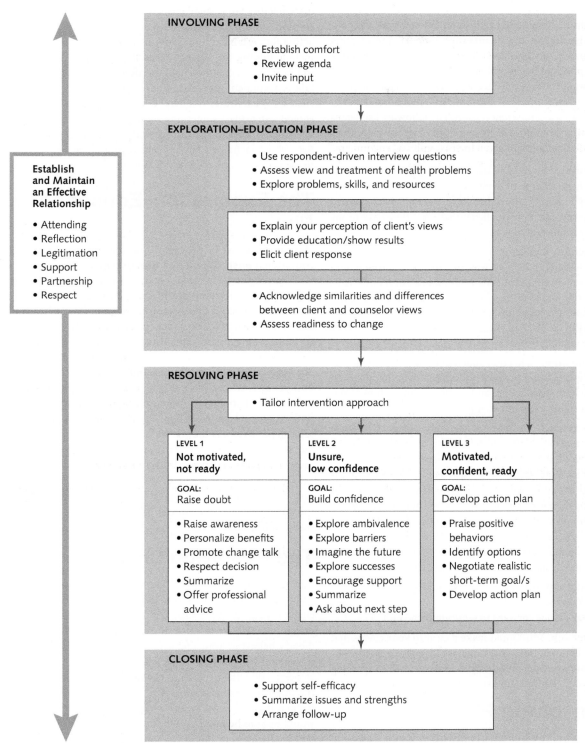

Source: K. Bauer, D. Liou, and C. Sokolik, *Nutrition Counseling and Education Skill Development* (Belmont, CA: Wadsworth/Cengage Learning, 2012).

Relationship-Building Skills

Relationship-building skills lay the foundation for making connections, developing and maintaining rapport, and creating trust. A trusting relationship is essential for clients to feel free to discuss personal issues and to be open to hearing the messages you want to convey. In fact, a productive relationship can in itself be an instrument of change and should be continually nurtured during a counseling session. The following list details the relationship-building skills emphasized in the algorithm, with special consideration given to cross-cultural encounters.

1. **Attending.** You need to use attentive behavior and listen actively in order to understand your clients' needs clearly. Also, you want to show that you are genuinely concerned and to indicate to your clients that what they have to say is very important to you.

2. **Reflection.** Reflection statements provide a vehicle for expressing empathy—a way to express, accurately and with sensitivity, that you understand someone's feelings and the meaning of those feelings. Empathy is not the same as sympathy. Sympathy is "I feel sorry for you." Empathy is "If I put myself in your shoes, I see where you're coming from."

3. **Legitimation.** Reflection statements acknowledge a person's feelings; legitimation responses affirm that it is normal to have such feelings and reactions. For example, "You have a right to feel upset. Anyone would."

4. **Show respect.** Counselors can show respect through words and body language that convey unconditional positive regard for their clients and a sincere interest in their welfare. Clients are more likely to feel free to express their thoughts and explain their actions if providers are not judging their actions. Do not criticize cultural differences. Be open to understanding divergent ideas and perspectives. Respect can also be shown through compliments. For example, "I really admire how your family was able to escape . . . and make a life for yourselves in California."

5. **Personal support.** Your clients should know you want to help. Your words and body language should convey the message "I look forward to working with you."

6. **Partnership.** You should make it clear to your clients that a number of options and strategies for solving their problems are available and that you look forward to working with your clients to find strategies that work for them.

The Involving Phase

Because first impressions tend to be lasting impressions, you want your greeting to convey a sense of warmth and caring. Begin interactions in a formal manner and refrain from using first names or nicknames because this could be considered disrespectful. Some small talk can aid in the development of a comfortable atmosphere and would be the expected course of action for certain cultural groups. Topics for small talk could include finding the office, the country of origin, or adapting to U.S. living. A common opening after the greeting and small talk is asking an open-ended question in a curious manner, such as "What brings you here today?" During this phase, you should also explain something about your program and/or the counseling process, indicating what you can and cannot do. Set a short agenda for the session so your client knows what to expect.

The Exploration–Education Phase

During this phase of the algorithm, the counselor provides educational interventions and uses respondent-driven interview questions (refer to Table 15-13 and to Table 4-9 on page 129) to understand nutritional concerns, while focusing on identifying skills and resources that can be used to find solutions. The first four components of the LEARN guidelines in Table 15-14—listen, explain your perceptions of workable strategies and your client's beliefs about treatment, acknowledge and discuss differences and similarities, and recommend options and strategies—provide a framework for discussing treatment strategies. After coming to the recommended options and strategies of the LEARN guidelines, the counselor needs to assess the client's motivational level for implementing any of the strategies. There are a number of ways to assess readiness to make changes,[3] but for people with limited English-speaking skills, the simplest method is simply to ask how they feel about working on a way to implement any of the strategies—in other words, whether they are ready, not ready, or not sure.

The Resolving Phase

The assessment of readiness is important because the algorithm takes into consideration the motivational level of your client. If your client is clearly not ready to make changes, your major goal will be to raise doubt about his or her present dietary behavior. Your major tasks are to raise awareness of the health/diet problems related to his or her dietary pattern, to personalize the benefits of change, to ask questions about the importance of changing (e.g., "What do you believe will happen if you do not change what foods you eat?" or "What would have to be different for you to believe that it is important to change your diet?"), to summarize what has been discussed, to offer professional advice, and to express support if your client decides he or she is ready to make changes. Respect your client's decision. If his or her condition is life-threatening, consider seeking the aid of a respected community elder to help negotiate changes.

Clients who are unsure of their readiness to take action need something to shift the balance in favor of making a change. Your goal will be to build confidence by exploring their ambivalence. Some strategies for exploring ambivalence are examining pros and cons and asking questions such as "What are your barriers to making the recommended dietary changes?" or "What would need to be different for you to feel you are able to make changes in your diet?" If the barriers are cultural, use the last component of the LEARN guidelines to negotiate making the recommended dietary changes more acceptable, such as eating the foods at a certain time of the day or mixing them with the client's acceptable foods. At the end of your discussion, summarize and ask, "What's next?" Set some modest goals, if appropriate.

Clients who clearly indicate that they are ready to make dietary changes are ready to set goals and develop action plans for implementing the goals. Goals should be worked out jointly between client and counselor.

The Closing Phase

Review what occurred during the session, summarize issues, identify strengths, support self-efficacy, and restate goals. Plan for the next counseling encounter, which could be a phone call, an e-mail, a text, or a counseling session.

CHAPTER **SUMMARY** . . . .

Gaining Cultural Competence

▶ Differences between cultures occur on many levels, such as communication, sense of time, family practices, beliefs about the cause of illness, and healing beliefs.

▶ Gaining cultural competence in community health care means developing attitudes, skills, and levels of awareness that enable one to provide culturally appropriate, respectful, and relevant interventions.

▶ The foundation of cultural competence is development of an awareness of one's own cultural matrix and an understanding that cultural beliefs influence our behavior and our conscious and unconscious thoughts.

▶ Culture strongly influences food behavior, and interventions need to be culturally appropriate as well as nutritionally sound.

Terms and Concepts Related to Cultural Competence

▶ Culture is shared history, consisting of "the integrated pattern of thoughts, communications, actions, customs, beliefs, values, and institutions associated, wholly or partially, with racial, ethnic, or linguistic groups, as well as with religious, spiritual, biological, geographical, or sociological characteristics."

▶ Diversity consists of differences among groups of people. The term *cross-cultural* denotes interaction between or among individuals who represent distinctly different cultures. People tend to be ethnocentric.

▶ *Ethnicity* is a property of a group that consists of its sharing cultural traditions, having a common linguistic heritage, and originating from the same land. *Acculturation* is the process of adopting the beliefs, values, and behaviors of another culture.

▶ There is a compelling need for community health professionals to gain cultural and linguistic expertise. The reasons include demographic diversity and projected population shifts; increased utilization of traditional therapies; disparities in the health status of various racial and ethnic groups; underrepresentation of health care providers from culturally and linguistically diverse groups; and legislative, regulatory, and accreditation mandates.

Cultural Competence Models

▶ In the cultural competence continuum model, the process of gaining cultural competence is envisioned as a succession of six stages from cultural destructiveness to cultural proficiency. The continuum provides a visual guide for assessing individual or agency progress (see Table 15-3).

▶ The Campinha-Bacote cultural competence model views cultural competence as a process rather than an end result. This model views cultural awareness, cultural skill, cultural knowledge, cultural encounters, and cultural desire as the five interdependent constructs of cultural competence. The pivotal construct in the process of becoming culturally competent is the cultural encounter.

Cross-Cultural Communication

▶ Successfully working with individuals from substantially different cultures and developing cross-cultural programming require culturally sensitive communication, negotiation, and education skills.

▶ Cultural orientation has a major impact on values and beliefs (see Table 15-6).

Culturally Appropriate Intervention Strategies

▶ Learning about the food habits, health beliefs, and behaviors of specific cultural groups can help community nutrition practitioners identify resources and find ways to build on community strengths to find solutions to problems related to health and nutrition.

▶ Explanatory models are useful for assessment, and the LEARN guidelines provide a framework for negotiating a culturally sensitive treatment plan to address a given illness episode. Listen with sympathy and understanding to a client's perception of a problem. Explain your perceptions of the problem. Acknowledge and discuss differences and similarities. Recommend treatment that is relevant, concise, and practical. Negotiate agreement.

Essential Organizational Elements of Cultural Competence

▶ Health care delivery organizations have a responsibility to provide appropriate care that is sensitive to cultural norms, values, and beliefs of individuals; linguistically accessible; and physically available.

SUMMARY **QUESTIONS** . . . .

1. Identify and explain five reasons that community nutrition practitioners should strive for cultural competence.
2. Identify and explain the components of the cultural competence continuum model and the Campinha-Bacote cultural competence model.
3. What factors should be taken into consideration when searching for and utilizing the services of an interpreter?
4. What are the hoped-for advantages of using an explanatory model for investigating perceptions regarding origin and treatment of an illness?
5. What are the essential organizational elements of cultural competence?
6. Cultural Values Activity. By yourself or with a group, review the following statements. Indicate if you believe they are cultural truths of Americans. Put an X in the appropriate box.

AMERICAN VALUE	VALUE OF OTHERS	CULTURAL TRUTH
❑	❑	Change is inevitable and desirable
❑	❑	Obligation to the group
❑	❑	Equality and egalitarianism are social ideals
❑	❑	Directness and openness are virtues
❑	❑	Appreciation for aesthetics
❑	❑	Self-help is preferred to dependence
❑	❑	Behave according to status
❑	❑	The individual is more important than the group
❑	❑	The future is more important than the past
❑	❑	Indirectness, saving face is valued
❑	❑	Competition and free enterprise are best for economic development
❑	❑	Informality is desirable in social interactions
❑	❑	Action is better than contemplation

AMERICAN VALUE	VALUE OF OTHERS	CULTURAL TRUTH
❏	❏	Harmony is valued
❏	❏	Cause-and-effect logic helps us make sense of human existence
❏	❏	Problem solving is the best approach to dealing with reality
❏	❏	Formality is valued
❏	❏	The practical is more important to deal with than the abstract, ideal, or intellectual
❏	❏	Socialism is valued
❏	❏	Improving material existence benefits human beings more than spiritual improvement
❏	❏	Tradition is valued

INTERNET RESOURCES

Culturally and Linguistically Appropriate Services (CLAS)
http://clas.uiuc.edu/aboutclas.html
Provides culturally and linguistically appropriate reviewed materials and practices that meet the dual criteria of (1) effectiveness and (2) cultural and linguistic appropriateness.

Diversity Rx
www.diversityrx.org
Addresses state and federal laws, multicultural health best practices overview, and interpreter services.

EthnoMed
http://ethnomed.org
Contains information about cultural beliefs, medical issues, and other issues.

Food and Nutrition Information Center
http://fnic.nal.usda.gov
USDA site that provides background and practical resources for those working with various ethnic/cultural groups.

Islamic Food and Nutrition Council of America (IFANCA)
www.ifanca.org
Describes the foods appropriate under Muslim law for halal consumers.

National Center for Cultural Competence
http://nccc.georgetown.edu
Cultural competence self-assessments for individuals and organizations.

Office of Minority Health
www.minorityhealth.hhs.gov
OMH Resource Center is a one-stop shop for minority health literature, research, and referrals.

Orthodox Union
www.oukosher.org
Questions and answers about kosher food and kosher supervision of food production.

Pacer Center
www.pacer.org
Provides information for enhancing the quality of life of children and young adults with disabilities.

CHAPTER 16

Principles of Nutrition Education

Chapter Revision by Virginia B. Gray, PhD, RD

LEARNING **OBJECTIVES**

After you have read and studied this chapter, you will be able to:

- Write clear, measureable instructional objectives.
- Use formative research in planning and evaluation of instructional materials targeted at a particular audience.
- Use the three levels of intervention to develop nutrition education plans that build awareness, change lifestyles, and create supportive environments.
- Develop age-appropriate nutrition education activities that support application of lesson content.
- Link nutrition education plans to behavior change theories.

- Design nutrition messages.
- Suggest means of evaluating nutrition education activities.
- Describe three basic principles of effective writing.

This chapter addresses such issues as educational theories and techniques, educational materials development, educational needs of diverse populations, presenting an educational session for a group, and lay and technical writing, which have been designated by the Accreditation Council for Education in Nutrition and Dietetics (ACEND) as Foundation Knowledge and Learning Outcomes for dietetics education.

CHAPTER **OUTLINE**

Something to think about...

"To cease smoking is the easiest thing I ever did. I ought to know because I've done it a thousand times."

—*MARK TWAIN*

For a complete list of references, please access the MindTap Reader within your MindTap course.

Introduction

Consumers are bombarded daily with dozens of health messages. Some are short and sweet: "Let's Move!" "Got Milk?" Others are complex and require time to process and understand. For example, an article in a consumer health magazine titled "Vitamin D in the Spotlight" describes research related to vitamin D and the risk of several chronic diseases and takes 15 minutes to read and study.[1] Growing interest in nutrition and health, in combination with increased access to information, have led to a complex nutrition information environment. Working within this complex environment requires more than a solid grasp of nutrition science (though this is important!).

What makes an effective nutrition education program? Think about a new behavior you have worked to adopt, or a habit you have worked to stop. What helped you or hindered you from making changes? For many people, learning about health benefits or harms of a behavior does not result in lasting behavior change. Instead, knowledge *plus* skill development, increased motivation, and environmental supports can work together to promote lasting change. Developing skills in this multifaceted approach to nutrition education is important for those planning nutrition education programs.[2]

This chapter describes how the community nutritionist develops the nutrition education component of an intervention. **Nutrition education** is an instructional method that promotes healthful behaviors by imparting information that individuals can use to make informed decisions about food, dietary habits, and health.[3] This chapter discusses the principles of nutrition education. Two major topics from previous chapters are particularly relevant here: the target population—what they think, feel, believe, want, and do—and entrepreneurship.

Nutrition education Any set of learning experiences designed to facilitate the voluntary adoption of eating and other nutrition-related behaviors conducive to health and well-being.

Applying Educational Principles to Program Design

Nutrition and health behaviors are complex issues. Individuals and groups can possess very different combinations of background, culture, health risks, health beliefs, motivators, learning style, environment, goals, and expectations.[4] An effective nutrition intervention program integrates good instructional design and learning principles and uses media that facilitate a high degree of individualization. Furthermore, nutrition education that is effective targets not only changes in knowledge, but also seeks to change motivation and attitudes. Furthermore, it provides opportunities to develop skills and practice them, thus promoting behavior change. In addition, nutrition education efforts can also incorporate strategies to change environments in which people are making health decisions. These three types of activities should be familiar to you. Recall the three levels of intervention discussed in Chapter 5 on Program Planning (Step 1: Build Awareness; Step 2: Change Lifestyles; and Step 3: Create a Supportive Environment). **Table 16-1** provides example strategies to use in applying these three types of changes to a Client-Centered Nutrition Education approach.

Educational research shows that the effect of an intervention on the target population's knowledge and behavior depends on the intervention's application of six basic educational principles: consonance, relevance, individualization, feedback, reinforcement, and facilitation.[5] **Table 16-2** offers examples of methods for applying these principles to the development of effective nutrition education interventions.

Step 1: Enhancing Motivation: "Why Change"

Explore feelings, attitudes, and beliefs about behaviors:
• Increase client awareness about behaviors through self-assessment activities such as food checklists or physical activity records.
• Explore pros and cons of behaviors to help participants explore and resolve ambivalence about trying a new behavior.
• Address social norms by discussing the impact of peers and media on behavior choices.
• Provide opportunities for clients to think about perceived benefits and barriers for behaviors.
• Help clients overcome barriers and increase self-confidence, or self-efficacy, to make a change.

Step 2: Providing Information and Skills to Act: "How to Change"

Incorporate activities that may help clients gain skills:
• Discuss relevant nutrition-related information.
• Build skills in food preparation and cooking.
• Practice critical thinking skills to help clients make healthy choices.
• Provide opportunities for clients to practice setting realistic goals.
• Encourage self-monitoring of food intake and physical activity in order to increase clients' sense of control over eating and activity behaviors.

Step 3: Creating a Support System

• Discuss how to develop a positive change support system. (Example: Identifying an exercise buddy)
• Map out places in the community to exercise or find inexpensive fruits and vegetables.

Source: Adapted from Client-Centered Nutrition Education toolkit, developed by the Texas Department of State Health Services to enhance nutrition education provided to WIC participants in Texas. The resources in this toolkit encourage WIC nutritionists to move beyond knowledge to facilitate behavior change. The full toolkit is available at *www.dshs.state.tx.us/wichd/nut/ccne.aspx*.

TABLE 16-1 Example Strategies for Enhancing Motivation, Providing Information and Skills to Act, and Creating a Support System in Client-Centered Nutrition Education

CRITERIA	DESCRIPTION	EXAMPLE
Consonance	Degree of fit between program and its objectives, or degree to which communication is directed toward accomplishing the intended outcome	In intervention to improve proper self-monitoring of blood glucose, teaching benefits of monitoring without showing how to monitor would be insufficient.
Relevance	Degree to which intervention is geared to clients, including reading level and visual acuity	Program should be tailored to clients' knowledge, beliefs, circumstances, and prior experience, determined by pretests, baseline questionnaires, or interviews.
Individualization	Allows clients to have personal questions answered or instructions paced according to individual learning progress	Because clients learn in different ways and at different rates, a program is more likely to be effective if the education is tailored to individual needs.
Feedback	Helps clients learn by providing a measuring stick to determine how much progress they are making	Feedback can be based on achieved learning objectives (such as increased knowledge about a given subject) or outcomes (such as increased adherence to a prescribed diet).
Reinforcement	Components of the program (other than feedback) designed to reward the desired behavior	Praise and congratulations are very effective in rewarding changed behavior.
Facilitation	Measures taken to accomplish desired actions or eliminate obstacles	For example, a weekly food diary sheet facilitates a client's ability to record actual food intake.

TABLE 16-2 Applications of Educational Principles to Program Design

Source: Adapted from R. Patterson, ed., *Changing Patient Behavior: Improving Outcomes in Health and Disease Management* (San Francisco: Jossey-Bass, 2001), 16–17.

Learning across the Lifespan

People of any age learn best if they have the prerequisite knowledge, if content is broken into small pieces, if what they learn is practiced and reinforced, and if the content seems relevant.[6] It is also important to consider that people's learning needs, preferences, and abilities change as they age.[7] Consider the tips listed in **Table 16-3** for teaching across the lifespan. Although children and adults learn in many of the same ways, there are some aspects of adult learning that are important to consider, as discussed in the next section. **Adult education** is a generic term that refers to formal, informal, vocational, and continuing education for the purpose of learning.[8] For adults, learning is an intentional, purposeful activity. Adult learners approach learning differently from the way children do, and they have different motivations for learning.

Adult education The process whereby adults learn and achieve changes in knowledge, attitudes, values, or skills.

Adult Learners Food and nutrition practitioners who provide education for adults need to know how adults learn best and to be familiar with ways to enhance instructional effectiveness in this age group. The basic principles guiding adult education are that (1) adult roles, responsibilities, and previous experiences influence learning; (2) adult

TABLE 16-3 Tips to Consider When Teaching across the Lifespan

Children

• Keep your message short, clear, and simple.
• Emphasize positive points; avoid negative or judgmental statements.
• Relate the message to the child's interests. Make learning fun!
• Make practical, concrete suggestions.
• Involve the child (ask questions, relate to his or her experiences and activities).
• Show the child how to, not why.

Adolescents

• Relate to the adolescent's interests.
• Consider the impact of peer pressure.
• Consider the client's rebelliousness and attitudes toward authority.
• Address his or her insecurities about physical changes.
• Discuss mood changes and impulsiveness.
• Tie teaching concepts to adolescent concerns, such as appearance and athletic performance.

Pregnant Women

• Relate present needs to the expected performance during labor and delivery and a healthy outcome.
• Address her anxieties and concerns.
• Consider the impact of the physiological, psychological, and emotional changes taking place.
• Acknowledge her needs.

Adults

• Acknowledge and relate to the client's needs and concerns.
• Consider his or her prior experiences with and knowledge of the subjects discussed.
• Personalize your interaction to the client's current health profile.
• Provide an opportunity to practice using knowledge and skills.

Older Adults

• Address any anxieties and concerns associated with isolation, chronic disease, and economic constraints.
• Consider the impact of chronic conditions and diseases on the client's ability to communicate and his or her attention span.
• Relate to a client's needs with empathy.
• Consider your recommendations in the context of the client's quality of life.
• Provide an opportunity to practice using knowledge and skills.

Source: Adapted from *Beyond Nutrition Counseling: Achieving Positive Outcomes through Nutrition Therapy* (American Dietetic Association, 1996).

learning is constantly occurring; and (3) the role of the adult educator is to facilitate this continuous learning process.

Adult learners learn best when the subject matter is tied directly to their own realm of experience, and their learning is facilitated when they can make connections between their past experiences (a parent died of cancer) and their current concerns (whether eating a high-fiber diet will protect them from cancer).[9] Adults are motivated to learn by the relevance of the topic to their lives.[10] They are more likely to stick with lifestyle changes if they make specific goals ("I will eat at least one vegetable for a snack every day" vs. "I will eat more vegetables") and do not attempt to change too many things at once. Also, making a goal is not enough: a practical plan for achieving it is also important.[11] Adults retain new information best when they are actively involved in problem-solving exercises and hands-on learning that enable them to assimilate, practice, and use the information in meaningful ways.[12] In short, an effective program takes into account the learning style and motivations of the target population.[13] **Table 16-4** provides a summary of points to consider when providing educational experiences for adult learners.[14]

What we know about adult learners suggests the following recommendations for nutrition educators:

- Make learning problem-centered and meaningful to the learner's life situations.
- Make information concrete; adults prefer concrete knowledge rather than abstract information. Define all abstract terms.

TABLE 16-4

Providing Learner-Centered Educational Experiences for Adult Learners

Many of the following are considerations for all types and ages of learners but should be carefully addressed when working with adults.

Create an Environment That Supports Learning

Physical Dimensions

- Geographically convenient location
- Easy-to-locate classroom or meeting room
- Furniture of appropriate size
- Adequate heat and light

Psychological, Sociological Dimensions

- Appropriate location for topic being presented to audience
- Friendly, open manner of the instructor
- Instructor respects learners.
- Opportunities for learners to get to know each other are provided.
- Guidelines and procedures allow all learners equal opportunity to participate in learning.

Preparing the Learning Episode

- Assess learners' needs.
- Assess learners' interests.
- Assess learners' abilities/previous knowledge.
- Encourage learner participation in establishing goals and content of the learning experience.

Providing Instruction

- Encourage high learner-interactive participation.
- Emphasize material that learners perceive as relevant.
- Use repetition and plan time for learner "practice."
- Use a variety of teaching methods.
- Use instructional resources that "fit" learners' needs.
- Plan audio-visuals that all can see and easily interpret.
- Provide frequent feedback.

Source: Adapted from E. J. Hitch and J. P. Youatt, *Communicating Family and Consumer Sciences* (Tinley Park, IL: Goodheart-Willcox Company, 1995), 59.

- Make learning a collaboration between the educator and the learner. Use the adult learners' experiences as educational resources. Adults do not learn well with a lecture style of teaching; instead, invite learners to dialogue with their peers and share their personal experiences and knowledge.
- Encourage participatory approaches to learning, such as small-group discussion and responding to questions. Ask open-ended questions to draw out what the adults already know about the topic you are teaching.
- Seize the "teachable moments." Adults who are in a transition phase in their lives, such as pregnancy, midlife, or older adult years, are generally more open to learning. Identify these specific life transitions and utilize them as opportunities for learning.
- Increase the adult learners' sense of self-worth by validating their experiences. Provide plenty of evaluation information and use positive feedback.
- Establish a positive learning environment. Ensure that the physical environment is attractive, comfortable, and well ventilated. Minimize distracting sounds.
- Recognize individual and cultural differences because they affect learning styles.[15]

To ensure successful educational interventions, it is imperative to study your potential audience, learning what motivates them, what they want, and what they need.[16] Research your target population by (1) reviewing the literature, (2) conducting formative research (e.g., one-on-one interviews or focus groups), and (3) asking representatives from the audience to help you with the planning and development of the program or material.[17] When using interviews and focus groups with members of the target audience, the following questions may be helpful in designing the intervention:

- How does what you eat affect you?
- What motivates you to choose healthy foods?
- What keeps you from eating healthy foods?
- Describe your current knowledge and skills related to choosing and preparing healthy foods.
- About which nutrition topics are you most interested in learning?
- What types of nutrition-related learning experiences would be most helpful to you?

These questions are based on the health belief model, and allow the nutrition educator to gain an understanding of (1) how the audience perceives healthy eating (i.e., perceived benefits and perceived threats), (2) how the audience perceives their ability to eat healthy (i.e., self-efficacy), and (3) nutrition-related interests. Reviewing the literature, integrating a theory-based approach, and involving the audience in planning the intervention will help foster a successful experience for the learner as well as the educator.

Developing a Nutrition Education Plan

The nutrition education plan outlines the strategy for disseminating the intervention's key messages to the target population. A strong plan also provides opportunities for program participants to practice skills and to develop specific plans for applying information. In addition, nutrition education plans may include an intervention that intends to create a supportive environment, in an effort to foster a particular health behavior. Consider the National Fruit and Vegetable Program message: "Fruits & Veggies—More Matters." Fruits & Veggies—More Matters is a national media program designed to get Americans to eat more servings of fruits and vegetables daily. The program aims to do this by engaging all three levels of intervention. First, the program increases public awareness of the importance of eating a diet rich in fruits and vegetables every day for better health (Step 1: Build Awareness). Second, the program provides consumers with tips for including more servings of fruits and vegetables into their daily routines, thus providing skills for behavior change (Step 2: Change Lifestyles). Lastly, the program increases the availability of fruits and vegetables at home, school, work, and other places where food is served (Step 3: Create a Supportive Environment).[18]

In addition to messages that promote consumer behavior changes, nutrition messages may also inform, educate, or advocate for policy changes to support healthy eating. When community nutritionists lobby legislators for more funding to support a statewide network of food banks and soup kitchens, they use nutrition messages to educate legislators about food insecurity and inform them of the consequences of malnutrition among young children.

The nutrition education plan is a written document that describes the needs of the target population, the goals and objectives for intervention activities, the program format, the lesson plans (including instructional materials such as handouts and videos), the nutrition messages to be imparted to the target population, the marketing plan, any partnerships that will support program development or delivery, and the evaluation instruments.[19] These aspects of the plan are often organized into a manual that can be used by staff who work with the program. Having a detailed nutrition education plan can prevent confusion, especially when new staff members join the team or a substitute instructor must be found on short notice.

A nutrition education plan is developed for each intervention target group. **Table 16-5** illustrates the similarities among nutrition education plans developed for individuals, communities, and systems. Nutrition education plans for individuals and communities are identical, the same activities being appropriate to both types of interventions. At the systems level, the nutrition education plan might properly be called a strategy. System-level strategies do not require formal lesson plans or program identifiers such as logos or action figures, but they may draw on these program elements to reinforce key messages. A marketing plan is just as crucial to system-level activities as to those aimed at individuals and communities. See the Internet Resources at the end of the chapter to learn more about statewide plans to promote nutrition and reduce obesity.

Developing Lesson Plans Nutrition educators have opportunities to provide nutrition education in many different settings. However, food and nutrition practitioners are usually not trained as teachers, and they rarely have all the skills needed to develop effective, interesting, and creative lesson plans.[20] However, nutrition practitioners can gain these skills by observing effective nutrition education in action.

	TARGET GROUP		
ACTIVITY	**INDIVIDUALS**	**COMMUNITIES**	**SYSTEMS**
Assess needs.	✓	✓	✓
Set goals and objectives.	✓	✓	✓
Specify the format.	✓	✓	✓
Develop a lesson plan.	✓	✓	
Specify nutrition messages.	✓	✓	✓
Choose program identifiers.	✓	✓	
Develop a marketing plan.	✓	✓	✓
Specify partnerships.	✓	✓	✓
Conduct evaluation research.	✓	✓	✓

TABLE 16-5 Activities Related to Developing a Nutrition Education Plan

Jaime Schwartz Cohen

ENTREPRENEUR
IN ACTION

At Ketchum Public Relations in New York City, Jaime Schwartz Cohen, MS, RD, works with food companies and commodity boards to develop strategic nutrition education programs that communicate science-based messages to consumers, the media, and health influencers. Says Jaime: "Digital and social platforms have provided us with new channels to share nutrition information. The important lesson for nutrition educators in the digital age is to recognize how powerful websites, blogs, and social networking can be for communicating nutrition information, and also for engaging with your audience. Another lesson is to consider the format of the information. A handout with paragraphs of information may be factual, but it may not be the most effective way to communicate nutrition messages, especially since people are now used to images, emoji, and information in 140 characters or less. No matter what aspect of community nutrition you are involved in, social media tools and channels can help you educate your audience." Find out what she has to say about the importance of networking online at *www.cengagebrain.com*.

Also, remembering to integrate literature that not only supports the content of lessons but also provides evidence of effective educational strategies for a particular target audience is important. Lastly, remembering to plan nutrition education activities with a base in behavior change theories (review Chapter 3) can enhance the effectiveness of a nutrition education plan. In sum, an effective lesson plan is evidence-based (content *and* strategy), application oriented, and straightforward for whoever is delivering the lesson.

The first step in developing a lesson plan is to know your target audience, the setting, and the content. Consider the following principles when you are developing your lesson plan.[21]

- Your lesson plan should be centered on the learner's interests, needs, and motivation. This information should be available to you if you have done a complete assessment of your target audience.
- When learning is related to real-life situations, learners can readily identify with the situation. The examples that you provide should be directly related to the learners' lives and experiences.
- Adults learn best when they are involved in the process. Ask them at the beginning of class what they expect to learn. People learn by doing and by being involved in solving the problem at hand.

Structuring Your Knowledge The first component of lesson writing is to identify the major concept that you are communicating. To attempt to design a lesson plan without organizing the main and related concepts within the subject matter is similar to putting the cart before the horse. It won't go anywhere. To help educators structure their knowledge, researchers have identified several questions that educators should ask themselves before creating a lesson plan.[22] Three of these questions are:

- What is the telling question? Ask yourself: What am I trying to teach? Have I identified the major concept to be taught, and what do I need to know about it? Here are two examples of telling questions in nutrition: What are calcium-rich foods and how are they important for health? What are *trans* fatty acids and why should they be limited?
- What are the key concepts? Once you have defined the telling question, list the concepts you plan to define and teach about. For example, if your telling question is "What are calcium-rich foods and how are they important for health?," some of the key concepts you will want to define are dairy sources of calcium, plant sources of calcium, and other alternative sources of calcium, such as calcium-fortified soymilk. You will also want to explain the benefits of calcium and provide practical approaches for achieving optimal intakes.
- What teaching methods are best suited to your audience? Consider your audience. For example, face-to-face instruction may not be how today's technology-savvy young adults want to learn about healthful eating. What teaching method would you like to use to teach this lesson? Is the lesson more conducive to a group discussion with related activities? Or is a lecture more appropriate for the target audience? Would demonstrations be more useful? Choosing the most effective teaching method is important in building knowledge,

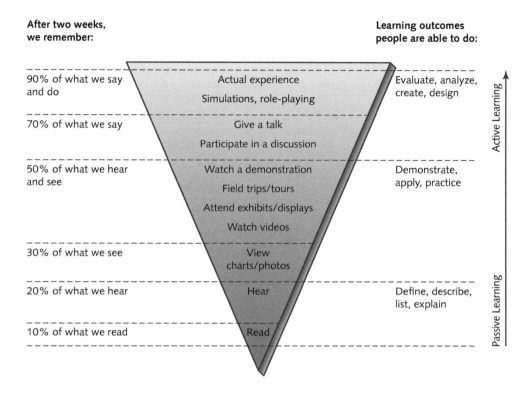

After two weeks,
we remember:

90% of what we say
and do

70% of what we say

50% of what we hear
and see

30% of what we see

20% of what we hear

10% of what we read

Actual experience
Simulations, role-playing

Give a talk
Participate in a discussion

Watch a demonstration
Field trips/tours
Attend exhibits/displays
Watch videos

View
charts/photos

Hear

Read

Learning outcomes
people are able to do:

Evaluate, analyze,
create, design

Demonstrate,
apply, practice

Define, describe,
list, explain

Active Learning

Passive Learning

FIGURE 16-1 The Cone of Experience: From Passive Learning to Active Learning

Source: Adapted from Edgar Dale's Cone of Experience, *Audio-Visual Methods in Teaching*, 3rd ed. (New York: Holt, Rinehart, and Winston, 1969).

skills, and motivation. Consider using some of the active learning experiences cited in **Figure 16-1**. Again, using a behavior change theory at this point will help you to create lesson strategies that connect with the audience's beliefs, values, and perceptions.

Writing Instructional Objectives

Developing useful lesson plans is based on writing effective objectives. Ask yourself, "What will the learner be able to do as a result of the learning experience?" Effective specific instructional objectives should (1) concentrate on the learner and not the teacher, (2) clearly communicate a specific instructional intent, (3) be stated in terms of the *end product* (the learning outcomes) and not in terms of the process of learning, and (4) describe one type of learning outcome per objective that is specific in describing learners' performance (**Table 16-6**).[23] Consider developing objectives that affect a variety of types of change. The Client-Centered Nutrition Education toolkit, a resource of the Texas Department of State Health Services, suggests developing objectives that affect participants in three areas: the head (cognitive/knowledge change), hands (skills/behavior change), and heart (affective/motivational change).[24]

Components of a Lesson Plan

Planning of lessons should not be done haphazardly. Certain essential elements should always be part of your plan: objectives, body of the lesson, activities, and evaluation. A common format used to structure lesson plans follows.[25]

1. **Lesson Title.** Every lesson should have a title. Choose a catchy title when you can, but be sure it is not ambiguous. A title is a one-sentence (limit it to 10 words) summary of your topic.
2. **Target Audience.** In order to maximize the usefulness of your lesson plan, clearly identify the target audience, their grade or educational level, and any other important characteristics that may affect development of the plan.

TABLE 16-6 Characteristics of Effective Objectives That Are Measurable and Attainable and Common Mistakes to Avoid

CHARACTERISTICS OF EFFECTIVE OBJECTIVES	COMMON MISTAKES TO AVOID	EXAMPLES OF INCORRECTLY STATED OBJECTIVES	EXAMPLES OF WELL-STATED OBJECTIVES
Concentrate on the learner.	Avoid describing the teacher's performance.	Demonstrates to students how to read a nutrition label.	At the end of the demonstration, students are expected to: Identify the serving size on the nutrition label.
Clearly communicate your intent using verbs such as *write, define, list, identify, compare, draw, differentiate.*[a]	Avoid using broad terms such as *grasp, believe, have faith, internalize, enjoy, see, love, realize.*	Sees the value of breastfeeding.	At the end of the session, students will be able to: Identify three benefits of breastfeeding.
State objectives in terms of the expected learning outcomes rather than in terms of procedure.	Avoid terms such as *increase, gain, improve, add, develop.*	Gains knowledge of fiber.	At the end of the session, students will be able to: Differentiate between low- and high-fiber foods.
Include one specific learning outcome that describes the behavior of the learner as a result of the learning experience.	Avoid including *two active verbs* in one objective.	*Understands* how to count carbohydrate grams and *applies* the knowledge effectively.	Upon completion of the class, students will be able to: Apply the knowledge of counting carbohydrates effectively.

[a] Verbs used with general objectives: *understand, know, learn, comprehend, apply, use, interpret, evaluate, demonstrate.* Verbs used with specific objectives: *write, identify, compare, describe, list, state, differentiate, distinguish, explain.*

Source: Adapted from R. AbuSabha, *Effective Nutrition Education for Behavior Change* (Clarksville, MD: Wolf Rinke Associates, 1998), 81–82.

3. **Duration.** Identify the duration of the lesson (e.g., two hours).

4. **Lesson Goal.** This is the goal for the class, a statement of what will be accomplished or learned. A general goal for a lesson plan on fruit and vegetable consumption might be "increase perceived benefits of consuming fruits and vegetables with each meal."

5. **Learning Objectives.** Identify the expected learning outcomes using measurable statements, as discussed earlier.

6. **Procedure.** Describe in detail your plan for the lesson, such as how the goals and objectives will be accomplished. Your lesson plan should include an introduction, a body, and a conclusion.

   - *Introduction.* Describe how the instructor will introduce the class. What activity, story, or segment will be used to start the session? Be sure that the introduction is interesting enough to grab the attention of the audience. Help learners make a connection with their own experiences.

   - *Body of the Lesson.* The body of the lesson should contain two pieces of information: background and the way the lesson is organized. It is helpful to provide background on the subject matter, along with references to familiarize future instructors with the major concepts and give them the opportunity to obtain further information when they need it. In addition, the instructor needs to know the organization of the lesson: what to do first, when to introduce an activity, and so on.

   - *Closure.* In one or two sentences, summarize the lesson. For example, if the lesson is about the grains food group and is targeted to children in the third grade, you may close your lesson with the following sentence: "Remind learners that whole-grain breads, cereals, rice, and pasta are important in our diet because they contain many vitamins and minerals that are essential to energy and good health." Then ask learners to identify a whole-grain food they learned about in the lesson that they would like to try.

7. **Learning Experiences or Activities.** List the different activities you expect the instructor and/or the learners to be involved with during the educational session. Activities may include showing slides or a video, group discussion, a cooking

activity, an application activity, or a virtual learning experience using the Internet. Be creative with the activity and aim to involve learners in applying the principles learned. Remember that participants are more likely to apply knowledge that they have practiced using (rather than just hearing it).

8. **Method of Evaluation.** Describe how the instructor will assess whether the expected outcomes have been achieved. Provide learners with experiences and/or tests designed to apply and evaluate what has been learned. Creative assignments, knowledge tests, exams, and homework are all methods of evaluating learners' performance. For longer-term programs, methods of assessing dietary changes may be included. In addition, be sure to include an evaluation of the educator's performance to assess how well the information was presented.

9. **Materials Needed.** List all of the necessary materials for use by the educator and those needed by the learner. Plan to include as many of these materials in the lesson plan as possible (e.g., all PowerPoint slides and handouts).

Creating a "Lesson-at-a-Glance" is a great way to summarize a lesson. It helps organize thoughts during the lesson planning process. In addition, the "Lesson-at-a-Glance" can serve as a helpful resource for a new instructor in gaining a sense of a lesson. See **Figure 16-2** for an example "Lesson-at-a-Glance" used in the introductory lesson of *Whole Grains in Child Nutrition Programs*, a resource of the Institute of Child Nutrition. This resource is targeted at school nutrition staff and intends to build knowledge and skills related to integration of whole grains in child nutrition programs.

LESSON-AT-A-GLANCE
Lesson 1: Identifying Whole Grains

Time	Topic	Task	Materials
Set-up	**Lesson Preparation**	• Set up classroom for Lesson 1. • Lead Activity: Opener.	• See Preparation Checklist. • **Activity: Opener**
10 minutes	**Introduction**	• Introduce lesson and present objectives. • Administer Lesson 1 Pre-Assessment.	• Lesson 1 Pre-Assessment

Objective 1: Identify the health benefits of consuming whole grains.

10 minutes	**Health Benefits of Whole Grains**	• Discuss the health benefits of consuming whole grains. • Refer to *Fact Sheet: Health Benefits of Whole Grains*.	• *Fact Sheet: Health Benefits of Whole Grains*

Objective 2: Define "whole grain."
Objective 3: Identify whole grains.

15 minutes	**Identifying Whole Grains**	• Define "whole grain." • Discuss common and usual names for whole grains. • Discuss Standards of Identity for whole grains. • Lead Activity: Identifying Whole Grains. • Refer to *Fact Sheet: What is a Whole Grain?*	• Sample whole-grain products (or names of whole-grain products on index cards) • **Activity: Identifying Whole Grains** • *Identifying Whole Grains Activity Sheet* • *Fact Sheet: What is a Whole Grain?*
10 minutes	**Lesson Summary**	• Discuss how lesson objectives were achieved. • Administer Lesson 1 Post-Assessment. • Summarize lesson.	• Lesson 1 Post-Assessment

FIGURE 16-2

Example "Lesson-at-a-Glance" Used in the *Whole Grains in Child Nutrition Programs* Trainer's Manual

Source: *Whole Grains in Child Nutrition Programs* resource is available at the Institute of Child Nutrition website at *www.nfsmi.org*. Used with permission from the Institute of Child Nutrition.

PROGRAMS IN **ACTION**

Making Healthy Eating Fun for Students

Providing students with information alone will not necessarily get them to change their health-related behavior. In order to reach students and catalyze change, education should be fun, integrated, and behaviorally based (the F.I.B. approach).[1] Furthermore, changes in the environment can enhance effectiveness of educational efforts. For example, environmental changes may change food access (such as by increasing access to fruits and vegetables). Environmental approaches may also endeavor to change social norms (such as by using marketing approaches to change attitudes and norms related to milk consumption). Students learn well when they are having fun, are actively participating in their education, and are surrounded by healthy environments.

School-based programs are able to provide children with knowledge and skills, as well as with the environment, motivation, services, and support to develop and maintain healthy behaviors.[2] Schools are uniquely positioned to offer an integrated environment that reinforces classroom learning with action.

It has been recommended that healthy eating programs in schools both provide instruction for students and integrate nutrition education into school nutrition services (e.g., school lunch programs).[3] Because children may not fully understand nutrition concepts, education should offer experiences such as increased exposure and opportunities to select healthy foods.[4] In nutrition education, the school cafeteria is the logical testing ground for information, a place where students can "practice" newly learned eating habits.[5] School nutrition service can reinforce healthy eating messages through changes in the menu and in individual food items to support classroom learning.

The Milk Matters program integrated classroom learning about calcium consumption and dietary fat with a schoolwide campaign that involved foodservice, faculty, and other staff. The use of a well-known national nutrition campaign, the Got Milk? milk mustache program, piqued the interest of students, teachers, and parents.

Goals, Objectives, and Rationale for the Intervention

The primary goals of the Milk Matters program were to increase elementary school low-fat and fat-free milk consumption at lunch and to inform students of the benefits of drinking milk. The program strategy involved incorporating fun, behavioral-based nutrition education into the school setting. The target audience for this program was the 142 students, kindergarten through sixth grade, at the Divide County School in northwest North Dakota.

The Milk Matters campaign was developed to address two separate issues: calcium consumption and a lack of interest in drinking milk at lunchtime. A USDA study showed that approximately half of all elementary school students consume inadequate amounts of calcium. Because childhood is a critical period for bone development, boosting calcium intake at school became a priority for the campaign. Poor acceptance of milk in the cafeteria was also a major concern. School personnel noticed that students were dumping out more low-fat and fat-free milk—approximately four gallons a day—than when foodservice had been serving higher-fat milk.

The area's public health nutritionist planned a program in cooperation with the local public health unit and the elementary school to increase consumption of lower-fat milk. Resources were limited, necessitating the expansion of partnerships with organizations like the Midwest Dairy Council, which had access to effective and fun national nutrition messages.

Methodology

The Milk Matters campaign incorporated educational, promotional, and environmental elements. The nutritionist conducted an in-service for the teachers to inform them of plans and activities. Photographs of several teachers with "milk mustaches" were taken and posted in the school. Each teacher received a packet of materials outlining the daily activities for the week, including classroom presentations by the nutritionist, daily milk trivia questions, art projects, coloring sheets, and a video on milk from the Dairy Council. Children were asked, through a newsletter to parents, to bring in an empty fat-free or low-fat carton, as a way to encourage families to try lower-fat milk. Each student who brought a carton received a Got Milk? poster of his or her choice. School cooks wore cow aprons to integrate the Milk Matters program into the lunchroom. A contest among classes promoted increased milk consumption at lunch; the winning class was photographed with milk mustaches.

Results

Milk Matters was a great success. Students loved being photographed with milk mustaches. Dumping of milk was eliminated completely during the week of the Milk Matters campaign. The parent newsletter was highly successful; 92% of students brought an empty fat-free or low-fat milk container to school. School personnel continued to monitor the amount of milk dumped. The average amount of leftover milk was cut in half.

Lessons Learned

- Programs like this can easily be replicated through partnerships among public health units, schools, and local dairy councils.

- Schools appreciate nutrition education programs that provide students with an integrated curriculum that links to public health concerns.

Source: Adapted from *Community Nutritionary* (White Plains, NY: Dannon Institute, 2003). Used with permission.

Nutrition Education to Reduce CHD Risk: Case Study 1

This section describes the development of lesson plans for the Heartworks for Women program, a health promotion activity designed to help individuals (women) reduce their CHD risk. The senior manager responsible for developing, implementing, and evaluating the intervention for reducing CHD risk among women (Case Study 1) reviews the proposed intervention activities.

As described in Chapter 5, the Heartworks for Women program has two goals: (1) to educate individuals about the contributions of diet to CHD risk and (2) to build skills related to heart-healthy cooking and eating. Specific objectives are as follows:

- Increase awareness of the relationship of diet to CHD risk so that by the end of the course, the percentage of participants who can name two dietary factors that raise total blood cholesterol will increase to 75% from 25%.
- Increase knowledge of dietary sources of saturated and *trans* fat so that by the end of the course, the percentage of participants who can name three major sources of dietary fat that contribute to heart disease will increase to 75% from 30%.
- Increase knowledge of heart-healthy cooking methods so that by the end of the course, the percentage of participants who can describe and use five heart-healthy cooking methods will increase to 75% from 60%.
- Increase label-reading skills so that by the end of the course, the percentage of participants who can specify accurately the saturated and *trans* fat content of foods using the nutrition information provided on food labels will increase to 75% from 20%.

Using these objectives as a guide, the community nutritionist sketches a rough outline of the program sessions (see Table 5-6 on page 163). The sessions for the program are organized as follows:

Session 1: Getting Started
Session 2: Looking for Fat in All the Right Places
Session 3: Choosing Heart-Healthy Protein Foods
Session 4: Dairy Goes Low-Fat
Session 5: Focus on Fruits and Vegetables
Session 6: Reading Food Labels
Session 7: Grocery Shopping Made Easy
Session 8: Reading Restaurant Menus

The outline shows the link between the program objectives and the individual sessions. In this manner, the community nutritionist can be certain that any information that must be imparted to participants to meet the program objectives has been included in the program outline.

▶ **THINK LIKE A COMMUNITY NUTRITIONIST**

Read the Programs in Action feature on the previous page. Make a list of strategies used in the Milk Matters program. Then identify the level of intervention for each. Why is it important that this campaign targeted more than one level of intervention? How would it have been different if it had only focused on building awareness?

Developing Lesson Plans to Reduce CHD Risk

The community nutritionist considers the instructional method (e.g., group sessions or one-on-one counseling) best suited for teaching heart-healthy cooking skills in the Heartworks for Women program. She chooses to present the material in group sessions, knowing that the participants will learn from one another.[26] Moreover, a program consisting mainly of group sessions is more likely to fit within the budget because group sessions tend to be less costly than individual counseling. She develops objectives, selects instructional materials, and specifies other materials (such as goal sheets) required for each lesson. **Table 16-7** shows this information for the first two sessions.

She must decide whether to develop nutrition education materials herself, use existing materials, or do both. To save time, she reviews existing programs and their nutrition education materials to determine whether they can be used or adapted for this population. For example, in Session 1, which describes the major risk factors for CHD, the community nutritionist elects to develop her own handout on homocysteine because she cannot locate one, but she plans to use an existing brochure that describes other leading CHD risk factors. In Session 2, she plans to use a dietary fats chart developed by a leading food company and used widely in nutrition counseling. For Session 3, which will demonstrate a variety of protein options and healthy cooking methods, she decides to use the flyer *10 Tips for Choosing Protein* and other materials from the *10 Tips Nutrition Education Series* produced by the USDA Center for Nutrition Policy and Promotion.[27] In the selection of program materials, factors such as the cost of purchasing existing educational programs and materials must be weighed against the time required to produce educational materials in-house and the cost of duplicating materials for participants. Check the Internet Resources at the end of the chapter for a list of websites that provide nutrition handouts and other useful educational tools.

Specifying the Nutrition Messages
Nutrition messages should be specified for each lesson plan. The messages should convey a simple, easy-to-understand concept related to heart-healthy eating and cooking: "Choose low-fat dairy products," "Choose lean cuts of meat," and so forth. One or two of these messages may be used in the nutrition education plan developed for the community- or systems-level interventions. The nutrition message for Session 5—"More Matters: Eat five or more servings of fruits and vegetables every day"—does

TABLE 16-7 Case Study 1: Lesson Plans for the First Two Sessions of the Heartworks for Women Program

SESSION	TITLE	SESSION OBJECTIVES	INSTRUCTIONAL MATERIALS	LEARNING ACTIVITIES	NUTRITION MESSAGES
1	Getting Started	At the end of the session, participants will be able to: • Describe the program's two goals and four objectives. • Describe five major risk factors for CHD.	• Participant information form • Description of course goals and objectives • Handout: "Is Homocysteine a Risk Factor for Heart Disease?" • Handout: "Recipe for Summer Salsa and Baked Pita Chips" • Brochure: "Get the Facts about Heart Health"	• CHD and nutrition knowledge pretest • Handout: "Am I Ready for Change?" • Taste test = Summer Salsa and Baked Pita Chips (a heart-healthy recipe)	• Diets high in saturated fat and *trans* fat raise total blood cholesterol. • High blood cholesterol levels are a risk factor for CHD. • Heart-healthy cooking is easy and enjoyable.
2	Looking for Fat in All the Right Places	• Define four types of dietary fats. • Describe the major food sources of dietary fat. • Describe the major sources of solid fat in the typical U.S. diet.	• Handout: "Definitions of Fats" • Handout: "Dietary Fats Chart" • Handout: Goal Sheet	• Dietary Fats Quiz • Completion of goal sheet: Reducing saturated fat and *trans* fat intake	• Choose heart-healthy foods more often than foods high in saturated fat and *trans* fat.

double-duty: It is used in the individual session for the Heartworks for Women program, and it is a key nutrition message used in the media campaign to build awareness among women. More detailed information about nutrition messages is given later in this chapter.

Conducting Formative Evaluation

Formative evaluation should be conducted throughout the program design process. Examples of formative evaluation research include the focus group sessions held early in the design phase (described on page 638) and additional focus group testing of dietary messages and program instructional materials, such as the handout on homocysteine for Session 1 and the dietary fats chart for Session 2. Here, the community nutritionist invites members of the target population to review these materials for reading level and ease of understanding. In other words, the target population helps determine whether the materials are appropriate and useful.

Formative evaluation The process of testing and assessing certain elements of a program before it is implemented fully.

Health literacy is increasingly vital to help people manage their own health by navigating a complex health care system and applying the vast amount of health and nutrition information available for improving health outcomes. However, many people lack health literacy.[28] Differences in the ability to read and understand materials related to personal nutrition and health appear to contribute to health disparities. People with low health literacy are less likely to use preventive care, and more likely to be hospitalized and have poor disease outcomes.[29–31] Furthermore, among older adults, the risk of faster physical decline increases with poor health literacy.[32]

Health literacy The degree to which individuals have the capacity to obtain, process, and understand basic health information, tools, and services needed to make appropriate health decisions.

Educational materials such as brochures, fact sheets, and handouts should be checked for reading grade level using an online tool, a word processor's readability formula, or a formula such as the Fry Index or SMOG grading test (see Appendix C and the list of Internet Resources at the end of this chapter). For educational resources and information on health literacy, visit *http://healthliteracy.worlded.org* for links to reliable online sources that have health information in easy-to-read formats.

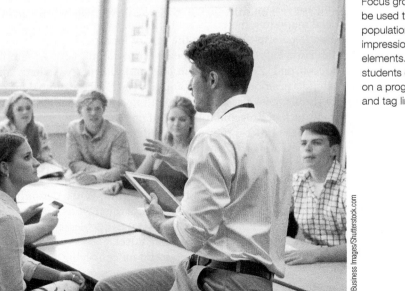

Focus group sessions can be used to obtain the target population's opinions and impressions about program elements. Here, college students offer their views on a program's name, logo, and tag line.

Monkey Business Images/Shutterstock.com

At least one trial run of the program should be completed to ensure that the lesson activities fit within the designated time frame, that the dietary messages are understandable and appropriate for the target population, and that the nutrition education plan is sufficiently detailed to curtail glitches. The results of formative evaluation are used to change and improve program delivery.

Designing Nutrition and Health Messages

Consumers process nutrition and health messages at different levels, depending on their interest in the topic and their past experience with similar messages. Their responses to nutrition and health messages can be viewed as a continuum. On one end is a state of mindless passivity, wherein consumers pay little attention to the message; at the other end is the state of active attention, where consumers respond to the message by thinking about it and considering what it might mean for their own health and well-being.[33] The important question is, how can nutrition messages be formulated to influence consumer behavior? This section describes several general ideas for designing nutrition and health messages.

General Ideas for Designing Messages

Developing and communicating clear, accurate, and precise messages is a key part of nutrition education.[34] Furthermore, these messages need to be ones that the target audience finds relevant and motivating, and that they can act upon. Formative research methods provide insights to guide message development and testing. For example, the Iowa Nutrition Network developed messages to encourage physical activity in children and used a process of testing with parents and children to match audience needs with the campaign. The "Play Your Way – One Hour a Day" campaign encourages elementary school children to be active for one hour a day, with the theme that being active does not necessarily involve sports, gyms, or equipment. In addition, the Iowa Nutrition Network developed a campaign focused on encouraging fruits and vegetables as snacks; classroom lessons and social marketing materials are included. Key messages in the "Pick a Better Snack" campaign (**Figure 16-3**) focus on the ease of incorporating fruit and vegetable snacks ("Wash. Bite. How Easy Is That?" appears on social marketing materials promoting apples and broccoli, and "Zero to Snack in 1 Second. How Easy Is That?" appears on social marketing materials promoting bananas and carrots).[35] These campaigns provide examples that convey simple messages and that intend to address commonly perceived barriers to healthy eating: lack of time and difficulty of preparation.

Children process information differently from the way adults do. A common mistake when presenting information to children has been to assume that children will reject a behavior portrayed as unhealthful or bad (e.g., skipping breakfast or snacking on junk food all day).[36] Sometimes a behavior is appealing to children and teenagers precisely *because* it is portrayed as bad or unhealthful! When designing messages for children and teenagers, go directly to the source: Ask them which messages they respond to and what type of messages they prefer. Also, start early. Messages directed to children and adolescents have the potential for a lasting effect.[37]

Clarity of information is important for conveying actionable messages. Whenever possible, avoid using qualifiers such as *perhaps*, *may*, and *maybe* that express uncertainty. Consumers prefer straightforward statements such as "Diets high in saturated fats and *trans* fats raise blood cholesterol levels" rather than tentative statements such as "A diet

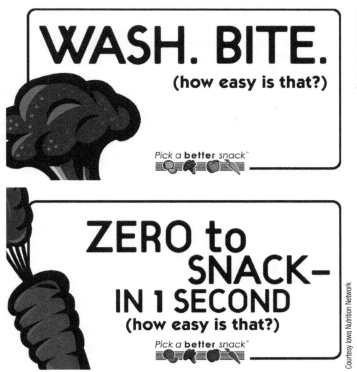

Courtesy Iowa Nutrition Network

FIGURE 16-3

Marketing Messages Used in the "Pick a Better Snack" Campaign

Source: *http://idph.iowa.gov/ inn/pick-a-better-snack.*

high in fat may increase blood cholesterol levels." Of course, the challenge for community nutritionists is deciding when strong, clear statements about research findings can be made and when more conservative statements are appropriate.

Looking back at messages around fat consumption in the 1980s and 1990s has provided insight on the pitfalls of messages that lack clarity. Many such messages focused heavily on dietary fat reduction, but were not clear in telling consumers what to consume in the place of fat. In that era, Americans began to consume less fat, but often replaced fat in the diet with refined carbohydrates and sugar. A key lesson was learned: make food-based recommendations to help consumers select healthy foods.[38,39] For example, instead of "eat less saturated fat," food-based guidance to promote healthy fats and to discourage high intakes of saturated and *trans* fats is more clear. In recent years, we have learned to adapt marketing techniques to promote behavior change. The International Food Information Council Foundation (IFIC) used a marketing model to design a toolkit known as "A New Nutrition Conversation with Consumers" that equips nutrition professionals with skills for understanding an audience and for developing consumer-friendly messages. Inherent to the consumer orientation, the tools acknowledge that message designers must know what consumers know, believe, value, and do. The tools use a stepwise process that solicits consumer input. In Step 1, the issue (or central idea to convey) is defined. Initial message concepts are then developed (Step 2). Step 3 involves assessing message concepts, using target audience feedback.[40] Then messages are fine-tuned (Step 4) and validated (Step 5). (For more information on these steps, visit the IFIC website.)

The New Nutrition Conversation with Consumers toolkit suggests the following take-home messages for developing consumer messages that work:

- "Use these pointers to develop insightful messages that affect consumer behavior." Using the steps outlined above, messages will be tailored to consumer interests and needs.

Amanda Archibald

ENTREPRENEUR IN ACTION

Amanda Archibald's strong appreciation of food from growing up and working in Europe, coupled with an excellent foundation in basic culinary arts, influenced her interest in community nutrition. She believes that we help people help themselves by giving them the right tools, including access to healthy foods *and* the knowledge of how to bring nourishment to the table. Amanda trains health care professionals and educators regarding the translation of nutrition advice into culinary experiences and recipes that are meaningful, doable, and healthful. Says Amanda: "The gateway from the field to the table is the kitchen, and the skill set is cooking. Nutrition is the science, but cooking is the translation. Giving a can of beans to someone has no meaning, unless you can relate how to translate that can into nourishment. It's a critical, life-saving skill set for you and for the people who look to you for expert guidance." Find out more about Amanda online at *www.cengagebrain.com*.

- "Speak in a language that is straightforward, relevant, and compelling to the audience." Information must connect with the lives of your audience.
- "Show consumers how to incorporate nutrition knowledge into everyday life by providing practical, easy-to-implement strategies." Action-based messages that provide specific ideas for implementation can motivate change.
- "Customize messages by giving specific reasons, meaningful to the audience, for changing behaviors. For example, talk about the benefits of taste, convenience, fun, culture, or feeling good." Do not connect healthy eating only with reduction of disease risk. Also connect with other reasons people eat the foods they select!
- "Offer choices for making behavior changes. Consumers are empowered when they can make their own choices." Provide options![41]

Using these tips, messages can be developed for a variety of audiences and programs. Continually seeking input from the intended audience will improve relevance of messages to the lives of target audience members.

Conducting Summative Evaluation

Summative evaluation
Research conducted at the end of a program that helps determine whether the program was effective and how it might be improved.

Summative evaluation, which is designed in the planning stage but conducted at the end of the program, provides information about the effectiveness of the program.[42] Summative evaluation is designed to obtain data about the participants' reaction to all aspects of the program, including the topics covered, the instructors or presenters, any instructional materials, the program activities (e.g., cooking demonstrations and taste tests), the physical arrangements for the program (including the location, room temperature, and availability of parking), registration procedures, advertising and promotion, and any other aspect of the program. Participants are asked to rate these program elements, perhaps scoring their assessment on a five-point rating scale. They may be asked to explain, in their own words, what aspects of the program they liked most or least and to suggest ways in which the program can be improved.[43] Summative evaluation can also assess changes in knowledge, attitudes and motivation, skills, and behaviors that occur among program participants. A variety of data collection methods may be used (including surveys, focus groups, interviews, and assessments of dietary behavior). For example, a survey may be used to assess changes in knowledge related to sources of healthy fats among adults in a nutrition education class focused on heart health. Among parents whose children attend a school implementing a healthy snack campaign, focus groups may be used to identify changes in parental motivation to offer healthy snacks to their children. A food frequency questionnaire may be used to assess changes in fruit and vegetable consumption among employees participating in a worksite wellness program focused on fruits and vegetables. As with formative evaluation, the data obtained from summative evaluation are used to improve the program's delivery and effectiveness and to make the program an inviting place for learning.[44] See Chapter 5 for more discussion of various types of program evaluation, including formative, process, impact, outcome, structure, and fiscal evaluation.

Entrepreneurship in Nutrition Education

Creativity and innovation—the twin elements of entrepreneurship—can be applied to many aspects of nutrition education, from the development of action figures and logos to the use of communications media such as the Internet, DVD, online blogs, and podcasts ready for download to personal computers and portable media players.[45] Program planning is definitely a good venue for practicing entrepreneurship. Consider a smoking reduction program integrated into an overall plan to reduce CHD risk. The program focuses on smokers—a target population that contributes the lion's share toward the costs of treating heart attacks and stroke—but in a new way. Rather than trying to get smokers to quit smoking altogether, the program is designed to build positive health behaviors in other areas of their lives (e.g., eating heart-healthy foods, taking a walk five days a week, and learning to manage stress). The program's goals are to help smokers to cut down on the number of cigarettes smoked and to reduce their CHD risk by adopting some of the positive health behaviors seen typically in nonsmokers. Before this program idea can be implemented, however, many questions must be asked: Has this approach been tried before? Does evidence from the literature indicate that it will work? Are there sufficient data to support making dietary and physical activity recommendations to smokers? What do the experts in this area think about this approach? What is the theoretical framework that supports this approach? If the approach has never been tried, should it be undertaken as a formal, scientific study? Some of these questions fall into the policy arena, but all must be addressed before program development can move forward.

Examine Mark Twain's comment at the beginning of this chapter. It highlights a perpetual problem in the field of health promotion: How can we help consumers change their behavior? One approach to motivating consumers is to design effective nutrition messages and programs, while keeping in mind the integration of three levels of intervention. Building awareness is important, but not enough. To change lifestyles, knowledge is not enough; it must be applied with skill-based practice and reinforced with motivational techniques. Lastly, considering physical and social environments will help you to understand how to most effectively promote healthy lifestyles within the context of your audience's lives.

case study

Developing a Nutrition Education Plan for Older Adults at Congregate Feeding Sites
by Virginia B. Gray, PhD, RD

Scenario

You are a nutrition consultant who specializes in developing nutrition education materials. You have recently been hired as a consultant for the local Agency on Aging to develop a new nutrition education program for use at local congregate feeding programs. The setting is urban, and the audience is ethnically diverse (primarily African American and Latino). Nutrition education activities take place once a month at congregate feeding sites. In your first contract, you are asked to develop lesson plans for four months of nutrition programming (four lessons delivered once a month). Each lesson will be approximately 20 minutes in length and will take place right before the midday meal service.

In this case study, you will use literature and formative evaluation data to develop topics and objectives for the four lessons. Then, you will develop a full outline for one selected lesson. Throughout this text, you have learned about three levels of intervention in communities:

- Level 1: Build awareness
- Level 2: Change lifestyles
- Level 3: Create a supportive environment

As you are working on this case study, remember to include strategies that address each of the three levels of intervention.

Learning Outcomes

- Review literature to identify nutrition education strategies that have been successful in similar settings.
- Use formative evaluation findings to guide development of clear, relevant, and measureable instructional objectives.
- Use the three levels of intervention to design nutrition education activities that build awareness, change lifestyles, and create a supportive environment.
- Identify activities that promote practicing skills gained during nutrition education sessions.
- Identify methods of evaluating nutrition education outcomes.

Foundation: Acquisition of Knowledge and Skills

1. Investigate the Older Americans Act Nutrition Program. Who does it serve, and what are the requirements for nutrition education?
2. Review the Client-Centered Nutrition Education materials available on the Texas Department of State Health Services website at *www.dshs.state.tx.us/wichd/nut/ccne.aspx*. The five modules on this website describe a client-centered approach to nutrition education. These modules provide tips for developing a positive nutrition education environment that provides hands-on application opportunities.
3. Conduct a literature review and identify at least two research articles that discuss nutrition education strategies used at congregate feeding sites. Particularly, look for research that identifies effective strategies for providing nutrition education to this audience.

Step 1: *Identify Relevant Information and Uncertainties*

After reviewing the literature, you decide to use formative assessment methods to help you understand the audience. First, you review recent nutrition screening checklists collected at the local congregate feeding sites. You notice that about 30% of program participants have either diabetes or heart disease. You also notice that about 25% of participants report problems chewing food. Food diaries are available for a subsample of participants, and you notice high intakes of grains, fruits, and vegetables, and low intakes of dairy and protein foods.

After reviewing the checklists and food diaries, you decide to visit several feeding sites and informally talk to participants to learn more about their nutrition-related knowledge, beliefs, values, and behaviors. In your interviews, you learn that many participants know they should eat more protein and consume more fluids, but they have not been successful in changing these behaviors. Participants report being inactive and express little motivation for changing their activity levels. Lastly, participants are concerned about their health-related quality of life. Participants report needing simple-to-implement nutrition tips, and enjoy sharing their life experiences in educational settings. They express positive impacts of participation in the congregate meals program, indicating they enjoy both the food and the social atmosphere.

1. After reviewing the formative assessment data, make a list of priorities for your nutrition education program. Which issues would be priorities, and why?
2. Connect your program with a behavior change theory. Explain why you have chosen the particular theory you select. How will using a behavior change theory impact development of your program?
3. What else would you want to know about your audience? Make a list of additional information you would like to gather, and indicate how you would gather it.

Step 2: *Interpret Information*

Now you are ready to begin planning your program.
1. First, create a name for your program. Then, determine a topic for each of the four lessons. Write a goal for each of the four lessons.
2. Next, develop objectives for each lesson. Refer to the chapter on program planning to recall types of objectives needed for promoting a change in behavior (such as knowledge, attitude/motivation, skill, and behavior). For example, if one of your lessons is focused on hydration, you may choose to include an objective aimed at creating awareness about the need for fluids, particularly among

older adults. You may include an objective aimed at motivation to consume fluids, and one aimed at skills for monitoring fluid intake. Lastly, you would want to include an objective aimed at actual changes in fluid intakes.

Note: Consider using the "Tips for Writing Learning Objectives" available in the Client-Centered Nutrition Education toolkit available at *www.dshs.state.tx.us/ wichd/nut/pdf/CCNEtoolkitM4Tips.pdf*. These tips encourage you to consider writing objectives that affect the head (cognitive/knowledge change), hands (skills/ behavior change), and heart (affective/motivational change). Keep in mind the behavior change theory you identified in Step 1 as you write your objectives.

Step 3: *Draw and Implement Conclusions*

Select one of your proposed lessons to develop into a full lesson outline, using the table at right.

1. Insert the objectives you developed in Step 2 into the chart.
2. Then indicate the time, topics and content, practical activities, and materials needed to accomplish the objectives. For each activity, indicate whether it is intended to build awareness (intervention level 1), change lifestyles (intervention level 2), or create a supportive environment (intervention level 3), remembering to integrate all three levels into your plan.

TIME	TOPIC/ CONTENT	ACTIVITY AND LEVEL OF INTERVENTION	MATERIALS NEEDED
Learning Objective 1:			
Learning Objective 2:			
Learning Objective 3:			

Step 4: *Engage in Continuous Improvement*

Remember that a great way to check to see if your objectives are measureable is to develop evaluation strategies for each. For each objective in the lesson plan you developed in Step 3, indicate how you will evaluate it.

PROFESSIONAL **FOCUS**

Being an Effective Writer

The written word, Rudyard Kipling once observed, is "the most powerful drug used by mankind." It inspires, educates, and engages us. Because it is so powerful, we want to be sure that we can express ourselves well, regardless of the audience for whom we are writing or the topic being discussed.

But how do you become a good writer? Any number of strategies, some of which are described here, can help you improve your writing, but one of the most important steps you can take is to practice. To learn to express yourself clearly and concisely, you must practice, practice, practice. Fortunately, most of us have ample opportunity to practice our craft. Our job or school requires us to write many types of documents: business letters, informal memos, reports, study proposals, scientific articles, fact sheets for the general public, and project updates, to name just a few. Mastering the basic principles of grammar and syntax is also important. Knowing how to use these tools properly will serve you well in all writing situations.

Three Basic Rules of Writing

Although there are different types of writing—for example, professional and business writing versus copy writing for an advertisement—several basic principles apply:

1. *Know what you want to say.* A well-known fiction writer once remarked, "I don't find writing particularly difficult; it's figuring out what I want to say that's so hard!" If you don't know what you want to tell the reader, your writing will meander around and leave the reader bewildered and dissatisfied. Your first step, then, is to decide what point or points you want to make. Jot them down before you begin to write your article or report. Once you clarify in your own mind precisely what it is that you want to say, the writing itself will flow more smoothly and the reader will follow your thinking more easily.

2. *Eliminate clutter.* "The secret of good writing is to strip every sentence to its clearest components."[1] Every word in every sentence must serve a useful purpose. If it doesn't, mark it out. Consider the approach used by Franklin D. Roosevelt to convert a federal government memo into plain English. The original blackout memo read as follows:[2]

> Such preparations shall be made as will completely obscure all Federal buildings and non-Federal buildings occupied by the Federal government during an air raid for any period of time from visibility by reason of internal or external illumination.

"Tell them," Roosevelt said, "that in buildings where they have to keep the work going to put something across the windows." By changing gobbledygook into plain English, Roosevelt made the memo simple and direct—and comprehensible. This strategy is important in all types of writing. Consider the following statement from one computer company's "customer bulletin": "Management is given enhanced decision participation in key areas of information system resources." What on earth does that mean? It might mean, "The more you know about your system, the better it will work," or it could mean something else.[3] The wording is so jumbled that the customer can't be sure what the company is trying to tell her and will probably take her business elsewhere as a result.

Whenever possible, eliminate clutter and jargon. To free your writing from clutter, clear your head of clutter. Clear writing comes from clear thinking.

3. *Edit, edit, edit.* A well-written piece does not occur by accident. It is crafted through diligent editing. Writers often edit their manuscripts eight, nine, ten, or more times. Editing pares the piece to the bare bones. It makes the writing stronger, tighter, and more precise. For more tips on editing manuscripts, see William Zinsser's book *On Writing Well.* Zinsser says that he is "always amazed at how much clutter can still be profitably cut."[4]

Reading and Writing

Russell Baker, who won the Pulitzer Prize for his book *Growing Up*, was asked to write a piece about punctuation as part of a series on writing published by the International Paper Company. Baker began his piece by saying, "When you write, you make a sound in the reader's head. It can be a dull mumble—that's why so much government prose makes you sleepy—or it can be a joyful noise, a sly whisper, a throb of passion."

He went on to speak of the importance of punctuation in letting your voice speak to the reader. "Punctuation," he wrote, "plays the role of body language. It helps readers hear you the way you want to be heard."[5]

How can you learn to master the rules of punctuation and the principles of writing? Read. The more you read, the better you write. The better you write, the better you can communicate. The better you communicate, the better you inform, inspire, and educate. To improve your writing skills, consider adding one or more of the following resources to your professional library:

- *On Writing Well* by W. Zinsser
- *The Elements of Style* by W. Strunk, Jr., and E. B. White
- *A Manual of Style* by The University of Chicago Press
- *The Elements of Grammar* by M. Shertzer
- *Fowler's Modern English Usage* by H. W. Fowler
- *A Writer's Reference* by D. Hacker
- *E-Writing: 21st Century Tools for Effective Communication* by D. Booher

Different Strokes for Different Folks

Not all writing assignments are the same. Some require the formal language of the scientific method, whereas others are meant to entertain (*and* inform). Choose a style, format, and tone of voice appropriate for the piece you are writing.

Writing for Professional Audiences

Materials written for professional groups must conform to a more rigorous, traditional format and style than those aimed at consumers. Scientific articles, for example, have specific subheadings and a formal tone (refer to the Professional Focus feature in Chapter 2). The best way to learn how to write these types of documents is to study published articles. Once again, editing is important. When possible, ask your colleagues to review your manuscripts. Their comments will help you identify places where your meaning is unclear.

Writing for the General Public

Writing for the general public is an important part of the community nutritionist's job. Newspaper and magazine articles, fact sheets, brochures, pamphlets, posters, and websites can all be used to teach and inform consumers. In addition to the basic writing principles outlined in the previous section, two things are important to bear in mind when writing for the general public:

1. *The most important sentence in any piece of writing is the first one.* If it doesn't engage readers and induce them to read further, your article or brochure is dead. Therefore, the lead sentence must capture the reader immediately. Consider this lead to an article about designer tomatoes: "Strap on your goggles, consumers, this one's getting messy."[6] The reader wonders instantly why tomatoes should be stirring up trouble. Or this lead from an article about dieting: "Dieters are a diverse group, but they share one common goal: to make their current diet their last one. Unfortunately, lasting results aren't what most get. In fact, the odds are overwhelming—9 to 1—that people

who've lost weight will gain it back."[7] Anyone who has tried to lose weight will find this lead enticing. In addition to capturing the reader's attention, the lead must do some work. It must provide a few details that tell the reader why the article was written and why she or he should read it.

2. *Know when to close.* Choosing an end point is as important as choosing a lead. A closing sentence works well when it surprises readers or makes them think about the article's topic. An article about the challenge of change concluded with this comment, made by a man who participated in Dean Ornish's lifestyle program for high-risk heart disease patients: "What Ornish has given me is that opening and an understanding of what members of the group have said many times: A longer life may be important, but a better life is of the essence."[8] This closing remark works because it is personal and thought-provoking.

CHAPTER **SUMMARY**

Applying Educational Principles to Program Design

▶ An effective nutrition intervention program integrates good instructional design and learning principles and uses media that facilitate a high degree of individualization.

▶ Educational research shows that the effect of an intervention on the target population's knowledge and behavior depends on the intervention's application of six basic educational principles: consonance, relevance, individualization, feedback, reinforcement, and facilitation (see Table 16-2).

▶ Nutrition education involves imparting knowledge, developing skills, and increasing motivation related to dietary habits. It can also include environmental supports to promote lasting change.

▶ People of any age learn best when they have the prerequisite knowledge, when content is broken down into small pieces, when what they have learned is used and reinforced, when they have an opportunity to practice what they have learned, and when the content seems relevant (see Table 16-4).

▶ The basic principles guiding adult education are that (1) adult roles, responsibilities, and previous experiences

influence learning; (2) adult learning is constantly occurring; and (3) the role of the adult educator is to facilitate this continuous learning process.

▶ When working with adult learners, make learning problem-centered and meaningful to the learner's life situations, offer concrete knowledge rather than abstract information, make learning a collaboration between the educator and the learner, encourage participatory approaches to learning, ask open-ended questions to draw out what the adults already know about the topic you are teaching, seize the "teachable moments," increase the adult learners' sense of self-worth by validating their experiences, establish a positive learning environment, and recognize individual and cultural differences because they affect learning styles.

▶ To ensure successful educational interventions, study your potential audience, learning what motivates them, what they want, and what they need. Research your target population by (1) reviewing the literature, (2) conducting formative research (one-on-one interviews or focus groups), and (3) asking representatives from the audience to help you with the planning and development of the program or material.

▶ **Developing a Nutrition Education Plan.** The nutrition education plan is a written document that describes the needs of the target population, the goals and objectives for intervention activities, the program format, the lesson plans, the nutrition messages to be imparted to the target population, the marketing plan, any partnerships that will support program development or delivery, and the evaluation instruments.

▶ **Developing Lesson Plans.** The first step in developing a lesson plan is to know your target audience, the setting, and the content. Your lesson plan should be centered on the learner's interests, needs, and motivation. When learning is related to real-life situations, learners can readily identify with the situation. Adults learn best when they are involved in the process. Using a behavior change theory at this point will help you to create lesson strategies that connect with the audience's beliefs, values, and perceptions.

- The first component of lesson writing is to identify the major concept that you are communicating.

- Developing useful lesson plans is based on writing effective objectives. Instructional objectives should (1) concentrate on the learner and not the teacher, (2) clearly communicate a specific instructional intent, (3) be stated in terms of the *end product* (the learning outcomes) and not in terms of the process of learning, and (4) include one type of learning outcome per objective to describe the learners' performance.

- Certain essential elements should always be part of your lesson plan: objectives, the body of the lesson, activities, and evaluation.

▶ Formative evaluation should be conducted throughout the program design process.

▶ Health literacy is increasingly vital to help people manage their own health by applying the vast amount of health and nutrition information available for improving health outcomes. Educational materials such as brochures, fact sheets, and handouts should be checked for reading grade level.

Designing Nutrition and Health Messages

▶ Consumers process nutrition and health messages at different levels, depending on their interest in the topic and their past experience with similar messages.

▶ Summative evaluation provides information about the effectiveness of a program. Summative evaluation is designed to obtain data about the participants' reactions to all aspects of the program, including the topics covered, the instructors or presenters, any instructional materials, the program activities, the physical arrangements for the program, registration procedures, and advertising and promotion. It also provides information on changes in knowledge, attitudes and motivation, skills, and behaviors among program participants.

SUMMARY **QUESTIONS**

1. Differentiate between the approaches you would use in teaching children versus teaching adults.
2. Imagine you are developing a school-based program to encourage milk consumption. Name one nutrition education strategy you could use related to each of the three levels of intervention (build awareness, change lifestyles, and create a supportive environment).
3. List and describe in detail the components of a well-developed lesson plan.
4. You have been asked to choose one of the *Dietary Guidelines* and translate it into practical information that consumers can understand and implement. What tips offered in the text will be helpful to you as you design effective nutrition messages for the consumer?
5. Differentiate between summative and formative evaluation. How are both important when planning and implementing nutrition education programs?
6. Describe three basic principles of effective writing.

INTERNET **RESOURCES** . . . .

National Agricultural Library's Food and Nutrition Information Center
https://fnic.nal.usda.gov/

Facilitated Dialogue Basics: Let's Dance
www.unce.unr.edu/publications/files/hn/2004/sp0421.pdf
Self-study guide for planning facilitated discussions using learner-centered education techniques.

Washington State Dairy Council's Nutrition Education Resources
www.eatsmart.org

Resources for Assessing Readability of Print Materials

Assessing and Developing Health Materials
www.hsph.harvard.edu/healthliteracy/practice/innovative-actions/

National Cancer Institute's Clear and Simple Method
www.nih.gov/clearcommunication/clearandsimple.htm

Multiple Readability Scores
www.online-utility.org/english/readability_test_and_improve.jsp

International Food Guides

Traditional Diets and Oldways' Heritage Pyramids
http://oldwayspt.org/resources/heritage-pyramids

USDA Ethnic and Cultural Resources
https://fnic.nal.usda.gov/professional-and-career-resources/ethnic-and-cultural-resources

USDA Special Audience MyPlate Resources
http://fnic.nal.usda.gov/dietary-guidance/myplate-and-historical-food-pyramid-resources/special-audience-myplate-resources

Examples of State-Wide Obesity Prevention Plans

California Obesity Prevention Plan
https://www.cdph.ca.gov/programs/COPP/Documents/COPP-ObesityPreventionPlan-2010.pdf.pdf

Minnesota Obesity Plan
www.health.state.mn.us/cdrr/obesity/pdfdocs/obesityplan20090112.pdf

New Jersey Obesity Prevention Action Plan
www.nj.gov/health/fhs/documents/obesity_prevention.pdf

North Carolina's Plan to Address Obesity: Healthy Weight and Healthy Communities
www.eatsmartmovemorenc.com/ESMMPlan/Texts/NC%20Obesity%20Prevention%20Plan%202013-2020_LowRes_FINAL.pdf

Wisconsin Nutrition, Physical Activity, and Obesity State Plan
https://www.dhs.wisconsin.gov/publications/p0/p00507.pdf

CHAPTER 17

Marketing Nutrition and Health Promotion

LEARNING **OBJECTIVES**

After you have read and studied this chapter, you will be able to:

- Develop a marketing plan.
- Conduct a situational analysis.
- Describe how to apply the four P's of marketing to the development of a marketing strategy.
- Explain how social marketing is used to promote community interventions.

This chapter addresses such issues as needs assessment, marketing theories and techniques, and current information technologies, which have been designated by the Accreditation Council for Education in Nutrition and Dietetics (ACEND) as Foundation Knowledge and Learning Outcomes for dietetics education.

CHAPTER **OUTLINE**

Something to think about... "I can give you a six-word formula for success: 'Think things through—then follow through."

—*EDWARD RICKENBACKER*

For a complete list of references, please access the MindTap Reader within your MindTap course.

Introduction

On her way home from work, a New York woman hears a familiar jingle on the car radio reminding her which soap to use for beautiful skin. Halfway around the world, in a remote Sri Lankan village, another woman hears a message on the community radio that teaches her about oral rehydration therapy for her child's diarrhea. Both of these women are part of a target audience for a well-planned marketing campaign. But whereas the New York woman is listening to traditional Madison Avenue marketing, the woman in Sri Lanka is a "consumer" receiving a message grounded in social marketing.[1] The same basic principles underlie both the commercial and the social approaches to marketing. The aim of both approaches is to persuade, convince, and strengthen the fit between the products, services, and programs offered and the needs of the population. As you will see, marketing is for everyone, regardless of job description. Whether you are a dietitian in private practice seeking referrals from physicians for new clients, a public health nutritionist developing nutrition education materials for pregnant teens, or a community nutritionist coordinating citywide screenings for hypertension, you can use marketing strategies. This chapter provides an overview of basic marketing principles and strategies.

What Is Marketing?

Buying and selling have a long history, but comprehensive and systematic marketing research evolved only in recent decades.[2] Peter Drucker, a management consultant, is credited with demonstrating the benefits of marketing to business. In the 1950s, he suggested that the primary focus of any business should be the consumer, not the product.[3]

Most people think that marketing means selling and promotion. Perhaps that is not too surprising, given that every day someone is trying to sell us something. But selling and promotion are only part of marketing. What, then, is marketing? **Marketing** is the process by which individuals and groups get what they need and want by creating and exchanging products and values with others.[4] Informally, marketing is the process of finding and keeping customers.[5] Many companies are very successful at commercial marketing, which employs powerful techniques for selecting, producing, distributing, promoting, and selling an enormous array of goods and services to a wide variety of people in every possible political, social, and economic context.[6]

Social marketing draws on many of the techniques and technologies of commercial marketing, but it seeks to increase the acceptability and desirability of an idea, a practice, a product, or all three among a certain group of people—the target population.[7] Social marketing, described in more detail later in this chapter, is a strategy for changing consumer behavior. It combines the best elements of consumer behavior theory with marketing tools and skills to help consumers change their beliefs, attitudes, values, actions, or behaviors.[8] Social marketing implies that individuals do new things or give up old things in exchange for benefits they hope to receive. Social marketing promotes ideas and behaviors as "products." In the nutrition arena, a social practice to be marketed, for example, is summed up in each of the following slogans: "Got Milk?" "Eat Fresh, Buy Local," "Fruits & Veggies—More Matters," and "Let's Move!" A social idea to be marketed is the theme "Heart-healthy foods taste great."

Marketing, whether commercial or social, is a tool for managing change. It helps companies, government agencies, nonprofit organizations, dietitians in private practice, and others recognize, define, interpret, and cope with changing consumer values, interests, lifestyles, and purchasing behaviors.[9] The purpose of marketing is to find a problem, need,

Marketing The process by which individuals and groups get what they need and want by creating and exchanging products and values with others.

Social marketing A method for changing consumer behavior; the design, implementation, and management of programs that seek to increase the acceptability of a social idea or practice among a target group.

or want (through marketing research) and to fashion a solution to it. The solution to the problem, need, or want is outlined in the marketing plan, which is described in the next section.

Develop a Marketing Plan

When completed, the marketing plan will outline the steps for achieving the goals and objectives of the overall intervention strategy and the program plan. It describes precisely how and in what form the nutrition and health messages will be delivered to the target population. **Figure 17-1** shows the steps the community nutritionist takes in developing a marketing plan.

First, determine the needs and wants of the target population because marketing starts with the customer.[10] Some ideas about their needs and wants can be gleaned from the community needs assessment and from focus group sessions held earlier in the program planning process. Additional information can be collected by asking questions of the target population: What are your perceptions about this nutritional problem or need? About this product or service? About this agency or organization? What products or services are you buying? What health benefits do you desire? The goal of this step is to build a knowledge base from which to develop a marketing strategy.[11]

Second, specify the benefits of the product or service to the target population. Remember, people generally want intangible things when they buy a product or service: safety, security, happiness, attractiveness, fun. Women who sign up for the Heartworks for Women program (Case Study 1 on page 645) may seek benefits such as reducing their risk of having a heart attack or stroke, learning new cooking skills, enjoying new recipes, and trying something new with a friend. It's the benefit that sells the product or service.[12]

Third, conduct a situational analysis. Analyze your potential **market** (those customers who share some common life characteristics), the environment in which your product or service will be positioned, and the competition.[13] Select a **target market**, which will be the primary, distinct customer group for your product, program, or service. In this step, you may be required to split your target population into smaller groups, each of which will respond differently to a given marketing strategy. For example, the target population for Case Study 2, which consists of independent older adults over the age of 75 years, may be very diverse, some having high incomes and personal computers with Internet access and others living near the poverty threshold. A marketing strategy that includes the Internet may reach the former but may or may not reach the latter.

Next, develop a marketing strategy for ensuring a good fit between the goals and resources of the organization and the needs and wants of the target population.[14] The marketing strategy specifies a target market and four distinct elements traditionally known as the four P's: product, place, price, and promotion.[15] For example, every time a consumer buys a box of Cheerios rather than a box of Corn Flakes, he or she makes the purchase at a competitive price in a grocery store, possibly because of a television advertisement. Such a sale was the result of a marketing strategy devised months before by the General Mills Corporation regarding the issues of product, place, price, and promotion. (These elements are described in a later section.) This phase requires setting goals and objectives to indicate what the marketing strategy is expected to accomplish.

Before the marketing plan can move forward, a budget and timetable must be developed. The budget accounts for all expenditures related to implementing the marketing

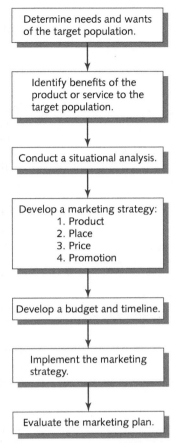

FIGURE 17-1 A Marketing Plan for Health Promotion
Source: Adapted from S. C. Parks and D. L. Moody, "A Marketing Model: Applications for Dietetic Professionals," *Journal of the American Dietetic Association* 86 (1986): 40; and J. C. Levinson and S. Godin, *The Guerrilla Marketing Handbook* (Boston: Houghton Mifflin, 1994), 5–7.

Market Potential customers for a product or service; a group of unique customers who share some characteristics.

Target market One particular market segment pinpointed as a primary customer group.

strategy, such as the cost of designing logos, websites, action figures, brochures, videos, and so forth, and printing all educational and promotional materials. The timetable specifies the marketing activities to be done each month both before the launch of the product, program, or service and after the launch, when the goal is to keep awareness high among the target market.

After all aspects of the marketing plan have been decided, implement the plan according to the original design and then evaluate its effectiveness. Did the marketing strategy reach the right audience at the right time with the right messages? Did the target market's beliefs, attitudes, actions, or behavior change? Use the results of the evaluation to make alterations to the marketing strategy and improve the positioning of the product or service in the marketplace.

Conduct a Situational Analysis

A situational analysis is a detailed assessment of the environment, including an evaluation of the consumer, the competition, and any other factors that may affect the program or business.[16] This step, which is critical to the ultimate success of the entire marketing plan, is sometimes referred to as a **SWOT** analysis (SWOT is an acronym for strengths, weaknesses, opportunities, and threats as shown in the box on the next page). Conducting such an analysis entails describing the present state of the business or agency, including its strengths and weaknesses, programs, and services, as well as the threats and opportunities present in the external environment (competition, pending legislation, and the like).[17]

> **SWOT** An acronym that stands for strengths, weaknesses, opportunities, and threats. A situational analysis technique often used in market research.

Get to Know Your Market The first step in the marketing process is the identification and analysis of all "consumers" of your product or service—your current and potential markets. Consumers can be categorized as one of three types: users of services, referral sources, and other decision makers.[18] The users of services are the clients themselves or potential clients. For example, the Special Supplemental Nutrition Program for Women, Infants, and Children (WIC) program identifies its users as low-income pregnant or breastfeeding women, infants, and children under five years of age. The National Dairy Council targets a different market—"leader groups," such as educators, dietitians, health teachers, and dental hygienists.[19] Users of the Heartworks for Women program are women aged 18 years and older.

Referral sources include anyone who refers clients or customers to you. They may include physicians, social workers, teachers, and former clients. Other decision makers are those who influence the client's decision to use a service or join a program. Such people include family members (spouses, parents) and third-party payers, among others. It is important to identify these three types of users for your particular setting. **Table 17-1** illustrates how consumers of the Heartworks for Women program are classified.

Market Research: Target Markets An inherent part of the situational analysis is to determine and target your clients or audiences. Each target market should be viewed as a separate and different audience. For example, dietitians in private practice might list the following as their target populations.[20]

- Overweight women between 20 and 40 years of age
- Athletic men
- People interested in sports nutrition
- People seeking healthful lifestyles
- Individuals wanting basic nutrition information
- Physicians for referrals
- Corporations to provide employee wellness workshops
- Local legislators to support zoning policies that promote health

SWOT Analysis

Identify **S**trengths, **W**eaknesses, **O**pportunities, and **T**hreats (SWOT) for your program. The presence of weaknesses and threats are gaps to be addressed in planning, while the absence of strengths or opportunities clarifies the need for further planning or development before action is taken.

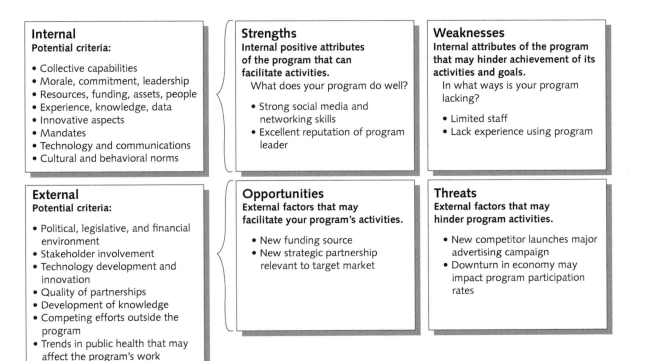

Internal
Potential criteria:

- Collective capabilities
- Morale, commitment, leadership
- Resources, funding, assets, people
- Experience, knowledge, data
- Innovative aspects
- Mandates
- Technology and communications
- Cultural and behavioral norms

Strengths
Internal positive attributes of the program that can facilitate activities.
  What does your program do well?

- Strong social media and networking skills
- Excellent reputation of program leader

Weaknesses
Internal attributes of the program that may hinder achievement of its activities and goals.
  In what ways is your program lacking?

- Limited staff
- Lack experience using program

External
Potential criteria:

- Political, legislative, and financial environment
- Stakeholder involvement
- Technology development and innovation
- Quality of partnerships
- Development of knowledge
- Competing efforts outside the program
- Trends in public health that may affect the program's work

Opportunities
External factors that may facilitate your program's activities.

- New funding source
- New strategic partnership relevant to target market

Threats
External factors that may hinder program activities.

- New competitor launches major advertising campaign
- Downturn in economy may impact program participation rates

Source: Adapted from Centers for Disease Control and Prevention, Communities of Practice Resource Kit, 2015.

TABLE 17-1

Worksheet to Identify Consumers: Case Study 1

TYPE	CONSUMERS	CHARACTERISTICS	BENEFITS
Users	Women living in the city of Jeffers	Age 18+ years	Improved quality of life; decreased risk of CHD; better health
Referral sources	Cardiologists, other physicians, social workers, former clients	Health care providers, coworkers	Delayed CHD development
Decision makers	Spouse/significant other, coworkers	Age 18+ years	Want spouse, significant other, or coworker to be "healthy"

Source: Adapted from C. B. Matthews, "Marketing Your Services: Strategies That Work," *ASHA Magazine* 30 (1988): 23.

Ideally, if resources are available, you should develop a specific marketing strategy for each target audience. Once a population group has been identified for targeting, it is important to determine its prevailing patterns of lifestyle, eating, drinking, working conditions, attitudes toward nutrition and health, and current and past state of health.[21]

Most programs and organizations find it unrealistic to serve the total target market effectively. For this reason, actual and potential markets should be divided further into distinct and homogeneous subgroups—a process called **market segmentation.** Market segmentation offers the following benefits:[22]

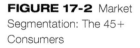

Market segmentation The separation of large groups of potential clients into smaller, distinct groups with similar characteristics and/or needs. Advantages include simpler, more accurate analysis of each group's needs and more customized delivery of service.

- A more precise definition of consumer needs and behavior patterns
- Improved identification of ways to provide services to population groups
- More efficient utilization of nutrition and health education resources through a better fit among products, programs, services, and consumers

As an example of market segmentation, consider as your potential market the population of adults aged 45 years or older—sometimes referred to as 45+ consumers. This total market can be divided into several more homogeneous parts, some of which are shown in **Figure 17-2**. Each of these segments can then be reached with a distinct marketing strategy (to be discussed shortly).

Market Research: Market Segmentation Market research enables community nutritionists to target specific groups for health promotion and disease prevention in terms of their geography, demography, and psychography. This type of analysis is helpful in many ways: (1) targeting those at risk; (2) carrying out strategic marketing planning; (3) developing marketing media strategies; (4) examining the feasibility of various promotional tools (e.g., direct mailing versus online distribution of nutrition education materials); and (5) determining the appropriate mix of nutrition programs and services to offer on the basis of demographics (such as concentration of women, infants, children, and older adults).

Four classes of variables are typically used for market segmentation:[23]

1. *Demographic segmentation* is the grouping of individuals on the basis of such variables as age, sex, income, occupation, education, family size, religion, race, marital status, and life-cycle stage.
2. *Geographical segmentation* is the grouping of people according to the location of their residence or work (region, county, census tract). This can be done on a simple geographical basis or according to other variables, such as population density or climate.
3. *Psychographic segmentation* is based on such criteria as personal values, attitudes, opinions, personality, lifestyle, and level of readiness for behavior change.
4. *Behavioristic segmentation* is based on such criteria as purchase frequency and occasion, benefits sought, and attitude toward product.

An understanding of demographics is essential to the development and targeting of nutrition and public health programs. Consider the public health agency or wellness

FIGURE 17-2 Market Segmentation: The 45+ Consumers

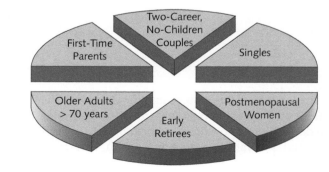

center with programs that promote such "products" as smoking cessation, heart-healthy diets, physical activity programs, maternal and infant care, cancer prevention, hypertension screening, diabetes education, infant mortality reduction, and AIDS prevention.[24] The community agency or wellness center must first analyze the demographics of the areas served by these programs in order to identify its clients. The information to categorize and examine includes:

- Total population of the area that the program is intended to serve
- Rate of change of the population
- Age and sex distribution
- Racial, ethnic, and religious composition
- Socioeconomic status
- Housing information
- Fertility patterns

Of these, age distribution of the population, trends over time, and fertility rates are particularly important to public health nutrition programs. Major segmentation variables for consumer markets are given in **Table 17-2**. **Figure 17-3** summarizes the steps required for market segmentation and target marketing.

Obviously, the situational analysis demands a significant amount of market research. This research includes the use of both primary (direct) and secondary (indirect) data. Primary data are new data collected for the first time through random-sampling surveys, questionnaires, and qualitative methods such as personal interviews and focus groups. **Table 17-3** describes six methods frequently used to collect primary data about a market.

Secondary data are those gathered by government agencies, private market research companies, and nonprofit organizations. Federal government sources of secondary data include the Bureau of Economic Analysis, Bureau of Justice Statistics, Bureau of Labor Statistics, Census Bureau, National Center for Health Statistics, National Technical Information Service, Social Security Administration, and U.S. Department of Agriculture. (Many of these were described in Chapter 4.) The *American Statistics Index, Statistical Abstract of the United States*, and *Survey of Current Business* are excellent sources of business and general economic statistics.

TABLE 17-2 Major Segmentation Variables for Consumer Markets

SEGMENTATION VARIABLES	EXAMPLES
Demographic	Age; Gender; Household Income; Education Level; Generation (Baby Boomer, Gen X, etc.); Marital Status; Race/Ethnicity/Nationality; Occupation; Social Class (middle class, etc.)
Geographic	Region (continent, country, state, neighborhood); Size of Metropolitan Area; Population Density (urban, suburban, rural); Climate
Psychographic	Lifestyles (values, attitudes, activities, opinions, interests); Personality (dependent, independent, leader, etc.)
Behavioral	• User Status: nonuser; ex-user; potential; first-time; regular • Purchase Occasion: regular occasion, special occasion • Usage Rate: light user, medium user, heavy user • Buyer Readiness Stage: unaware, aware, informed, interested, intending to buy, trial • Brand Loyalty: none, medium, strong, absolute • Benefits Sought: quality, service, economy, convenience, health, performance • Media Habits: TV, Internet (websites, social media), magazine, radio, newspaper

Source: Adapted from P. Kotler and A. Andreasen, *Strategic Marketing for Health Care Organizations* (Upper Saddle River, NJ: Prentice Hall, 1995). Used with permission.

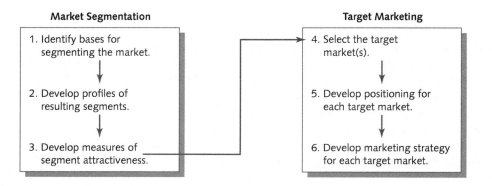

FIGURE 17-3 Steps in Market Segmentation and Target Marketing

Source: Adapted with permission from P. Kotler and R. N. Clarke, *Marketing for Health Care Organizations* (Upper Saddle River, NJ: Prentice-Hall, 1987), 234.

Private market research companies include A. C. Nielsen and America's Research Group, both of which conduct consumer behavior surveys. Some nonprofit groups, such as the Academy of Nutrition and Dietetics and other professional associations, are sources of secondary data. Directories such as *Dun & Bradstreet, Moody's Manuals,* and *Thomas Register* provide data on businesses in a given market area. The *Sales Management Annual Survey of Buying Power* provides local information on population, income, and retail establishments. If you can't locate the secondary data you require, consider working with a specialist or information broker who can provide research services for a fee.[25]

A number of vendors also provide information about various segments of a population based on demographics, geography, and psychographics. Each vendor has a clustering system that groups individuals on the basis of like characteristics. This technique uses the statistical method called *cluster analysis* to classify neighborhoods by their residents' demographics, attitudes, media habits, and buying patterns.

TABLE 17-3 Methods Used to Collect Primary Data

METHOD	DESCRIPTION
Mail survey	Tips to improve reliability: use homogeneous sample, keep length reasonable, pretest and rewrite as necessary.
Telephone survey	Can involve errors as in mail surveys. Helpful to ask: Is the true meaning of the question being reflected by the interviewer, or is it distorted? Is the wording of the question likely to elicit a biased response?
Internet survey	Gathers data from people who have e-mail accounts or visit a particular website; can obtain highly specific information about people who use the Internet.
Personal interview	A recommended supplement to mail or telephone surveys; helpful in observing subtle feedback that would otherwise be unavailable.
Consumer panel	Often used to test new products using the same persons in several tests; a problem is that panel members do not always represent the buying population and may not always give honest answers.
Focus group	Frequently used to gather information from small, homogeneous groups; allows the researcher to see how people view a product, intervention, or other issue; serves as a communications bridge between the researcher and the people the researcher is trying to reach; not to be used to persuade, convince, or reach a consensus.

Source: Adapted from P. Kotler and A. Andreasen, *Strategic Marketing for Health Care Organizations* (Upper Saddle River, NJ: Prentice Hall, 1995), p. 234. Used with permission.

Analyze the Environment and Watch for Trends

The next step in the situational analysis is to identify any external environmental factors or social trends that may influence the needs of the program or organization. Such issues include health care reform, legislative and regulatory changes, shifting demographics, and behavioral changes such as eating on the run and sedentary indoor lifestyles. For example, a declining birth rate and a growing population of older people are affecting the composition of many communities. Changes in the typical family, including older first-time parents, the high divorce rate, and increasing numbers of working mothers, also affect the needs of a given community.

The general age of the target area is influential in determining needed programs. In an area largely inhabited by people of retirement age, classes on prenatal nutrition counseling will have far less impact than, for instance, a class on heart-healthy cooking for one or two. Other significant trends include the aging of the baby boom generation and the increasing cultural and ethnic diversity of the population, which must be considered when developing or expanding any public health program.

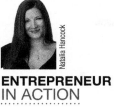

Natalia Hancock

ENTREPRENEUR IN ACTION

Natalia Hancock, RD, created her niche out of her strengths. She recognized that, unlike many, she loved to cook. With her degree in culinary nutrition, Natalia has been bringing healthy cuisine to various communities for the past 10 years.

After working as a clinical dietitian for three years, she joined CulinArt Inc., a boutique dining service company, as its nutrition specialist. There, she was able to combine her culinary and nutrition backgrounds, creating and implementing healthy food programs in a wide range of foodservice operations and training chefs on nutrition and healthy cooking. She next worked as culinary nutritionist at the Rouge Tomate restaurant in New York City and at SPE Certified, where she applied her extensive knowledge in nutrition and culinary arts. Today she works as a personal chef meeting the specific dietary needs of clients across New York City. Find out what she has to say about entrepreneurship online at *www.cengagebrain.com*.

Analyze the Competition

Once you have a thorough understanding of your consumers, you must determine how your existing competitors are positioned in the marketplace. What are their strengths and weaknesses? What is the attitude of your target market toward the competition? **Table 17-4** shows the results of such an analysis completed by a community nutritionist who specializes in cardiovascular disease.

Your aim is to find a **market niche** for your program or service in which your strengths can be matched with the needs of your particular target market. To satisfy those needs, you must know and understand your target audience so well that your service provides the perfect fit and "sells" itself, setting you apart from other providers in the same market and improving your **competitive edge**. Examples of competitive edges include your area of expertise, professional image, size, location, and customer service. You will want your

Market niche The particular area of service or the particular product suited to the specific clients to be reached. The underlying philosophy is that you cannot be all things to all people, so you must find the spot that fits your objectives and goals and enables you to meet a particular unmet need.

Competitive edge An advantage over others who are in the business, gained through use of business strategies, market research, expert management, new product development, or other sound business techniques.

TABLE 17-4

Worksheet for Analyzing the Competition

COMPETITOR	STRENGTHS	WEAKNESSES	MY COMPETITIVE ADVANTAGE
Wellness center	Great location; personable staff	Large and diverse; no known specialty; little follow-up after program completion	I specialize in cardiovascular nutrition counseling; I provide six months of follow-up (phone calls, e-mail, e-newsletter, blog).
Sports medicine clinic	Personable staff; good programming in sports nutrition; good name recognition	Outdated brochures and videos; nearly impossible to find parking	I maintain up-to-date educational resources; I travel to the client in my "Nutritionist-on-Wheels" mobile.

Source: Adapted from C. B. Matthews, "Marketing Your Services: Strategies That Work," *ASHA Magazine* 30 (1988): 23.

▶ **THINK LIKE A COMMUNITY** NUTRITIONIST

When analyzing the competition related to a health behavior, "outside of the box" thinking is required. For example, a competitor to physical activity among children could be video games and other electronic activities. For each of the following health behaviors, list one or more competitors:

- Physical activity among adults
- Soda consumption among children
- Cooking fresh foods at home among families
- Fruit and vegetable consumption among children
- Milk consumption among adolescents
- Healthy snacks after sporting events among children

Marketing mix Four universal elements of marketing that are often called the "four P's"— product, price, place, and promotion.

Product Encompasses the range of services offered.

target market to perceive that it can benefit from using your services rather than those of your competition.

Develop a Marketing Strategy

The four elements of the marketing strategy— product, place, price, and promotion—are usually referred to as the **marketing mix**. The development of the appropriate marketing mix should result directly from the previous step of the marketing process—analysis of the consumer, environment, and competition. Once the needs of the target audience have been identified and analyzed, the set of four P's can be constructed. The primary focus of the four P's is the identified target market, as shown in **Figure 17-4**. Successful marketers get the right product, service, or program to the right place at the right time for the right price.[26]

Product The term **product** refers to all the characteristics of the product or service that are to be exchanged with the target market. Characteristics such as style, special features, packaging, quality, and brand name must be designed to fit the needs and preferences of the target market. From a marketing standpoint, the product or service—whether it's a new automobile, a diet soft drink, or a nutrition class for a congregate meal site—is viewed as a collection of tangible and intangible attributes that may be offered to a market to satisfy a want or need.[27]

In community nutrition, the product is often a service to be delivered. These services should be of high quality, tailored to fit the needs of the target market, and adapted to

FIGURE 17-4 The Four P's of the Marketing Mix

Source: Adapted with permission of the author from M. Ward, *Marketing Strategies: A Resource for Registered Dietitians* (Binghamton, NY: Niles & Phipps, 1984), p. 11.

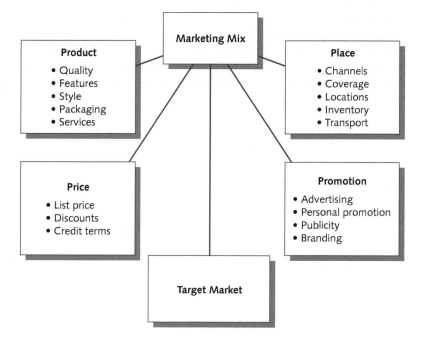

Marketing Mix

Product
- Quality
- Features
- Style
- Packaging
- Services

Place
- Channels
- Coverage
- Locations
- Inventory
- Transport

Price
- List price
- Discounts
- Credit terms

Promotion
- Advertising
- Personal promotion
- Publicity
- Branding

Target Market

be congruent with the consumers' social characteristics (e.g., culture, ethnicity, or language skills). A group of dietitians in private practice delineated their services as including individual counseling for modified diets, weight reduction, sports nutrition, normal nutrition, prenatal diets, and eating disorders; group programs and workshops on nutrition topics; consulting services to schools, health care facilities, supermarkets, health spas, and restaurants; and the teaching of courses at community colleges and universities.[28]

Place **Place** is the actual physical (or online) location where the exchange takes place. Accessibility, convenience, and comfort for the client are the criteria to consider. Are your hours of operation convenient and flexible? Is parking available? Place also includes the channels of distribution required to deliver the service or product to the consumer. The distribution channels are the intermediaries—individuals, facilities, or

ENTREPRENEUR IN ACTION

As an author, professional speaker, and small business owner, Lucille Beseler, RD, CDE, has extensive expertise in pediatric and adolescent nutrition. She founded the Family Nutrition Center in Florida with the vision of improving the nutritional health of families and children. Many of her entrepreneurial projects have come her way through networking. At first, she advertised her services by going door to door to pediatricians and discovered that they were excited about referring their patients to someone. Eventually other physicians referred clients to her based on her reputation and because she was listed as a provider on a number of insurance plans. Says Lucille: "My business has evolved over the last few years, much as I have. Reinventing yourself is imperative for success. Don't be afraid of making mistakes. My favorite quote is from Danny Kaye: 'Life is a great big canvas, and you should throw all the paint on it that you can.'" Learn more about her experiences at *www.cengagebrain.com*.

agencies—that control or influence the consumer's choice of service or product.[29] Health providers, employers, school boards, voluntary health organizations, shopping malls, and commercial retailers are a few of the important intermediaries for community nutritionists. They are viewed as channels for reaching identified target markets.

In other instances, distribution channels are more like "gatekeepers"—you cannot reach your target except by going through them. Physicians, parents, media program directors, corporate executives, members of Congress, and insurance company decision makers can all be gatekeepers, depending on the service being offered and the target audience. The overall marketing strategy may include one approach for the client and a different approach to reach the intermediary or gatekeeper.

Distribution channels vary depending on the target market and the service provided. Because third-party reimbursement by insurance companies for nutrition services usually requires a physician referral, a dietitian in private practice may want to target obstetricians, cardiologists, or other medical practice groups identified as distribution channels. Another approach the dietitian might take is to target insurance companies or state legislators in an effort to enhance the current third-party reimbursement system. A wellness program dietitian might identify corporate executives or employers as distribution channels because approval for a wellness program usually rests with a company's management.

Price **Price** includes both tangible costs (fee for service) and intangible commodities (time, effort, and inconvenience) that the consumer must bear in the marketing exchange. Once you understand what the consumer perceives as the costs involved in adopting a health behavior or participating in a given program, you have a better chance of influencing the exchange. You may do this by persuading the consumer that the benefits to be received outweigh the perceived costs. Alternatively, incentives (money, groceries, gifts, or personal recognition) can be offered to increase motivation and facilitate consumer participation. Likewise, costs can be reduced (less waiting time) or prices discounted to certain groups (older adults, students). Any of these tactics can considerably reduce the "price" consumers perceive themselves as paying for the program or service.

Place Where the product is available.

Price Encompasses the monetary and intangible value of the product.

Promotion Persuasive communication aimed at targeted users.

Promotion

The last P in the marketing mix—**promotion**—consists of the agency's or organization's informative or persuasive communication with the target market. What do you want to say? To whom do you want to say it? When do you want to say it?[30] The communication messages are designed to have a measurable effect on the knowledge, attitude, and/or behavior of the target market.[31] The medium, message content, and message format are chosen to complement the target market's communication needs.[32]

Promotion has four general objectives:[33]

- To inform and educate consumers about the existence of a product or service and its capabilities (what the community program has to offer)
- To remind present and former users of the product's continuing existence (e.g., prenatal nutrition counseling)
- To persuade prospective purchasers that the product is worth buying (improved health status, other benefits)
- To inform consumers about where and how to obtain and use the product (accessibility, location, and time)

Although people often assume that promotion is limited to advertising, promotion actually includes much more than advertising, as shown in **Table 17-5**. As one author has noted:

> Marketers generally agree that although mass media approaches are appropriate for developing consumer awareness in the short term, face-to-face programs such as workplace encounters are more effective (though not always cost-effective) in changing behavior in the long term. In designing any communication policy, the marketer commonly considers the effects that may be achievable through the use of a mix of approaches, capitalizing on the strengths of each.[34]

Advertising Any paid form of nonpersonal presentation and promotion of ideas, goods, or services by an identified sponsor.

The four most common promotional tools are advertising, sales promotion, personal promotion, and public relations.

Advertising is standardized communication in print or electronic media that is purchased.[35] Examples of advertising media include telephone directory yellow pages,

TABLE 17-5

Promotional Tools

PERSONAL PROMOTION AIDS	MEDIA AND PUBLIC EVENTS	GRAPHIC/PRINT MATERIALS
One-to-one communication	Public relations	Logos
Networking	Publicity	Brochures
Business cards	Press releases	Flyers
Letters	Press kits	Portfolios
Résumés	Media interviews	Proposals
Letters of reference	News conferences	Posters and signs
Use of a name	Special events	Banners
Seminars	Cooking demonstrations	Multi-image slideshows on laptops
Workshops	Celebrities	DVDs
Consulting	Advertising	Blogs
Public speaking	Classified ads	YouTube
Writing	Yellow Page ads	Multimedia presentations
	Websites	Computer graphics
	Blogs	Giveaways (T-shirts, mugs, gym
	Social networking	bags, product samples)
	YouTube	Internet websites
	Social media	Statement stuffers
	Direct mail	Catalogs
	Contests	Screen savers
	Trade shows	

Source: Adapted from K. K. Helm, *The Competitive Edge: Advanced Marketing Strategies for Dietetics Professionals*, 3rd ed. (Philadelphia: Wolters Kluwer/Lippincott Williams & Wilkins, 2010); J. Kremer and J. D. McComas, *High-Impact Marketing on a Low-Impact Budget* (Rocklin, CA: Prima, 1997), 237–92.

billboards, newspapers, radio, trade and professional journals, magazines, and the Internet. The role of advertising is to communicate a concise and targeted message that ultimately stimulates action by the carefully defined audience. Advertising can reach large numbers of people in many locations and can help build image. In advertising, you control the nature and timing of the message because you are buying the time or space. Which media you choose will depend on the characteristics of your target market, the size of your budget, and the goals of your advertising campaign. The advantages and limitations of the major media categories are listed in **Table 17-6**. The Professional Focus feature on page 225 of Chapter 6 offers tips for working with the media.

Sales promotion consists of such things as coupons, free samples, point-of-purchase materials, and trade catalogs. The use of these materials as part of the promotion strategy encourages potential consumers to purchase or use a particular product or service.

Personal promotion or **communication** can be done through small group meetings, counseling sessions and nutrition classes, formal presentations to organizations or community groups, displays and booths at health fairs and related conferences, and telephone conversations, personal meetings, or online communication with the public and other professionals (such as your referral sources). Unlike the standardized message presented in advertising, the message presented in personal promotion can be tailored to fit the needs of the particular individual or group. Personal promotion also offers other advantages:[36]

- Direct contact provides positive feedback to the listener through both the verbal communications and the nonverbal gestures of the communicator.
- The interpersonal contact facilitates the transfer of the message better than other methods.

Sales promotion
Short-term incentives to encourage purchases or sales of a product or service.

Personal promotion/communication Oral presentation in a conversation with one or more prospective purchasers for the purpose of making sales or building goodwill.

MEDIUM	ADVANTAGES	LIMITATIONS
Newspapers	Flexibility; timeliness; good local market coverage; broad acceptance; high believability	Short life; poor reproduction quality; small "pass-along" audience
Television	Combines sight, sound, and motion; appealing to the senses; high attention; high reach	High absolute cost; high clutter; fleeting exposure; less audience selectivity
Direct mail	Audience selectivity; flexibility; no ad competition within the same medium; personalization	Relatively high cost; "junk mail" image
Radio	Mass use; high geographical and demographic selectivity; low cost	Audio presentation only; lower attention than television; nonstandardized rate structures; fleeting exposure
Magazines	High geographical and demographic selectivity; credibility and prestige; high-quality reproduction; long life; good pass-along readership	Long ad purchase lead time; some waste circulation; no guarantee of position
Outdoor	Flexibility; high repeat exposure; low cost; low competition	No audience selectivity; creative limitations
Internet/online marketing • e-mail • e-zine • podcast • blog	Low cost; high selectivity; personal; is interactive one-on-one marketing	Not always statistically representative; can't verify user identity

TABLE 17-6

Advantages and Limitations of Major Media Categories

Source: Adapted from P. Kotler, J. Shalowitz, and R. J. Stevens, *Strategic Marketing for Health Care Organizations: Building a Customer-Driven Health System* (San Francisco: Jossey-Bass, 2008); J. Sterne, *World Wide Web Marketing* (New York: Wiley, 1995), 239–68.

- The communicator can ensure comprehension by asking questions and monitoring responses.
- The communicator has an opportunity to probe for resistance to change and then is in a position to address each issue.
- The listener may believe that someone is now in a position to monitor his behavior and thus hold him accountable for it.

Public relations An organized effort to promote a favorable image of a person or product through news coverage or goodwill (free services, charitable work, etc.).

Public relations, or publicity, is used to create a positive image of an individual or organization in the mind of the consumer. The Academy of Nutrition and Dietetics receives publicity every March during National Nutrition Month activities. Personal branding is the process of "creating a world of meaning and relevancy for others to know what is genuinely unique about you."[37] See the accompanying box for examples of Academy members who have had success in branding their services. See the Professional Focus feature on Social Media later in this chapter for additional tools for building a brand image and expanding public relations.

Brand-Name Dietetics

Nancy Clark, MS, RD, sports nutritionist, is showcased on the Wheaties box advertising the Summer 2004 Olympics.

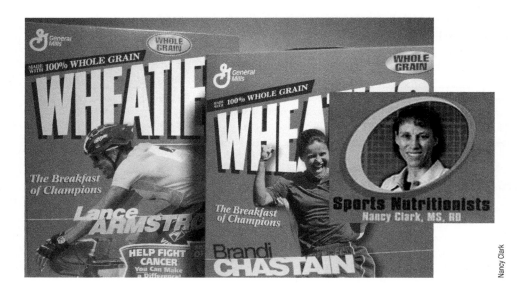

Nancy Clark

For most grocery shoppers, choosing a store is a relatively straightforward process, with cost and convenience being paramount; however, once inside, shoppers have a vast array of choices to make between many similar products by different manufacturers. Cost can be the primary factor in deciding which product to purchase, but many shoppers make purchases based on the brands themselves. The same process is used when selecting a provider of health-related services, such as a community nutritionist. *Branding*—what a product or service stands for and is designed to do—is established and understood among consumers to help them make decisions as to what goods and services they will purchase. Much like the branding of consumer products, dietetics professionals must establish a strong **brand image**, defined by the American Marketing Association as "a mirror reflection of the brand personality or product being marketed; it is what people believe about a brand: their thoughts, feelings, expectations."

Brand image A mirror reflection of the brand personality or product being marketed; it is what people believe about a brand: their thoughts, feelings, and expectations.

Branding Works

Several members of the Academy of Nutrition and Dietetics have had success in branding their services by blogging, podcasting, and participating in social media sites. Getting one's name out there is one way to establish a brand. Nancy Clark, MS, RD, sports nutritionist and author of *Nancy Clark's Sports Nutrition Guidebook*, adds her name to all her products, including her books and website. Similarly, Becky Dorner, RD, president of Becky Dorner and Associates, says that her company uses its logo on all marketing pieces, as well as on its website, letterhead, note cards, envelopes, publication flyers, quarterly newsletter, consulting services brochure, ads, manuals, and books—and on the company's e-zine, which reaches more than 3,000 long-term-care health professionals across the United States. According to Dorner, an eye-catching logo and a memorable name are of the essence.

Other members have found that discovering a niche market is an effective means for brand creation. Sylvia E. Meléndez-Klinger, MS, RD, of Hispanic Foods Communication, discovered that the Hispanic market was virtually untapped. "There are so few dietitians with my food industry marketing experience," Meléndez-Klinger explains. "It helped to have a great education, be bilingual, and have a great knowledge of many of the Hispanic cultures, having lived in Mexico, Puerto Rico, Spain, and Central America." Cathy Leman, RD, owner of NutriFit, found her combination of being a personal trainer and a dietitian, as well as marketing specifically to women, to be an effective means of differentiating herself among dietitians and personal trainers.

Accepting speaking engagements is also recommended as a means of establishing oneself as a brand. "My name has become associated with reliable, helpful sports nutrition information," says Clark. "This helps me to get asked to be a speaker at professional and lay organizations, as well as an author of articles for magazines." Similarly, Meléndez-Klinger rarely turns down an opportunity to speak in front of an audience, but she also recommends networking, becoming a media spokesperson, and volunteering as additional ways to become known.

There are many branding and marketing communications specialists—several focused specifically on health care services—that can help you create your brand and market your services. However, even without using such services, with the right combination of patience, enthusiasm, and savvy, success is within your reach.

Source: Excerpted from K. Stein, "Brand Name Dietetics," *Journal of the American Dietetic Association* 104 (2004): 1530–33.

Publicity Tools Publicity tools include articles in newsletters or local newspapers, informational brochures and newsletters, radio and television interviews, other forms of public speaking, displays, posters, Internet websites, blogs, podcasts, participation in social media sites, and other tools that present a favorable image of the organization or professional to the target market.

Public service announcements (PSAs) can also be used as a form of publicity. They offer the advantage of being free of charge and have the potential of reaching a large audience. PSAs are brief messages—often only 30 to 60 seconds in length—used to promote programs, activities, and services of federal, state, or local governments and the activities of nonprofit organizations when they are regarded as serving a community interest. A nutrition message can be a PSA with credit given to the organization submitting it. *PSA Research* offers an online information library of public service advertising with access to reviews of PSA campaigns to affect health behaviors.

Here are five tips for creating effective PSAs:[38]

- Produce announcements of professional quality. One professional PSA is better than several low-quality ones.

- Get the audience involved. Sound effects, questions, repetition, and humor are sometimes more effective at grabbing the attention of the audience than the factual approach.
- Market the service offered, not just the PSA topic. Offer a brochure, a toll-free information hotline, or a screening service.
- Simplify the response action needed. Advertise a local phone number or an easy-to-remember post office box number or web address.
- Develop and nurture a good rapport with the television and radio public service directors. They may be able to improve the PSA's production quality and increase scheduled air time.

Two additional promotional tools deserve mention: direct mail/e-mail and word-of-mouth referrals. Many marketers develop brochures, newsletters, fliers, and other promotional items that are mailed or e-mailed to specific targeted groups or geographical areas. Others claim that the word-of-mouth referral—having associates and clients do some of the promoting for you—is one of the most important promotional strategies. A successful program or service will generate its own word-of-mouth publicity because satisfied consumers will tell others about the program and may encourage their participation. The promotional strategies used by individuals or organizations will vary with the populations they are trying to reach, the goals of the program, and the resources available for promoting it.

Monitor and Evaluate

Evaluation is the key to the success of any marketing program. Evaluation methods include tracking changes in volume or net profit, referral sources, and customer satisfaction.[39] In this step of the marketing process, you need to ask the following questions: Are you accomplishing your goals? Who benefited from the service? What changes in knowledge, attitudes, and practices occurred? What are the actual costs of providing the service? What changes are warranted to make the service more effective in the future? For example, once you understand the profile of clients who were successful with a given program, your promotional efforts can be targeted more effectively.

If your marketing plan included a thorough situational analysis and you carefully translated these results into a marketing mix for your targeted audience, a periodic assessment may be all that is needed. Marketing is an ongoing process, however, and situations change—sometimes affecting your marketing strategy. If so, you may need to reevaluate your objectives. Are they still achievable? Do you need to take an alternative direction? Should you redirect your strategy?

In *Guerilla Marketing*, J. C. Levinson cautions against abandoning your marketing plan once it begins generating favorable results. Instead, he advises an ongoing commitment to your marketing orientation and continued investment in your marketing strategy. He offers "ten truths you must never forget":[40]

1. The market is continually changing.
2. People forget quickly.
3. Your competition won't quit.
4. Marketing strengthens your identity.
5. Marketing is essential to survival and growth.
6. Marketing enables you to keep your customers.
7. Marketing maintains morale.
8. Your marketing program gives you an advantage over competitors who have ceased to market.
9. Marketing allows your business to continue operating.
10. You stand to lose out on the money, time, and effort you've invested.

Social Marketing: Community Campaigns for Change

Social marketing makes a comprehensive effort to influence the acceptability of social ideas in a population, usually for the purpose of changing behavior.[41] Health ideas such as cardiovascular fitness, heart-healthy eating, and cancer screenings can be "sold" in the same way as presidential candidates or toothpaste.[42] Examples of social marketing include the public service messages produced by electronic and print media, such as messages intended to change behavior related to smoking, driving safely, reducing risks for cancer, consuming enough calcium, and similar concerns. **Table 17-7** presents examples of recent health promotion campaigns using social marketing techniques.

Whereas traditional marketing seeks to satisfy the needs and wants of targeted consumers, social marketing aims to change their attitudes and/or behavior. To do so, the marketing process must be followed in its entirety (**Figure 17-5**).[43] Marketers identify four types of behavior change, listed here in order of increasing difficulty:

- *Cognitive change.* A change in knowledge is the easiest to market, but there appears to be little connection between knowledge change and behavior change. Examples include campaigns to explain the nutritional value of different foods and campaigns to expand awareness of government programs such as the Supplemental Nutrition Assistance Program (SNAP) or WIC.
- *Action change.* This kind of change is more difficult to achieve than cognitive change because the individual must first understand the reason for change and then invest something of value (time, money, or energy) to make the change. Screening programs for hypertension, hypercholesterolemia, or breast cancer involve this type of change.
- *Behavior change.* This type of change is more difficult to achieve than either cognitive change or action change because it costs the consumer more in terms of personal involvement on a *continuing* basis—for example, the adoption of a diet with plenty of fruits, vegetables, and whole grains, or the addition of regular physical activity to one's lifestyle.
- *Value change.* This type of change is the most difficult to market. Examples include sustainable food system strategies intended to persuade communities to decrease the size of their ecological footprint and population control strategies designed to persuade families to have fewer children.

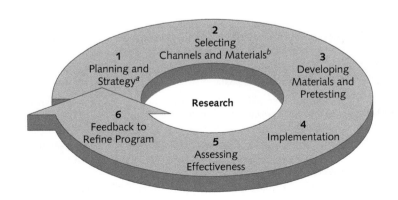

FIGURE 17-5 The Six Steps of Social Marketing See Chapter 5 for details regarding the program planning, implementation, and evaluation process.

[a] See the Social Marketing Planning Process box on page 678.

[b] Channels = The routes or methods used to reach the target audience.

Source: P. Kotler, J. Shalowitz, and R. J. Stevens, *Strategic Marketing for Health Care Organizations: Building a Customer-Driven Health System* (San Francisco: Jossey-Bass, 2008).

TABLE 17-7 Examples of Health Promotion Campaigns Using Social Marketing Techniques

HEALTH BEHAVIOR	SOCIAL MARKETING CAMPAIGN	PURPOSE	READ MORE ABOUT THE CAMPAIGN
Breastfeeding	National WIC Breastfeeding Promotion Project	Increase the number of breastfeeding women, increase the average duration of breastfeeding among WIC program participants, increase the number of referrals to WIC for breastfeeding support and technical assistance, and increase acceptance and support for breastfeeding among the general public.	*www.fns.usda.gov/wic/ breastfeeding-promotion- and-support-wic*
Achieving optimal calcium intake	Best Bones Forever	Educate and encourage girls age 9–12 to establish lifelong healthy habits, especially increased calcium consumption and bone-strengthening activities, to build and maintain strong bones.	*www.bestbonesforever.org*
	Calcium: Select to Protect Campaign	Increase calcium consumption in limited-resource African American and Hispanic children during their formative years using educational materials that are science-based, culturally sensitive, and suitable for low-literacy audiences.	*www.njsnap-ed.org/social/ index*
Consuming a healthy diet	National Fruit and Vegetable Program	A national partnership to increase consumption of fruits and vegetables by all Americans.	*www.fns.usda.gov/ffvp/fresh- fruit-and-vegetable-program*
	Pick a Better Snack & Act	Emphasize fruit and vegetable choices for snacks and the importance of daily physical activity.	*http://idph.iowa.gov/inn/ pick-a-better-snack*
Getting regular physical activity	VERB™ It's what you do.	Increase and maintain physical activity among tweens (youth age 9–13).	*www.cdc.gov/ youthcampaign*
	America On the Move	Empower individuals to take control of their health by making and sustaining small measurable changes to their daily eating and activity routines.	*www.active.com/articles/ america-on-the-move-small- steps-to-being-fit*
Getting regular physical activity and consuming a healthy diet	CDC's LEAN Works! (**L**eading **E**mployees to **A**ctivity and **N**utrition)	Provide interactive tools and evidence-based resources to design effective worksite obesity prevention and control programs.	*www.cdc.gov/ workplacehealthpromotion*
	Let's Move!	Combat child obesity by creating a healthy start for children; empowering parents and caregivers; providing healthy food in schools; improving access to healthy, affordable foods; and increasing physical activity.	*www.letsmove.gov*
	We Can! (**W**ays to **E**nhance **C**hildren's **A**ctivity & **N**utrition)	Designed for families and communities to help children maintain a healthy weight by *improving* food choices, *increasing* physical activity, and *reducing* screen time.	*www.nhlbi.nih.gov/health/ educational/wecan*
	Sisters Together: Move More, Eat Better	Designed to encourage black women age 18 and over to maintain a healthy weight by becoming more physically active and eating healthier foods.	*www.win.niddk.nih.gov/ sisters/index.htm*
	You Can! Steps to Healthier Aging	Designed to increase the number of older adults who are active and healthy.	*http://nutritionandaging.fiu .edu/You_Can/index.asp*
Access to healthy foods at school	California Project Lean (**L**eaders **E**ncouraging **A**ctivity and **N**utrition)	Increase healthy eating and physical activity to reduce the prevalence of obesity and chronic diseases.	*www.californiaprojectlean.org*
Practicing food safety	Be Food Safe Fight BAC!®	Be Food Safe builds on Fight BAC!'s successful, long-standing four messages of Clean, Separate, Cook, and Chill.	*www.befoodsafe.gov www.fightbac.org*

Social marketing goes beyond advertising. It seeks to bring about changes in the behavior of the target audience as well as in its attitudes and knowledge (see the box on the next page).[44] Social marketing can be applied to a wide variety of social problems but is particularly appropriate in three situations:[45]

1. When new research data and information on practices need to be disseminated to improve people's lives. Examples include campaigns for cancer prevention, breastfeeding promotion, and childhood immunization.
2. When countermarketing is needed to offset the negative effects of a practice or the promotional efforts of companies for products that are potentially harmful—for example, cigarettes, alcoholic beverages, or (in developing countries) infant formula.
3. When activation is needed to move people from intention to action—for example, motivating people to lose weight, be physically active, increase fruit and vegetable or calcium intakes, or floss their teeth. Without movement, there is no marketing.[46]

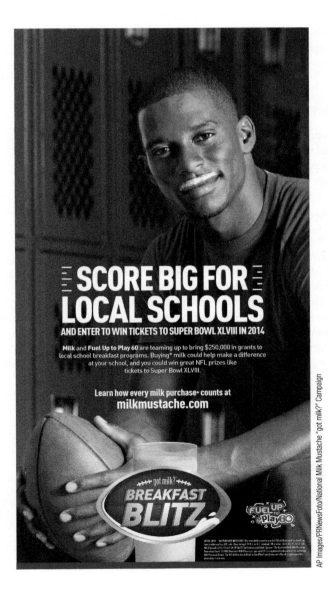

Think about novel ways to reach your target population. This ad features one of several celebrities who helped promote the "Got Milk?" message. For this ad, the *Got Milk?* Campaign joined with the *Fuel Up to Play 60* program to promote milk as part of a healthy breakfast in local school breakfast programs. NFL wide receiver Victor Cruz sports a milk mustache to show how milk helps him fuel his day.

AP Images/PRNewsFoto/National Milk Mustache "got milk?" Campaign

> ## Social Marketing Planning Process

The main components of a social marketing plan are the *problem/health issue, target audience, behavior*, and *strategy for change*. The following sample questions can help you move through the social marketing planning process. Answers may be found by collecting secondary data (review of the literature for existing studies, health statistics, etc.) or by conducting primary data collection, as discussed in Chapter 4.

Social Marketing Plan Component and Questions to Ask and Answer

 I. Problem/health issue. How can we define the problem?

1. What is the problem we need to address?
2. What factors contribute to the problem? What causes or contributes to those factors?
3. Who is affected by the problem?
4. Who is most likely to change?
5. What evidence demonstrates there is a health problem? Do you have evidence to show the burden of the health problem in your community?

II. Target audience. Who is affected by the problem and how can they be reached?

1. Who is the most appropriate audience for your intervention?
2. What are some meaningful ways to distinguish one group from another?
3. Which audiences are your partners and stakeholders interested in reaching?
4. Which audiences fit in with your organization's priorities?

III. Behavior. What do we want the audience to do?

1. What is the current behavior of your target audience?
2. What specific behavior are you going to address with your intervention?
3. What is the most realistic behavior change for the target audience to adopt?
4. What behavior can you feasibly try to change?
5. Will a change in this behavior actually affect the problem?
6. What will the audience like about the new behavior? What are the consequences of change?
7. What might keep the audience from adopting the new behavior?
8. Are there environmental factors that play a role? What are they?
9. Are there policies or standards (e.g., government laws or corporate policies) that either help or hinder the behavior change?
10. What recommendations or guidelines (i.e., *Healthy People 2020* objectives, clinical guidelines) exist related to this behavior?
11. What makes the audience's current behavior easy? What makes the target behavior difficult?
12. Is it a measurable behavior? Is it observable?

IV. Strategies for change. How can we get the target audience to adopt the desired behavior(s)?

1. What strategies were used in interventions that have similar goals? Who was the target audience of those other interventions? How are the audiences similar to or different from your target audience?
2. Which strategies are promising?
3. Which strategies have not worked in the past?
4. Are there strategies that have been fully evaluated or draw on a base of evidence?

5. Does the audience believe they can do the behavior (self-efficacy)?

6. Where are they along the stages-of-change model: no intention to change, thinking about changing, maintaining the healthy behavior already? (See Chapter 3.)

7. What social supports exist to help your audience adopt the behavior?

8. What things keep them from doing the behavior (barriers/costs)?

9. Who would be a credible source of information to the audience about the health topic or about the behavior?

Source: Adapted from Social Marketing for Nutrition and Physical Activity; *www.cdc.gov/nccdphp/dnpao/socialmarketing/index.html.*

Social Marketing at the Community Level

The Pawtucket Heart Health Program (PHHP) is presented here as an example of how marketing principles can be used in the planning, implementation, and evaluation of a community-wide social marketing campaign.

The Pawtucket "Know Your Cholesterol" campaign was one of the earliest cholesterol awareness and screening efforts.[48] The following objectives for the campaign were formulated on the basis of national random sampling data for both the general population and physicians:

- Increase physician education on blood cholesterol and heart disease
- Increase awareness among the general population of blood cholesterol as a risk factor for coronary heart disease
- Increase numbers of people knowing their cholesterol level as a result of attending PHHP-sponsored screening, counseling, and referral events (SCOREs)
- Increase numbers of people showing reductions in their blood cholesterol level at two-month follow-up measurements

In segmenting the community of Pawtucket, Rhode Island, adults were a primary focus because demographics (gender and age) showed that awareness levels were equivalent for men and women in the national sample. Cardiologists, family practice physicians, and physicians in general practice were targeted for direct-mail educational packages and grand rounds presentations on blood cholesterol and heart disease at the community hospital. Middle-aged men who had had previous contact with the PHHP were also the focus of a direct-mail and telemarketing campaign to attend SCOREs during the campaign period.

Early program development steps included a pilot test of a self-help "nutrition kit" on lowering cholesterol levels and pretesting the SCORE protocol at the community hospital. Promotional tools selected to reach the general and targeted audiences included newspapers; print media distributed through worksites, churches, and schools; direct mail and telemarketing; and SCORE delivery at worksites, churches, and various other community locations. In order to avoid spillover into the control community, television and radio were not used.

In the marketing mix, SCOREs were initially priced at $5 per person for both an initial and a follow-up measurement. The researchers reasoned that people who had already paid for a second measurement would be more likely to have a follow-up test than if they had to pay for it separately. Price reductions and specials were also offered. Promotional publicity strategies included the "kick-off" SCORE at a St. Patrick's Day parade and six weekly advice columns in the local newspaper.

Results showed that 1,439 adults attended 39 SCOREs. Sixty percent were identified as having elevated serum cholesterol levels. Two months after the campaign, 72.3% of these

The "5 P's" of social marketing are:[47]

- *Product:* the behavior or health idea that the campaign planners would like the targeted individuals to adopt.
- *Price:* the costs associated with "buying" the product (e.g., money, time [inconvenience]).
- *Place:* the distribution channels used to make the product available to target audiences.
- *Promotion:* the efforts taken to ensure that the target audience is aware of the campaign.
- *Positioning:* the efforts to place the product so as to maximize benefits and minimize costs.

persons had returned for a second measurement. Nearly 60% of this group had reduced their serum cholesterol levels.

The essential components of the campaign's marketing strategy were integrated into the ongoing activities of the PHHP. During the first two years following the campaign, over 10,000 persons had their blood cholesterol level measured, were given information on dietary management of high serum cholesterol, and were referred to physicians when necessary. A later survey of local physicians showed that they were more aggressive in initiating either diet or drug therapy than physicians in the neighboring community or those who had participated in the national survey. The local physicians cited as the major reason for changing their practice the increase in patient requests for blood cholesterol measurements and/or nutrition information. The researchers concluded that informed consumers had influenced changes in their physicians' treatment of high serum cholesterol levels. Their overall conclusion was that "a well-functioning marketing operation can lead to more effective and efficient use of resources and improved consumer satisfaction. . . . **Health marketing** has the potential of reaching the largest possible group of people at the least cost with the most effective, consumer-satisfying program."[49] Check the Internet Resources related to social marketing at the end of the chapter.

Health marketing Health promotion programs that are developed to satisfy consumer needs, are strategically planned to reach as broad an audience as is in need of the program, and thereby enhance the organization's ability to effect population-wide changes in targeted risk behaviors.

PROGRAMS IN **ACTION**

Motivating Children to Change Their Eating and Activity Habits

Many children do not eat a healthful daily diet or get the physical activity they need to avoid nutrition-related chronic diseases and to promote lifelong health. Children eat less than the recommended number of daily servings of fruits and vegetables.[1] A majority of children in this country eat too much fat, especially saturated fat.[2] Only about half of young people regularly participate in vigorous physical activity.[3] One in four children in the United States is overweight.[4] Children do not always have the chance to reap the benefits of a lifestyle marked by a good diet and adequate physical activity. Children spend more time watching television in a year than they spend in school,[5] many school systems are limiting or eliminating physical education,[6] and food industry advertising may influence children to choose foods high in solid fat and/or added sugar.[7,8]

As we noted earlier in the chapter, social marketing seeks to bring about changes in the behavior of a target audience, as well as in its attitudes and knowledge. Social marketing is highly applicable when countermarketing is needed to offset the negative effects of a practice (e.g., lack of physical activity) or the advertising campaigns of companies for certain products (e.g., high-fat or high-sugar snacks for children). Eat Well & Keep Moving applied the principles of social marketing in the development of a program to improve the nutrition status and health of children.

Goals and Objectives

The goals of the research phase of Eat Well & Keep Moving were to decrease students' consumption of total and saturated fat, to increase their intake of fruits and vegetables, to reduce television viewing, and to increase moderate and vigorous physical activity.

Target Audience

The target audience was 479 fourth- and fifth-grade students in six intervention and eight matched control elementary schools in Baltimore. Eighty-five percent of participating students received free/reduced-price school lunch; over 90% were African American.

Rationale for the Intervention

Unlike traditional health curricula, Eat Well & Keep Moving was a multifaceted program encompassing all aspects of the learning environment, from the classroom, cafeteria, and gymnasium to the school hallways, the home, and even community centers. This varied approach helped reinforce important messages about nutrition and physical activity, and it increased the chance that students would eat well and be physically active throughout their lives.

Methodology

The research phase of Eat Well & Keep Moving was conducted in collaboration with the Baltimore City Department of Education. It was taught by classroom teachers over the course of two years. Using the interdisciplinary approach, the curriculum was integrated into the core subjects of math, science, language arts, and social studies. Thirteen lessons on nutrition and health-related fitness concepts were taught each year. Four of the classroom lessons involved children practicing a "safe workout" routine while learning concepts related to nutrition and physical activity. To further integrate nutrition and physical activity, five supplementary physical education lessons were taught, using nutrition and food as the themes of the activities. Modules that were developed as extensions of classroom lessons provided opportunities for students to participate in activities related to program goals. These included Freeze My TV to reduce television viewing, 3 at School and 5 a Day to promote consumption of fruits and vegetables, and Walking Clubs to promote physical activity and fitness. Educational materials established links to school foodservice, using the cafeteria as a learning laboratory for nutrition. To reinforce concepts at home, families received nutrition and fitness information through newsletters and other vehicles. Teachers were motivated through a wellness session that was part of their teacher training.

Results

Fourteen Baltimore elementary schools successfully participated in the four-year demonstration program. Students rated the lessons and activities highly, and 100% of responding teachers said that they would utilize the program again. Diet was evaluated with 24-hour recall measures. Longitudinal data collected from 479 students demonstrated significant decreases in percent of total calories from fat and saturated fat, a significant increase in fruit and vegetable consumption, and a marginal reduction in television viewing. Student knowledge on nutrition and healthful activity also increased significantly.

Since September 1997, schools involved in the study and the Baltimore Department of Education have sustained Eat Well & Keep Moving on their own. To date, personnel in 65 Baltimore elementary schools have been trained, and 40 schools have been implementing the program.

Lessons Learned

For a program to be successful, those who develop its components must consider the school constituents' needs, constraints, and motivations. Program designers should obtain inputs not only from teachers, foodservice staff, and principals but also from students and parents. Keeping the program inexpensive to implement helps, too.

Source: From *Community Nutritionary* (White Plains, NY: Dannon Institute, Fall 2001). Used with permission. For more information about the Awards for Excellence in Community Nutrition, go to *www.dannon-institute.org*.

A Marketing Plan for Heartworks for Women: Case Study 1

Team 2—the team responsible for the nutrition intervention activities in the Heartworks for Women program—reviewed the results of the community needs assessment (see **Table 5-1** on page 153), the goals and objectives for the intervention strategy (see page 156), and the program objectives (see page 163). The following needs and wants of the target population were identified in the community needs assessment and in focus group discussions: want to stop smoking (one participant's view: "I want to get this monkey off my back");

want to feel better; want to look better; don't want to have a heart attack (one participant remarked, "My mother died of a heart attack at the age of 44. She was shopping at the mall and just went like that. I don't want that to happen to me"). Some women wanted better health and more information about heart-healthy cooking (one participant said, "I just buy whatever is convenient to cook. Junk food is quick and easy").

The benefits of the Heartworks for Women program, shown in Table 17-1, addressed these needs and wants. The results of the situational analysis revealed one major target segment: working women (64% of the total market), who were mostly aged 25–58 years. Two smaller segments were university/college students (20%), aged 18–24 years; and an "other" category (16%), which included stay-at-home mothers, retirees, and other women who did not work outside the home or go to school. The latter group had two main age segments: 18–30 years and 55+ years. Drawing on an analysis of the broad environment in which these women live and work, team 2 found both positive and negative elements in the environment. On the positive side, smoking was not allowed in government buildings, and many women were aware of heart-healthy eating messages in the media. On the negative side, the media seldom present women, especially middle-aged women, as fit and active. Competition for the Heartworks for Women program included weight management programs offered by all private health/fitness clubs and counseling provided by 11 dietitians in private practice in the areas of weight management and cholesterol reduction.

The objectives for the marketing strategy were designed to meet the broad goals outlined for the Heartworks for Women program: (1) increase women's awareness of the relationship of diet to CHD risk and (2) build skills related to heart-healthy eating and cooking. Specific objectives of the marketing strategy for the program are as follows:

- The Heartworks for Women program will be offered in 60 companies within the city by the end of one year.
- The Heartworks for Women program will be offered in all five universities and colleges within the city by the end of one year.
- At least 100,000 women living in the city of Jeffers will be exposed to Heartworks for Women messages through the following channels: advertising (city bus), flyers, promotional brochures, posters, radio interviews, newspaper articles, and the Internet website.

The marketing mix for the Heartworks for Women program is shown in **Figure 17-6**. It focuses on worksites and universities/colleges as the primary gates for delivering program messages and promoting the program. Partnerships with local private health/fitness clubs provide another opportunity for boosting the program's visibility in the community. The program will be promoted through flyers, brochures, posters in company cafeterias, press releases related to special events, a painted city bus, the Internet website, and the Mother/ Daughter Walk. The program will be priced competitively at $60 per participant.

The projected budget for the marketing strategy must take into account both staff time for designing materials and the cost of printing and copying promotional materials such as flyers and posters. (Additional information about the projected budget for the marketing strategy is presented in the next chapter.) The timeline allows team 2 to schedule all marketing activities prior to the program launch date. An example of a timetable is shown in **Figure 17-7**. Of course, in real life, the timetable is considerably larger than this because it shows all activities for the program, including those designed to sustain awareness and increase participation over the life of the program.

As with all other aspects of program planning, the marketing strategy must be evaluated. In this example, the summative evaluation conducted six months after the launch determined that only 35 companies had signed on for the program, and most of these were large companies with a human resources department and more than 200 employees.

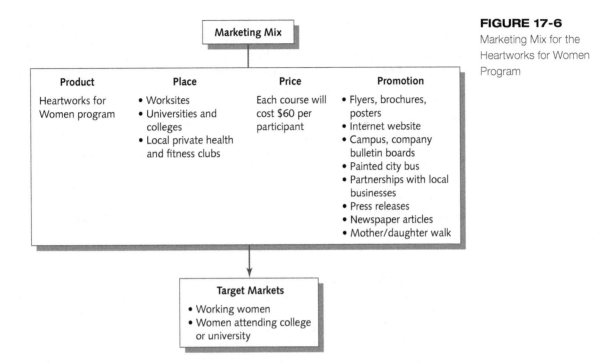

FIGURE 17-6

Marketing Mix for the
Heartworks for Women
Program

Team 2 realized that two changes should be made in the marketing strategy. First, an important segment of the target group—women who worked in light-manufacturing companies with no human resources department and fewer than 100 employees—were not aware of the program. Thus, the marketing strategy and the program format had to be redesigned to be more attractive to this group. For example, rather than offering a full eight-session course, small companies were offered only two or three 45-minute sessions, each held over the lunch hour. Each individual session cost only $5 per participant. The

Launch

Marketing Tool	Jan.	Feb.	Mar.	Apr.	May	Jun.	Jul.	Aug.	Sept.	Oct.	Nov.	Dec.
Bulletin boards												
Campus			✔	✔	✔			✔	✔	✔		
Worksite			✔	✔	→							→
Flyers			✔	✔				✔	✔			
Brochures			✔	→								→
City bus				✔	→							→
Internet website			✔	→								→
Mother/daughter walk									✔			
Press releases				✔					✔			
Radio announcement				✔					✔			
Newspaper articles				✔					✔			

FIGURE 17-7

Marketing Timetable
for the Heartworks for
Women Program

marketing mix was changed accordingly. Second, the decision to paint a city bus with the program logo and one nutrition message had been made early in the planning process, after team 2 learned of the success of this approach in another city. However, the chosen bus route was one that included a small mall and two large residential sections in an affluent part of town. Team 2 decided to choose another bus route, one that circulated through two industrial parks that featured light-manufacturing businesses. This bus route would provide more program visibility for women in the target market and for small companies, which were more difficult to recruit to the program than large companies. Adjustments in the marketing strategy would be made again in another six months when another evaluation was to occur.

Entrepreneurship Leads the Way

The challenge for the current decade will be to use the marketing strategies described in this chapter to remind consumers of the benefits of good health and to motivate them to make behavior changes. The important thing is to stay focused on the needs and wants of the "consumer" of health promotion activities. Remember, too, that consumers are a diverse lot, and broad target groups such as men age 18–49 years or teenagers or post-menopausal women no longer describe today's consumer market. Consumers can and should be grouped into smaller, better-defined categories. In today's marketplace, the Internet makes one-to-one marketing feasible. Even mass marketing, a successful marketing tool of the past, is giving way to selective, targeted marketing. Tomorrow's consumer promises to be an independent thinker, highly educated and sophisticated, demanding, a seeker of innovation, and a pursuer of wellness.[50] Marketing will help you capture this changing profile, and entrepreneurship will help you plan for it.

PROFESSIONAL FOCUS

Social Media for Nutrition Professionals

By Nicole Geurin, MPH, RD, and Jessica Anderson

What Is Social Media?

Social media, not to be confused with social networking, is a broad category of websites that allow users to interact and share information with each other. Because there is no limit to the number of social media sites that can be created, nor to the number of people who can view, join, or subscribe to a given site, there is significant opportunity for professional growth among social media users. Some of the most popular social media sites include Facebook, Twitter, LinkedIn, YouTube, WordPress, and TypePad. Facebook and LinkedIn are two social networking sites that can dramatically affect one's professional connections and can also be linked to the user's other social media accounts. If you have not already done so, make the choice now to learn how to use social media to your advantage. You will soon find yourself networking with peers and potential employers and clients in an expansive, dynamic environment.

The Benefits of Social Media

According to current estimates, 82% of the population in developed nations used the Internet regularly in 2015.[1] Nutrition professionals who know how to use social media effectively have access to the many benefits of interacting with this vast population. Social media can function as a networking tool, a means for educating others, and an avenue for learning and inspiration among professionals. Using social media can lead to job opportunities and can cultivate beneficial professional relationships between nutrition professionals. One registered dietitian shares her experience with social media:

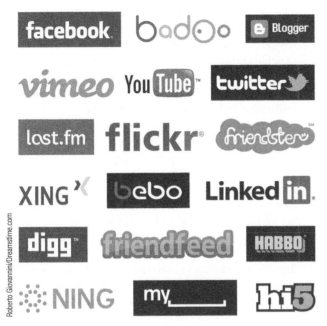

Roberto Giovannini/Dreamstime.com

I have made many connections, primarily through Twitter, that have led to amazing opportunities for me. Very early on when I started tweeting (in '09), an editor from the Food Network reached out to me, and I have been blogging for the Food Network's Healthy Eats blog ever since. I have also worked with a handful of book authors whom I met through social media, and have contributed to books (including a cookbook and both Operation Beautiful books). My "social media for dietitians" knowledge has allowed me to speak at two annual conferences about the topic to encourage other registered dietitians to use social media.[2]

Registered dietitians and nutrition professionals can use social media as an educational tool by creating online resources for clients, peers, or the general public. According to the Pew Research Center's Internet and American Life Project, 83% of adult Internet users search for health information online.[3] Nutrition professionals who understand how to use social media are in an excellent position to share their nutritional expertise with Internet users.

Because blogs have grown substantially in popularity over the years, bloggers have greater visibility in their prospective industries than their nonblogging peers.[4] According to data compiled by the Centers for Disease Control and Prevention, 60% of Internet users, or 150.4 million people, were blog readers in 2014.[5] Many health professionals, including registered dietitians, create blogs to chronicle their personal experience with certain health conditions or to share their expertise. Coincidentally, Internet users with health or medical conditions tend to seek blogs or websites created by those who have had similar experiences.[6] Thus, social media allows nutrition professionals to have a positive influence in many people's lives.

In addition to educating others, nutrition professionals can use social media to learn and to become inspired. All health professionals have a responsibility to continue learning once they've entered the field. With this in mind, other blogs and websites can serve as a source of new information. Also, nutrition professionals should tap into their readership as a source of inspiration. Polling your readers regarding their current health and nutrition concerns, their favorite recipes, or their level of understanding can reveal which topics you, as a blogger, might consider writing about in the future.[7]

Getting Started

Those who have yet to use any form of social media in a professional capacity should first open user accounts with larger sites, such as Facebook and LinkedIn.[8] It is worth noting that Facebook permits users to create a Facebook business page, a more professional take on the traditional personal Facebook account. No matter your current level of knowledge, don't let yourself become discouraged. Allotting a certain amount of time each day or week for social media exploration and learning is a great way to take responsibility for developing your online presence. It is perfectly acceptable to start with just one site while you gain familiarity with it.

If you already use multiple social media sites, consider linking them or opening accounts with new sites that can supplement your existing accounts. In between blog posts, bloggers can submit and receive short updates via Twitter. Using Flickr, bloggers and their readers can post relevant photos, such as a quick picture of a recipe readers have tried or anything else relevant to the content of the blog. Keep in mind the importance, however, of maintaining a consistent image across your various social media accounts. If you keep a personal social networking account, it is to your benefit to make it visible only to members of your personal network.

Before you jump in and create a website or blog, consider this short list of tips:

- Do choose a unique and visually appealing layout for your blog or website.
- Do post frequently. One post per week is sufficient, including shorter posts using Twitter or Flickr.
- Do be succinct; too lengthy a post may bore your readers.
- Do maintain a consistent image online if you use more than one social media site.
- Do be genuine. Originality will attract an audience and differentiate your blog from others that may focus on a similar topic.[9]
- Do have a goal in mind before you start, and choose a topic you are passionate about. Blogging just to blog will leave you uninspired in no time.

Know Your Terms and Tools

- **Social media**: A broad category of websites that allow users to interact and contribute content. Social media sites include blogs, social networking sites, and video- and image-sharing websites.
- **Social networking**: The term used to describe the formation of personal or professional relationships among users of social media websites.
- *Twitter.com*: A specific website that facilitates social networking. Members of the website post short (140 characters or less) thoughts, questions, or comments and gather responses from members of their social network.
- *Facebook.com*: A specific social networking website. Members create a profile, to which they can add photographs and personal information. Although originally used for personal social networking, Facebook has increased in popularity among businesses and professionals.
- *LinkedIn.com*: A social media site used for social networking among professionals. Members' profiles include information regarding work experience, education, and professional affiliations.
- *YouTube.com*: A social media website used for sharing videos. Users may post videos for public viewing on the site and receive feedback in the form of ratings and comments.
- **Weblog** (a.k.a. "blog"): A type of social media website. In contrast to a traditional website, a weblog's contents are not static. Bloggers post new content frequently and interact with their readers.
- **Blogging software**: Programs that allow users to post and manage online content are referred to as blogging software. Some of the most popular blogging software sites include:
  - *www.WordPress.com*
  - *www.Blogger.com*
  - *www.TypePad.com*
- **Niche:** In social media terms, a niche is a group of people who are interested in a particular topic and are likely to find your blog or website. Choosing and researching a niche is arguably the most important step and should be completed before creating your blog or website.[10] Social media users who create a blog without a specific target audience in mind will lack a clear vision of whom they are writing for and, as a result, may struggle to establish a following.
- **Keywords**: Words or phrases that describe what the Internet user is searching for are referred to as keywords. Every niche, by definition, has certain interests and will use particular words to search the Internet for content. Programs such as Google AdWords Keyword Tool and SEO Book Keyword Suggestion Tool monitor search engine results and allow blog developers to research commonly used keywords. Deliberately using the appropriate keywords in your blog content will allow readers to find your blog when they perform Internet searches.[11] For example, according to Google AdWords, a blogger who wants to reach individuals interested in managing their blood cholesterol levels should include keywords such as "LDL cholesterol," "lower cholesterol," "high-cholesterol foods," and "cholesterol-lowering foods," as these are the most frequently searched phrases among this niche.
- **Search engine optimization (SEO)**: Search engine optimization is the process of designing one's blog or website and its content in such a way that allows search engines to find it easily. Two major search engines, Yahoo and Google, provide search results for 151 million searches each day. To compile results for Internet users, search engines "crawl" the World Wide Web to gather content, which is categorized and organized based on the keywords found within.[12] Bloggers who strategically use keywords in their content improve their chances of inclusion in the first page of search results, a place every blogger wants to be. In addition to the use of keywords, the use of a web hosting service and registering with blog and website directories are two other examples of SEO.
- **Directories**: Blog and website directories are categorized lists Internet users can browse to find blogs or websites that interest them. Also, search engines may crawl directories to update their search result offerings.[13] Bloggers can register with multiple directories; a few to start with include *BlogCatalog.com*, *StumbleUpon.com*, *DMOZ.org*, Yahoo Directory, *Digg.com*, and *Technorati.com*. Nutrition professionals who use a blog or website to promote their services can also register with Google Places, an online directory for local businesses.[14]
- **RSS**: RSS, or "really simple syndication," is a tool recognized for saving readers' time. Instead of individually checking favorite websites or blogs for updates, new content is collected and posted to the reader's homepage of choice.[15] Most blogging software programs provide an automatic RSS feature, making it easy for bloggers to offer an RSS feed to their readers.

Developing Your Brand and Establishing Readership

A brand is the idea or image that represents your business. You can develop your brand by choosing physical representations, such as logos and slogans, and by cultivating professional relationships with your readers, clients, and peers. Using consistent colors and images in your blog or website layout will allow readers to associate these things with your brand. Investing time in online professional relationships with your readers will reinforce your image as a credible, reliable source.

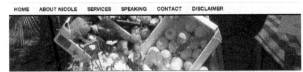

Nicole Geurin, MPH, RD

Bringing the science and joys of nutrition to life.

| HOME | ABOUT NICOLE | SERVICES | SPEAKING | CONTACT | DISCLAIMER |

← Q&A with the Dietitian: Low-Sodium Lunch and Snack Ideas   Sleep More to Eat Less →

5 MORE Healthy Meals in 5 Minutes or Less

Posted on October 24, 2011 | 3 Comments

My original 5 Healthy Meals in 5 Minutes or Less were so popular, I decided to make a sequel. These 5 MORE Healthy Meals in 5 Minutes or Less feature all-new recipes that are just as fast, healthy and delicious. They include:

- Fruit-Infused Oatmeal
- Shrimp and Zucchini Saute
- Black Bean and Corn Salsa
- Grilled Fish Tacos
- Grilled Bananas

These recipes use the microwave, a George Foreman grill, or the stove for quick, healthy cooking. Enjoy! Check out Nicole's entire collection of healthy recipes here.

Share this: 📧 Email   🖨 Print   📘 Facebook 2   🐦 Twitter 3   ⊞ More

NICOLE GEURIN, MPH, RD

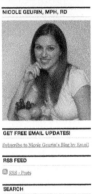

The George Foreman Grill is great for fast and healthy meals!

GET FREE EMAIL UPDATES!

Subscribe to Nicole Geurin's Blog by Email

RSS FEED

🔲 RSS - Posts

SEARCH

[ ] (Search)

CATEGORIES

Nicole Geurin

One of a blogger's best self-promotion strategies is to find readers rather than waiting for them to find you. Your exchanges with readers will contribute to your online reputation. Begin by conducting searches using the same keywords you found in your niche research. From your search results, choose blogs or websites that feature forums. A forum is a discussion board where readers share their thoughts and ask questions about blog content. By joining relevant forums, you can interact with members of your target niche, who may one day become readers of your blog.

In addition to major search engines, blog directories can also be useful tools for locating forums. Participate in popular forums that receive at least 50–100 posts per day. This helps to ensure there will be enough Internet traffic to make it worth the time you will invest participating in a given forum. Spend a few days or weeks getting acquainted with regular users on the forums you have chosen. This will demonstrate your sincerity in forming professional relationships. If possible, use signature links to sign your name in your forum post, as this will provide a link to your blog. Not all forums allow this, so be sure to check before you begin using any given forum.[16]

Conclusion

As the population of nutrition professionals in social media continues to grow, both opportunities and competition will increase online. For this reason, now is the time to start utilizing social media. Once you have made the commitment, the most important first step is simply to start. There is always more to know and improvements to be made as a social media user, but with an open mind and a willingness to learn from mistakes, social media can become invaluable to the nutrition professional. As you begin, remind yourself of your reasons for using social media, be it building a clientele, finding employment, networking with other nutrition professionals, educating others, or any other reason. Keep these goals in mind and acknowledge that although achieving them will take time, it will be well worth the effort.

case study

Marketing Nutrition and Health Promotion

By Alison Barkman, MS, RD, CDN, Alice Fornari, EdD, RD, and Alessandra Sarcona, MS, RD, CSSD

Scenario

You are an RD running a weight-loss and healthy eating program at a local endocrinologist's office. This three-month program consists of once-weekly private, one-on-one nutrition counseling sessions with you, as well as once-weekly group meetings where you lead a discussion on a topic relevant to healthy eating and physical activity. It costs $600 to enroll in the three-month program. Currently, you have 20 clients enrolled, all direct referrals from the endocrinologist's practice. The program is designed to appeal to both men and women, ages 18 and up.

The endocrinologist would like to grow this wellness program and expand it beyond her own client pool. Not only do you have to market the program to attract new clients but also create marketing tools that will keep current clients interested and possibly spur them to re-enroll beyond three months if needed. This takes time, and you are the only RD managing the program, plus counseling clients.

You need to consider your competition. This includes not only other dietitians in your area but weight-loss companies that are well known and cheaper, such as Weight Watchers. One advantage is that your program may be covered by some insurance plans, mostly for cases where clients have diabetes.

Another consideration is that you have little experience with marketing. You do know how powerful marketing can be to help build the practice. You have a limited budget that will not allow for advertising on TV, radio, or in local newspapers. In addition, the endocrinologist does not use or understand social media such as Facebook. She feels the program can grow successfully by word-of-mouth alone and that marketing may not be necessary. You must figure out a way to create buzz about the program to get potential clients in the door within budgetary constraints.

Learning Outcomes

- Create a marketing plan that helps identify your target audience and tools to reach them effectively.
- Identify marketing tools that are inexpensive, yet effective, so you do not waste your time or limited budget.
- Identify barriers in reaching your target audience.
- Identify the benefits of having a weight-loss program run by an RD in an endocrinologist's practice that will make it more attractive to potential clients versus other commercial programs.

Foundation: Acquisition of Knowledge and Skills

1. Review the *Journal of the Academy of Nutrition and Dietetics* May 2009 supplement titled *Marketing Yourself—Enhance Your Profile and Advance Your Career* (vol. 109, no. 5). If you are a member of the Academy of Nutrition and Dietetics, this can be accessed via their website, *www.eatright.org*. Specifically, review the following articles from the supplement:
   a. "Blogs, Podcasts, and Wikis: The New Names in Information Dissemination"
   b. "Showcasing Your Expertise: Creating a Video for the Web"
   c. "Networking Moves Online"
2. Access various marketing fact sheets for registered dietitians on the Nutrition 411 website: *www.nutrition411.com*.

Look under Career Development → Entrepreneur Tools to find a list of marketing tip sheets and entrepreneurial tools for RDs.
3. Review the Social Marketing for Nutrition and Physical Activity web course (go to *www.cdc.gov* and search for "Social Marketing for Nutrition and Physical Activity").

Step 1: *Identify Relevant Information and Uncertainties*

1. Using the information in Figure 17-1 ("A Marketing Plan for Health Promotion") and in the section "Develop a Marketing Plan" in your text, briefly outline a marketing plan for your weight-loss program. Be sure to provide some detail for each step of the marketing plan as it relates to this case study (e.g., define your target population; actually list benefits of the program; outline details of a strengths, weaknesses, opportunities, and threats [SWOT] analysis as it relates to your program).
2. What are your challenges in marketing this weight-loss program? What are some things you may be unsure of in this marketing process?
3. Create a chart outlining the four P's of the marketing mix using examples from your text. Go beyond details provided in the case study; be creative in sketching out the details of each "P." Refer to Figure 17-4 ("The Four P's of the Marketing Mix").

Step 2: *Interpret Information*

1. Using information from your text about brand image, identify a "brand image" for your weight-loss program. Be creative in coming up with a name for the program, potential slogan, brand logo, and other branding ideas.
2. What marketing tools will you use? Consult your text and the three websites listed at the beginning of this case study. Also use any of your own knowledge on topics such as social media (e.g., Facebook, Twitter). List each marketing tool and your rationale for choosing that particular tool. Be sure to include a mix of traditional marketing tools and new ones such as social media. For each tool:
   a. Explain what the tool is and why you are using it.
   b. What audience do you plan to target with this tool?
   c. Draft an example of the actual tool, or an outline of what content will be included in the tool.
   d. How do you plan to measure the success of this tool?

Step 3: *Draw and Implement Conclusions*

1. Using information you provided in Step 1 and 2 answers so far, plus additional ideas you may have, outline a timeline for rolling out your marketing plan from the planning phase, through implementation, to monitoring and evaluation. Write your timeline in terms of steps (e.g., Step 1, Step 2, etc.).
2. Using information under "Marketing to Your Clients" on the Nutrition 411 website, identify some tools you will use for current clients to keep them interested in

the program and returning for more nutrition services as needed.

Step 4: *Engage in Continuous Improvement*

Describe how you will evaluate and measure the success of your program and your return on investment (ROI) for each marketing tool used in order to determine whether they are cost-effective enough to be used again. Brainstorm ideas on your own and consult Step 5 ("Evaluation") of the Social Marketing for Nutrition and Physical Activity web course.

CHAPTER **SUMMARY**

What Is Marketing?

▶ The purpose of marketing is to find a problem, need, or want (through marketing research) and to fashion a solution to it.

▶ When completed, a marketing plan will outline the steps for achieving the goals and objectives of the intervention strategy and program plan (see Figure 17-1). First, select a target market. Next, determine the needs and wants of the target population. Conduct a situational analysis, or SWOT (strengths, weaknesses, opportunities, and threats) analysis.

▶ Develop a marketing strategy for ensuring a good fit between the goals and resources of the organization and the needs and wants of the target population. The four

elements of the marketing strategy are often called the "four P's" of the marketing mix—product, price, place, and promotion.

Social Marketing: Community Campaigns for Change

▶ Social marketing seeks to increase the acceptability of an idea, a practice, a product, or all three among a certain group of people, known as the target population. Social marketing is a strategy for changing consumer behavior; its premise is that individuals do new things or give up old things in exchange for benefits they hope to receive.

● The main components of a social marketing plan are the problem or health issue, target audience, behavior, and strategy for change.

SUMMARY **QUESTIONS**

1. Compare and contrast the goals of traditional marketing and social marketing and provide an example of each.
2. Discuss the steps that the community nutritionist takes in developing a marketing plan.
3. Define market segmentation and illustrate how it is used effectively to market nutrition interventions.
4. Describe methods for collecting both primary and secondary data for a situational analysis.
5. Based on a specific community nutrition program, product, or service:
   a. Identify your target market.
   b. Describe an appropriate marketing mix for your target market.
   c. Develop a marketing strategy to promote the program, product, or service.

INTERNET **RESOURCES**

Social Marketing Resources

Hispanic Health Council, Inc.
www.hispanichealth.com/hhc

CDC Social Marketing Resources
www.cdc.gov/nccdphp/dnpao/socialmarketing/index
.html

Prevention Institute
www.preventioninstitute.org

Case Studies in Social Marketing
www.cdc.gov/nccdphp/DNPAO/socialmarketing/
casestudies.html

Tools of Change
www.toolsofchange.com/en/home/

Turning Point Collaborative
http://socialmarketingcollaborative.org/index.html

Public Service Announcements
www.psaresearch.com

Social Media Toolkit
www.cdc.gov/socialmedia/Tools/guidelines/pdf/
SocialMediaToolkit_BM.pdf

CHAPTER 18

Managing Community Nutrition Programs

LEARNING **OBJECTIVES**

After you have read and studied this chapter, you will be able to:

- Differentiate between strategic and operational planning.
- Describe the four functions of management.
- Describe methods to coordinate an organization's activities.
- Outline methods for obtaining peak performance from employees.

This chapter addresses such issues as strategic management, program planning and documentation of appropriate activities, human resource management, budget preparation, time management, informatics, and current information technologies, which have been designated by the Accreditation Council for Education in Nutrition and Dietetics (ACEND) as Foundation Knowledge and Learning Outcomes for dietetics education.

CHAPTER **OUTLINE**

Something to think about...

"Do you want to be a positive influence in the world? First, get your own life in order. Ground yourself in the single principle so that your behavior is wholesome and effective. If you do that, you will earn respect and be a powerful influence. Your behavior influences others through a ripple effect. A ripple effect works because everyone influences everyone else. Powerful people are powerful influences.
If your life works, you influence your family.
If your family works, your family influences the community.
If your community works, your community influences the nation.
If your nation works, your nation influences the world.
If your world works, the ripple effect spreads throughout the cosmos."

—*LAO TZU, TAO TE CHING (The Tao of Leadership)*

For a complete list of references, please access the MindTap Reader within your MindTap course.

Management The process of achieving organizational goals through engaging in the four major functions of planning, organizing, leading, and controlling.

Introduction

Community nutritionists must be good planners and managers. One of the past presidents of the Academy of Nutrition and Dietetics, Judith L. Dodd, said this about dietitians' need for management expertise: "It's not enough to have technical knowledge. Other skills are necessary, whether you want to call them leadership skills or communication skills or simply survival skills. We must know how to communicate, how to negotiate, how to persuade, and how to work with various groups within any of our market environments."[1] In other words, community nutritionists must have good management skills. **Management** is the process of achieving organizational goals through planning, organizing, leading, and controlling.[2] In this chapter, we examine the functions of management and consider how they are used by community nutritionists. In the following chapter, we review the principles of grant writing because community nutritionists often seek extramural funding for program activities.

The Four Functions of Management

The main activities and responsibilities of managers can be grouped into four areas, or functions, as shown in **Figure 18-1**. *Planning* is the forward-looking aspect of a manager's job; it involves setting goals and objectives and deciding how best to achieve them. *Organizing* focuses on distributing and arranging human and nonhuman resources so that plans can be carried out successfully. *Leading* involves influencing others to carry out the work required to reach the organization's goals. *Controlling* consists of regulating certain organizational activities to ensure that they meet established standards and goals. This section describes each management function.

Planning

A colossal marketing blunder made headlines around the world in the spring of 1993. Hoover, a subsidiary of the Maytag Corporation, launched a promotional campaign in Ireland and Britain in which consumers who purchased any of its household appliances

FIGURE 18-1 The Four Functions of Management
Source: K. M. Bartol and D. C. Martin, *Management*, p. 7. Copyright 1991 by McGraw-Hill, Inc. Used with permission of the McGraw-Hill Companies.

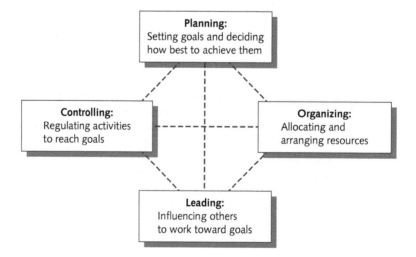

(worth at least $150 U.S.) were offered two free return plane tickets to Europe or the United States (valued at about $500 U.S.). Hoover's aim was to stimulate interest in its products, a feat it readily achieved. For reasons not entirely clear, Hoover's management failed to anticipate the number of customers who would accept the promotion's restrictions (such as inconvenient departure times) and demand the promised air tickets. The result was a $30 million loss, the firing of three top executives, and a place in management textbooks as "one of the great marketing gaffes of all time."[3]

What is the lesson in this story for community nutritionists? In two words: plan ahead. To those of us standing outside the Hoover snafu, it seems incredible that no one foresaw the shortfall between anticipated revenues and actual expenses. What happened on the inside may never be fully known. Regardless, the magnitude of the event suggests a glitch in the planning process—failure of managers to calculate accurately the direct and indirect costs associated with the promotional campaign.

For the manager or managerial team, **planning** involves deciding what to do and when, where, and how to do it. It focuses on future events and on finding solutions to problems. Planning is ongoing. It involves performing a number of activities in a logical sequence and considering a variety of solutions before a plan of action is chosen.[4]

Types of Planning

There are different types of planning, including **strategic planning**, **operational planning**, and **project management**. Strategic planning is broad in scope and addresses the organization's overall goals. Strategic planning occurs over a period of several years and is usually undertaken by the organization's senior managers. It focuses on formulating objectives; assessing past, current, and future conditions, trends, and events; evaluating the organization's strengths and weaknesses; and making decisions about the appropriate course of action. The Academy of Nutrition and Dietetics' strategic plan includes the three strategic goals listed in the box that follows. The plan allows for flexibility and innovation while providing direction for the organization in its mission to empower members to be the nation's food and nutrition leaders.[5]

The strategic plan guides the development of operational plans. Operational planning is short-term planning typically done by midlevel managers. It deals with specific actions, expenditures, and controls and with the timing of these activities in a formal, structured process.[6] After setting policy as a major strategic initiative in its 1996–1999 strategic plan, for example, the Academy of Nutrition and Dietetics set into motion an operational plan to obtain data it could use in meeting its policy goal. It commissioned the Lewin Group to determine the cost savings associated with medical nutrition therapy services and then launched its first public relations campaign to educate policymakers about the study findings.[7]

Another type of planning is project management. Community nutritionists who implement diabetes education programs, conduct citywide hypertension screenings, and assess the iron status of inner-city school children are all involved in project management. You have participated in project management through the case study activities in this book. Project management involves coordinating a set of activities that are typically limited to one program or intervention. It requires setting goals and objectives and outlining the project's **critical path**, the series of tasks and activities that will take the longest time to complete. Any delay in the activities on this path will delay the project's completion.[8] Managers work to spot and then remove bottlenecks, thus improving work flow along the critical path.[9] Refer to the case study later in this chapter for a discussion of the critical path for the Heartworks for Women program.

Planning Deciding what to do and when, where, and how to do it. Planning facilitates finding solutions to problems and is the basis for good management.

Strategic planning Long-term planning that addresses an organization's overall goals.

Operational planning Short-term planning that focuses on the activities and actions required to meet the organization's goals.

Project management A plan that coordinates a limited set of activities around a single program or intervention.

Critical path In a complex project, the series of tasks that takes the longest amount of time to complete.

Values, Goals, and Strategies of the Academy's Strategic Plan[a]

Vision

Optimizing health through food and nutrition.

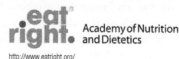

http://www.eatright.org/

Mission

Empowering members to be food and nutrition leaders.

Values

- *Customer Focus*—Meet the needs and exceed the expectations of all customers
- *Integrity*—Act ethically with accountability for lifelong learning, commitment to excellence, and professionalism
- *Innovation*—Embrace change with creativity and strategic thinking
- *Social Responsibility*—Make decisions with consideration for inclusivity as well as environmental, economic, and social implications
- *Diversity*—Recognize and respect differences in culture, ethnicity, age, gender, race, creed, religion, sexual orientation, physical ability, politics, and socioeconomic characteristics

Goal 1: The public trusts and chooses registered dietitian nutritionists as food, nutrition, and health experts.	**Goal 2:** Academy members optimize the health of individuals and populations they serve.	**Goal 3:** Members and prospective members view the Academy as vital to professional success.
Outcomes and Measures	**Outcomes and Measures**	**Outcomes and Measures**
1. Increases in members' perception of Academy achievement of strategic goals	1. Increases in members' perception of Academy achievement of strategic goals	1. Increases in members' perception of Academy achievement of strategic goals
2. Increases in visibility of the Academy to media and consumers, via *www.eatright.org* and other media outlets (online, print, and broadcast)	2. Increases in Affiliate Advocacy, Dietetic Practice Group, Academy Committee and Academy Employee Engagement Indices	2. Increases in Academy membership over time
3. Maintenance or increases in consumer-rated credibility of RDNs, NDTRs, and the Academy	3. Increases in level of collaboration (e.g., more engagement) that strengthens relevant partnerships to promote legislative efforts, including more influential partners, members of Congress and federal agencies[b]	3. Increases in membership market share of nutrition and dietetics practitioners, and students in accredited programs
4. Increases in number of RDN and NDTR appointments to external organizations	4. Increases in utilization of the EAL, an Academy member benefit	4. Increases in perceived value of Academy membership
5. Increases in number of invitations to present Academy initiatives to external medical and other health care disciplines and their organizations		5. Increases in the diversity of nutrition and dietetics professionals
		6. Increases in utilization of *www.eatrightPRO.org*, an Academy member benefit
		7. Increases in the number of nutrition and dietetics practitioners
		8. Increases in enrollment in supervised practice programs

[a] The Academy has identified a fourth goal: Goal 4: Members collaborate across disciplines with international food and nutrition communities; available at *www.eatright.org/strategicplan.*

[b] The Academy has identified several priority food and nutrition issues in which Academy members can make a significant impact. They include aging, child nutrition, food and food safety, health literacy and nutrition advancement, medical nutrition therapy and Medicare/Medicaid, nutrition monitoring and research, and obesity/overweight/healthy weight management.

Source: Academy of Nutrition and Dietetics, 2014–2015 Strategic Plan; used with permission. The Academy of Nutrition and Dietetics strategic plan is subject to change.

Organizing

Organizing is the process by which carefully formulated plans are carried out. Managers must arrange and group human and nonhuman resources into workable units to achieve organizational goals. Thus, certain structures must be in place to guide employees in their activities and decision making. Imagine the confusion that would result if you had a problem and didn't know who your supervisor was! In this section, we describe organization structures and how people are managed as part of the process of organizing.

Organization Structures Just as a building's layout—the arrangement of offices, windows, hallways, restrooms, and stairwells—affects the way people work, so does an organization's structure.[10] The organization structure is the formal pattern of interactions and activities designed by management to link the tasks that employees perform to achieve the organization's goals. The word *formal* is used intentionally here to distinguish management's official operating structure from the informal patterns of interaction that exist in all organizations.[11] In developing the organization structure, managers consider how to assign tasks and responsibilities, how to define jobs, how to group individual employees to carry out certain tasks, and how to institute mechanisms for reporting on progress.

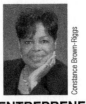

Constance Brown-Riggs

ENTREPRENEUR IN ACTION

As owner of CBR Nutrition Enterprises, Constance Brown-Riggs, MSEd, RD, CDE, CDN, is a recognized expert on the subject of nutrition, diabetes, and the cultural issues that impact the health of African Americans with diabetes. Says Constance: "As a registered dietitian, a certified diabetes educator in private practice, and a national speaker, I've had the opportunity to work with thousands of individuals—responding to their questions, clearing their confusion, easing their fears, and helping them create action plans for living well with diabetes. 'Diversify' is the operative word for a successful full-time private practice. My specialty is diabetes—and everything I do supports that mission. As an author, my books, articles, and educational tools have afforded me the opportunity to shorten the cultural distance between African Americans with diabetes and their health care providers. As a consultant to industry, I've had the opportunity to ensure that people with diabetes receive credible information." She also writes a blog, Diabetes: Don't Claim It! Manage It! (*www.eatingsoulfully.com/blog*). Find out more sage advice about developing your own career at *www.cengagebrain.com*.

In organizing their employees, managers may find an organization chart helpful. Organization charts give employees information about the major functions of departments, relationships among departments, channels of supervision, lines of authority, and certain position titles within units.[12] According to the organization chart for a typical public health department (shown in **Figure 18-2**), the community nutritionist who coordinates the

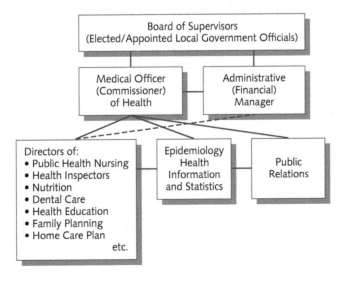

FIGURE 18-2

Organization Chart for a Hypothetical Local Health Department

Source: J. M. Last, *Public Health and Human Ecology* (Stamford, CT: Appleton & Lange, 1998), p. 323. Reprinted by permission of the author.

maternal, infant, and childcare programs reports to the department manager, the director of nutrition, who in turn reports to the medical health officer. Nontraditional organization charts, in which employees have roughly the same rank, also exist. A "web" format, such as the one shown in **Figure 18-3**, exhibits no strict hierarchy of authority. This format has the advantage of promoting teamwork and consensual decision making, but it can create confusion about authority and responsibility. This design seems to work well in small companies and organizations.

Organization charts help establish lines of communication and procedures, but they do not depict rigid systems. An organization's informal structure, depicted humorously in **Figure 18-4**, is often quite powerful and sometimes paints a more realistic picture of how the organization actually works. The informal structure arises spontaneously from employees' interactions, brief alliances, and friendships with coworkers throughout the organization.[13]

Another essential dimension of organization structure is departmentalization, or the manner in which employees are clustered into units, units into departments, and departments into divisions or other larger categories. Departmentalization directly affects how managers carry out their duties, supervise their employees, and monitor group dynamics and perspectives. An important aspect of departmentalization is the **span of management**, or **span of control**—that is, the number of subordinates who report directly to a specific manager.[14] Deciding how many employees should report to a single manager is not a trivial decision. When a manager must supervise a large number of employees directly, he or she may feel overwhelmed and have difficulty coordinating tasks and keeping on schedule; with too few employees to supervise, he or she may feel underutilized and disaffected. The ideal span of management has not been identified precisely. Some researchers argue that the range is about 5 to 25 employees, depending on the level of organization; theoretically, lower-level managers can supervise more employees directly than managers higher in the hierarchy. Napoleon once remarked, "No man can command more than five distinct bodies in the same theater of war." Most management experts now recommend that each manager directly supervise only three to seven subordinates.[15]

Organization charts
A line diagram that depicts the broad outlines of an organization's structure and suggests the reporting relationships among employees.

Span of management or **span of control** The number of subordinates who report directly to a specific manager.

FIGURE 18-3

Nontraditional Organization Chart for Nutrition in Action In this nontraditional organization structure, employees have roughly the same rank and there is no strict hierarchy of authority.

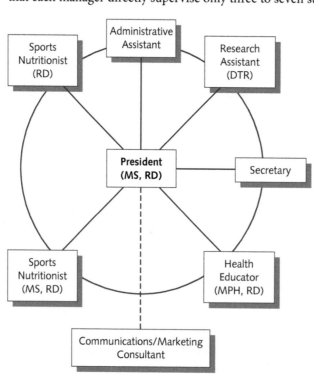

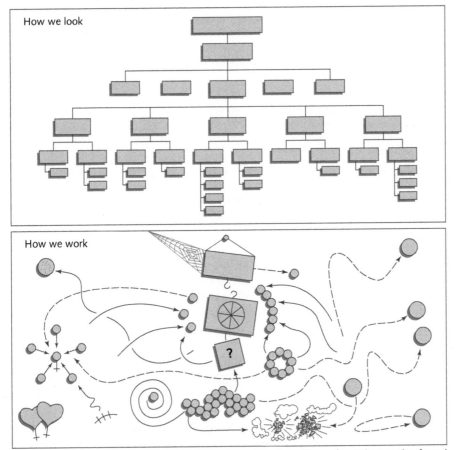

FIGURE 18-4 The Typical Organization Chart on Paper and in Practice

Source: *Organizational Behavior: Concepts and Applications*, 4th ed. by Gray/Starke. © 1988. Reprinted by permission of Prentice-Hall, Inc., Upper Saddle River, NJ.

How an organization looks on paper differs from how it really works. Whereas the formal organization structure shows the lines of authority and how communications should travel, the informal organization reveals the actual patterns of social interaction between employees in different units of the organization.

Another method of coordinating an organization's activities is through **delegation**, or the assignment of part of a manager's work to others. "Everyone knows about delegating, but not too many people do it, and fewer still do it well."[16] The inability to delegate work to others has felled many a fast-track manager.[17] Some people do the work themselves because they don't realize they can delegate it, don't know how to get the most out of a computer, or don't appreciate how delegating work enables them to work more efficiently. **Table 18-1** gives tips on how managers can delegate some activities to their employees.

Line and staff relationships also help clarify an organization's structure. A person in a **line position** has direct responsibility for achieving the organization's goals and objectives. The term *staff* is commonly used to refer to the groups of employees who work in a particular unit or department—for example, the director of nutrition in a public health department is said to supervise the nutrition staff. In management practice, however, *staff* has a particular meaning. An employee in a **staff position** assists those in line positions. To some extent, the concept of line and staff positions is a holdover from eighteenth- and nineteenth-century management theory, but the terms are still used today in many organizations to help employees identify individuals who have the authority and responsibility for fulfilling the organization's mandate.

Delegation The assignment to others of part of a manager's work, along with both the responsibility and the authority necessary to achieve the expected results.

Line position A position with the authority and responsibility to achieve the organization's main goals and objectives.

Staff position A position whose primary purpose is to assist those in line positions.

TABLE 18-1 Tips for Delegating Your Work to Others

- The first step to take when delegating your work to subordinates is to evaluate their skill levels and the difficulty of the task. The trick is to select the employee with the appropriate skills who will find the task challenging but not frustrating.

- Once you have chosen the best employee, give him or her all the information needed to do the job well. Be honest about the work; if it's drudgery, say so.

- Do these three things to ensure success:
  1. Give the employee responsibility for completing the project or task.
  2. Hold the employee accountable for the results.
  3. Provide the employee with the authority to make needed decisions, direct others to help with the project, and carry out actions as required.

- Make sure the employee has the necessary materials, equipment, time, and funds to complete the project.

- Evaluate the employee's progress periodically and be prepared to accept a less-than-perfect result.

Source: Adapted from L. Baum, "Delegating Your Way to Job Survival," *Business Week* (November 2, 1987), 206.

Job design The specification of tasks and activities associated with a particular job.

Job analysis The systematic collection and recording of information about a job's purpose, its major duties, the conditions under which it is performed, and the knowledge, skills, and abilities needed to perform the job effectively.

Job Design and Analysis

Managers in community nutrition are responsible for **job design**—that is, for determining the various duties associated with each job in their area. They sometimes need to conduct a **job analysis** to determine the purpose of a job, the skill set and educational background required to carry it out, and the manner in which the employee holding that job interacts with others. The formal outcome of a job analysis is the preparation of a job description.[18]

A job description helps employees understand what is expected of them and to whom they report. Although there is no standard format, most job descriptions include the items shown in **Table 18-2**.[19] The job description serves as a basis for rating and classifying jobs, setting wages and salaries, and conducting performance appraisals (described later). It helps organizations comply with the accrediting, contractual, legal, and regulatory directives of the government or other institutions, and it provides a basis for decisions about promotions and training. In addition, it can be adapted for use in recruiting and hiring prospective employees. For example, the text of a position announcement to be published in a newspaper or journal can be taken from the job description. A sample job description for a nutritionist with the FirstRate Spa and Health Resort is given in **Figure 18-5**.

Human Resource Management

Paying attention to the people who produce a product or service is what human resource management is all about. Community nutritionists report being involved in several aspects of managing people, including recruiting

TABLE 18-2 Components of a Job Description

- **Job title.** The job title clarifies the position and its skill level (e.g., director, supervisor, assistant, or secretary).

- **Immediate supervisor.** The job description states the position and title of the immediate supervisor.

- **Job summary.** The job summary is a short statement of the purpose of the job and its major tasks and activities.

- **Job duties.** This section of the job description is a detailed statement of the specific duties of the job and how these duties are carried out.

- **Job specifications.** This is a list of minimum hiring requirements, usually derived from the job analysis; it includes the skill requirements for the job, such as educational level, licensure requirements, and experience (usually expressed in years), and any specific knowledge, advanced training, manual skills, and communication skills (both oral and written) required to do the job. The physical demands of the job, if any, including working conditions and job hazards, are included here.

Source: Adapted from J. G. Liebler and C. R. McConnell, *Management Principles for Health Care Professionals*, 5th ed. (Sudbury, MA: Jones and Bartlett, 2008).

FIGURE 18-5 Sample Job Description

FirstRate Spa and Health Resort
Department of Human Resources

Position Title: Community nutritionist

Responsible to: Director of health promotion

Responsibilities: Under the general direction of the director of health promotion, the nutritionist is responsible for developing, implementing, and evaluating the spa's risk reduction programs.

Job Duties: The nutritionist has the following duties and responsibilities:
- Develops, implements, and evaluates the spa's risk reduction programs in the areas of smoking cessation, blood cholesterol reduction, stress management, and diabetes control.
- Assists the director in developing marketing strategies for the risk reduction program.
- Assists the director in developing budgets.
- Tracks program revenue and expenses.
- Works with other spa nutritionists and staff to develop marketing tools and teaching/instructional aids.
- Participates as required in coordinating research projects.

Qualifications and Experience: The nutritionist should have the following qualifications and experience:
- A university degree in nutrition
- Certification as a registered dietitian nutritionist (RD/RDN)
- Two years of experience teaching community-based courses or programs

Skills: The nutritionist should have the following skills:
- Demonstrated ability to write and give presentations
- Experience using spreadsheet, web design, and weblog software, social media, and teleconferencing tools is desirable
- Experience using evidence-based guidelines is desirable
- Ability to work with people of all ages and backgrounds

Date: June 2016

people for the organization and evaluating the performance of their employees.[20] Both of these activities are described in the next paragraphs.

Staffing Staffing is the set of human resource activities designed to recruit individuals to help meet the organization's goals and objectives. Recruitment has two distinct phases: attracting applicants and hiring candidates.[21] Both direct and indirect recruiting strategies are used to attract applicants. Direct methods include placing "Help Wanted" ads in print or online newspapers, job sites, and journals, sending personalized letters to potential applicants, and participating in job recruitment fairs. Indirect recruiting strategies include activities that keep the organization's name in the public's eye, such as collaborative projects with other institutions and training sessions for professionals.

An important aspect of recruiting is **affirmative action**, which includes all activities designed to ensure and increase equal employment opportunities for groups protected by federal laws and regulations. A significant law in this area is Title VII of the Civil Rights Act of 1964, which forbids employment discrimination on the basis of gender, race, color, religion, or national origin. Most organizations have some type of affirmative action plan that details its goals and policies related to hiring, training, and promoting

Affirmative action Any activity undertaken by employers to increase equal employment opportunities for groups protected by federal equal employment opportunity (EEO) laws and regulations.

protected groups. In fact, organizations with federal contracts exceeding $50,000 and with 50 or more employees must file an affirmative action plan with the Department of Labor's Office of Federal Contract Compliance Programs; others may develop such plans on a voluntary basis.[22]

The hiring process involves conducting job interviews with potential candidates, screening applicants, selecting the best candidate, checking references, and, finally, offering the position. In some cases, two or three suitable candidates will be invited back for interviews with key managers in other departments or divisions before a final candidate is chosen.

Evaluating Job Performance Providing feedback to employees about their performance is essential to maintaining good working relationships and can occur informally at any time. In the daily course of solving unexpected problems and reviewing the progress on a project, managers in community nutrition have ample opportunity to update their employees about their performance. In fact, the best managers spend up to 40% of their time in face-to-face interactions with their employees that allow time for performance feedback.[23]

---

66 *Employees want to hear from management, and they want management to listen to them.* 99

—D. Keith Denton

Performance appraisal A manager's formal review of an employee's performance on the job.

The **performance appraisal** is a formal method of providing feedback to an employee. It is designed to influence the employee in a positive, constructive manner and involves defining the organization's expectations for employee performance and discussing how the employee's recent performance compares with those expectations. The performance appraisal is used to help define future performance goals, determine training needs and merit pay increases, and assess the employee's potential for advancement. Because employees are often uneasy about the review process, managers must take care to be objective in their rating of performance. One way to reduce employees' discomfort is to let them know in advance how the process works and what to expect during the performance appraisal interview. Employees are most likely to have a favorable impression of the process when they are aware of the evaluation criteria used, have an opportunity to participate in the process, and are able to discuss their career development.[24]

The performance appraisal interview is a good time for reviewing and changing both organizational and personal goals. Managers who spend time helping subordinates develop their personal goals are more likely to achieve their organization's goals because setting challenging personal goals is linked strongly with performance.[25]

The key to conducting a good performance appraisal interview is to start with clear objectives, focus on observable behavior, and avoid vague, subjective statements of a personal nature. Consult **Table 18-3** for a list of questions that can be used in talking about performance and giving constructive criticism.[26]

Leading

Leading is the management function that involves influencing others to achieve the organization's goals and objectives. It focuses on the horizon, asking what and why, whereas managing focuses on the bottom line, asking how and when.[27] (Reread the Professional Focus feature on leadership that appears in Chapter 11.) Organizations need strong leaders *and* good managers.

Use the process outlined here to offer constructive criticism to your employees without making them defensive. These questions can be used in a performance appraisal interview, but they lend themselves to many other job-related discussions. Most people questioned in this manner make specific suggestions to improve their performance.

TABLE 18-3 How to Provide Constructive Criticism

- **Initiate.** "How would you rate your performance during the last six months?" or "How do you feel about your performance during the last quarter?"

- **Listen.** If you get a general response like "Fine," or "Pretty good," or "8 on a 10-point scale," follow up with a more focused question: "What in particular comes to mind?" or "What have you been particularly pleased with?" Your objective is to discuss a positive topic raised by the employee.

- **Focus.** "You mentioned that you were particularly satisfied with … Let's talk further about that aspect of your job."

- **"How" probe.** "How did you approach … ?" or "What method did you use?"

- **"Why" probe.** "How did you happen to choose that approach?" or "What was your rationale for that method?"

- **"Results" probe.** "How has it worked out for you?" or "What results have you achieved?"

- **Plan.** "Knowing what you know now, what would you have done differently?" or "What changes would you make if you worked on this again?"

Source: J. G. Goodale, "Seven Ways to Improve Performance Appraisals," *HRMagazine* 38 (1993): 79.

Motivating Employees An important function of managers is to motivate their employees to "get the job done." Barcy Fox, a vice president with Maritz Performance Improvement Company, comments, "Your employees aren't you. What works for you won't work for them. What motivates you to pursue a goal won't motivate them. Until you grasp that, you won't set attainable goals for your workers."[28] There is no single strategy for motivating employees to perform, and opinions differ on exactly what managers need to do to stimulate motivation. Peter Drucker, a well-known management consultant and author, argued that managers can do four things to obtain peak performance from their employees:[29]

- *Set high standards and stick to them.* Employees become demoralized when managers do not hold themselves to the same high standards set for other workers in the organization. Employees are stimulated to work hard with managers who expect a lot of themselves, believe in excellence, and set a good example.
- *Put the right person in the right job.* Employees take pride in meeting a challenge and doing a job well. Their sense of accomplishment enhances their performance. Underutilizing employees' skills destroys their motivation.
- *Keep employees informed about their performance.* Employees should be able to control, measure, and evaluate their own performance. To do this, they need to know and understand the standard against which their performance is being compared. The job description and performance appraisal interview help keep employees informed about what managers expect of them. Keep in mind the unwritten rule of managing people: Put praise in writing. But when you must reprimand an employee, do so verbally and in private.
- *Allow employees to be a part of the process.* One means of motivating employees is to give them a managerial vision, a sense of how their work contributes to the success of the project, program, or organization. In a sense, a manager cannot "give" his own vision to his employees, but he can allow them to help mold and shape the vision, thereby making it theirs as well as his.

Communicating with Employees

Communicating is a critical managerial activity that can take many forms. Verbal communication is the written or oral use of words to communicate messages. Written communications can take the form of reports, résumés, telephone and e-mail messages, memoranda, procedure manuals, policy manuals, and letters. Oral communications, or the spoken word, usually take place in forums such as telephone conversations, committee meetings, and formal presentations. Good managers are skilled in both of these areas (review the Professional Focus features in Chapter 3 ["Being an Effective Speaker"] and Chapter 16 ["Being an Effective Writer"]). Nonverbal communication in the form of gestures, facial expressions, and so-called body language is also important. Tone of voice—the *way* something is said, as opposed to *what* is said—sometimes relays information more effectively than the words themselves. Even the placement of office furniture communicates certain elements of attitude and style. Reportedly, nonverbal communication accounts for between 65 and 93% of what actually gets communicated.[30]

Becoming a good communicator means paying attention to people and events, observing the nuances of nonverbal and verbal communication, and becoming a good listener. Open communication in an organization does not occur by accident. It results from the daily use of certain techniques and skills that promote communication. Merck, a pharmaceutical company, uses an approach called face-to-face communication. The four rules on which this communication is built are listed in **Table 18-4**.[31] Communicating effectively with coworkers is a skill that, like other skills described in this book, can be acquired with practice and determination.

The team leader for the Heartworks for Women course in Case Study 1, for example, learns of a conflict between two staff members—each believes that she is the main liaison with the design company hired to prepare the marketing materials. The liaison has a key role in keeping the project on schedule and also has the opportunity to become involved in the organization's other marketing campaigns. The team leader determines, first, that the design company will want to deal with only one staff member and, second, that the rivalry between these two staff members has been friendly but has the potential to be disruptive. She schedules a meeting with the two of them, asking them to think about the problem and how it might be resolved. During the meeting, the three of them talk about the liaison's role, the responsibilities and activities of each staff member, and certain projects "in the works" within the department. The leader aims to keep the discussion open and amiable. She succeeds in getting the more senior staff person to agree to allow the junior staff person, who has worked with the design company previously, to serve as liaison; she gives the

TABLE 18-4 Four Rules of Face-to-Face Communication

- **Be candid.** Any questions or comments that arise during face-to-face interactions (be they performance appraisal interviews or committee meetings) should be addressed truthfully. If appropriate, indicate that you cannot answer the question because of its confidential nature. If you do not know the answer to a question, say so.

- **Be prepared.** Ask participants to submit questions or topics for discussion several weeks or days before the meeting is scheduled to occur. Organize an agenda, preferably a written one. This strategy has the advantage of ensuring that topics of interest to you and your employees are covered. If you develop a written agenda, distribute it to the participants before the meeting so that they can arrive prepared.

- **Encourage participation.** Conduct the face-to-face meeting in a relaxed and friendly atmosphere where people feel comfortable expressing their ideas.

- **Focus on listening, not judging.** When sensitive topics arise, try not to appear upset or judgmental. Listen carefully to questions and the discussion they prompt. Pay attention to nonverbal cues and group dynamics. The essence of good communications is simple: Treat others with respect.

Source: Adapted from Merck's face-to-face communication, in D. K. Denton, *Recruitment, Retention, and Employee Relations* (Westport, CT: Quorum Books, 1992), 158–59.

senior staff person the responsibility for developing the website content and some design elements. The leader's role in this communication process is to help the staff members appreciate each other's skills and contribution to the organization.

Controlling

Controlling is the management function concerned with regulating organizational activities so that performance meets accepted organizational standards and goals.[32] The controlling function involves determining which activities need control, establishing standards, measuring performance, and correcting deviations. Managers set up control systems—mechanisms for ensuring that resources, quality of products and services, client satisfaction, and other activities are regulated properly. Such controls help managers cope with the uncertainties that arise when plans go awry. An unforeseen reduction in the public health department's budget, for example, might force the manager of the nutrition division to reallocate personnel and impose tighter spending controls.

Community nutritionists often have responsibility for program and departmental budgets and for managing information. The Academy of Nutrition and Dietetics' role delineation study determined that managers in community or public health programs were responsible for preparing financial analyses and reports, controlling program costs, monitoring a program's financial performance, documenting a program's operations, and making decisions about capital expenditures.[33] Even entry-level community nutritionists are expected to be able to define basic financial terms, read and understand financial reports, maintain cost control of materials and projects, and, in some settings, develop plans to generate revenue.[34] Strong management skills enable community nutritionists to detect irregularities in client service or cost overruns and to handle complex projects and programs. Two aspects of the control process are described in the following paragraphs.

Financial and Budgetary Control The primary tools of financial control are two types of financial statements: balance sheets and income statements. The **balance sheet** lists the organization's assets and liabilities. Assets include cash, accounts receivable (sales of a product or service for which payment has not yet been received), inventories, and items such as buildings, machinery, and equipment. Liabilities include accounts payable (bills that must be paid to outside suppliers and the like), short- and long-term loans, and shareholders' equity such as common stock. (Government agencies and most small, independent companies do not have shareholders' equity.) The **income statement** summarizes the organization's operations over a specific time period, such as a quarter or a year. It generally lists revenues (the assets derived from selling goods and services) and expenses (the costs incurred in producing the revenues). The difference between revenues and expenses is the organization's profit or loss—sometimes called the *bottom line*.

Financial control is typically managed through an operating budget, which is "a plan for the accomplishment of programs related to objectives and goals within a definite time period, including an estimate of resources required, together with an estimate of the resources available."[35] Budgets can be planned for the organization as a whole or for subunits such as divisions, departments, and programs. **Budgeting** is closely linked to planning. It is the process of stating in quantitative terms (usually dollars) the planned organizational activities for a given period of time. Although the terms *budgeting* and *accounting* are sometimes used interchangeably, they are not the same thing. Accounting is a purely financial activity, whereas budgeting is both a financial and a program planning activity.

Because all expenses of an organization—everything from pencils and paper clips to salaries and benefits—must be accounted for, the budgeting process requires considerable

Balance sheet A financial statement that depicts, at given intervals (such as monthly), an organization's assets and the claims against those assets (liabilities) at that time.

Income statement A financial statement that summarizes the organization's financial position over a specified period, such as a quarter or a year.

Budgeting The process of stating in quantitative terms, usually dollars, the planned organizational activities for a given period of time.

planning and managing. It usually begins with a review of the previous budget period and proceeds to the development of a new budget. Most programs and projects receive a monthly budgetary review. The primary areas to be examined include total project funding, expenditures to date, current estimated cost to complete the project, anticipated profit or loss, and an explanation of any deviations from the planned budget expenditure. Periodic status summaries help managers control resources and adhere to the planning schedule.[36] The internal approval process for a new budget can involve bargaining, compromise, and outright competition for scarce resources. Managers who can justify their budget requests are more likely to be successful in getting funds appropriated for their program's projects and activities.

Information Management In the course of your community work, you will need to collect, organize, retrieve, and analyze many types of data and information. At the very least, you will need to know about the health and nutrition status of the population in your district, the demographic profile of your client base, how people in your community use your organization's programs and services, how cost-effective your programs are, and what expenses your staff incurred in carrying out their program activities. To this end, **nutrition informatics** can be used in community nutrition practice to guide decision making, develop programs and services, evaluate outcomes, and improve professional practice. Nutrition informatics is evident in the computer application areas provided in **Table 18-5**.[37]

At this point, a distinction must be made between data and information. **Data** are unanalyzed facts and figures. For example, a survey of infants in your community shows that over the past 12 months, 36 out of 478 infants had birthweights less than 2,500 grams. These data don't mean much on their own; to be meaningful, they must be transformed

Nutrition informatics The effective retrieval, organization, storage, and optimum use of information, data, and knowledge for food- and nutrition-related problem solving and decision making.

Data Unanalyzed facts and figures.

TABLE 18-5 Nutrition Informatics: Utilization of Computer Applications and Technology in the Nutrition Field

PRACTICE AREA	EXAMPLES
Clinical Nutrition	Electronic health records; documentation of nutrition care process; access to evidence-based guidelines and protocols; nutritional analysis of menus, patient's dietary intake, enteral feedings, and modified diets; use of personal digital assistants (PDAs), smartphones, or similar devices
Communication	Data-sharing networks with other departments; e-mail and chat communications; listserv networking; websites; other e-communication methods (podcasts, blogs, YouTube)
Community Nutrition	Collection and analysis of needs assessment data on individuals and populations; identification and retrieval of relevant global, national, state, and local health-related population data and information sources to guide program planning and evaluation; use of program design models and evaluation tools; grant management; financial management and reimbursement systems; multimedia education and training systems; and computer-based diet instruction (e.g., web-based programs)
Foodservice Management	Budgeting; financial management; purchasing and inventory management; recipe and menu planning; food procurement, preparation, and delivery
Research	Statistical computation and reporting of study results, use of electronic library databases, and other sources of electronic reference documents

Source: Adapted from American Dietetic Association, "HOD Backgrounder: Nutrition Informatics," Fall 2008; see also *www.eatrightpro.org/resources/advocacy/quality-health-care/hitech-act*.

into **information**. For example, by processing the data further (perhaps converting the data to percentages or calculating the mean weights), the manager can compare these figures with those from previous reporting years. A change in the figures may signal the need to reassess program goals and reallocate resources to help prevent low birthweight.

The primary purpose of information is to help managers make decisions. Information is a decision support tool in that it helps managers answer these questions: What do we want to do? How do we do it? Did we do what we said we were going to do? The first question addresses the planning function of management, the second the organizing function, and the third the controlling function. Managers begin the decision-making process by organizing the data into usable information. Then they specify the means by which the data are to be analyzed. This analysis usually involves sorting, formatting, extracting, and transforming the data via certain statistical methods. Finally, managers interpret the output and prepare reports that summarize the information. Decisions are then based on the figures in the reports.[38] Of course, managers' decisions are only as good as their information. Constant vigilance is required to prevent GIGO (garbage in/garbage out) syndrome.

Computers make the processing of information both simpler and more complex. It is simpler because many aspects of data analysis are carried out on computers and not by hand. It is more complex because one must choose from hundreds of computer systems and software programs. Because computers can produce reams of data very quickly, managers are apt to become overwhelmed by the magnitude and diversity of the data available to them.

To be useful, information must be:[39]

1. *Relevant*. Although it is sometimes difficult to know precisely what information is needed, managers should try to identify the information most likely to help in making decisions.
2. *Accurate*. If information is inaccurate or incorrect, the quality of the decision will certainly be questionable.
3. *Timely*. Information must be available when it is needed.
4. *Complete*. Information must cover all of the areas important to the decision-making process.
5. *Concise*. Information should be concise, providing a summary of the items central to the decision.

Information Data that have been analyzed or processed into a form that is meaningful for decision makers. Information may include qualitative or quantitative data, scientific papers, evidence-based practice guidelines, public health resource databases, current news, research findings, and more.

Management Issues for Heartworks for Women: Case Study 1

The development and design of the Heartworks for Women program has spanned several chapters in this text, beginning in Chapter 4. We have discussed how it fits into a larger intervention strategy, the choice of program format and nutrition messages, and the elements of the marketing plan. In this section, we describe three management issues related to the program: the critical path, the budget, and grantsmanship.

The Critical Path

The community nutritionist who leads team 2—the team responsible for the nutrition intervention activities for the Heartworks for Women program, as discussed in Chapter 5—develops a timeline early in the planning stages, when the program plan (also described in Chapter 5) is outlined. A variety of formats can be used for this activity. Figure 17-7 on page 683 is one example of a timetable and shows key marketing activities for the Heartworks for Women program. (In reality, the marketing timetable would be developed after the timeline showing the critical path.) Because the program will be launched the following April, the team 2 leader lays out the paths that must be completed to ensure that all program elements have been finalized before the launch date. She plots a timeline, shown in **Figure 18-6**. The critical path consists of the steps involved in program design and evaluation—a process estimated to take seven months. Two minor paths—developing the marketing plan and testing the appropriateness of the nutrition messages for the target population—are estimated to require several months as well. Any glitches in finalizing the program will produce delays in finalizing the marketing plan. For example, some elements of the marketing plan will be incomplete if the nutrition messages aren't finalized on time.

Several milestones appear on the timetable: early June, when program planning begins; August 1, when the formative evaluation has been completed; December 31, when the program must be finalized; January 15, when the marketing plan is finalized; and April 18, the date of the launch. These are the points at which major tasks must be completed on time or the program launch date will be delayed.

Once the timeline has been developed, what is the next step for the community nutritionist? First, she shares it with her team members to confirm that it is reasonable and that all activities have been accounted for. Next, she breaks down each path into a group of activities that can be monitored. For example, the program launch requires that the following tasks be completed: Choose and confirm the date, location, and time for the launch; prepare a list of invitees; develop and send invitations; prepare and send press releases; prepare and finalize all advertising about the launch; choose a menu; arrange for delivery of food and beverages; outline the launch program (e.g., opening remarks); contact guest speakers and send a confirmation letter to each of them; arrange for any decorating of the facility; and arrange interviews with the media. Completion dates for these activities are also determined.

FIGURE 18-6

Timeline for Determining the Critical Path for the Heartworks for Women Program: Case Study 1

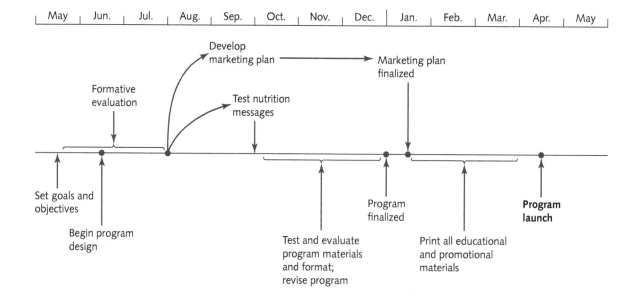

PROGRAMS IN **ACTION**

The Better Health Restaurant Challenge

Public and private partnerships can advance nutrition education efforts by helping to ensure the delivery of consistent messages. Perhaps most important, such partnerships can combine resources to achieve an effective nutrition education program—more than any one party may be able to accomplish alone.[1]

A variety of partners can become involved and provide leadership for the design and development of health promotion and chronic disease prevention programs. Coalition building can take place among community-based nutrition and health professionals, opinion leaders, and local businesses. It is important to involve the food industry in the implementation of prevention programs. Voluntary community and health organizations involved in disease prevention work include the American Cancer Society, the American Heart Association, and numerous others. Such volunteer organizations are often effective in promoting community-based nutrition and dietary interventions and risk-reduction programs.[2]

An increasing proportion of food dollars is spent on foods eaten or purchased away from home. Portion sizes of foods prepared away from home often exceed those recommended in the MyPlate Food Guide—three-cup portions of pasta and nine-ounce cooked portions of meat are not unusual. Furthermore, estimating portion sizes when eating out is difficult—even for nutrition students. Balanced meals—with appropriate portions from at least three food groups—can be difficult to find. Foods tend to be prepared with generous amounts of fat. Additionally, healthier items are limited or may not be on the menu.

Consumers want healthy menu options. The availability of healthy foods in restaurants helps individuals eat more responsibly. Sales of menu items that are promoted as healthy have been shown to increase during special programs and campaigns.

Partnerships and coalitions can be a highly effective way to coordinate healthy-eating programs in the community. They extend and enhance individual resources as partners work together to deliver consistent nutrition messages. A partnership between health providers and restaurants is a win–win situation for the partners and for the community: The health provider's message is reinforced in local restaurants, the restaurant's name and reputation are enhanced, and consumers have access to healthy food when dining out.

The Better Health Restaurant Challenge (BHRC) demonstrates how health professionals, HMOs, restaurants, consumers, and health organizations can benefit from partnership. The month-long challenge was an annual contest to determine the best-tasting heart-healthy restaurant menu items in the Minneapolis/St. Paul area. The program was sponsored by Health-Partners, a large Minnesota-based managed-care organization. Health organizations such as the American Heart Association and the American Cancer Society received a financial contribution from HealthPartners on behalf of winning restaurants.

Goals and Objectives

The goals of the BHRC were to increase the availability of tasty, healthy menu items in restaurants and to increase restaurant patrons' selection of healthy menu items, even among diners who would not ordinarily do so. To achieve these goals, program objectives included promoting participating restaurants, menu items, HealthPartners, and heart-healthy eating to the community; encouraging the long-term availability of healthy menu items; providing healthy dining options in a variety of eating establishments; and increasing consumer and restaurant participation in the BHRC.

Methodology

Restaurants in the Minneapolis area were contacted by mail and telephone to acquaint them with the program and interest them in participating. Dietitians from HealthPartners also attended trade shows and restaurant association meetings to solicit participants. (In the first years of the program, dietitians cold-called area restaurants. Many restaurants now call on their own to sign up.)

Participating restaurants agreed to work with HealthPartners' registered dietitians to create at least two heart-healthy menu items, to train restaurant staff to promote the healthy items, to keep at least one heart-healthy item on the menu for one month, and to extend a 20% discount on heart-healthy food items to members of HealthPartners. Participating restaurants and their menu items were widely promoted by HealthPartners through the media and extensive advertising.

HealthPartners and its dietitians developed and funded numerous materials, including point-of-purchase promotions of the healthy menu items. They also created ballots so that diners could rate the healthier menu items based on taste; the ballots were passed out by restaurant staff to diners who ordered the healthy items. The slogan to encourage diners to participate in the BHRC was "Enjoy Being a Food Critic? We Savor Your Opinion."

Restaurants with the highest overall taste ratings were declared winners. Winners in the nine categories in which diners voted were announced to the media.

Results

The number of restaurants and locations participating in the BHRC has more than tripled since the program's inception. Over that same period, the number of different menu items has increased from 60 to 280.

Approximately 14,000 diners completed ballots. Over half reported that items tasted better than expected. The average taste rating was 4.13 out of 5. An overwhelming majority of diners said that they would order the heart-healthy item again and that the BHRC program increased the likelihood of their ordering healthier menu items in the future. Over 90% of participating restaurants kept their healthy menu items on the menu after the program ended.

Lessons Learned

Treating diners as food critics increased participation, as did the challenge's focus on foods that taste good. Big advertising budgets are not necessary. Partners such as the local chapter of the American Heart Association, area hospitals, and even community leaders can help get the word out.

Source: Adapted from *Community Nutritionary* (White Plains, NY: Dannon Institute, Fall 2001). Used with permission. For more information about the Awards for Excellence in Community Nutrition, go to *www.dannon-institute.org.*

The Operating Budget The operating budget is a statement of the financial plan for the program. It outlines the revenues and expenses related to the program's operation. Revenues for the Heartworks for Women program will be derived from the enrollment fees for individual participants and the sales of merchandise such as coffee mugs and T-shirts, as shown in **Table 18-6**. Some expenses, such as the design of

TABLE 18-6

Sample Operating Budget for the Heartworks for Women Program

Revenue		
Program income ($60/participant		$270,000
× 75 participants/worksite		
× 60 worksites)		
Sales of merchandise		4,500
	Total revenue:	$274,500
Expenses		
Direct expenses		
Personnel—salaries		$163,500
Telephone/Internet		4,250
Equipment		2,000
Travel		1,575
Postage		3,500
Office supplies		8,000
Instructional materials		5,500
Advertising and promotion		10,000
Design		3,750
Printing		3,000
	Total direct expenses	$205,075
Indirect expenses		
Personnel—benefits (28.7%)		$ 46,925
Rent		7,800
Utilities		1,200
Equipment depreciation		7,200
Maintenance and repairs		2,000
Janitorial services		4,300
	Total indirect expenses:	$69,425
	Total expenses:	$274,500
	Net revenue (expenses):	$0

the program logo and printing of educational materials, are directly related to the program; others, such as office rent and electricity, contribute indirectly to the program's costs. At the beginning of the fiscal year, the operating budget has a zero balance (net revenue minus total expenses). Expenses will be offset by anticipated revenue. Any discrepancies in either revenue or expenses will be reflected in the operating budget's monthly net balance.

Extramural Funding Early in the planning process, the team 2 leader identifies several activities for which extramural funding might be obtained. She perceives that some expenses related to the launch, such as the costs of printing banners and balloons and providing food for invitees, could be underwritten, as might the costs of printing program manuals and training materials. She sets a target figure of about $8,000 and begins networking in her community. She contacts two colleagues whose organizations have sponsored health promotion activities in the past—the manager of a leading supermarket and a registered dietitian who is the district sales representative for a national drug company—who agree to provide financial support for these activities on behalf of their organizations. She expands her network to include the owner of a popular ladies' dress shop, who is interested in "doing some community work." This contact proves profitable—the owner of the dress shop is willing to contribute $1,000 toward the launch. Other commitments are confirmed over a period of several months. The team 2 leader assures all grantors that their contributions will be acknowledged publicly and negotiates such details as the amount of the grant and the timing of the payment.

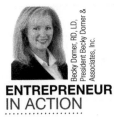

Becky Dorner, RD, LD, President Becky Dorner & Associates, Inc.

ENTREPRENEUR IN ACTION

Becky Dorner's career has focused primarily on improving nutrition care for older adults. As part of her quest to achieve this mission, in 1983 she developed Nutrition Consulting Services, Inc., a consulting practice that places registered dietitian nutritionists (RDNs) and nutrition and dietetic technicians registered (NDTRs) in settings that care for older adults. Says Becky: "As an entrepreneur, you can create the future based on your personal vision, mission, goals, and strategic plan. Entrepreneurialism is really all about serving others and building relationships with your clients, staff, colleagues, and constituents. After more than 30 years in business, my mission to improve care and quality of life for older adults continues through education and empowerment of health care professionals. Being an entrepreneur can be extremely challenging. If you have not had formal education in business or marketing, learn as much as you can. Develop a network of colleagues you can share ideas with on a regular basis. Find a mentor or coach to help you hone in on what you truly want to achieve, define your goals, and keep your focus to achieve them." Find out more about Becky online at *www.cengagebrain.com*.

The Business of Community Nutrition

Whether you work in the public or the private sector, you need strong management skills. You must be able to set a direction for your business or program; define goals and objectives; organize the delivery of your product or service; motivate people to help your organization reach its goals; allocate materials, equipment, personnel, and funds to your operations; control data systems; and provide leadership. More than ever before, management and leadership skills are needed to gain a competitive edge in what has become an increasingly competitive health care environment. As you move into the community with your ideas, products, and nutrition services, keep these four strategies for success in mind:[40]

- Continually assess the competitive environment.
- Continually assess your strengths.
- Build organizational skills.
- Build managerial (people and process) skills.

PROFESSIONAL **FOCUS**

Time Management

Time is a nonrenewable resource, a precious commodity. "Time is life," writes Alan Lakein in his best-selling book *How to Get Control of Your Time and Your Life*.[1] "It is irreversible and irreplaceable. To waste your time is to waste your life, but to master your time is to master your life and make the most of it."

Many of us have difficulty deciding how to spend our time. Every day we must choose among dozens of activities and duties, all competing for our time and attention: family, friends, work, school, shopping, sports, television, movies, hobbies. The list is endless. Given that we all have a limited amount of time available each day, how can we choose from the multitude of options that surround us? The key to effective time management, argues Lakein, is *control*.

Control Is Essential

Control means recognizing that it is easy to become overwhelmed by the number of decisions we face about how we spend our time. The secret to controlling time effectively is making conscious decisions about which activities deserve our attention and effort—and which don't. Taking control of your time means *planning* how you will spend it. Planning starts with deciding what your priorities are.

Where the Action Should Be

Stephen Covey, author of *The 7 Habits of Highly Effective People*, writes that the essence of good time management can be summarized in the following phrase: Organize and execute (in other words, *plan*) around priorities. The time management matrix, shown in **Figure 18-7**, demonstrates how most people spend their time.[2]

Covey defines activities as either "urgent" or "important." Urgent activities demand immediate attention. Important activities are those that will yield long-term results; they require a more proactive approach than urgent activities. Look at the time management matrix. Quadrant 1 activities are both urgent and important. These activities are called "crises" or "problems." All of us have to deal with Quadrant 1 activities at times. The problem with focusing constantly on Quadrant 1 activities, though, is that doing so tends to lead to stress, burnout, and a sense that we are always putting out brushfires.

Some people spend quite a bit of their time in Quadrant 3, thinking that they are in Quadrant 1. They are reacting to things that are urgent and appear important but that actually yield short-term results. People who spend their time in Quadrant 3 are likely to feel out of control. Covey believes that people who devote most of their time to Quadrant 3 and 4 activities lead irresponsible lives because they do not manage themselves and their actions.

Highly effective people spend their time in Quadrant 2 activities, such as those listed in Figure 18-7. It is through these activities that we accomplish the truly important things in life.

It's as Easy as ABC

The first step in taking control of your time is setting priorities—determining those things that are most important to you. Lakein calls this process the ABC Priority System: "A" activities have a high value, "B" items a medium value, and "C" items a low value.

Take three minutes to write down all of the things you should accomplish, or would like to accomplish, in the next three months. These activities probably fall into several categories: personal, family, community, social, school, career, financial, and spiritual goals. Don't hesitate to include some things

FIGURE 18-7 Time Management Matrix™

Source: Adapted from *The 7 Habits of Highly Effective People*, p. 151, by Stephen R. Covey.

Time Management		Urgent	Not Urgent
	Important	**1** Crises Deadlines Pressing problems Emergencies Some meetings Necessary appointments	**2** Long-range planning Productive meetings Relationship-building & networking New project development Professional development Personal health & relaxation
	Not Important	**3** Some meetings Some mail Some calls Some reports Needless interruptions	**4** Busy work Junk mail Spam mail Certain calls Mindless activities

that are off the wall. Now, for each item, assign a priority of A, B, or C. Remember, the A activities are those with the highest value in your life. In addition, rank each activity within each category: A-1, A-2, and so on; B-1, B-2, and so on.

Your A activities are top priorities, the items you want to find time for. The key to finding time for them lies not in prioritizing the activities on your schedule but in scheduling your priorities. In other words, if your A-1 activity is learning Japanese, then schedule time for it, even if you can spend only 10 or 15 minutes a day.

Keep three things in mind as you carry out this task. First, only you can decide what your priorities are. No one else can do this for you. Second, your A list will probably change over time and should be reviewed periodically. What is important to you now may not be important to you in six months. Finally, because planning in advance is the best thing you can do for yourself, write down your priorities. "A daily plan, in writing, is the single most effective time management strategy, yet only 1 person in 10 does it. The other nine will always go home muttering to themselves, 'Where did the day go?'"[3]

The Top Ten Time Wasters

People from different jobs and disciplines have similar problems managing time. A survey of 40 sales representatives and 50 engineering managers from 14 countries identified the following activities as the top time wasters:[4]

- Telephone interruptions
- Drop-in visitors
- Meetings (scheduled and unscheduled)
- Crises
- Lack of objectives, priorities, and deadlines
- Cluttered desk and personal disorganization
- Ineffective delegation
- Attempting too much at once
- Indecision and procrastination
- Lack of self-discipline

These are not the only time bandits by any means. Paperwork and e-mail messaging, inadequate staffing, too much socializing, and travel all undermine our ability to manage time well. The key to managing these time wasters is to take control of them. Schedule your telephone calls for certain periods of the day, and do not accept interruptions during "quiet" times unless an emergency arises. Minimize interruptions from colleagues and visitors. Attend only meetings that are directly related to your work.

Learn to Say No

When you set your priorities—that is, when you say yes to one thing—you must say no to something else. You will always be saying no to something. You can never do everything that you want to do or everything that everyone else wants you to do! The key to managing your time effectively is to learn to say no, firmly and courteously. Sometimes this can be difficult, for a task that is a B or C priority for you may be an A priority for someone important to you. When this happens, take a moment to consider the consequences for you, the other person, and your mutual relationship if you say no. In many cases, you can reach a compromise and maintain goodwill by deciding together how to rank an activity.

Work Smarter, Not Harder

It is a myth that the harder you work, the more you accomplish. Many workaholics fall into this trap. They are more attuned to time spent working than to time spent working effectively. Avoid the trap of thinking that time spent working is automatically time spent valuably. "If it is not quality time and quality work, you are wasting time."[5]

Mastering the principles of good time management can take several months or even years. If you experience difficulty achieving control of your time, don't give up. Keep working at it. Although your progress may seem slow, you are further along than if you had never begun this challenging process at all.

CHAPTER **SUMMARY**

The Four Functions of Management

▶ Management is the process of achieving organizational goals through planning, organizing, leading, and controlling.

▶ **Planning** is the forward-looking aspect of a manager's job; it involves setting goals and objectives and deciding how best to achieve them. Planning facilitates finding solutions to problems and is the basis for good management. Strategic planning is broad in scope and addresses the organization's overall goals. Operational planning is short-term planning that focuses on the activities and actions required to meet the organization's goals.

▶ **Organizing** focuses on distributing and arranging human and nonhuman resources so that plans can be carried out successfully.

▶ **Leading** is the management function that involves influencing others to achieve the organization's goals and objectives.

▶ **Controlling** consists of regulating activities to ensure that they meet established standards and goals. The controlling function involves determining which activities need control, establishing standards, measuring performance, and correcting deviations.

- Financial control is typically managed through an operating budget. Budgeting is the process of stating in quantitative terms, usually dollars, the planned organizational activities for a given period of time.

- Nutrition informatics is the effective retrieval, organization, storage, and optimum use of information, data, and knowledge for problem solving and decision making.

▶ Whether you work in the public or the private sector, you must be able to set a direction for your business or program; define goals and objectives; organize the delivery of your product or service; motivate people to help your organization reach its goals; allocate materials, equipment, personnel, and funds to your operations; control data systems; and provide leadership.

SUMMARY QUESTIONS

1. Describe the four functions of management.
2. Differentiate between strategic planning and operational planning.
3. Discuss some ways that you can provide constructive criticism to your employees during a performance appraisal interview.
4. As a manager, what types of things can you do to obtain peak performance from your employees?
5. Define nutrition informatics and describe examples of its utilization in community nutrition practice.

INTERNET RESOURCES

Association for Healthcare Foodservice
http://healthcarefoodservice.org

Business Tools
www.score.org

Federal Citizen Information Center
http://publications.usa.gov/USAPubs.php

Informatics Reference List
www.eatright.org/informatics

Institute of Child Nutrition
www.nfsmi.org

School Nutrition Association
https://schoolnutrition.org

Links to Business and Management Magazines
www.brint.com/magazine.htm#ISJbus

U.S. Department of Labor Employment and Training Administration
www.doleta.gov

Free Management Library
http://managementhelp.org

BusinessUSA
http://business.usa.gov

CHAPTER 19

Building Grantsmanship Skills

Carol Byrd-Bredbenner, PhD, RD, FAND

LEARNING **OBJECTIVES**

After you have read and studied this chapter, you will be able to:

- Outline the general process for preparing a grant proposal.
- Conduct the foundational work needed to generate a grant proposal.
- Develop a grant proposal.
- Analyze grant proposals and identify their strengths and weaknesses.
- Create Logic Models for grant proposals.

This chapter addresses such issues as written communications and technical writing, documenting appropriately a variety of activities, preparation of a budget, and current information technologies, which have been designated by the Accreditation Council for Education in Nutrition and Dietetics (ACEND) as Foundation Knowledge and Learning Outcomes for dietetics education.

CHAPTER **OUTLINE**

Something to think about...

"Determine that the thing can and shall be done and then find the way."

—*ABRAHAM LINCOLN*

For a complete list of references, please access the MindTap Reader within your MindTap course.

Introduction

Community nutritionists increasingly find themselves seeking extramural funding for program activities and interventions. Perhaps extra funds are needed for printing banners and T-shirts, publishing a newsletter, underwriting the advertising costs for a program launch, buying food supplies for a cooking demonstration, marketing nutrition messages on a local television station, developing and evaluating new program materials, or expanding services. Annually, grants totaling over $150 billion are distributed by public and private groups. These grants are vital in helping today's organizations fund many of their important projects, which often exceed the resources they have available. To capture grant dollars for their organizations, grant seekers will find that well-honed grantsmanship skills (proposal seeking, writing, and management abilities) are essential.

Although you may not realize it, you have been creating proposals that resulted in awards of services, goods, and money throughout your life. Babies present a compelling argument for attention every time they cry. As children grow and mature, they may use their rapidly developing verbal and reasoning skills to explain why they require an increased allowance or how their communication needs warrant the purchase of a cell phone. In fact, both a child's informal request and a formal grant proposal submitted to a public or private grant sponsor are designed to achieve the same goal: convince a decision maker to provide the services, goods, and/or money the recipient needs to achieve the objectives stated in the proposal.

Proposals range in length from a single page to more than a hundred pages. Regardless of the length, the development of proposals can be divided into three main steps: laying the foundation, building the grant proposal, and assembling the final product. The fourth step, reviewing the grant proposal, is completed by the grant reviewers selected by the grant sponsor. The final step is putting the proposal into action if it is funded or revising it in hopes of future success.

Laying the Foundation for a Grant

Writing a grant is a lot like building a house. To build a house that will be sound and pass the reviews of building inspectors, builders must first lay a solid foundation. The grant proposals deemed most worthy of funding by grant review panels also grow out of a solid foundation. The foundation work for grant writing includes generating ideas, describing goals, and identifying funding sources and potential collaborators.

Generate Ideas

Proposal preparation begins with an idea. Ideas can be generated in a variety of ways, including noting a legislative initiative, reading the implications for research included at the ends of many journal articles, observing societal trends or needs in the community, brainstorming with colleagues, and reviewing statistical data such as census figures or morbidity and mortality rates and causes. Ideas also may come from a grant sponsor (see the section, later in this chapter, on identifying funding sources).

In community nutrition, the ideas that lead to grant proposals often are related to a desire to better understand the parameters affecting dietary behaviors and/or a desire to improve dietary behaviors. As ideas gel, they become goals such as the following:

- Gather baseline data. Examples: Survey adult women to determine their ability to use the nutrition facts given on food labels to make dietary planning decisions. Examine the effect that television food advertisements have on children's food preferences.

- Create a nutrition education intervention based on a new learning theory or innovative teaching method, and assess its effectiveness. Examples: Assess the effectiveness of a series of nutrition classes based on the Transtheoretical Model on lowering the dietary fat intake of cardiac bypass patients. Compare the impact of nutrition education comic books and nutrition website activities on teens' vitamin C and vitamin A intake. Evaluate the impact of a social marketing campaign to increase iron intake on blood lead levels in urban children. Evaluate the impact of a web-based, self-paced instructional program focusing on common problems in feeding children and on parents' comfort and satisfaction in dealing with these problems.
- Provide a service and evaluate its impact. Examples: Evaluate the impact of participation in the School Breakfast Program on school tardiness and absence rates. Distribute nutritious foods to pregnant women and assess the impact of these foods on maternal weight gain, infant birthweight, and length of gestation. Compare bone density changes in women who received vouchers for calcium-rich foods with those in women who continued eating their regular diet and received calcium supplements. Determine the relationship between the availability of nutrition peer counselors in college dorms and the rate of problems with weight gain and weight loss among residents.

Once an idea is formulated, the next step is to review the literature for *at least* the last five years and preferably more. In your search of the literature, you should address all facets of the idea, keeping in mind that many facets may not be directly related to nutrition. For example, let's say your idea is to design a school-based nutrition education class series and determine its impact on teens' calcium intake. A literature search for this project should include investigating current studies on teen calcium needs and intake levels; factors affecting teens' intake of calcium-rich foods; preferences of teens and teachers with regard to learning activities; physical and emotional developmental characteristics of teens; and learning theory applied to teen education programs, especially those aimed at changing health and nutrition behavior.

Surveying the literature is a worthwhile investment of time. It enables grant seekers to assess the value of an idea and adjust its focus to describe their goals more clearly.

- Grant seekers may find that someone else thought of the idea first. If so, the grant seeker should think about how the idea differs from or complements existing resources or activities. For example, several well-designed, effective curricula addressing calcium intake may already be available. In that case, the grant seeker may decide to narrow the focus of the idea to implement one of these existing curricula and evaluate its impact rather than also developing a curriculum.
- Grant seekers may discover that the idea is too narrow. For instance, they may learn that the main barrier to getting teen girls to increase their milk intake is that the girls believe they'll gain weight. If so, the grant seeker might choose to widen the focus of the idea to include healthful, low-fat choices and fat trade-offs from all the food groups.
- Grant seekers may find that they should alter their focus if they discover that the need for programs that help teens control their portion sizes hasn't been addressed effectively. Alternatively, they might discover that the face-to-face instruction they were planning isn't how today's technology-savvy teens want to learn about healthful eating.

Not only will the literature search help grant seekers to more fully develop and refine an idea and describe their goals, it will also help identify other professionals who could be sources of valuable advice and/or potential collaborators. And the literature search will provide the background data required to write a compelling needs statement for the proposal. When the literature search nears completion, grant seekers should be able to describe the following, clearly and concisely, in two or three minutes: their idea, the uniqueness of the proposed project, and why it is likely to succeed. This preparedness will help them when the time comes to contact potential collaborators and grant sponsors.

Key to Success The most successful grant writers are up to date in their subject-matter area. They read key journals regularly and are well informed about current trends and activities. The time needed to complete a literature review can be substantial if the idea is in a new area. In recent years, however, online abstracts and journals and Internet search engines have greatly facilitated the task of locating and retrieving pertinent resources. Also, keep in mind that grant seekers can reap long-term benefits from the literature review by focusing their work on a particular subject-matter area (e.g., diabetes or weight control) and/or audience (e.g., children or women) over the course of several years. Once the initial time investment has been made in developing an expertise in a subject-matter area and/or audience, only a small time investment is needed weekly or monthly to remain abreast of new developments. Moreover, focusing one's work helps to develop a track record of working in a particular topic, which in turn establishes one's credibility as an authority on the topic.

Describe Goals

Goals are broad statements describing desired long-range improvements. The four broad goal statements in *Healthy People 2020* are good examples of how to state goals:

- Attain high-quality, longer lives free of preventable disease, disability, injury, and premature death.
- Achieve health equity, eliminate disparities, and improve the health of all groups.
- Create social and physical environments that promote good health for all.
- Promote quality of life, healthy development, and healthy behaviors across all life stages.

Note that the goals grant seekers set are likely to be less expansive than the *Healthy People 2020* goals because grant seekers are setting goals for their organizations, not for the entire nation.

In community nutrition, there are so many worthwhile goals and vital needs that it is sometimes difficult to know which should be addressed first. However, perceptive grant seekers know that they improve their chances of receiving funding if they focus on addressing important goals that can be achieved with the combined finite resources available from their organization and the grant sponsor. *Healthy People 2020* goals and objectives, along with the following questions, can help grant seekers narrow the list of possible goals. If a question can be accurately answered "yes," proceed to the next question. Otherwise, seriously consider adjusting the goal.

1. Are the goal and the need(s) it will fulfill congruent with the grant seeker's mission? Most employers have a mission statement that describes the broad scope of their work. A review of the organization's mission statement can help grant seekers quickly determine whether a goal is appropriate to pursue. For example, the mission statement in **Figure 19-1** clearly indicates that the ABC Institute's mission is to help people improve their lives through educational processes.* Thus, grants designed to deliver prenatal care to teenage girls would not be an appropriate pursuit for a grant seeker employed by the ABC Institute. However, the grant seeker might collaborate with other organizations, such as a hospital that could provide the obstetrical care,

---

* *Note:* Figures 19-1 through 19-3 and 19-5 through 19-14 were developed for illustrative purposes only. Figures 19-5 through 19-14 are a composite of several actual grant proposals; these figures are not from an actual proposal.

FIGURE 19-1

Example of an
Organization Mission
Statement

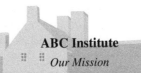

ABC Institute

Our Mission

The mission of the ABC Institute is to help the diverse population of
this state adapt to a rapidly changing society and improve their lives
through an educational process that uses science-based knowledge
focusing on issues and needs related to nutrition, food safety, health,
and agricultural sustainability.

and propose to provide only nutrition counseling and education to the pregnant teens.
If the answer to question 1 is clearly "no," then the goal is not an appropriate one for
the grant seeker's organization to address.

2. Is working to meet this goal a priority of the grant seeker's organization? If not, think
carefully before proceeding to work on this goal and the need(s) it will fulfill. For
success (and sometimes to gain permission to work on the goal), it is important to
have the organization's support.

3. Is it possible to achieve the goal in a timely manner? Some goals and needs are
extremely difficult to address. Before deciding to tackle such a goal, think carefully
about the commitment, time frame, funding, and other resources that will be
required. Weigh the required inputs against the possibility of meeting several other
needs instead with the same time, money, and energy. It may be more worthwhile to
focus the organization's efforts in a way that generates the greatest community impact
and likelihood for success than on needs arising from virtually intractable problems.

4. Does the goal align with an objective stated in *Healthy People 2020*? *Healthy People
2020* is our nation's health agenda. It can serve as the foundation for all work in
community nutrition related to health promotion and disease prevention. If the
goal is not part of *Healthy People 2020* objectives, or similar state or local policy
documents, community nutritionists should consider whether other, more critical
or more widespread needs should be addressed.

5. Would working to achieve the goal meet the needs of a substantial number of people?
Is their need severe? If this need is not met in the near future, are the long-term
consequences likely to be severe? If the answer to all of these questions is "no," there
are probably other goals and needs that are more important for the grant seeker's
organization to address. However, if the need is severe in the short term or long
term for even a small proportion of the population, grant seekers should consider
addressing it.

6. Have those in need been consulted to determine whether they are interested in having
this need addressed? If not, consider why. Perhaps they are not aware of their need,
distrust those who have offered help in the past, or do not see this need as a problem.
The reason for their lack of interest may indicate that a different need must be met
before the proposed need is addressed. If those in need are interested in having the
need attended to, grant seekers should think about whether their organization is
willing to work collaboratively with them using a community-based participatory
research (CBPR) approach. If not, the likelihood of successfully achieving the goal
and meeting their need is limited.

CBPR can help grant seekers and program developers create community nutrition interventions that address key needs of the community. CBPR is "a collaborative approach to research that equitably involves all partners in the research process and recognizes the unique strengths that each brings. CBPR begins with a research topic of importance to the community and has the aim of combining knowledge with action and achieving social change to improve health outcomes and eliminate health disparities."[1]

Once the goals have been selected, the grant seeker is ready to write clearly defined, specific goals that will meet important needs and answer important questions. When a project's goals are too broad or poorly defined, it is difficult to establish measurable objectives, create an evaluation plan, or develop a proposal budget and time schedule.

In today's world, it is still possible to find grants specifically designed to establish or enhance a community service, such as distributing food packages or providing nutrition counseling. However, more and more grant sponsors also want to know what impact their funds had on the community. For example, a grant sponsor is likely to want to know more than the fact that the $50,000 it gave was used to buy fresh produce that was distributed throughout the year to 29 limited-resource families. The sponsor might also want to know that participation in the food packages program was associated with improved growth patterns among toddlers or that participants had fewer school or work absences due to infections. Because of this increasing need to demonstrate the impact of grant dollars, it is often helpful to begin by stating grant goals in the form of precisely worded questions, as shown in **Table 19-1**. In this table, the question on the right is just one example of how the question on the left can be made more specific. For practice, try to write a different, more precise question for each of the questions that are too broad.

Note that the questions in the right column of the table can easily be converted to a goal statement. For instance, the first could be rephrased as "Determine whether a weight-loss clinic that incorporates behavior modification techniques helps obese women decrease their intake of simple carbohydrates." Try to write a goal statement for each item in Table 19-1.

TABLE 19-1 Framing Broad versus Precise Goal-Related Questions

TOO BROAD	MORE PRECISE
Does nutrition education change people's food patterns?	Can a weight-loss clinic that incorporates behavior modification techniques help obese women to decrease their intake of simple carbohydrates?
Can counseling sessions improve blood lipid levels?	Do counseling sessions geared to a teen's stage of change for fat intake lead to lower LDL values?
Does poor personal hygiene increase the rate of foodborne illness?	Can the rate of school absences due to gastrointestinal distress be reduced by having middle school children wash their hands with warm soapy water before eating lunch?
Does poor diet reduce the effectiveness of education?	Is regular participation in the School Breakfast Program associated with increased reading scores in third-grade children?
Are women who participate in WIC better nourished?	Do pregnant women who participate in WIC for at least five months before delivery give birth to fewer low-birthweight and/or preterm infants?
Can social marketing campaigns reduce health care costs?	Can a social marketing campaign promoting increased physical activity levels reverse the trend toward increased body weight and related disease among residents in Green County?
Do Nutrition Facts labels help people eat better diets?	Can an interactive online presentation that teaches women with type 1 diabetes mellitus how to use nutrition labels improve their hemoglobin A_{1c} (HbA_{1c}) levels?

Key to Success Successful grant seekers choose worthwhile goals that match their organization's mission and interests, and address important needs that can be met in a meaningful and timely manner. They also sharply focus their goals. They know that most grants have a finite dollar amount and time frame, and they are well aware of the resources their own employer has available for the proposed project. Therefore, to stay within the parameters of the grant and the grant seeker's resources (such as available personnel or office space), successful grant seekers divide multifaceted projects into manageable pieces and then decide which pieces to work on first.

Identify Funding Sources

Finding a funding source generally takes two forms: generating an idea in response to a grant sponsor's request or finding a grant sponsor to fund the grant seeker's idea.

- The grant seeker generates an idea in response to a grant sponsor's request for proposals (RFP) or request for quotation (RFQ). Both an RFP and an RFQ invite grant seekers to submit proposals. An RFP (also called a Request for Applications [RFA] or Funding Opportunity Announcement [FOA]) tends to be much less specific in regard to the activities that can be proposed (**Figure 19-2**), whereas an RFQ tends to be very specific about the activities that the grant recipient must engage in. That is, the issuers of RFQs are looking to award a contract for work they specified and want grant seekers to provide a cost estimate for that work (**Figure 19-3**).

FIGURE 19-2 Two Sample Requests for Proposals (RFPs) Note the general nature of an RFP.

Good Health Foundation

The Good Health Foundation operates under the laws of the state. Only nonprofit organizations are eligible to receive a Good Health Foundation grant. Grant recipients must submit an annual progress report and audited financial statement of the expenditures of the foundation grant. The Good Health Foundation invites eligible applicants to submit grant proposals that:

- Support community nutrition education programs for children and young adults that improve their health and development.
- Provide nutrition counseling for pregnant women and mothers of infants so that they can assist their children in developing good nutritional practices at an early age.
- Train persons to work as educators and demonstrators of good nutritional practices.
- Promote dissemination of information regarding healthful nutritional practices.

Federal Government Agency—Brand New Research Initiative

99.0 Improving Nutrition and Food Handling for Optimal Health

Investigators are encouraged to contact the Program Director at (000) 000-0000 regarding questions about the suitability of research topics (or at *programdirector.gov* to arrange a telephone consultation).

- Standard research project awards for this program are not likely to exceed a total budget (including indirect costs) of $300,000 for three to four years of support.
- Program Deadline: November 15

The consumption of a nutritious diet is important for maintaining health and decreasing the risk for chronic diseases. There is a need to improve understanding of the role of foods and their components (e.g., phytochemicals) in promoting health. The primary objective of this program is to support research that contributes to our understanding of appropriate dietary practices throughout the life cycle and factors that affect these requirements such as gender. Studies to determine the effects of dietary components on immune function are encouraged. In addition, new insights are needed about factors that affect the attitudes and behavior of consumers toward food.

The following areas of research will be emphasized: (a) nutritional requirements including metabolism and utilization for all age groups; (b) effect of community projects on lowering the incidence of obesity through increased physical activity; (c) identification of obstacles to adopting healthful food habits, with particular emphasis on factors affecting consumer attitudes and behavior; (d) development of recommendations for interventions to improve nutrition status; and (e) improvement of safe food handling behaviors among those at increased risk for foodborne illness. Support will not be provided for research on dietary requirements as related to therapies for infectious diseases, cancer, and alcohol-related disorders.

FIGURE 19-3

A Sample Request
for Quotation (RFQ)
Note that this RFQ is
much more specific
than the sample RFPs
in Figure 19-2.

The XYZ Government agency seeks a researcher with established expertise in the evaluation of classroom nutrition education materials to conduct a study to assess the use and effectiveness of the Healthy Eating Kit as an instructional resource in high schools. Information from the study will be used to revise the Kit; develop future nutrition education classroom materials; and document the nutrition-related subject matter, types of lessons, and hands-on activities that are of greatest interest to teachers and have the most impact on students. The Kit will be assessed by brief interviews of 150 teachers that focus primarily on questions from the evaluation form included in the Kit and in-depth qualitative interviews of 30 teachers. In-depth interviews will focus on the effectiveness of the Kit in communicating with culturally diverse youth, methods for adapting the Kit for use with younger children, and suggestions for communicating nutrition topics in the future. Study participants may be recruited through the evaluation forms returned to the XYZ Government Agency, State Departments of Education, and advertisements in professional journals. Efforts must be made to represent all geographic regions in the United States, culturally diverse student segments, and urban, suburban, and rural areas.

- The grant seeker generates an idea for which he or she seeks an appropriate grant sponsor. Regardless of the goal and need, there is probably a government or community agency, industry trade group, food or drug company, or local business willing to support the program or intervention activities. According to some, "If you can find an effective solution to a pressing community problem, you can find funders to help you implement it."[2] The challenge is to find the grant sponsor who is willing to fund the proposal.

Many types of grants are available (**Figure 19-4**). How do community nutritionists find out these grants? They network with colleagues to learn about upcoming funding opportunities; they contact granting agencies for information about RFPs; and they call local businesses to seek small grants to support community projects. In the United States, grant funding usually comes from government agencies, foundations and community trusts, and business and industrial organizations (**Table 19-2**). The Internet Resources section at the end of this chapter lists websites of potential funding sources.

When grant seekers begin to explore potential grant sponsors, they should think about each facet of the project.[3] For example, say the goal is to determine the effect of early intervention on the incidence of type 2 diabetes mellitus in overweight teenage boys. Grant seekers should ask themselves:

- Will the project provide nutrition education to the boys or training to physical education teachers who work with the boys? If so, the grant seekers could try a sponsor that funds after-school projects or in-service training for teachers.
- Will the project use exercise equipment? If so, the grant seekers could try sporting goods manufacturers or athletic shoe manufacturers.
- Will the project involve the use of monitoring equipment? If so, they might try a pedometer maker or pharmaceutical company that markets glucose monitoring supplies.
- Will the project include a community awareness component? If so, it would make sense to try a sponsor that funds social marketing campaigns or a nonprofit organization that works to raise awareness about health issues.
- Will the project involve providing more low-calorie, fiber-rich foods such as fresh produce and whole grains? If so, they might try a supermarket chain, produce association, or grain trade group.
- Is this a demonstration project? If so, grant seekers could try a local foundation or municipal government.

FIGURE 19-4 Types of Grants

Block grant: A grant from the federal government to states or local communities for broad purposes as authorized by legislation. Recipients have great flexibility in distributing such funds as long as the basic purposes are fulfilled. The federal block grant areas are maternal and child health, community services, social services, preventive health and health services, and primary care.

Capitation grant: A grant made to an institution to provide a dependable support base, usually for training purposes. The amount of the grant is dependent on the size of enrollment or number of people served.

Categorical grant: A grant similar to a block grant, except funds must be expended within specific categories, such as maternal and childcare. Funds available may be based on a specific formula (see *Formula grant* below).

Challenge grant: A grant that serves as a magnet to attract additional funding.

Conference grant: A grant awarded to support the costs of meetings, symposia, or special seminars.

Demonstration grant: A grant, usually of limited duration, made to establish or demonstrate the feasibility of a theory or an approach.

Equipment grant: A grant that provides money to purchase equipment.

Formula grant: A grant in which funds are provided to specified grantees based on a specific formula, prescribed in legislation or regulation, rather than based on an individual project review. The formula is usually based on such factors as population, enrollment, per capita income, morbidity and mortality, or a specific need. Capitation grants are one type of formula grant, and block grants usually are awarded based on a formula.

Matching grant: A grant that requires the grant recipient to match the money provided with cash or in-kind gifts (such as donated products, supplies, equipment, services) from another source.

Planning grant: A grant made to support planning, developing, designing, and establishing the means for performing research or accomplishing other approved objectives.

Project grant: The most common form of grant, made to support a discrete, specified project to be performed by the named investigator(s) in an area representing his or her specific interest and competencies.

Research grant: A grant made to support investigation or experimentation aimed at the discovery and interpretation of facts, the revision of accepted theories in light of new facts, or the application of new or revised theories.

Service grant: A grant that supports cost of organizing, establishing, providing, or expanding the delivery of health or other essential services to a specified community or area. This also may be done through a block grant.

Training grant: A grant awarded to an organization to support costs of training students, personnel, or prospective employees in research, or in the techniques or practices pertinent to the delivery of health services in the particular area of concern.

Once grant seekers have identified a potential grant sponsor, they must decide whether to compete for it. According to the old adage, "It takes two to tango." Nowhere is this truer than with procuring grant funds. For success, the needs of the grant seeker must be in tune with the needs and interests of the funding source—that is, the proposal must clearly demonstrate how the grant seeker's goals complement those of the grant sponsor. The following questions can help grant seekers decide whether to compete for a grant from a particular grant sponsor.

1. Do the grant sponsor's funding priorities include the project's goals? If not, can the project's goals be easily revised to be congruent? Even the most eloquently written proposal is unlikely to be funded if its goals do not match those of the grant sponsor.

TABLE 19-2 Types of Funding Agencies

TYPE	EXAMPLES
Federal	National Institutes of Health (e.g., National Cancer Institute; National Institute on Aging; National Heart, Lung, and Blood Institute); Department of Health and Human Services (e.g., Food and Drug Administration); U.S. Agency for International Development; U.S. Department of Agriculture (e.g., National Institute of Food and Agriculture)
State and local	Department of education, department of human services, health department, arts council, local school district
Foundations	Ford Foundation, Spencer Foundation, Rockefeller Foundation, International Life Sciences Institute, International Nutrition Foundation, March of Dimes, Robert Wood Johnson Foundation
Nonprofit organizations	American Diabetes Association, American Heart Association, Academy of Nutrition and Dietetics, American Cancer Society, local civic groups
Industry	Pharmaceutical companies, trade associations, commodity groups, local supermarkets
Institutional	Local universities and hospitals

2. Are sufficient grant funds available for the grant seeker's organization to achieve the goals in a successful and timely manner? If not, ask whether your organization is willing and/or able to provide sufficient resources to augment grant funds. Is there another organization that could serve as a partner and furnish some funds? If grant funds combined with resources from the grant seeker's organization and partners are insufficient, the likelihood of achieving the goals is very low.

3. What will this grant sponsor fund (e.g., personnel, travel, or office supplies)? Is that what is needed? Every proposal has specific needs. If the grant sponsor is not able to support those needs, the grant objectives cannot be achieved. Let's say the project is one that would require travel to several states to train dietitians to use a teaching kit, but the sponsor won't fund travel. If face-to-face instruction is essential, this sponsor is not a good match unless travel funds are available elsewhere. Alternatively, if face-to-face instruction is not essential, the proposal could be revised to use other methods of training, such as web conferencing or a self-instructional manual, which would be eligible for funding.

4. Who is eligible to apply for this grant? Some grants are limited to specific types of organizations such as nonprofit agencies, accredited universities, or outpatient clinics. If the grant seeker's organization is not eligible, an alternative may be to collaborate with another organization that is.

5. Can the grant seeker's organization meet any special requirements of the grant sponsor? For example, some grants may require audited quarterly financial reports. Some require the grant recipient to match grant funds dollar for dollar. If the organization cannot meet the special requirements, other funding sources will need to be considered.

6. When is the grant application due? Can the grant seeker's organization respond in time? If not, when will this grant opportunity be available again? Writing a grant proposal, depending on the sponsor's requirements and the applicant's prior experience and readiness, can take as long as six months. Thus, grant seekers must honestly assess prior time commitments and how much time will be required to

generate a thoughtful, well-written proposal. Proposals that arrive after the due date are almost always discarded. And hastily written proposals may establish a negative reputation for the grant seeker and his or her organization.

7. What are the guidelines for writing this proposal? What forms and format are required? Every grant sponsor publishes some type of proposal-writing guidelines; some are extremely specific, others more general. For success, it is essential that grant seekers follow such guidelines, forms, and formats exactly. In addition, grant seekers need to be certain to use the forms provided by the sponsor; trying to revise the forms to better fit one's proposal will create extra work (and frustration) for grant reviewers, who are expecting to find information presented in a specific way. Many grant sponsors will discard proposals that are not prepared according to their instructions. Even though proposal guidelines, forms, and formats vary from sponsor to sponsor, you will see below that the elements in proposals tend to be quite similar across grant sponsors.

8. Is information available on the types of projects the sponsor has funded in the past? Many grant sponsors publish abstracts of projects they have funded. Increasingly, the abstracts are available on their websites. Reviewing these can help grant seekers determine how well their idea is likely to be received. They may find that their project is too similar to grants already funded to reveal anything new. On the other hand, they may learn that the sponsor says it has six funding priorities but seems to fund only two priorities. Grant seekers also may want to contact a few grant recipients and ask them to share their experiences and insights related to procuring a grant from this sponsor and how they would approach this activity differently next time. Some may be willing to share a copy of their winning proposals.

9. What are the credentials of the grant reviewers? Some sponsors reveal the names of past reviewers, but many do not. However, nearly all sponsors will indicate the general background of reviewers. Knowing the reviewers' level of expertise can help grant seekers determine the level of detail and documentation to use in their proposal. For example, if dietitians and physicians are to review the proposal, grant seekers will be able to use precise medical terminology, which might not be appropriate if the reviewers have a nonmedical background. If the sponsor does reveal the names of past reviewers, grant seekers might ask them to share their insights on how the review process worked, pitfalls to avoid, and general advice.

10. Is it possible to contact the sponsor before preparing the proposal? Most government sponsors and some private sponsors welcome inquiries (see Figure 19-2 on page 719). Contacting the sponsor before preparing a proposal can save grant seekers and the sponsor time. Moreover, it helps to verify the accuracy of the information in the call for proposals—sometimes changes occur after the RFPs or RFQs are printed. After carefully reading the call for proposals, reviewing past funded projects, and speaking with reviewers, grant seekers may still have questions or need more information on how to fine-tune project goals to be fully congruent with the grant sponsor's priorities. For example, if the sponsor seems to be funding only two of its six priorities—and the two are not the priority area the proposal will be in—grant seekers might ask why. It could be that the sponsor did not receive any worthy proposals in other areas or that the two priorities funded are its top priorities.

Key to Success The most successful grant seekers select a grant sponsor before writing a proposal. They understand the value of doing their homework so that they do not waste time writing a proposal for a sponsor that is unlikely to fund work in the area proposed. They also know that it is essential to follow the grant guidelines, forms, and formats exactly and to observe all deadlines. In addition, they write the proposal using terminology familiar to the grant reviewers—after all, it is the reviewers who will make funding recommendations to the sponsor. Even successful grant writers experience failure; but they capitalize on the time invested in writing a proposal by preparing it using word processing software. This way, they can easily cut, paste, and reformat the proposal for other grant sponsors or revise it for the same sponsor for the next funding cycle.

Another Key to Success   The most successful grant seekers avoid "chasing" grants. That is, they keep their work focused and do not jump from topic to topic just to capture the latest stream of grant funding. Unfocused grant chasers usually feel frustrated because they are constantly changing gears and trying to develop expertise in many, often unrelated areas. In addition, without a history of successful related projects, grant chasers will have difficulty demonstrating to grant reviewers that they can deliver the work proposed. Keeping work focused does not mean that one is forever locked into a single topic or audience. Successful grant seekers can and do change gears, but the progression is usually an evolutionary one. That is, their work naturally branches into new areas as science progresses, community demographics change, or new problems arise. For instance, a professional working with type 2 diabetes mellitus (DM) treatment in adults may branch into prevention of this disease in children. Or, because this disease is a risk factor for cardiovascular disease (CVD), this professional may branch into CVD prevention work. Alternatively, because obesity is a risk factor for this type of DM, this professional's work may branch into weight-control programming for teens. Grant seekers who *do* want to make an abrupt or radical change in their focus, however, can increase their chances of success by working with collaborators to generate a history of successful work in the new focus area.

Identify Potential Collaborators

It is possible to complete the work in some grant proposals alone, but one person usually does not have all the expertise or time needed to complete all the proposed tasks. For instance, depending on the project, a community nutritionist may need the expertise of a statistician, epidemiologist, or physician to complement his or her nutrition expertise. Collaboration is the rule rather than the exception.

Collaborators may come from within the grant seeker's organization or from outside. For example, if the organization is not eligible to apply for a particular grant, it will need to partner with another organization that is eligible. Collaboration with other organizations is important when one organization lacks expertise in an area vital to the proposal. Collaborating may be critical to success for novice grant seekers or those who are changing their focus. Increasingly, government grant sponsors are requiring—or giving bonus points to—proposals that are multidisciplinary and/or multi-institutional, thus making collaboration essential. Often, proposals that reflect a multidisciplinary approach to a problem are highly rated.[4]

Collaboration can greatly improve a proposed project. A well-conceived and well-managed collaboration plan gives grant seekers the opportunity to assemble a team that can effectively and efficiently achieve the project goals. The best collaborators are those who know what is expected of them and when, are excited about and committed to the project, and are willing to follow through on all their responsibilities related to the project. A clear system of frequent communication with all collaborators will help keep everyone on track and moving toward achieving the project goals in a timely manner. Collaborative efforts that are poorly managed or lack teamwork and open communication will hinder success. See the Professional Focus feature on page 748 for more about the benefits of teamwork.

Community nutritionists can find collaborators by networking with colleagues and corresponding with individuals identified via the literature search who are working on similar projects. Before inviting someone to be a collaborator, explain the project's objectives, time frame, and budget and gauge his or her interest and ability to participate. You also may want to interview a few references to learn more about the potential collaborator's prior performance record.

Key to Success Select collaborators carefully and try to get them involved as early in the grant-writing process as possible. Make certain every collaborator knows and agrees to the duties involved, timelines, budget allocation, and sequence of names on publications before the project begins. Keep all collaborators informed of the progress of the grant application.

Building the Proposal

Throughout the grant-writing process, keep in mind that the goal is to write a clear, complete, concise, and compelling document that will persuade the grant sponsor to award the grant seeker a portion of its finite resources. The most successful grant proposals demonstrate that the proposed project matches the sponsor's priorities; that it is among the most worthwhile, well planned, sound, and likely to succeed of all the proposal alternatives; and that it is in the hands of qualified professionals who are committed to seeing the project through to completion.

Components of a Proposal

The components of a proposal vary from one grant sponsor to another (carefully check the sponsor's instructions!), but they generally include the items discussed below. Note that the sequence of these items is the order in which they usually appear in a proposal; however, they are not necessarily written in this sequence. For example, the transmittal letter frequently is written last, and the abstract should not be written until after the proposal is in final form.

Letters of Intent Increasingly, grant sponsors are encouraging or requiring grant seekers to submit a letter of intent prior to submitting a full proposal. In some cases, the grant sponsor wishes to receive only a very brief letter of intent stating that the grant seeker intends to submit a proposal in response to a specific grant program. This type of letter of intent helps the grant sponsor determine how many proposals it will receive, estimate the time it will need to spend processing the proposals, and determine the number of grant reviewers it is likely to need. Often, grant sponsors do not send a reply to this type of letter of intent.

In other cases, grant sponsors indicate that the letter of intent is a preproposal that includes a synopsis of most or all of the parts of a full proposal. This type of letter of intent should give the grant sponsor a clear picture of the type of proposal a grant seeker intends to submit. Using this type of letter of intent, the grant sponsor can get an idea about whether the proposal is suitable for its grant program. Most grant sponsors respond to this type of letter of intent and indicate to the grant seeker whether or not it should submit a full proposal.

The letter of intent should be sent, by the due date, to the individual specified on the call for proposals. This letter should include all of the information requested and should indicate how the grant sponsor can contact the grant seeker.

Transmittal Letter The transmittal letter is a brief, friendly communication addressed to the individual designated on the call for proposals. As shown in **Figure 19-5**, this letter should indicate the reason for submitting the proposal. That is, is the proposal in response to a call for proposals, is it in response to an invitation to submit a full proposal after submitting a preproposal or letter of intent, or is it an unsolicited proposal? Some grant sponsors have several grant programs under way simultaneously, so grant seekers must clearly indicate the grant program to which they are submitting the proposal. The transmittal letter also should state the name of the proposal and, if submitted as hard copies, the number of copies enclosed. And grant seekers must be sure to indicate how the grant sponsor can contact them.

Title Page Many grant sponsors, especially government agencies, have a specific form that must serve as the title page. If the grant sponsor does not have a specific form or provide information on how to set up the title page, include the following information on the title page: project title; the grant program the proposal is being submitted to; proposed start and end dates of the project; funds requested; the project director's name, address, phone number, fax number, and e-mail address; the legal name of the organization to which the award should be made; and the authorized organizational representative's name, title, address, telephone number, fax number, and e-mail address (**Figure 19-6**). Note that some of the information from the transmittal letter is repeated on the title page—it is important that this information appears in *both* places. Keep in mind that reviewers will see the title page, only the individual designated to receive the proposal submission is likely to see the transmittal letter.

FIGURE 19-5

Proposal Transmittal Letter

January 11, 20XX

Federal Government Agency
Brand New Research Initiative
Proposal Services Unit
Room 000 Canal Place
000 Main Street, N.W.
Washington, DC 00000

Dear Sir or Madam,

My colleagues and I are pleased to submit the enclosed proposal, *Improving Safe Food-Handling Behaviors of Immunocompromised Adults*, in response to the Federal Government Agency's Brand New Research Initiative call for proposals, category 99.0, Improving Nutrition and Food Handling for Optimal Health. The proposal requests $185,289 for a two-year project. Enclosed please find the original and 19 copies of this proposal, as specified in the Request for Proposals.

If you have questions or need additional information, please contact me. I am looking forward to your reply.

Sincerely,

Greta Grantwriter

Greta Grantwriter, Ph.D., R.D.
Nutrition Services Director
Super State University
000 Elm Street
University City, USA 00000
Phone: 222-222-0000
Fax: 222-222-1111
E-mail: grantwriter@superuniversity.edu

Project Title: Improving Safe Food-Handling Behaviors of Immunocompromised Adults
Grant Program: Federal Government Agency's Brand New Research Initiative, category 99.0, Improving Nutrition and Food Handling for Optimal Health
Proposed Start Date: September 15, 20XX
Proposed End Date: September 14, 20XX
Funds Requested: $185,289

Project Director:
Greta Grantwriter, Ph.D., R.D.
Nutrition Services Director
Super State University
000 Elm Street
University City, USA 00000
Phone: 222-222-0000
Fax: 222-222-1111
E-mail: grantwriter@superuniversity.edu

The award should be made to:
Super State University

Authorized Organizational Representative:
Joseph Jones, Dean of Research
Office of Research & Sponsored Programs
00 University Plaza
University City, USA 00000
Phone: 222-222-2222
Fax: 222-222-3333
E-mail: authorizedorganizationalrep@superuniversity.edu

FIGURE 19-6 Sample Proposal Title Page When No Form or Format Is Specified

The proposal title should be brief, specific, and informative. It should set the stage for the proposal and quickly and accurately inform the grant reviewers about what they will be reading. Note that some sponsors impose a limit on the number of characters (and spaces) permitted.

Abstract The proposal abstract or summary outlines the proposed project and appears at the beginning of the proposal. The abstract is usually limited to one page or a specified number of words. Some sponsors provide a structure that must be used. Regardless of the limitations, the abstract should contain a needs statement (why the project is important and needs to be done) and should describe the main goals of the project. A sample abstract is shown in **Figure 19-7**. Note that some grant sponsors may instruct grant seekers also to describe the project methods, time frame, and budget in the abstract.

It is best to write the abstract after the final proposal draft is complete to ensure that no key information is omitted. Nevertheless, do not let the abstract be an afterthought. Be sure to allow sufficient time to write it carefully because the abstract is usually the first part of the proposal that reviewers read. Grant reviewers form their initial impression of a project from the abstract, which means the abstract can be critical to success. If the abstract does not convince reviewers that the project is well matched to the sponsor's priorities or does not address an important need, the grant reviewer may be inclined to spend little time on the proposal and rate it poorly.

After writing the abstract, grant seekers should ask these questions:

1. Does the abstract succinctly summarize all the important elements of the project?
2. Is it prepared according to the format specified in the call for proposals?
3. Will it create in the grant reviewer's mind an accurate, complete picture of what is being proposed and why?

FIGURE 19-7 Sample Abstract

Improving Safe Food-Handling Behaviors of Immunocompromised Adults

Foodborne disease caused by microbial pathogens remains a significant public health problem in the 21st century. Each year, contaminated food causes approximately 1,000 reported foodborne disease outbreaks and an estimated 48 million illnesses, 128,000 hospitalizations, and 3,000 deaths. Costs for treating victims of foodborne illnesses top $152 billion—this does not include the cost of lost productivity and total societal burden of chronic, long-term consequences of some foodborne illnesses. A primary contributor to the high rate of foodborne illness in this country is that many consumers are simply unaware of the vital role they play in preventing foodborne illness. In reality, food mishandling in home kitchens likely causes a significant amount of illness. Further exacerbating the rate of foodborne illness is that recent generations have not been taught about safe food handling at school or at home. As a result, a large proportion of adults have limited food preparation experience, have never learned basic principles of food safety, and thus lack the critical knowledge needed to help them proactively protect themselves and their families. For most people, a bout with foodborne illness is a relatively short-lived, minor inconvenience. But, for the one-quarter of the U.S. population "at increased risk" (e.g., persons with weakened immune systems due to disease [e.g., HIV/AIDS] or pharmaceutical or radiological treatments; pregnant women and their fetuses; lactating mothers; infants and young children; preschool children in daycare; and older adults), foodborne illness can be debilitating, even deadly. The high rate and exorbitant cost of foodborne disease, coupled with the devastating effects it can have on the nutrition status and overall health of individuals with weakened immune systems, clearly indicates a need for an effective, behaviorally focused, and audience-specific food safety education program. Previous work by the applicant indicates that immunocompromised adults and their caregivers prefer food safety information that addresses key foodborne illness prevention measures and issues in the context of their value to them and delivers this education via interactive, online instruction. Thus, the objectives of this project are to: (a) develop a behaviorally focused food safety intervention program that is responsive to the documented needs and interests related to food safety education of immunocompromised adults and their caregivers and is based on the Health Belief Model; (b) evaluate the effectiveness of the intervention program in effecting positive food safety behavior change and reducing foodborne illness risk; (c) refine the intervention program; and (d) disseminate the program to health professionals. This project will span 24 months. The budget request is $185,289.

When a grant seeker is able to answer "yes" to all of these questions, he or she should have a colleague read the abstract and then ask the colleague to describe the project. If the colleague misses any major points, the grant seeker would be wise to check to be certain that the abstract is complete and clear.

Grant Narrative

The grant narrative includes these sections: needs statement, goals and objectives, and methods. Some grant sponsors indicate that the time and activity charts from the methods section, along with the capability statements, should be included in the grant narrative; others indicate that they should appear in another section.

Needs Statement

This section includes a clear, concise, and well-supported problem statement (or needs assessment), with a review of the current literature related to the problem. The literature review should establish the grant seeker's familiarity with and expertise in every facet of the study. Pilot-test data and/or needs assessment data can be included, too. The introduction should clearly demonstrate that the problem described represents a gap between what currently exists or is known and what could (or should) exist or be known. It should build a convincing case that the proposed project will help bridge that gap and extend the current knowledge base. The most successful grant proposals convey a sense of urgency regarding the problem and its resolution (i.e., the goals of the project).

Figure 19-8 shows a sample needs statement. The introduction and literature review found in many journal articles provide other helpful examples.

When evaluating a needs statement, ask the following questions. If any are answered "no," the needs statement must be revised until every question can be answered "yes."

1. Does the needs statement demonstrate a clear understanding of the problem or need and why it is significant to address at this time?
2. Does the needs statement explicitly describe the focus (goals) of the proposed project and provide a conceptually sound rationale for the focus?
3. Is it clear that the proposed project is feasible, that it is different from prior work, and that it will resolve a significant, timely problem or meet a pressing need?

FIGURE 19-8 Grant Narrative: Improving Safe Food-Handling Behaviors of Immunocompromised Adults

---

Improving Safe Food-Handling Behaviors of Immunocompromised Adults

NEEDS STATEMENT

Foodborne disease caused by microbial pathogens remains a significant public health problem in the 21st century, so much so that it is one of the priorities in the *Healthy People 2020* initiative (1).* In addition, the *Dietary Guidelines for Americans* highlight the importance of food safety (2). Headline news stories focusing on widespread outbreaks of foodborne illness caused by lapses in personal hygiene or emerging pathogens are vivid reminders that the food that nourishes and sustains us also can be debilitating, and in some cases deadly (3). Each year contaminated food causes approximately 1,000 reported foodborne disease outbreaks and an estimated 48 million illnesses, 128,000 hospitalizations, and 3,000 deaths (4). Costs for treating victims of foodborne illnesses top $152 billion—this does not include the cost of lost productivity and total societal burden of chronic, long-term consequences of some foodborne illnesses (5). In addition, these costs do not account for the vast majority of foodborne disease cases caused by mishandling of food at home that go unreported (4–7) because consumers believe they have the "flu" (8).

A primary contributor to the high rate of foodborne illness in this country is that very few consumers believe foodborne illness originates in their homes—almost two-thirds never questioned whether someone in their household with "flu-like" symptoms (i.e., fever, chills, and nausea) could actually have had a foodborne disease caused by foods prepared at home (9–10). Concomitantly, many consumers do not understand the magnitude of the control they have in their own kitchen to reduce the risk of acquiring microbial foodborne illness (3).

Further exacerbating the rate of foodborne illness is that recent generations have not learned about safe food handling and food preparation in school (11–12). Increasing numbers of working mothers and growing reliance on frozen meals, restaurant dining, and take-out foods have decreased opportunities for children to learn safe food handling via observation. As a result, a large proportion of adults have limited food preparation experience, have never learned basic principles of food safety, and thus lack the critical knowledge needed to help them proactively protect themselves and their families (3, 13–18).

The importance of foodborne illness as a current public health concern is underscored by the increasing numbers of "at risk" or highly susceptible populations (19). One-quarter of the United States population is considered at increased risk for foodborne illness (1). Those considered "at risk" include persons with weakened immune systems due to disease (e.g., HIV/AIDS) or pharmaceutical or radiological treatments; pregnant women and their fetuses; lactating mothers; infants and young children; preschool children in daycare; and older adults (8). Others who may be at a disproportionately greater risk include those living in institutional settings and financially disadvantaged individuals such as homeless persons and migrant farmworkers (9).

The high rate and exorbitant cost of foodborne disease, coupled with the devastating effects it can have on the nutrition status and overall health of individuals with weakened immune systems, clearly indicates a need for an effective, theory-driven, behaviorally focused food safety education program for these individuals and their caregivers. Although a wide variety of food safety educational efforts initiated by the FDA and USDA have been launched in recent years, the target audience for these efforts has been very broadly defined (e.g., American consumers). That is, the same message and delivery mode is used to reach everyone regardless of personal needs and/or interests. Food safety education is most likely to be effective if the messages are tailored to the needs and interests of a specific audience (20–22).

* The numbers in parentheses in this sample narrative refer the grant reviewer to the proposal's bibliography. The style used to note references in the text and the bibliographic referencing style may be specified in the call for proposals. If it is not, citations should be presented in an accepted journal format, including the title and complete reference. Authors should be listed in the same order as they appeared on the published paper.

1

---

4. Does the needs statement's organization logically and methodically build a case for the proposed solution (objectives)?
5. Does the needs statement indicate how this project will build on previous work completed by the grant seeker or others?
6. Are current, reputable references such as refereed journal articles, statistical data, and reference books cited?
7. Does the needs statement explain why this particular grant sponsor should be interested in this proposal?
8. Does the needs statement convey a sense of urgency regarding the problem (need) and its resolution?
9. Is the needs statement interesting enough to compel the grant reviewer to continue reading?
10. Does the length of the needs statement conform to the sponsor's instructions?

FIGURE 19-8 Grant Narrative: Improving Safe Food-Handling Behaviors of Immunocompromised Adults—*continued*

Findings of 17 focus group interviews (*n* = 97) conducted by the grant applicant to document the needs and interests related to food safety education of immunocompromised adults and their caregivers revealed that these individuals wanted food safety information that specifically addressed key foodborne illness prevention measures and issues in the context of their value to immunocompromised individuals. They also indicated that the preferred delivery mode for food safety education is via interactive, online instructional modules, dedicated chat rooms, and monthly e-mail or voice mail food safety tips and news (23). Currently, food safety education targeted to this population and delivered in the manner they prefer does not exist.

GOALS AND OBJECTIVES

The goal of this project, like that of the grant sponsor, is to improve the safe food-handling behaviors of those at increased risk for foodborne illness, specifically immunocompromised adults and their caregivers. The project objectives are:

1. To develop a theory-driven, behaviorally focused food safety intervention program that is responsive to the needs, interests, and delivery mode preferences of immunocompromised adults and their caregivers that will enable them to increase their food safety knowledge, develop more positive attitudes toward practicing safe food handling, and improve their food safety self-efficacy and self-reported food safety practices.
2. To evaluate the effectiveness of the food safety intervention program on improving food safety knowledge, attitudes, self-efficacy, and self-reported food safety practices.
3. To revise the food safety education intervention program based on the findings of the evaluation study.
4. To make health professionals throughout the region aware of the food safety intervention program and encourage them to promote the program to their patients.

METHODS

Project Design. This project has two primary phases: intervention lesson development and intervention lesson summative and impact evaluation.

Intervention Lesson Development. The intervention program to be developed will include six online, interactive, 15-minute lessons focusing on food safety for immunocompromised adults. The lessons will be online because research indicates that computer-based learning can heighten learner interest and motivation, meet the needs of learners with varying learning styles, increase achievement levels, and shorten learning time (24–29). In addition, focus group data collected by the applicant revealed that immunocompromised adults and their caregivers preferred computer-based learning because it is convenient, provides constant interaction, and is under their direct control. Another important feature of computer-based learning is that it permits features that are not possible in printed materials (e.g., links to other websites, animation, video, narration), allows the use of full color graphics at no extra production costs, and can be updated more cost-effectively and easily than printed matter.

Each lesson will include a brief introduction, the lesson itself, and a brief conclusion. The introduction will be designed to "grab" the attention of the participants and will include interactive quizzes, games, and short video clips. Each lesson will focus on one aspect of food safety. (Figure 0 summarizes the primary generalization addressed and change process(es) emphasized in each lesson.) All lessons will have a strong visual component (e.g., simulation of bacteria growth rate in the danger zone; demonstration of how cross-contamination occurs). Lesson conclusions will reiterate important points and provide participants with concrete methods for immediately applying the lesson's content. At the end of each lesson, participants will be able to print out fact sheets that summarize the lesson and post questions to the project staff.

2

For practice, read the needs statement in Figure 19-8 carefully and answer the ten questions listed on the previous two pages. For any question answered "no," grant seekers should think about how to improve the needs statement.

Goals and Objectives The project's goals and objectives describe what the grant seeker plans to achieve. Goals tend to be broad, general-purpose statements or ideals, such as "to improve the food-handling practices of immunocompromised adults and their caregivers." The project objectives are much more specific and measurable than goals. They specify what will have been accomplished when the project is completed. See the goals and objectives section in Figure 19-8. Also refer to the section on program goals and objectives in Chapter 5 on pages 153–156.

FIGURE 19-8 Grant Narrative: Improving Safe Food-Handling Behaviors of Immunocompromised Adults—*continued*

Lesson development procedures are described below in a stepwise fashion.

1. Develop plan for the lesson series by creating (a) a conceptual outline of the specific subject matter to be included, (b) generalizations to be addressed, and (c) objectives that reflect expected learner outcomes.
2. Partition outline into lessons (i.e., single topics in the conceptual outline). Create map to show the links or interrelationships between lessons.
3. Create storyboard for each lesson. Transform storyboard into a multimedia format as each lesson storyboard is complete (i.e., text is written and accompanying images and sounds assembled).
4. Conduct formative evaluation of each lesson as soon as the lesson is transformed into a multimedia format. The cognitive response method will gauge learner reactions and satisfaction (i.e., learners will verbalize the thoughts, feelings, and ideas that come to mind immediately after exposure to each screen). This means of inquiry was selected because it has proved useful in evaluating food and nutrition education materials (30). The formative evaluation of each lesson will involve three to five dietetic interns and three to five immunocompromised adults and/or caregivers of these adults. Formative evaluation data will be analyzed and needed refinements identified.
5. Link lessons in the series using the map created in Step 2 above.

The Health Belief Model will guide the development of the lessons. This model was chosen because it provides a framework for understanding why individuals are (or are not) motivated to follow heath care advice and perform health-protective behaviors.

Intervention Lesson Summative and Impact Evaluation. When the intervention program is complete, summative and impact evaluation will occur as follows.

Sample. Study participants will be recruited from adults (age 18 and above) with weakened immune systems due to disease (e.g., HIV/AIDS) or pharmaceutical or radiological treatments who are receiving outpatient treatment from the Super State University Health Care System during spring 20XX and caregivers of immunocompromised adults. The University Health Care System includes 11 hospitals (two specialize in cancer treatment; one is recognized as the premier treatment center for HIV/AIDS in the tri-state metropolitan area) and has nearly 1,700 physicians on staff. The attending physicians of eligible adults will receive information about the study and will be asked to encourage their patients to enroll. Enrollment invitation posters and flyers will be distributed to all physician offices and placed in key areas of each hospital in the system. Interested patients and caregivers will have the option of contacting project staff via telephone, e-mail, texting, fax, or letter. One hundred individuals will be recruited to participate in each of the four study groups. Immunocompromised adults and their caregivers often experience greater than normal time pressures due to increased need for medical interventions. Thus, to increase the likelihood of their participation in this project, each treatment group participant who completes all phases of the study will receive $50 and an instant-read food thermometer. Control group participants who complete all study phases will receive $10 and an instant-read food thermometer.

Study Design. A Solomon 4-Group experimental design will be used (31). This research design includes a pre/post treatment group, post-only treatment group, pre/post control group, and post-only control group. Participants will be randomly assigned to the study groups. The pre/post treatment group will complete the pretest and posttest and participate in the six intervention lessons. The post-only treatment group will complete the posttest and participate in the six intervention lessons. The pre/post control group will complete the pretest and posttest while the post-only control group will complete only the posttest. Those in the control groups will have the opportunity to complete the lessons after the posttest data are collected. The Solomon 4-Group design was selected because it maintains a great deal of internal and external validity (31). To assess the long-term effectiveness of the intervention lessons, a follow-up posttest will be administered approximately six months after the posttest to all study groups.

Participants in the treatment groups will be instructed that one intervention lesson will be posted at one-week intervals, for a total of six weeks. They will receive an e-mail and/or voice mail notification when each lesson is posted. Each lesson will be available for a one-week period during which participants will complete it at a time convenient to their schedules. One week after each lesson is posted, the project staff will host a

3

Once all the objectives are written, the grant seeker should place them in a logical sequence. For example, if the project objectives will be addressed in phases, the grant seeker should place them in chronological order. If some objectives are more important than others, they should be presented from most important to least important.

Although the goals and objectives section tends to be short (half a page or less), the importance of thoughtfully and precisely constructed goals and objectives cannot be over-emphasized. The goals and objectives are the heart of the proposal—*they are the reason one seeks a grant sponsor's help.* "When sponsors fund your projects, they are literally 'buying' your objectives."[5]

FIGURE 19-8 Grant Narrative: Improving Safe Food-Handling Behaviors of Immunocompromised Adults—*continued*

one-hour chat room discussion that will address questions participants posted to researchers about the lesson's content and offer an opportunity to discuss related issues. Each chat room session will be scheduled at three different times (one weekday, one weekend day, and one weekday evening). A six-week intervention period was chosen because the applicant's previous research revealed that this is a sufficient intervention time for individuals to significantly improve their food safety knowledge, attitudes, self-efficacy, and reported practices (32). After completing the lesson series and chat rooms that accompany each lesson, the participants will have the opportunity to post questions to the researchers and/or engage in monthly chat rooms for the next six months. They also will receive monthly e-mail, text message, and/or voice mail food safety tips and news. The food safety lessons will remain available for them to consult if they desire.

Questionnaires. Two self-report questionnaires will be used in this study. The first will collect demographic data. The second, the Food Safety Questionnaire–Model 2 (FSQ) (33), developed and validated previously by the applicant, is a highly reliable 55-item objective instrument that assesses food safety knowledge, attitudes, and reported food-handling behaviors and consumption of foods at high risk for bacterial contamination.

The pretest will be administered via mail or e-mail one week before the first intervention lesson is posted. The pre/post treatment and pre/post control groups will complete both study questionnaires during the pretest. The posttest will be administered one week after the last intervention lesson. All study groups will complete the FSQ during the posttest. The post-only treatment and post-only control groups also will complete the demographics questionnaires during the posttest. Approximately six months after the posttest, the study groups again will complete the FSQ. To minimize potential learning effects of the questionnaires, the purpose of the questionnaires will not be discussed with study participants and feedback on participant performance on the questionnaires will not be provided. To protect participant confidentiality, only key project staff will have access to data collected, and upon completion of the study all identifying characteristics will be stripped from the data files.

Data Analysis. Analysis of variance on the posttest scores will be conducted to determine whether pretesting affected posttest performance. Analysis of covariance, with pretest scores serving as the covariate, will be conducted to determine the impact of the interventions on knowledge, attitudes, and reported behaviors.

Intervention Program Revisions and Dissemination. The summative and impact evaluation data will be reviewed to determine needed lesson refinements. The lessons will be revised and posted permanently on the university's website.

To extend the impact of this project and enhance its value, the findings of the study and availability of the free online program will be disseminated via the media; professional organization publications and conferences; university publications distributed to alumni, faculty, and students; appropriate electronic listservs, discussion groups, and electronic bulletin boards; and the university's website and food- and nutrition-related websites. All health care professionals employed by the applicant institution will be made aware of these products through e-mail advisories sent to the faculty directors of these programs. The availability of this program also will be noted in the research presentations and journal articles that result from this project. The results of this project will be further disseminated by presentations at health and nutrition professional meetings (e.g., Academy of Nutrition and Dietetics, American Public Health Association) and in journal articles and related educational publications (e.g., *Journal of Nutrition Education and Behavior, Journal of Food Protection*).

4

A grant seeker should ask the following questions to assess the quality of the project goals and objectives. It will be important to revise project goals and objectives until all of these questions can be answered "yes."

1. Is each objective clearly and logically related to the sponsor's goal(s) and priorities?
2. Is each objective clearly and logically related to the goal and mission of the grant seeker's organization?
3. Does the grant seeker's organization have the skill, personnel, and resources to achieve each goal in a timely and cost-efficient manner?
4. Does each objective contribute to meeting the project goals?
5. Does each objective provide a realistic, feasible, attainable, and manageable solution to the problem or need?
6. Is the list of objectives complete? That is, do the objectives address all of the project's major activities?

7. Do the objectives clearly describe what will be different when the project is completed? For example, will people gain new skills that will improve their health? Will a more effective nutrition intervention program be available? Will we discover how to deliver community nutrition services more effectively?
8. Do the objectives clearly indicate what must be measured to determine progress toward meeting each objective? Is it clear that the grant seeker will know when each objective has been reached?
9. Are the objectives presented in a logical sequence?
10. Does each objective use an action verb?
11. Are the objectives written so clearly and precisely that writing the evaluation section will be a simple task?

Methods The methods section (sometimes called project description) describes in detail the procedures for achieving the study's objectives, justifies those procedures, and explains why the plan is likely to work. A full account of how the objectives will be achieved usually includes describing the project design, how success will be measured (e.g., through an evaluation plan), the participants (or sample) who will be involved, the sequence and time frame of activities (time and activity charts), and the duties and capabilities of the project staff.

Many grant sponsors place more emphasis on this part of the proposal than on other parts—this is where the grant seeker must convince the sponsor that he or she knows how to achieve the project's objectives. Explanations are bolstered by citing pertinent past work that the grant seeker or others have completed and by highlighting innovative or unique features of the present project.

It is important that the methods section clearly describes all the resources needed to complete the project activities. This description will make it easier to construct the budget and justify every proposed expense.

Project Design This section describes the overall organization of the proposed project. The sample proposal in Figure 19-8 indicates that this project has two primary phases: intervention lesson development and intervention lesson summative and impact evaluation. Both are described in detail.

Participants (Sample) If people will be involved in the project (for example, answering questions or participating in classes), grant seekers need to provide a complete description of their characteristics (e.g., women with osteoporosis or preschoolers who are overweight), how many will be involved, how they will be involved and/or what they will be asked to do, and how participants will be recruited. If participants will be assigned to various groups (e.g., experimental vs. control), grant seekers should explain how the assignments will be made (e.g., randomly or as whole classrooms).

To strengthen a proposal, grant seekers can indicate how accessible participants with the desired characteristics are to them. For instance, if the grant seeker is a weight-loss counselor and proposes a weight-control intervention, he or she could indicate the number of clients coming to the organization's clinic each month who might agree to participate. If participants will be offered an incentive to secure their participation, grant seekers should be sure to explain why the incentive is needed, what the incentive will be, and when it will be awarded. Many grant sponsors realize that recruiting participants can be a challenge and that incentives are sometimes necessary. However, it is a good idea to verify that the sponsor will fund an incentive before including it in a proposal. Note that any time grant seekers propose to work with people, they will need to comply with their institution's institutional review board (IRB) policy on dealing with human subjects (see the accompanying box, "Basic Principles of the Protection of Human Subjects").

Basic Principles of the Protection of Human Subjects

Scientific research has produced substantial social benefits, but it has raised some troubling ethical questions, too. Public attention focused on these questions after reported abuses of human subjects in biomedical experiments, especially during World War II. During the Nuremberg War Crimes Tribunals, the Nuremberg Code was drafted as a set of standards by which to judge physicians and scientists who had conducted biomedical experiments on concentration camp prisoners. This code became the prototype for many later codes designed to ensure that research involving human subjects would be conducted ethically. (*Note:* Human subjects are living individuals about whom a researcher obtains data by intervention or interaction with the individual or identifiable private data.)

The code consists of rules that guide researchers or the reviewers of research in their work. Sometimes, however, these rules are inadequate, conflicting, and/or difficult to interpret or apply. Thus, in 1978, the National Commission for the Protection of Human Subjects met to articulate the ethical principles that could be used to formulate, criticize, and interpret rules. This commission's report, *The Belmont Report: Ethical Principles and Guidelines for the Protection of Human Subjects of Research*, describes three fundamental ethical principles for acceptable conduct of research with human subjects: respect for persons, beneficence, and justice.

- Respect for persons recognizes the personal dignity and autonomy of individuals. It also requires special protection of vulnerable groups, such as children and prisoners. Researchers must get full consent from individuals before including them as research subjects. Before giving full consent, subjects must be informed about the research purpose and procedures, as well as its risks and benefits. Subjects must have a chance to ask questions and must be able to withdraw from the research at any time.
- Beneficence is the obligation to protect persons from harm by maximizing benefits and minimizing possible risks. The appropriateness of involving vulnerable populations must be clearly demonstrated, and the consent process must thoroughly disclose risks and benefits.
- Justice requires that the benefits and burdens of research be distributed fairly. Subjects should not be selected simply because they are readily available or because they are vulnerable as a consequence of illness, age, or socioeconomic condition. Research should not overburden individuals already burdened by their environments or conditions.

In community nutrition, our work nearly always involves human subjects. Sometimes community nutrition work is limited to practice; at other times it involves research; at still other times it is a combination of research and practice. The term *practice* tends to refer to interventions designed solely to enhance the patient or client well-being and to have a reasonable expectation of success. The purpose of medical or behavioral practice is to provide diagnosis, preventive treatment, or therapy to individuals. On the other hand, the term *research* refers to any systematic gathering and analysis of information designed to develop or contribute to generalizable knowledge (expressed, for example, in theories, principles, and statements of relationships, or shared at public meetings or in publications). Research includes:

- Interviews, surveys, tests, or observations that are designed to gather nonpublic information about individuals or groups.
- Studies of existing data, either public or private, where the identity of individuals is known.
- Studies designed to change participants' physical or psychological states or environments.

Whenever human subjects are involved in research of any type, the *Belmont Report's* principles should guide the researchers' actions. Keep in mind that the protection of human subjects is important in all types of research, from behavioral to biomedical. Most colleges, universities, and hospitals, as well as many other organizations, have an institutional review board (IRB) that is responsible for educating researchers about the protection of human subjects and for approving research involving humans.

Source: Adapted from Department of Health, Education, and Welfare, Office of the Secretary, the National Commission for the Protection of Human Subjects of Biomedical and Behavioral Research, *The Belmont Report: Ethical Principles and Guidelines for the Protection of Human Subjects of Research* (April 18, 1979).

Evaluation Plan (Study Design) An evaluation plan explains how the grant seeker proposes to measure the outcomes or impact of the project. That is, how will the grant seeker determine that the objectives have been met?

Many grant sponsors have long required an evaluation plan—they want to know whether the granted funds are having the desired impact. In other words, they want evidence that they are getting their money's worth! Even if the sponsor does not require evaluation as a condition of funding, it is a good idea to include one. That's because programs without an evaluation plan cannot demonstrate their impact and thus often have difficulty sustaining their funding, especially during an economic downturn. Furthermore, if grant seekers genuinely want to achieve the goals set, a well-designed and well-executed evaluation plan will help them track the project's progress and its strengths as well as pinpoint weaknesses and indicate new directions for future work.

When planning an evaluation, grant seekers need to review the call for proposals very carefully to see whether the sponsor requires the plan to include special methods. For example, the sponsor may require that a specific test be used to measure blood glucose levels or may specify the use of a particular software package to report data. For large, complex projects that involve numerous staff working in more than one organization, a management plan also may be a required part of the evaluation plan. For ideas on how to evaluate projects, review journal articles summarizing similar projects.

Recall that there are four types of evaluation: formative, process, summative, and impact. *Formative evaluation* is the process of testing and assessing program elements before the program is fully implemented. *Process evaluation* occurs during the program implementation to be certain the program is implemented as intended. *Summative evaluation* occurs at the end of a program to document its success and the extent to which project objectives were achieved. Finally, *impact evaluation* measures the overall worth and value of the program. In community nutrition, it tells us to what extent participants improved their knowledge, attitudes, values, skills, and/or health behaviors and physiological parameters. It also indicates the changes that have occurred in social, economic, civic, environmental, and/or regulatory/legislative conditions. Grant seekers need to consider carefully how each of these evaluation types will be addressed in the evaluation plan.

To create the evaluation plan, grant seekers begin by asking, "What questions do we want to answer as a result of the evaluation?" For instance, during formative evaluation they may want to learn how people respond to a fact sheet design or whether the contents are accurate. As a part of the summative and impact evaluation, they may want to know how much program participants learned about a topic, the amount their bone density increased, or how their intake of fruits and vegetables changed. This question is easy to answer when the project objectives are written in measurable terms. If answering this question is difficult, the grant seeker should revisit the project objectives and fine-tune them until they are expressed in clear, precise, measurable terms and clearly state the questions he or she wants to answer as a result of the evaluation. Then the grant seeker can use answers to the questions below to write the evaluation plan in three parts: measurements, data analysis, and dissemination.

1. What specific information is needed to generate those answers?
2. What is the source of the information?
3. How will the information be gathered? Specifically, what data instruments are needed to generate the data?
4. What evaluation design will be used?
5. What analyses will be conducted?

Measurements There are many ways to measure intervention outcomes, including tests, questionnaires, surveys, clinical examinations, food recalls, personal logs or memos, checklists, observational rating cards used by program staff or experts, and program records (such as daily activity reports and e-mail files). In any one study, there are often several methods for gathering the same information, and depending on the circumstances, some methods are better than others. Let's say you want to determine dietitians' understanding of genetics. To find out, you could create a questionnaire or use an existing one. Then you could interview each person face-to-face or by phone, or you could survey them by mail or online. Dietary intake could be assessed via a food frequency form, 24-hour recall, or three-day food record or in several other ways.

The measures selected to generate needed information will depend on several factors, including the purpose and scope of the evaluation, resources available for evaluation (such as personnel time, money, and skill), instrument choices available, measurement precision needed, and burden to participants (such as the time they must spend and the commitment they must make). The best measurement choices are feasible, justifiable, valid, and reliable. **Feasible measures** fit resource constraints, yield measurements that are suitably precise, are manageable, and are not overly burdensome to study participants. (For example, a 14-day weighed food record probably isn't feasible in a study of preschool eating patterns.) **Justifiable measures** are among the best choices available to measure a particular characteristic, are as safe and nonintrusive as possible, and are truly necessary and within the project's scope. **Valid measures** actually measure what they are intended to measure. **Reliable measures** are just that; they give similar results each time they are used. Many excellent research design resources are available that can provide more detail on choosing feasible, justifiable, valid, and reliable measures for community nutrition programs, as shown in the accompanying feature, "Research Design Resources for the Community Nutritionist."

The measurements section will flow most logically if it is written in the same sequence as that in which the objectives appear in the grant narrative. The grant seeker can further increase clarity by describing the interrelationships among the project activities. This section of the proposal should have the following characteristics:

- Provide sufficient detail about how the grant seeker will measure progress toward meeting each objective to demonstrate the technical soundness of the measurements selected, his or her in-depth understanding of the method, and his or her credibility as an evaluator. A critical discussion of the feasibility, justifiability, validity, and reliability of the instrument, along with the advantages associated with the method and how any disadvantages will be overcome, helps demonstrate the technical soundness of the proposed measures.
- Describe the procedure for administering the measurement in a stepwise fashion. If it is a complex or confusing procedure, consider including a diagram. Example: The participants will be placed in a private room, instructed to change into a paper robe and slippers, and weighed on a calibrated balance-beam scale.

Feasible measures Fit resource constraints, yield measurements that are suitably precise, are manageable, and are not overly burdensome to study participants.

Justifiable measures Among the best choices available to measure a particular characteristic, are as safe and nonintrusive as possible, and are truly necessary and within the project's scope.

Valid measures Measure what they are intended to measure.

Reliable measures Give similar results each time they are used.

Research Design Resources for the Community Nutritionist

Research: Successful Approaches, edited by E. R. Monsen, 3rd ed. (Chicago: American Dietetic Association, 2008).

A comprehensive guide to planning, executing, presenting, and evaluating various types of research. Includes topics such as evidence-based practice, behavioral theory-based research, and research methods in complementary and alternative medicine.

The Practice of Social Research, by E. Babbie, 15th ed. (Belmont, CA: Wadsworth, 2016).

An authoritative research methods text with a broad set of topics, including illustrative examples such as welfare and poverty, gender issues, the AIDS epidemic, and more.

Research Design: Qualitative, Quantitative, and Mixed Methods Approaches, edited by J. Cresswell, 4th ed. (Thousand Oaks, CA: Sage, 2014).

An authoritative handbook on research and evaluation methods designed for researchers in health sciences.

Research in Education, by J. W. Best and J. V. Kahn, 10th ed. (Boston: Allyn and Bacon, 2005).

A reference book covering topics such as identifying problems, forming hypotheses, constructing and using data-gathering tools, designing research studies, and employing statistical procedures to analyze data.

Health Behavior and Health Education: Theory, Research, and Practice, edited by K. Glanz, B. K. Rimer, and K. Viswanath, 5th ed. (Hoboken, NJ: Wiley, 2015).

A textbook that provides information on health behavior theories and research practice, drawing on fields such as cognitive psychology, marketing, and communications to explain a range of factors affecting health behavior in diverse populations.

Planning, Implementing, and Evaluating Health Promotion Programs: A Primer, by J. F. McKenzie, B. L. Neiger, and R. Thackeray, 6th ed. (San Francisco: Pearson Education, 2013).

A comprehensive text providing information needed to plan, implement, and evaluate health promotion programs in a variety of settings, with discussion of needs assessment, how to acquire needs assessment data, and how to apply theory to practice.

- Describe how the measurements have been used previously. Indicate the grant seeker's experience with these measures. Example: The project director developed and validated the Nutrition Attitude Scale with individuals having characteristics similar to those of participants in the proposed study sample. The scale yielded highly reliable results (Cronbach's alpha reliability coefficient = 0.89).
- Describe who will collect the data and how they will be trained. Example: Three dietetics graduate research assistants will be trained to be observers who can uniformly complete the observation checklist. This training will include a detailed review of the recipe and observation instrument, preparation of the recipe several times, role-playing practice sessions, analysis of the practice sessions highlighting inconsistencies, and further practice sessions to achieve uniformity. Each observer also will gain field practice by completing practice observations with a minimum of five individuals who have characteristics similar to those of the study participants. During the field practice, the observers and project director will simultaneously observe the same individuals. An observer will be considered ready to collect data when the interrater reliability rate for

the observer and project director is a minimum of 90%. Dr. Harris, a senior project associate, is nationally known for his evaluation expertise and will conduct all phases of the observer training.

- Indicate where the data will be collected. Example: Each person will individually participate in a face-to-face interview with a trained interviewer in a room relatively free of distractions.
- Indicate how the data will be recorded. Example: The interviewer will take notes during the interviews, and the interviews will be audiotaped for later transcription. Example: The questionnaire is a pencil-and-paper, self-report, objective instrument designed to measure attitudes toward eating whole grains.
- Indicate how participant confidentiality will be protected. Example: All study questionnaires will be kept in a locked file cabinet in the project director's office. Once data are transcribed into computer files, all identifying data will be removed and the paper questionnaires will be shredded.

Data Analysis The data analysis section describes how the data collected will be analyzed to determine the success of the project. It is a good idea to consult a statistician during preparation of the proposal, and periodically throughout the project, to ensure that the data collected will be valid, usable, and generalizable and can be interpreted to provide answers to study questions. Example: Frequencies, percentages, and means will be calculated to determine the participants' scores on knowledge about nutrition label reading, their attitudes toward diet and health, and their label usage behaviors.

Dissemination The purpose of this section is to describe how interested audiences will learn about the project and its outcomes. The dissemination section should explain why dissemination activities are important for the project; concisely describe a feasible, effective, and suitable dissemination plan; and indicate who will be responsible for this task.

Dissemination offers many benefits to both the sponsor and the grant recipient. For instance, members of the public learn more about the sponsor and its priorities. They become aware of the priorities, mission, and activities of the organization receiving the funds. This increased awareness can lead to other funding opportunities, help locate new clients and collaborators, and enhance information sharing among colleagues. It also helps build the reputation of the grant recipient.

Unfortunately, many worthwhile projects are funded and completed without anyone except those involved knowing about their outcomes. Increasingly, grant sponsors are requiring grant seekers to declare, either in the methods section or in a special dissemination section, specifically how they will disseminate information generated from the project.

The methods section in Figure 19-8 is an example of how this section might be written for the objectives stated earlier in the figure. Note how the example details the manner in which each project objective will be achieved and indicates why the grant seeker selected that method. Also note how the flow of this section parallels the sequence in which the objectives are presented earlier in the figure and addresses each of the items in the bulleted list on pages 736–738. Many journal articles provide other excellent examples of how to develop the methods section.

Time and Activity Chart A time and activity chart breaks the entire project into manageable steps that clearly show grant reviewers how the project will proceed. This chart can take several forms. Two common formats appear in **Figures 19-9** and **19-10**. All formats of these charts should chronologically list all steps that must be taken to complete

Task	Time to Complete	Start Date	End Date	Personnel Responsible[a]
Lesson Development and Evaluation				
1. Develop plan for lesson series, conceptual outline, generalizations, and objectives.	8 weeks	9/15/17	11/15/17	PD, SAs, RA
2. Partition outline into lessons. Create map of lesson links.	2 weeks	11/15/17	11/30/17	PD, SAs, RA
3a. Create storyboard for each lesson (complete research, writing, image selection/creation, and preparation of all materials for Step 3b).	30 weeks	12/1/17	6/15/18	PD, SAs, RA
3b. Transform storyboards into multimedia as each lesson is completed.	30 weeks	3/1/18	8/15/18	PD, RA, CPT
4a. Conduct formative evaluation of each lesson as it is completed.	22 weeks	3/15/18	8/31/18	PD, RA
4b. Refine lessons.	22 weeks	4/1/18	9/15/18	PD, SAs, RA, CPT, CE
5. Link lessons as the formative evaluation concludes for the lesson series.	2 weeks	9/1/18	9/15/18	PD, SAs, RA, CPT
6. Recruit study participants.	8 weeks	9/15/18	11/15/18	RA

[a] PD = Project Director; SAs = Senior Associates; RA = Research Assistant; CPT = Computer Programming Team; CE = Copy Editor.

FIGURE 19-9 Time and Activity Chart This incomplete sample chart for the proposal in Figure 19-8 shows what activities will occur, when they will occur, and who is responsible. For practice, finish this chart using the proposal in Figure 19-8.

the project and should indicate when work on each step will begin and end. Note in Figure 19-9 how the chart also shows the duration of the activity and who is responsible for the work. Figure 19-10 reveals how project activities overlap. If proposal page limitations permit, consider submitting charts formatted like both Figures 19-9 and 19-10. If there is room for only one, choose a format like Figure 19-9 because it also reveals who is responsible for completing each task, which can greatly facilitate writing the budget narrative. Time and activity charts often appear in the methods section; however, some grant sponsors instruct applicants to place them in a separate section or in an appendix.

Accurate, neatly constructed time and activity charts are essential to all but the simplest grant proposals. These charts not only guide the grant seeker's work if the grant is funded but also help convince grant reviewers that the grant seeker understands the process involved in reaching the proposed goals and objectives.

Capability The capability section establishes the credibility of the grant seeker, including project staff, and the organization's ability to complete the proposed project with expertise, on time, and within the budget. It is essential for the grant seeker to convince reviewers of his or her capabilities in this section *and* throughout the entire proposal. The quality of the proposal itself will tell reviewers a great deal about the grant seeker—it will indicate whether he or she thinks clearly and logically, expresses thoughts cogently and succinctly, has technical skill, analyzes data objectively and accurately, interprets results

Task	Year: 2017				Year: 2018												Year: 2019								
	9	10	11	12	1	2	3	4	5	6	7	8	9	10	11	12	1	2	3	4	5	6	7	8	9
Lesson Development and Evaluation																									
1. Develop plan for lesson series, conceptual outline, generalizations, and objectives.	|---		-|																						
2. Partition outline into lessons. Create map of lesson links.			|																						
3a. Create storyboard for each lesson.				|---	---	---	---	---	---	-|															
3b. Transform storyboards into multimedia as each lesson is completed.							|---	---	---	---	---	-|													
4a. Conduct formative evaluation of each lesson as it is completed.								|---	---	---	---	---													
4b. Refine lessons.									|---	---	---	---	-|												
5. Link lessons as the formative evaluation concludes for the lesson series.													|												
6. Recruit study participants.													|---	-|											

FIGURE 19-10 Time and Activity Chart

This incomplete sample chart for the proposal in Figure 19-8 shows the overlap among activities. For practice, finish this chart using the proposal in Figure 19-8.

correctly and conservatively, and discriminates between significant and inconsequential information.

The capability section should describe the grant-seeking organization's goals and philosophy (mission), activities, success stories, and distinguishing characteristics that make it uniquely qualified to carry out the proposed project. It also describes the facilities, equipment, reference materials, support personnel, and any other resources that are key to the success of the proposed project. In some cases, the organization's capability statement appears in the proposal introduction to establish why the organization is proposing a particular program and how it is uniquely qualified to deliver the program with excellence.

The credibility and capability of project staff can be established by including curricula vitae (résumés) for all key project personnel and/or a brief (one page or less) personal statement describing in narrative form each person's training and expertise, previous experience with projects and grants like the one proposed, and role in the proposed project. Many grant sponsors set limits on the length, content, and/or style of curricula vitae. In addition, they may instruct grant seekers to place curricula vitae in a different location, such as in an appendix. Whenever possible, it is helpful to weave the project staff's expertise (or that of the organization) into the proposal's needs statement or methods section. This technique builds credibility and indicates to grant reviewers that the applicant has a proven record of accomplishment. Note in Figure 19-8 how the writer took the opportunity to begin establishing her expertise by citing prior work ("focus group data collected by the applicant revealed that . . ."; "the applicant's previous research revealed that . . ."; and "the questionnaire developed and validated previously by the applicant").

For success, the project director (or principal investigator) must clearly have the expertise needed to direct all the activities of the grant. If the project director lacks expertise, a co-director can provide complementary expertise. For multiphase, complex projects, an interdisciplinary team usually is needed. Teams that have a successful track record of working together are much more credible than teams hastily assembled to compete for a newly announced grant.

Budget

The budget is one of the most important parts of the proposal. It not only describes the expected cost of the project but also demonstrates the grant seeker's planning and management expertise. Incomplete, inflated, or inadequate budgets signal inexperience and/or incompetence.

To begin, grant seekers should carefully review the grant guidelines to determine exactly which expenses can be charged and which are excluded. In addition, they need to determine exactly how the grant sponsor wants the budget presented. Some grant sponsors provide forms that must be used. Others list the budget categories that must be included. Still others offer little direction regarding the budget. Next, grant seekers need to scrutinize the grant narrative and list all anticipated expenses, being sure to build in some flexibility to cover unanticipated events, cost increases, and salary raises. Grant seekers also need to remember that all project costs must be incurred during the proposed period of time. Paying for expenses that occurred prior to the grant period (including costs associated with proposal preparation) is rarely allowed. In addition, prepaying people for work that will occur after the grant ends or buying supplies, materials, postage, and the like to be used after the grant ends is rarely permitted. In nearly all cases, all costs must be auditable (i.e., receipts are needed).

The most successful grant proposals have budgets that are totally consistent with their grant narrative—that is, every budgeted expense is clearly related to the project goals, objectives, and methods. No budget item should make grant reviewers wonder why it is included. For instance, if participants will be offered incentives, grant seekers need to be sure to describe them in the grant narrative. If the incentives are not described, the reviewers will wonder about their purpose and expense—and about the grant seeker's skill as a grant manager. To be certain that the budget and grant narrative are clearly linked, grant seekers should analyze the narrative carefully and list all anticipated expenses. Then, once the budget is constructed, they need to examine each expense and verify that the need for the expense is clearly justified in the grant narrative.

The importance of an accurate budget cannot be overstated. Grant seekers who overextend their resources, propose to do too much in a funding period, or underestimate their costs will appear unqualified and inexperienced to seasoned grant reviewers. If somehow the grant seeker does receive the grant in spite of such underestimates, the insufficient resources, time, and money will cause a great deal of frustration and anxiety and may result in a failure to achieve the proposed goals.

Budget Categories Budgets are usually divided into two main categories: direct costs and indirect costs. Some also require cost sharing, which includes cash or in-kind gifts (e.g., donated products, supplies, equipment, and services).

Direct Costs Direct costs are concrete project expenditures that are directly listed line by line (i.e., they are line items). Direct costs usually include personnel (i.e., salaries, wages, consultant fees, and fringe benefits), equipment, supplies, and travel (**Figure 19-11**).

FIGURE 19-11 Budget
This incomplete sample budget for the proposal in Figure 19-8 lists each anticipated financial cost. For practice, finish this budget using the proposal in Figure 19-8.

```
YEAR 1

DIRECT COSTS
A. Salaries and Wages
   1. Senior Personnel
      a. 1 Project Director (PD): Greta Grantwriter              $17,271
      b. 2 Senior Associates (SAs): John Smith and Margaret Anderson  $23,832
   2. Other Personnel
      a. 1 Research Assistant                                     $4,500
      b. 1 Copy Editor                                            $1,400
      c. 1 Computer Programming Team                             $25,000
B. Fringe Benefits                                              $13,321
C. Total Salaries, Wages, and Fringe Benefits                  $85,324
D. Equipment                                                    $3,000
E. Materials and Supplies                                       $1,000
F. Travel                                                         $263
G. All Other Direct Costs                                         $530
H. Total Direct Costs (Items C to G)                           $90,117

INDIRECT COSTS (23% of direct costs)                           $22,530

TOTAL COST                                                    $112,647

YEAR 2

DIRECT COSTS
A. Salaries and Wages
   1. Senior Personnel
      a. 1 Project Director (PD): Greta Grantwriter              $9,673
      b. ...
```

Indirect Costs Indirect costs are also called overhead, administrative costs, or facilities and administrative costs. Indirect costs are real costs associated with a grant that usually are not specifically listed on budgets, primarily because they tend to be difficult to price individually. They may include the costs of administering the grant, facility and equipment usage, and utilities. Because it is hard to estimate the extra costs the grant recipient will incur in administering the grant, indirect costs are usually calculated as a percentage of the direct costs. As you can see in Figure 19-11, indirect costs were calculated as 23% of the direct costs.

The percentage charged for indirect costs varies with the grant-seeking organization and the grant sponsor. Organizations that frequently receive federal grants usually have an approved federal indirect costs percentage rate. The percentage of indirect costs that grant sponsors will pay ranges from zero to the full federal indirect cost rate. Grant seekers need to be sure to check the grant guidelines or call the grant sponsor to determine how much they can charge for indirect costs. If the grant sponsor does not pay indirect costs, grant seekers can estimate the administrative costs of the project and list them as direct costs. For example, a grant seeker could estimate the cost of renting workspace and the percentage of a payroll clerk's time that will be devoted to this project and list them as direct-cost line items.

Some people erroneously view indirect costs as an unwarranted windfall to the grant recipient's organization. However, indirect costs are indeed actual costs that must be incurred by the grant-seeking organization if the grant is to be completed successfully. For example, the grant recipient's organization must administer the grant; these administrative duties are likely to increase the work of nongrant staff (e.g., the payroll department will need to pay and keep records for new grant-paid employees; the accounting department will have the added responsibility of processing purchasing requests for items used in the grant and of auditing grant expenditures). Sometimes the increase is so great that administrative departments need to hire extra help or pay overtime. Also, to do the work of the grant, staff will need to use facilities, equipment, and utilities, thereby making them unavailable or less accessible to employees doing nongrant work. Remember that if indirect costs are not covered by the grant sponsor, these costs nearly always must be drawn from the grant-seeking organization's other resources. Thus, if a grant sponsor will not pay indirect costs, the grant-seeking organization must assess whether it is able to bear the burden of the additional indirect costs it will incur in the course of completing the project funded by the grant.

Cost Sharing   Cost sharing, which is also called *matching* or *cost matching*, occurs when the grant-seeking organization agrees to pay certain costs (by contributing cash or in-kind goods or services) of the project. For instance, an organization may agree to contribute the cost of office space, incentives, photocopying, a percentage of a worker's time, and/or indirect costs. Grant seekers should check the grant guidelines or call the sponsor to determine whether cost sharing is required and, if so, how much of the grant costs must be matched. If cost sharing is required, the grant-seeking organization usually is required to contribute (or match) a percentage of the funds requested. For example, some grant sponsors require that the grant seeker contribute $1 for every dollar they award (a 100% match). Others may require the grant seeker to contribute more or less than a dollar for every dollar they award. **Figure 19-12** shows a sample budget for an RFP that required a minimum of a 100% match.

FIGURE 19-12

Cost-Sharing Budget
This incomplete sample cost-sharing budget for the proposal in Figure 19-8 lists each anticipated financial cost. For practice, finish this budget using the proposal in Figure 19-8.

YEAR 1

DIRECT COSTS

	Amount Requested	Cost Sharing	Total Amount
A. Salaries and Wages			
1. Senior Personnel			
a. 1 Project Director (PD): Greta Grantwriter	$7,271	$10,000	$17,271
b. 2 Senior Associates (SAs): John Smith and Margaret Anderson	$11,000	$12,832	$23,832
2. Other Personnel			
a. 1 Research Assistant	$4,500	$0	$4,500
b. 1 Copy Editor	$0	$1,400	$1,400
c. 1 Computer Programming Team	$25,000	$0	$25,000
B. Fringe Benefits	$3,000	10,321	$13,321
C. Total Salaries, Wages, and Fringe Benefits	$50,771	$34,553	$85,324
D. Equipment	$3,000	$0	$3,000
E. Materials and Supplies	$1,000	$0	$1,000
F. Travel	$263	$0	$263
G. All Other Direct Costs	$530	$0	$530
H. Total Direct Costs (Items C to G)	$55,564	$34,553	$90,117
INDIRECT COSTS (23%)	$0	$22,530	$22,530
TOTAL COST	$55,564	$57,083	$112,647

YEAR 2

DIRECT COSTS
	Amount Requested	Cost Sharing	Total Amount
A. Salaries and Wages			
1. Senior Personnel			
a. 1 Project Director (PD): Greta Grantwriter	$5,000	$4,673	$9,673
b. ...			

Budget Narrative The budget narrative follows the budget in the proposal. Its purpose is to explain or justify all expenditures. It is wise to include a budget narrative even if the grant sponsor does not request one. The narrative may be as extensive as the one shown in **Figure 19-13**, which explains all the expenses in Figure 19-11. Alternatively, it could be quite brief, as shown in **Figure 19-14**. The most useful budget narratives show the basis for all calculations. For example, instead of just saying that fringe benefits equal $13,321, give explicit calculations like those shown in Figure 19-13.

FIGURE 19-13

Budget Narrative
This incomplete sample budget narrative for the proposal in Figure 19-8 describes each anticipated financial cost and how it was derived. For practice, finish this narrative using the proposal in Figure 19-8 and the budget completed in Figure 19-11.

YEAR 1

DIRECT COSTS

A. Salaries and Wages
  1. Senior Personnel
   a. 1 Project Director (PD): Greta Grantwriter: 20% time for a total of $17,271. Responsibilities include: serving as instructional design expert for the design of all lessons; overseeing all lessons including development of outline, generalizations, and objectives; direction of partitioning of outline into lessons; creation of map of all lessons; creation of storyboards for each lesson; directing transformation of storyboards for all lessons into multimedia as each is completed; working with programming team to develop online lesson structure; overseeing formative evaluation of each lesson as it is completed; identifying refinements needed in all lessons based on formative evaluation results; overseeing refinement of all lessons.
   b. 2 Senior Associates (SAs): John Smith and Margaret Anderson: 15% time each for a grand total of $23,832. Responsibilities of each include: developing outline, generalizations, and objectives for three lessons; partitioning developed outline into lessons; creating map of the lessons; creating storyboards for the lessons (completing research, writing, image identification); identifying refinements needed in lessons based on formative evaluation results.
  2. Other Personnel
   a. 1 Research Assistant: 10% time for a total of $4,500. Responsibilities include: assisting PD and SAs to create storyboards for each lesson (gathering research materials, locating, and/or creating images); working with programming team to transform storyboards for all lessons into multimedia as each is completed; conducting formative evaluation; identifying refinements needed in all lessons based on formative evaluation results.
   b. 1 Copy Editor: The copy editor will edit all written portions of the lessons under the direction of PD: 40 hours @ average rate of $35 per hour = $1,400.
   c. 1 Computer Programming Team: The computer programming team will transform storyboards into multimedia as each lesson is completed, refine lessons, link lessons, make CD-ROM masters. $2,500/month x 10 months = $25,000.
B. Fringe Benefits: Fringe Benefits are 24% for 1 Project Director, 2 Senior Associates, and 1 Research Assistant @ 0.24 x ($17,271 + $23,832 + $4,500) for a total of $10,945. Fringe Benefits are 9% for 1 Copy Editor and 1 Computer Programming Team 0.09 x ($1,400 + $25,000) for a total of $2,376. Total Fringe Benefits equal $13,321 ($10,945 + $2,376).
C. Total Salaries, Wages, and Fringe Benefits: Total Salaries, Wages, and Fringe Benefits = $85,324 [$72,003 (Total Salaries and Wages) + $13,321 (Total Fringe Benefits)].
D. Equipment
  1. Multimedia-capable computer hardware with scanner: Equipment to be used by Research Assistant for storyboard work @ $3,000.
E. Materials and Supplies
  1. **Research Articles:** (i.e., cost for article reprints from online sources for research for each lesson) Estimated 20 articles x 6 lessons @ $2.50 each = $250.
  2. **Storyboard Creation Materials:** (i.e., cost of clip art, office supplies) Estimated at $125 per lesson x 6 lessons = $750.
F. Travel
  Mileage to meetings with Computer Programming Team ($0.35/mile x 10 trips x 75 mile average round trip). Total mileage cost equals $263.
G. All Other Direct Costs
  1. Telephone: Telephone costs are estimated to be $15 per month ($15 x 12 months) for a total cost of $180.
  2. Printing & Copying: Miscellaneous copying: $50.
  3. Duplicated CD-ROMs: 100 copies for formative evaluation @ $3.00/CD = $300.
H. Total Direct Costs
  Total costs for C through G above equal $90,117.

INDIRECT COSTS
Indirect Costs equal $22,530 (23% of total direct costs)

TOTAL COST
Total Direct and Indirect Costs equal $112,647 ($90,117 + 22,530).

YEAR 2

A. Salaries and Wages
  1. Senior Personnel
   a. 1 Project Director (PD): Greta Grantwriter: 10% time for a total of $9,673. Responsibilities include: …

```
YEAR 1

DIRECT COSTS
A. Salaries and Wages
   1. Senior Personnel
      a. 1 Project Director (PD): Greta Grantwriter          $17,271ᵃ
      b. 2 Senior Associates (SAs): John Smith and Margaret Anderson   $23,832ᵇ
   2. Other Personnel
      a. 1 Research Assistant                                $4,500ᶜ
      b. 1 Copy Editor                                       $1,400ᵈ
      c. 1 Computer Programming Team                         $25,000ᵉ
B. Fringe Benefits                                           $13,321ᶠ
C. Total Salaries, Wages, and Fringe Benefits               $85,324
D. Equipment                                                 $3,000ᵍ

Budget Narrative
ᵃ 20% time for a total of $17,271.
ᵇ 15% time each for a grand total of $23,832.
ᶜ 10% time for a total of $4,500.
ᵈ 40 hours @ average rate of $35 per hour = $1,400.
ᵉ $2,500/month x 10 months = $25,000.
ᶠ Fringe Benefits are 24% for Project Director, Senior Associates, and Research
Assistant and 9% for Copy Editor and Computer Programming Team.
ᵍ Multimedia-capable computer hardware with scanner.
```

FIGURE 19-14

Budget
This incomplete sample budget with brief budget narrative for the proposal in Figure 19-8 lists each anticipated financial cost. For practice, finish this budget using the proposal in Figure 19-8.

Appendixes Appendixes are placed at the end of the proposal. They should contain carefully selected materials that directly support the proposal. Appendixes may include strong letters of support and endorsements from individuals critical to the project's success, assurances of cooperation between institutions and subcontractors, reprints of articles published by the project staff, data collection questionnaires, organization charts, financial statements, and recent annual reports. In some proposals, curricula vitae from all key project personnel are included in the appendixes; in others they are placed elsewhere.

Appendixes should not be used to get around the page limits set by the grant sponsor. Keep in mind that grant reviewers are very busy and may skip over the appendixes. Some grant sponsors do not forward appendixes to reviewers. Therefore, the grant seeker should be certain that all the information reviewers need to make an informed decision about the proposal is included in the grant narrative.

Assembling the Final Product

When all parts of the proposal are finished, the next step is to assemble them into a complete package and review them using a word processor's spelling and grammar checker. The grant seeker should carefully proofread the proposal to find obvious errors as well as to identify ways to refine the proposal further. Next, the grant seeker needs to format the proposal in an inviting, professional style, following all instructions provided by the grant sponsor, and give it to conscientious colleagues who will supply thorough, honest feedback. Using this feedback to refine the proposal can lead to important and valuable improvements. Once the proposal is finished, it is time to make the specified number of copies and send it to the designated address before the deadline passes.

Keys to Success The most inviting and easy-to-read proposals tend to have these characteristics. However, keep in mind that some grant sponsors may specify different characteristics (e.g., a certain font size or style, binding style).

- The writing is clear, cohesive, and highly readable (i.e., in the active voice, with sentences of varying length but none more than 30 words long).
- Appropriate vocabulary is used, any terms likely to be unknown to reviewers are defined, and jargon is avoided.
- For grants submitted as hard copies, paper is white, 20-pound bond, of standard letter size.
- Margins are 1 inch (top, bottom, and sides).
- Typeface is 12-point serif (such as Times Roman).
- Pages are numbered.
- Bold headings and subheadings are used to guide the reader to each section.
- The right margin is ragged (not justified).
- Upper- and lowercase letters are used (not all uppercase).
- Italics, bolding, and underlining are used sparingly.
- Paragraphs are indented five spaces.
- White space is used to break up the pages. For example, double spacing between paragraphs helps increase white space and makes the document appear inviting and readable.
- For hard copies, the document is bound with only a staple in the upper left-hand corner.
- Illustrations, graphs, and charts are clear and enhance understanding.

Review of the Grant Proposal

After receiving a grant proposal, grant sponsors usually send grant seekers a note confirming that they received the proposal and indicating approximately when they plan to announce which proposals will be funded. If the grant seeker does not receive a letter within a few weeks of submitting the proposal, he or she should contact the individual designated on the call for proposals by phone, e-mail, or letter to confirm that the proposal was received and ask when a funding decision is likely to be made. Keep in mind that making funding decisions sometimes takes longer than the grant sponsor originally planned. However, if the grant seeker does not receive a funding decision (or a notice that the decisions have been delayed) within a few weeks of the date provided by the grant sponsor, the grant seeker should contact the individual designated on the call for proposals and politely ask when a funding decision is likely to be made.

After receiving a grant proposal, the grant sponsor organizes the proposals submitted and distributes them to grant reviewers. The job of grant reviewers is to review each proposal, compare it to the sponsor's priorities and criteria, judge the relative merit of the project and its likelihood for success, assess whether the project staff and organization can deliver what is proposed within the time frame specified, and evaluate the adequacy of the budget. In many ways, the reviewers are stewards of the grant sponsor's funds, and most take their responsibilities very seriously. Grant seekers are most likely to get the

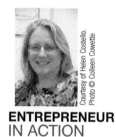

Courtesy of Helen Costello.
Photo © Colleen Cowette

ENTREPRENEUR
IN ACTION

As program manager for the *Recipe for Success* community food programs at the New Hampshire Food Bank, Helen Costello, MS, RD, LD, uses her dietetics, science, and policy backgrounds to achieve success with programs that help individuals alleviate their food insecurity. Many elements of entrepreneurship make the programs successful: a solid and shared vision; strong networking; some calculated risk taking; and, most importantly, assembling a great team with the same vision to get the job done. Working in the nonprofit sector is deeply rewarding, says Helen. Find out more about her sage advice on looking for resource opportunities everywhere at *www.cengagebrain.com*.

best review possible when they prepare their proposals carefully and thoughtfully and observe all the instructions provided by the grant sponsor.

Everyone hopes that his or her grant proposals are fully funded the first time around. Sometimes, however, grant sponsors will contact an applicant and ask him or her to modify the proposal (e.g., by reducing the budget, trimming away some objectives, or increasing the number of participants). When this happens, the grant seeker will need to analyze the proposal carefully and decide whether the changes are feasible and how they will be made. It is important for both grant sponsor and grant seeker to understand clearly the work that will be completed before the grant is awarded.

Successful grant seekers will need to apply their management and budgeting skills carefully so that they will achieve grant goals expertly, on budget, and on schedule. Remember, the proposal is what the sponsor is buying, so it is important for the grant recipient to deliver the product promised. If the grant recipient needs or wants to diverge from the proposal, he or she will probably need to renegotiate with the grant sponsor. Grant recipients should carefully review all the rules governing the grant before accepting it.

Learning that a grant wasn't funded isn't good news, but it's not necessarily bad news, either. That's because many grant proposals can be revised and resubmitted for consideration in the next go-round. In fact, many funded grants are resubmissions. Remember that in grant writing, "failure often precedes success."

The most common reasons for proposals not to be funded are that there were problems with planning and time management, the proposal did not follow the guidelines or was submitted after the deadline, the proposal lacked a well-conceived plan of action or idea, and/or the proposal had errors in the budget estimates. In many cases, a proposal is rejected because it does not match the grant sponsor's funding priorities. A "generic" proposal sent out to several grant sponsors is *not* recommended—every proposal should be tailored to the specific sponsor's priorities and guidelines.

Most government grant sponsors and some private grant sponsors provide grant seekers with a written summary of the reviewers' comments. These summaries can help all applicants—successful and unsuccessful—learn how to improve future proposals. Grant seekers use these comments to rework a rejected proposal and put it in a more competitive position next time. Another great way to improve grant-writing skills and better understand the review process is to become a reviewer. Grant sponsors do recruit reviewers, so grant seekers should consider sending them a letter along with copies of their curricula vitae.

There is no doubt that grant writing takes considerable time and effort, but the rewards of success are worth it! The most successful grant seekers demonstrate four critical qualities: (1) diligence in researching and identifying grant sponsors, (2) creativity in matching project goals with those of sponsors, (3) attentiveness to detail in proposal preparation, and (4) persistence in revising proposals and resubmitting them to potential grant sponsors.

The Logic Model

As discussed in Chapter 5, the Logic Model provides a framework for planning, implementing, managing, and evaluating community nutrition programs.[6] It can be very useful for grant proposal writers because, like a road map, it graphically shows where you are and what you'll need to get to where you want to be. In addition, some grant sponsors now require proposals to include a planning model like the Logic Model.

▶ **THINK LIKE A COMMUNITY NUTRITIONIST**

After a proposal is funded, the Logic Model will help you stay on track and achieve the goals that were proposed. By regularly updating the project's Logic Model and sharing it with project personnel, everyone will know how the project is progressing and see the importance of their role in achieving its goals.[7] To develop your skills, try completing the Logic Model in **Figure 19-15** using the proposal found in Figure 19-8. Also, visit *www.uwex.edu/ces/pdande/evaluation/* to learn more about this planning model.

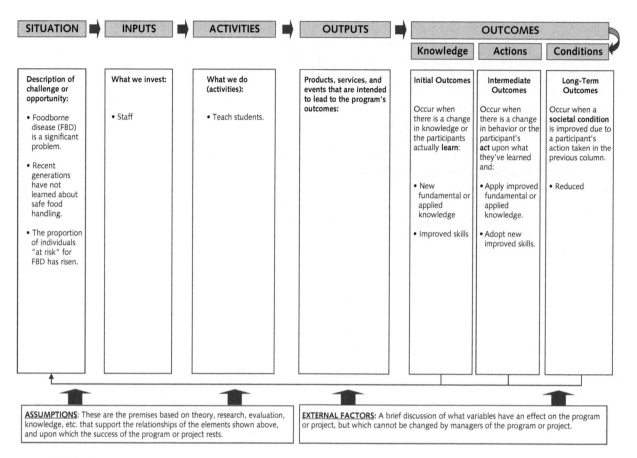

FIGURE 19-15 Logic Model for the Proposal in Figure 19-8
For practice, complete this model using the proposal in Figure 19-8.
Source: Adapted from Generic Logic Model for NIFA Reporting; available at *http://nifa.usda.gov/sites/default/files/resource/Generic%20Logic%20 Model%20for%20NIFA%20Reporting.pdf.*

Teamwork Gets Results

At the end of the day, you bet on people, not on strategies.
—Larry Bossidy, CEO, AlliedSignal, as cited in N. M. Tichy's *The Leadership Engine*

Few things are accomplished in community nutrition without teamwork. Community nutritionists often work in teams to lobby state legislators, plan mass media campaigns, identify perceived needs in the community, design programs, and raise awareness about a nutritional problem. When the Arizona Department of Health Services designed a program to help the staff at childcare facilities learn how to meet the needs of children with special health care needs, they used a team approach. The course instructors for Project CHANCE included a parent of a child with special health care needs, a nutritionist, an occupational therapist, and a director of a childcare facility.[1] Each member of the teaching team brought personal insights and experiences to the discussion of how to meet the nutritional needs of children with cerebral palsy, cystic fibrosis, epilepsy, cleft palate, and other challenges.

A team is a *small number of people* with *complementary skills* who are committed to a *common purpose* for which they hold

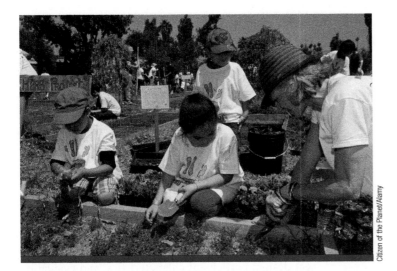

Achieving a team's goals requires the cooperation of every team member. Here, children participate in a garden-to-table activity of the Healthy Kids Challenge® (HKC)—a nonprofit health initiative providing training, support, and resources for schools and community youth programs. HKC seeks to raise awareness and encourage healthy changes in the eating and physical activity habits of children using interactive activities that promote wellness. For example, on a Fruit and Veggies Field Trip to a local farm, farmers' market, or grocery store, children can learn more about fresh fruits and vegetables. For more information, visit *www.healthykidschallenge.com*.

Citizen of the Planet/Alamy

themselves *mutually accountable*.[2] Each aspect of this definition is important. A team has a minimum of two members. Twelve members is a size that allows team members to interact easily with one another. Large groups can be unwieldy to manage and direct.[3]

The people on the team should be selected carefully so that the team has balance, variety, and essential expertise.[4] When pulling a team together, prepare a list of potential team members. Think about their similarities and differences. A strong team consists of people with different problem-solving styles and methods of organizing information. Consider diversity of age, sex, educational training, and the like among team members. Diversity ensures a wealth of ideas and views.

Select team members who offer the expertise you believe will be needed to help achieve a goal or solve a problem. If you are developing a restaurant program, for example, you might want team members with expertise in nutrition, foodservice, marketing, and communications. If you are planning an intervention to address a nutrition problem such as hypertension, include someone from the target population—someone who can speak personally about hypertension—on the team.

"The heart of any team is a shared commitment by the members to their collective performance."[5] Achieving the team's goals requires the cooperation of every team member. In other words, a team probably won't be successful in meeting its goals if one or more members don't participate fully. Successful teams are those whose members decide how they will work together and know what goal they are working toward.

Team members are mutually accountable for results. They are willing as individuals to assume responsibility for the portion of the work assigned to them. They are active participants, not passive bench sitters. They prepare in advance for meetings, contribute their ideas, and evaluate themselves.

Most teams have a single leader or captain, but some teams have a "rotating leader"—that is, the team leadership shifts among team members. The team leader is responsible for preparing the meeting agenda, raising important issues, asking questions, keeping the discussion on friendly terms, maintaining order during the meeting, steering the team toward its goal, and recording the team's accomplishments. Diplomacy and humor are two tools the team leader can use to keep the team on track. Much like the football coach or symphony conductor, the team leader's main role is to help team members work together effectively.

Because teams are composed of individuals with different backgrounds, perspectives, ideas, and opinions, conflicts can arise. Thus, team leaders must be able to deal with conflict, a by-product of how people interact in groups. Conflict often has a negative connotation and typically is viewed as a signal that something is wrong. Most people, in fact, try to avoid conflict at all costs. Yet conflict is inevitable in any relationship. It can arise from competition among workers for scarce resources, from questions about authority relationships, from pressures arising outside the organization, and even from solutions developed for dealing with previous conflicts. The problem in most organizations and work groups is that conflicts are avoided and left unresolved. When this occurs, team members are likely to be defensive and hostile and to suspect that they can't trust one another.[6]

To handle conflict positively, team leaders should remember that conflict usually emerges because of differences in attitudes, values, beliefs, and feelings. Appreciating and being sensitive to such differences helps establish a climate of cooperation. Next, team leaders work to pinpoint the underlying cause of the conflict. Finally, they resolve the differences through open negotiation. If necessary, rules and procedures are changed to address the underlying problem. At all times, leaders work to ensure that team members feel their complaints and concerns are perceived as legitimate. The trick to managing a team on which there are strong differences of opinion is to work toward finding common ground.[7]

CHAPTER **SUMMARY** ....

Laying the Foundation for a Grant

▶ Grants are vital in helping today's organizations fund many of their important projects, which often exceed the resources they have available.

▶ A formal grant proposal submitted to a grant sponsor is designed to convince a decision maker to provide the services, goods, and/or money the recipient needs to achieve the objectives stated in the proposal.

▶ Development of proposals can be divided into three main steps: laying the foundation, building the grant proposal, and assembling the final product. The fourth step, reviewing the grant proposal, is completed by the grant reviewers. The final step is putting the proposal into action if it is funded or revising it in hopes of future success.

▶ The foundation work for grant writing includes generating ideas, describing goals, and identifying funding sources and potential collaborators.

- Once an idea is formulated, the next step is to review the literature to assess the value of an idea, adjust its focus to describe goals more clearly, help identify potential collaborators, and provide the background data required to write a compelling needs statement for the proposal.

- When the literature search nears completion, grant seekers should be able to describe the following, clearly and concisely, in two or three minutes: their idea, the uniqueness of the proposed project, and why it is likely to succeed.

- The next step is to describe goals. *Healthy People 2020* can serve as the foundation for all work in community nutrition related to health promotion and disease prevention.

- A community-based participatory research (CBPR) approach can help grant seekers and program developers create community nutrition interventions that address key needs of the community.

- Finding a funding source generally takes two forms: generating an idea in response to a grant sponsor's request (request for proposals [RFP] or request for quotation [RFQ]), or finding a grant sponsor to fund the grant seeker's idea.

- For success, the needs of the grant seeker must be in tune with the needs and interests of the funding source, and it is essential to follow the grant guidelines, forms, and formats exactly and to observe all deadlines.

Building the Proposal

▶ The components of a proposal vary from one grant sponsor to another, but they generally include the following items: letter of intent; transmittal letter; title page; proposal abstract; grant narrative with needs statement, goals and objectives, and methods; project design; participant characteristics; and evaluation plan that includes measurements, data analysis, and dissemination.

- A time and activity chart breaks the entire project into manageable steps that clearly show grant reviewers how the project will proceed.

- A capability section establishes the credibility of the grant seeker, including project staff, and the organization's ability to complete the proposed project with expertise, on time, and within the budget.

- Budgets are usually divided into two main categories: direct costs and indirect costs. Some also require cost sharing, which includes cash or in-kind gifts. Every budgeted expense should be related to the project goals, objectives, and methods.

- The budget narrative follows the budget in the proposal and explains or justifies all expenditures.

- Appendixes are placed at the end of the proposal. They should contain carefully selected materials that directly support the proposal. A Logic Model provides a framework for planning, implementing, managing, and evaluating programs and may be required.

▶ The job of grant reviewers is to review each proposal, compare it to the sponsor's priorities and criteria, judge the relative merit of the project and its likelihood for success, assess whether the project staff and organization can deliver what is proposed within the time frame specified, and evaluate the adequacy of the budget.

- The most common reasons for proposals not to be funded are that there were problems with planning and time management, the proposal did not follow the guidelines or was submitted after the deadline, the proposal lacked a well-conceived plan of action or idea, and/or the proposal had errors in the budget estimates. In many cases, a proposal is rejected because it does not match the grant sponsor's funding priorities.

- The most successful grant seekers demonstrate four critical qualities: (1) diligence in researching and identifying grant sponsors, (2) creativity in matching project goals with those of sponsors, (3) attentiveness to detail in proposal preparation, and (4) persistence in revising proposals and resubmitting them to potential grant sponsors.

SUMMARY **QUESTIONS**

1. What are the foundational steps in generating a grant proposal?
2. List several questions that can help grant seekers decide whether to compete for a grant from a particular grant sponsor, and explain how these questions are relevant.
3. What are the characteristics of the best collaborators for grant writing? Discuss the advantages and disadvantages of working with collaborators.
4. Describe the different components that are included in the methods section of a grant proposal.
5. Differentiate between direct and indirect costs and give examples of each.

INTERNET **RESOURCES**

Agency for Healthcare Research and Quality
www.ahrq.gov

American Federation for Aging Research
www.afar.org

Centers for Disease Control and Prevention/Funding
www.cdc.gov

Canadian Foundation for Dietetic Research
www.cfdr.ca

Department of Agriculture
www.usda.gov

Department of Education
www.ed.gov

Department of Health and Human Services
www.hhs.gov/asfr/ogapa/index.html

Economic Research Service Research on Food Assistance and Nutrition
www.ers.usda.gov

The Foundation Center
www.foundationcenter.org

The Grantsmanship Center
www.tgci.com

Henry J. Kaiser Family Foundation
http://kff.org

Life Sciences Research Foundation
www.lsrf.org

National Center for Advancing Translational Sciences
http://ncats.nih.gov

National Dairy Council
www.nationaldairycouncil.org

National Institute of Food and Agriculture
http://nifa.usda.gov

National Institutes of Health
www.nih.gov

National Science Foundation
www.nsf.gov

Office of Research on Women's Health
http://orwh.od.nih.gov

Robert Wood Johnson Foundation
www.rwjf.org

Nutrition Assessment and Screening

For a complete list of references, please access the MindTap Reader within your MindTap course.

A-1 How to Plot Measures on a Growth Chart

FIGURE A1-1 How to Plot Measures on a Growth Chart

You can assess the growth of infants and children by plotting their measurements on a percentile graph. Percentile graphs divide the measures of a population into 100 equal divisions so that half of the population falls at or above the 50th percentile and half falls below. Using percentiles allows for comparisons among people of the same age and gender. To plot measures on a growth chart, follow these steps:

- Select the appropriate chart based on age and gender. For this example, use the accompanying chart, which gives percentiles for weight for girls from birth to 36 months.

- Locate the infant's age along the horizontal axis at the bottom of the chart (in this example, six months).

- Locate the infant's weight in pounds or kilograms along the vertical axis of the chart (in this example, 17 pounds or 7.7 kilograms).

- Mark the chart where the age and weight lines intersect (shown here with a black dot) and read off the percentile.

Source: E. Whitney and S. Rolfes, *Understanding Nutrition*, 14th ed. (Belmont, CA: Wadsworth, 2016), 511.

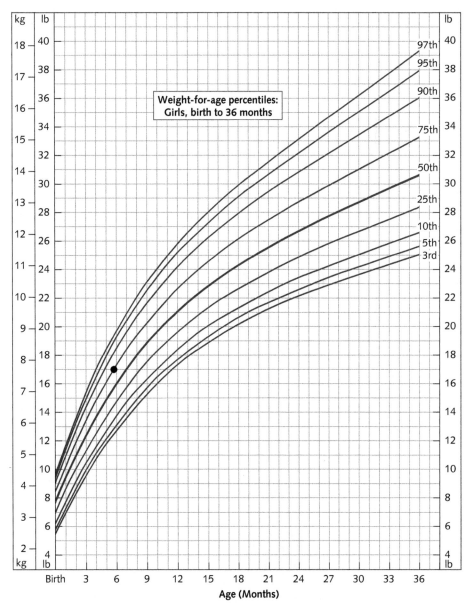

Weight-for-age percentiles: Girls, birth to 36 months

This six-month-old infant is at the 75th percentile. Her pediatrician will weigh her again over the next few months and expect the growth curve to follow the same percentile throughout the first year. In general, dramatic changes or measures much above the 80th percentile or much below the 10th percentile may be cause for concern.

A-2 Assessment of Children's Growth Status

Several indices for assessing growth are derived from a child's height, weight, and age. The actual values for height, weight, and age are plotted on a nomogram or growth chart as shown in **Figure A1-1**, which makes it possible to compare a particular child's height and weight for age with a standard. The percentile curves (e.g., 5th, 10th, 25th, 50th, 75th, 90th, and 95th) for the reference population are displayed on growth charts. In 2006, the World Health Organization (WHO) released new international growth standards for children. There are growth standards for infants to one year, and for children up to five years.

Similar to the 2000 CDC growth charts, these standards describe weight-for-age, length (or stature)-for-age, weight-for-length (or stature), and body mass index-for-age. The charts are available at *www.cdc.gov/growthcharts* or *www.who.int/childgrowth/standards/en*.

CDC recommends that health care providers:

- Use the WHO Child Growth Standards to monitor growth for infants and children from birth to two years of age (**Figure A2-1**).
- Use the CDC growth charts for children age two years and older in the U.S. (**Figure A2-2**).

FIGURE A2-1 WHO Growth Charts for Girls, Birth to 24 Months

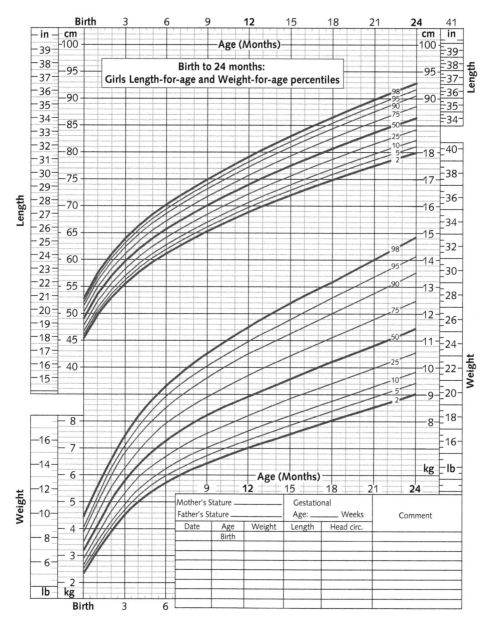

FIGURE A2-1 WHO Growth Charts for Girls, Birth to 24 Months—*continued*

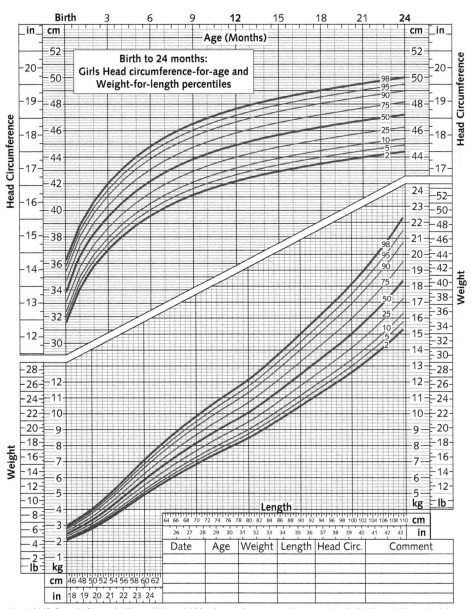

Note: WHO Growth Charts for Boys, Birth to 24 Months can be accessed at *www.who.int/childgrowth/standards/en*.

Source: Published by the Centers for Disease Control and Prevention, November 1, 2009; WHO Child Growth Standards (*http://www.who.int/childgrowth/en*).

The CDC growth charts describe how the average child grows but do not indicate how children should grow for the best health outcome.[1] The recommendation to use the 2006 WHO international growth charts recognizes that breastfeeding is the recommended standard for infant feeding. In the WHO charts, the healthy breastfed infant is intended to be the standard against which all other infants are compared; 100% of the reference population of infants for the WHO Child Growth Standards were breastfed for 12 months and were predominantly breastfed for at least four months. In contrast, approximately 50% of the infants in the CDC growth chart data set had ever been breastfed.[2] The physical growth charts for girls from birth to 24 months are shown in Figure A2-1. When using the WHO growth charts, values of two standard deviations above and below the median, or the 2.3rd and 97.7th percentiles (labeled as the 2nd and 98th percentiles on the growth charts in Figure A2-1), are recommended for identification of children whose growth might be indicative of adverse health conditions. A discussion of indices derived from growth measurements is given here.

Stature/Length-for-Age

Low stature-for-age is defined as a stature-for-age value below the 5th percentile. In other words, low stature-for-age reflects a child's failure to achieve for a given age group distribution a height that conforms to standards established for a well-nourished, healthy population of children. Low stature-for-age is sometimes referred to as growth stunting, which may be the consequence of poor nutrition, a high frequency of infections, or both.

Although shortness in an individual child may be a normal reflection of the child's genetic heritage, a high prevalence rate of growth stunting reflects poor socioeconomic conditions. In some developing countries, the prevalence rate is as high as 60–70%. In developed countries, the rate is about 2–5%.[3] The prevalence of stunting is highest during the second or third year of life.[4]

Weight-for-Length/Stature

Low weight-for-length, or thinness, is defined as a weight-for-length value below the 5th percentile. This indicator is a sensitive index of current nutrition status and is often associated with recent severe disease. Between the ages of 1 and 10 years, the indicator is relatively independent of age. It is relatively independent of ethnic groups, particularly among children age one to five years.[5]

Weight-for-length differentiates between nutritional stunting, when a child's weight may be appropriate for her height, and wasting, when weight is very low for height owing to reductions in both tissue and fat mass. The prevalence of low weight-for-length is usually less than 5% except during periods of famine, war, or other extreme conditions. A prevalence rate greater than 5% indicates the presence of serious nutritional problems.

At the other end of the spectrum, a high weight-for-length (a value greater than the 95th percentile) correlates well with obesity. It typically indicates excess food consumption, low activity levels, or both.

Weight-for-Age

Weight-for-age is a composite index of stature-for-age and weight-for-length. In children age six months to about seven years, weight-for-age is an indicator of acute malnutrition. It is widely used to assess protein-energy malnutrition and overnutrition. However, one limitation of using weight-for-age as an indicator of protein-energy malnutrition is that it does not consider height differences. For example, a child who has low weight-for-age may be genetically short with proportionally low height and low weight, rather than too thin with a low weight for height. As a result, the prevalence of protein-energy malnutrition in small children may be overstated if only this indicator is used.[6] Weight-for-age is most useful in clinical settings where repeated measurements of the indicator are used to evaluate children who are not gaining weight.[7]

Body Mass Index (BMI)-for-Age

BMI-for-age is an anthropometric index of weight and height combined with age. BMI-for-age charts for boys and girls age 2 to 20 years are a major addition to the CDC Pediatric Growth Charts and are used to classify children and adolescents as underweight, overweight, or obese. For children, BMI is gender specific and age specific.

The recommendations are to classify BMI-for-age at or above the 95th percentile as obese and between the 85th and 95th percentile as overweight.[8] The cutoff for underweight of less than the 5th percentile is based on recommendations by the World Health Organization Expert Committee on Physical Status.[9] Figure A2-2 plots a child's measurements on the BMI-for-age, weight-for-age, and stature-for-age charts.

Example

Angelica is a 13-year-old girl with intermittent weight and height measurements since age two. Her measurements have been plotted on the BMI-for-age, weight-for-age, and stature-for-age charts.

AGE	WEIGHT (LB)	STATURE (IN)	BMI
2	23.25	33	15
3	28.5	36.25	15.2
4	36.5	39.25	16.7
7	60	46	19.9
11	94.5	52.5	24.1
13	143	60.25	27.7

The BMI-for-age chart shows a steady increase in BMI-for-age from age two to four. By age seven, Angelica's BMI-for-age was slightly above the 95th percentile, and it remains in this channel or above to the present, indicating that she is obese. Her stature-for-age has consistently been below the 50th percentile, whereas after age three her weight has been consistently above the 50th percentile. At age 13, it is above the 90th percentile. We see that Angelica is slightly shorter than other girls her age, while her weight is higher.

FIGURE A2-2   BMI-for-Age, Weight-for-Age, and Stature-for-Age

Girls: 2 to 20 years, BMI-for-Age Percentiles

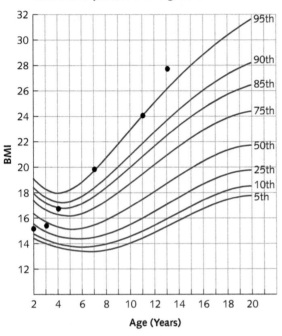

Girls: 2 to 20 years, Stature-for-Age and Weight-for-Age Percentiles

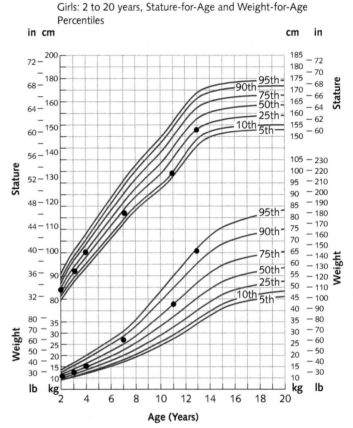

Note: CDC Growth Charts for Boys, 2 to 20 Years can be accessed at *www.cdc.gov/growthcharts*.

Source: Developed (2000) by the National Center for Health Statistics in collaboration with the National Center for Chronic Disease Prevention and Health Promotion.

Complementary Nutrition and Health Therapies

For a complete list of references, please access the MindTap Reader within your MindTap course.

Paralleling a paradigm shift from "sickness" to "wellness" is an expansive interest in and use of *complementary and alternative medicine (CAM)*—whether it be acupuncture, herbs, or chiropractic. **Table B-1** lists the seven major categories of complementary and alternative medicine. Many of the CAM therapies defined in the glossary that follows are called "holistic," which means that the health care provider considers the whole person, including physical, mental, emotional, and spiritual health. In the past two decades, a National Center for Complementary and Alternative Medicine was established at the National Institutes of Health, courses on complementary medicine were introduced into medical schools, and herbs and supplements became best-sellers for national pharmaceutical and supermarket chains. See **Table B-2** for a list of herbs thought to be effective and those that should be avoided.

A number of important factors have led to the current proliferation of alternative health therapies, such as an interest in returning to a more natural lifestyle, dissatisfaction with the current state of Western health care, the unwanted side effects of prescription drugs, the spiraling cost and disarray of managed health care, and aging baby boomers who want a better quality of health. As members of the Academy of Nutrition and Dietetics, food and nutrition practitioners serve the public through the promotion of optimal nutrition, health, and well-being.[1] Therefore, the implications for the nutrition and dietetics profession are noteworthy. Clients and others may ask for your opinion on various alternative therapies, and you will want to inquire about the use of CAM therapies by clients and educate them about the state of scientific knowledge with regard to alternative nutrition and health therapies.

TABLE B-1 Classification and Examples of Complementary and Alternative Medical (CAM) Practices

I. **Mind–Body Medicine**

Involves behavioral, psychological, social, and spiritual approaches to health. Examples include yoga, psychotherapy, art therapy, tai chi, hypnosis, dance therapy, meditation, biofeedback, music therapy, imagery, support groups, humor therapy, and prayer.

II. **Alternative Medical Systems**

Involves complete systems of theory and practice that have been developed outside the Western biomedical approach. It is divided into four subcategories:
A. Acupuncture and Oriental medicine; examples include acupuncture, herbal formulas, and tai chi
B. Traditional indigenous systems; examples include American Indian medicine, ayurvedic medicine, traditional African medicine, traditional Aboriginal medicine, and Central and South American practices
C. Unconventional Western systems; examples include homeopathy, Cayce-based systems, and orthomolecular medicine
D. Naturopathy

III. **Lifestyle and Disease Prevention**

This category involves theories and practices designed to prevent the development of illness, identify and treat risk factors, or support the healing and recovery process. To be classified as CAM, the lifestyle therapies for behavior change, dietary change, exercise, stress management, and addiction control must be based on a nonorthodox system of medicine or be applied in unconventional ways.

IV. **Biologically Based Therapies**

Includes natural and biologically based practices, interventions, and products. Many overlap with conventional medicine's use of dietary supplements. There are four subcategories as shown below:
A. Individual herbs; examples include ginkgo biloba, garlic, ginseng, echinacea, saw palmetto, ginger, green tea, and psyllium
B. Special diet therapies; examples include Pritikin, Omish, Gerson, vegetarian, fasting, macrobiotic, Mediterranean, Paleolithic, Atkins, and natural hygiene
C. Orthomolecular medicine; this subcategory refers to products used as nutritional supplements for preventive or therapeutic purposes; they are usually used in combinations and at high doses (e.g., ascorbic acid, carotenes, tocopherols, niacinamide, choline, lysine, boron, melatonin, dehydroepiandrosterone [DHEA], amino acids, carnitine, probiotics, glucosamine sulfate, and chondroitin sulfate)
D. Pharmacological, biological, and instrumental interventions; includes products and procedures applied in an unconventional way (e.g., cartilage, enzyme therapies, hyperbaric oxygen, bee pollen, cell therapy, and iridology).

TABLE B-1 Classification and Examples of Complementary and Alternative Medical (CAM) Practices—*continued*

V. Manipulative and Body-Based Systems

Refers to systems that are based on manipulation and/or movement of the body. There are three subcategories:
A. Chiropractic medicine
B. Massage and bodywork (e.g., Swedish massage, applied kinesiology, reflexology, rolfing, and polarity)
C. Unconventional physical therapies (e.g., colonics, hydrotherapy, and heat and electrotherapies)

VI. Biofield

Involves systems that use subtle energy fields in and around the body for medical purposes; examples include therapeutic touch, healing touch, and reiki.

VII. Bioelectromagnetics
Refers to the unconventional use of electromagnetic fields for medical purposes.

Source: Adapted from National Institutes of Health, National Center for Complementary and Alternative Medicine, *Classification of Complementary and Alternative Medical Practices: General Information Package* (Silver Spring, MD: Office of Alternative Medicine Clearinghouse, 1998).

TABLE B-2 Selected Herbs and Their Common Uses and Risks

COMMON NAME	CLAIMS AND USES	RISKS[a]
Aloe (gel)	Promote wound healing	Generally considered safe
Black cohosh (roots)	Ease menopause symptoms	May cause clotting in blood vessels of eye; change curvature of cornea
Chamomile (flowers)	Relieve indigestion	Generally considered safe
Chaparral (leaves/twigs)	Slow aging; "cleanse" blood; heal wounds; treat acne	Acute, toxic hepatitis; liver damage
Cinnamon (bark)	Relieve indigestion; lower blood glucose and blood lipids	May have a blood-thinning effect; not safe for pregnant women or those taking diabetes medication
Comfrey (leafy plant)	Soothe nerves	Liver damage
Echinacea (roots)	Alleviate symptoms of colds, flus, and infections; promote wound healing; boost immunity	Generally considered safe; may cause headaches, dizziness, and nausea
Ephedra (stems)	Promote weight loss	Rapid heart rate, tremors, seizures, insomnia, headaches, and hypertension
Feverfew (leaves)	Prevent migraine headaches	Generally considered safe; may cause mouth irritation, swelling, ulcers, and GI distress
Garlic (bulbs)	Lower blood lipids and blood pressure	Generally considered safe; may cause garlic breath, body odor, gas, and GI distress; inhibits blood clotting
Ginger (roots)	Prevent motion sickness and nausea	Generally considered safe
Ginkgo biloba (tree leaves)	Improve memory; relieve vertigo	Generally considered safe; may cause headache, GI distress, and dizziness
Ginseng (roots)	Boost immunity; increase endurance	Generally considered safe; may cause insomnia and high blood pressure
Goldenseal (roots)	Relieve indigestion; treat urinary infections	Generally considered safe; not safe for people with hypertension or heart disease
Kava (roots)	Relieve anxiety; promote relaxation	Liver failure
Saw palmetto (ripe fruits)	Relieve symptoms of enlarged prostate; diuretic; enhance sexual vigor	Generally considered safe; may cause nausea, vomiting, and diarrhea
St. John's wort (leaves and tops)	Relieve depression and anxiety	Generally considered safe; may cause fatigue and GI distress
Tumeric (roots)	Reduce inflammation; relieve heartburn	Generally considered safe; may cause indigestion; not safe for people with gallbladder disease

continued

TABLE B-2 Selected Herbs and Their Common Uses and Risks—*continued*

COMMON NAME	CLAIMS AND USES	RISKS[a]
Valerian (roots)	Calm nerves; improve sleep	Long-term use associated with liver damage
Yohimbe (tree bark)	Enhance "male performance"	Kidney failure; seizures

[a] Allergies are always a possible risk. Call your physician or the FDA Med Alert hotline at 800-332-1088 if you experience adverse effects.

Sources: S. Foster and V. E. Tyler, *Tyler's Honest Herbal: A Sensible Guide to the Use of Herbs and Related Remedies* (New York: Haworth Press, 1999); adapted from E. Whitney and S. Rolfes, *Understanding Nutrition*, 12th ed. (Belmont, CA: Wadsworth/Cengage Learning, 2011).

Glossary of Complementary and Alternative Medicine Therapies

Additional information about the following therapies can be found at *www.nccam.nih.gov*.

Acupuncture A technique that involves piercing the skin with long, thin needles at specific anatomical points to stimulate, disperse, and regulate the flow of *chi*, or vital energy, and relieve pain or illness. Acupuncture sometimes uses heat, pressure, friction, suction, or electromagnetic energy to stimulate the points.

Aromatherapy A technique that uses essential oils (the volatile oils distilled from plants) to enhance physical, psychological, and spiritual health. The oils are inhaled, massaged into the skin in diluted form, or used in baths.

Ayurveda (EYE-your-VAY-dah) A traditional Hindu system of improving health. In this approach, illness is a state of imbalance among the body's systems and can be detected through procedures involving reading the pulse and checking the tongue. It uses herbs, diet, meditation, massage, and yoga to stimulate the body to make its own natural drugs.

Bioelectromagnetic medical applications The use of electrical energy, magnetic energy, or both to stimulate bone repair, wound healing, and tissue regeneration.

Biofeedback The use of special devices to convey information about heart rate, blood pressure, skin temperature, muscle relaxation, and the like, to enable a person to learn how to consciously control these medically important functions.

Chelation therapy The use of ethylenediamine tetraacetic acid (EDTA) to bind with metallic ions, thus healing the body by removing toxic metals.

Chinese (Oriental) medicine Practitioners use methods—including acupuncture, herbal medicine, massage, moxibustion (heat therapy), and nutrition and lifestyle counseling—to treat a broad range of acute and chronic diseases.

Chiropractic A manual healing method of manipulating or adjusting vertebrae to relieve musculoskeletal pain suspected of causing problems with internal organs.

Guided imagery A technique that guides clients to achieve a desired physical, emotional, or spiritual state by visualizing themselves in that state.

Herbal medicine The use of plants to treat disease or improve health; also known as *phytotherapy*.

Homeopathic medicine A practice based on the theory that "like cures like"—that is, that substances that cause symptoms in healthy people can cure those symptoms when given in very dilute amounts.

Hypnotherapy A technique that uses hypnosis and the power of suggestion to improve health behaviors and relieve pain.

Iridology The study of changes in the iris of the eye and their relationships to disease.

Massage therapy A method in which the therapist manually kneads muscles to reduce tension, increase blood circulation, improve joint mobility, and promote healing.

Meditation A self-directed technique of relaxing the body and calming the mind.

Naturopathic medicine A system that integrates traditional medicine with herbal medicine, clinical nutrition, homeopathy, acupuncture, hydrotherapy, and manipulative therapy.

Orthomolecular medicine The use of large doses of vitamins to treat chronic disease.

Ozone therapy The use of ozone gas to enhance the body's immune system.

Qi gong (chée GUNG) A Chinese system that combines movement, meditation, and breathing techniques to enhance the flow of *qi* (vital energy) in the body.

Reflexology Manipulation of specific areas on the feet and hands that correspond to a particular organ or zone in the upper body.

Therapeutic touch A technique that uses graceful, sweeping movements of the hands, a few inches from the body, to scan the patient's energy flow, replenish it when necessary, release congestion or obstruction, and generally restore balance.

The SMOG Readability Formula[*]

For a complete list of references, please access the MindTap Reader within your MindTap course.

To calculate the SMOG reading grade level, begin with the entire written work that is being assessed and follow these four steps:

1. Count off 10 consecutive sentences near the beginning, in the middle, and near the end of the text.
2. From this sample of 30 sentences, circle all of the words containing three or more syllables (polysyllabic), including repetitions of the same word, and total the number of words circled.
3. Estimate the square root of the total number of polysyllabic words counted. This is done by finding the nearest perfect square and taking its square root.
4. Finally, add a constant of three to the square root. This number gives the SMOG grade, or the reading grade level that a person must have reached if he or she is to fully understand the text being assessed.

A few additional guidelines will help to clarify these directions:

- A sentence is defined as a string of words punctuated with a period (.), an exclamation point (!), or a question mark (?).
- Hyphenated words are considered as one word.
- Numbers that are written out should also be considered, and if in numeric form in the text, they should be pronounced to determine if they are polysyllabic.
- Proper nouns, if polysyllabic, should be counted, too.
- Abbreviations should be read as unabbreviated to determine if they are polysyllabic.

Not all pamphlets, fact sheets, or other printed materials contain 30 sentences. To test a text that has fewer than 30 sentences:

1. Count all of the polysyllabic words in the text.
2. Count the number of sentences.
3. Find the average number of polysyllabic words per sentence as follows:

$$\text{Average} = \frac{\text{Total number of polysyllabic words}}{\text{Total number of sentences}}$$

4. Multiply that average by the number of sentences *short of 30*.
5. Add that figure to the total number of polysyllabic words.
6. Find the square root and add the constant of 3.

[*] Sources: U.S. Department of Health and Human Services, Public Health Service, *Pretesting in Health Communications*, NIH Pub. No. 84–1493 (Bethesda, MD: National Cancer Institute, 1984), 43–45; and American Cancer Society, *Cancer Facts & Figures 2011* (Atlanta: American Cancer Society, 2011).

Perhaps the quickest way to administer the SMOG grading test is by using the SMOG Conversion Table. Simply count the number of polysyllabic words in your chain of 30 sentences and look up the approximate grade level on the chart shown on page 762.

An example of how to use the SMOG Readability Formula is provided below. The SMOG Conversion Table is shown on page 762.

In Controlling Cancer—You Make a Difference

The key is ACTION. You can help protect yourself against cancer. Act promptly to:

Prevent some cancers through simple changes in lifestyle.
Find out about early detection tests in your home.
Gain peace of mind through regular medical checkups.

Cancers You Should Know About

Lung cancer is the number one cancer among men in deaths (85,600) and second in number of new cases each year (115,060). Rapidly increasing rates are due mainly to cigarette smoking. By not smoking, you can largely prevent lung cancer. The risk is reduced by smoking less and by using lower tar and nicotine brands. But quitting altogether is by far the most effective safeguard. The American Cancer Society offers Quit Smoking Clinics and self-help materials.

Prostate cancer is first in the number of new cases each year (240,890) and second in deaths (33,720). It occurs mainly in men over 60. A regular rectal exam of the prostate by your doctor is the best protection.

Colorectal cancer is third in cancer deaths for men (25,250) and third in new cases (49,000). When it is found early, chances of cure are good. A regular general physical usually includes a digital examination of the rectum and a guaiac slide test of a stool specimen to check for invisible blood. Now there are also Do-It-Yourself Guaiac Slides for home use. Ask your doctor about them. After you reach the age of 40, your regular check-up may include a "Procto," in which the rectum and part of the colon are inspected through a hollow, lighted tube.

A Check-Up Pays Off

Be sure to have a regular, general physical including an oral exam. It is your best guarantee of good health.

How Cancer Works

If we know something about how cancer works, we can act more effectively to protect ourselves against the disease. Here are the basics:

1. Cancer spreads; time counts—Cancer is uncontrolled growth of abnormal cells. It begins small and, if unchecked, spreads. If detected in an early, local stage, the chances for cure are best.
2. Risk increases with age—This is not a reason to worry, but a signal to have more regular thorough physical check-ups. Your doctor or clinic can advise you on what tests to get and how often they should be performed.
3. What you can do—Don't smoke and you will sharply reduce your chances of getting lung cancer. Avoid too much sun, a major cause of skin cancer. Learn cancer's Seven Warning Signals, listed on the back of this leaflet, and see your doctor promptly if they persist. Pain usually is a late symptom of cancer; don't wait for it.

Unproven Remedies

Beware of unproven cancer remedies. They may sound appealing, but they are usually worthless. Relying on them can delay good treatment until it is too late. Check with your doctor or the American Cancer Society.

More Information

For more information of any kind about cancer—free of cost—contact your local unit of the American Cancer Society.

Know Cancer's Seven Warning Signals

1. Change in bowel or bladder habits.
2. A sore that does not heal.
3. Unusual bleeding or discharge.
4. Thickening or lump in breast or elsewhere.
5. Indigestion or difficulty in swallowing.
6. Obvious change in wart or mole.
7. Nagging cough or hoarseness.

If you have a warning signal, see your doctor.

(This pamphlet is from the American Cancer Society.)

We have calculated the reading grade level for this example. Compare your results to ours, then check both with the SMOG Conversion Table:

Readability Test Calculations

Total number of polysyllabic words	= 38
Nearest perfect square	= 36
Square root	= 6
Constant	= 3
SMOG reading grade level	= 9

SMOG Conversion Table[a]

TOTAL POLYSYLLABIC WORD COUNTS	APPROXIMATE GRADE LEVEL (+1.5 GRADES)
0–2	4
3–6	5
7–12	6
13–20	7
21–30	8
31–42	9
43–56	10
57–72	11
73–90	12
91–110	13
111–132	14
133–156	15
157–182	16
183–210	17
211–240	18

[a] Developed by Harold C. McGraw, Office of Educational Research, Baltimore County Schools, Towson, Maryland.

Part One: Community Needs Assessment Assignment

by Virginia B. Gray, PhD, RD

For a complete list of references, please access the MindTap Reader within your MindTap course.

Introduction

Successful community nutrition programs are based on understanding both the needs and desires of the community. In this assignment, you will practice planning and carrying out a community needs assessment, using the steps described in Chapter 4: Community Needs Assessment.

Step 1: Set the parameters of the assessment.

Defining the community of interest is an important first step in a community needs assessment. As discussed in Chapter 4, there are times in which a community needs assessment investigates the needs of a given community (e.g., geographical area), and then a target audience is selected based on needs and desires of the community and available resources to meet them. At other times, the target audience is decided at the outset.

For this assignment, you are to select a target population at the beginning to help focus your investigation. Being specific will ensure that you are able to obtain needed data to meet the needs of your audience. In selecting a target population, you may consider needs you have noticed in your community. For example, imagine you are a volunteer with a local organization serving congregate meals to older adults and you have noticed that the older adults served often mention experiencing constipation. Or you may have a young family member who participates in youth sports, and you notice that children are commonly refueling on high-sugar, low-protein "junk" foods after games.

Some potential target audiences you might select for this assignment include:

- Low-income pregnant women (you may further specify a particular race or ethnicity)
- School children living in a food desert
- Older adults participating in home-delivered meals or a congregate feeding program
- Parents of children involved in youth sports
- Food-insecure students on a college campus
- Homeless individuals seeking meals at a local shelter

Note: It is recommended that you select a target population in or near the community in which you live, as this will facilitate collection of new data when necessary.

1. Describe your target population.
2. State the overall goal(s) of conducting the needs assessment. What is the purpose of the assessment? Your goal(s) should communicate a broad overview of what you intend to accomplish by conducting the needs assessment.
3. Now write objectives for your needs assessment. These objectives should be specific and measurable, and will determine the types of data you collect as a part of your needs assessment.

Step 2: Develop a data collection plan.

In this step, you create a data collection plan, thinking of the three categories of needs assessment data: community data, community environment and background conditions, and individuals who represent the target population. *Note:*

- Refer to Table 4-2 for examples of types and sources of community data to collect.
- Refer to Table 4-3 for examples of types and sources of data about the community environment and background conditions.
- Refer to Table 4-4 for examples of types and sources of data to collect about the target population.

First, make a list of the types of data you would like to collect in the first column of the table on the next page. In the second column, indicate if there are existing sources for retrieving the needed data or if you would have to collect new data. Then use the third column to indicate the source of data (for existing data) or how you would collect the data (for new data). For example, you might include "belief in link between diet and health" as a type of data related to the target audience. You may indicate you would collect these data directly from the target audience, using a focus group and/or survey.

In your plan, be sure to include at least one of each of the following sources of data:

- Existing data
- Relevant literature related to nutrition status of the target population, health beliefs of the target audience, and effective nutrition interventions among similar audiences
- Key informant(s)
- Direct assessment of the target audience

TYPE OF DATA	EXISTING DATA OR NEW DATA?	SOURCE OF DATA (FOR EXISTING DATA) OR HOW TO COLLECT DATA (FOR NEW DATA)
COMMUNITY DATA		
COMMUNITY ENVIRONMENT AND BACKGROUND CONDITIONS		
TARGET POPULATION		

Note: As you are developing a plan for data collection, be sure to address the objectives you set for the community needs assessment in Step 1.

Step 3: Collect data.

In this step, you collect data about the community, about the community environment and background conditions, and about individuals who represent the target population. Use the chart you created in Step 2 to guide your data collection; then create a new chart to summarize the data you collect.

Check to ensure that you have met the objectives you set for the needs assessment in Step 1.

Step 4: Analyze and interpret the data.

Reflect on what you learned in Step 3.

- What did you learn about the community (demographics, health statistics, economic level, etc.)?
- What did you learn about the community environment and background conditions (food availability, resources, social and cultural norms, policies, etc.)?
- What did you learn about the target population's needs, wants, motivations, attitudes, etc.?
- What does the nutrition literature say about your target population's nutrition status and health beliefs? What does the literature say about effective means of intervention?

Your job in this step is to relate the needs of the target population to the broader community setting (resources and characteristics).

After reflecting on the questions listed in Step 4, create a summary that indicates:

- A description of the nutrition status of the target population. Remember to focus on the most prevalent needs and concerns, and to relate needs and wants of the target audience to the broader community environment and background conditions.
- Community and target audience resources that might be used to address needs.
- Barriers and facilitators related to community needs and wants.

Step 5: Share the findings of the assessment.

Make a list of key people with whom you would share findings of the assessment. Remember to involve those who provided input as you were gathering data. Also, consider key stakeholders and organizations who will be affected by the plan of action you take in response to the community needs assessment.

Step 6: Set priorities.

Table 4-14 provides guidance related to setting priorities for action based on community needs assessment data. After reviewing the table, look back at the data you collected in Step 3. Choose one or two priorities for action. For each priority, indicate the following:

- Nutrition priority to be addressed (indicate the priority and why you chose it)
- Relationship with national nutrition priorities (consider *Dietary Guidelines for Americans* and/or *Healthy People 2020*)

Step 7: Choose a plan of action.

After completing the needs assessment, you are ready to develop a plan of action. Indicate which issues you will address and how you will address them. There are many options for action after investigating community needs. The community nutritionist may:

- Use community assessment findings to advocate for a change in policy.
- Organize a workshop or conference with community leaders and stakeholders to explore future actions.

- Alter an existing program by developing new educational materials, enlarging a marketing campaign, or changing the mechanism for delivering the program.
- Develop a new program to address the nutritional needs of the target population.

Write a summary of the plan of action you propose based on the needs assessment findings. Connect this plan with community needs and wants and with available resources.

Part Two: Community Needs Assessment Assignment

Adapted from an assignment completed by Jenny Mei, Kristin Mahood, and Sarah Walatka, MS, Nutritional Science students at California State University Long Beach (CSULB)

Step 1: Set the parameters of the assessment.

Target population: The target population for this needs assessment is participants in a fitness-focused wellness program (Beach Community Wellness Program) developed by CSULB Kinesiology faculty in partnership with the City of Long Beach Department of Health and Human Services. Participants in the program are primarily Hispanic (Spanish-speaking), though the program also includes Caucasians, African Americans, and Asians. The program takes place in a low-income, underserved neighborhood in Southern California.

Goal of needs assessment: The goal of the needs assessment is to determine nutrition-related needs and wants of participants in the Beach Community Wellness Program. These data are intended to direct development of a nutrition-focused piece to add to an existing fitness-focused wellness program.

Objectives of needs assessment:

- To assess patterns of food consumption among participants in Beach Community Wellness Program (BCWP)
- To assess typical consumption of foods (vegetable, fruit, grain, protein, dairy, dessert-type foods, and sweetened beverages) at meals and snacks among participants in BCWP
- To obtain data on sources of nutrition information used by participants in BCWP
- To assess perceived level of confidence related to healthy food selection, purchase, and preparation among participants in BCWP
- To assess perceptions of healthy eating among participants in BCWP
- To assess status of enrollment in a food supplementation program among participants in BCWP

Step 2: Develop a data collection plan.

Table D-1 portrays existing and new data needs for three categories of data: community data, community environment and background conditions, and target population data.

Step 3: Collect data.

Data collection for this assignment included: (1) a review of literature focused on needs of the target audience, (2) demographic and population health data (**Table D-2**), (3) food availability data (**Tables D-3** and **D-4**), and (4) new data collected by surveying and interviewing the target population (**Tables D-5** through **D-8**). Additional qualitative data obtained by open-ended survey questions, an oral survey, and key informant interviews are also presented.

Literature review: As the rates of obesity and chronic disease increase, nutrition remains a critical concern for all Americans, especially for the rapidly growing Latino population in the United States. Potential health issues and concerns have been well documented in past literature. Despite the Latino health paradox that points to lower overall death rates in some Latino populations,[1] Latinos still have a high risk for chronic conditions and diseases such as type 2 diabetes[2,3] and obesity[4] due to many challenges in prevention and treatment. The prevalence of major cardiovascular risk factors and diseases among Latinos is well documented, such as smoking, hypercholesterolemia, diabetes, obesity, and hypertension.[5] Culturally relevant communication and building rapport are important considerations when developing interventions among Latinos. Taking cultural beliefs and values into consideration, such as the belief that disease is a punishment for sins, can improve the effectiveness of care for Latinos.[6]

Assessing the nutrition status of Latinos is complex, as characteristics such as the level of acculturation and socioeconomic status have pronounced effects. One study found that as a whole, Latinos consumed at least one additional serving of fruits and vegetables per day compared to their non-Hispanic white counterparts.[7] However, increased acculturation levels were associated with having fewer than recommended servings of fruits and vegetables. This study also found that less acculturated Latinos consumed less fat and more fiber, and had a higher intake of protein; vitamins A, C, E, and B_6; folate;

TABLE D-1 Needs Assessment Data Needs

TYPE OF DATA	EXISTING DATA OR NEW DATA?	SOURCE OF DATA (FOR EXISTING DATA) OR HOW TO COLLECT DATA (FOR NEW DATA)
COMMUNITY DATA		
Demographic data	Existing data	Census, LB CHA[a]
Income data	Existing data	Census, LB CHA[a]
Health data	Existing data	Census, LB CHA[a]
COMMUNITY ENVIRONMENT AND BACKGROUND CONDITIONS		
Food stores in the area	New data	Google maps and drive around community
Resources available in community	New data	Internet search
Nutrition counseling/education classes available in the community	Existing data	WIC[a], LBDHHS[a]
TARGET POPULATION DATA		
Habits/behaviors: eating, food choices, location, shopping, cooking methods, dining out, consumption of food groups	New data	Survey with target audience
Nutrition topics on nutrition/health concerns	New data	Survey with target audience
Population's definition of health/belief of health	New data	Oral interviews with target audience
Barriers to and motivators of eating healthy	New data	Key informant interviews; survey and oral interviews with target audience
Needs and perceptions of target audience related to food habits	New data	Key informant interviews; oral interviews with target audience

[a] The following abbreviations appear in this table: LB CHA, Long Beach Community Health Assessment; WIC, Special Supplemental Nutrition Program for Women, Infants, and Children; and LBDHHS, Long Beach Department of Health and Human Services.

calcium; potassium; and magnesium. Ayala et al. (2005) found that acculturation significantly influenced eating and shopping habits in Latino women. Higher acculturation to the Anglo-American culture was associated with eating out more for lunch and dinner, eating fast food, and having less difficulty reading nutrition labels. The study found that participants all shopped at supermarkets, grocery stores, and discount/bulk stores, but the latter was the most popular due to cost, availability, and familiarity, especially for less acculturated Latinos.[8] Acculturation and culture must be taken into account when assessing nutrition among Latinos, as these factors influence food choices and patterns.

Food patterns are also heavily influenced by social and economic factors. Socioeconomic barriers make improving diet quality and health difficult for many lower-income Latino families. Knapp et al. (1985) found that intake of vitamin C was affected by socioeconomic status in Mexican Americans.[9] Findings from a study on low-income Latino families showed that food insecurity and obesity are prevalent.[10] Participation of low-income families in food assistance programs such as the Supplemental Nutrition Assistance Program (SNAP) has been found to correlate with a lower diet quality.[11] A study found that stressful events reduced fruit and vegetable intake.[12]

The same study also highlighted the fact that home availability of fruits and vegetables is an important factor related to increasing intake. The literature supports that lower socioeconomic status imposes negative influences on diet quality and nutrition.

In a needs assessment conducted through a collaborative effort of four major nonprofit hospitals in Long Beach, the following health data were presented. The 90805 zip code where the BCWP is located was placed in the highest need category, and was referred to as a "vulnerable zip code."[13] The incidence of hospitalization due to heart disease in this zip code was 185.4 out of every hundred thousand, the second highest of all zip codes in Long Beach. Fast-food consumption in vulnerable zip codes was higher compared to healthier zip codes, with 62% of the people in those zip codes consuming fast food two to three times per week and 26% consuming fast food four or more times per week. About one-third (37%) who needed Cal-Fresh, the food assistance program in California, did not get assistance. In Long Beach overall, poor nutrition and lack of exercise were two of the top five social issues for adults. The overall obesity rate in Long Beach is 40.7%. The final adult health priorities stated were chronic diseases (diabetes, hypertension), overweight and obesity, and preventative care.

TABLE D-2 Demographic/Population Health Data

	ZIP CODE[a]—90805	CITY[a,b,c]—LONG BEACH	STATE[b,c,d]—CALIFORNIA
Population	92,627	462,257	38,332,521
Population by race/ethnicity:			
Hispanic/Latino	> 50%	40.8%	37.6%
White	1–14%	29.4%	57.6%
African American/black	14–21%	13.0%	6.2%
Asian	1–14%	12.6%	13.0%
Two or more races	NA	2.7%	4.9%
Native Hawaiian/Pacific Islander	NA	1.1%	0.4%
American Indian	NA	0.3%	1.0%
Other	NA	0.2%	NA
Population by age:			
< 18 years	31.4%	24.9%	25%
18–24 years	12.2%	11.7%	38.7% (18–44 years)
25–44 years	29.0%	30.5%	
45–64 years	20.7%	23.6%	24.9%
65+ years	6.7%	9.3%	11.4%
Life expectancy (age in years)	76.8	78.6	75.9
Median household income	$33,157	$52,711	$61,094
Families below poverty level		19.1%	13.7%
Receiving SNAP benefits		17,764 (10.8%)	1,012,610 (8.1%)
Education status < high school	39%	11.2%	10.2%
# Lead poison cases 2000–2011	21	115	
Hospitalization rate per 10,000 population	1,635	1,437	
Diagnosed diabetes with high hospitalization rate	21.7–24.3%		
Homicide by firearm per 100,000 population	> 6.4		4.2
% Fifth graders overweight/obese	59%	52%	
Top leading causes of death:			
Disease of the heart		29%	25%
Malignant neoplasms		22%	24%
Chronic lower respiratory disease		6%	6%
Cerebrovascular disease		6%	6%
Other		37%	39%
Heart disease hospitalization rate by race (per 10,000):			
African American/black		303	
Hispanic/Latino		168	
Asian/Pacific Islander		152	
White		125	
Heart disease hospitalization rate	185.4 (per 10,000)	22.7% (South Bay SPA)	40.4%
Death rate for cancer by race (per 10,000):			
African American/black		226.6	222.4
Hispanic/Latino		132.8	132.9
Asian/Pacific Islander		147.8	121
White		158.7	175.3

continued

TABLE D-2 Demographic/Population Health Data—*continued*

	ZIP CODE[a]—90805	CITY[a,b,c]—LONG BEACH	STATE[b,c,d]—CALIFORNIA
Diagnosed with diabetes, prediabetes, or sugar diabetes	23.3%	10.1% (South Bay SPA)	8.4%
Diabetes hospitalization rates by race:			
African American/black		64.9%	
Hispanic/Latino		35.4%	
Asian/Pacific Islander		22.9%	
White		17%	
Diabetes hospitalization rates by age (in years):			
0–14		3.1%	
15–29		9.5%	
30–44		12.8%	
44–59		33.4%	
60+		41.1%	
Consumed five servings of fruits and vegetables per day		14.5%	
Had access to high-quality fruits and vegetables		92.8%	
Consumed fast food one or more times per week		46.3%	

[a] City of Long Beach Department of Human and Health Services, *Community Health Assessment* (2013); available at *http://www.longbeach.gov/health/media-library/documents/planning-and-research/reports/community-health-assessment/community-health-assessment/*.

[b] United States Census Bureau, *Long Beach California Quick Facts 2007–2013* (2014); retrieved from *http://quickfacts.census.gov/qfd/states/06/0643000.html*.

[c] UCLA Center for Health Policy Research, *California Healthy Survey Interview* (2012); retrieved from *http://ask.chis.ucla.edu/main/DQ3/geographic.asp*.

[d] California Department of Public Health, *Prevalence of Diabetes in California Counties 2003* (2015); retrieved from *http://www.cdph.ca.gov/Pages/DEFAULT.aspx*.

TABLE D-3 Food Stores within 2.5 Miles of Beach Community Wellness Program

El Puerco Rancho Market
6583 Atlantic Ave
Long Beach, CA 90805
562-423-2775
0.7 mi from Houghton Park
Fresh produce: Yes
Accepts SNAP/WIC: Yes

Thai Number One Market
5927 Cherry Ave
Long Beach, CA 90805
562-422-6915
1.5 mi from Houghton Park
Fresh produce: Yes
Accepts SNAP/WIC: Yes

3 Brothers Market
16200 Hunsaker Ave
Paramount, CA 90723
562-529-2864
1.7 mi from Houghton Park

Young's Market Co LLC
6432 North Paramount Blvd
Long Beach, CA 90805
562-428-7035
2.1 mi from Houghton Park

Super Bargain 99 Cent Store
6583 Atlantic Ave
Long Beach, CA 90805
0.7 mi from Houghton Park
Fresh produce: Yes
Accepts SNAP/WIC: Yes

Food 4 Less
6700 Cherry Ave
Long Beach, CA 90805
562-220-2373
1.7 mi from Houghton Park
Fresh produce: Yes
Accepts SNAP/WIC: Yes

El Nuevo Guadalajara Market
6792 Long Beach Blvd
Long Beach, CA 90805
310-537-1539
1.9 mi from Houghton Park

WinCo Foods
3400 East South St
Lakewood, CA 90805
562-529-5658
2.3 mi from Houghton Park
Fresh produce: Yes

Big Saver Foods
1313 East Artesia Blvd
Long Beach, CA 90805
562-423-2800
0.9 mi from Houghton Park
Fresh produce: Yes
Accepts SNAP/WIC: Yes

Superior Grocers
5450 Cherry Ave
Long Beach, CA 90805
562-634-6700
1.7 mi from Houghton Park

London Market
6350 Long Beach Blvd
Long Beach, CA 90805
562-728-4226
1.9 mi from Houghton Park

Safeway
4550 Atlantic Ave
Long Beach, CA 90807
562-984-1421
2.4 mi from Houghton Park
Bus available
Fresh produce: Yes

TABLE D-3 Food Stores within 2.5 Miles of Beach Community Wellness Program—*continued*

Vons	**Northgate Markets**
4550 Atlantic Ave	4700 Cherry Ave
Long Beach, CA 90807	Long Beach, CA 90807
562-984-1421	562-423-1300
2.4 mi from Houghton Park	2.4 mi from Houghton Park
Bus available	
Fresh produce: Yes	

TABLE D-4 Farmers' Markets in Long Beach

Greener Good North Long Beach Farmers' Market	**Long Beach Uptown Farmers' Market**	**Compton Blue Line Farmers' Market**
Artesia Blvd and Atlantic Ave	4600 Atlantic Ave	101 East Palmer St
Long Beach, CA 90805	Long Beach, CA 90807	Compton, CA 90220
310-766-3246	562-983-1665	310-761-1474
Time: Fridays, 3:00–7:00 PM	**Time:** Thursdays, 3:00–6:00 PM	**Time:** Thursdays, 11:00 AM–7:00 PM
Bellflower Farmers' Market	**Federal Nutrition Benefits:**	**Federal Nutrition Benefits:**
Oak St and Clark Ave	**WIC:** Yes	**WIC:** Yes
Bellflower, CA 90706	**WIC Cash Value Voucher:** Yes	**WIC Cash Value Voucher:** No
Time: Mondays, 9:00 AM–1:00 PM	**SFMNP:** Yes	**SFMNP:** No
Federal Nutrition Benefits:	**SNAP:** Yes	**SNAP:** Yes
WIC: No	**Products:** Baked goods; canned or preserved fruits/vegetables; eggs; fresh/dried herbs; fresh fruits; fresh vegetables; honey; juices/nonalcoholic ciders; nuts; prepared foods (for immediate consumption)	**Products:** Baked goods; coffee/tea; fish/seafood; fresh fruits; fresh vegetables; honey; juices/nonalcoholic ciders; nuts; prepared foods (for immediate consumption); soap/body care products
WIC Cash Value Voucher: No		
SFMNP: No		
SNAP: No		
Old MacDonald's Farmers' Market		
5000 East Spring St		
Long Beach, CA 90815		
818-859-2001		
Time: Sundays, 8:30 AM–3:00 PM		

TABLE D-5 Reported Eating Patterns among Beach Community Wellness Program Nutrition Participants ($n = 14$)

HOW OFTEN DO YOU:	RARELY (0–1 TIMES) *n* (%)	OCCASIONALLY (2–3 TIMES) *n* (%)	OFTEN (4+ TIMES) *n* (%)
Eat a meal at a fast-food restaurant in a week?	7 (50%)	7 (50%)	0
Eat a meal at a sit-down restaurant in a week?	10 (71%)	2 (14%)	1 (7%)
Prepare meals at home to bring to work/school in a week?	2 (14%)	0	11 (77%)
Purchase food at a convenience store in a week (i.e., 7-11, liquor stores, gas stations)?	12 (86%)	2 (14%)	0
Purchase food at a grocery store in a month?	1 (7%)	3 (21%)	9 (64%)

TABLE D-6 Reported Consumption of Food Groups in a Typical Day by Meal among Beach Community Wellness Program Nutrition Participants (n = 14)

	BREAKFAST	LUNCH	DINNER	SNACK	NONE
Includes a vegetable (fresh, canned, frozen, processed)	43% (6)	64% (9)	50% (7)	50% (7)	7% (1)
Includes a fruit (fresh, canned, dried, or frozen)	79% (11)	36% (5)	36% (5)	64% (9)	7% (1)
Includes a grain (rice, pasta, bread, tortilla, oats)	50% (7)	64% (9)	57% (8)	57% (8)	—
Includes a protein (meat, fish, tofu, poultry, beans)	21% (3)	71% (10)	50% (7)	7% (1)	—
Includes dairy (milk, cheese, yogurt)	79% (11)	29% (4)	43% (6)	21% (3)	—
Includes a dessert-type food (flan, pan dulce, cookies, candy, cake/pie)	14% (2)	21% (3)	43% (6)	43% (6)	7% (1)
Includes a sweetened beverage (juice, soda, energy drink)	21% (3)	36% (5)	29% (4)	—	36% (5)
Includes processed foods (frozen meals, prepackaged snack foods)	—	7% (1)	14% (2)	36% (5)	50% (7)

TABLE D-7 Reported Sources of Nutrition Information among Beach Community Wellness Program Nutrition Participants (n = 14)

SOURCE OF INFORMATION	n
Family	6
Books	6
Internet blogs	6
TV	5
Doctor	4
Friends	3
Magazines	3
School	2
Social media	2
News articles	1
Work	0
Dietitian	0
Other	2

Note: Participants circled all sources that applied, so many indicated more than one source.

TABLE D-8 Perceived Confidence Levels among Participants Related to Food Planning, Preparation, and Purchasing among Beach Community Wellness Program Nutrition Participants ($n = 14$)

	NOT CONFIDENT n (%)	SLIGHTLY CONFIDENT n (%)	MODERATELY CONFIDENT n (%)	VERY CONFIDENT n (%)
Following recipes	2 (14%)	6 (43%)	5 (36%)	1 (7%)
Preparing healthy meals for you and/or your family	—	2 (14%)	6 (43%)	6 (43%)
Choosing healthy food while dining out	2 (14%)	4 (29%)	7 (50%)	1 (7%)
Purchasing healthy foods at the grocery store	—	1 (7%)	10 (71%)	3 (21%)
Staying within budget when purchasing healthy foods	—	3 (21%)	10 (71%)	1 (7%)
Using nutrition labels to select healthy foods	2 (14%)	5 (36%)	4 (29%)	3 (21%)
Planning healthy meals for you and/or your family	—	2 (14%)	6 (43%)	6 (43%)
Finding reliable nutrition information	—	4 (29%)	8 (57%)	2 (14%)

Participant enrollment in a food assistance/supplementation program (SNAP/CalFresh/food stamps): yes, 31% ($n = 4$); no, 69% ($n = 9$).

Participants listed the following barriers to healthy eating at home/work/school/social settings:

- Lack of information and time
- Work
- No money
- Being away from home (work, social settings)
- Cravings
- Bad habits

Participants listed the following factors at home/work/school/social settings that help them to make healthy eating choices:

- Preparing at home
- Being at home
- Thinking about health
- Eating fruits and vegetables
- Healthy eating during week
- Healthy recipes
- Change bad habits

Participants listed the following topics of interest for nutrition classes:

- Eating for strength/energy
- Portion sizes (how much is needed of each food group per day)
- Eating for heart health (cholesterol specifically was mentioned)
- How to find healthy food in a grocery store
- Is juice healthy?
- Using the "rainbow" concept to encourage children to eat colorful vegetables
- Eating for weight control
- How to balance the diet (specifically talked about meat, how often to include it, etc.)
- What is an appropriate schedule for eating? How often? What time (does late eating make a difference)?

When asked, "What is 'healthy'?", participants listed:

- Feeling good
- Balance, including fruits and vegetables
- Eating the right portions

When asked, "How does what you eat affect you?", participants mentioned:

- Chronic diseases (diabetes, cholesterol, "acid")
- Mental effects (depression and "nerves")
- Headaches
- "Sobre todo el peso" ("Above all, weight")

Interviews with key informants (directors of BCWP fitness-focused classes) indicated that the target audience is very interested in learning about nutrition, and many members of the target audience have been approaching fitness leaders with nutrition-related questions. They anticipate the audience to be eager to learn and to enjoy hands-on learning activities.

Step 4: Analyze and interpret the data.

As is consistent with the area code of 90805 in which the program is located,[14] the majority of the BCWP participants are Hispanic/Latino, with many being Spanish-speaking only. Research has indicated that acculturation scores relate to the ability to read nutrition labels among Southern California Latino women.[15] Furthermore, research has shown that those who were more acculturated to the U.S. lifestyle would benefit from tips on healthy eating while dining out and those less acculturated would benefit from shopping habit interventions including supermarket tours.[16] The target population survey reflected similar needs, with half of participants having low confidence in using nutrition labels to select healthy foods, and 43% having low confidence in choosing healthy foods while dining out. Being able to select healthy foods while dining out and grocery shopping is important, since 50% of participants consume fast food more than once a week and 69% report visiting a grocery store four or more times in one month. In addition, 57% responded with no or slight confidence in following recipes, but many (86%) were at least moderately confident in planning and preparing healthy meals for themselves and/or their families.

Four participants (31%) are enrolled in a food assistance/supplementation program. Research has shown that SNAP participants have a lower dietary quality score than nonparticipants[17] and that Mexican Americans have lower vitamin A, vitamin C, and calcium intakes than Anglo Americans.[18]

During the discussion questions, BCWP participants expressed that they were interested in learning about eating for weight control and heart health. In the city of Long Beach, the rate of hospitalization for diabetes for Hispanic/Latinos is 35.4%, and the rate of residents who have been diagnosed with diabetes, prediabetes, or "sugar diabetes" in area code 90805 is 23.3%, almost one-fourth.[19] Caballero (2011) states that Hispanic/Latinos may have fears of type 2 diabetes and its treatment, which could be due to lack of knowledge.[20] In addition, the Hispanic/Latino heart disease hospitalization rate for Long Beach is 168 per 10,000 population.[21] Nutrition for children was another topic about which the target audience expressed interest in learning. Available data substantiate the need for nutrition education focused on children, with 59% of fifth graders overweight or obese in area code 90805, which is 7% higher than for the City of Long Beach as a whole.[22] **Table D-9** presents a summary of salient data from the needs assessment.

Step 5: Share the findings of the assessment.

Findings of the assessment will be shared with:

- Faculty and students providing the fitness portion of BCWP
- Local Department of Health and Human Services Health Promotion Coordinators
- Funders of BCWP
- Local city council members
- Nutrition graduate students planning the nutrition intervention

TABLE D-9 Summary of Salient Needs Assessment Data

	EXISTING DATA	NEW DATA
Race Hispanic/Latino	> 50% (area code 90805)	~99%
Enrolled in food assistance/supplementation programs	10.8% (Long Beach city)	31% (4)
Consume fast food > 1×/week	46.3% (Long Beach city)	50% (7)
Fruit and/or vegetable consumption:		
Consume no fruits and/or vegetables		7% (1)
Consume five servings of fruits and vegetables per day	14.5% (Long Beach city)	
Grocery store 4+ times/month		69%
Access to high quality fruits and vegetables	92.8% (Long Beach city)	
Low confidence in:		
Following recipes		57% (8)
Choosing healthy foods while dining out	Evidence in Ayala, 2005	43% (6)
Using nutrition labels to select healthy foods	Evidence in Ayala, 2005	50% (7)
Consume dessert food or sugary beverage		50% (7) = 1×/day
Diagnosed pre-/diabetes	23.3% (area code 90805)	
Hispanic/Latino diabetes hospitalization	35.4% (Long Beach city)	
Hispanic/Latino heart disease hospital rate	168:10,000 (Long Beach city)	
% Fifth graders overweight/obese	59% (area code 90805)	

Step 6: Set priorities.

Nutrition priorities to be addressed: Selection and preparation of healthy foods, with a focus on: (1) use of nutrition labels, (2) selecting foods in grocery stores and restaurants, and (3) preparation of nutrient-rich meals and snacks.

Justification: Survey results indicate that the target audience has low confidence in following recipes, choosing healthy foods while dining out, and using nutrition labels. Participants expressed interest in learning how to plan a balanced diet and how to select healthy foods while shopping. Furthermore, participants expressed that preparing foods at home helps them to eat healthier. Prior research has shown group-based cooking and nutrition classes among Latinos to be helpful in promoting healthy eating habits,[23] and that interventions including a grocery store tour may decrease the total number of calories and calories per dollar purchased in Spanish-speaking, low-income families.[24]

The program will coordinate with the following national nutrition priorities:

- *Dietary Guidelines for Americans*[25]

  - Improve nutrition literacy and cooking skills, including safe food-handling skills, and empower and motivate the population, especially families with children, to prepare and consume healthy foods at home.

- *Healthy People 2020*[26]

  - NWS-14 Increase the contribution of fruits to the diets of the population aged two years and older.
  - NWS-15 Increase the variety and contribution of vegetables to the diets of the population aged two years and older.

- NWS-17 Reduce consumption of calories from solid fats and added sugars in the population aged two years and older.
- HC/HIT-1 Improve the health literacy of the population.

Step 7: Choose a plan of action.

In response to the findings of the needs assessment, a 12-session (two one-hour lessons offered twice a week for six weeks) nutrition education and cooking class is proposed. In order to determine nutrition topics for BCWP, the following factors are considered:

- First, the time allotted for each lesson as well as the length of the total program must be considered. Two one-hour-long lessons will be taught per week on each topic, one on Wednesday and one on Friday.
- The need for lessons to be provided in English and Spanish must be taken into account.
- Data from the needs assessment will be used to determine the particular needs and interests of the population.

Six nutrition lesson topics will form the basis for the lessons, summarized in **Table D-10**. Participants will be provided with recipes and other informative handouts in Spanish and English.

Note: The Beach Community Wellness Program is directed by Dr. Christine Galvan and Dr. Ayla Donlin, faculty members in the Department of Kinesiology at California State University Long Beach. Dr. Virginia Gray directs the nutrition component of BCWP; graduate students in Dr. Gray's Advanced Community Nutrition class completed a needs assessment to guide development of the nutrition component of BCWP in spring 2015.

TABLE D-10 Summary of Lesson Topics and Activities Proposed for Nutrition Component of Beach Community Wellness Program

LESSON NUMBER	LESSON TITLE	TOPIC(S)	COOKING/SHOPPING ACTIVITY
Lesson 1	Balanced Nutrition	Portion sizes, food groups, intuitive eating	Healthy stuffed baked potatoes (with beans and vegetables)
Lesson 2	Exploring Nutrition Labels	Using nutrition labels	Vegetable quesadillas
Lesson 3	Functions of Foods and Disease Prevention	Functions of nutrients, benefits of variety and color in foods, eating for weight control and disease prevention	Whole-grain pasta salad with vegetables
Lesson 4	Grocery Shopping and Eating Out	Meal planning, making grocery lists, shopping on a budget, making healthy choices while dining out	Grocery store tour
Lesson 5	Nutrition for Children and Older Adults	Nutrition needs and appropriate foods for children and older adults	Healthy fruit and vegetable smoothie
Lesson 6	Cooking with Veggies	Nutrient-rich vegetables (unfamiliar vegetables participants identify and express interest in preparing during the shopping market tour will be featured)	Kale and Brussels sprouts salad

Index

Note: Page numbers in *italics* indicate tables or figures.

INVENTING
MODERN AMERICA

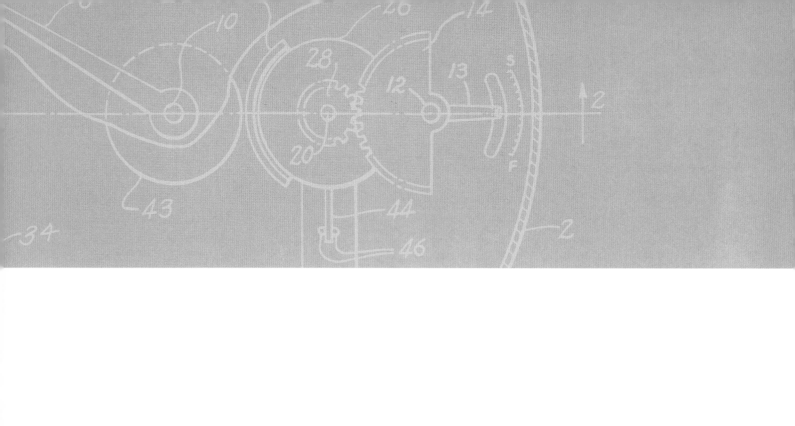

INVENTING MODERN AMERICA

From the Microwave to the Mouse

Text by **David E. Brown**

Foreword by **Lester C. Thurow**

Introductions by **James Burke**

A Publication of the Lemelson-MIT Program
for Invention and Innovation

The MIT Press

Cambridge, Massachusetts

London, England

First MIT Press paperback edition, 2003

©2002 Massachusetts Institute of Technology

This book was set in Scala Sans and Officina Sans by The MIT Press
and printed and bound in the United States of America.

Library of Congress Cataloging-in-Publication Data
Brown, David E.
    Inventing Modern America: from the microwave to the mouse / text
by David E. Brown ; foreword by Lester C. Thurow ; introductions by
James Burke.
        p. cm.
"A publication of the Lemelson-MIT program for invention and inno-
vation." Includes bibliographical references and index.
ISBN 0-262-02508-6 (hc.: alk. paper), 0-262-52349-3 (pb)
    1. Inventions—United States—History—20th century. 2. Inventors—
United States—Biography. I. Title.

T20 .B76 2002
609.73'09'04—dc21   2001044768

10 9 8 7 6 5 4 3 2

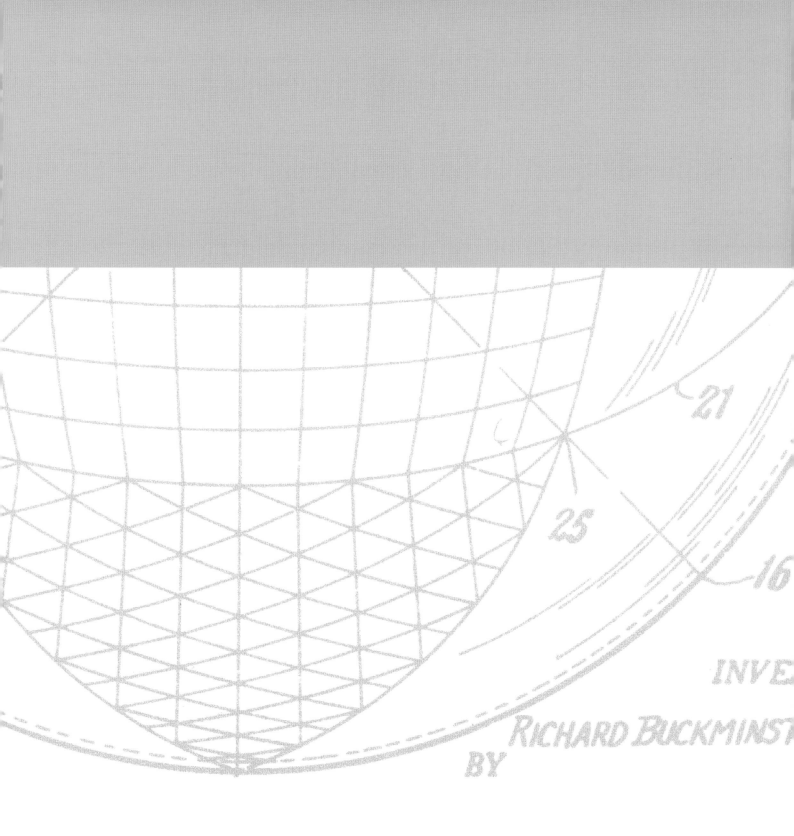

21

25

16

INVE

BY RICHARD BUCKMINST

CONTENTS

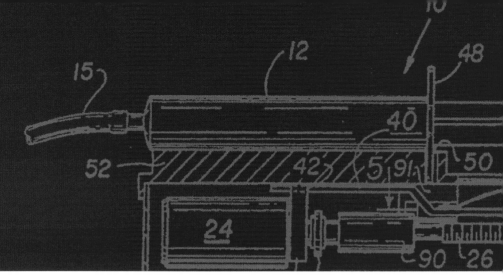

FOREWORD

Lester C. Thurow

Our advance from caves to cyberspace is a history of technical progress. The invention of tools allowed early humans to compete with animals far stronger and faster than they. With humankind's first great technological leap, the domestication of animals and the development of farming, a nomadic hunter-gatherer way of life came to an end. Settled permanent villages emerged. Eventually agriculture had advanced to a point where it could generate food surpluses large enough to feed substantial populations and those villages became cities.

Once everyone did not have to work full time as a farmer, some individuals could devote their time to learning. With the invention of writing and reading, humans took a second great technological leap forward. Knowledge could be saved from one generation to the next. It did not depend upon fallible human memories. It did not depend upon direct person-to-person contact. Knowledge could be accumulated. Information could be sent from one place to another. The dissemination of knowledge was speeded up. Henceforth no one would have to reinvent the wheel. They could read about the wheel. One human being could stand on the technological shoulders of another. With the gradual accumulation of knowledge, civilizations would emerge. The monuments of ancient Egypt still symbolize the glory of these ancient civilizations and their inventions.

For most of human history technical progress has occurred very slowly. Often it has even contracted. Fifteenth-century China was more technologically advanced than nineteenth-century China. For almost fifteen hundred years, in what we know as the Dark Ages, European per capita incomes were below the peaks achieved during the Roman Era. But even in these dark times technical progress did not stop—the human animal is inventive and its inventiveness cannot be stopped. The compass, the rudder, gunpowder, and the horse collar appeared in this era. But social disorganization meant that newly developed technologies spread slowly and that old technologies were little used. Ancient Romans knew how to make and use chemical fertilizers. The farmers of the Dark Ages did not. Crop yields per hectare fell dramatically. Cities shrank and disappeared. At the depth of the Dark Ages, the largest cities in Europe were less than one percent as large as Imperial Rome at its peak. Literacy rates plunged.

Over time, technological leadership has moved from one part of the world to another. In ancient times it was found in Egypt and the Euphrates River Valley, then it moved on to Greece and Rome. During Europe's Dark Ages, the Western center of learning and innovation moved to the Islamic world, where modern numbers were invented.

In the fifteenth century, before Columbus landed in America, China was the world's technology leader. It produced more iron and steel than eighteenth-century Europe would. China had gunpowder, the compass, and the rudder. It had put an armada with 28,000 troops on the east coast of Africa with ships four times as big as those of Columbus. It had moveable type and paper. It had the plow and threshing machine. And, believe it or not, it knew how to drill for natural gas. To this day there is a debate as to how many "European" inventions are really technologies that slowly moved from China, where they had been invented much earlier.

But the long European downturn eventually ended. The Renaissance began. In the fifteenth century the printing press (probably invented twice—once in Germany and earlier in China) made it feasible for everyone to participate in the cultural revolution that we know as literacy and numeracy. Books became cheap; it was no longer just the elite who could afford reading materials. The door was open for everyone to learn what others had already learned.

Most of what we think of as technical progress has happened in the last 200 years. With the invention, or more accurately perfection, of the steam engine (ancient Egyptian temple doors were opened and shut with the pressure of steam), the industrial age arrived. What was developed as a device to pump water out of coal mines caused a revolution in transportation (the railroad) and powered the development of a system of industrial factories (first in textiles and then elsewhere).

Eight thousand years of agriculture as the dominant human economic activity had come to an end. Ninety-eight percent of Americans worked on the farm in 1800. Today only two percent are full-time farmers.

If one wanted to be rich as an individual, company, or nation, one had to play the industrial game. Prior to the steam engine, differences in per capita income between countries were small. Everyone depended upon agriculture for their wealth. But with the first industrial revolution it was possible to raise per capita Gross Domestic Products far above the levels afforded by agriculture.

Some countries made that leap into the industrial age. Others did not. What we call the first world and the third world came into existence. Everyone knew about the new technologies, but some countries had the social organization to leap into this new world and some did not. Two hundred years later some countries are still struggling to make it into the industrial age.

At the end of the nineteenth century one great idea and one great discovery changed the nature of technical progress. This great discovery was that electricity could be harnessed (with lightning and static electricity, the existence of electricity had been known for a long time) and used. Electricity replaced lamp oil in lighting, the steam engine in transportation—and allowed the telegraph to be invented. Communication at the speed of horse and rider (the pony express) was replaced by communication at the speed of light. At the beginning of the twenty-first century it is impossible even to conceive of modern life without electricity.

The great idea (a German idea that arose in the course of developing their chemical engineering industries at the end of the nineteenth century) was that systematic investments in research and development based upon academic science could lead to much faster rates of technological progress. In the nineteenth century the world's technological leaders were to be found in Great Britain. Today we would call them great industrial tinkerers. Bessemer, for example, never knew—chemically speaking—what was going on inside his blast furnaces as he made steel. He just found by experimentation what worked and what did not work. By contrast, in the twentieth century most inventions sprang from systematic scientific investments in research and development (R&D).

The industrial research and development laboratory, our great research universities, government research budgets (the National Science Foundation, the National Institutes of Health), and government laboratories all flowed from this great German idea. Invention still depended upon creative individuals, but the scientific platforms upon which they worked had to be socially created and supported. Technical progress had been systematized and was no longer just the product of fortunate accidents. It came to be seen as the normal condition of human kind. To the ancient Egyptians, Greeks, or Romans, forever advancing technical progress—something we all assume to be true—would have been a concept impossible to comprehend.

Based upon systematic investments in R&D, Germany became the world's technological leader in the first half of the twentieth century. Its scientists, or those closely related (Werner Heisenberg, Niels Bohr, Albert Einstein), and its inventions (V-2 rockets during World War II) were ahead of those in the rest of the world. Until the 1940s, if one wanted the best scientific education, one went to Germany. World War II led to the eclipse of German science and the rise of American science. To a great extent this shift was led by the brilliant individuals who moved from Europe to the United States (such as Einstein and Enrico Fermi).

Today scientific understanding, engineering advances, invention, innovation (bringing a product to market), and the widespread use of new products in human life are seen as a logical, linear process. Sometimes they are: Einstein's theory of the equivalence of mass and energy, $E=mc^2$, led to the development of atomic weapons. But often they are not. Invention often comes before scientific understanding, and this leads to the search for the principles that make those inventions possible. Steel was made long before we understood the scientific principles of how iron became steel. Selective breeding of plants (replanting the seeds of the most prolific, hardiest plants) occurred long before genetics was understood.

What seems useless is often found to be useful. Often this depends on complementary technological developments. Bell Laboratories' lawyers did not want to patent the laser because they could think of no uses for it. Today, nothing is more ubiquitous than the laser—for correcting your eyesight, playing your music, and transmitting your telephone calls.

In the end, invention is a mysterious process. It almost always involves hard work and countless dead ends. Luck often plays a role. But in the end the "Eureka!" of the inventor reflects reality. Something not known, or not possible, has become both known and possible.

Inventions and innovations do not occur evenly in human history. Long periods with little activity are interspersed with periods of intense technological creativity. Historians see these latter periods as technological revolutions, as with the agricultural revolution 8,000 years ago, the steam revolution at the end of the eighteenth century, and the electrification revolution at the end of the nineteenth century. Today we are in the midst of what I believe will come to be called the third industrial revolution. This revolution is based upon rapid advances in six technologies—microelectronics, computers, telecommunications, new man-made materials, robotics, and biotechnology—and the interactions between them.

The interactions are probably even more important than the leaps. When physics and microelectronics met biology, for example, robotic microelectronic analyzers allowed the sequencing of the human genome to be completed six years earlier than expected. At the same time, biology was informing physics and electrical engineering: for example, researchers began building computers based on molecular, not electronic, principles.

Whenever there is a profound change in the way we understand the world—and biotechnology should be seen as the Newtonian and Einstein revolutions in physics compressed into a 50-year period—there is a period of ferment, invention, and innovation. Old production modes are suddenly replaced with new ones (e-commerce replaces the neighborhood store). Never-before-seen technologies (the Internet) change how humans live their lives.

In the short run, technical progress and economic progress are not identical. The deployment of knowledge requires social organization, and often that key ingredient is absent. That is why Imperial Rome had a much higher level of economic activity and standard of living than the Dark Ages, even though the Dark Ages had technologies not available to the Romans.

But in the long run, technical progress and economic progress move on parallel tracks. Without technical progress, even in a perfectly organized society, economic progress would quickly stagnate. All of the investments that could profitably be made would have been made and there would be nothing new in which to invest. Improvements in standards of living would come to a halt.

This book celebrates the technical advancements that make human progress possible. It presents snapshots of the twentieth-century innovation that led us to where we are, and it is a peek into the torrent of inventiveness that is appearing at the start of the twenty-first century.

These stories do not look at the whole process. They look at inventions and not the scientific discoveries that made those inventions possible. This is not a book about Nobel Prize winners. The book also does not focus on innovation—the hard process of bringing a product to market and making it into something that humans want to use. Persuading Americans to use a garbage disposal was not easy (how could one put garbage in the sink where one was washing one's dishes?). In fact, it took the dishwasher to make the garbage disposal a common household appliance (dishes were now not washed where garbage was deposited).

Some inventors are innovators. Ford invented the assembly line and built a company and a product based upon what he invented. Most inventors, however, are not. Philo Farnsworth invented the television but no company or TV set bears his name. Conversely, most innovators are not inventors. Carnegie built America's steel industry but he did not invent the technologies that he used.

This book springs out of the Lemelson-MIT Program, based at the Massachusetts Institute of Technology, which every year awards the world's largest single prize for invention, the $500,000 Lemelson-MIT Prize, to an American inventor.

The aim of this prize (inspired and financed by Jerome and Dorothy Lemelson nearly a decade ago) is to bang the drum for American invention and to provide role models for young Americans. They, too, might become inventors when they grow up.

Many of the world's greatest inventions were not American—the jet engine came from Great Britain, the printing press from Germany, the wheelbarrow from China, the World Wide Web from Europe. This book focuses on American inventors, not because the country has a monopoly on inventing, but because it is designed to help Americans understand the process of invention and to excite and stimulate them to become more inventive.

At the same time, it is worth focusing on American inventiveness at the turn of the twenty-first century. Other nations now look to the American model to find ways to increase their inventiveness. It explains why the European and Japanese newspapers that were writing about the end of the American century a decade ago are today writing about the difficulties of keeping up with new American technologies. The technological revolution now under way is not the whole answer to this turnaround in American economic success (American firms did some very rapid learning about total quality management, just-in-time inventories, and design for manufacturability from the Japanese in the late 1980s and early 1990s), but it is a large part of the answer.

Perhaps there is another justification. Americans have not always been the world's technological leaders. In the nineteenth century that honor was held by Great Britain, and in the first half of the twentieth century it was held by Germany. Technology and American leadership have only come together in the last 50 years. What has been gained can be lost. Understanding how those who gave us that leadership came to be creative can perhaps help us keep the creativity going far into the twenty-first century.

The inventions and inventors in this book were picked both because they have contributed to raising human standards of living and because they are interesting—good fun, if you like. Some of them have contributed to making human life longer and healthier—medical devices, water purification, the traffic signal. Some of them helped make life more fun—TV, video games, the outboard engine. Some are ubiquitous—plastics, the computer mouse. Some serve the human desire to wan-

der—the auto assembly line. But they have all contributed to making us what we are.

This book is first and foremost a tribute to American ingenuity and inventiveness. Second, it may help us understand the conditions under which ingenuity occurs. Third, it is designed to provide role models for tomorrow's inventors; wishing to become Steve Wozniak (inventor of the Apple computer) is no more outlandish than wishing to become Babe Ruth. Fourth, it is a natural outcome of the invention outreach initiatives of the Lemelson-MIT Program.

This book is not meant to be a comprehensive listing of twentieth-century American inventors, and it certainly does not reflect our judgment as to who are the 35 most important inventors. They were selected because they have made important contributions and because their stories are interesting; they are inspiring individuals. Some have been picked because we hope they will surprise the reader. Their stories are ones you don't already know.

The book includes profiles of the inventors, organized into five main categories: medicine and healthcare, consumer products, transportation, energy and the environment, and computing and telecommunications. Science historian James Burke has written an introduction to each section. Burke's introductions are designed to lay the groundwork and provide a historical context for each section.

We want readers to have fun with this book. We want them to say, "I could do something like that too." We want readers to set out on great voyages of intellectual discovery themselves. And just as those who set out on the great voyages of geographic discovery aren't always remembered in history, most of the inventors in these pages won't be found in the history books. But these inventors have had courage and perserverance not to discover, but rather to invent, a new world. We hope you enjoy the journey.

To journey further on line, visit:
www.inventingmodernamerica.com

INVENTING
MODERN AMERICA

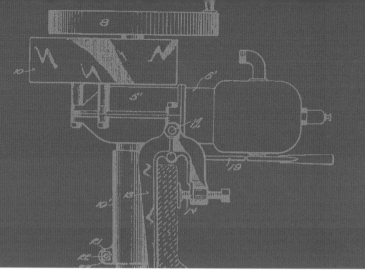

INTRODUCTION

James Burke

It is ironic that the United States should be the most technologically innovative country in the world, with an annual patent rate running at about 70,000 (not to mention the hundreds of thousands of unpatented inventions)—and more than six million patents issued since the Founding Fathers opened the U.S. Patent Office in 1790. The irony is that it was the rediscovery of America by Columbus that triggered it all.

The sixteenth-century canonical authorities (the Bible and Aristotle) made no mention of the new continent, so what was it doing there? Over the following hundred years the avalanche of new plants and animals (such as pineapples and turkeys and potatoes) flooding into Europe from the New World (and none of these had been included in the canonical lists, either) brought a crisis of intellectual confidence. If the classical Greek knowledge on which everyone relied was wrong, then what was right? Things became even more perturbed in the sixteenth century when Copernicus's *De Revolutionibus* turned everything upside down when his heliocentric system removed the Earth from the center of the cosmos. As the contemporary English poet John Donne later understated it: "The new philosophy calls all in doubt."

In an effort to find a more secure way to generate trustworthy knowledge, the seventeenth-century French engineer René Descartes produced two rules: Doubt everything that is not self-evident, and reduce all problems and structures to their simplest, irreducible components, so as to understand how they work.

Methodical doubt and reductionism laid the foundation of scientific thought and fail-proof technological practice, and triggered four centuries of innovation that modern inventors such as those in this book can now draw on. By the early twenty-first century, Cartesian thought had generated hundreds of scientific and technological disciplines, each working according to natural laws discovered by the same Cartesian process. Before Descartes we had lived by the simple axiom *credo ut intelligam* (faith brings comprehension). Descartes reversed it: *intelligo ut credam* (when I have examined the proposition for traps I'll get back to you).

As any scientist will agree, reductionism requires unremitting attention to detail. Some modern fields of endeavor, such as genetics or particle physics, involve mind-numbing patience and months of routine analysis before even the smallest advance can be achieved. Thomas Edison, the inventor's inventor, defined genius as "99 percent perspiration and 1 percent inspiration." He was speaking from experience. To arrive at the right filament for his light bulb Edison and his trusty assistants tested thousands of materials over many months. Recognizing this requirement for exhaustive investigation, Edison systematized the process with the world's first research lab in his Menlo Park, New Jersey, establishment, and brought the innovative production technique down to a fine art: a minor invention every ten days and a "big trick" every six months or so. A colleague of Edison's, Nikola Tesla, summed him up: "If Edison had a needle to find in a haystack he would proceed at once with the diligence of a bee to examine straw after straw until he found it."

Thanks to the kind of human ingenuity celebrated in this book, innovation has brought us to the threshold of transition from a culture of scarcity to one of abundance, in which we may have the technology to release the awesome potential of more than six billion imaginative brains around the planet. Each of those brains is adept at (perhaps even designed for) thinking in the fundamentally innovative mode celebrated in this book. The kind of thinking that causes one and one to make three: an evolutionarily valuable characteristic, since it permits the brain to run scenarios, to bring together the various elements of any situation, predict the likely outcome, and make a decision based on that prediction.

All of the inventors in this book do this, in some way or another. And, while in no way detracting from their brilliance, or that of the thousands of innovative minds that preceded them both in America and elsewhere, perhaps their greatest contribution has been to develop the tools and provide the opportunity for any other human brain to do the kind of innovative thinking they have done.

We can all be all inventors, just like the ones in this book. They show the way.

MEDICINE AND HEALTHCARE

INTRODUCTION

The first group of inventors featured in this book displays the same talents for attention to detail as the early reductionists. They all work in the world of medicine. Not surprisingly, reductionism has brought astonishing developments in this (literally) life-and-death field of study. Medicine, as our inventors' biographies show, has a history of dogged application mixed with moments of wonderful serendipity. In 1928 Alexander Fleming returned from holiday to his London hospital to find a mold growing on the unwashed lab dishes he had left stacked in the sink. The mold spores had come in through a window accidentally left open, the air had stayed at exactly the right temperature and humidity for the right number of days for the mold to grow, and the lab cleaner happened to have not washed up. This combination of events made Fleming's discovery of penicillin possible.

Similar periods of application interrupted by serendipitous flashes have enlivened the work of our first group of inventors. On one occasion, a patch of seaweed inspired a novel method for growing artificial human tissue. In the case of Mary-Claire King, her discovery of the marker for the gene related to breast cancer came only after years of unremitting step-by-step analysis.

In every case, there was also a defining moment of insight, when all of the inventors say they suddenly saw the answer to the problem. Each time, the innovative moment came when they were able to look at things in an unconventional way. Thomas Fogarty unexpectedly understood the relevance to his cardiovascular work of a technique he often used to tie fishing flies. Raymond Damadian's MRI scanner came out of a realization that a way of using a magnetic field to analyze physical substances could be employed to provide pictures of the inside of a living human body.

The other common characteristic of this group is (naturally enough, given their specialty) an abiding desire to help people. As twenty-first-century American science and technology offers greater and greater insight into the workings of the human body, opportunities will proliferate for minds like these to use the widening pool of knowledge to help them achieve the goal they share: to better the human condition.

—JB

RAYMOND **DAMADIAN**

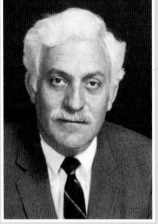

At some point in June of 1977, the huge, heavy, complicated machine that Dr. Raymond Damadian and his assistants were building needed a nickname. Since the seven years they had spent building and rebuilding it had been full of struggle, adversity, and near-failure, Damadian gave it a name that reflected the courage and dedication that went into it: Indomitable. Less than a month later, the machine was switched on and, over the course of five hours, it delivered the first magnetic resonance image (MRI) of a living human.

That first MRI, a relatively crude picture of the chest of one of Damadian's assistants, ushered in a new era in medical imaging. Today, MRI machines are used at every hospital to produce safe, noninvasive images that detect cancer and other diseases, guide surgeons, and reveal some of the body's secrets. Indomitable, the machine that started it all, has found a permanent home in the collection of the Smithsonian Institution.

The story of Damadian's invention begins with his research into one of those secrets. As a postdoctoral student in the 1960s, he was trying to find out how the kidney moved sodium it had absorbed back into the body. Most people assumed that there was a "sodium pump" in the kidney, but no one had found it or come up with an alternative explanation for the process. Damadian searched for a pump for five years before concluding that one did not exist. So he began reexamining how the body's cells work, specifically how water helps sodium and potassium move into and out of them. In 1969, he was discussing his research with a physicist and physician, Freeman Cope, who had measured sodium in cells with a device called a nuclear magnetic resonance (NMR) spectrometer, and hoped to measure potassium. Damadian was intrigued by the method and offered to help.

The phenomenon of nuclear magnetic resonance (NMR) had been discovered in 1937 by the physicist Isidor Rabi. His research, later refined by physicists Felix Bloch and Edward Purcell, revealed a fundamental property of physics. When radio waves were aimed at atomic nuclei in a strong magnetic field and then turned off, the nuclei emitted consistent, measurable amounts of energy for a short period of time. That period of time—called the relaxation

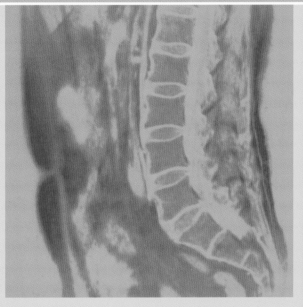

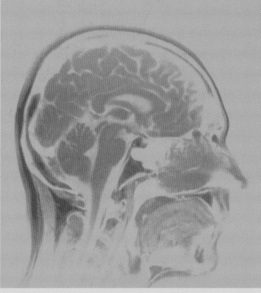

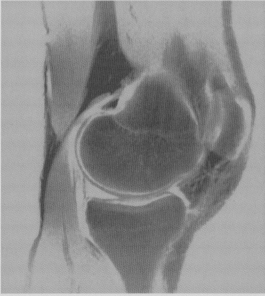

Originally conceived as a method for detecting cancer, the MRI has become the standard for diagnostic imaging, producing pictures of the body's internal structure and organs with unparalleled detail.

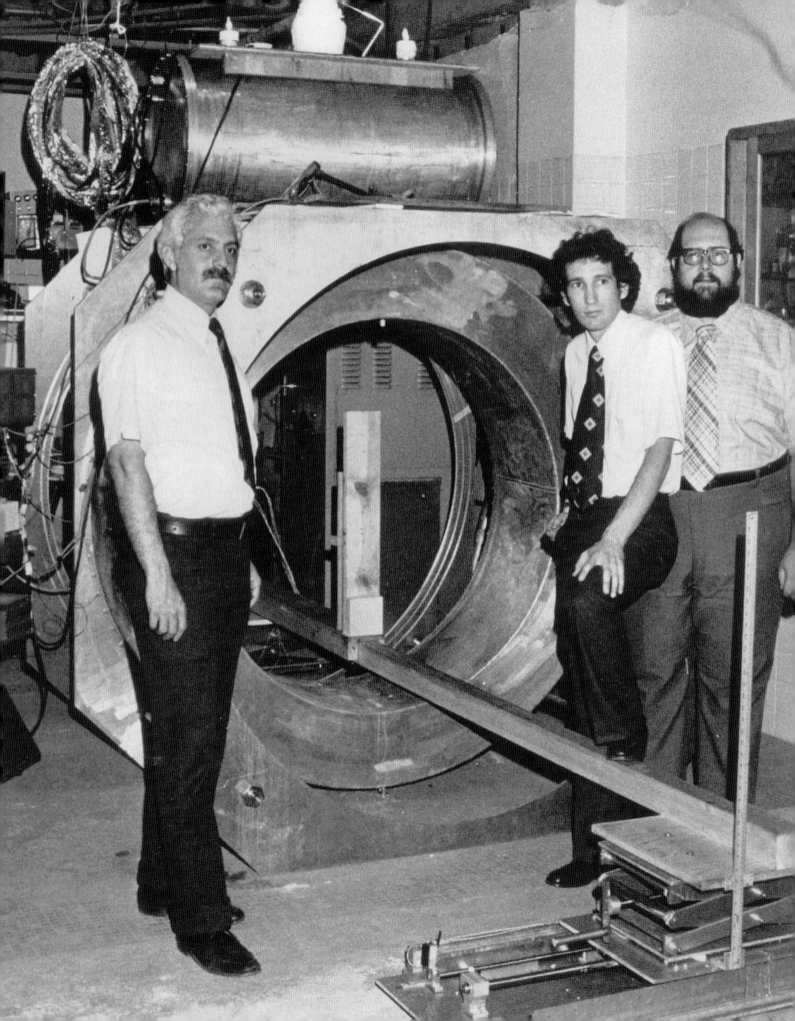

rate—differed for different substances. Soon scientists were using NMR to determine the physical properties of all kinds of things. Until Damadian and Cope, though, no one had used NMR to probe the workings of living cells.

The two scientists traveled to a NMR lab in Pennsylvania to examine a potassium-rich strain of bacteria. They inserted a sample into the NMR machine—essentially a large magnet equipped with an antenna that emitted radio waves—and saw an oscilloscope signal that revealed the bacteria's potassium levels. Damadian was awed by this result, something he could barely have replicated in a lab. "It had a profound effect on me," he said. "It was doing chemistry by wireless electronics."

A few days later Damadian had a vision of where NMR could lead. "If you could ever get this technology to provide the chemistry of the human body the way it does for the chemist," he said, "you could spark an unprecedented revolution in medicine." For one thing, Damadian realized that cancerous cells have a different proportion of sodium and potassium than healthy ones. If NMR could detect that difference—and he thought it could—then a doctor could diagnose cancer early and without surgery.

In June 1970, Damadian took the first step in doing just that. Working with healthy and cancerous tissue samples from rats, he successfully used NMR to detect which was which. He also realized that each type of tissue, whether healthy or not, had a different relaxation rate, so NMR scanning was not limited to detecting disease—it could provide a basic window into the body. The next year, he published his findings in the journal

Science, and in 1972 filed for a patent. The patent was awarded in 1974, the first covering the technology.

There was a personal note to his quest for a successful imaging technique: For several years in the 1960s, Damadian had been plagued with abdominal pain. After several doctors failed to find its cause, Damadian decided that there should—and could—be a better way to examine the body. Also, as a child he had witnessed his grandmother succumb to a slow and painful battle with breast cancer, inspiring a lifelong quest to conquer the disease.

Born in 1936 in New York, Damadian grew up in Forest Hills, Queens, surrounded by high-achieving peers. He was a prodigy at the violin, attended the Juilliard School of Music, and dreamed of becoming a solo violinist. At 15, Damadian realized that very few people are good enough to be professional musicians, so he gave up studying music and accepted a scholarship to the University of Wisconsin. He soon decided to become a doctor, and in 1960 graduated from the Albert Einstein College of Medicine in the Bronx. The combination of science and medicine—as well as a fierce fighting spirit picked up as a tennis player—would serve him well.

The 1971 article in *Science* should have been Damadian's finest hour, an announcement of a new way of seeing the body. Instead, it was the beginning of years of dismissal and ridicule by his peers, as well as cutthroat competition. His ideas of using technology from the world of physics to probe the body were completely new, and his long-range vision of using NMR to detect disease struck many scientists as wild and improbable.

Raymond Damadian, Larry Minkoff, and Michael Goldsmith

stand next to their just-completed magnetic resonance imaging

(MRI) machine, called Indomitable.

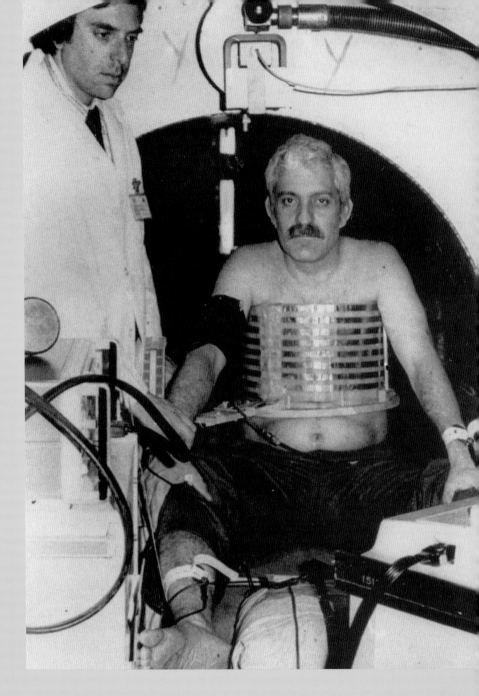

In May 1977, Damadian wrapped himself in a cardboard antenna and became the first test subject of the first MRI machine. The test was unsuccessful; the inventor was too big for the antenna.

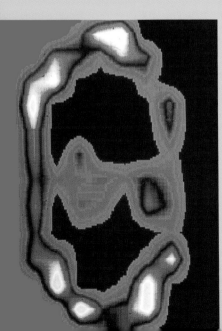

On July 2, 1977, the slimmer Larry Minkoff entered Indomitable. For five hours, Damadian and Michael Goldsmith recorded the machine's readings; they later created this digital image of Minkoff's chest from the data.

In his lab at the Downstate Medical Center in Brooklyn, Damadian assembled a small group of assistants and began exploring how to make a machine that could use NMR to scan a human. Several challenges faced them. First, they needed to build a magnet big enough for a human to fit in; only a handful of magnets that large existed, for use in nuclear physics research. They also had to find a way to focus the NMR and move it over a human body; the machine Damadian had used in his cancer cell study was designed to analyze small quantities of a single substance, so it didn't need a sharp focus or have to move.

Working on a shoestring budget, Damadian and his assistants built a large superconducting magnet and its liquid helium cooling system, often working into the early morning winding miles of wire and searching for helium leaks. He devised a method for focusing the NMR's radio waves, so as a human was moved through the device, different parts of the body could be seen. Since no one had built a large, focused NMR device before, the team constantly had to break new technical ground, experimenting to find the best way to make almost every part of the machine.

Through much of the 1970s, Damadian's main competition came from Paul Lauterbur, a chemist at the State University of New York in Stony Brook. In 1973, Lauterbur used NMR to scan the interior of a small clam—the first living creature to be imaged. He also developed a different way to focus the machine's signal, a method that gained wide use. Although Damadian thought of him as his rival, the two eventually shared the National Medal of Technology (1988) for their achievements.

In May 1977, Damadian thought Indomitable was ready to be tested. He volunteered himself as a subject, although no one knew what effects were possible from prolonged exposure to a strong magnetic field. Wrapped in a cardboard antenna, he lay down in the machine as it was switched on. But there was no NMR signal from his body; he was too big for the device. Two months later, on July 2, 1977, his slimmer assistant, Larry Minkoff, entered Indomitable. Damadian and his colleagues slowly read NMR signals from different levels of Minkoff's chest, plotting their values on a piece of graph paper. After almost five hours, Minkoff emerged to see a cross-section of his own chest, drawn in pencil. (A computer would be used later to replot and enhance the image.) It was the first scan of a human.

Three years later, Damadian's company, Fonar, built the first commercial MRI scanner. (Because of the negative publicity then surrounding all things nuclear, "nuclear magnetic resonance" was shortened to "magnetic resonance," hence MRI.) Scan time had been reduced considerably, and the image's resolution was many times higher than Indomitable's first effort. While Damadian had met with intense criticism for years, MRI machines became common (and soon essential) features of every good hospital.

Success breeds competition, and Damadian's small company soon found itself out-spent and out-marketed by Hitachi, Philips, and General Electric, among others. By the 1990s, Fonar had only a one percent market share. But Damadian is a firm believer in the power of the U.S. patent system, and he began to challenge other MRI makers. Many companies settled out of court, but GE—which had rejected his ideas in the 1970s, then began working on its own version of a scanner—fought his patent. In 1997, the Supreme Court upheld a judgment against GE, ordering it to pay Damadian damages of $128.7 million. After almost three decades of effort, his pioneering work had been validated not only in hospitals around the world, but also in the nation's highest court.

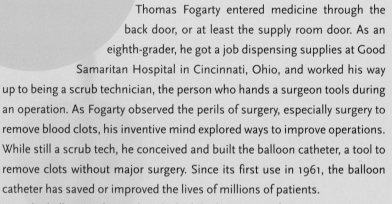

THOMAS
FOGARTY

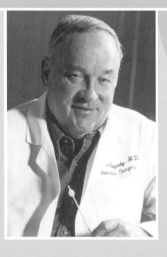

Thomas Fogarty entered medicine through the back door, or at least the supply room door. As an eighth-grader, he got a job dispensing supplies at Good Samaritan Hospital in Cincinnati, Ohio, and worked his way up to being a scrub technician, the person who hands a surgeon tools during an operation. As Fogarty observed the perils of surgery, especially surgery to remove blood clots, his inventive mind explored ways to improve operations. While still a scrub tech, he conceived and built the balloon catheter, a tool to remove clots without major surgery. Since its first use in 1961, the balloon catheter has saved or improved the lives of millions of patients.

The balloon catheter also marked the beginning of noninvasive surgery. By minimizing trauma to the patient and reducing time spent under anesthesia, surgical procedures such as blood clot removal became much safer and more cost-effective. Noninvasive procedures are now the standard of care for many health problems that once required lengthy surgery.

Fogarty showed his inventiveness at an early age. He was born in Cincinnati in 1934; his father, a railroad engineer, died when Fogarty was just eight years old. Fogarty took an active role in the family, taking care of things his father might have. "If my mother needed things fixed," he remembers, "she would call on me." It wasn't much of a stretch for Fogarty: "I just had a natural inclination and inquisitive nature about building things," he says. "I looked at things and just naturally thought, 'Okay, how can I make this better?'" His first mechanical explorations were with soapbox derby cars and model airplanes. Fogarty's planes were so good that he sold them to other kids in the neighborhood. He eventually graduated to more complex machines, devising, for example, an automatic clutch for a friend's motor scooter.

With money tight in his family, Fogarty went to work when he was 14 years old. Devoting time to work and mechanical tinkering, and having little interest in his classes, he did not do well in high school. However, by the time he was a senior, Fogarty knew he wanted to be a doctor. With the recommendation of a family priest, he was admitted to Xavier College in Cincinnati, although

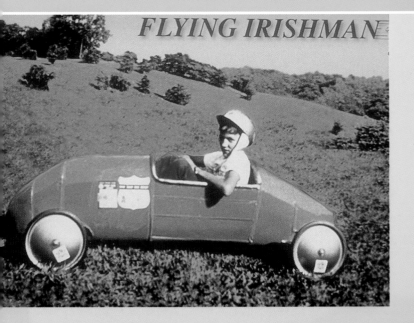

Thomas Fogarty's inventiveness first surfaced in the soapbox derby cars he designed and raced in Cincinnati in the 1940s. He soon moved on to modifying model airplane engines and motorized scooters. He is shown here in his "Flying Irishman," a go-cart that he built.

Fogarty's first medical device was the balloon embolectomy catheter—which he made by tying a small balloon to the end of a urethral catheter. It is inserted into a blocked blood vessel and then inflated and pulled back out, bringing a clot, or embolism, with it.

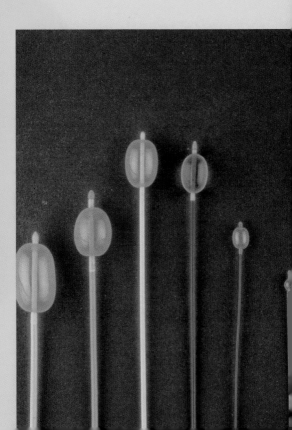

he was immediately put on academic probation. (He quickly learned how to study.) Fogarty needed three jobs and the financial help of a mentor, Dr. Jack Cranley, to get through college. He kept his scrub technician job and also worked as an X-ray technician and an orderly on the night shift.

It was as a scrub tech during college that Fogarty began to think about better ways to perform various surgical procedures. "I had a chance to see what worked and what didn't work," he says. "One of the things that didn't work was the way they took care of blockages in arteries and veins." At the time, the procedure for removing a clot was dangerous and not particularly successful. "They would make incisions that were horrendously long and open up the whole artery to try to take the clot out," he says. "That would end up with a 9- to 12-hour operation, with in-cisions in both legs and the abdomen. And it often didn't work, patients died or they had amputations."

Fogarty considered different ways to make the procedure better—especially how to avoid the long incisions. His first idea was to use a modified catheter. Inserted through a small incision, a catheter could get to the clot without much trauma to the patient. And Fogarty had an idea of how to get the clot out once the catheter was there.

Fogarty's scheme was straightforward. He started with a urethral catheter, which is flexible but strong enough to be pushed through a blood clot. Then he added a small balloon made from a finger of a latex glove, which could be inflated with saline once it was past the clot. The balloon expands to the size of the artery and is then pulled back out, bringing with it the clot.

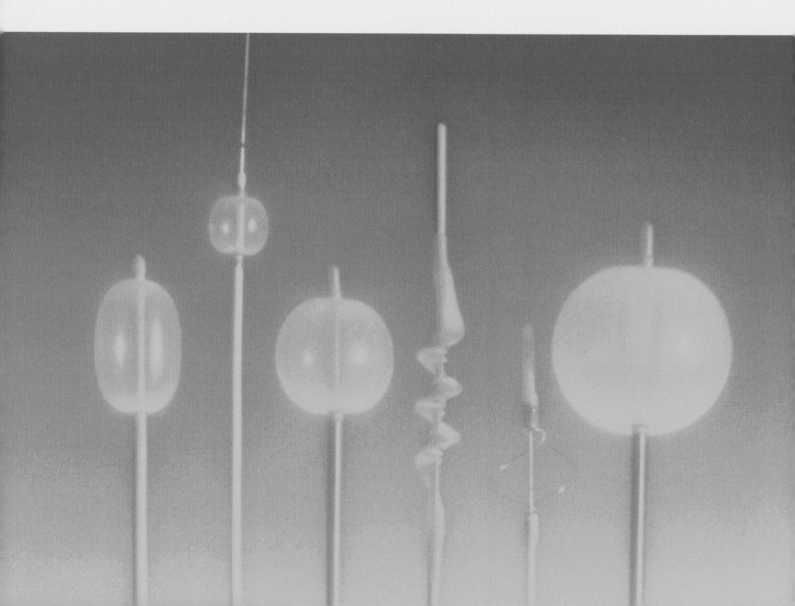

"You can feel the resistance, or the drag on the artery wall," Fogarty explains. "You adjust the volume of the balloon so you've got continual traction."

There was one main challenge in building such a device. "There was no way to attach the balloon," Fogarty says. The catheter was made of vinyl and the balloon of latex, and no glue available would hold the two together. Fortunately, one of Fogarty's hobbies was fly fishing, and he applied the sport's skill of precise hand-tying to the task. "I'd always tied flies and made lures," he remembers, "so it was just a natural thing."

With the balloon attached to the catheter, Fogarty began testing his device. First, he filled glass tubes with blood from a blood bank and let it clot, then inserted his catheter and pulled the clot out. He then tried the catheter on cadavers during autopsies. In 1961, his balloon embolectomy catheter—named for the clot-removal procedure performed—was used for the first time on a human patient. As Fogarty watched, a small incision was made and the catheter was threaded up the patient's blocked artery. When inflated and pulled back out, it did indeed bring the clot with it. Today, the procedure takes about an hour and is done under local anesthesia.

Transforming that single working catheter into the tool that thousands of surgeons now use took several years. When Fogarty was finishing his cardiovascular surgery residency at the University of Oregon, he spent a lot of time making catheters by hand for his colleagues. General acceptance, though, was harder to come by. A paper detailing the catheter's successes in surgery was rejected by three major journals and finally pub-lished in a smaller publication's "technique" section. "Traditional wisdom said that this was going to damage the artery," Fogarty explains. "A lot of people would say, 'This is crazy. Only someone that didn't know anything would suggest this.'"

Building catheters by hand was not a practical long-term strategy, but no medical equipment company seemed to be interested in making them. Eventually, Fogarty got to know Al Starr, a cardiac surgeon who had developed the first artificial heart valve used in humans. Starr recognized the catheter's utility and convinced his heart valve manufacturer to make them. Tens of thousands of Fogarty's catheters have been sold since, including several variants for different kinds of clots.

After Fogarty completed his residency and became a cardiovascular surgeon, he continued to invent new medical devices. He holds more than 70 patents, and some 20 companies have been founded to build his devices. One of the most successful of these products is the Fogarty Stent-Graft, an ingenious fix for the difficult problem of abdominal aortic aneurysms. As some people get older, their arteries become clogged with fatty deposits, weakening the vessel. Over time, this can cause the blood vessel to balloon, and eventually rupture. The traditional surgery to fix it, by removing the weakened part of the aorta, is dangerous, with a mortality rate of five percent or more.

Rather than removing the bad part of the vessel, Fogarty's idea was to strengthen it with an implant: a stent, a thin polyester tube that grabs on to the blood vessel with metal "rings." The method begins with an inflatable catheter, which transports the stent to the weakened portion of the vessel. Once it is

Some of Fogarty's catheters: from left, balloon embolectomy catheter, thru lumen embolectomy catheter, venous thrombectomy catheter, adherent clot catheter, graft thrombectomy catheter, and occlusion balloon catheter. Some 20 million people have been treated with these kinds of catheters.

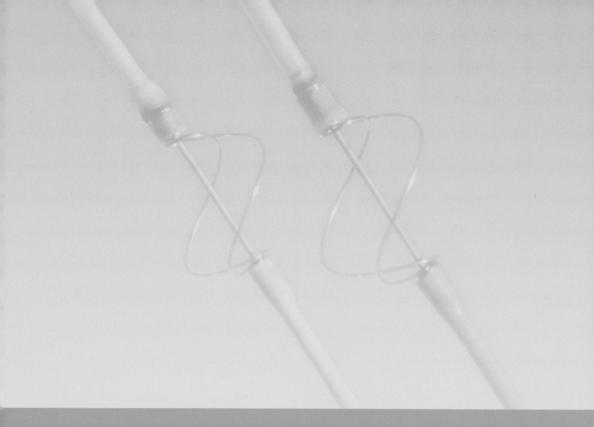

The graft thrombectomy catheter.

"I had no concept that [noninvasive surgery]

would reach the magnitude that it has."

aligned with the help of X-rays, the balloon is inflated and the stent expands to the size of the artery. After the stent is affixed permanently to the artery wall, blood flows normally and the aneurysm is bypassed.

The Fogarty Engineering company is currently developing several new medical devices, including a minimally invasive method for taking biopsies to test for breast cancer. Fogarty himself continues his work as a top cardiovascular surgeon, helps run several other medical equipment and research companies, and presides over the Thomas Fogarty Winery, 325 acres in the coastal hills west of Palo Alto that produce 15,000 bottles of premium wine each year.

When Fogarty built his first balloon catheter, he says, "I had no concept that [noninvasive surgery] would reach the magnitude that it has." Yet the movement toward noninvasive techniques is a logical extension of the concerns he wrestled with back in 1960, as he watched both surgeons and patients struggle with the dangers of blood clot surgery. "If you look at the issues I was trying to solve at that time," he explains, "they are the same issues applied to all these other things we do noninvasively. We minimize the anesthesia, we minimize the tissue trauma, and we shorten the recovery. Those were the things I felt I had to do. And those are the things we now do with everything that's less invasive."

In addition to creating medical inventions, Fogarty is a respected cardiovascular surgeon and also a vintner, operating a small winery in the hills outside of Palo Alto, California.

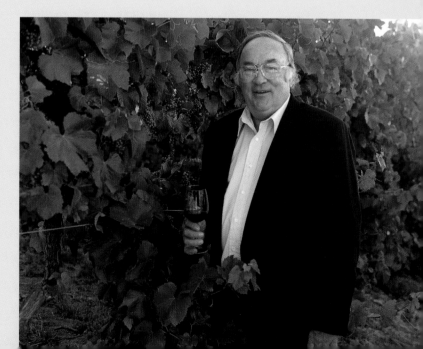

WILSON **GREATBATCH**

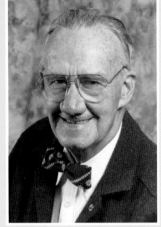

A tiny mistake led to the invention of the pacemaker, a device that has helped millions of people lead longer and more active lives. In 1958, Wilson Greatbatch was building a small device to record the sounds a heart makes. He reached into a box full of resistors—small electronic components color-coded with their resistance value—and pulled the wrong one out. "I misread the colors and got a brown-black-green [resistor] instead of brown-black-orange," he recalls. The finished device did something odd: It sent out a short pulse of electricity at an interval of one second. This was not useful for capturing heart sounds, but the mistake happened to be exactly what Greatbatch was looking for.

Seven years earlier, while working at the Cornell University Psychology Department's animal behavior farm, measuring sheep's and goats' vital signs, Greatbatch got into a lunchtime conversation with two surgeons. They told him about a condition called heart block, when a nerve fails to send the electrical impulses that makes the heart's muscles work to its lower chambers. This causes an irregular heartbeat and can lead to death. Doctors had already discovered that a quick jolt of electricity to the heart could substitute for the natural process, but the equipment for this was bulky and delivered a painful 100-volt shock to the patient's chest. When the surgeons described the problem to Greatbatch, he later wrote, "I knew immediately that I could build a much better and smaller implantable device." The problem was that no equipment was small enough for the task; transistors, the small semiconductors that replaced vacuum tubes, weren't widely available yet, and the batteries of the time were too big.

By 1958, things had changed. Transistors had hit the market, and Greatbatch was using one in the small oscillator he was making. When he saw the short pulse of electricity it made, he recalled, "I stared at the thing in disbelief, realizing this was *exactly* the properties of a pacemaker." At the time, Greatbatch was a member of a group of local engineers interested in medical technology.

Wilson Greatbatch's first pacemaker consisted of a simple transistor circuit and 10 batteries. Later pacemakers would have much better batteries, improved casings, and more sophisticated electronics.

In the late 1960s, Greatbatch turned his attention to powering pacemakers and introduced the small lithium batteries that still run millions of the devices. Here he displays an early pacemaker and a schematic of its circuit.

He was called to the local hospital to try to fix a problem a surgeon, Dr. William C. Chardack, was having with some equipment. Greatbatch couldn't help with the problem, but while he was there, he described his idea for a transistor-based pacemaker. "Chardack looked at me strangely and walked up and down the lab a couple of times," Greatbatch wrote, "and then said, 'If you can do that, you can save 10,000 lives a year.'"

Greatbatch finished a prototype pacemaker three weeks later. At the hospital, Chardack and a team of surgeons caused heart block in a dog by tying off the relevant nerve. Then Greatbatch touched the wires of his pacemaker to the slowly beating blocked heart. "Dr. Chardack looked at the pacemaker pattern on the oscilloscope," Greatbatch remembers, "and then said, 'Well I'll be damned!'" The dog's heart was beating normally.

That first working pacemaker was a culmination of Greatbatch's long interest in electronics. Born in 1919, he grew up in modest circumstances in Buffalo, New York, the son of a grocer and a contractor. From an early age, he was fascinated with radio, and in his teens he built a short-wave receiver, then joined the Sea Scouts, partly to use their transmitter. He also used his radio skills in World War II, where he served as a radioman on a destroyer. Later, he was stationed on an aircraft carrier and tended its electronics while also flying combat missions as a rear gunner. After the war, Greatbatch returned to New York and earned a degree in electrical engineering at Cornell, where he was also exposed to other disciplines, including physics and chemistry. Although his education was paid for in part by the G.I. Bill, Greatbatch's finances were tight—he had three of his five children by the time he finished Cornell—so he took jobs with the university. After working on Cornell's radio telescope, he settled into the animal behavior farm, where the idea for the pacemaker was born.

Greatbatch's dog pacemaker was far from the first attempt at a viable, reliable pacemaker for humans. Although Greatbatch didn't know it, several people had already tried. In 1918, an American doctor named Albert Hyman suggested that electrical pulses could shock a heart back to life. In 1933, an electrical engineer, William Kouwenhoven, demonstrated that electric shocks could restore a heart's normal rhythm. In 1952, Paul Zoll, a doctor who had worked with Kouwenhoven, built an external pacemaker; it worked, but not for long, and it was a bulky, awkward device. A few years later, in 1957, Minnesota physician Walton Lillehei and Earl Bakken, a local electronics repairman,

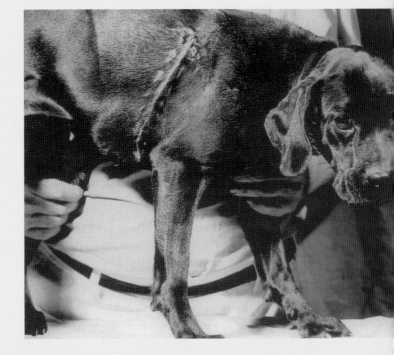

On May 7, 1958, Greatbatch's device was implanted in a dog— and it worked. Later, he wrote, "I seriously doubt if anything I ever do will ever give me the elation—when my electronic design controlled a living heart."

After the success of his first, experimental pacemaker, Greatbatch quit his job and worked to improve the design. He set up this workshop in a barn behind his house; his wife helped build and test the devices, using two ovens set up in their bedroom.

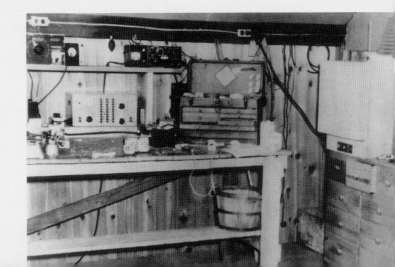

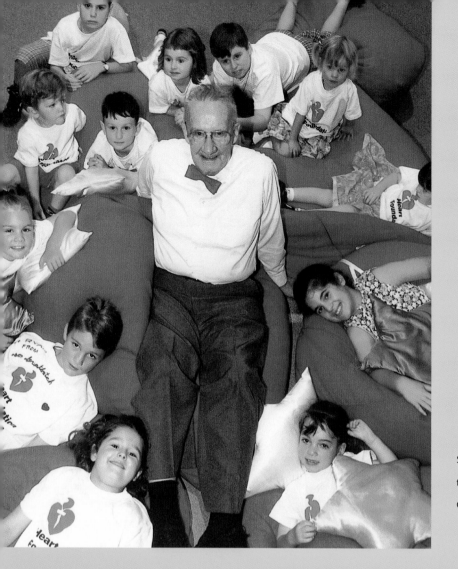

Since the first pacemaker was implanted in a person in 1960, the devices have extended and saved millions of lives. Here, Greatbatch poses with a group of children who have pacemakers.

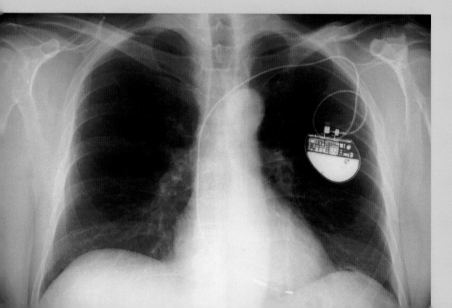

Today's pacemakers contain small but sophisticated computers that monitor the heart and turn the devices on or off or adjusting their impulses as the situation warrants.

built a portable, battery-powered pacemaker, about a foot square. Although their device also worked, its size and the fact that it worked externally made it only a short-term solution to heart problems.

It wasn't just technology that got in the way of the creation of the pacemaker. In the early 1930s Hyman built an "artificial pacemaker" that successfully revived several patients with a condition called Stokes-Adams syndrome. In contrast to the positive reaction to Greatbatch's pacemaker, many people criticized Hyman for intervening in a "natural" death. Others were horrified that doctors would meddle with the heart, the symbol of man's soul.

With the advent of open-heart surgery in the early 1950s, these objections fell by the wayside. After seeing his pacemaker work, Greatbatch set out to make one that could be implanted in humans. He quit his job at Cornell and began working in a barn behind his house, building pacemakers by hand. He hand-soldered the components together—some circuitry, a couple of transistors, and a zinc-mercury battery—and encased the unit in epoxy and silicone. Two ovens were set up in his bedroom to bake the transistors, and his wife, Eleanor, would test each one by tapping it with a pencil. By 1960, he had made about 50 pacemakers, and Dr. Chardack and others started implanting them in human patients. The first recipient lived for 18 months; another led a normal, healthy life into the 1990s.

Those first pacemakers were simple and vulnerable devices. Because of short battery life and the toll exacted by the hostile environment of the body, they usually lasted just two years. In the late 1960s, Greatbatch began working on a new battery. There were two promising kinds: lithium and plutonium. The latter would have lasted as long as a human could live, but the idea was scrapped because plutonium is toxic and radioactive. Greatbatch had greater success with lithium batteries. Not only were they a reliable source of power, they also solved a bigger problem: The earlier mercury-zinc batteries produced a small amount of gas, so the epoxy covering of the pacemaker had to be slightly permeable, which accelerated the decay of the pacemaker. Pacemakers made with gasless lithium batteries could be completely sealed in metal, greatly increasing their durability. Since the 1970s, lithium batteries produced or licensed by Greatbatch's company (which was later run by one of his sons) have powered some 90 percent of all pacemakers. Other pacemaker advances pioneered by Greatbatch

and others include units that sense when the heart needs help, and how much.

Throughout his career, Greatbatch, a deeply religious man, strove to uphold a strong ethical code. When he received a patent for the pacemaker, he quickly licensed the technology to another company that could get the devices out to doctors and patients much faster—although the financial return for him was lessened. Greatbatch made it a policy of his various companies to pay for employees' children's college education. And he and his wife have donated millions of dollars to schools and other causes.

Since his work on improving pacemaker batteries, Greatbatch's interests have ranged far and wide. During the oil crisis of the 1970s, he bred a strain of poplar tree that produced a great deal of wood, which he hoped to use as a source of wood alcohol for fuel. He cloned flowers and other plants, and built a solar-powered canoe. In the past decade, Greatbatch has been involved in the fight against AIDS. He and the Cornell scientist John Sanford have received three patents for methods of inhibiting the replication of the AIDS virus and a similar virus found in cats.

Still, Greatbatch's crowning achievement will always be the implantable pacemaker. Dr. Chardack's guess that it could save 10,000 lives a year proved to be an underestimate—more than three million pacemakers have been implanted since 1960. And Greatbatch knew from the moment the dog's heart was shocked into a normal rhythm that something significant had happened. In 1959, he wrote in his lab notebook, "I seriously doubt anything I ever do will ever give me the elation I felt that day when my own two-cubic-inch piece of electronic design controlled a living heart."

DEAN KAMEN

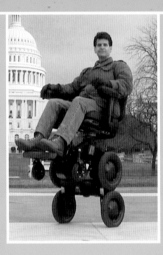

If Dean Kamen had gotten his way as a young man growing up on Long Island, he would have spent his days contemplating esoteric matters. "My hobby was thinking," he says. "It was mostly abstract thinking, trying to understand the universe at a very abstract level." When the financial realities of the world became clear, however, Kamen chose what seemed to him the most obvious path to wealth: He'd become an inventor. Although for many people invention is a surefire way to lose money, not make it, Kamen's creative mind produced medical devices that have been extremely successful and, more important, have improved thousands of people's lives. These inventions include the first portable infusion pump, for delivering precise amounts of drugs to patients; a wearable insulin pump for diabetics; and a portable dialysis machine, which has freed kidney patients from frequent visits to the doctor.

Kamen's realization that abstract thinking wasn't going to turn into a career came to him after graduating from high school. He asked himself, "What am I going to do to make a lot of money?" His answer was, "I could invent something that people want." Kamen's first opportunity came that summer, while he was working for a company that produced audiovisual shows. The equipment the company relied on was clunky and out-of-date; although a new generation of electronics had just come out, it was still controlled with switches and relays. Kamen bought $400 worth of solid-state parts, and over the course of a couple of months he taught himself how they worked, then built a small box that controlled the show in more active and creative ways. He sold the box for $2,000, and then began building them for other companies and museums like the Hayden Planetarium at the American Museum of Natural History in New York City. As he began attending the Worcester Polytechnic Institute (WPI) in Massachusetts, Kamen founded his first company, to make the control systems. By the end of his freshman year, Kamen had sold $60,000 worth of them, all built in his parents' basement.

"The universe is a big playground...."

One of the first things Kamen did with the earnings from his first

invention was to outfit his parents' basement as a machine

shop. Kamen still does hands-on engineering work in his shop,

though it has grown larger and more sophisticated.

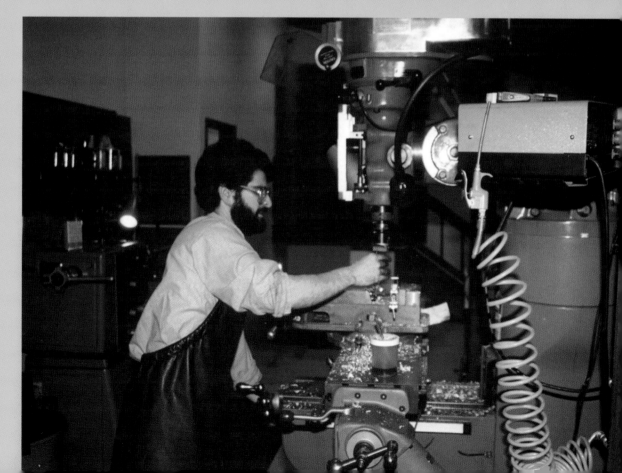

One of Dean Kamen's latest creations harnesses the power of the microprocessor and the gyroscope to solve some of the mobility problems of people who use wheelchairs. Equipped with high-speed microprocessors, a gyroscope, and two independent axles, his Independence 3000 Ibot Transporter, or simply Ibot, can roll up a curb, over sand, and even climb stairs.

Two events inspired Kamen's Ibot. First, he saw a young man struggling to get his wheelchair up a street curb. "It just seemed to me that the fundamental issue was the world has not been architected for people that are sitting down at 39 inches," he told MSNBC's John Hockenberry. The second event happened in his shower—when he stepped out of it one day, he slipped and had to grab a wall to regain his balance. He had already been thinking about how he might use the latest generation of Pentium microprocessors and he now realized he could use their computing power in combination with gyroscopes and small motors to re-create the body's power of balance.

The Ibot can do many things a wheelchair cannot. Its sturdy motor-driven wheels move independently and can raise themselves up to negotiate a curb or stairs. As in a modern all-wheel-drive car, the computer-monitored and -controlled drivetrain automatically adjusts itself to roll over sand, grass, and other irregular surfaces. The Ibot's gyroscopes provide it with a sense of balance; together with its Pentium chips and motors, it reacts to changes in position or weight to keep things stably rolling. Its sense of balance is so good that the Ibot can rear itself up on its back wheels, raising its user to standing height.

Rechargeable batteries keep the Ibot moving all day, and since mechanical or computer failure could be disastrous for its user, backup systems are built in. The Ibot is currently being built and tested by a subsidiary of Johnson & Johnson.

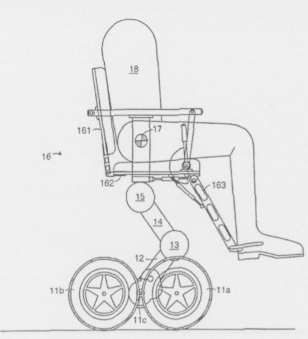

The Ibot, known to the patent office as a "transportation vehicle with stability enhancement."

One of Dean Kamen's most recent inventions is the Independence 3000 Ibot Transporter, or simply the Ibot. Using gyroscopes and microprocessors to help maintain its balance, the Ibot can negotiate stairs and curbs, as well as bring its user to a standing height.

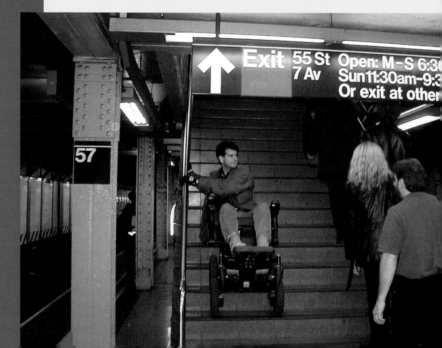

With his earnings, Kamen outfitted the basement with electronics and equipment like lathes and milling machines. At WPI, he was a passionate student of physics but neglected his grades to pursue ideas that interested him. He eventually dropped out.

Inspiration for his next invention came from his brother, who was a medical student at Harvard concentrating on the care of newborns. "He'd come home from med school frustrated," Kamen remembers. "He'd say, 'They have these pumps that are made for adults but I can't deliver microliters of stuff into these babies.'" Building a better pump didn't sound too difficult, so the 20-year-old Kamen got to work. "The conceptual idea of the pump wasn't very hard," he remembers, "but making a device that is going to have lethal, toxic amounts of drug in it that has to work right all the time—that turned out to be more challenging than I thought." A new kind of microchip that required very little power had recently come out and Kamen used it to put together a circuit that controlled a small pump connected to a syringe. The portable pump delivered precisely measured doses of drugs to a patient throughout the day.

A few months later, Kamen's brother showed the pump to a doctor at Harvard, who was immediately excited by it. Between that doctor's enthusiasm and a paper published in the *New England Journal of Medicine*, Kamen was soon flooded with orders. His second business was born, and he put his mother, his younger brother, and his brother's friends to work in the basement workshop, assembling pumps as fast as they could.

Although he enjoyed the technical challenge of making the pump, initially Kamen didn't realize how rewarding his invention could be. "It never occurred to me that people would say, 'Without this my daughter wouldn't be alive,' or 'My mother wouldn't be home,'" he says. "It was *very* gratifying to make things that really helped people." As more and more doctors began ordering his pump, the talkative and inquisitive Kamen built his knowledge of what devices the medical industry needed. "I'd deliver this equipment to different doctors," he remembers, "and my questions to them were always the same: What do you do with this? What else can I do to it? What else do you need? They would always have some unsolved problem."

The next problem that Kamen worked on was delivering insulin to diabetics. When diabetics inject themselves with insulin, their blood sugar can vary widely. Using the same principles as his first pump, Kamen built a portable, wearable device that delivered small, customized quantities of insulin, freeing diabetics from their injection regimen and smoothing out the peaks and valleys of their blood sugar level. The pump was released in 1978.

In 1979, Kamen moved his 20-person company to Manchester, New Hampshire, and three years later he sold it to a large medical equipment manufacturer for tens of millions of dollars. At age 31, Kamen was financially secure and free to do whatever he wanted. He founded another company, DEKA, and developed a new generation of insulin pumps, which are still considered the state of the art. He bought and renovated several nineteenth-century mill buildings on the Manchester riverfront to house the company. And he continued his hobby of collecting antique engines and machinery, some of which are displayed in his office.

Although the engines are often beautiful, his interest in antique technology is not merely aesthetic. For Kamen, there are lessons to be learned from the scientific and technical past. "I think most engineers are worried about how current they can stay," he says. By contrast, one of DEKA's recent products, a kidney dialysis machine that can be used at home, works around physical laws discovered in the seventeenth and eighteenth centuries. (The machine also weighs in at just 22 pounds, one-seventh the bulk of previous dialysis equipment.)

Kamen's current projects include the Ibot, an "advanced mobility system" that could replace the wheelchair. He is also looking at a long-ignored, early-nineteenth-century engine technology, the Stirling Engine, as a way to create small electrical generating systems. The engine, he says, "can be scaled to very small size, it can be used locally, and it doesn't make pollution. Its flexibility in fuel is just awesome." With the electric power industry freshly deregulated, he adds, the engine could "revolutionize the way people think about making and distributing electricity."

In early 2001, news of another Kamen invention caused a sensation. After word of the mystery creation, known as "Ginger" or "IT," was leaked to the press, feverish speculation about what "IT" might be ensued. Many people believe "Ginger" will be a personal scooter powered by hydrogen or a Stirling Engine, and Amazon.com founder Jeff Bezos was quoted as saying it would be "revolutionary." IT, whatever it is, is expected to be unveiled in 2002.

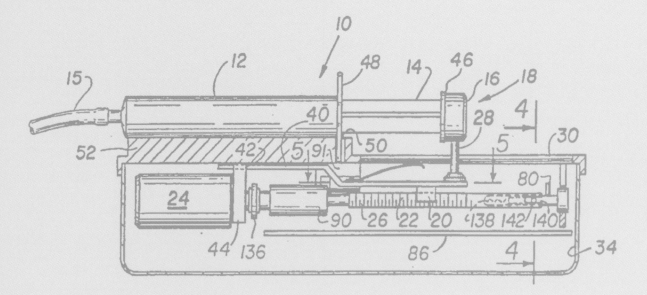

A lightweight kidney dialysis system, patented in 1994.

Kamen's first patent was awarded in 1975 for a portable pump
that delivered precise amounts of medication to a patient.

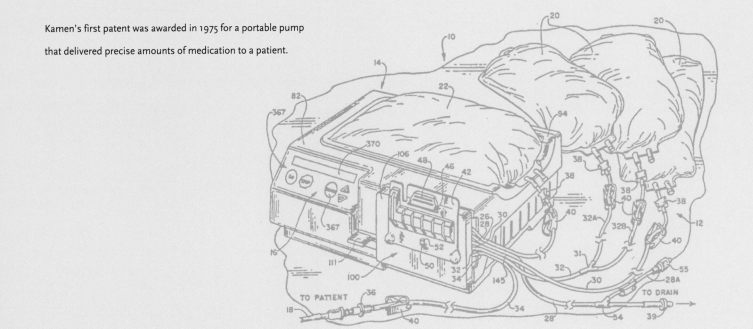

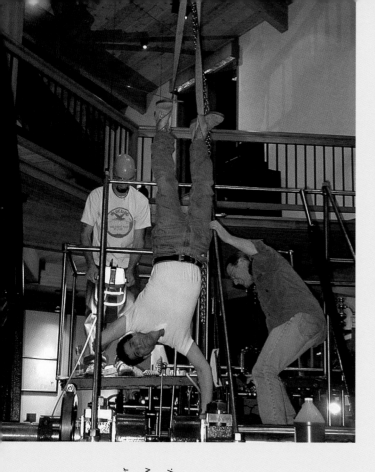

Kamen hangs upside-down in the foyer of his home in order to work on a large, antique engine. His office in Manchester, New Hampshire, includes many other pieces of vintage machinery.

Much of Kamen's attention these days goes to an invention that is not physical at all. In 1989, he started FIRST (For Inspiration and Recognition of Science and Technology), an organization dedicated to developing an interest in technology among high school students. Each year, FIRST partners teams of students with engineers to build robots that compete with each other in regional and national tournaments. The results are auditoriums full of passionate kids shouting encouragement at their robots.

Like many people, Kamen was disturbed by the relative lack of scientific education in American schools. But he didn't focus on the teaching. "I looked at the decay at a cultural level," he explains. "In America you get what you celebrate. Kids will play basketball with chicken-wire hoops because they have desire, they have passion." So FIRST creates a kind of sports for the mind. Its raucous competitions, Kamen continues, "create models and heroes for these kids." A few years ago, Lego joined with FIRST to begin another competition based around its robotics kits. Thousands of students are now involved with the program. All of this pleases Kamen. "The universe is a big playground," he says. "It's fun to be here if you know some of the rules."

MARY-CLAIRE **KING**

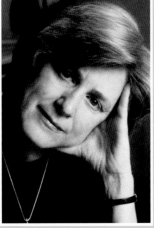

Breast cancer strikes more people today than ever before, for reasons ranging from diet to changes in childbearing practices and the use of hormones at menopause. According to the National Cancer Institute, a girl born today in the United States has a one-in-eight chance of eventually being diagnosed with breast cancer if she lives to the age of 95. In 1990, geneticist Mary-Claire King proved that breast cancer can be inherited in some families by mapping the chromosomal location of a gene that leads to about five percent of all cases of the disease—the first time breast cancer had been associated with a single gene. Finding a gene responsible for hereditary breast cancer—and demonstrating how other such genes might be found—holds many promises for women and men with breast cancer. It allows people at high risk to be screened for mutations in the gene; if a mutation is found, the woman who carries it can pursue preventative measures such as frequent mammograms and even preventive surgery. The discovery could also lead to more focused cancer therapies and, ultimately, prevention.

Born in Wilmette, Illinois, in 1946, Mary-Claire King grew up in a traditional family. Her father worked at Standard Oil while her mother took care of the household, including Mary-Claire and her brother. Mary-Claire became interested and skilled in puzzles as a child, an interest that led to a love for mathematics. Because she was so skilled at math, she continued studying it when she enrolled in Carleton College. King knew that studying math could open up all kinds of academic avenues. The question of how to combine mathematics with biological science—an interest sparked by the death of a childhood friend from cancer—was answered by genetics, a discipline in its infancy when she began her doctoral studies at the University of California at Berkeley in 1969.

King had difficulty translating her ideas—such as studying mutations caused by environmental chemicals—into results. Frustrated, she complained to Berkeley biochemist Allan Wilson, a founder of the field of molecular evolution. He told her, "If everyone whose experiments failed stopped

Genetic trails lead to Argentina's missing children

Paula Lavallen was abducted when she was 22 months old. When she was returned to her grandmother's house more than 6 years later, she walked straight to her old bedroom and asked where her doll was.

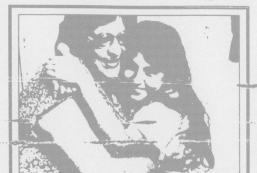

By Simson L. Garfinkel
Special to the Globe

When Paula Lavallen showed up with her birth certificate and medical documents for her first day of Argentine kindergarten, something was plainly wrong.

Although her parents were not poor, the documents indicated that no medical personnel was present at her birth. And the birth certificate was signed by a military doctor who had visited her home several hours after Paula's birth.

"The birth certificate was obviously phony," said American geneticist Mary-Claire King, who was called to Argentina to investigate the case. Other documents were suspicious, King said; for example, Paula's health had been excellent at birth, even though she had allegedly received no prenatal or postpartum care, and she seemed much older than what her documents reported.

Mayol, a human rights group made up of mothers of young men and women who had "disappeared," along with their small children, between 1976 and 1983, during the rule of Argentina's brutal military dictatorship. In 1984, a government comission documented 8,961 such disappearances.

Many of the disappeared were in their early 20s, said King, a professor of epidemiology at the University of California at Berkeley. Many were women, perhaps a third of them pregnant. Often kidnapped mothers were killed after they gave birth. Other women were kidnapped with infant children in their arms.

Whenever the Grandmothers learned of a child who was suspected of being a kidnap victim – perhaps from an attending midwife, or others in kidnapping – they put the information into their files and waited. Today, they say they know of 208 children who disappeared during the military regime. Although some of the children were abandoned, they say, many were adopted by military families.

---

doing science, there wouldn't be any science." Wilson's attitude reassured her, and she soon began doing her doctoral research with him.

This work eventually landed her on the cover of the prestigious journal *Science*. She searched for differences in the genetic code of chimpanzees and humans. Although most people thought there should be significant variation between the species, considering the differences between a living chimp and a human, "I couldn't find any differences," King recalled. There was a difference of only one percent between human and chimpanzee DNA. She and others in the Wilson lab used this data to calculate when chimpanzee and human evolution diverged; the answer was about 5 million years ago, far more recently than in previous estimates.

King began researching the genetics of breast cancer in 1974. The fact that breast cancer ran in some families was recognized as far back as Roman times; the idea was rekindled by clinicians in the nineteenth century. In the 1920s, statisticians began to investigate and write about it. By the 1970s, there was extensive statistical data, but little molecular data, about inherited cancers.

King and her graduate students evaluated the cancer histories of some 1,500 women; about 15 percent of those came from families with a history of breast cancer over several generations. Her team collected blood from families with the highest incidence of breast cancer and used genetic markers to track cancer across generations in each family. A genetic marker is an identifiable stretch of DNA that identifies a specific region on a chromosome. At the time, geneticists had identified only about 30 markers, which limited King's work. In the early 1980s,

that number increased to more than 100, allowing the search to be much more specific.

In the 1980s, King applied genetic analysis to a very different subject: identifying the children of *los desaparecidos*, "the disappeared," in Argentina. A group of military generals had taken power in that country after the fall of Isabel Peron's government in 1976. Over the next several years, some 15,000 of their political opponents were kidnapped and killed. Their victims' small children—and the newborn children of kidnapped pregnant women—were often given to childless families of the military or police, or to those involved with the government. Although these children's parents had been killed, their grandparents, especially their grandmothers, began demonstrating for their return in a plaza in front of the government's headquarters in Buenos Aires. The grandmothers also collected information about the children of the disappeared.

In 1983, after the Argentinean military dictatorship was replaced by a democratically elected government, the grandmothers came to America looking for help. They knew where some of the children were, but since all the witnesses to the kidnappings were dead, they didn't know how to prove who was related to whom. Mary-Claire King agreed to tackle the problem. She traveled to Argentina and took blood samples from as many relatives as possible as well as the children suspected of being kidnapped. King compared children's and surviving relatives' blood samples for proteins that are highly variable among individuals—the same proteins that cause humans to reject transplanted organs. With this test, which provided a 99.9 percent level of accuracy, she identified the natural family of Paula Eva Logares, an eight-year-old girl. Since then, some 70 children

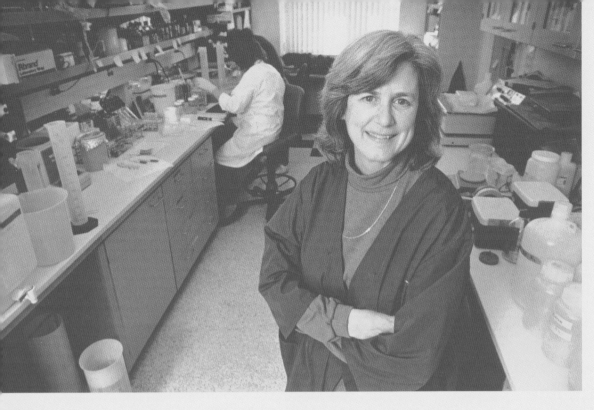

In 1990, Mary-Claire King found the general location of a gene responsible for about five percent of all breast cancer. The discovery came after years of laboratory work tracking hundreds of genetic "markers."

THE POLYMERASE CHAIN REACTION

The key to current genetic research is the polymerase chain reaction method (PCR), created in the early 1980s by Kary Mullis. PCR allows scientists to take a small, individual strand of DNA and multiply it millions of times in just a few hours. This abundance of DNA allows researchers to delve more quickly into the mysteries of genetics, lets doctors better diagnose patients, and helps police officers to identify suspects through genetic "fingerprints."

Here's how it works: The fragment or strand of DNA one wants to duplicate is placed in a test tube. When the tube is heated, the twin strands of the DNA separate. Then primers—

short segments of DNA—are added. When the mixture cools, the primers attach to the strands in question. Then a large amount of the four individual nucleotides that make up DNA are added to the test tube, along with an enzyme called a DNA polymerase. When the tube is heated again, to 75 degrees Celsius, the polymerase "reads" the DNA sequence and harnesses the individual nucleotides to duplicate it.

When this cycle is finished, there are two new strands of DNA in the test tube, one of each of the original paired strands. As the simple process is repeated, the number of strands in-

have been returned to their relatives; about 150 children are still to be reunited.

Also in the 1980s, genetic technology had gotten a big boost. A new technique, the polymerase chain reaction, allowed researchers to quickly make millions of copies of the DNA they were studying. This enormously increased the number of markers available, from a few hundred to many thousands, making King's search for breast cancer genes much more precise.

King's team laboriously examined these markers one by one, trying to determine if they tracked disease in a cancer-suffering family. In August 1990, they tested their 183rd marker. King found that several families—but not all of them—shared this marker. Looking at some of the data, King thought she might have found the right location for the gene, but wasn't sure.

Then one of her students, Beth Newman, suggested that they include the age at which the people had first been diagnosed with breast cancer, since cancers that occurred at an early age were more likely to be inherited. With this, King said, "everything fell into place." The marker she had found tracked disease in families with the youngest patients; after that, the correspondence was weaker. Women with the still hypothetical, but now mapped, gene had an 85 percent chance of developing breast cancer over their lifetime; to them, it was potentially life-saving news.

King announced her findings at a genetics conference in October 1990. The news sent shock waves throughout the research community. Immediately, other scientists rushed to verify her research. There was still a huge amount of work to do:

King had identified only the marker for the breast cancer gene (which she named BRCA1), not the gene itself. In the marked stretch of chromosome, there were some 50 million pieces of genetic code—pairs of the bases that make up DNA. The race to find the exact gene had begun; with King's research pointing the way, anyone could find it.

One of the first results of this new wave of study was the discovery by the French geneticist Gilbert Lenoir that the same markers tracked ovarian cancer in some families. Then, in the summer of 1994, a team of scientists that included Roger Wiseman, Andy Futreal, and Mark Skolnick found BRCA1. Since then, another breast cancer gene (BRCA2) has been found, and research continues on other genetic causes of cancer.

The discovery of BRCA1 and BRCA2 has led to genetic screening for people from families with a history of breast cancer. For many people, it is important to know how high their real risk for cancer is. Those who do harbor mutations in one of these genes know to watch much more closely for signs of cancer; some have chosen to undergo phrophylactic surgery. The isolation of the breast cancer gene also holds the possibility for gene-targeted therapy, where an outside agent enters the body's cells to alter the consequences of losing the critical gene. Although effective therapy based on these genes against a disease as complicated as breast or ovarian cancer is still years away, it is King's work that has opened the door.

creases exponentially, doubling each time. In about three hours, the test tube will contain millions of copies of the DNA.

With the creation of PCR, scientists could make endless, perfect copies of any bit of DNA they were interested in. Suddenly, the limitations of time (it took a long time to isolate a bit of DNA) and supply were gone. PCR has not only allowed larger scale genetic investigations, like the Human Genome Project, but the simple method has also brought the cost of DNA analysis way down, allowing for much more precise medical testing in labs all over the world.

ROBERT **LANGER**

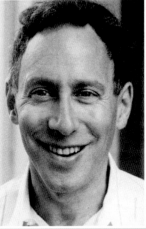

When chemical engineer Robert Langer began working at Children's Hospital in Boston in 1974, the synthetic materials being used for medical procedures were fairly primitive. If doctors needed to fashion an artificial heart valve, for example, they searched for an off-the-shelf material that had the elasticity of the actual heart. They found it in a ladies' girdle.

Over the past 25 years, Langer has introduced several new medical materials that not only are far more sophisticated than a girdle's polyurethane, they also work much better. Langer's most notable advances have come in the field of drug delivery, where he created several polymers and other systems that can administer precise doses of drugs to the right part of the body. His polymer research also led him to tissue engineering, the manufacture of replacement skin, cartilage, and bone. Today, Langer and other scientists are working to grow whole organs in the lab, from the bladder to the liver.

Born in 1948, Robert Langer grew up in Albany, New York. His interest in chemistry was sparked when he received a Gilbert chemistry set as a teenager. "I just was fascinated playing with [the chemistry set]," he remembers, "seeing the colors change when I mixed different things together." Since he was good at math and science, Langer was encouraged to study engineering, and he enrolled at Cornell University. The only subject that really interested him, though, was chemistry, so he concentrated on chemical engineering. He earned his bachelor's degree in 1970, then a doctorate at Massachusetts Institute of Technology in 1974.

Langer received about 20 job offers when he finished his graduate work, but none of them really appealed to him. When he was offered a postdoctoral fellowship with Dr. Judah

Michael Cima, John Santini, and Robert Langer display a silicon wafer holding several of their programmable drug-delivery chips. Each chip contains dozens of tiny reservoirs for drugs; once implanted, the device can release precise amounts of medicine.

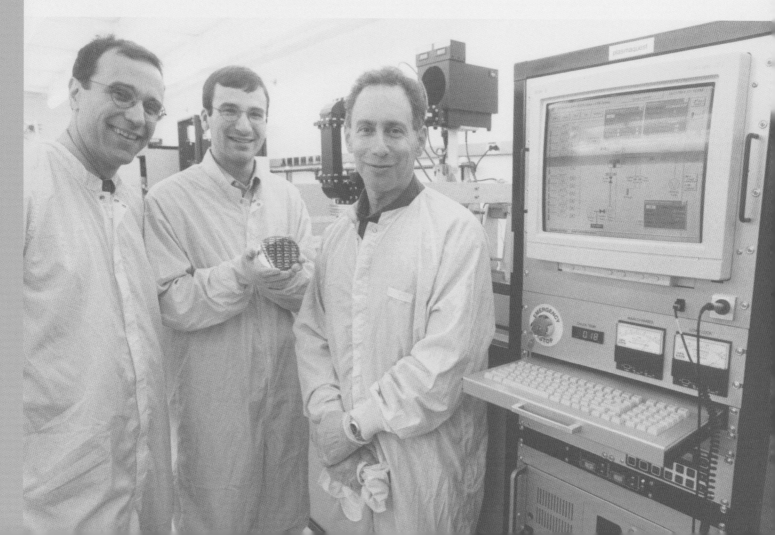

Folkman, who was doing cancer research at Boston Children's Hospital, he jumped at the chance. It was an odd position for a chemical engineer; while today it is not uncommon for engineers to work in medical research, it was almost unheard of at that time. "People thought I was nuts, and they probably thought Judah Folkman was nuts, too," Langer says.

Dr. Folkman's lab proved a fertile environment for Langer. "I started getting a lot of ideas about how you could apply chemical engineering to medical problems," he recalls. One of the areas he began exploring was drug delivery. At the time, few people were exploring the science of gradual or controlled delivery of drugs into the body. Pharmaceutical companies had figured out how to time-release small-molecule drugs by encasing them in wax that broke down over time; the best known example of this is the Contac cold capsule, which contains hundreds of encapsulated "pellets" with its active ingredients.

Langer thought that synthetic polymers, which he had worked with in school, could hold a new solution to delivering drugs—especially those, such as steroids and hormones, with larger molecules. Although synthetic materials had already revolutionized plastics, fabrics, and other industries, there was little or no original work being done in creating polymers ex-

pressly for medical applications. In addition to the girdle material used in heart valves, Langer notes that one type of breast implant was made from an industrial lubricant while another came from mattress stuffing.

The engineer's first invention to come out of this investigation, conducted with Dr. Folkman, was a polymer structure that could slowly release almost any kind of drug molecule. "We were able to create a very complex, tortuous, porous network in the polymer," Langer says. Drug molecules "wanted" to get out of the polymer, but the difficult internal structure made their progress slow. He compares the process to driving in Boston, a notoriously difficult activity. Since one could measure the drug molecule's progress, the polymer acted as an accurate and gradual way to release drugs into a patient.

After the success of this complex polymer, Langer knew that he could create custom materials with almost any kind of molecular properties. "I thought we could come up with a strategy where we could ask what you really want from a biomaterial and then design it from scratch, take it from first prin-

Since 1974, Robert Langer has been applying his chemical engineering skills to medical problems, especially the challenge of delivering drugs in precise doses over a period of time.

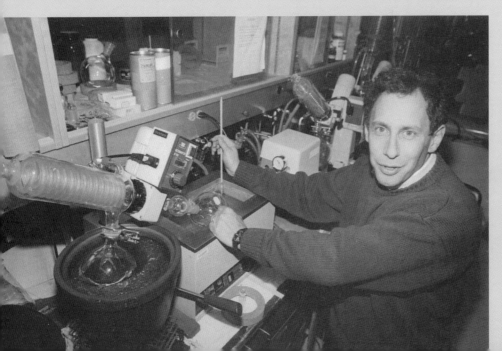

ciples," he says. Langer and his students at MIT, where he has taught since 1977, decided to try to make a polymer that would degrade over time—a property that would gradually release encased drugs. They succeeded with a type of polymer called a polyanhydride.

When Langer first made polyanhydrides, he wasn't sure what their specific applications might be. Then Dr. Henry Brem of Johns Hopkins University approached him with an idea for using the new polymer to treat brain cancer. Chemotherapy for brain cancer was a dangerous process. The human body protects the brain with the so-called blood-brain barrier, which keeps most drugs and other harmful substances out of it. The traditional way to get around the barrier is to load the body with large amounts of drugs, a small portion of which will reach the brain. Cancer drugs, however, are highly toxic, and this method could damage the kidney, liver, and spleen.

Langer and Brem devised a drug-delivery system that not only minimized the amount of drugs in the body, but also concentrated them directly at the point of disease. They created a small wafer of polyanhydrides and BCNU, the drug used to fight brain cancer. A brain surgeon would remove as much of a cancerous tumor as possible, then implant up to eight of the dime-sized wafers into the brain. The polyanhydride biodegrades over the course of a month, slowly releasing the drug right at the affected area of the brain.

When the Food and Drug Administration approved Brem's and Langer's drug wafer in 1996, it was the first new treatment for brain cancer in 23 years. One recent study of its effectiveness showed that five times more patients survived over two years than with conventional treatment.

Biodegradable polymers also led Langer into a different area of research: tissue engineering. He and Dr. Joseph Vacanti of Harvard University began working on growing human skin in the lab in the 1980s. Skin cells were grown on a two-dimensional frame made of polyanhydrides. As the cells multiplied and became a coherent tissue, the polymer frame biodegraded, leaving only the tissue. Working in two dimensions was limiting—they were able to grow only tissues about 1/16th of an inch thick. When they tried to make them thicker, the tissue on the inside couldn't get enough oxygen or nutrients.

In 1986, Dr. Vacanti was watching seaweed wave in the water off Cape Cod when inspiration struck: If they could create a polymer frame that mimicked the branching structure of the seaweed, they might be able to create three-dimensional tissues. Langer made just such a framework, and it did work. One researcher has already grown bladder tissue using the technique, and Langer and others have created working liver tissue. Someday, Langer says, they may be able to create whole, functioning organs for use in humans.

Recently, Langer has been working on an even more sophisticated drug-delivery system. While watching a documentary on how computer chips are made, he realized he might use a similar technique to precisely deliver drugs. Working with computer engineer and MIT professor Michael Cima and then graduate student John Santini, he designed a device that could both store and release minute quantities of medicines. On a chip the size of a dime, there are 34 small reservoirs for drugs, sealed on both sides with gold plates. A microprocessor can send an electrical impulse to an individual reservoir. The interaction of the gold, electricity, and a chloride solution around the chip causes the gold plate to corrode, releasing the drug. The chip can be programmed to open the reservoirs in any order, at any time, allowing for precise and complex drug-delivery protocols. Although the prototype has just 34 reservoirs, the chip at its current size could eventually contain 1,000 microdoses of drugs, even more if the chip was bigger or the reservoirs smaller.

The next challenge Langer is facing is gene therapy, the introduction of DNA into the human body to combat various diseases. Until now, most attempts have used viruses to deliver the DNA to the body's cells. There are obvious dangers in using viruses as a delivery system; in 1999, one patient died during a trial of this kind of gene therapy. Langer's method concentrates on benign polymers. He and his collaborators are trying to create a polymer small enough to move through the wall of a cell and that also has chemical characteristics that will make it stop at a certain part of the cell, where it will release a payload of DNA.

Although the fields Langer has helped create—biomedical polymers and tissue engineering—are barely 25 years old, they have already benefited millions of people. As more and more engineers, doctors, and researchers join the fields, how medicine works may be fundamentally changed. All of this helps Langer pursue his original goal: "I was always interested in doing things that I thought would help people."

ROSALYN **YALOW**

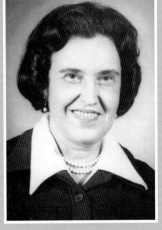

Rosalyn Yalow's path to her 1977 Nobel Prize in Medicine was not an easy one. As a woman, she was discouraged or prevented from pursuing her education. And even when she and her longtime collaborator, Dr. Solomon Berson, made a huge breakthrough in studying diabetes, scientific publications wouldn't print their conclusions, considering them too revolutionary. It was that breakthrough, though, that led to their invention of radioimmunoassay (RIA), an extremely sensitive method for measuring substances in the body. RIA led to major medical discoveries and is now used in research and medical labs all over the world.

Rosalyn Yalow was born Rosalyn Sussman in 1921 in New York City, where she has remained for all but a few years of her life. Her father ran a small business on the Lower East Side of Manhattan selling paper and twine; during the depression, her mother did sewing work at home to make ends meet. Although neither of her parents had a high school education, they always encouraged her academic pursuits. Yalow's love for knowledge was clear very early; she began reading before kindergarten, and she and her brother would walk to the library once a week to trade in their just-read books for fresh ones. Her legendary stubbornness was also evident from a young age. "Perhaps the earliest memories I have are of being a stubborn, determined child," she wrote. "My mother has told me that it was fortunate I chose to do acceptable things, for if I had chosen otherwise no one could have deflected me from my path."

When Yalow began attending Hunter College, New York's public women's college, she fell in love with physics. "In the late 1930s," she wrote, "physics, and in particular nuclear physics, was the most interesting field in the world. It seemed as if every experiment brought a Nobel Prize." Yalow was such a driven student that Hunter created a physics program just for her.

When she graduated from college in 1941, Yalow's options were limited—very few graduate programs in physics would admit women. As she looked for some way to continue her education, she was offered a part-time job as a secretary for a biochemist at Columbia University; she would be able to take some graduate courses there, as long as she learned to take shorthand. She

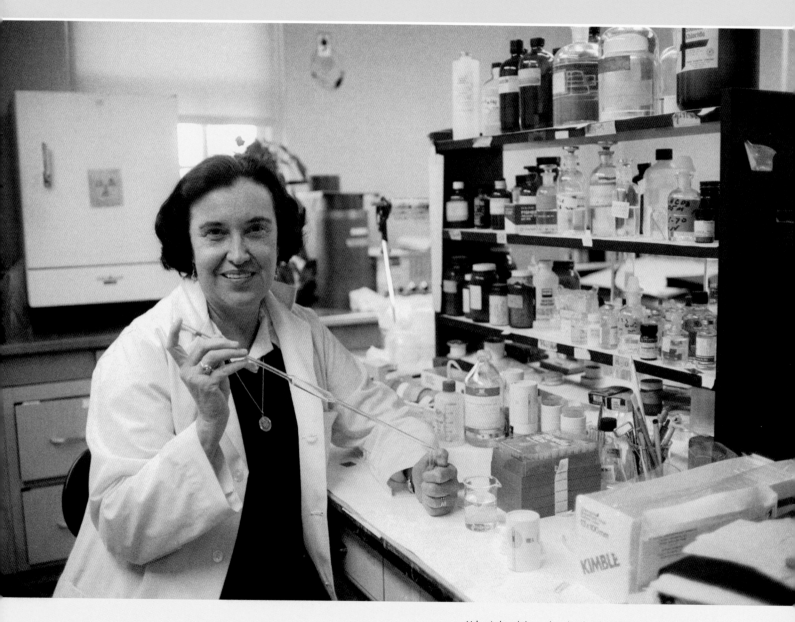

Yalow's breakthrough—the development of radioimmunoassay,

a highly sensitive technique for measuring substances in the body—

came in the late 1950s. She continued working as a researcher, and

later as a professor, until her retirement in 1991.

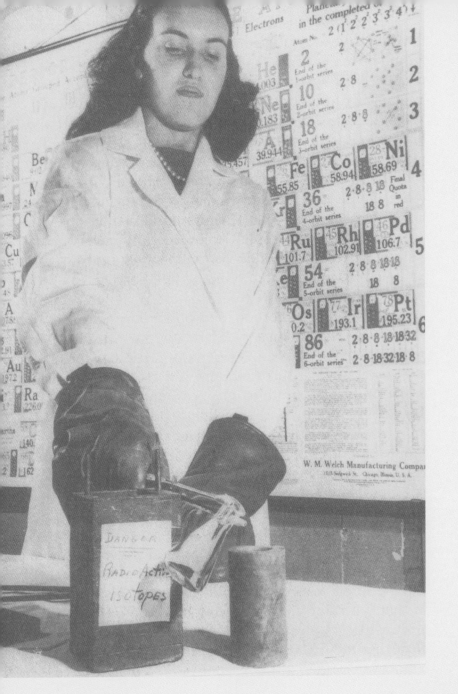

Rosalyn Yalow built the Bronx Veterans Administration Hospital's nuclear medicine research program almost from scratch. Here she prepares an "atomic cocktail" of radioactive isotopes in 1948, her second year at the hospital.

soon enrolled in secretarial school. But the country was preparing for World War II, and suddenly male graduate students were in short supply. Yalow was finally offered a place at the University of Illinois, and she tore up her stenography books.

Things were not much easier in Illinois. Yalow was shocked to discover that she was the only woman in a class of 400. (On the brighter side, on the first day of class she met fellow physics student Aaron Yalow, whom she would marry in 1943.) And Yalow's course work in physics at Hunter had been minimal—less than any of the other graduate students. She set to work, taking undergraduate courses to catch up and graduate courses, while also teaching physics to freshmen. She received three As and an A- in an optics laboratory; the chairman of the department declared, "that A- confirms that women do not do well at laboratory work."

Yalow earned her doctorate in 1945 and returned to New York. While she was teaching physics to returning veterans at Hunter College, Aaron Yalow began working as a radiation physicist. Soon, he introduced Rosalyn to Dr. Edith Quimby at Columbia's medical school, who was researching the medical applications of radioactive isotopes—artificially made, unstable variants of elements like carbon and iodine. Quimby had just the job for her: She called up a colleague at the Veterans Administration hospital in the Bronx, and Yalow was soon working in its brand-new nuclear medicine program.

The era when Yalow began working at the V.A. was one of high hopes for nuclear physics. Although most people were horrified by the atomic bombs dropped on Hiroshima and Nagasaki, some worked to apply nuclear physics in technologies that would benefit mankind. President Eisenhower announced the "Atoms for Peace" program, part of which was Project Plowshare, an attempt to find peaceful uses for nuclear bombs. Weapons scientists proposed using bombs to dig harbors, release underground deposits of fossil fuel, and create a new canal through Panama, among other things. (The dangers of radioactive fallout kept any of these from happening.) On the medical side, many researchers were exploring the uses of radioactive isotopes to treat cancer and other diseases.

Yalow built the V.A.'s radioisotope research program almost from scratch. Working out of what had been a janitor's closet, she built her own equipment and began clinical research. By 1950, she knew she needed a partner with medical knowledge to complement her work on the physics side. That partner was Solomon Berson, a young doctor whom Yalow later called "the smartest person I had ever met." Their close and productive professional relationship would last until his death in 1972.

Yalow and Berson began to use radioisotopes to measure the hidden workings of the human body. This led them to look closer at the endocrine system, which is composed of the endocrine glands (the thyroid, adrenals, ovaries, testes, and others) and the hormones they produce. The endocrine disorder that affects the most people is diabetes. Diabetics are not able correctly to process insulin, a hormone that keeps a person's blood sugar in check. No one knew exactly what happened to insulin in a diabetic; Yalow and Berson spent hours discussing the problem in their office, where they had positioned their desks head-to-head so they could speak directly to each other.

The two researchers thought that radioactive isotopes might help reveal how insulin (and thus diabetes) worked. By tagging an individual substance, in this case insulin, with a radioactive isotope of iodine, they could track the otherwise invisible hormone by measuring its radioactivity. When they injected tagged insulin into diabetics, they observed something unexpected: Their insulin became bound with a larger molecule, gamma globulin. Yalow and Berson determined that the gamma globulin was an antibody, a protein the body's immune system produces to protect us from invaders such as viruses and bacteria. When a diabetic was injected with synthetic insulin, they discovered, the body was treating it as an invader, preventing it from doing its usual job. This groundbreaking study was published in 1956, and it led to the development of synthetic insulin that is not attacked by the immune system.

Even more significant than what they found was how they found it. Buried in the middle of their paper on insulin was a description of their new method for measuring the insulin, a method that they eventually called radioimmunoassay (RIA). The basic principle of RIA works for a number of substances, from hormones like insulin to enzymes, vitamins, viruses, and drugs. First, a researcher tags a known sample of a hormone or other substance with a radioactive isotope. Then, that hormone is mixed with its naturally occurring antibody to form a solution of hormone-antibody pairs. This solution is combined with a quantity of a patient's blood, which contains an unknown quantity of the hormone being tested for. Antibodies "prefer" nonradioactive versions of the hormone they were made to match up with, so after a period of time they let go of the tagged hormones and pair up with the natural ones in the patient's blood. A researcher then separates out all the hormone-antibody pairs (both radioactive and not) from the solution. By calculating the difference in radioactivity of this group of pairs with the original tagged group, one can measure how many radioactive hormones were replaced by natural ones—which is to say, how many hormones were originally in the patient's blood.

This may seem like a complicated procedure for a simple result, but before RIA it was essentially impossible to measure substances as tiny as insulin. And RIA is extremely sensitive; it can measure very low concentrations of these substances, which is important because they generally occur in the body in very small quantities. Insights from RIA testing have led to new treatments for diabetes, mental retardation, and other conditions.

In the 40 years since its invention, RIA has become one of the basic methods of medical testing and research and has

WOMEN IN SCIENCE

Rosalyn Yalow wasn't the only woman scientist who found opportunity during World War II. Graduate schools, university faculties, and military and civilian research labs suffered a severe shortage of able-bodied and able-minded scientists as much of the young male population of the country enlisted or was drafted into the armed services. And, just as industrial jobs were famously filled by "Rosie the Riveter," women quickly replaced men in scientific fields. The war was one of the first cracks in the all-male—or at least almost all-male—surface of science. For many women, however, wartime gains were temporary. "When the men returned to civilian life," notes historian Martha Bailey, "the women were expected to return home."

While the end of the war curtailed many women scientists' budding careers, it didn't end all of them—four of the 11 women who have ever been awarded a Nobel Prize for science received some career boost from World War II. And the war also had profound effects on science in general—effects that would help open its ranks to a much more diverse group. Many disciplines and technologies were introduced or matured then, including nuclear physics, advanced medicine, and computing, and these fields required a large number of new workers, too many to be filled only by men. Another barrier the war helped demolish was one of cultural expectations: Most people assumed that scientists were men, often lone geniuses. As thousands of women and men entered scientific and technical professions for the first time, science was demystified. "A profession that had been cohesive, homogeneous, and populated in the hundreds," writes Vivian Gornick in *Women in Science*, "now exploded with uncontrollable multiplicity into a pluralism that soon numbered in the hundreds of thousands."

Even though the stage was set for science to become diverse, it would take decades before it really happened. Throughout the 1950s and 1960s, many women were thwarted from entering scientific careers, some by outright discrimination, some by the effects of the "old-boy" network, and some by ingrained attitudes toward women's roles in society. (Many women were asked if

been adopted by virtually every medical lab in the world. Variations on the basic method have also been developed to measure an even broader range of things: The standard test for HIV, for example, is done with a nonradioactive version of Yalow's and Berson's groundbreaking invention. And while the two researchers knew in 1956 that radioimmunoassay was an important medical advance, they never considered making money from their invention. "We never thought of patenting RIA," Yalow told Eugene Straus, her friend and biographer. "Patents are about keeping things away from people. . . . We wanted others to be able to use RIA."

they intended to marry, Bailey notes, or when they were going to start a family, implying their employment might be temporary.) Antinepotism rules kept wives and husbands from working at the same university, usually dooming the wife to a temporary position, a job at a lesser institution, or no job at all.

Progress in bringing women into science careers speeded up in the late 1960s and 1970s, as a wide range of social attitudes shifted and the generation of women born after World War II—women who had internalized new definitions of what science is, and what work should be—came of age. Efforts to achieve equality in the workplace (and throughout society) slowly paid off, as more and more women became scientists or pursued other professions. Between 1966 and 1996, the proportion of women earning bachelor's degrees in science or engineering jumped from 24.8 percent of the total to 47.1 percent. The number of female science and engineering Ph.D.s saw an even greater jump: from 8 percent to 31.8 percent.

While many women going into science during the twentieth century aimed toward university jobs, this boom in science education has led to more diverse goals and opportunities, notes Catherine Didion, executive director of the Association for Women in Science. "Today, a lot of technical and scientific women are moving into entrepreneurial and small businesses, such as smaller firms supporting biotech, engineering consulting firms, places where you need a degree but one has a lot more control over one's day and how it's spent. Women are seeing those degrees as a tool for more than just academic careers, which wasn't the case even two decades ago."

CONSUMER PRODUCTS

INTRODUCTION

In the late nineteenth century German engineer Wilhelm Maybach, at the time working with the Daimler car company, put together the new perfume pump spray with the new gasoline and came up with what we now call the carburetor.

Maybach is a good example of what may be the most fundamental of all elements in the magic process of invention: the moment when two things are brought together, by an innovative mind, in a new way that causes one and one to equal three (the result being more than the sum of the parts). Sometimes, as in the case of one of our inventors in this group, the different parts of the equation are quite bizarre: Percy Spencer's microwave oven owes its existence, as much as anything, perhaps, to the coming together of a magnetron and a chocolate bar.

The best-laid plans often go awry and generate innovation. In 1852 British chemist William Perkin went looking for artificial quinine in coal tar. After weeks of noodling he came up with a dark sludge that was definitely not quinine. On throwing it into the sink, Perkin discovered he had unintentionally invented the world's first artificial aniline dye.

The same kind of off-center result came out of the work of Stephanie Kwolek, when she decided to grapple with an impending gasoline shortage by finding a way to make tires lighter and stronger (to save weight and fuel). As you'll see, that wasn't all she found.

Daydreams also do the trick. The great German chemist Kekulé von Stradonitz said he conceived of the benzene ring while dozing on a London bus, where he dreamed about serpents eating their own tails. There's no suggestion here that

Philo T. Farnsworth was asleep on the job, but the image of a hayfield at harvest time seems to have figured large in his invention of the line-scan system fundamental to every television set.

Sometimes, a basic principle will find innovative application in many different fields and circumstances. The seventeenth-century discovery of the vacuum created just such a situation. It gave rise, among many other things, to ventilators for hospitals, the barometer and weather forecasting, Galvani's research into electricity (leading Volta to the battery), and Newcomen's pre-Watt steam engine. Taking a principle, and seeing what it can be made to do, is one technique adopted here by Jerome Lemelson, who proves his talents in the matter with a list of over 500 patents.

Curiosity is a powerful driver of inventive thinking. In 1304 the medieval monk Dietrich of Freiberg virtually started the modern study of optics with his investigations into why the rainbow looked as it did. His sheer curiosity (there was no possible practical application for the research at the time) led him to shine light through simulated raindrops made of small flasks filled with water and to come close to understanding the mechanisms involved.

The feeling that inventive opportunities lie out there waiting to be identified was well expressed by one of our inventors, Jacob Rabinow: "I was willing to bet lunches for years that *something* inside the Post Office could be automated." As a result of that hunch, your mail is now sorted by machines.

Jerome Lemelson believed that inventors are powered by an insatiable curiosity and that they best satisfy this by working alone. In some way or other, however, all the inventors in this group have come to experience what can be the stultifying effect of corporate or bureaucratic institutions. As has often been said, a camel is a horse designed by committee. This problem has existed since prehistoric stone weapons and tools generated the first top-down hunt-planning hierarchy and the "standard operating procedure" that has so often since stifled the innovative spark.

Ironically, institutionalized thinking is all too often the result of innovative thinking in the first place. The first clay-tablet writing in early Mesopotamia made possible a level of organization that immediately required laws. In next to no time this produced a legal system every bit as cumbersome as the one with which we suffer today. The institutional problem arises in the first place because when an innovation makes life better for both the individual and the group, which is the aim of every innovator, one reaction is frequently to confine the new idea or the process, so as to protect it from any interference that might limit its beneficial effects. All too soon those responsible for this happy state of affairs become more interested in protecting the idea from any input at all, fearing it might rock the boat. This in turn often generates an attitude expressed as: "This is how we do things here," which can render further innovative thinking impossible.

Jerome Lemelson also once said that the work of the inventor-entrepreneur is essential to the well-being of the United States. Innovation generates jobs. In the 1930s the U.S. Department of Labor identified 80 different types of work (education, medicine, engineering, secretarial, and so on). Today, seven decades of innovation later, the number of types of work has risen to over 800. The U.S. marketplace has exploded beyond anything that could have been imagined in the 1930s, and we stand at the threshold of an e-commerce global consumer goods revolution that will dwarf all that went before. The requirement to satisfy that market with innovations will be well-nigh insatiable. Minds like those of this group of inventors will have much to occupy themselves with for the foreseeable future.

—JB

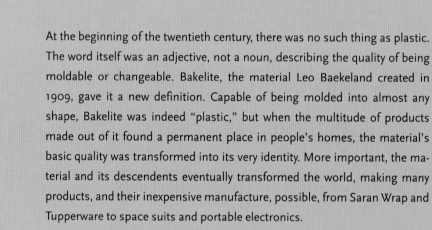

At the beginning of the twentieth century, there was no such thing as plastic. The word itself was an adjective, not a noun, describing the quality of being moldable or changeable. Bakelite, the material Leo Baekeland created in 1909, gave it a new definition. Capable of being molded into almost any shape, Bakelite was indeed "plastic," but when the multitude of products made out of it found a permanent place in people's homes, the material's basic quality was transformed into its very identity. More important, the material and its descendents eventually transformed the world, making many products, and their inexpensive manufacture, possible, from Saran Wrap and Tupperware to space suits and portable electronics.

Born in Ghent, Belgium, in 1863, Leo Baekeland was the son of an illiterate shoemaker who hoped the boy would continue his trade. The young Baekeland, however, had broader interests, notably chemistry, and he excelled at his studies. At the age of 16 he won a scholarship to the University of Ghent, and by the time he was 21 he had a doctorate in electrochemistry. A few years later he became a professor of physics there.

Baekeland was also an avid photographer, and in the 1880s he began looking at ways to improve the photographic process. At that time, photographs were made on "dry plates"; pieces of glass coated with a light-sensitive emulsion were exposed, then immersed in a chemical "developer" in a darkroom. Baekeland invented a dry plate that had the developing chemicals built-in—when immersed in water, the plate would develop itself. For this he received his first patents, and in 1888 he founded a company to manufacture the plates. The business soon interfered with Baekeland's academic career, and he was faced with a choice between the two—a decision complicated by his engagement to the daughter of the head of his physics department.

In 1889, Baekeland and his bride, Celine, sailed to the United States on their honeymoon. While in New York, he met with the owners of a photographic company and decided to work for them, abandoning both teaching and Belgium. In the 1890s, he began working on a new

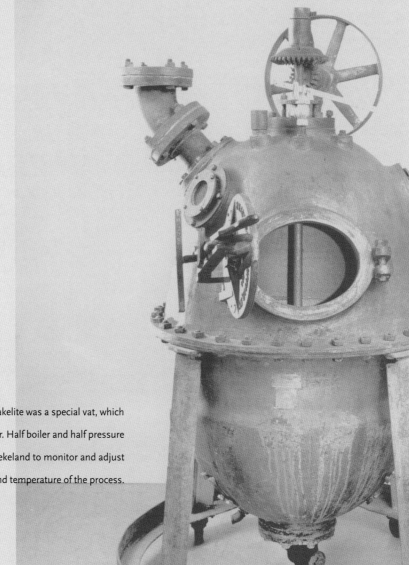

The key to manufacturing Bakelite was a special vat, which Baekeland dubbed the Bakelizer. Half boiler and half pressure cooker, the device allowed Baekeland to monitor and adjust the pressure and temperature of the process.

Leo Baekeland intended for his plastic to change what things were made of. But as with many technologies, Bakelite had an unintended consequence: It also changed what things looked like. The almost infinitely moldable plastic was perfect for the aesthetic styles—Art Deco, Streamline, Modernism—just being introduced.

The basic properties of Bakelite encouraged a streamlined look. Until moldable plastic came on the scene, many products were made by joining pieces of wood or metal or other materials—so things had right angles and seams. By contrast, to make something out of Bakelite one poured the resinous plastic into a mold. To ensure that it flowed smoothly, designers had to avoid sharp angles and edges in their molds. The results were products with smooth, gentle curves.

Bakelite also became popular just as a new discipline was emerging: the professional designer. Previously, product design had been the job of engineers, or craftsmen, or no one at all. This changed in the late 1920s and 1930s, as schools such as the Bauhaus began to teach design. One of the beliefs of this first generation of modern designers was that "form follows function"—that a product's design should reflect what it does. Fancy materials and decorations were eliminated, while shapes were simplified. And in their rejection of previous styles, modern designers embraced the "machine age"—they celebrated all things man-made, especially synthetic materials.

One of Bakelite's most far-reaching impacts is easy to overlook. When first introduced, it was seen as a cheap imitation of "real" materials like wood—in fact, many early Bakelite products came in mottled brown, to imitate wood. As ever more elaborate and colorful goods were made with it, though, Bakelite became a "real" material itself. Designers were finally free to create purely synthetic goods, and they never looked back.

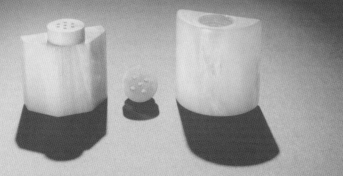

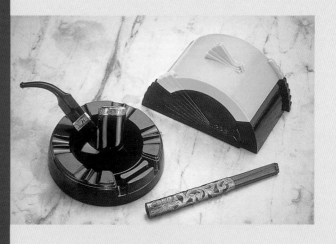

Advertisements called Bakelite the "Material of a Thousand Uses." Today, Bakelite is best known for its role in consumer products of the 1930s, especially brightly colored plastic housewares and jewelry.

kind of photographic paper, and through careful experiments and much trial and error, he invented one that was much slower than previous papers—so slow that photographers were able to use it under artificial light in a darkroom, where they had much more control over the results. Baekeland's paper, which he named Velox, appealed to the new market of amateur photographers and achieved great popularity. The Eastman Kodak Company, already a photography giant, saw it as competition and purchased the rights to the paper for $750,000—a huge sum for the time.

One requirement of Baekeland's agreement with Eastman Kodak was that he not work on anything photographic. With that part of his career cut short and a great deal of money in the bank, Baekeland bought a large estate in Yonkers, New York, where he set up his own research laboratory. There he turned his attention to a problem other chemists were attacking: inventing an artificial substitute for shellac.

Shellac, a resin harvested from a Southeast Asian beetle, was used as an electrical insulator, among other things. As America began to use electric power on a large scale, demand for shellac outstripped the supply, and prices went up. The race was on to find a substitute, a material that wouldn't conduct electricity and was plastic—easy to shape.

People had been pursuing such a material for years. In the eighteenth and nineteenth centuries, powdered horns and hooves were molded into snuff boxes and other goods. In the 1840s, the vulcanization process turned natural rubber into a more durable and moldable material. And in the 1860s, as the world faced an ivory shortage owing in part to a craze for billiards, the American John Wesley Hyatt created celluloid, made from plant fiber and camphor. It could be permanently molded into any shape, and it found a market as a substitute for ivory, bone, and other materials. But celluloid was flammable—billiard balls made from it would occasionally explode—and perceived as a cheap substitute for better materials.

Baekeland focused his research on finding a material that was purely synthetic—using no natural materials. In 1904, he and his assistant, Nathaniel Turlow, began investigating the products of combining two chemicals, formaldehyde and phenol, a product of coal tar. Thirty years earlier, a German chemist had worked with the two chemicals in pursuit of a synthetic dye, but the odd and unmanageable resin they produced was not of interest to him. By the turn of the century, other researchers had combined formaldehyde with casein, a substance derived from milk, to make an early plastic, but its use was limited.

Baekeland methodically studied each variable that went into the reaction between phenol and formaldehyde—from the proportion of chemicals to heat and pressure, as well as the effect of added solvents. The process usually created a useless goo, sometimes too brittle and sometimes too spongy. Baekeland's breakthrough came in 1907, when he learned to control the gases given off by the chemical reaction. In a complicated apparatus that was half boiler, half pressure cooker (it was later dubbed the Bakelizer), Baekeland sped up the reaction with heat and kept the gases in check with pressure.

It took several steps to turn the translucent solution that came out of the Bakelizer into Bakelite. First, it was allowed to cool and harden, then it was ground into a powder. A filler composed of wood powder, cotton, asbestos, or other materials was added, as were other chemicals necessary to the next stage. When heated, the mixture turned into a resin that was again allowed to cool, then ground up. This powder was Bakelite, ready to be put into a mold, then set in place forever with the application of heat and pressure. The final product was "a magnificent and hard mass," in Baekeland's words, impervious to heat, electricity, and most solvents. In his lab book, he wrote, "Unless I am very much mistaken this invention will prove important in the future." The chemist soon filed two patents covering the process, the first of many protecting his invention.

Almost two more years of research and refinement passed before Baekeland was ready to announce his invention. In February 1909, he presented Bakelite to the New York chapter of the American Chemical Society, showing off several items made from it. The assembled chemists gave him an ovation, and the era of plastics was underway. At first, Baekeland envisioned Bakelite as an industrial material, to be used for electrical insulators, floor tiles, and chemical- and fire-resistant coatings, among other things. Its "use for such fancy articles [knobs, buttons, handles]," he told the American Chemical Society, "has not much appealed to my efforts as long as there are so many more important applications for engineering purposes."

The electrical industry eagerly adopted Bakelite, using it for sockets, fuses, switches, and other small molded components. By the early 1920s, the new radio and automobile industries were using it, too. The material was flexible, durable, and colorful

With the small fortune he made from selling a photo paper he invented, Leo Baekeland set up a lab in a New York suburb. In 1904, he and his assistant began experimenting with the chemicals that would eventually become Bakelite, the first modern plastic.

(dyes could be added to produce vibrant hues such as yellow, orange, and red), and it suggested progress to the consumer.

Meanwhile, Baekeland had entered a long patent war with other chemical firms, which had started to manufacture Bakelite knock-offs almost as soon as the invention was announced. One strategy of Baekeland's company—the General Bakelite Corporation—was to brand products with a logo. A more successful approach was taking competitors to court; after a long battle, Baekeland orchestrated a merger of plastics manufacturers. In 1939 he sold the company to Union Carbide and retired to Florida. He died in 1945.

As the 1920s went on, an increasing number of products were made out of Bakelite. Radios and telephones were the most visible of them, but the material soon entered almost every consumer niche. Indeed, the product's slogan was "The Material of a Thousand Uses." There was Bakelite jewelry, kitchenware, cigarette cases, cabinets, lamps, toothbrushes, and fountain pens. Even after America plunged into the depression, sales of Bakelite products remained strong. Not only were they colorful, durable, and attractive, but mass production made them inexpensive.

Bakelite remained popular until World War II, when production lines were switched over to war materials, not consumer goods. It was also losing its technological edge. In the 1930s, DuPont had introduced its first synthetics, including Lucite, Plexiglas, and Nylon; after the war, these and other new plastics took over the market.

Today, of course, plastics define the look and feel of almost everything we touch. And a new wave of plastics, including some that (surprisingly) conduct electricity, will make synthetics an even more fundamental part of the material world. With Bakelite now known more as a collectible than a material that changed the world, it's easy to forget that the plastics revolution began with Leo Baekeland's research in a vat called the Bakelizer.

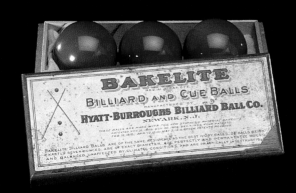

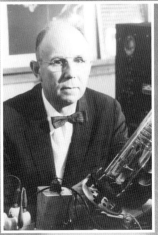

Harold Edgerton's business was stopping time. With high-speed cameras and flash equipment of his own invention, Edgerton photographed the events of a split second—a thousandth of a second, even a millionth of a second. By capturing those tiny moments of time he revealed, often for the first time, how things work. In his pictures, a hummingbird's wings stop; a drop of milk becomes a beautiful, crown-shaped splash; a golf ball deforms on impact; and a nuclear explosion expands, microsecond by microsecond, into a huge fireball.

Edgerton's photographs and equipment were important to science and business, revealing in sharp detail the smallest increments of industrial and natural processes. But his images were even more appealing to the public, which was thrilled to see the hidden world they unveiled. His pictures were first published in *Life* magazine and elsewhere in the mid-1930s, a time of great technological change and hope. Atomic science was beginning to explore the innermost workings of the universe, while new electronics, drugs, and other technologies were improving the quality of Americans' lives. Edgerton's photographs were a kind of proof that this new world was understandable, that science and technology could help us comprehend previously mysterious events. They were also often beautiful; many of his photographs are now in major museum collections.

The man who opened these hidden realms to public view had humble beginnings. Edgerton, who was known to most people as "Doc," was born in 1903 in Fremont, a small Nebraska farming town. His father held a succession of jobs, including president of a local bank, school principal, lawyer, and Washington, D.C., correspondent for a newspaper in Lincoln, Nebraska. Eventually, the family settled down in Aurora, Nebraska, population 3,000. The young Edgerton became interested in all kinds of mechanical things, from cars and motorcycles to engines and electrical equipment. When he was in high school, he went to Aurora's electrical plant and asked for a job. The future inventor was hired to sweep the floors. His mechanical talents soon

With the electronic flash he developed for industrial use, Harold Edgerton could capture even the briefest of moments.

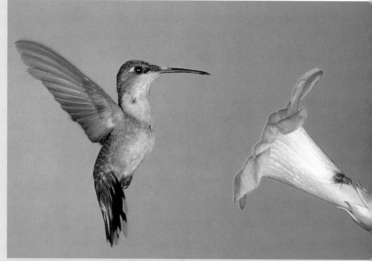

Hummingbird, late 1940s

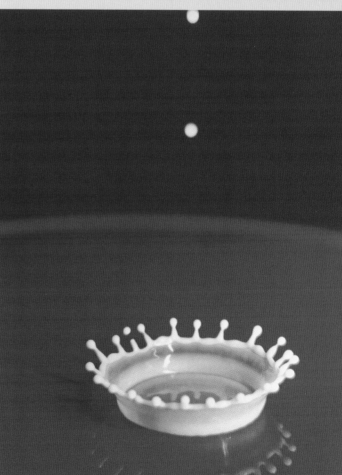

Milk-drop Coronet, 1957

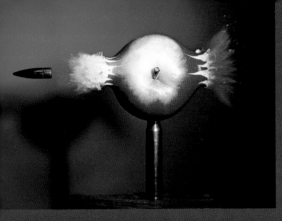

Shooting the Apple, 1964

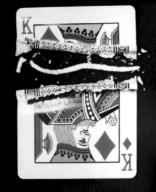

Cutting the Card Quickly, 1964

Desmore Shute Bends the Shaft, 1938

became clear, though, and in the early 1920s, when many of the firm's repairman were still in the military, Edgerton fixed electrical equipment and even strung power lines on the Nebraska prairie. Around this time, Edgerton was introduced to photography. His uncle, Frank Edgerton, ran a photo studio in Fremont, and there Harold learned how to make and print pictures.

After high school, Edgerton earned a degree in electrical engineering at the University of Nebraska, then applied to the Massachusetts Institute of Technology in 1925. Edgerton was accepted, but before classes began he was offered a place in a one-year research program to work on large electrical motors at General Electric's huge facility in Schenectady, New York. The next year he finally entered MIT, where he remained until his death in 1990.

At MIT, Edgerton studied how large surges of electricity, like those caused by lightning, affected a particular kind of electric motor. But there was a problem: The motor turned far too fast for him to see what was happening. A few years earlier, he had noticed that a thyratron—a mercury gas–filled tube that emitted regular pulses of light—had made the blades of a moving fan seem to rotate very slowly. Edgerton set up a mercury tube next to the electric motor and synchronized its pulses

with the speed of the motor, so that each flash of light occurred when the motor was in the same position. It worked perfectly; when Edgerton turned the mercury tube on, the moving parts of the motor seemed to be standing still. He was able to capture this on film, using a movie camera.

What Edgerton had used was a stroboscope, a device that fools the human eye into thinking that a moving object is still. It works, Edgerton explained, because "eyes aren't designed for speed." When we see a split-second image, our brain retains it for a moment. This is how movies work: Motion picture film contains a sequence of still images, each of which pauses for a split second before the next moves into view, at a speed of 24 frames per second. A shutter blocks the frames from view as they move. The brain retains each image until the next appears, giving the impression of continuous movement. Edgerton's stroboscope allowed him to see only the "frames" created by its flashes of light. When properly synchronized with the motor, it hid its motion from view.

Edgerton knew his stroboscope could be used to examine machinery in any number of industries, not just his electric motor. He soon formed a partnership with two colleagues from MIT, Kenneth Germeshausen and Herbert Grier. The three began using stroboscopes to let businesses closely examine their

Wes Fesler Kicking a Football, 1934

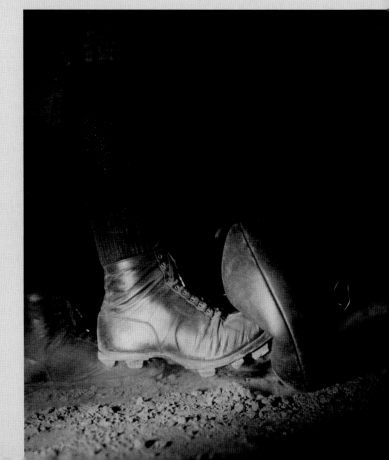

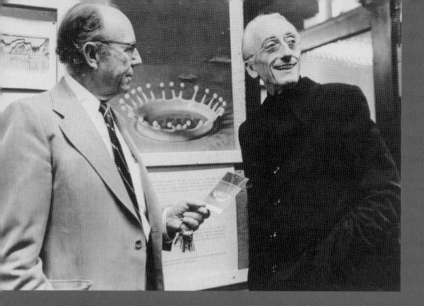

Edgerton chats with Jacques Cousteau, with whom he collaborated on undersea photography expeditions.

"The trick to education," he said, "is to not let them know they're learning something until it's too late."

manufacturing processes. After a piece of equipment was filmed, the movie could be watched in extreme slow motion, and faults invisible to the naked eye suddenly became prominent.

One day, an MIT professor dropped by Edgerton's lab to see his stroboscopes and wondered what would happen if they were aimed at something besides a motor. "I suddenly realized, hey, there are a lot of things in the world that move," Edgerton remembered. "I looked around and there was a faucet right next to where I worked. So I just moved the strobe and took a picture of water coming out of a faucet." The results were amazing. Under the stroboscope, a seemingly smooth stream of water turned out to be made up of many individual drops strung together. Edgerton began aiming his camera and stroboscope at all kinds of action—the splash of a drop of milk, the wings of a hummingbird, a light bulb being smashed with a hammer.

By the late 1930s, Edgerton's pictures were becoming known to the public. (There was even a short film made about his work, *Quicker 'n a Wink,* which won an Oscar in 1940.) At the same time, photojournalists were adopting his electronic flash, using it to capture sports action and other moving subjects with extraordinary clarity.

When the United States entered World War II, Edgerton was asked to work on the problem of nighttime aerial surveil-lance. The army was using 50-pound bombs full of explosive powder to illuminate the night sky and take pictures of enemy territory. The bombs were dangerous and unreliable, and their use was limited. Edgerton and his partners built an electronic flash that put out far more light than anything they had made before; it could light up a square mile of land from 2,000 feet up. The flash was finally used in June 1944, to photograph the German army the night before D day. The photos confirmed that the Germans weren't ready for the massive Allied attack; after that success, the flashes were used in Europe until the end of the war.

Edgerton's next big challenge came in the late 1940s, when the company he formed with Germeshausen and Grier was asked to photograph a nuclear explosion. There was no camera capable of capturing such a detonation, which lasted only a few ten-thousandths of a second. His solution was the Rapatronic camera, whose shutter was actually a rapidly changing mag-netic field that, in concert with a pair of polarizing filters, could let light in or keep it out. A magnetic field can change much faster than a mechanical shutter can move, allowing Edgerton's camera to capture exposures of a millionth of a second; its pic-tures revealed the glowing, bulbous form at the beginning of an atomic explosion.

But military work was only a small part of Edgerton's activities. He continued to photograph split-second action, and in the 1960s he made two of his most famous images: a bullet at the moment it sliced through a playing card, and an apple exploding on both sides as a bullet passed through it. Edgerton also applied his photographic skills to the completely different realm of the undersea world. In 1953, the famous underwater explorer Jacques Costeau enlisted his help in photographing the Deep Scattering Layer, a previously unexamined layer of living marine organisms. Later, Edgerton and Costeau used time-lapse photography to watch the graceful and surprising movements of some of the seafloor's slowest-moving creatures, starfish.

Edgerton was known almost as much for his teaching style as for his photographs. He was a firm believer in experiment, and he urged his students to learn by doing, no matter what the outcome. "Most of the things you do in life are a failure," Edgerton told them. "Then you find what the failures are and you don't do it that way the next time." His lectures were always packed, as students crowded in to see his stroboscopes stop time. This was all part of his plan. "The trick to education," he said, "is to not let them know they're learning something until it's too late."

Self-portrait with Balloon and Bullet, 1959

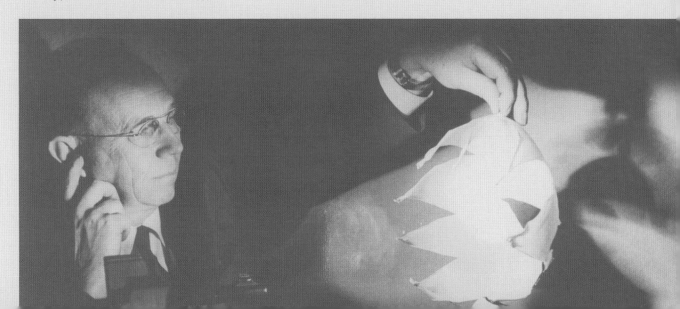

PHILO T.
FARNSWORTH

Television was conceived not in a labora-
tory or on a university campus, but in a hay field in rural
Utah. It was there, as he harvested hay row by row, that 14-year-old
Philo T. Farnsworth thought of scanning and displaying a moving image line by
line. Although there had been earlier attempts at broadcasting moving pictures, it is
Farnsworth's system that underlies the television found in almost every home.

Since Farnsworth was not the first to think of sending moving images through a wire or by
radio waves, and because years passed before he could build the system he envisioned during that harvest, it is hard to say exactly who invented television. Scientists in Europe and the United States pursued
the elusive means to transmit live, moving images for almost 50 years. A German scientist discovered how to
use a spinning disk to scan a moving image in 1884. An English inventor suggested using a cathode ray tube to
display an electronic image in 1907. In the 1920s, researchers working independently in America and England used
spinning disks to capture and display moving images. And in some ways television is simply the logical conclusion
to two of the defining inventions of the nineteenth century: photography, which recorded images, and the telegraph,
which transmitted information.

Still, the hundreds of millions of televisions in use today do have one inventor in common—Philo T.
Farnsworth, who was born in 1906 to a Mormon family near Beaver City, Utah. In 1919, the Farnsworths moved to
a ranch near Rigby, Utah. It was a decidedly rural place—every day Philo rode the four miles to the local schoolhouse on horseback. But the twentieth century had already come to Rigby, in the form of electricity. The new
technology fascinated Farnsworth. He soon figured out how the ranch's power system worked and began
building small electric motors in an attic workshop. And Farnsworth discovered he had a goal: to become an inventor, like Thomas Edison and Alexander Graham Bell.

In 1921, Farnsworth entered high school, but he found he wasn't challenged by his science class. He was moved to the senior chemistry class, and he began studying after
school with the chemistry teacher, Justin Tolman. He learned physics and fixed
radios in his spare time and read all the books and magazines about
science and mechanics he could find. In 1922, one of those
magazines ran a story on "Pictures That

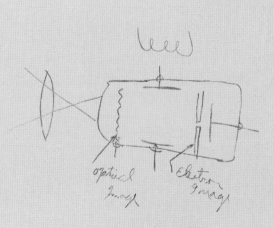

Previous attempts at television involved spinning mechanical disks. Philo Farnsworth's breakthrough was in devising an electronic method for capturing an image, which could then be transmitted and re-created on a cathode ray tube screen.

Could Fly through the Air," which speculated on a technoloci- cal marriage between motion pictures and radio.

The story described some of the early research into televi- sion, which focused on a mechanical system invented in 1884 by Paul Nipkow, an inventor in Berlin. A spiral pattern of small holes was punched into a metal disk. When a motor spun the disk, an image in front of it would be broken up into a sequence of small parts—something like pixels on a computer screen— as light passed through the holes. The small bits of light struck a light-sensitive surface that created electric signals based on the strength of the light. The signals could then be sent through a wire to a neon bulb behind an identical spinning disk. The process then worked in reverse: the light passed through the disk's holes and formed an image on a screen on the other side. In the 1920s, two scientists, Charles Jenkins in the United States and John Logie Baird in England, worked on refining Nip- kow's method. Both managed to create and transmit moving images along with sound, although the pictures were crude and

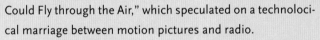

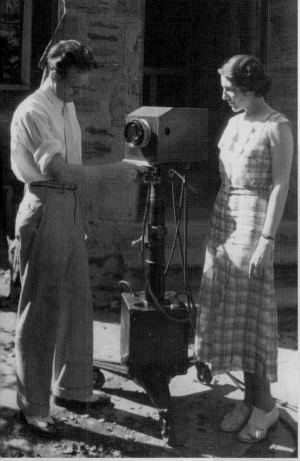

In 1934, Farnsworth and his colleagues, including secretary Mabel Bernstein, traveled to Philadelphia to demonstrate television. For three weeks, live performances were broadcast to an auditorium. Thousands of people came to see the new technology.

Farnsworth transmitted his first televised image in 1927, two years before this photo was taken. A long-running patent dispute with RCA prevented him from ever capitalizing on his technical triumphs.

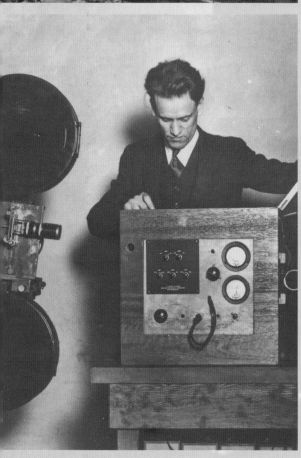

fuzzy. Baird even broadcast television (or "televisor," as he called it) programs through the BBC beginning in 1929.

As Farnsworth learned more about the spinning-disk system, he was sure it would never be practical—the disks could never spin fast enough to produce a clear and consistent image. He thought of a better way to do it while he was harvesting hay on the family ranch. As Farnsworth moved his harvesting machine down straight row after straight row of hay, he envisioned a television system that worked in similarly straight lines. Electrons, he thought, could be used to scan an image line by line, then reassembled back into an image after they were transmitted.

In 1922, Farnsworth sketched out his plans for television on a blackboard for Justin Tolman. Even as he refined the scheme over the next several years, the basic idea remained. A camera lens focused an image on a light-sensitive surface; then, a beam of electrons guided by a magnetic field moved horizontally over the image, scanning it. The beam was moved down a small amount and the process was repeated. The number of electrons released by the light-sensitive surface depended on the strength of the image on it; these electrons were directed into the "image dissector," a special kind of vacuum tube Farnsworth had designed. The electrons were then transmitted to the receiver, where a similar system guided the beams of electrons, moving horizontally and then vertically line by line, to the inside surface of special kind of glass vacuum tube called a cathode ray tube. The surface was coated with a material that glowed when the electrons hit it, to create an image. Thus Farnsworth created electronic television.

In 1926, Farnsworth told George Everson, a professional fund-raiser he was working for, about his invention. Impressed, Everson staked him $6,000 to build his television. Farnsworth and his friend Cliff Gardner, along with their wives, moved to Los Angeles to get to work. It wasn't easy to build a television, they soon found. Everything had to be made from scratch; once, the Los Angeles Police Department showed up to destroy the alcohol still they thought Farnsworth was building.

The operation moved up to San Francisco the next year, and on September 7, 1927, it was ready for a test. Farnsworth, his wife, Pem, and George Everson watched the display tube in one room while Gardner placed a glass slide with a straight line painted on it in front of the camera in the other. It worked—the line was clearly visible, and when Gardner turned it 90 degrees, the first television audience saw it move. In his notebook, Farnsworth wrote, "The received line picture was evident." In a telegram to a business partner, Everson was more enthusiastic: "The damned thing works!"

Farnsworth was not the only person trying to make an electronic television, however. The man most interested in TV was probably David Sarnoff, the president of the Radio Corporation of America (RCA). Through the aggressive purchase and enforcement of patents, RCA had a virtual monopoly on the radio industry in America. With many of those patents due to expire soon and the obvious appeal of images to go along with sound, Sarnoff was eager to have a television technology of his own. In 1930, he hired Vladimir Zworykin, who had been working on the spinning-disk kind of television throughout the 1920s. Before Zworykin came to RCA's lab in New Jersey, Sarnoff sent him to look at Farnsworth's work in San Francisco. It was far ahead of what Zworykin had achieved; he is reported to have said, "this is a beautiful instrument. I wish I'd invented it." Aspects of it were to show up in his work for RCA.

Not long after Zworykin's visit, Sarnoff himself came out to Farnsworth's San Francisco lab, although only when the inventor was out of town. He was impressed, too, and offered $100,000 for the business. After Everson turned down the lowball figure, Sarnoff said, "Then there's nothing here we'll need."

Even after the depression brought America's economy to a halt, Farnsworth's and RCA's television work continued. But RCA took the competition to the courtroom as well as the lab. The corporation sued Farnsworth for patent infringement, claiming that Zworykin had invented Farnsworth's system in 1923. The hearings dragged on for months. Farnsworth's old teacher Julian Tolman was even called to testify about the drawings on the chalkboard back in 1922. In the end, Farnsworth's priority of invention was confirmed, but RCA was not easily defeated. Their appeals dragged the matter out for years, while their monopoly position let them discourage radio manufacturers from dealing with Farnsworth.

Still, there were other victories for Farnsworth. In 1934, the Franklin Institute in Philadelphia invited him to demonstrate television; for three weeks, performances by politicians, vaudevillians, athletes, and others were broadcast to an auditorium. Thousands of people showed up to watch. And in 1936, using technology licensed from Farnsworth, the German government broadcast the Olympic Games. Although it was to a very small number of receivers—and in the service of Nazi propaganda— this was the first live broadcast of a major event.

The "official" debut of television in the United States came at the 1939 World's Fair in New York, when David Sarnoff announced RCA's sets and its first broadcasts. However, RCA still didn't have any patents on its television equipment; later that year, it entered a $1 million licensing agreement with Farnsworth, the first time RCA had ever had to license another company's technology.

The spread of television was curtailed by World War II. The five-year disruption also ruined Farnsworth's chances of really competing with RCA. In 1947, just as the economy was getting back to normal, his key patents expired. That year, 6,000 TV sets were sold; by 1952, there were 22 million sets in American homes.

Farnsworth kept developing related technologies, though. He helped work on radar as well as video scanners and amplifiers. He also devoted much time and money to chasing another Holy Grail: generating power through nuclear fusion. Although he invested much time and money, nothing came of this obsessive pursuit. Farnsworth died in 1971.

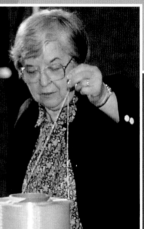

STEPHANIE KWOLEK

An odd, cloudy batch of polymers that DuPont chemist Stephanie Kwolek mixed up in 1964 might have seemed like a mistake to another researcher. Usually, a polymer solution was clear and viscous. This one was thin and cloudy, almost as if it were contaminated. But Kwolek was more intrigued than disappointed, and she continued to work with the chemicals. Her diligence paid off—that milky batch of chemicals led to the development of Kevlar, a super-strong, super-stiff fiber that has saved thousands of lives.

Kevlar is now virtually synonymous with high-tech materials. Heat-resistant, five times as strong as steel, and lighter than fiberglass, it is used in hundreds of products, from protective gloves, helmets, and boots to tires, brake pads, and cables. It's used on spacecraft and to build bridges. Its most famous role, though, is in bulletproof vests, which contain several layers of a fabric woven from Kevlar fiber. When a bullet hits a vest, its thousands of pounds of force are spread out among individual Kevlar fibers. Because they are so strong and stiff, the fibers absorb a great amount of energy very quickly. According to the International Association of Chiefs of Police DuPont Kevlar Survivors Club, based in Alexandria, Virginia, at least 2,000 lives have been saved by the bullet-stopping fiber.

The introduction of Kevlar ushered in a new era of products dependent on synthetic materials. Consumers now take it for granted that materials like carbon fiber, Teflon, high-performance epoxies, and new metal alloys, as well as Kevlar, will make things stronger, lighter, and more durable. In many products, such as sports equipment or protective clothing, it's rare to find something made without new materials.

With such a big role in the invention of one of the world's best-known synthetic fibers, it's ironic that Kwolek didn't intend to become a chemist. She wanted to be a doctor.

Stephanie Kwolek was born in New Kensington, Pennsylvania, in 1923. Although her father died when she was only ten years old, he had an early influence on her interest in science. "I remember trudging through the woods near my house with him and looking for snakes and other animals," she says.

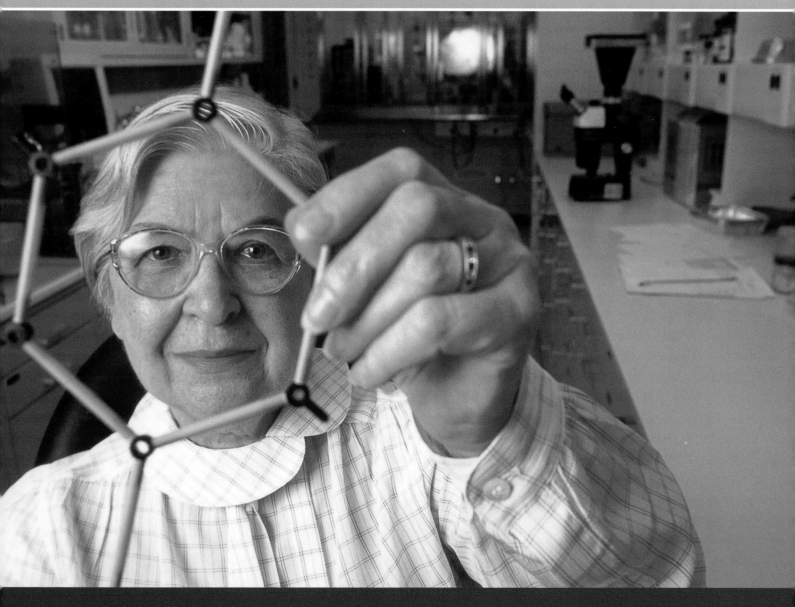

"I seem to see things that other people did not see.

If things don't work out I don't just throw them out, I struggle

over them, to try and see if there's something there."

In 1964, Stephanie Kwolek investigated a curious polymer

solution in her Dupont lab; that polymer eventually became Kevlar,

a fiber five times as strong as steel and lighter than fiberglass.

Here, Kwolek is shown holding a model of a Kevlar molecule.

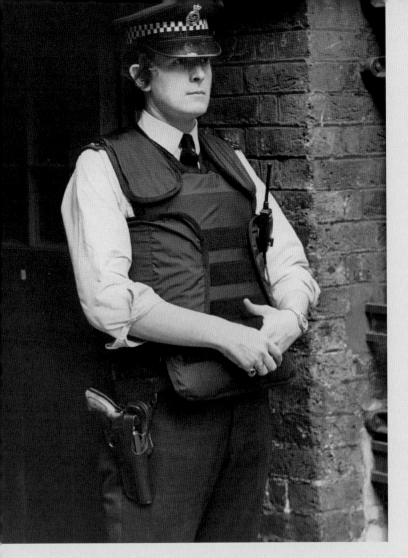

The most famous application of Kevlar is in bulletproof vests, which are made of layers of fabric woven from strands of the super-strong fiber. The thousands of Kevlar fibers in a vest absorb and distribute the force of a bullet.

BULLETPROOF SPORTS EQUIPMENT

The qualities of Kevlar that make it a great material for protective gear—stiffness, strength, durability—are also perfect for many kinds of sporting equipment. While DuPont and Stephanie Kwolek may not have envisioned Kevlar-reinforced cricket bats or archery gauntlets when they introduced the material in 1971, it has proved versatile enough to work as well for a kayak as it does in a bulletproof vest. What follows is a selection of sporting equipment enhanced with Kevlar. And although many sports have already adopted the material, each year equipment designers find new uses for the super-strong fiber.

Archery

Eagle Classic Archery in England makes a 100 percent Kevlar gauntlet, to protect against the serious cuts or splinters that an errant or damaged arrow can produce.

Bicycling

Bicycle tires reinforced with Kevlar are resistant to punctures and last many miles more than traditional tires. Kevlar beads—the strips that bind tire to rim—replace steel ones, reducing the weight of the tires. Also available are Kevlar strips to mount inside regular tires, to guard against "snake bites" and other punctures.

"We also studied the various wild plants and leaves and seeds." At the same time, she adds, "I was very much interested in designing fashions. That interest came from my mother. I spent many hours creating clothes for my dolls." It was a happy coincidence that the group she later joined at DuPont was devoted to fibers and textiles.

Kwolek's mother supported the family through the depression, and when Kwolek graduated from Margaret Morrison Carnegie College (now Carnegie Mellon University) in 1946, she realized she couldn't afford to study medicine. Kwolek had majored in chemistry, and she decided to get a job in that field to save enough money to eventually go to medical school. She knew that DuPont was the leading chemical company; fortunately, Dr. Hale Charch, the inventor of moisture-proof cellophane and later a mentor to Kwolek, was interviewing prospective chemists. After some forceful insistence on Kwolek's part, Charch offered her a job on the spot, and she soon joined DuPont's Buffalo, New York, research facility.

Technical fields like chemistry had just opened up to women. During World War II, women had entered the work force in unprecedented numbers. When the war ended, many men weren't available, since they had spent the previous five years fighting, not studying. Kwolek was also lucky to sign up with Dr. Charch; under his leadership, she notes, DuPont hired more women than many other companies. Still, women were a minority in the field, and in the company. Her first promotion at DuPont came after 15 years—"far too long," she later told a reporter.

When Kwolek began working at DuPont in 1946, the first synthetic fiber, nylon, was only about eight years old. With a team of chemists called the Pioneering Research Laboratory, she began exploring new polymer fibers. Before Kevlar, she had contributed to the creation of Orlon, Lycra, and Spandex, as well as DuPont's first high-performance fiber, Nomex, which is used in firefighters' protective clothing. Kwolek also explored new ways to make these fibers, which until that time required very high temperatures. These new methods allowed her team to make and test hundreds of thousands of new polymers.

In 1964, her group decided to search for a new high-performance fiber. They had a specific use in mind for it: There were predictions of a coming gasoline shortage, and they thought that a strong, lightweight fiber could be used to reinforce car tires; cars using lighter, stiffer tires would consume less gasoline. "A number of people had been asked to take up this project and no one seemed to be particularly interested," Kwolek explains. "So I was asked if I would do it." She started out working with two "aromatic" polymers—molecules with benzene rings in them. Kwolek knew from working on

Canoeing and Kayaking

Kevlar has become one of the standard materials used in the manufacture of canoes and kayaks. It is especially useful in river and sea kayaks, which often collide with rocks. Kevlar's stiffness makes the watercraft strong, but it has more give than carbon fiber, allowing for an easier journey.

Hockey

The Kevlar in a hockey stick and blade reduces vibrations when hitting the puck, lowers weight, and increases strength.

Hunting

The Wise Hunter company recently introduced a line of camouflage hunting pants and chaps that incorporate Kevlar, to protect against venomous snake bites.

Tennis

The graphite racquet, introduced around 1980, was one of the biggest advances in the sport in the twentieth century. The addition of Kevlar to the graphite—in about a 20/80 ratio—has since increased racquets' stiffness and durability and reduced vibration.

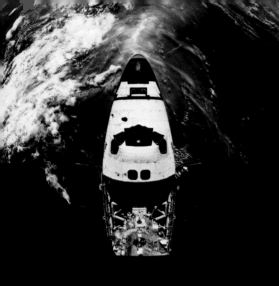

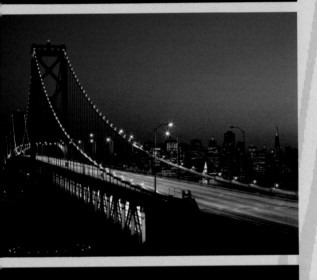

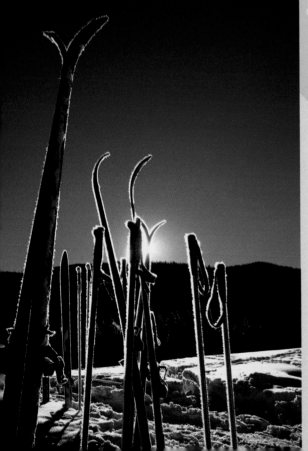

Kevlar has found hundreds of uses since its introduction in 1971, including use in space shuttle components and space suits; for suspension bridge cables; and for strengthening sports equipment such as skis.

Nomex that this kind of polymer was resistant to high temperatures and she thought these molecules might provide greater stiffness.

"In the course of that work I made a discovery," she says modestly. Under specific conditions, these polymers would form liquid crystals in a solution, which no polymer had ever done before. And instead of the usual "bent" polymer molecules—she likens them to spaghetti—these were straight, like match sticks. When the cloudy solution was "spun"—forced through the tiny holes of a device called a spinneret—the straight fibers lined up parallel to each other. This made the new fiber very stiff and very strong.

At first, though, it was not easy for Kwolek to get the polymer solution into the spinneret. "That solution was very different from the standard polymer solution," she recalls. "It had a lot of strange features about it. I think someone who wasn't thinking very much or just wasn't aware or took less interest in it, would have thrown it out." Kwolek filtered it to see if the cloudy solution was contaminated. It wasn't. Still, she continues, "when I submitted it for spinning, the guy refused to spin it. He said it would plug up the holes of his spinneret, because he assumed that [it had] solid particles. So it was a while before he consented to spinning it. I think either I wore him down or else he felt sorry for me. It spun beautifully."

The results of this first spinning were, for Kwolek, unbelievable. When a chemist spins a fiber, she sends it to a lab to test its strength, stiffness, and other properties. This new fiber came back from the lab with a stiffness at least nine times greater than anything she'd made before. "I was very hesitant about telling anyone," she says. "I didn't want to be embarrassed if someone had made a mistake. So I sent the fiber down several times. The numbers always came back in the same vicinity." Only then did she announce her results, and DuPont realized it had a fiber with great potential. After much more work and refinement by the group, Kevlar was introduced in 1971. The fiber has since found more than 200 applications, and brings DuPont hundreds of millions of dollars in sales each year.

As for Kwolek's dream of becoming a doctor, after a couple of years at DuPont she realized that the temporary job she'd taken to save some money was the right one for her. "I love doing chemistry," she says. "And I love making discoveries." Her careful, dedicated approach to research helped her succeed throughout her 40-year career at DuPont. "I'm very conscientious," Kwolek explains. "And I discovered over the years that I seem to see things that other people did not see. If things don't work out I don't just throw them out, I struggle over them, to try and see if there's something there."

It was just that will to carefully observe, struggle, and stay the course that led to her famous fiber. Today, police officers and others whose lives depend on Kevlar often come up to her to tell of their experiences. One Virginia police officer even had Kwolek autograph his bulletproof vest, which had stopped a 9 mm bullet and saved his life. "I feel very humble," she says. "I feel very lucky. So many people work all their lives and they don't make a discovery that's of benefit to other people."

JEROME **LEMELSON**

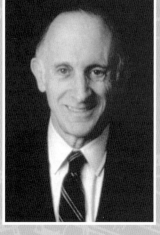

Few people have invented as many things, or invented for as long, as Jerome Lemelson. Over a period of more than 40 years he received, on average, one patent every month. Only a handful of people hold more U.S. patents than he, and perhaps no one in as many different fields. Many of the products we encounter every day are either based on his ideas or made with machines he helped create, from camcorders and the Walkman to industrial robots and the bar code scanner. Lemelson was also a true believer in the power of the individual inventor, devoting much of his time not only to defending his own patents but also to encouraging other people's work.

Lemelson was curious and inventive even as a child. Growing up in Staten Island, New York, where he was born in 1923, he developed a fascination with model airplanes. By the time he was a teenager, he was designing his own planes, which he flew in competitions in the still open fields of the borough. He was also learning to identify problems inventions could solve: For his father, who was a doctor, he built a tongue depressor with a built-in light, to illuminate the backs of patients' mouths.

His fascination with planes led Lemelson to enlist in the Air Force during World War II. Bad eyesight prevented him from becoming a pilot; instead, he became an engineer. After the war, he studied aeronautical and industrial engineering at New York University, where he did research for the Air Force. Between 1947 and 1951, he was part of Project Squid, which developed rocket and jet engines for improved versions of the missiles Germany used during the war.

Lemelson continued working as an aeronautical engineer after college, but he was also filling notebooks with ideas for new inventions. He applied for his first patent in 1949, for a typewriter eraser that attached to the machine with a magnet. The patent was denied—someone had already invented it. Six years later, his first patent was awarded, for a toy cap, a variation on the propeller beanie. By the end of the 1950s he had given up his engineering job to invent full time.

PATENTED APR 1 5 1975

3,877,207

SHEET 2 OF 2

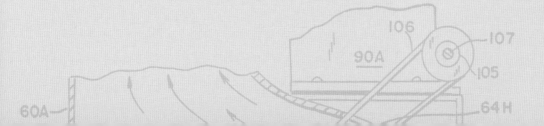

93

81A

63 67 68

68

70
69
80

86
98
79

97
62

94Z
60

81
61

95

81B

94
90
93

99
86
64

26

100
72
71

88 87
84

89 65
66 83

82

FIG.3

In 1995, Jerome Lemelson dedicated the Jerome and Dorothy Lemelson Center for the Study of Invention and Innovation at the Smithsonian Institution. Its mission, in part, is to encourage invention in young people and to foster an appreciation for the central role invention plays in the United States.

106
107

90A

105

60A
64 H

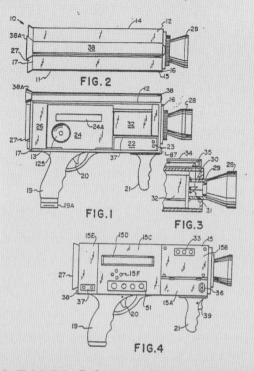

FIG. 2

FIG.1

FIG.3

FIG.4

He often worked 18 hours a day, with ideas coming one af-ter another. Regularly, Lemelson would wake up in the middle of the night to jot down an invention that had come to him during sleep. During his early years, Lemelson couldn't afford a drafts-man, so he did his own patent drawings. The earnings of his wife, Dorothy, an interior decorator, helped support the family.

Many of Lemelson's early patents were for toys, since that industry depended on a constant stream of new products and was accustomed to licensing outsiders' ideas. But he was also inventing much more complex devices. The first of these was an industrial robot that could perform many tasks. Inspiration for the robot came during a 1951 demonstration of an automatic lathe that was programmed with punch cards. "I thought, 'Gee, here's a principle I can apply to many different fields,'" Lemel-son recalled. In a 150-page patent application he filed on Christ-mas Eve 1954, he described a computer-controlled robot that

THE LEMELSON FOUNDATION

Throughout his career, Jerome Lemelson devoted time to the cause of invention and innovation in the United States. As the earnings from his many inventions accumulated, Lemelson began thinking about how to use that money to encourage American inventors and to teach schoolchildren about the excitement of invention and engineering. "We must convince our nation's young people that the field of invention can be far more rewarding—financially and in other respects—than most of them think," he declared.

In 1993, he and his wife, Dorothy, created the Lemelson Foun-dation to develop and fund programs devoted to invention at several American institutions. Major programs supported by the Foundation include:

Massachusetts Institute of Technology, Cambridge, Massachusetts
To celebrate excellence in innovation, the Massachusetts Institute of Technology administers the Lemelson-MIT Program, which presents inspiring inventor-innovator role models through annual awards including the world's largest for invention—the $500,000 Lemelson-MIT Prize—and educational outreach activities. The foundation also supports the teaching and training of tomorrow's innovators through the Jerome & Dorothy Lemelson Professor-

ship and several "E-Team" courses on product development and entrepreneurship.

The Smithsonian's National Museum of American History, Washington, D.C.
Established in 1995, the Lemelson Center for the Study of Inven-tion and Innovation is dedicated to exploring invention in history and encouraging inventive creativity in young people. The center offers lectures, conferences, publications, exhibits, educational programs, and curricular materials in both conventional and elec-tronic form and supports oral and video history projects, fellow-ships, and internships. The Lemelson Foundation also supports the Museum's Hands-on Science Center, which is part of the "Sci-ence in American Life" exhibition.

Hampshire College, Amherst, Massachusetts
The Lemelson Assistive Technology Development Center (LATDC) at Hampshire College is one of the only centers of its kind in the nation. Its mission is to provide students with an experiential ed-ucation in design, invention, and entrepreneurship through the use of assistive technology and universal design. LATDC achieves

could perform a variety of industrial tasks, including assembling, welding, riveting, and painting. Although "computers took up a whole room in those days," he noted, "I believed that computers would come down in size." They did come down in size, of course, and industrial robots have become standard tools in the manufacture of many products.

Lemelson's robots had to see what they were doing, and out of that necessity came his most lucrative invention, "machine vision." By converting the image from a video camera into raw data, a computer could see with great accuracy. The system could help a robot—or any other machine—tell if all of a product's parts were there, if there were defects in it, what color it was, or any number of other things. Today, this concept is applied to all automated precision manufacturing. The production of silicon chips, for example involves quickly verifying that all of a chip's connections are valid, a process that would take a

person with a microscope days to do by hand. Machine vision is also used by car manufacturers and in the aerospace industry; all of the space shuttle's heat-resistant tiles, for example, are checked with such a system.

Industrial robots and machine vision were both intended to make manufacturing easier, more flexible, and more efficient. In the early 1960s, Lemelson received patents for an automatic warehousing system with the same aim. The system he outlined is familiar to anyone who has been in a modern warehouse: Computer-controlled and -guided forklifts and cranes fetch or stack pallets of goods, delivering inventory exactly when it's needed. In 1964 Lemelson had his first big success at licensing his patents when he sold the system to an Ohio company for $100,000.

While many of Lemelson's patents were focused on the way things are made, he also created products people use every

this through a combination of courses, activities, internships, and collaborations with business and nonprofit organizations, and through teams of students who design, develop, and make available equipment for people with disabilities.

National Collegiate Inventors and Innovators Alliance, Hadley, Massachusetts

The National Collegiate Inventors and Innovators Alliance (NCIIA) is an alliance of faculty and students at over 175 colleges and universities nationwide working to advance the teaching of invention and innovation in American higher education. Its mission is to nurture a new generation of innovators by promoting curricula designed to teach creativity, invention, and entrepreneurship, and to support independent teams of student innovators. The NCIIA provides grants for curriculum development and commercialization of technology-based products, as well as conferences and workshops designed to disseminate curricular innovation.

University of Nevada, Reno, Nevada

The foundation helped establish a center at the university to augment its "E-Team" program in the electrical engineering curricu-

lum and to promote invention, innovation, and entrepreneurship in courses.

E-Teams

A common thread running through the foundation programs is "E-Teams," students working in teams to design and develop new ideas and, in some cases, to pursue their commercialization. (The "E" is for excellence and entrepreneurship.) Recent studies show that new businesses launched by multiple cofounders have a greater chance of success than those started by individuals. These results suggest that one element of academic programs aimed at preparing students for careers in business and industry should be teams of students identifying and developing a solution to a practical problem or market need, and undertaking the steps necessary to translate that solution into a commercial product.

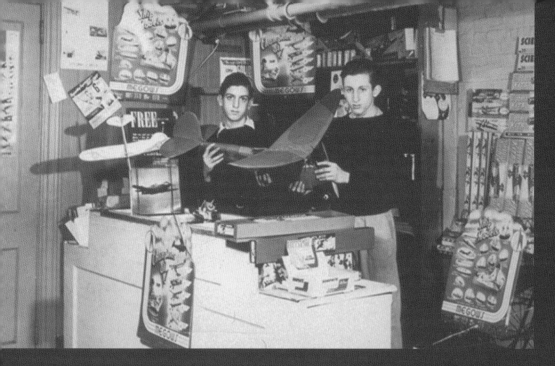

As a young man, Lemelson was fascinated by model airplanes, which he designed and built from scratch. In this picture from the 1940s, Lemelson (right) and his brother Howard display a homemade aircraft.

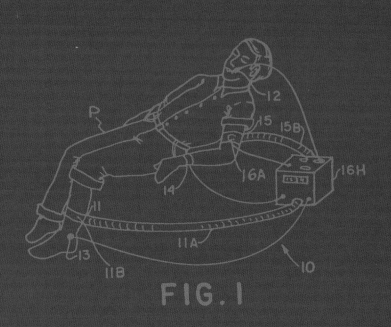

FIG. 1

Lemelson (left) with Howard and "Pete," the dog from the "Our Gang" comedies, in Atlantic City, New Jersey, 1933.

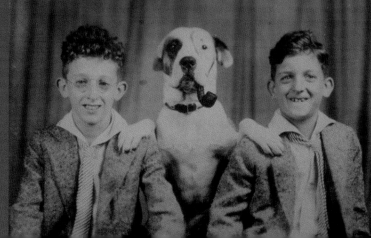

day. Some of his patents, for example, cover technologies used in camcorders, VCRs, and fax machines. Lemelson's invention with the most far-reaching cultural impact may be his magnetic tape drive mechanism. Lemelson had first thought of using magnetic tape to store electronic images in the 1950s, when he and his wife were wading through the stacks of documentation at the United States Patent Office. More than a decade later, he created a miniature tape drive for the audiocassette format developed by Philips in the early 1960s. Sony licensed the patent in 1974 and five years later used it in the Walkman. That portable tape player changed how people listened to music and, as the first piece of electronics that millions of people carried around with them, it opened the way for the dozens of portable devices we use today, from the cell phone to personal digital assistants.

While the Sony licensing deal was straightforward, it was rarely that easy for Lemelson to control the use of his patents. He first encountered patent infringement, a problem many individual inventors face, in the 1950s. One of the toys he thought of was a mask to be printed on the back of a cereal box and cut out by kids. Kellogg's rejected the idea, so Lemelson was shocked three years later when he found masks printed on the back of Corn Flakes boxes. He sued, but at that time judges were not sympathetic to patent infringement cases, and Lemelson lost.

In the decades following his cereal box defeat, Lemelson became more vigilant in defending his patents, an effort that paid off in the late 1980s. One outgrowth of his work on machine vision had been the bar code scanner, which was part of his patent applications in the 1950s. By the time the final patents were issued in the 1980s, many manufacturers, notably automakers and electronics companies, had adopted the idea. In 1992 and 1993, Lemelson made licensing deals with most of the companies using bar codes in their factories.

The income Lemelson generated from his patents allowed him to expand his efforts at encouraging future inventors. For Lemelson, active independent inventors were the key to America's continuing industrial success. "Unless we get more of our young people interested in engineering and technology, our country will face serious problems," he said. "Engineers and designers are the front-line soldiers in any economic battle." Dorothy Lemelson adds that "he always wanted to celebrate invention. So when he was able, financially, to think about it, he sat down with [his sons], and they said, 'You've been want-

ing to do these things all your life, now's the time to do it. Go for it.' And he did." In the 1990s, Lemelson and his wife established the Lemelson Foundation to increase awareness of the importance of invention to the nation's economy and culture. A private philanthropy, the foundation's purpose is to stimulate the U.S. economy and secure its position in the global marketplace by creating the next generation of inventors, innovators, and entrepreneurs whose ideas will provide the basis for new companies and job creation in the twenty-first century.

Unfortunately, Jerome Lemelson was able to see only some of the results of his philanthropy before he died of cancer in 1997. Even in his last year, though, he continued inventing. In fact, the 40 patent applications he made that year alone broke even his own record for quantity, and they helped establish him as one of history's most prolific inventors. "He had an ability to take things that weren't connected at all and see the relationships between them and see what they could become," Dorothy Lemelson remembers. "I realize he saw the world we're living in [today]. In the 1950s, in his head, he saw the world that was to come."

Lemelson (right), Howard (center), and a friend experiment with an air-powered model airplane. From 1947 to 1951, Lemelson worked for the Air Force developing jet and rocket engines.

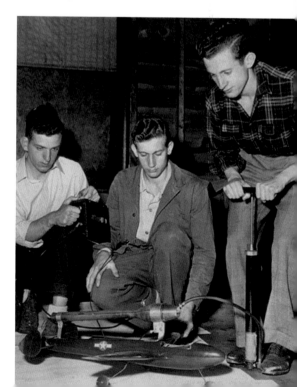

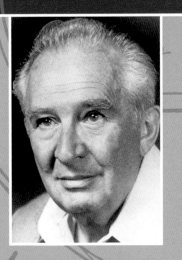

JACOB **RABINOW**

For lifelong inventor Jacob Rabinow there was as much beauty in inventing as there was in art. A successful invention, the engineer once said, "is like a good poem. . . . It does the thing it's supposed to do with a minimum number of parts."

Rabinow pursued this kind of poetry all his life, from his first invention at the age of nine until his death, at age 89, in 1999. He eventually received 230 patents, covering an extraordinarily wide range of technologies. He built the first magnetic disk storage system for computers, letter-sorting machines for the Post Office, a self-adjusting clock used for decades in most American cars, the first practical optical character-recognition system, and missile guidance systems that are still used today. There are thousands of other ideas in his notebooks, some that weren't patented because others had thought of them first (unbeknownst to him), but most because there simply wasn't enough time.

That first invention came in Siberia, where Rabinow's family had moved from Kharkov, Russia, when the threat of civil war had become too great. The Russian Revolution indeed began, and the Russian army would sometimes come through his Siberian town. Rabinow was keenly interested in their equipment. (He was also an avid reader of Jules Verne's science fiction.) One day, Rabinow and his brother made a small machine that could throw rocks, building it out of a couple of posts and some twisted rope. It worked, but an adult gave the young inventor some bad news: He had reinvented a Roman *ballista*, a 2,000-year-old technology. ("I didn't know there were Romans," he later said.)

Rabinow's father died of typhus not long after the Communists closed down his shoe factory. The family fled to China in 1919, and from there moved to Brooklyn, New York, in 1921. Rabinow's mother worked making corsets, and he attended public school, where he continued to be fascinated by engineering and dreamed of becoming an inventor. But people told Rabinow that he would never become an engineer in America because he was Jewish. He listened to them, and he graduated from the City College of New York with a degree in "straight" science. Rabinow wasn't satisfied with this for long, though; after graduation, in the middle of the depression, he decided, "If I'll starve, I'll starve doing something I like." With some borrowed money and savings from working in a radio shop, Rabinow went back to City College and earned a masters degree in engineering.

In 1938 Rabinow got a job at the National Bureau of Standards (now the National Institute of Standards and Technology), performing the mundane task of calibrating water meters. His inventiveness was soon noted by his superiors, and as America began to prepare for World War II, Rabinow started working on something much more interesting: fuses for bombs and missiles.

An armed bomb is a dangerous thing; the trick is to activate it when it's safely away from the people firing it. The device that does this is called a fuse. Although the technology for arming conventional shells already existed, missiles were new, and the old techniques didn't work. Rabinow's first fuse consisted of four sets of weights. To activate a missile, the force of acceleration would move the weights one after the other, until a circuit was completed. If the missile was simply mishandled or dropped only one set of weights would move, and the missile would not arm.

It was much more difficult to make a fuse smart enough to arm and detonate a missile only when it was close enough to its target to damage it. (Earlier proximity fuses, as they're called, worked either on contact with a target, which limited the damage they could do, or with timers, which often made them explode too early.) Rabinow's major contribution to proximity fuses was to realize that the shock wave created by an aircraft traveling faster than the speed of sound could be used to trigger a missile. Later, he was asked to work on the problem of keeping a missile's radar antenna straight even as the missile wobbled. A modified version of the gyroscope mounting system he invented is still used in Sidewinder missiles.

Rabinow was a constant, even compulsive inventor. One of his favorite sayings was, "We all curse at first, but inventors fix." Any mechanical challenge or shortcoming at work or home was grounds for working on a new

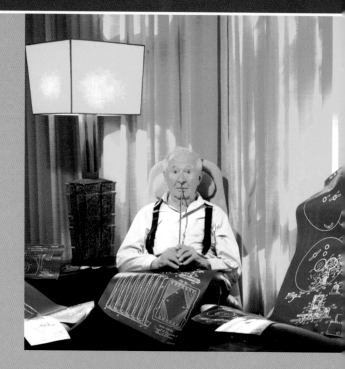

Rabinow received some 230 patents during his life, ranging from industrial devices such as automatic mail-sorters and character recognition systems to pick-proof locks and a new method for hanging pictures.

Jacob Rabinow loved talking about his inventions and about invention in general. He returned again and again to certain themes, such as the moment of invention, the art of invention, and the importance of cultivating American innovation. Here are some samples of Rabinow's wisdom.

On inventing

"People are so carried away with their own brilliance that it is hard for them to believe that the world is filled with equally brilliant people. One gains tremendous respect for the human race when one sits in the Patent Office Search Room for a day and looks through the tremendous variety of ideas on any subject one can possibly conceive."

"If you want to be different, you better be good. If you want to make a really different product, it better be very good."

"The feeling I get when I see [an elegant device] is exactly like that of a person who likes art and sees a great painting for the first time."

"Inventing is a hell of a lot of fun if you don't have to make a living at it."

On working without official permission

"Things that are done illegally are done efficiently."

On designing weapons

"You may wonder how I can talk so coldly about designing weapons, throwing bombs, and killing people. . . . I think that of all the things mankind has done and is doing now, the most obscene, the most vile, the most terrible, the most cruel by far is war. And yet, I am not a pacifist, even though I had seen war and death when I was a young boy in Siberia and know what it is like to be terribly frightened. I think it is better to kill than to be murdered in cold blood. I think it is necessary to fight despotism and sometimes it is necessary to fight in self-defense."

On invention in America

"Invention is culturally driven, and American culture today is not a strong driver. If a country wants great inventors, it has to make sure that inventors are encouraged, rewarded, liked, made heroes."

On the joys of inventing

"It would be wonderful if all inventors started by being very rich, so that selling or licensing a patent would make relatively little difference to them. Unfortunately, that does not happen often. Although I have known one or two inventors who were very rich, I have met thousands who aren't. They were not rich in money, but there are other riches. There is excitement in seeing a glimpse of the future, leaving something better than you found it, of leaving a scratch on history."

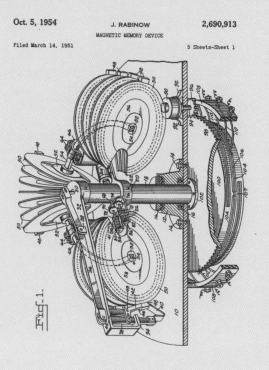

Fig. 1.

INVENTOR.
JACOB RABINOW
BY
G. J. Kesemich + A. W. Dew
ATTORNEYS

Rabinow's magnetic memory device was a precursor to the modern hard disk drive, featuring spinning, magnetically charged disks that held data.

device. When a short friend complained that her feet didn't reach the ground from a Washington, D.C., theater seat, Rabinow whipped up a portable stool whose legs folded up into a modified hardcover book. At home, he noticed how hard it was to read the label on a rotating record album, so he created a spinning prism device that would make the label seem to be standing still. He even created a new way to hang pictures that wouldn't damage his walls.

While these fixes for everyday life pleased Rabinow, he was even better at envisioning solutions to complicated problems. In 1945, his wife, Gladys, gave him a Swiss watch as a birthday present. Although it was an excellent watch, like all timepieces made then it slowed down after a while. Rabinow opened up his new watch—scratching its nice case in the process—and discovered a small lever that would speed up or slow down the watch. He adjusted the watch, but a year later it slowed down again. Although watchmaking had been one of the most advanced crafts skills for centuries, no one had figured out how to make a watch that could automatically adjust itself. Rabinow set to work, and made a very small limiting device that adjusted a watch's speed when the time was reset—a watch owner would never even know he was fixing the speed.

Rabinow's first moneymaking invention was the self-regulating clock, which adjusted itself as it slowed down. Watchmakers didn't want to admit their products were less than perfect, so Rabinow sold the idea to carmakers.

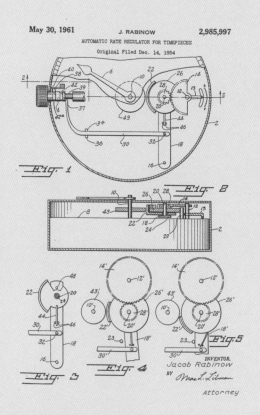

Fig. 1
Fig. 2
Fig. 3
Fig. 4
Fig. 5

INVENTOR.
Jacob Rabinow
BY
Mom L. Libman

Attorney

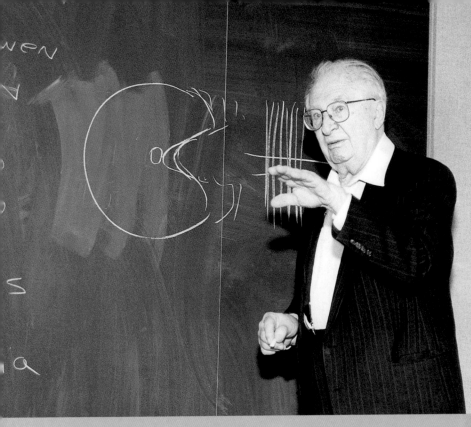

Jacob Rabinow always enjoyed discussing inventions, and especially his inventions. Here he illustrates the principles behind the "magnetic memory device" he invented in 1951.

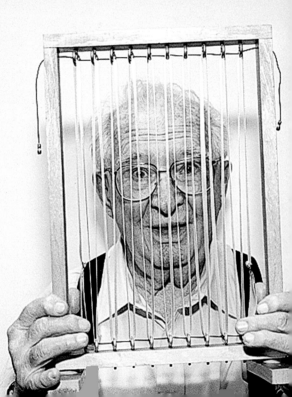

One of Rabinow's inventions was a new kind of Venetian blind—no design problem was too small for him to address.

The watch industry did not accept Rabinow's advance easily. To call a new watch "self-adjusting" implied that older watches weren't as good—which they weren't. Eventually, Rabinow's device was licensed to automobile clock makers, since it was almost impossible to get to the workings of a car's clock to adjust it. This turned out to be Rabinow's most lucrative invention—he netted one cent for every clock made, about $20,000 a year.

Rabinow was particularly intrigued by problems others thought were impossible. "I had once heard the U.S. Postmaster General say that the Post Office could not be automated," he recalled in his 1990 book *Inventing for Fun and Profit*. "I was willing to bet lunches for a year that something could be done." He had already done some work for the Census Bureau designing a punch-card sorting machine and thought he could translate some of that experience to the task of sorting millions of letters a day. The system he invented was complicated, involving custom keyboards, sorting trays with built-in mechanical "memory," vacuum devices to lift the letters, and intricate "roller coasters" to move the trays. And it worked; Rabinow's system, finished in the 1960s, was only recently replaced by newer technology.

A key aspect to sorting mail was recognizing the often irregular letters in the address. After working on a system for automatically selecting microfilm documents, Rabinow realized he could make a machine that could read—or at least recognize individual letters. A character was projected onto a piece of film; behind that film was a spinning disk printed with each character of the alphabet. By means of light-sensitive photocells, each character was compared with the ones on the disk, until a match was found.

The secret to Rabinow's Optical Character Recognition (OCR) system was that it didn't try to match each letter exactly. "If a character is printed perfectly," he wrote, "any reading system works." But when a character is poorly printed, it's nearly impossible to come up with a perfect match. So Rabinow's machine used a "best match" approach, deciding that a character was an A, for example, because it was more like an A than anything else. The system wasn't 100 percent accurate, but it was close, and far better than anything else on the market. Although the first OCR system was very slow—it read a character a second—refinements eventually allowed it to read up to 14,000 characters a second. The "best match" system is still used for character recognition, and the principle has been successfully applied to other fields.

Rabinow's belief in the power and importance of invention was not limited to his own work. He seized on any opportunity to talk about innovation and the state of invention in the United States, which he was very worried about. In the 1980s, he contributed several articles to scientific magazines that not only detailed his own approach to invention ("You have to realize that invention is an art form") but also declared the need for a better attitude toward innovation and small inventors. "Let's support the small inventor," he wrote, "not because he's going to save the country, but because he will keep the big guys honest." Although he officially retired from the National Institute of Standards and Technology in 1989, he continued to advise the agency and helped it plan a museum of American technology. He also continued to invent, and he spent much of his later life solving a pet problem, one first posed to him by an NBS colleage in 1938: creating a pick-proof lock.

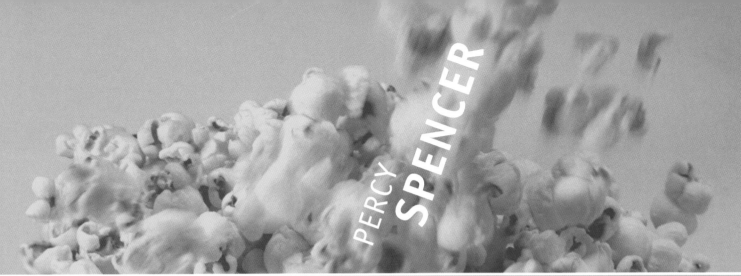

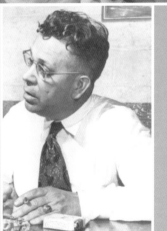

The microwave oven began with a sticky mess in the pocket of Percy Spencer's lab coat. One day in 1946, he was testing a magnetron—the tube that powers radar systems—at the Raytheon Company, where he worked. When he reached into his pocket for the chocolate bar he had been carrying around, he found it had melted. Although many people would have assumed that the chocolate had melted from body heat, Spencer guessed that the culprit was microwaves emitted by the magnetron.

To test this hypothesis, Spencer sent an assistant out for a bag of popcorn. When the kernels were held up in front of the magnetron, they exploded all over the lab. The next morning, Spencer conducted another experiment. He took an old tea kettle and cut a hole in its side. Then he put an uncooked egg in it, aimed the magnetron at the kettle's hole, and powered it up. A skeptical colleague peered into the kettle just as the egg exploded—the yolk had gotten so hot that its steam burst open the shell. By 1947, Raytheon had built the first microwave oven, and in 1949 Spencer received a patent for his new "method of preparing food."

During his youth, Spencer would have seemed an unlikely candidate for inventive greatness. Born in 1894 in the small town of Howland, Maine, Spencer's early life was full of tragedy. His father died when Spencer was just 18 months old, and his mother left home soon after that, leaving him to his aunt and uncle. When he was seven, that uncle died, too. The small family's modest circumstances prevented Spencer from completing school; when he was just 12, he began working at the local spool mill.

When he was 16, Spencer took a job that set him on a different course. The local paper mill was buying its first electrical system, and although the teenager knew nothing about electricity, he was hired to help install it. Within two years, he was a full-fledged electrician, having learned by trial and error. In 1912, inspired by the story of how a wireless radio operator had helped save many passengers on the *Titanic*, Spencer joined the navy to learn radio. After his tour of duty (and an education at the Naval Radio School), he joined a company that was making radio equipment for soldiers fighting World War I.

Barely 21 years old, Spencer threw himself into the work, logging long hours not only building radios but also trying to figure them out. "Many's the time the gang would come back in the morning and find Percy still there," a coworker recalled to *Reader's Digest* in 1958. "He had stayed up all night just to find out how things worked."

In the late 1920s, Spencer joined Raytheon, which had been founded a few years earlier by Vannevar Bush and two other scientists. (Bush would later lead the Manhattan Project, which built the first atomic bomb.) Although the company's first product, a refrigerator, was a flop, it soon became known for its new invention, the radio tube. Through the 1920s and 1930s, Spencer worked on new kinds of radio tubes, often in collaboration with physicists at the Massachusetts Institute of Technology. "Spencer became one of the best tube designers in the world," one of those physicists told *Reader's Digest*. "He could make a working tube out of a sardine can." One of his tubes eventually became part of the modern television camera.

When World War II began in Europe in 1939, Raytheon, like many companies in the United States, shifted its focus to military work. In 1941 Spencer began working to improve a top-secret project of the British: radar.

Radar, short for "radio detection and ranging," was an extremely important invention. It allowed the British to "see" enemy planes and ships from a great distance, even at night or in bad weather. The idea behind the technology is fairly simple. Microwaves, which are electromagnetic waves shorter than radio waves but longer than the waves that make up visible light, are transmitted into the air. When they hit an object, such as a plane, they are reflected back. An antenna picks up these reflected waves, and by measuring the time between transmission and reception, one can determine exactly where the object is. Repeating the process reveals what direction the object is moving in, and how fast.

The heart of a radar system is the magnetron, a tube that produces and emits microwaves. The magnetrons designed by the British were "awkward and impractical," according to Spencer. Although thousands of them were

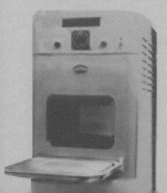

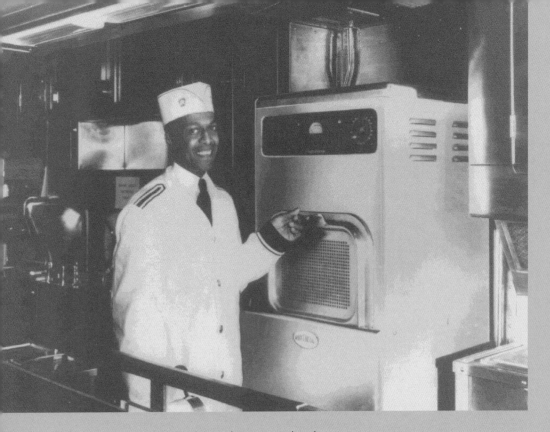

The first microwave ovens were large and expensive and used mainly in institutional kitchens: cruise ships, resorts, and trains.

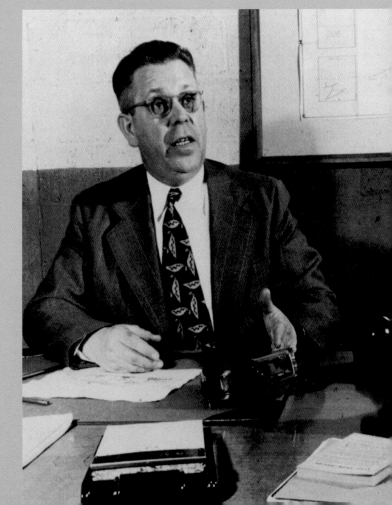

The core of a microwave oven is a magnetron (sitting on Spencer's desk), a tube that creates a high-frequency electromagnetic field.

needed, it could take a machinist a week to build just one magnetron. Spencer was given the task of speeding up this process. Using the British design, his workers at Raytheon were able to make about 100 a day. Still, that wasn't nearly enough. So Spencer redesigned the magnetron, creating a model that was much easier to build. Soon, Raytheon was producing 2,600 magnetrons a day.

Spencer's redesigned magnetron also led to more sensitive radar systems; when his system was installed in U.S. bombers, it could detect an object as small as a German submarine's periscope. For his radar work, the navy awarded him the Distinguished Public Service Award, its highest honor for a civilian.

This extensive experience with magnetrons let Spencer quickly see why his chocolate bar had melted. And while other scientists had noticed that microwaves could make things heat up, only Spencer thought to use them to cook food. It was a conceptual leap, since microwaves heat food in a completely different way than conventional ovens.

Normal cooking works by thermal conduction—the heat produced by gas, electricity, or fire starts at the outside of the food and moves in, "conducted" by the food itself. Microwave cooking, on the other hand, does not begin with heat. Microwaves move freely through food (and many other substances); as they do, they excite the molecules in water and fat. The excited molecules vibrate, which produces friction between them. That friction, in turn, produces heat, which actually cooks the food. (It's a myth that microwaves cook from the inside out; they simply cook everything at once.)

Raytheon's first microwave oven, called the "Radarange," was huge and primitive—essentially a large, liquid-cooled magnetron pointed directly into a metal box. About the size of a refrigerator, weighing hundreds of pounds, and priced at $2,000 to $3,000, the few that sold went to restaurants, the military, and railroads. In the 1950s, Raytheon and the Tappan company produced a smaller model for $1,295; this also failed commercially.

Success came only after Japanese engineers had shrunk the magnetron to a size that would fit in a small box. In 1967, the Amana appliance company (which Raytheon had bought a couple of years earlier) introduced the first compact microwave oven. At $495, it was affordable for many families. And although the new methods of cooking frightened a lot of people, by 1975 microwave ovens were outselling gas ranges.

While microwaves may never replace conventional ovens, Spencer's accidental invention has made its way into some 90 percent of the kitchens in America.

TRANSPORTATION

INTRODUCTION

Although the quote is often attributed to Isaac Newton, it was in fact the thirteenth-century English cleric and noodler Roger Bacon who said, of innovative thinkers like himself: "We stand on the shoulders of giants." In different ways, this group of change-makers represents that view of invention: What comes from their endeavors is only the latest improvement in a long historical series of gradual development. This is not to denigrate in any way the essential value of any single innovation. Far from it. In one sense, the latest high-tech plasma torch or electrophoretic technique is part of a continuum that started with the first flint tool. No invention comes, like Minerva, fully formed from the brow of Zeus. Each represents the final piece of a local section of a jigsaw puzzle. Even the great Thomas Edison might have failed in his light-bulb efforts had it not been for a newly developed air pump from the lab of German chemist Hermann Sprengel. That pump made possible the high vacuum inside Edison's bulb on which the consequent longevity of his burning filament depended.

The innovative continuum reaching back into history is comprehensive in scope. One example of a sequence taken from it will illustrate the point: The cams used in medieval gearing mechanisms (working mills of all kinds) were later adapted as pegs on the surface of a cylinder spun by waterpower to trigger devices that would automate the motion of automata or control and direct the flow of fountains in Renaissance water gardens. One of the most famous was at the Villa d'Este in Tivoli, outside Rome, where cam-controlled machinery caused statues to move, music to be played, and fountains to weave fantastic patterns in spray. Failure of the pumps used to lift the well water required for the gardens led to investigation by such luminaries as Galileo Galilei and his pupil Evangelista Torricelli, whose subsequent discovery of air pressure and then of the vacuum would eventually make possible James Watt's improved steam engine, which used the combination of vacuum inside a cylinder and air pressure outside it to move the cylinder piston up and down. The steam engine in turn made possible the locomotive, in one form developed by the Swedish inventor John Ericsson, who went on to fame (if not fortune) as the designer of the *Monitor* and the first American ironclads. By the time these had developed into late-nineteenth-century all-metal ships, their navigators were beginning to have problems with the effect of an iron hull on their compasses. This problem was solved through the adoption of the gyrocompass, which depends for its accuracy on inertia rather than magnetism. And by a touch of the serendipity with which innovation is rife, the gyrocompass was developed by Elmer Sperry (who appears in this book), one of the many inventors whose technology was a direct descendant of the medieval millwheel.

This group of inventors, however, shares another, particularly American, aspect. All belong to a "can-do" American tradition first formally noted in a British Parliamentary Committee report of 1841, which warned parliamentarians of the real danger that one day the mighty British industrial machine would be overtaken by that of the United States, thanks to "the American system of manufacture," of which Henry Ford is a prime example. From the early years of the Republic, without the restrictive old European craft practices to hold them back, Americans embraced the use of labor-saving machinery as did no other Western nation. They were encouraged in this by a scarce labor market. When most male immigrants headed away from the coast to buy cheap land and become farmers, the only readily available labor pool left in the East was made up of women without craft experience. So, machines were developed that could operate in semiautomatic mode, requiring only unskilled (female) machine-minders.

This readiness to adapt to circumstance is one of America's most enduring characteristics and is what makes the American social environment more amenable to innovation than any other, because America sees change as an opportunity rather than a threat. This attitude is rooted in America's past. The frontier was no place for the suffocating grip of accepted practices. Self-help was the only way out of most local problems, and resulted in such great inventions as barbed wire.

The Victorian writer and reformer Samuel Smiles made the innovative loner a hero, less in his native Britain than in America. Smiles's biographies of engineers helped create the role model of the individual problem-solver working to improve the daily life of ordinary people. In the nineteenth century great innovative effort was expended on matters relating to transportation, as the country grew and expanded: railroads, automobiles, bridges. Much in the same vein, in the twentieth century this group of inventors' efforts ranged from essential but everyday necessities like the traffic signal, to exotic examples of derring-do such as the solar-powered airplane, to the grand scale of the interplanetary launch vehicle.

This group of inventors also belongs to the tradition, born of the American system of manufacture, of helping to provide society with a democracy of possessions. Ford took a production-line concept originating with the British Royal Navy (and at the time not taken up elsewhere in British industry) to make automobiles that would be cheap enough for everybody to own. Ole Evinrude upgraded ordinary people's leisure time with an affordable outboard motor. By such unglamorous advances is the quality of life enhanced.

—JB

OLE **EVINRUDE**

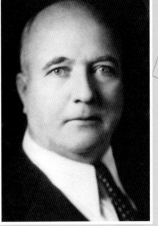

On a hot August afternoon in 1906, Ole Evinrude went for a lakeside picnic with some friends and his fiancée, Bess Cary. The party had rowed two and a half miles out to a small island in the Wisconsin lake when Bess said that she'd really like some ice cream. Evinrude, already devoted to his future wife and business partner, jumped back in the boat and rowed to shore to fetch some. As he struggled in the heat on the five-mile round trip, he had an idea: Someone should invent a motor for his boat. That someone, it turned out, was Evinrude himself. He already had experience building small gasoline engines, and by the next summer he had built his first outboard motor, the prototype for hundreds of thousands of motors that have changed the face of aquatic transportation.

Until that moment of ice cream–inspired invention, Ole Evinrude's life had been typical of the late-nineteenth-century immigrant experience. The first of his parents' 11 children, he was born in 1877 on a small farm in Norway, about 60 miles from Oslo. His father was a practical and frugal farmer; his mother, who tended the farmhouse and the children, was descended from a family of blacksmiths. Evinrude's earliest memories from Norway were, appropriately, of local marine activity. "What I remember first in my life is the lake nearby," he said later, "playing on its shores and watching the boats." When he was five years old, Evinrude's family moved to America. His second memory is of that voyage from Norway: "My mother and grandmother were constantly fishing me out of the engine room, only to have me dash back again. I couldn't possibly stay away from the engines." The family settled near a lake in Wisconsin, where there was already a sizable Scandinavian community. The young Evinrude helped out on the farm his father was homesteading and also attended two local schools—one taught in English, the other in Norwegian. But he stopped going after the third grade; he was needed on the farm, and he was also far ahead of his classmates. "I could do all the problems in the book up to the eighth grade," he recalled.

As Evinrude grew up, his thoughts remained with boats and engines. One of his uncles was a sailor, and on visits to the family he taught the boy how to distinguish the different kinds of ships. With money saved up from a job sorting tobacco, Evinrude subscribed to a magazine devoted to science and mechanics. Before he was 16, Evinrude tried to build his own sailboat, carving its parts out of scrap lumber. But when his father found the pieces in their woodshed, he threw them into the fire, feeling that they were a waste of money and time. Undaunted, Evinrude started his boat over, this time hiding the parts around the farm. When his father was away for a few days, a little after Evinrude's 16th birthday, he assembled them into an 18-foot sloop.

This time, his father wasn't angry. He recognized his son's dedication and skill, and (after Evinrude began charging tourists a quarter for a sail on the lake that summer) his business sense, too. When the season was over, Evinrude took his earnings and set out for Madison, where he apprenticed at a farm machinery shop. With the job paying just $2.50 a week and room and board costing $3.50, his boating earnings turned out to be essential.

For the next several years, Evinrude worked in different kinds of factories throughout the industrial Midwest. He toiled in a steel rolling mill, made machine tools, and began working with the then new gasoline engine. In 1900, at the age of 23, Evinrude returned to Wisconsin, taking a job as a pattern-maker at a Milwaukee machine shop. At the same time, he was carrying on his own experiments with internal combustion engines, even firing one up in his boarding house room. Evinrude's landlady forced him to relocate his workshop to a nearby shed, where he managed to build a horseless carriage. Local accounts described that contraption as a "fearsome thing, with a bark like a sea lion and an exhaust that fogged the whole street with smoke."

Bess Cary lived next door to Evinrude's shed workshop, and the two developed a friendship. When Evinrude and another man founded a company to manufacture small engines, Bess typed their correspondence. The engine company was successful at first, selling 50 portable engines to the government. (It was those portable engines that helped Evinrude see the possibility

Evinrude's first motor was a simple machine: a small gasoline engine was mounted on top of a driveshaft that turned a propeller. A standard clamp attached the motor to the back of any boat.

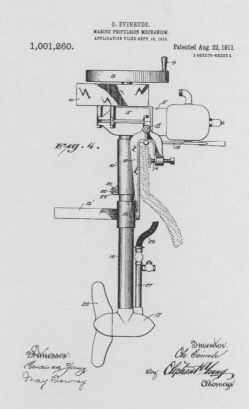

of a small motor for his row boat.) Bess and Ole did even better: In November 1906 they were married.

Evinrude's first company failed within a year or two, and
in a very short time he went through two other failed motor
companies. With a wife (and soon a son, Ralph) to support,
Evinrude went back to the more reliable occupation of pattern-
making, with Bess once again taking care of the business
correspondence. He was soon running a successful pattern
shop, yet in his few spare evening hours (and even when he was
bed-ridden with rheumatism) he would turn to his idea for a
portable boat motor.

The design Evinrude came up with was simple: A single-
cylinder gasoline engine turned a long, slender driveshaft, at
the bottom of which was a propeller. A clamp would hold the
motor to the flat back end of a boat. In the summer of 1907, he
proudly showed his first motor to his wife. She chastised him
for wasting the family's money on such a thing and declared
that it looked like a coffee grinder.

Bess Evinrude also saw the potential of her husband's invention, however. She encouraged him to refine the design, and
when one of Evinrude's employees put that engine on a boat the
next summer and put-putted around a local lake, her intuition
proved right: He returned with orders for 10 of them.

Evinrude was not the first person to think of the outboard
motor. In 1896, a New York company sold 25 "portable boat motors," and in 1905 a Detroit inventor, Cameron Waterman, began building his own motors, selling some 3,000 of them in
1907. But Evinrude's motor was more reliable, simpler to build,
and the first to be well promoted.

Evinrude began producing his motor in larger quantities in
1909, and by 1911 had entered into a partnership to found the
Evinrude Detachable Row Boat Motor Company. Perhaps more
important, in 1909, he advertised the motor for the first time,
with a slogan written by Bess: "Don't Row! Throw the Oars Away!
Use an Evinrude Motor." The ad was perfectly suited to the era.
With new technologies such as electricity and the automobile, it
was finally possible for people to be free of the drudgery of manual labor. And as Evinrude had learned on that quest for ice
cream, there was considerable boating labor to be freed from.

The ad campaign went national in 1911. That year, the company sold about 1,000 outboards; 4,650 were sold in 1912, and
9,412 in 1913. It seemed that Evinrude had found some permanent industrial success. But the effort to keep the business go-

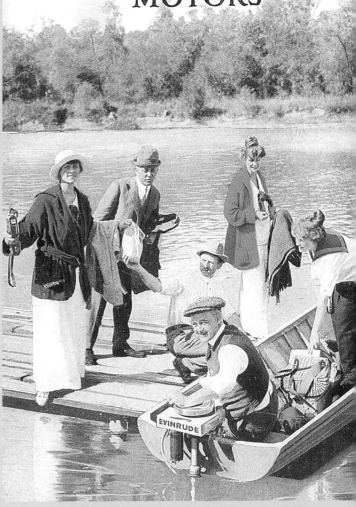

EVINRUDE
MOTORS

Inspiration for building an outboard motor struck Ole Evinrude
on a hot summer day, when he grew tired of rowing to an island
where he was picnicking.

ing had taken a serious toll on Bess Evinrude's health, and in early 1914, Ole sold his share of the company to his partner. Bess, Ole, and Ralph drove around the United States, settling in Florida and then New Orleans, where her health slowly improved.

Although Evinrude had agreed not to compete with his company for five years, by 1917 he was designing a new and better outboard motor. When the five years were up, he offered his new design—a lightweight two-cylinder engine made of aluminum—to Chris Meyer, his former partner. Meyer didn't want to give up on the proven success of the old model, however, and declined to buy Evinrude's new design. It was a fatal mistake; Evinrude started another company, Elto, and in 1920 began selling the new motor. It was a quick success, while the older Evinrude motor slowly lost market share.

The Elto engine had to compete with more than its Evinrude ancestor. In the five years of Ole Evinrude's exile, the outboard market had changed. Speed was becoming more important than simply getting around, and the new Johnson Motor Company's engines could propel a boat at up to 16 miles per hour, versus the Elto's 10 mph. The three companies were highly competitive, with Johnson and Elto continually refining their motors. In 1929, Elto merged with the old Evinrude company and another competitor to form the Outboard Motors Corporation (OMC). Six years later, during the depths of the depression, OMC bought Johnson, consolidating the industry.

In 1933, Bess Evinrude passed away, ending not only a marriage but also Ole Evinrude's most successful business partnership. He died a year later, a few months before his son orchestrated the purchase of Johnson. Ralph Evinrude led the company through the depression and on to greater success. Today, the Evinrude and Johnson brands live on as part of the Boats and Outboard Engines Division of Bombardier Motor Corporation of America, almost a century after its founder first grew tired of rowing.

When Evinrude's wife Bess fell ill, Evinrude left the outboard motor business. Idleness did not suit him, though, and he designed a lighter and more powerful motor. When Evinrude's original company rejected the motor, he founded a new firm, Elto.

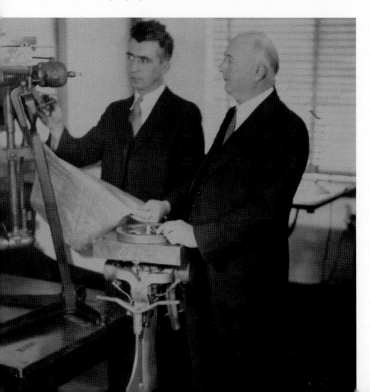

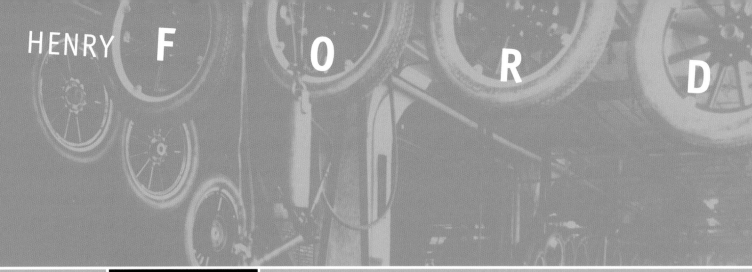

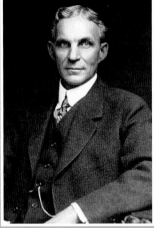

Henry Ford wasn't the first person to build an automobile. He was not even the first person to build an automobile in Detroit. Ford's genius wasn't in being there first, but in doing it best. The car that he introduced in 1908, the Model T, was better engineered, more reliable, and less expensive than its competitors. And the Model T was uniquely suited to Ford's real innovation: the moving assembly line. First introduced in 1913 and reaching its peak at Ford's River Rouge plant in the late 1920s, the assembly line changed forever how cars—and most other products—were made in America. With the new manufacturing process, Ford's workers could build a complete car in 93 minutes.

As befits an almost mythical giant of industry, the story of Ford's childhood and rise to car-making dominance is heroic. Ford was born in 1863 in the small town of Dearborn, Michigan. His father, William, was a farmer and carpenter who had emigrated from Ireland in the 1840s, fleeing that country's devastating potato famine. His mother, Mary, died in childbirth when Ford was 13. The Ford family farm was fairly prosperous, and Henry's childhood was typical for a boy in rural America. At the age of 7, he began attending the one-room school a mile away, while also tending to chores on the farm. In his own accounts of his youth, Ford described his fascination with machinery, learning how to fix clocks and watches and even traveling from farm to farm collecting timepieces to work on. He also spent considerable time tinkering with farm machinery.

When Ford was 16, he left the farm and moved to Detroit to apprentice at a machine shop. There he learned to use specialized machine tools to make all kinds of metal goods, from valves to fire hydrants. After three years he returned to Dearborn, where he fixed and demonstrated the new steam-powered tractors that were just arriving in Michigan. In 1888 he married Clara Bryant, and they settled on a small farm where Henry also ran a sawmill. They would not stay for long; three years later, Henry was offered a job with the Edison Illuminating Company in Detroit, and the couple moved to the city.

In early 1896, Ford was talking with some other engineers at Edison. A recent issue of a magazine had described how to build a gasoline engine and

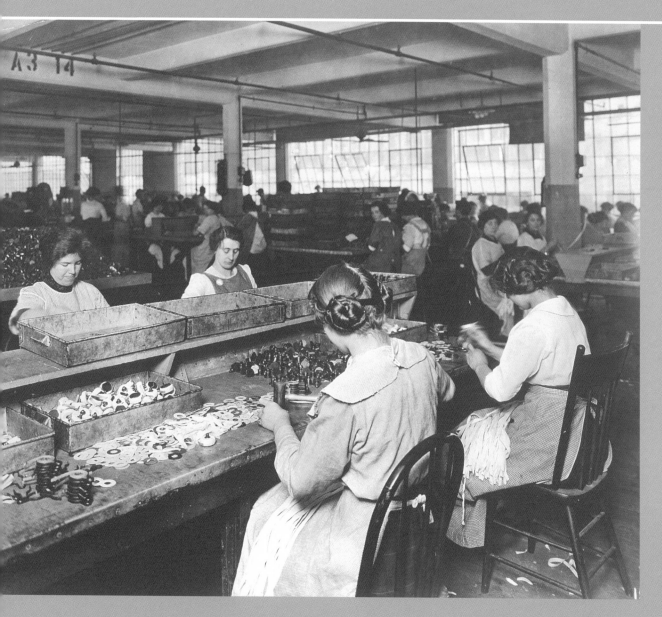

Ford's first assembly line made magnetos, a part of the Model T's ignition system. Each worker performed a specific task, over and over again.

Ford declared, "I want to build one of those." The engine featured was probably a version of the Otto engine, invented in Germany in 1876. About ten years later, two Germans, Karl Benz and Gottlieb Daimler, had independently adapted the engine to a carriage, creating the first self-propelled gasoline vehicles. By the time Ford saw the magazine story, automobiles were being made in Germany, France, and the United States.

In March 1896, Charles King, a friend of Ford's, wheeled his horseless carriage onto the streets of Detroit. Ford bicycled alongside as King accelerated to five miles per hour. But Ford was also working on his own automobile, which he completed that June. The Quadricycle had a two-cylinder gas engine, rode on four large bicycle wheels, and was steered, like a boat, with a tiller. After having to tear down a wall of his garage workshop to get it out, he, Clara, and their new son, Edsel, motored around the streets of Detroit.

Ford left the Edison company and helped found two automobile companies, both of which failed. Like many early carmakers, he also raced his own cars, and in 1901, Ford upset the speed-record-holding French champion. The fame the victory brought helped Ford start another company, and for the next several years he and his partners built ever more refined automobiles.

The Ford Motor Company was just one of thousands of small operations producing cars. Almost all of these cars were produced by hand, with skilled mechanics spending hours or days casting and altering parts and coachmakers custom-building chassis and bodies. These hand-made cars were expensive, the playthings of the rich. Ford sensed that there was a much larger market for the automobile, and by 1906 he was designing cars that could be sold at a reasonable price.

The result of this work was the Model T, unveiled in 1908. The new car had many advances—among them a cylinder block cast as one piece, an electric ignition system, and an enclosed body. Although at $825 it wasn't the cheapest car on the market, the Model T was a great value and orders flooded in. Ford sold almost 19,000 cars in 1909–1910, a figure that would jump to 78,440 during 1911–1912.

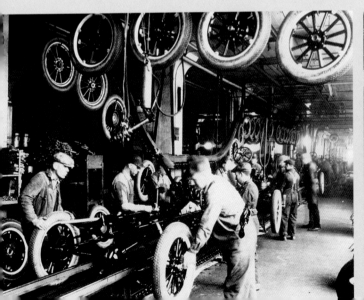

When it was fully up and running, Henry Ford's assembly line reduced the time it took to build a Model T from 14 hours to 93 minutes.

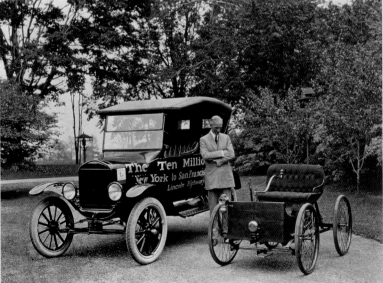

By 1924, the Ford Motor Company had sold ten million Model T's. A special car was driven from New York to San Francisco to commemorate the milestone. Here, Ford stands with that car and a model of his first, the 1896 Quadricycle.

The company could sell as many cars as it made. Assembling a car, though, was still a complicated process, requiring about 14 hours of skilled labor. More efficient manufacturing was needed. First, Ford made sure that every component made was identical, so no one had to waste time refitting or reshaping parts. He also hired Frederick Taylor, an efficiency expert, who carefully observed how people worked and suggested faster ways to do things.

Efficient mass production had been a dream of Ford's for a long time. "The way to make automobiles," he explained to a lawyer in 1903, "is to make them all alike . . . just as one pin is like another pin when it comes from a pin factory." Four years later he announced, "I will build a motor car for the great multitude. . . . It will be so low in price that no man making a good salary will be unable to own one—and enjoy with his family the blessing of hours of pleasure in God's great open spaces."

A worker typically built an entire component, like the ignition system's magneto, by himself, moving about the factory floor to collect its parts. In 1913, Ford introduced another way to do it. Inspired by the continuously moving racks of animal carcasses in a slaughterhouse, he devised a moving assembly line. A worker stayed in one place and did just one or two things to components moving by on a conveyor belt. The first assembly line was for magnetos, a component of the electrical system; one man would bolt a part on, then the component would move to the next man, who would add another part. In about 13 minutes, a complete magneto emerged.

After Ford built another moving assembly line for engines, a problem arose: The engines were being built much faster than the chassis and bodies. The logical next step was to install moving assembly lines throughout the factory. Every worker now stood in place and added a bolt or a part or something similarly small. The bodies moved along hung from chains; when done, they were lowered onto the chassis, complete with engine and interior, which were built on another line. The new process was almost 90 percent more efficient than the old way; at its peak, Ford was producing a Model T every 93 minutes.

Highly efficient production allowed Ford to cut prices, and then cut them some more, to a low of about $360 for a basic car. Although the profit margin on a single car was small, the huge volume of sales more than made up for it. Ford became one of the richest men in the world. In 1914, those profits allowed Ford to take one of his most famous actions, raising his workers' daily wages to $5, almost twice what he had been paying them. His rationale was that all of his workers should be able to afford the cars they built. Ford received great press, and many of his workers did indeed buy Ford cars.

In 1927, when the company introduced the Model A, Ford took the principles of control over production to an unprecedented level. He had bought coal mines in Kentucky, iron mines in Michigan, and a rubber plantation in Brazil in order to become independent of almost all outside suppliers. At the company's new River Rouge factory near Detroit, Ford built not only an assembly line but also blast furnaces to turn the iron and coal into steel, and a plant to turn the rubber into tires. The ideal of the self-sufficient operation that Ford may have learned as a boy on his family's homesteaded farm was finally realized in the world's biggest industrial complex.

The River Rouge plant was Ford's last great triumph. He spent his later years battling for control within the company and resisting, sometimes violently, attempts at unionization. Ford also turned to philanthropic causes. Ford built vocationally oriented schools for rural children, sponsored a homespun radio show, and built Greenfield Village, a mock small town that recreated America's agrarian and small-industrial past. He died in 1947, two years after his grandson, Henry Ford II, assumed control of the company. Today, Ford is still run by the family; William Clay Ford, Jr., was named chairman in 1999 and has since been credited with making the company "greener."

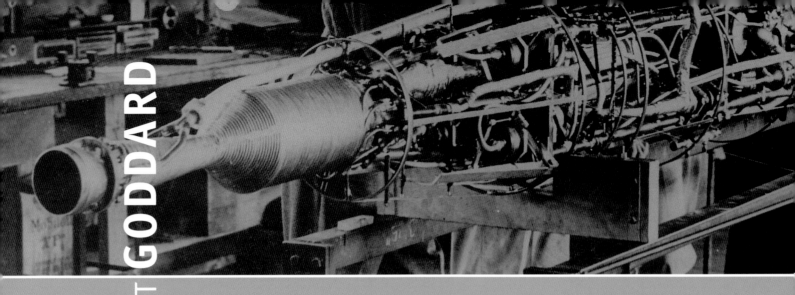

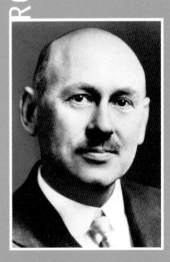

On October 19, 1899, Robert Goddard climbed a cherry tree in his yard and had a vision that would define his career and eventually send men to the moon. A year after being enthralled by H. G. Wells's interplanetary science-fiction tale *The War of the Worlds*, the 17-year-old Goddard imagined traveling through space himself. "As I looked to the fields at the east," he later wrote, "I imagined how wonderful it would be to make some device which had even the *possibility* of ascending to Mars."

Although Goddard's idea that day of how get to Mars was wrong—it involved using centrifugal force—the epiphany changed him. "I was a different boy when I descended the tree," he continued. "Existence at last seemed very purposive." Goddard pursued that vision for the next 45 years, building and launching rockets and devising the basic concepts of rocketry and space flight—concepts used in all succeeding rockets, from Germany's V-2 missiles of World War II, to the Saturn V that took men to the moon, to the boosters that launch satellites today.

Although his ascent into the cherry tree was a turning point in Goddard's career, it was far from his first thought of flight. Born in 1882 to parents whose roots in America went back to Puritan settlers, Robert Goddard grew up in a house where scientific and technological progress was always prized. His father, Nahum Goddard, was an occasional inventor and early adopter of late-nineteenth-century advances such as electricity. Goddard himself began experimenting at an early age; when he was just five, he tried using static electricity and zinc from a battery to enable him to jump very high, and in high school he attempted to melt aluminum to create a balloon. (Neither experiment worked.)

Goddard's investigations became more focused, and more successful, in college. Beginning as an undergraduate at the Worcester Polytechnic Institute, Goddard worked to understand the challenges of flight, especially rocket flight. He continued his education at Clark University, where he earned his master's in 1910 and his doctorate in 1912. There were two main problems facing him: the general belief that nothing could be propelled in the vacuum of

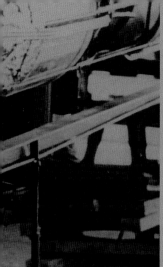

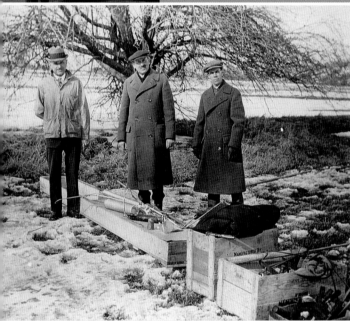

In December 1925, Robert Goddard fired the first liquid-fueled rocket that could lift its own weight—it moved about an inch. Four months later, he traveled to his aunt's farm in Auburn, Massachusetts, to set up a bigger rocket.

That rocket, seen here on its launch frame, emitted a flame and a steady roar and then began to rise, eventually reaching a height of 41 feet during its two-and-a-half-second flight.

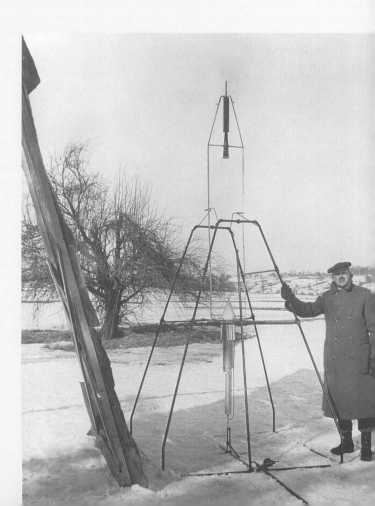

The press- and publicity-shy Goddard moved his research to Roswell, New Mexico, in 1930. His wife, Esther, filmed this launch of a rocket code-named Nell in August 1937.

space, and the limited power of black powder, the fuel then used for projectiles. In 1907 he proved mathematically that a rocket could work in a vacuum—Newton's third law of thermodynamics, "For every action there is an equal and opposite reaction," still applied. And in 1909 Goddard hit upon a solution to the problem of fuel. Liquid fuels, like liquid hydrogen and oxygen, could increase a rocket's power tenfold or more. Unfortunately, neither fuel was available at the time. (Unknown to Goddard, a Russian named Konstantin Tsiolkovsky, also keenly interested in space flight, had come up with a similar idea a few years earlier.)

In 1914, after recovering from tuberculosis, Goddard became a professor of physics at Clark University. That year he also received two patents, one for a rocket using liquid fuel, the other for a multistage rocket. The next year, he set up a vacuum chamber in his lab and ignited a rocket in it, proving empirically that an engine could work in the absence of air.

In the mid-1910s Goddard first confronted one of the major non-technical challenges that would plague much of his career: money. Rocketry was an expensive pursuit, and his experiments soon drained his resources. In 1917, he finally received a small grant ($5,000) from the Smithsonian Institution to continue his studies; the funds would continue through 1929. In 1919, he submitted a report detailing his expenditures and outlining his progress. The report also suggested, probably in jest, that one way to prove his theories was to send a rocket equipped with flash powder to the moon. When humans saw the flash, they'd know it worked. The report, "A Method of Reaching Extreme Altitudes," was published in late 1919, and reached the press in early 1920.

Goddard was unprepared for the reaction to his seemingly obscure paper. Journalists latched on to his idea to send a rocket to the moon, dubbing the scientist "Moon Man" and running headlines such as "Modern Jules Verne Invents Rocket to Reach Moon." The *New York Times* ran a skeptical editorial that attacked him personally: "Professor Goddard does not know the relation of action to reaction, and of the need to have something better than a vacuum against which to react. . . . Of course he only seems to lack the knowledge ladled out daily in high schools."

For the rest of his career, Goddard was publicity-shy, avoiding the press and working in out-of-the-way places. But he continued to work. Goddard spent the early 1920s designing and

refining rocket engines that used liquid fuel. In December 1925, he fired a rocket that could lift its own weight—a crucial test. It moved only about an inch, but, Goddard wrote, "it shows that a larger rocket constructed on the same plan could raise itself to considerable altitudes."

Four months later, on March 16, 1926, he journeyed to his aunt's farm in Auburn, Massachusetts. There he set up a larger liquid-fuel rocket, a thin, spindly looking device about ten feet tall. At the bottom of the rocket were tanks holding gasoline and liquid oxygen. Fuel lines ran to the top of the rocket frame, to a combustion chamber. The two fuels combined in the chamber and were ignited by a flame; the exhaust, expelled through a nozzle, provided thrust. That afternoon he lit the rocket; for a few seconds the engine just roared, then it slowly lifted off the ground. The world's first liquid-fueled rocket flew for about two and a half seconds and achieved a maximum height of 41 feet. In his notes, Goddard wrote, "It looked almost magical as it rose . . . as if it said: 'I've been here long enough. I think I'll be going somewhere else, if you don't mind.'"

It was a humble beginning for space flight, but more experiments, both successes and failures, followed. In 1930, Goddard moved his research to Roswell, New Mexico, to avoid prying eyes. There he devoted himself full-time to refining his rockets and soon introduced such innovations as gyroscopic stabilization and fins in the path of the rocket's blast to keep it stable. The rockets grew larger and faster, too. In 1935, one flew faster than the speed of sound, and two years later a rocket reached 9,000 feet, the highest launch of Goddard's career.

Goddard always believed that his rockets had important military uses. During World War I, he worked with the army to develop small rockets and launchers, innovations that eventually produced the bazooka. As World War II approached, he became worried about German rocket research; he knew German scientists had been eager followers of his work. When he approached the army about using his rockets as weapons, though, he was turned away. They did not see any practical potential in his inventions. Instead, Goddard was put to work designing jets to assist planes as they took off.

The German military, on the other hand, saw plenty of potential in rocketry. Led by Wernher von Braun, German scientists used Goddard's patents to design the V-2 rocket, a powerful weapon with a range of up to 200 miles. Flying extremely fast and at a great altitude, the V-2 was impossible to defend against.

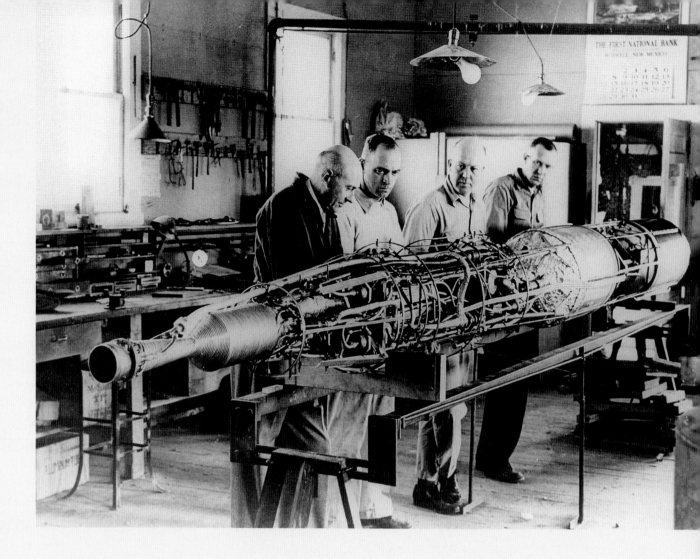

KONSTANTIN TSIOLKOVSKY—THE FATHER OF SPACE TRAVEL

Although Robert Goddard was a rocketry visionary, sending the world's first liquid-fueled rockets more than a mile into the sky, many of his ideas were first thought of by Konstantin Tsiolkovsky, a deaf schoolteacher working in provincial Russia. But while Tsiolkovsky developed some of these concepts first, he was interested not in rocket propulsion itself, but where it could take people. From the time he was a teenager, he dreamed of space flight and man's eventual life in space.

Born in Ijevskoe, Russia, in 1857, Tsiolkovsky was one of 18 children in a modest farm family. At the age of 10 he lost his hearing as a result of scarlet fever, which prevented him from finishing school. He continued to read on his own, though, and in 1880 he

became a math and physics teacher in a public school while continuing his investigations into both science and philosophy.

From the 1880s until his death in 1935, Tsiolkovsky published dozens of papers and books about his scientific ideas. His 1897 paper, "Exploration of Outer Space with Reactive Devices," laid out the basic idea of humans using rockets to travel through space. Six years later, he wrote a paper outlining spacecraft that used the reaction of liquid hydrogen and liquid oxygen for thrust—several years before Goddard made the same discovery.

Tsiolkovsky's work was always theoretical—he never built any of the rockets or ships he discussed. But his theories were far ahead of his time. In one paper, he drew a spacecraft that looks

The first rockets were launched against Paris and London in September 1944; before the war ended, about 1,100 V-2s were used, killing some 2,800 people.

Robert Goddard died in August 1945, just days before the end of the war. His work was continued by the army, however, which had finally seen the promise of rockets. In the years following the war, they launched 67 captured V-2s and began developing a new generation of missiles. The V-2 tests led to the Redstone and Jupiter rockets, which in turn led to the massive, multistage Saturn rocket that powered America's Apollo launches.

Recognition for Goddard's pioneering achievements did come, but only long after he died. Today he is widely regarded as the father of rocketry, and NASA's first space flight research facility, the Goddard Space Flight Center, located in Greenbelt, Maryland, was named after him. Even the *New York Times* eventually came around. On July 17, 1969, three days before Neil Armstrong and Buzz Aldrin walked on the moon, the paper's editorial page noted "it is now definitely established that a rocket can function in a vacuum as well as in an atmosphere. The *Times* regrets the error."

A late-model rocket without its casing sits on its assembly frame in Roswell in 1940. Goddard, at far left, inspects it with three of his colleagues: Nils Ljungquist, Albert Kisk, and Charles Mansur.

remarkably modern: An astronaut sits at the front of a long rocket filled with hydrogen and oxygen. He conceived of steering vanes much like Goddard's later versions, pressurized cabins and space suits, gyroscopic stabilization, and air locks to permit entering and leaving a ship. He also had a vision for permanent human outposts in space, including space stations that spun to simulate gravity and closed biological systems that could provide food and oxygen.

After the Russian Revolution in 1917, other scientists began to notice and pursue some of his ideas. When the Soviet space program was in its heyday, from the launch of Sputnik in 1957 through the Soyuz missions of the 1970s, Tsiolkovsky was a na-

tional hero. It is still remarkable how many of his ideas and predictions have become reality—the U.S. space shuttles, for example, rely on essentially the same kind of engine he sketched out in 1903, and the International Space Station has confirmed his early vision of a habitat continuously orbiting the Earth.

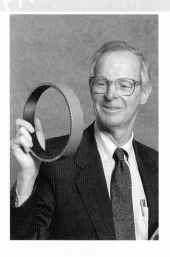

Anyone who happened to be on the English Channel on the morning of June 12, 1979, must have done a double take. Moving slowly through the air, just a few feet above the choppy waters, was one of the oddest looking flying machines ever built. Almost 100 feet wide and sheathed in a shiny, semitransparent skin, the craft, called the *Gossamer Albatross*, had a big propeller at its back but no engine to speak of. Instead, in an enclosed pod hanging beneath its huge wing, was Bryan Allen, a bicycle racer, furiously pedaling to make the improbable craft go. After almost three hours of physical effort, and covering more than 22 miles, Allen gently landed the plane on the beaches of England. The *Albatross*'s inventor, Paul MacCready, who had been in a boat following the slow, tense journey from the shores of France, rushed to join the celebration.

Men have dreamed of flying under their own power for thousands of years. A Greek myth tells of Icarus, whose father Daedalus built wings of feathers and wax so the two of them could fly like birds. The dream was revived in the Renaissance, when Leonardo da Vinci sketched complicated machines that would allow men to fly. After the Wright Brothers built their first airplane in 1903, the search for a way to fly without a motor entered a new phase. Throughout the twentieth century, experimenters built a succession of human-powered planes, most of which never left the ground.

Although he didn't begin building a human-powered airplane until he was 51 years old, Paul MacCready had been involved with flight for most of his life. As a boy growing up in New Haven, Connecticut, he was fascinated with butterflies and moths, and his interests soon included model airplanes, too. His first model plane came from a kit, but after that he was building his own, from balsa wood and microfilm and glue. He didn't build only standard aircraft. "For some reason I got interested in a variety of things," he says. "Ornithopters, autogyros, helicopters, indoor models, outdoor models. Nobody seemed to be quite as motivated for the new and strange as I was."

Paul MacCready's second human-powered airplane, the
Gossamer Albatross, flew across the English Channel in June 1979,
pedaled and piloted by Bryan Allen.

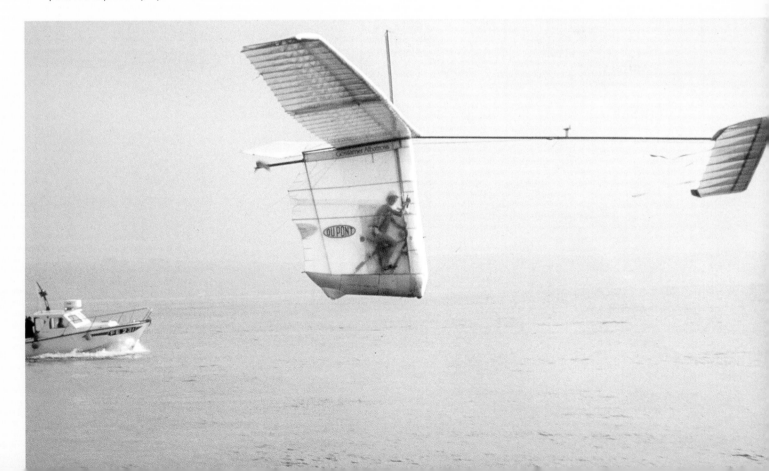

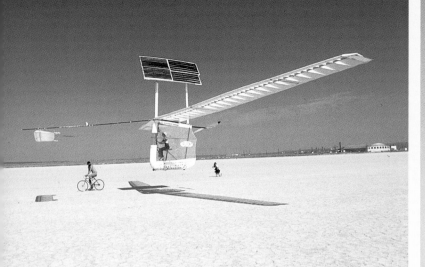

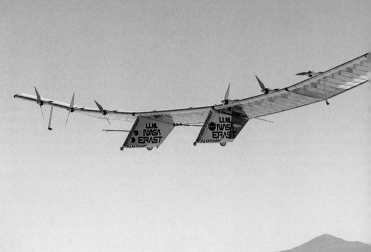

After the success of the *Albatross*, MacCready began to work on the challenge of solar-powered flight. His first solar plane was the *Gossamer Penguin*, here on a test flight at NASA's Dryden Flight Research Center.

The *Pathfinder*, a lightweight, solar-powered, remotely piloted flying wing made its first flight in 1994. Though it flew at only 15 to 20 mph, it could stay in the air for great lengths of time and in 1997 reached an altitude of 71,500 feet.

FLYING A DINOSAUR

Paul MacCready has made a career of flying things that shouldn't fly. The aviation challenge he took up in 1984, though, was very different from the flights of the *Gossamer Albatross* and the *Pathfinder*. Rather than exploring a new way to fly, he and his team at AeroVironment set out to resurrect a 65-million-year-old flyer, the pterodactyl.

Pterosaurs, or flying dinosaurs, were the first large creatures to fly and may be the ancestors of today's birds. In 1972, paleontologists in Texas discovered the well-preserved fossils of the largest pterosaur known, *Quetzalcoatlus northropi*, which had a wingspan of 36 feet. In 1980, MacCready heard about the fossil, went to see it, and came away amazed that it could fly at all; its large size pushed its flight to the edge of physical possibility. By 1983, after more study, he became convinced that he could build an air-worthy model of *Quetzalcoatlus*.

The money to build such a flying dinosaur came in 1984, in the form of a commission from the Smithsonian's National Air and Space Museum, which was preparing to make an IMAX movie, *On the Wing*, relating manned and natural flight. With sponsorship from the Smithsonian and the Johnson Wax Company, MacCready got to work.

Figuring out how a pterodactyl flew was a difficult task. The dinosaurs had no tails, so how they steered and maintained stability was a bit of a mystery. (It was "like trying to fly an arrow with the tail feathers in front," according to the director of the project.) Making a model's wings flap realistically and with enough power to lift it was an even bigger challenge. Technology and intensive aerodynamic study came to the rescue. MacCready's team used lightweight carbon-fiber tubes to build a skeleton, small motors to control its wings, and a sophisticated computer

After winning several model plane competitions, Mac-Cready graduated to sailplanes, gliders built to soar and maneuver in the wind. "It's a very scientific sort of hobby," he recently told an interviewer. "It's not just like going out and rowing a boat. You get involved in the science of the vehicle, because the vehicle has to be efficient." When he was 23, he won the U.S. National Soaring Championship.

During World War II MacCready trained to be a navy pilot, but he never flew in combat. After the war, he returned to his education, though, he recognizes now, he struggled with a mild form of dyslexia. In 1947 he earned a degree in physics at Yale, then went on to receive his Ph.D. in aeronautics from the California Institute of Technology in 1952. Although flying was still one of his great passions, MacCready didn't want to join a big aeronautics or engineering firm. "There were already enough brilliantly qualified people working in aerospace," he says, "and the typical projects were big things where they'd hire another acre of engineers and they'd work on something where in seven years it would fly. It's kind of hard to get motivated." In a smaller operation, he adds, "a person can make a much greater contribution to society." After CalTech he cofounded Meteorology Research, a company that pioneered weather modification, including cloud seeding. In 1970 he left to start another company, AeroVironment, to focus on new energy sources such as solar and wind power.

It was bad news that got MacCready working on human-powered flight. He had guaranteed a loan for a relative's business. It failed, and he was stuck with a $100,000 debt. Daydreaming one day in 1976, he recalled that there was a cash prize for a successful human-powered flight: the Kremer Prize, with an award of £50,000. With the British pound worth about two dollars at the time, he remembers, "the Kremer Prize, in which I'd had no interest, was just about equal to my debt. Suddenly human-powered flight seemed important."

MacCready began thinking of ways to build a plane that could win the prize, which required flying around a figure-eight course. (Other human-powered planes had flown, but they couldn't make turns.) The Aha! moment, as he calls it, came on a family vacation. On the side of the road, MacCready watched hawks and vultures in flight, calculating their flight speed and turning radius. He began thinking about how scaling—making something bigger or smaller—affects a wing's aerodynamic lift.

In 1986, MacCready built and flew a lifelike model of a pterodactyl, complete with beak, 18-foot wingspan, and a light coat of fur.

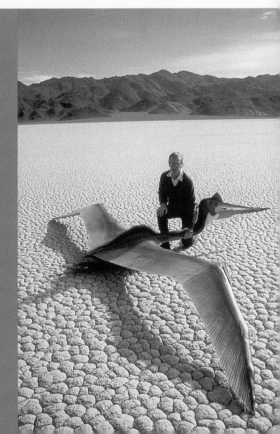

to control their flapping. The model pterodactyl's head and bill acted as a kind of rudder, and its wings were moved forward and back to give it lift and stability.

Their finished model, with an 18-foot wingspan and sporting fur and a realistic paint job, was tested in a wind tunnel and also mounted to the roof of a speeding van. In January 1986, after almost two years of work, experiment, and crashes, MacCready's pterosaur was ready to fly. With the flight team and a crew of IMAX filmmakers standing by, *Quetzalcoatlus* was launched into the blue sky above Death Valley, California. Soaring 500 feet into the air, the relic of the past gently glided through graceful turns above the craggy landscape, its re-created wings gently flapping and its long-billed head turning in the direction of its flight. Nothing, it seemed, is too ungainly or unlikely for MacCready to fly.

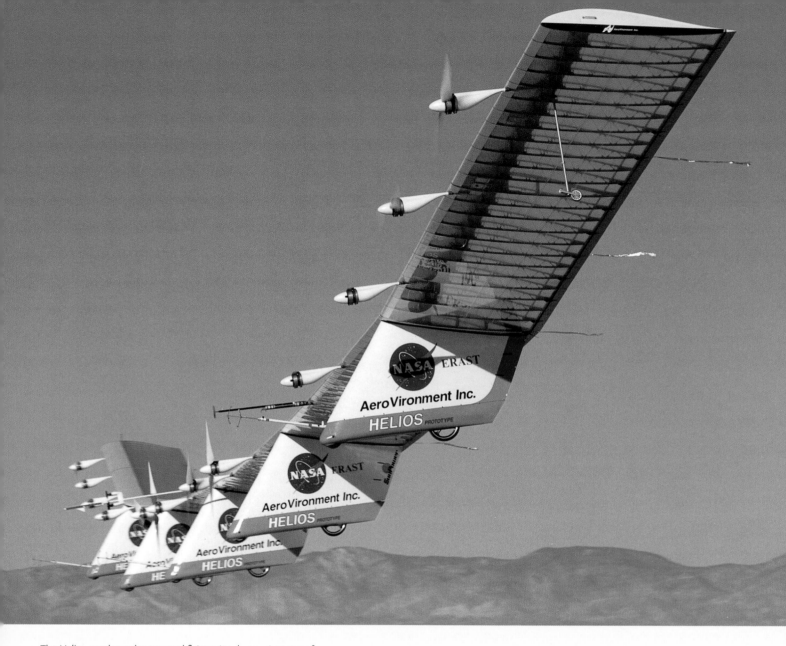

The *Helios*, another solar-powered flying wing, has a wingspan of
247 feet. It is meant to reach extremely high altitudes and stay
aloft for months at a time.

"For some reason I got interested in a variety of things," he says.
"Ornithopters, autogyros, helicopters, indoor models, outdoor
models. Nobody seemed to be quite as motivated for the new and
strange as I was."

He realized that as a wing is built bigger, it requires less power to keep it aloft. If built a lot bigger, it requires a lot less power. A very light, 96-foot-long wing (as big as a DC-9's) built like a hang glider's wing would only require about 0.4 horsepower to make it fly—about the power a good bicyclist can produce.

"I had the advantage of no background in aircraft structures," MacCready says. "So rather than being lured into doing airplane wings in standard ways, I just went back to fundamentals. How do you make a 96-foot wing that weighs practically nothing?" It took six months of sometimes nonstop work for MacCready and his team, made up of friends, colleagues, and family, to build the *Gossamer Condor*. They used simple materials that were light and could be fixed easily, including Mylar, piano wire, aluminum tubing, and lots of tape. When it was finished, the *Condor* weighed just 70 pounds, didn't look much like a plane, and didn't always act like one. (Bryan Allen, the pilot/engine, said flying it was "like pedaling a house.") On August 23, 1977, with Allen at the pedals, the *Condor* flew the Kremer course. Today, the *Gossamer Condor* hangs in the Smithsonian Institution's National Air and Space Museum, alongside the Wright Brothers' plane, the *Spirit of St. Louis,* and an Apollo Lander.

There was another prize to be won: The Kremer Prize's sponsor put up £100,000 for the first human-powered aircraft to cross the English Channel. With sponsorship from Dupont, which made his planes' Mylar skin, MacCready set about building a second plane, the *Gossamer Albatross*. Two years later the human-powered *Albatross* crossed the Channel.

From human power MacCready moved on to another challenge, harnessing the sun's energy. Building on the design and success of the first Gossamer planes, he constructed the *Gossamer Penguin*, which in 1980 became the world's first solar-powered airplane. The craft caught the eye of the Department of Defense, which wanted something that could stay up in the air for long periods of time. Eventually, the project was taken up by NASA, which was interested in creating an airborne platform for atmospheric observations. The unmanned *Pathfinder* soared to a height of 71,530 feet in 1997; its successor, the *Pathfinder Plus*, reached 80,201 feet in 1998. The next step in this evolution is the 200-foot-wide *Helios*, which might reach 100,000 feet and stay aloft for months at a time. MacCready envisions a fleet of these craft in the air permanently, serving as a high-performance communications platform.

In the late 1980s, MacCready applied his knowledge of solar power and aerodynamics at the ground level. Working with General Motors, he designed a solar-powered car, the Sunrayracer, for the World Solar Challenge race across Australia. Powered by 8,800 photovoltaic cells that covered its superaerodynamic body, the Sunrayer dominated the 1,867-mile race, winning by two full days and averaging 41 miles per hour. Although the light, low-slung car could never be called practical transportation, its success spurred GM's effort to create the Impact, the auto giant's first electric vehicle. The popularity of that prototype led to GM's EV-1, a production electric vehicle that can go from 0 to 60 mph in eight seconds.

MacCready is interested once again in model planes. For the past few years, he's been working on small aircraft with built-in cameras to send images back to the ground. "You are looking out as if you were a little creature inside," he explains. "You can soar with the birds. It's just like you're one of them." This new vehicle fits in perfectly with MacCready's interest in finding a balance between nature and technology. "The overall goal is a sustainable world," he says. "Not consuming nonreplenishable resources, not getting steadily more dependent on foreign oil, and not causing global climate change." How can a toylike plane that lets you fly with birds help reach those goals? "If I hadn't been doing the ornithopters 60 years ago there wouldn't have been a *Gossamer Condor* or *Albatross* or Impact car or a mandate in California on zero emission vehicles. It's a toy, but it's a pretty important toy."

The Sunrayer, a solar-powered car designed by MacCready and General Motors, won the first World Solar Challenge Race in 1987, averaging 41 mph over 1,867 miles.

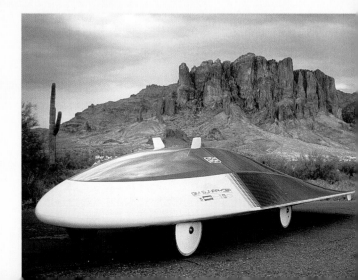

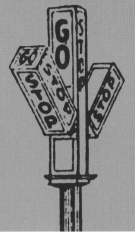

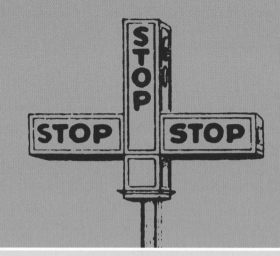

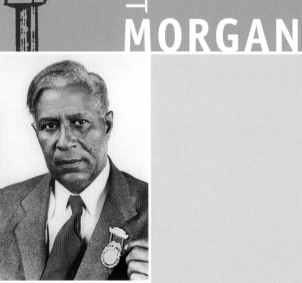

Most inventors wait for years or even their entire life for the chance to prove the value of their work. Not Garrett Morgan. On July 25, 1916, news came to the Cleveland businessman that disaster had struck—and Morgan had his chance. Thirty-two men building a tunnel beneath Lake Erie had been trapped by an explosion. The tunnel was full of debris, smoke, and toxic gases. Rescue parties had been sent in but had not returned. Morgan and his brother Frank rushed to the scene, equipped with a device he had invented four years earlier, the Safety Hood, a version of what is now called a gas mask.

His invention consisted of a large, heavy canvas hood fitted with small glass windows to see through. A long tube ran from the bottom of the hood to a pouch containing a sponge that could filter smoke, ammonia, and other dangerous substances from incoming air. (Morgan's inspiration for the hood and its long tube was seeing a circus elephant use its trunk to reach fresh air from inside a stifling hot big top.) The hood was big enough to hold enough air to breathe for at least 15 minutes, even when the filter was plugged up to keep dense smoke out.

Morgan and his brother donned Safety Hoods and entered the smoke-filled tunnel. After an agonizing wait, the two emerged, each carrying a worker on his back. Two other men joined them, and they went back into the tunnel for other survivors. Although many of the workers could not be saved, Morgan's rescue made him a hero in Cleveland, and his Safety Hood garnered national attention.

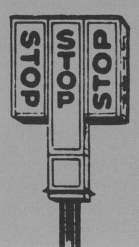

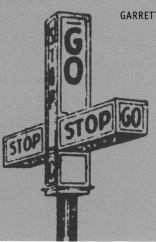

The Safety Hood was already known to fire departments around the country. In 1914 Morgan and his invention had won a gold medal at the Second International Exposition of Safety and Sanitation in New York, and testimonials of its usefulness had come from as far away as New Haven, Connecticut. But the wave of publicity following the Cleveland rescue was not necessarily a good thing. Garrett Morgan was black, and when white buyers of his hoods learned this, many canceled their orders. Morgan had known that the color of his skin might prevent people from buying his products; when he demonstrated the Safety Hood in New Orleans in 1914, he did so under an assumed name, "Big Chief" Mason, and claimed to be a "full-blooded Indian, from the Walpole Reservation in Canada." Although he had received a patent for the hood, he did not dare take public credit for the invention. However, when the Germans threatened to use chemical weapons during World War I, Morgan gave his patent to the U.S. government, which developed a gas mask based on his work.

Garrett Morgan was born in 1877 in Paris, Kentucky, to Sydney and Elizabeth Morgan, both former slaves. As a child, he attended a local school and worked on his parents' farm. Morgan dreamed of furthering his education, but in rural Kentucky there was little opportunity to do anything but farm. At the age of 14, he left home and headed north, working for a while in Cincinnati as a handyman, then moving to Cleveland in 1895. There he found work fixing sewing machines for a clothing manufacturer. Morgan worked for several sewing machine makers until 1907, when he had saved enough money to open his own shop selling and repairing sewing machines. It was the first of several businesses he would start.

Morgan's first big invention came two years later, after he had expanded his business to include a tailor's shop. (His wife was an accomplished seamstress.) He had noticed that sewing machine needles moved so fast that they sometimes scorched fabric. Morgan began to experiment with a variety of liquids that could polish a needle so it would sew smoothly and without friction. As he left his workshop one night after working with one such liquid, he wiped

Garrett Morgan's initial fortune came from selling hair-care products made specifically for the African American market. But while his work on the gas mask and traffic signal, among other things, was original, his cosmetic empire followed a path forged a few years before by Madame C. J. Walker, who may have been America's first black female millionaire.

Born Sarah Breedlove in rural Louisiana in 1867, Madame C. J. Walker—she adopted the last name and title during a brief marriage—worked as a washerwoman until 1905. That year, Walker claimed, she had a dream in which a treatment for African American women's hair was revealed to her. This treatment comprised a shampoo, a "hair grower," and a method for straightening hair. (Previously, many African American women straightened their hair with a flatiron.)

Madame Walker began selling her hair products in St. Louis in 1905, but she soon moved to Denver and gradually increased her business. One of the keys to Walker's success was her business model, which relied on door-to-door sales by a network of "Walker agents" that eventually spanned the entire country and parts of the Caribbean. This approach was successful for several reasons; for one, it allowed her to reach a commercially disenfranchised market, African American women. Face-to-face contact and personal demonstrations were also powerful enticements to buy her products. Many Walker customers also became agents, which helped business increase exponentially.

By the late 1910s, the Madame C. J. Walker Manufacturing Company had some 2,000 agents actively selling; her clients included celebrities such as Josephine Baker. Madame Walker's own fortune had increased beyond $1 million. Before she died in 1919, she made generous gifts to several philanthropic enterprises, including schools for African American girls. After Madame Walker's death, her daughter, A'Lelia, continued some of her mother's social activities, notably by holding an artists' and writers' salon in Walker's luxurious mansion in New York's Harlem. This salon, in part, helped kick-start the Harlem Renaissance, which flourished through the 1920s.

has hands dry on a piece of pony fur cloth. When Morgan returned, the fur had become straight and was sticking up. Intrigued, he applied the liquid to the wiry fur of a neighbor's dog. It, too, became straight. Next, Morgan tested it out on his own hair. It worked on humans, too, and Morgan soon christened the product G. A. Morgan Hair Refining Cream.

The G. A. Morgan Hair Refining Company was a big success. Morgan added several other products to its line, including hair dyes for men and women and a "hair-growing" cream. The company sold its goods by mail order and through a network of salespeople. With this business model, Morgan may have been emulating the success of Madame C. J. Walker, who had started a similar business a few years earlier in St. Louis. Walker and a small army of "agents" demonstrated and sold her hair straighteners and other beauty products door-to-door. Walker's products quickly became famous, and by the 1910s Madame C. J. Walker was a millionaire, one of the first African Americans to achieve such financial success.

While Morgan's hair-straightening cream didn't reach the level of success of Madame Walker's, it did make him one of Cleveland's most successful African American citizens. By the early 1920s, he was the proud owner of a new automobile, at a time when cars were still something of a novelty. The streets of Cleveland, as was the case in most American cities, were filled with horses, horse-drawn carriages, bicycles, pedestrians, and cars. One day in 1922, Morgan was driving his two young sons around town when they witnessed a horrible accident between a car and a horse-drawn carriage.

The shock of witnessing this accident quickly turned into a resolve to do something to prevent similar occurences. Efforts had already been made to control the flow of traffic. The most common solution was using a police officer to direct traffic, although that required a lot of labor and the officer was not visible over the roofs of cars. Some people had designed signals, but those usually had only "stop" and "go" settings. While these were useful, the inventor's granddaughter, Sandra Morgan, explains, "no one would know that the traffic pattern was about to change," which could lead to accidents.

Morgan's solution was the folding traffic signal. Mounted above traffic on a post, the signal had folding arms with "stop" and "go" written on their various sides. The arms folded into four different positions. When it was time for east-west traffic to move, for example, a traffic attendant would turn a crank at the

Garrett Morgan's first successful invention was a hair-straightening cream—he called it a "hair refiner"—which he sold by mail order and through a network of salespeople.

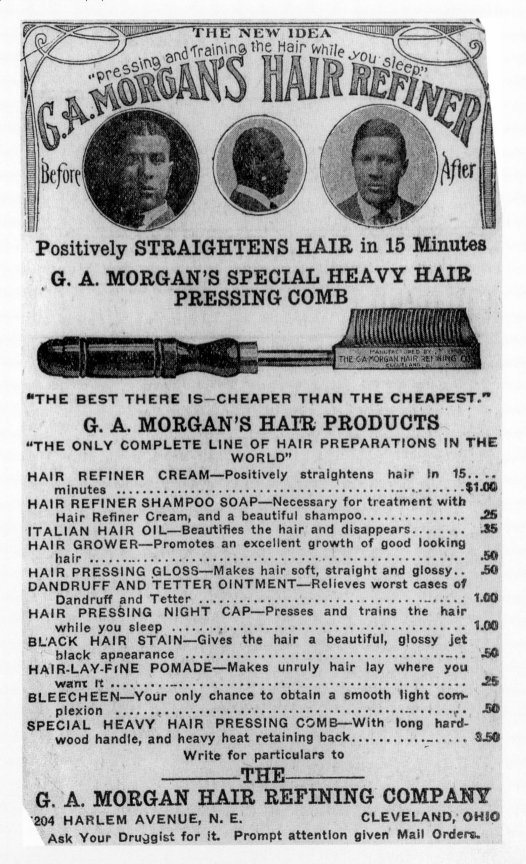

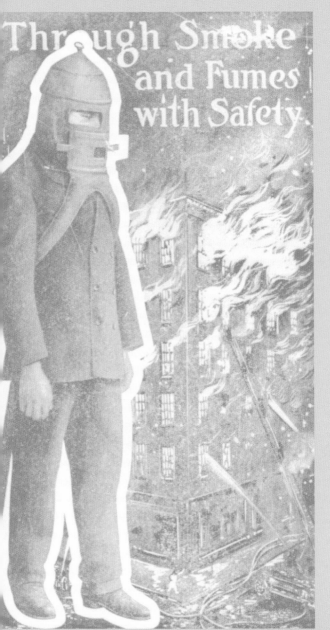

In 1912, Morgan invented the "safety hood," a forerunner of the gas mask. The hood completely covered a firefighter's head, to protect him from smoke and gases. Air was filtered through the hood's long "tail."

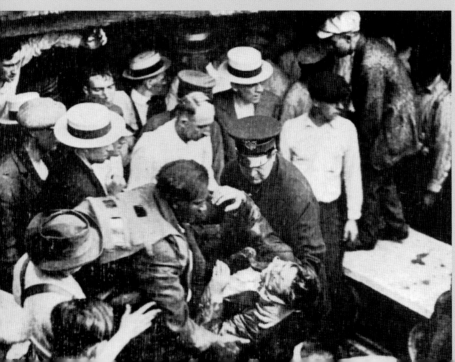

In July 1916, Morgan's safety hood was put to its greatest test, in a rescue of workers trapped in a mine beneath Lake Erie. Morgan and his brother donned hoods and rushed in to help; his action made him a hero.

base of the post and two signs saying "go" would be revealed. When north-south traffic needed to move, the folding signal would be rotated 90 degrees, and now three bold signs reading "stop" would face the east-west traffic. If pedestrians needed to cross, or traffic needed to be stopped for any reason, the sign could fold up to read "stop" in all four directions. Finally, the arms of the signal could be raised halfway between "go" and "stop," to indicate that motorists should proceed with caution. This was the ancestor of the yellow light in the middle of the modern traffic signal. A patent for the folding signal was issued in 1923, and Morgan soon sold the rights to General Electric for $40,000.

With the success of his hair products, the traffic signal, and his tailoring shop, among other ventures, Morgan had become a prominent and wealthy man. But he never forgot—or let others forget—that he had been born poor and had struggled against discrimination. "His big line was, 'I have not been well educated, but I am a graduate from the school of hard knocks and cruel treatment,'" recalls Sandra Morgan. And he always encouraged his children and grandchildren to pursue their education, insisting, "Work with your head, not with your hands."

Morgan's efforts at education and advancement were also directed at Cleveland's African American community. In 1920 he helped found a weekly newspaper, the *Cleveland Call*; in 1925 it became the *Call & Post*, and it is still published in several Ohio cities. In 1931 Morgan ran for a position on the Cleveland city council, and while he did not win, his candidacy established the black community as an important constituency. Although he faced several setbacks—the depression hit his business very hard, and in 1943 he lost most of his sight—he continued to both invent and work as a community leader until his death in 1963.

In 1922, after Morgan witnessed a horrible traffic accident, he turned his inventive mind to automobile safety. A year later, he was awarded the first patent for a traffic signal.

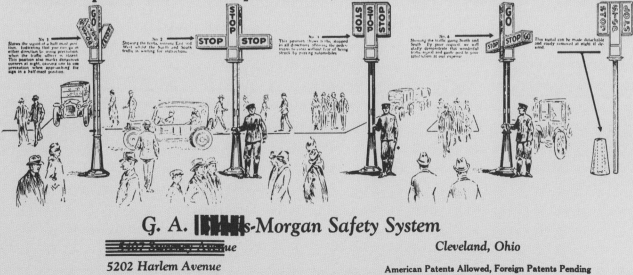

A better protection for the pedestrian, school children and R.R. crossing

G. A. ▮▮▮▮s-Morgan Safety System

5202 Harlem Avenue

Cleveland, Ohio

American Patents Allowed, Foreign Patents Pending

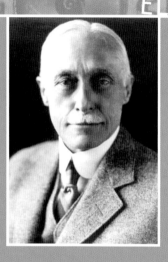

Sailors have been using magnetic compasses to find their way since the twelfth century, first with natural lodestone and later with magnetized needles. In the late nineteenth century, however, the invention of metal-hulled ships threatened this navigational necessity: All of that metal surrounding a compass made it erratic. The problem was worse in the submarines just being developed. And once the airplane was invented, it became clear that aerial navigation would pose an even more severe problem.

Around 1907, the engineer and lifelong inventor Elmer Sperry became interested in gyroscopes, which until then had been treated as a novelty. A gyroscope always spins in the direction of its original motion, until friction slows it down enough to make it unstable. Sperry used this property to create a gyroscopic compass that would always "point" north. He also used heavy gyroscopes to help ships resist rolling on high seas. His gyrocompass and gyrostabilizer were installed in large navy vessels and soon revolutionized marine navigation.

Sperry was born in the small town of Cortland, New York, in 1860. His mother died soon after his birth, and because his father had to earn a living—variously as a lumberman, a carpenter, a wagonmaker, and the owner of a traveling carnival—Elmer was raised by his aunt, Helen, on a farm outside Cortland. Like many other inventors of the late nineteenth and early twentieth centuries, Sperry acquired his mechanical education from farming—a small farmer needed to know his machines inside and out, to fix them and to improve them. Sperry's interests soon went beyond farm equipment; as a boy, he built model windmills and water wheels. At the age of six, he gave his aunt what may have been his first invention, a hand mill for grating horseradish.

In 1907, Sperry began to experiment with gyroscopes—especially their potential to stabilize automobiles. Within a couple of years, he had turned his attention to stabilizing ships; this 30-ton gyro wheel would eventually be installed in a 10,000-ton vessel.

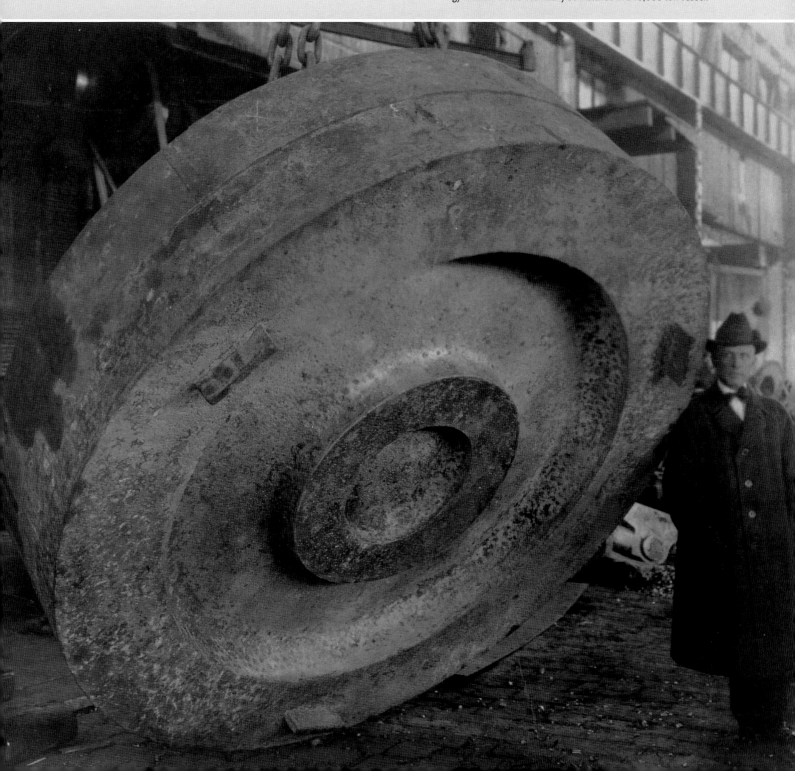

When he was about 10 years old, Sperry moved into Cortland with his grandparents. Although the town was small, it was an important stop on the railroad and boasted several industries. While he was a teenager, Sperry had the chance to observe the goings-on at the blacksmith's shop, the machine shop, the rail yard, and elsewhere. He also began working at some of these businesses, including the local foundry and the book bindery. When Sperry was 16, he helped build an electric dynamo at the foundry, and he traveled to the Centennial Exposition in Philadelphia where it was exhibited. The exposition was a great place for him to see the fruits of modern technology, including the Jacquard loom, which was controlled by punch cards.

After using gyroscopes to stabilize ships and compasses, Sperry turned to aviation and built a "gyropilot" from small gyroscopes. Here, the famous aviatrix Amelia Earhart poses with a 1930s version.

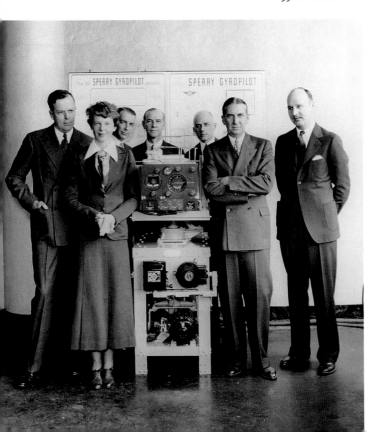

In Cortland, Sperry attended the local college for about two years, studying science and engineering, but he never got his degree. By the time he left the school in January 1880, however, his main interest had become clear: electricity. The announcement of Thomas Edison's incandescent light bulb in 1879 had excited him along with much of the country. That year, he had built his own dynamo and a new kind of arc lamp, and in 1880 he moved to Chicago to begin manufacturing them. He had high hopes; in 1883 he wrote, "Do you suppose for one moment that I am going to fail in great Chicago where one can turn a hundred ways—no sir."

The field of electricity and lighting was wide open when Sperry arrived in Chicago. For several years, his company was a success, selling lighting systems to cities and towns throughout the Midwest; his lights even adorned the tower of the Chicago Board of Trade. He was a better engineer than a businessman, though, and several of his companies struggled as technologies changed. From 1880 to 1910, Sperry was involved in a series of industries, including lighting, engines, rail cars, batteries, automobiles, and chemistry.

In 1907, for reasons that are not entirely clear, Sperry turned his attention to the gyroscope. The French physicist Jean-Bernard-Léon Foucault had built the first proper gyroscope in the 1850s: a heavy spinning wheel mounted in a frame that let it rotate in any direction. The gyroscope's most useful properties are its stability—the wheel will keep spinning in its initial direction—and its precession, the tendency to move at a right angle to any force exerted on it. One of the problems of capitalizing on these characteristics was that eventually friction would slow the wheel down. In 1890, an engineer solved this by building an electric motor to drive the wheel.

Sperry had been building automobiles for several years and thought to use a spinning gyroscope to stabilize a car. The theory was simple: If a car with a large horizontally spinning gyroscope (it was mounted beneath the seats) tipped, the angular force exerted by precession would resist the tip. He patented the idea, but could find no interest among carmakers.

Despite the rejection, Sperry still thought the idea was a good one, and he applied it next to ships. During an 1898 voyage to Europe, he had experienced an unpleasant effect of a rolling ship—seasickness. Using the same basic concept as his auto stabilizer, Sperry built a large, heavy gyroscope meant to be

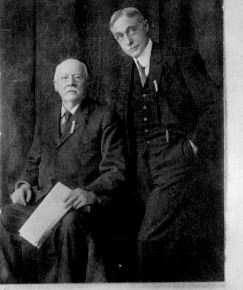

In Memory of the Evening of
April 15th 1884.

April 7th 1911.
Nathaniel S. Keith.   *Elmer A. Sperry,*

Elmer Sperry's early career was devoted to the burgeoning business of electricity. In April 1884, he helped found the American Institute of Electrical Engineers, now the IEEE; at Sperry's right is Nathaniel S. Keith, secretary of the group.

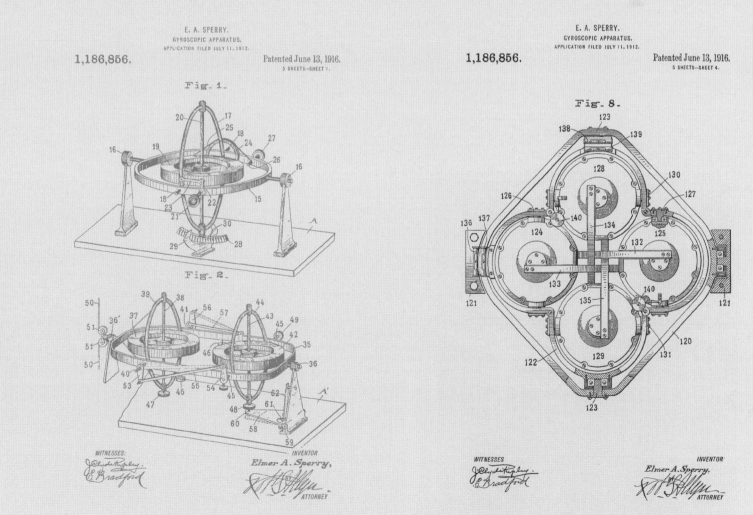

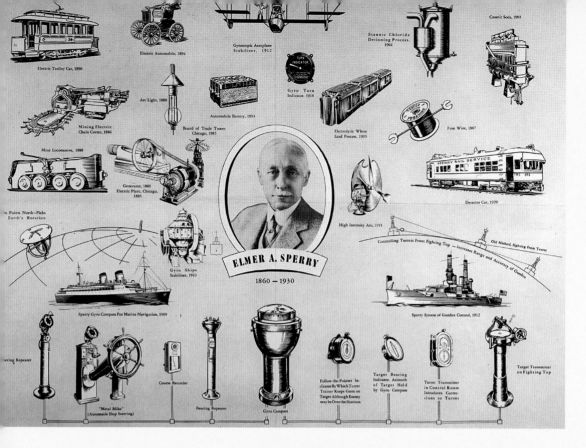

Sperry amassed more than 350 patents before his death in 1930.

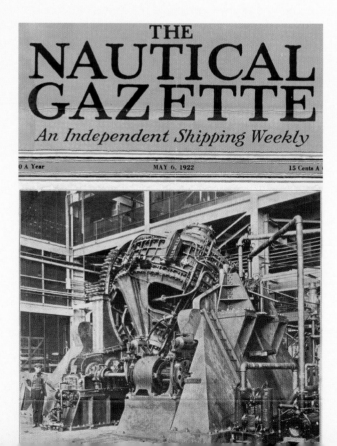

When this gyrostabilizer was built in 1922, it was the largest in the world, with a gyro wheel 12 feet across and weighing 109 tons.

mounted in the center of a ship. When a wave pushed the ship sideways, the gyroscope's precession would lessen the roll.

At least one other engineer had built a similar system, but Sperry added something new: a pendulum that acted as a sensor, picking up the first hint of a roll and activating motors that quickened the gyroscope's response. In 1911, after he had built several models of the gyrostabilizer, the U.S. Navy offered a ship to test a full-size system in. A four-thousand-pound gyroscope was installed, and the refitted ship was launched in 1912. The stabilizer worked well, eliminating minor roll and reducing a 30-degree roll to about six degrees.

At the same time he was designing the gyrostabilizer, Sperry was also working on a gyroscope-based compass. A German engineer concerned with the navigational difficulties of all-metal submarines had already begun pursuing a gyrocompass. Both he and Sperry began from an observation Foucault had made in 1852: that a spinning gyroscope initially aligned toward the north would always point north, even disregarding the rotation of the earth. Transforming this physical principle into a working compass took some engineering tricks, such as limiting its movement to two axes and automatically correcting for shifts as the gyro's position changed with regard to latitude. Sperry applied for a patent on his gyrocompass in 1911 and installed a working model in the same ship as his stabilizer. The two new navigational aids were further refined in the years leading up to World War I; by the time the United States entered the war, many of its ships were equipped with Sperry's inventions.

The problems of navigating ships paled in comparison to those of airplane flight. "Of all the vehicles on earth," Sperry wrote, "the airplane is . . . obsessed with motions, side pressure, skidding, accelerations, pressures, and strong centrifugal moments . . . all in endless variety and endless combination." Early airplanes, such as the Wright Brothers', depended on the pilot to control the plane through physical effort at every moment. This made long flights impossible, since the pilot would grow too tired to wrestle the controls. Another problem was that it was easy for pilots to grow disoriented, especially in clouds or at night, when they had no visual reference to the ground. Sperry used gyroscopes to address both problems.

He tackled the problem of control by designing a four-gyroscope stabilizer. As in a ship, when a plane tipped or rolled, the gyros would exert an opposing force. The plane stabilizer couldn't depend on the large gyroscopes suitable for ships; in-

stead, the movement of small gyros sent signals to motors attached to the elevators and other parts that controlled flight. Sperry's system flew for the first time in 1914; one observer noted that "this marvelous machine can recover lost equilibrium unaided by man." The next year, Sperry began working on gyroscopic instruments that would tell pilots if they were turning or climbing or diving. The gyros in the stabilizer could also indicate the true horizontal level—an "artificial horizon" that no pilot could confuse.

Sperry continued inventing long after he perfected his navigation systems, amassing more than 350 patents before his death in 1930. And while his work had advanced more industries than perhaps anyone except Edison, it was his gyroscopic work that would have the greatest impact. His autopilots, stabilizers, and gyrocompasses are still the basis for marine navigation, and it was the airplane gyrostabilizer, artificial horizon, and other flying instruments that allowed aviation to become an important mode of transportation. In the 1960s, his gyroscopic work was extended even further, as an essential part of the guidance systems in the American space program.

One of Sperry's patents was for this "calculator," a circular slide rule designed to look like a pocket watch.

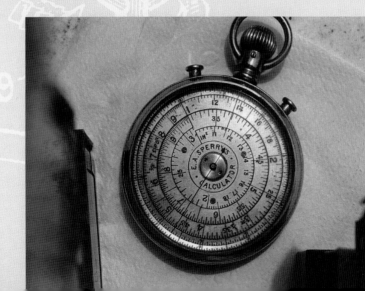

ENERGY AND ENVIRONMENT

INTRODUCTION

Much of the innovation for which America is famed has its roots in the reductionist approach to problem solving, which involves the inventive mind in identifying a specific issue, or need for improvement, and then focusing intensely on the search for a solution. This kind of thinking has to an extent generated the myth of the lonely genius (such as Leo Baekeland or Steve Wozniak) locked in a garage, surrounded by arcane gadgets, like some medieval alchemist, cut off in his magic isolation from the real world outside.

The first technological apotheosis of reductionism was probably the Industrial Revolution, and its inventors epitomized the isolated noodler at work. James Watt was totally immersed in finding how to keep his cylinder hot while it was being sprayed with cold water to condense the steam inside and cause the partial vacuum needed for piston movement. James Nielson (of hot blast fame) spent years working out the exact temperature of the hot air he wanted to inject into a furnace to obtain maximum smelting performance from inferior coal. Robert Fulton drove himself to exhaustion developing an engine that would coax out the extra knot of speed needed to make his steamboat commercially viable.

On a larger scale, the products of the Industrial Revolution were good examples of both the way in which reductionism isolates science and technology in separate silos, and also of the unexpected and sometimes unwelcome effects that happened when the work of those isolated innovators comes onto the market and interacts with inventions emerging from other, similarly isolated noodlers. The positive side of this interaction—

as, for instance, when steam power joined textile machinery to produce clothing everybody could afford; or when mass production generated the first steady year-round jobs and regular wages—was to raise the standard of living of the general populace. The negative side was that industrial innovations such as nineteenth-century production lines and automation brought millions from the villages and farms into the factory towns, and packed them into slum dwellings where they lived ankle-deep in sewage, easy prey to the cholera epidemics that ravaged so much of Europe and the American East Coast in the late nineteenth century. These events raised the consciousness of politicians and innovators and triggered the first of the great public health reforms and the inventions required to carry them out: new medical advances (America opened the first public health lab employing techniques and apparatus developed for the entirely new field of bacteriology), and improvements in sewerage technology (in Victorian England: Doulton's first glazed sewer pipes connected to Jennings's first patent ceramic flush toilets).

The modern world faces a continuation of this dual nature of innovative social effects, but on a global scale. Thanks to the twentieth-century drive to spread industrialization across the globe and then to raise world standards in public health, the planet has come under sustained pressure from both the effect of pollution and of uncontrolled population growth. A recent guess estimated one effect of this phenomenon to be a loss of 6,000 species every day, and forests are disappearing at the rate of one Switzerland-equivalent per year. Population levels are forecast to hit unsustainability before mid-century. Add ozone layer depletion and possible global warming to the mix, and the full-scale ramifications of what can sometimes go wrong with the reductionist approach become apparent: We may have spent several centuries not seeing the wood for the trees. Although reductionist innovation has brought most of us the highest material standard of living in history, it has done so only at a considerable, perhaps unacceptable environmental price.

One of the fundamental effects of invention has been to introduce once-for-all change. Innovation can never be wished out of existence. We live with the tools for change that our inventors gave us. In the long run, this has meant that some of the greatest inventors in history caused problems they could never have foreseen. But in the main, they also gave us the tools with which to find solutions to those problems.

This group of innovative thinkers represents a growing number of people concerned to apply this principle and to encourage us to "think globally, act locally." Their efforts range from pollution-free forms of energy, to environmentally friendly textile manufacture, to cheap water purification. Given the scale of our present worldwide ecological difficulties, there is still much to do.

—JB

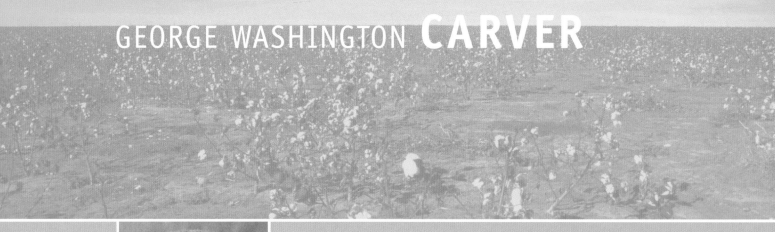

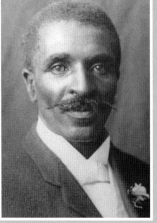

George Washington Carver was many things to many people. As someone who transformed himself from an orphaned ex-slave into a scientist and national hero, he was a living example of the American Dream. As a devout Christian, he was a symbol of religious faith. As one of the most famous African Americans of his time, he represented the possibility of advancement for people of any color. Carver's most important role, though, may have been as an agricultural scientist. Working at the Tuskegee Institute in Alabama, he helped revolutionize farming in the South, introducing alternative crops, the idea of crop rotation, and natural methods of fertilization, as well as inventing hundreds of products and uses for his favorite plants, the peanut and the sweet potato.

Carver, born in 1864, had an early childhood full of conflict and tragedy. His mother, Mary, was a slave owned by Moses and Susan Carver, farmers living near the small Missouri town of Diamond. Carver never knew his father, who is said to have died in an accident before his child's birth. Although the Civil War ended in April 1865, many rural areas of the South remained in turmoil. Sometime that year, a band of marauding "bushwhackers" kidnapped Carver and his mother and carried them off to Arkansas. Moses Carver sent an emissary to ransom them, although by the time he arrived Mary apparently had been sold and had disappeared; the young Carver was traded for a $300 racehorse.

After George was returned, the childless Carvers adopted him and his brother. Because he was sickly, George did chores around the house rather than work in the field. He also spent a great deal of time outside, where he developed his love for plants. In 1897, he remembered this time of his life: "Day after day I spent in the woods alone in order to collect my floral beauties and put them in my little garden I had hidden in brush not far from the house." Carver's skill at caring for flora soon earned him the nickname "plant doctor," and people would bring him their sick plants for treatment.

Carver's early education came from his adoptive mother and a single book, *Webster's Elementary Spelling Book*, which he read so many times, he later said, "I almost knew the book by heart." The local school would not ac-

When George Washington Carver joined Tuskegee University in 1896, most Southern farms grew only cotton. Carver championed alternative crops such as peanuts and soybeans, whose uses he demonstrated in his lab.

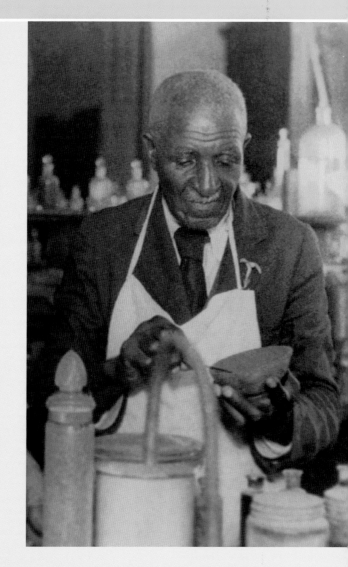

cept black students, so when he was 12 Carver moved to the nearby town of Neosho, Kansas, to begin school. There he lived with a black couple, Andrew and Mariah Watkins, and earned his keep by doing domestic chores and helping Mariah with her laundry business. After a year in Neosho, he went on to attend schools in several Kansas towns, eventually finishing high school and moving to Kansas City to learn shorthand and typing at a business school.

Clerical work could not satisfy Carver's thirst for knowledge, and in 1885 he applied to a college in Highland, Kansas. He was accepted, but when he showed up for class, school officials were shocked to find out that he was black, and they refused to let him in. A few years later, he moved to Winterset, Iowa, where he set up his own laundry business and became close friends with a white couple who urged Carver to try college again. In 1890 he entered Simpson College, where he discovered his talent for painting. A year later, his art teacher, who had noticed his detailed drawings of plants, persuaded him to study agriculture at what is now Iowa State University. He was the school's first African American student.

With his natural talent for plants, Carver thrived at Iowa State. After he graduated, he stayed on to teach and to study for his master's degree. He might have remained there if not for Booker T. Washington, a leader and educator who had founded the Tuskegee Institute, the leading college for African Americans. When Washington invited him to join the faculty at Tuskegee, Carver saw it as an opportunity to serve his race. "It has always been the one great ideal of my life to be of the greatest good to the greatest number of 'my people,'" he wrote Washington. "This line of education [agriculture] is the key to unlock the golden door of freedom to our people."

At the turn of the twentieth century, Southern agriculture was devoted primarily to cotton. But cotton is a destructive crop, draining nutrients from the soil. Also, any region devoted to one crop is at a greater danger of agricultural disaster, from plant diseases or insects. After more than a century of cotton growing, much Southern farmland was growing less productive, and many fields were ruined. This affected African American farmers more severely, since

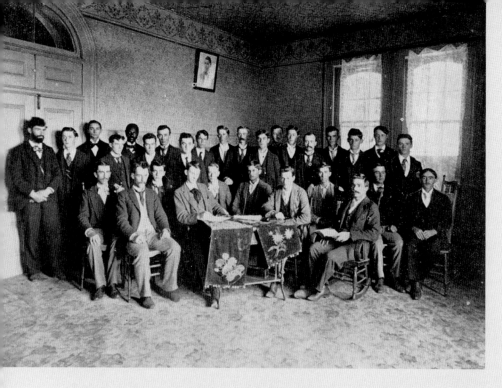

Encouraged by an art teacher who had noticed his drawings of plants, Carver began studying agriculture at Iowa State College in 1891. He was the college's first African American student.

While pursuing his master's degree at Iowa State, Carver was approached by Booker T. Washington, the founder of the Tuskegee Institute, the country's leading school for African Americans. In 1896, Carver accepted a position on Tuskegee's faculty, pictured here. He remained at Tuskegee for four decades. Carver is at the far left of the top row.

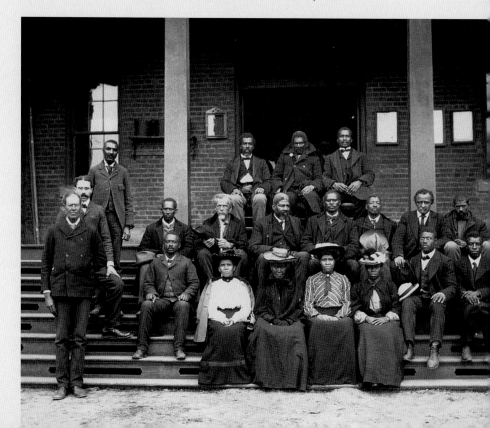

their farms were almost always smaller than those of whites, and were often rented rather than owned.

Carver thought that a scientific knowledge of agriculture could help meet these challenges. He also had a deep belief that man should work in concert with nature, paying attention to natural processes and being careful not to waste resources. At Tuskegee, Carver started by experimenting with new ways to work the local land, which was in poor condition, then began using the school as an educational pulpit to encourage local farmers to follow his example.

During Carver's years at Tuskegee, he promoted three agricultural innovations: organic fertilizing methods, crop rotation, and new crops that returned nutrients to the soil. By plowing the unused remains of a harvest under the soil, a farmer could create a kind of natural compost heap that acted as a highly effective fertilizer for the next crop. Rotating crops—alternating cotton and other crops from year to year—reduced cotton's destructive power. Carver's real passion, however, was exploring alternative crops: soybeans, pecans, the sweet potato, and, above all, the peanut.

The worst thing that cotton did to soil was rob it of nitrogen, an essential nutrient. Carver knew that peanuts and sweet potatoes replenished nitrogen; rotating these crops with cotton could heal the South's fragile soil. It would also lower the danger that insects like the boll weevil could destroy the region's economy.

Many farmers began testing Carver's ideas in their fields and found that he was right: Peanuts and sweet potatoes did restore the soil. But while the market for cotton was well established, demand was limited for these new crops. So in his laboratory Carver set to finding practical uses for them. Over the course of his four decades at Tuskegee, he created hundreds of products based on peanuts and sweet potatoes. From the peanut, he was able to make plastics, animal feed, oil, ink, paper, and stains, as well as many foods, from cheese and milk to meat substitutes, candy, and breakfast snacks. And from sweet potatoes he devised methods for making flour, glue, alcohol, syrup, and starch, among other things. In 1921, he was called to testify before the U.S. Congress when it was considering imposing taxes on peanut imports. He dazzled the legislators by exhibiting some of his peanut products, including mock oysters and a face cream.

Carver patented only three of his agricultural products: cosmetics, paints, and stains made from soybeans. His goal in agricultural research was not to get rich—he lived modestly and made a point of refusing money offered to him—but to improve the plight of farmers, especially African American farmers. A deeply religious man, he credited God for his many inventions, and would say, "God gave them to me. How can I sell them to someone else?"

His appearance in Congress and many favorable articles about him made Carver a famous man. In the 1920s, he began speaking to white youth groups in the South to improve race relations. As his amazing life story became widely known, he became an American folk hero.

When Carver died in 1943, his entire estate was given to the Tuskegee Institute to start the Carver Research Foundation for agriculture. Another permanent reminder of his life was established that same year. Just six months after he passed away, President Franklin Roosevelt dedicated the George Washington Carver National Monument, near Carver's childhood home in Diamond, Missouri. The honor was unprecedented—not only was it the first national monument to an African American, it was the first to anyone other than a U.S. president.

Among the hundreds of products Carver coaxed from peanuts and soybeans were dyes, paints, cleansers, charcoal, and fuel, as well as many different foodstuffs.

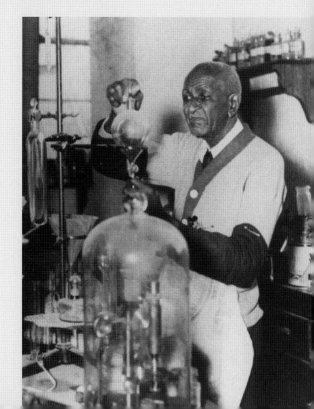

CARL DJERASSI

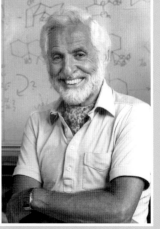

The world does not lack brilliant organic chemists, but few have had such a profound effect as Carl Djerassi. His synthesis in 1951 of artificial progesterone earned him the title of Father of the Pill. Before that, Djerassi had been instrumental in the creation of the first antihistamine and the first synthetic steroids. And his innovation continued when he became a director of research and a chemical entrepreneur, leading a team of scientists exploring the hormonal secrets of insects. This work led to new approaches to pest control that relied on mimicking natural chemicals rather than on dangerous neurotoxins.

Djerassi's interests outside the lab are even more diverse. He is a well-known collector of art, especially that of Paul Klee, as well as a patron who runs an artists' and writers' retreat on his ranch outside Santa Cruz, California. In the past few years, Djerassi has been breaking new educational ground by teaching scientific ethics through fiction writing, specifically the writing of "science in fiction," stories and novels revolving around the processes and customs of the scientific establishment. His own science-in-fiction novels have been well reviewed and well read; the first, *Cantor's Dilemma*, a novel about the fierce competition that drives star scientists, has sold more than 100,000 copies.

Djerassi, who was born in Vienna in 1923, had an eventful adolescence. His father was a doctor and his mother a dentist, although she, too, had been trained as a physician. Djerassi spent his first few years in Bulgaria, where his father was from, then returned to Vienna for his education. (The move back to Vienna was also due to his parents' divorce.) He was doing well in school and planning to go into medicine like his parents when, in March 1938, Nazi Germany occupied Austria. While many Austrian Jews thought they would be safe in their native country, Djerassi's father knew to take quick action. He temporarily remarried his ex-wife, to get her and his son Bulgarian passports. As foreigners, they could leave Austria; his mother traveled to England, while Djerassi went to Bulgaria with his father, where he enrolled in the American College (a high school) there. In September 1939, just after Germany invaded Poland, Djerassi and his mother were granted visas to the United States, and

Djerassi at his Syntex lab in Mexico City in 1951, working with his

assistant Arelina Gonzalez on synthetic progesterone.

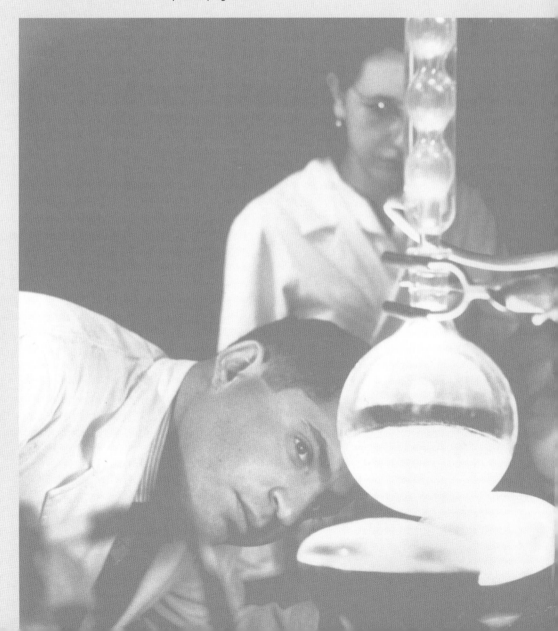

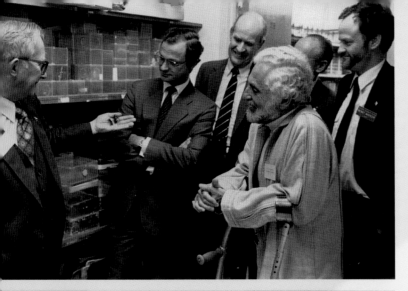

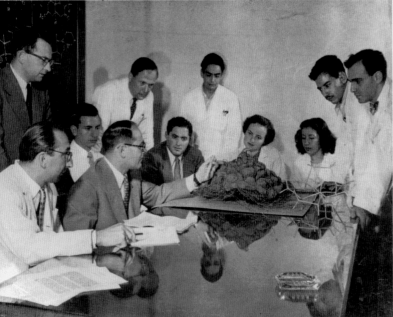

Carl XVI Gustaf, King of Sweden, at center, visited Djerassi's insect-control company Zoecon in 1984. Djerassi looks on as Gerardus Staal, Zoecon's director of biological research, shows the king two immobilized cockroaches.

In 1951, Carl Djerassi (center, seated) was the first person to make synthetic progesterone—a hormone that eventually led to the birth control pill. At a press conference, Djerassi and his colleagues examined the yamlike plant from which they extracted the chemical precursor to the hormone.

he pulled up roots again; the two of them soon arrived in New York, virtually penniless.

In America, Djerassi and his mother were again separated—she went to work in upstate New York, while he was taken in by a generous family in Newark, New Jersey. There he began his American education at a junior college, although he had not completed high school. Djerassi soon realized that he would need a more substantial education to get anywhere. He had no financial resources, so he took what he thought was a logical step: He wrote to Eleanor Roosevelt asking for help. Improbably, it worked. His letter was forwarded to the Institute for International Education, which secured him a scholarship at a tiny Presbyterian college in northwestern Missouri.

For a while, Djerassi supported himself by speaking at local churches on the conflict in Europe. The next year he moved on to Kenyon College in Ohio, where the 17-year-old set out to get his bachelor's degree in chemistry in just one year. Carrying heavy course loads through two semesters and a summer, Djerassi earned his degree in this seemingly impossible time frame.

The new graduate applied to many of the chemical companies in New Jersey (the center of the industry in the United States), and was soon hired by the Swiss pharmaceutical firm CIBA. Djerassi's rise was swift; during his first year there, he was involved in the creation of the first antihistamine and was credited as a coinventor on the patent and a coauthor of the article detailing the work. CIBA was also a leader in steroid research, and exposure to that science in the lab, as well as his reading of a seminal book on the subject, soon had Djerassi hooked. A disabling knee injury kept him out of World War II, allowing him to pursue a Ph.D. at the University of Wisconsin, which he earned in just two years.

Djerassi returned to CIBA for a few years, but in 1949 he was offered the chance to head a steroid research group in the Mexico City office of the Syntex company. At the time, Syntex was involved in the race to make a synthetic version of cortisone. Within two years, Djerassi and his colleagues had done it first, putting his Mexico City lab on the steroid research map.

The next challenge Djerassi turned to was making a form of progesterone that could be taken orally. Progesterone is produced naturally when a woman is pregnant; it prevents her from ovulating. In the 1920s, an Austrian endocrinologist had proposed that this hormone could be used as a contraceptive. But that is not why Djerassi was trying to synthesize it. Syntex was already the largest producer of progesterone, which was used to treat menstrual disorders and was thought to be a treatment for cervical cancer. But the hormone could be administered only by injection; this made it an expensive and not always practical treatment and limited its uses. An orally delivered version would avoid those problems.

On October 15, 1951, Djerassi's lab converted a precursor to synthetic progesterone—extracted from a yamlike plant— into norethindrone, which turned out to be much more active than the natural hormone as well as capable of being taken orally. "That was the Eureka part," Djerassi says. The lab's published research made its way to Gregory Pincus, a biologist looking into contraception, and John Rock, a doctor at Harvard. Using Djerassi's synthetic hormone, they developed the oral contraceptive pill, usually known as the Pill. Since its introduction in 1960, according to one of its manufacturers, some 80 percent of American women have used it.

By the mid-1960s, Djerassi's lab began investigating insect hormones. It was an exciting time for this research: Improved chemical and analytical techniques were allowing scientists to deeply explore insect endocrinology for the first time. One of the most exciting discoveries of the time was that a single hormone, ecdysone, governed insects' molting process. Syntex and several other labs worked to synthesize this complex steroid; Djerassi's team was one of the first to do it. (By this time Djerassi was the director of research at Syntex; he monitored others' work and assigned scientists' priorities, but he didn't do the actual synthesis.)

That success is "really what got us interested in insects," Djerassi explains. "But it was a chemical interest rather than biological." Eventually, he continues, having done this work, "we wondered, can we use it for something?" Djerassi hired two of the most distinguished endocrinologists in the United States, Herbert Röller and Carroll Williams, and began exploring what applications the research might have.

A discovery by Röller showed the way. He had found a "juvenile hormone" in insects that maintained their larval state. When this hormone is "turned off," the insect grows into an adult and is able to reproduce. If one could synthesize this hormone and continuously apply it, insect pests would never live to reproduce. "It would be the equivalent to using a human contraceptive in which you prevent the onset of puberty," Djerassi has noted. The lab was able to synthesize this hormone, and in

1968, Djerassi convinced Syntex to spin off this research division as a separate company, which he named Zoecon.

At the time, the pesticide DDT was being banned worldwide, even though, Djerassi notes, it had done much good for humans, if not for animals. "Chemophobia is to a very large extent propagated by the word pesticide, in its dirtiest sense," he says. Zoecon was formed to find alternative, "biorational" approaches to pest control, methods that would kill the insect but not humans or other, nontargeted animals. "Conceptually," Djerassi explains, "our approach to insects was very similar to Syntex's earlier approach to birth control."

By the early 1970s, Zoecon had developed a product, Altosid, based on insect juvenile hormones, which are part of a larger class of agents called insect growth inhibitors. "In many respects it was one of the ideal pest-control agents," Djerassi says, "in terms of being biodegradable, and being metabolized completely through innocuous things." Altosid was adopted in the fight against insects that do their damage as adults—fleas, cockroaches, and, most important, mosquitoes. Today, Altosid is common in many mosquito-control products. But Djerassi laments that most money for insect-control research, development, and treatment goes to commercial crop pests. "Malaria is one of the greatest killers of human beings," he says, "but there really is not much money in public health things."

For the past decade, Djerassi has dedicated much of his time to writing novels and stories that explore the culture and personalities of science as it is actually practiced. He has also begun teaching a writing seminar at the Stanford University School of Medicine, where prospective doctors can explore through fiction the ethical dilemmas of their future practice that often, according to Djerassi, "are not raised for reasons of discretion, embarrassment, or fear of retribution." Djerassi's latest novel, *No*, was recently published in paperback, and he is preparing a new book, *One Man's Pill*, an exploration of how his contraceptive discovery changed both him and the world.

SALLY FOX

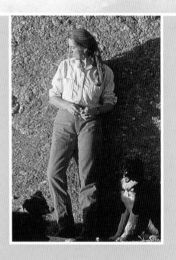

Sally Fox didn't invent colored cotton—it has always existed in nature. The Incas used it in their textiles. Khaki was first made in India from brown cotton. In the United States, slaves grew brown and green cotton in their own gardens, since they were forbidden from growing white cotton that they might sell.

When Fox introduced her own colored cotton to the world in 1989, though, she had done something no one had thought possible: created a naturally colored cotton that could be spun (made into thread) on a machine. Until then, colored cotton had suffered from short, weak fibers, which meant it had to be spun by hand, a slow and expensive task. The only cotton that was commercially viable was white cotton, which had been bred and refined to have long, strong fibers, perfect for machines to work with. But white cotton is not an environmentally friendly product. Before it becomes jeans, or sheets, or a shirt, it has to be bleached and then dyed, and both processes create large amounts of pollution. Fox Fibre, the brand name of Fox's cottons, required no bleaching or dyeing. Her first two colors—a celadon green and a warm reddish brown—were immediate sensations. For the first time, the textile industry and the public saw how environmentally friendly clothes could be. Orders for her cotton began pouring in.

Fox never imagined she would be a cotton revolutionary. But in many ways everything she had done before announcing her new cotton had been perfect training for the role. When she was 12, she fell in love with the process of spinning. With a spindle she bought with baby-sitting money, she created thread out of all sorts of materials, from the cotton in medicine bottles to her dog's hair. She was soon a master spinner. But Fox also dreamed of living and working far from cities. Until she was seven, she lived on the last acres of land her father's family had homesteaded in Woodside, California. "There were big expanses of land," she says. "When we moved from that into Menlo Park I never got over it. I always wanted to live in the country and have some means of supporting myself."

In high school, she discovered a new passion: entomology, the study of insects. An entomologist visiting from Kenya, Elizabeth Wangari, taught a

Each year, Fox examines the her main crops and test fields to
determine which plants exhibit new qualities and which should
be selected for the next year's planting.

By carefully selecting the best plants of a cotton crop, Sally Fox
gradually bred a new kind of cotton: colored and spinnable.

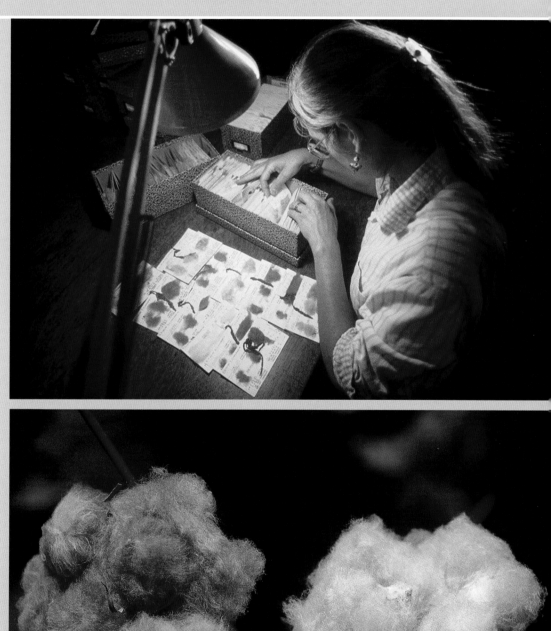

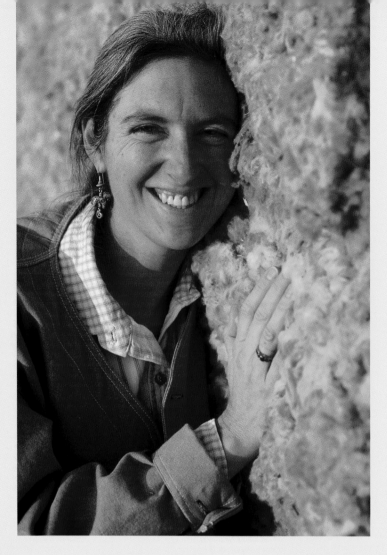

ARTIFICIAL SELECTION AND THE ORIGIN OF FOX FIBRE

The process of artificial selection in plants—choosing, over many generations, the most beneficial or fertile or beautiful examples—is as old as agriculture. Long before the age of industrial farming, all crop plants were the product of countless generations of careful selection, with farmers choosing to plant seeds from the strongest or most bountiful of their plants. Naturally occurring corn, for example, has an ear only an inch or two long, with small kernels; it was only through selection and cross-breeding over centuries that our modern food staple was created.

Although artificial selection has been around for millennia, the science behind it—genetics—was discovered only in the nineteenth century, by the Austrian botanist and monk Gregor Mendel. In carefully studying garden peas in his nursery, Mendel noticed that certain differences between generations—for example, in plant size or seed shape—were predictable, and he proposed that these traits were controlled during reproduction. Some differences had only two states—shrunken or nonshrunken, for instance—while others had more subtle variations. It is understood now that simple differences are controlled by one gene, while subtler changes are the result of combinations of genes. By breeding pea plants with specific characteristics—and isolating them from other plants—Mendel could produce plants that emphasized those qualities.

In her pursuit of machine-spinnable, naturally colored cotton, Sally Fox used the same basic ideas that Mendel developed (and which have been refined in the ensuing 135 years). Fox estab-

class on the subject and helped Fox get an internship at Zoecon, Carl Djerassi's company, which was developing natural ways to control insects. Wangari also encouraged her to go to college—Fox had wanted to start a hand-spinning business—where she studied biology and entomology.

After she graduated, Fox joined the Peace Corps and traveled to The Gambia, in West Africa, to help fight the pests and diseases that affected rice and peanuts. What she really learned there, though, was the dangers of pesticides. Europe and the United States had recently banned DDT and other chlorinated-hydrocarbon-based pesticides, and some European manufacturers had "donated" their large stocks to African countries—in unlabeled, leaking 55-gallon drums. It was an environmental disaster waiting to happen. The local men hired to administer the pesticide were instead selling bags of it at the market for people to use on household pests. Fox began giving safety classes on the pesticides' use, but she also became very ill from exposure to them. "It was so horrible that I actually had to leave" before her two-year assignment was finished, she says. "So I'm sort of a fanatic against pesticides."

When Fox began looking for work in the United States in the early 1980s, the farming industry had just entered a long economic depression, from which it has never fully recovered. The only job Fox could find in her field was as a pollinator for a cotton breeder searching for pest-resistant plants. She was bored by the job, since it took a year to see if new strains of cotton were better than old ones. One day she found a bag of seeds that produced cotton that was pest-resistant but brown. The breeder hadn't pursued these seeds, because he didn't think he could get rid of the color. Fox was intrigued. "I said, 'Why aren't we doing this?'" she remembers. "And he said, 'Why don't you do it?' So I went through the seeds and hand-spun each single one. I decided which ones were the easiest ones to spin and I planted those. That was the beginning."

For the next seven years—even after she stopped working for the cotton breeder—Fox tended her cotton plants, now growing in pots on her back porch. Each year, when the cotton bolls opened up, she would carefully select seeds from the plants with the best fibers and the best colors. She also cross-bred her cotton with white cotton, to produce a longer fiber, or staple. "I was an entomologist, and I hadn't read all the plant books saying you couldn't breed for longer staple," she says. Eventually she had two colored cottons that were stable—they didn't change when planted in the field—and were spinnable.

lished several characteristics she was looking for, including color, the length of the cotton fiber, the softness of the fiber, and the strength and pest-resistance of the plant.

Over a period of 10 years—or 10 generations of plants—she examined the cotton for these characteristics. Each generation's best plants were then bred, through pollination, with each other. The following year, a few of the plants would exhibit stronger qualities; those, in turn, would be selected out, bred, and grown. At a genetic level, each generation of these hand-selected plants had a combination of genes that better produced the characteristics Fox was looking for. Some of these qualities were linked—pest resistance always came with certain colors of cotton—while others were the result of combinations of independent genes.

Eventually, the qualities of Fox's plants were sufficiently different from their ancestor that she could essentially patent them and call them her own.

Genetic engineers are also working toward many of these same goals, such as stronger plants and bigger fruits—but they are using a much faster, although less well explored, means. By incorporating the actual sequences of DNA that code for beneficial characteristics in a certain plant—strawberries' frost resistance, for example—into another crop, they can speed up the processes of artificial selection and cross-breeding a thousand-fold and, in many cases, produce plants that no amount of breeding could ever make. These techniques, pioneered in agriculture, are also being applied to animals and even humans, in the budding science of gene therapy.

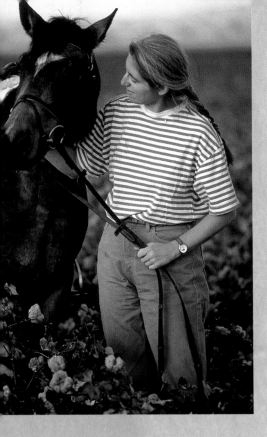

She applied for and won Plant Variety Protection Certificates for them, the plant equivalent of patents.

In 1989 she sold her first crop, 122 bushels of cotton, to a Japanese mill. American customers weren't far behind. Levi's began making "natural" jeans and other clothes. L.L. Bean, Land's End, and Esprit also placed big orders. Fox was running a $10 million business. She put together a network of cotton growers that produced hundreds of thousands of pounds of Fox Fibre cotton.

But Fox's natural cotton revolution has not been a smooth one. California's powerful cotton growers were afraid that her colored varieties would contaminate their own crops. They imposed strict rules on her operation, which forced her to move to Arizona in 1993. Six years later, Arizona cotton growers did the same thing, and Fox had to relocate again, this time to Northern California. Even worse for her business were the changes in the spinning industry. Between 1990 and 1995, most of the spinning mills in Japan and Europe closed, as well as many in the United States. "What was going on was the beginnings of globalization," Fox explains. "Everything was moving to Southeast Asia and South America." These mills wouldn't or couldn't process the relatively small quantities of cotton her farmers produced, and she lost her big customers.

Until the spinning industry moved to less-developed countries, Fox's cotton had a financial advantage over traditional cotton. It cost about $2 per pound of cotton to treat and dispose of the toxic waste from the cotton-dyeing process. However, many of the new, offshore mills weren't required to protect the environment, and didn't. On a recent trip to Hong Kong, Fox noticed a headline in the local newspaper: "Farmers Downstream from Denim Plant Lose Entire Crop." A dye plant had dumped its waste just when the rice harvest began, and killed some 300 acres of crops. "If it kills the plants like that," she asks, "What are the long-term effects?"

Through all of her cotton's ups and downs, Fox has continued to develop new colors. It takes about 10 years of careful selection from generation to generation to coax a usable variety of cotton from an initial cross-bred seed. "You get a color, and it's not a great plant, and it's not a great fiber, but it's a color," she says. "And then you keep at it until you get a better plant. You just work at it year after year." She has a new redwood color almost ready for market; combined with white cotton, it makes a shade of pink. She's also added a deeper "New Green" and the chocolate-toned "Buffalo" to the Fox Fibre line.

Fox now concentrates on smaller mills and smaller customers, and she is rebuilding her business and her network of growers. One new client is emblematic of her hopes for Fox Fibre. Two brothers in Mexico, she explains, want to rebuild their family's spinning business. Their grandfather had built a mill, then a dyeing plant, then a factory, and finally a store for the clothes he produced. By the time the brothers were in their twenties, though, the village's water supply had been destroyed by the dyes, and the mill shut down. With Fox's cotton, they hope to start the mill up again and to set an example for other mills in the area that it's possible to make textiles without destroying the local environment. "They're the kinds of people I dream of selling to," Fox says. "It can really make a difference."

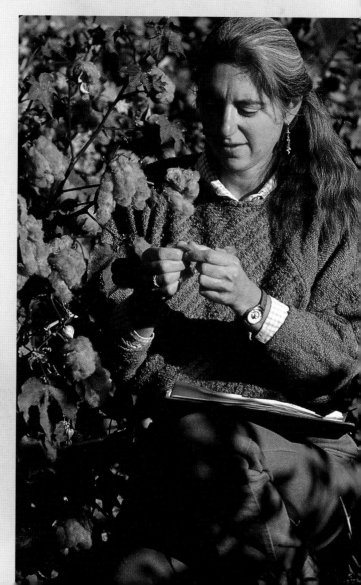

Selective breeding, a process that is thousands of years old, requires careful attention to each plant and a knowledge, acquired through experiment, of how plants can be cross-bred.

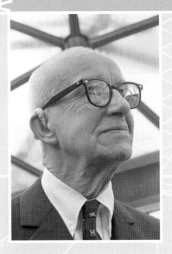

In 1927, R. Buckminster ("Bucky") Fuller was a failed businessman who was drinking too much, depressed about the death of his first daughter, and worried about how to take care of his family. That winter, while living in Chicago, he walked out to Lake Michigan to throw himself into its icy waters. "I said to myself, 'I've done the best I know how and it hasn't worked. I guess I'm just no good,'" he remembered. Fuller gave himself a choice: jump or think. He stood on the lakeshore for hours, finally deciding that he didn't have the right to kill himself. And so began Fuller's career as an inventor, thinker, and futurist.

From that point on, Fuller thought of his life as an experiment designed to discover what he could "do effectively on behalf of all humanity that could not be accomplished by great nations, great religions or private enterprise." He christened himself "Guinea Pig B" (B for Bucky) and started "thinking about our total planet Earth and thinking realistically about how to operate it on an enduringly sustainable basis as the magnificent human-passengered spaceship that it is." The results of Fuller's lifelong experiment include the geodesic dome, new types of houses and cars, and a new kind of geometry. Underlying all of his work was the profound realization he had come to that night in Chicago, that he could "find ways of giving human beings more energy-effective" systems and machines that would create a higher quality of living for everyone. "Under those more favorable physical circumstances," he wrote, "humans would dare to be less selfish and more genuinely thoughtful toward one another."

Anyone who had watched Fuller growing up would have been surprised at his desperate circumstances in 1927. Richard Buckminster Fuller, Jr., was born in 1895 to a wealthy and long-established Massachusetts family. Although his father died in 1907, Bucky had an active and fairly happy childhood.

Fig. 5.

INVENTOR.

RICHARD BUCKMINSTER FULLER

BY

The family spent its summers on a private island off the coast of Maine, and as a teenager he attended Milton Academy, a prestigious prep school. In 1913, like four generations of Fullers before him, he entered Harvard University.

Fuller never really fit into Harvard's rigid social structure, and he earned only a C average. At the end of his freshman year, he took the college money his mother had put away and went to New York City, where he spent all of it and more trying to romance a Ziegfeld Follies dancer. The university expelled him for "irresponsible conduct."

After getting kicked out of Harvard a second time, Fuller met and married Anne Hewlett, who also came from a venerable family. During World War I, his mother secured him an officer's commission in the navy by donating one of the family's boats. Fuller loved the navy; he patrolled the northeastern coast for much of the war, and later designed a mast-and-winch system to rescue seaplane pilots. After the war, he began working with his father-in-law on a concrete-block building system. Although their investors had high hopes, the American construction industry stuck to traditional techniques, and in 1927, with the company failing, Fuller was forced to quit. He was a new father, jobless, and broke when he walked out to Lake Michigan.

After his epiphany, Bucky Fuller resolved to think before he did anything. For a year he kept silent, speaking only when he was sure he had something important to say. He thought about what he could do to help people live better. He started with something he already knew a bit about, and which was also a basic human need: building shelter. And he had an idea for a new way to build. Fuller knew that while conventional buildings' strength came from compression—stacking bricks on top of each other—tension was far more efficient. Steel, for example, can support twenty times more weight suspended from it (as with the steel cables of a suspension bridge) than placed on top of it.

In 1929, Fuller unveiled the Dymaxion House, a residence unlike anything that had ever been built. (An advertising writer dreamed up the word Dymaxion, from "dynamic," "maximum," and "tension.") At the center of the house was a tall pole, the "mast," from which the body of the six-sided house

In 1959, Buckminster Fuller and his wife, Anne, built a geodesic dome that served as their home in Carbondale, Illinois, where he taught at Southern Illinois University.

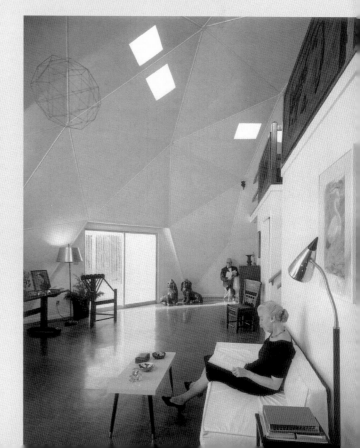

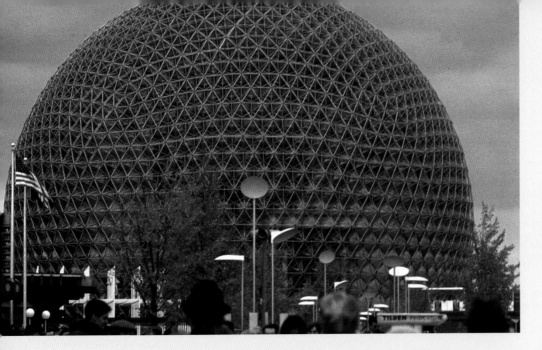

One of the largest geodesic domes in the world was built as
the United States Pavilion for Expo '67, a world's fair held in
Montreal. Today, the dome houses Biosphere, an ecologically
oriented science museum.

was suspended by steel cables. Inside, the space was split up into traditional, if oddly shaped, rooms: bedrooms, kitchen, living room. Fuller also included a "go-ahead-with-life" room, which incorporated a library, a radio, a television, a typewriter, and a drawing board. In his book *Bucky Works*, Fuller's longtime colleague J. Baldwin calls this room "nothing less than a personal multimedia center—in 1927!"

Fuller's Dymaxion House was designed to be a portable residence that a family could buy once (for approximately the cost of a high-end automobile), and then easily pack up and take with them when they moved. It was meant to be built from aluminum, a light, strong, and durable material. The whole thing would weigh only three tons, compared with the 150 tons of a normal building, and its hexagonal shape and the strength of steel tension would keep it sturdy and safe. While Fuller's radical house quickly captured the public's attention, the building industry was less enthusiastic. Because it was easy to build and used a minimum of standardized components, the Dymaxion House would be very affordable, but only if it were mass-produced, and mass production was the enemy of architects and builders. When one (and as it turned out, the only) Dymaxion House was built in 1945, thousands of orders poured in. But

Fuller was never an effective businessman, and his disagreements with stockholders and manufacturers doomed the project.

After the failure of the Dymaxion House, Fuller went back to doing research. He was thinking about geometry, specifically about a geometric system he had begun formulating in the 1930s. Just as he had done with his own life in 1927, Fuller was determined to start over from scratch. Instead of exploring the conventional—Euclid's abstract ideas of points and straight lines—Fuller looked to nature, examining how natural shapes can be broken down into smaller and smaller elements. The smallest element he ended up with was the tetrahedron—a pyramid with four equal sides, the most minimal enclosed space possible. "The tetrahedron is the basic structural system," he wrote, "and all structure in the universe is made up of tetrahedronal parts." From this starting point, Fuller constructed a new kind of geometry, a system he called "synergetics" (from "synergy" and "energetic").

In 1948, Fuller was looking for a way to apply these principles to making a building, and began thinking about making a dome-shaped structure. Humans had been using domelike buildings such as igloos and yurts for thousands of years. Fuller thought that a dome made with the tetrahedron as its basic building block would "have structural strength without any

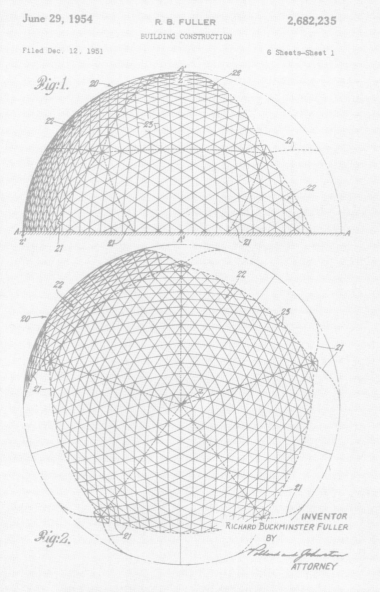

June 29, 1954   R. B. FULLER   2,682,235
BUILDING CONSTRUCTION

Filed Dec. 12, 1951   6 Sheets—Sheet 1

Fig:1.

Fig:2.

INVENTOR
RICHARD BUCKMINSTER FULLER
BY
ATTORNEY

Fuller was granted his first patent on the geodesic dome in 1954. In the application, he detailed the construction of "a frame of generally spherical form in which the main structural elements are interconnected in a geodesic pattern."

Fuller's first large dome was built for the Ford Motor Company's headquarters in Dearborn, Michigan, in 1953. The dome, which protected a round courtyard, weighed eight and a half tons—versus the 160-ton conventional structure Ford's engineers had proposed.

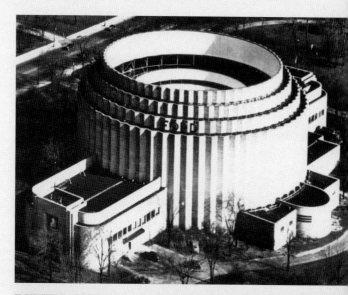

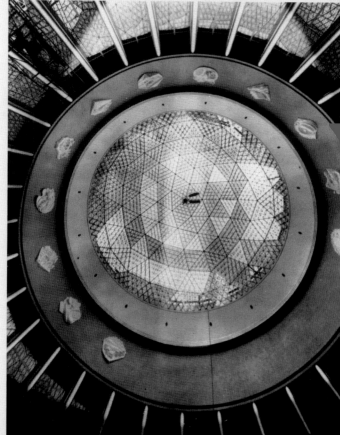

In 1985, three scientists, Robert Curl, Harold Kroto, and Richard Smalley, stumbled upon a molecule no one had seen before. In Kroto's investigations of how chains of carbon were formed in deep space, he enlisted the help of Smalley and Curl, who were experts in exotic chemistry. While experimenting with using a laser to vaporize carbon, they were left with some intriguing soot. At the conclusion of the experiment, they found that they had created a stable cluster of 60 carbon atoms. What was most intriguing about this cluster was its shape: The carbon atoms formed a spherical cage made of up hexagons and polygons. The sphere had a close resemblance to both Buckminster Fuller's geodesic domes and a soccer ball. The new molecule was officially named buckminster-fullerene, but it has a nickname that reflects both of its real world analogs: Buckyballs.

The discovery of fullerenes was exciting for several reasons. They represented a completely new form of carbon, in addition to diamond and graphite. A new form of molecule, especially one as prominent as carbon, promised all kinds of new and unforeseen applications. And Buckyballs were beautiful—symmetrical and strong, they seemed tantalizing proof of some kind of harmony in the design of the universe.

When other researchers found an easier way to make fullerenes in 1990, the race was on to find applications for the new molecule. Because fullerenes are round, some scientists thought they could serve as a lubricant, with each molecule acting as a ball bearing. Others looked into using Buckyballs as ion-rocket fuel and as superconductors.

A decade later, there are still no Buckyball-laden products on our shelves. But scientists have continued to open up new potential fields for the molecule. Current research is exploring their use in therapies for HIV (a modified buckyball fits perfectly into an HIV enzyme) and ALS, Lou Gehrig's Disease (buckyballs act as powerful antioxidants, slowing the progress of the fatal disease).

Research into fullerenes also led to the discovery of another form of carbon molecules: nanotubes, long chains of carbon that look like stretched-out Buckyballs. Nanotubes are strong and flexible and can be made in almost unlimited lengths. As happened 10 years ago, the sense of great possibilities for this new molecule is powerful. Richard Smalley told the *New York Times*, "[Buckyballs] are not nearly as interesting as the tubes. Bucky's biggest legacy has been to show us about the tubes."

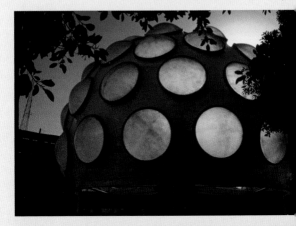

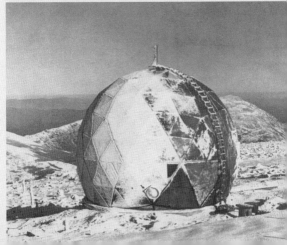

precedent in history." And a spherical building would enclose the maximum amount of space using the minimum amount of materials.

After working out the complicated mathematics involved, Fuller sketched out his first geodesic dome, made up of hundreds of interconnected triangles, each of which reinforced its neighbors through tension. In the summer of 1949, he and some students tried to build it, using aluminum slats from Venetian blinds. The slats were too flimsy, and the first dome collapsed into a twisted pile. Fuller was not discouraged. In 1950, he built a large dome in Montreal, and in 1953 he constructed a dome 50 feet in diameter at the Ford Motor Company's headquarters.

Thousands of people saw the Ford dome, and soon universities, businesses, and individuals were clamoring for a dome of their own. One of Fuller's biggest customers was the United States Air Force, which was setting up the Distant Early Warning system, a network of radar installations near the Arctic Circle that watched for an attack from the Soviet Union. Conditions in the Arctic were horrible, and some kind of shelter for the radar was needed. In response, Fuller designed the radome, a geodesic dome made from fiberglass struts that would not in-terfere with radar waves. The dome itself was perfect for the conditions: It could withstand very strong winds, and its non-metallic surface never iced up.

The simplicity, beauty, strength, and novelty of the geodesic dome captured the public's attention, and Fuller himself soon became a symbol of a future based on new, nondestructive technologies. Some 300,000 geodesic domes have been built, serving as restaurants, factories, and even private houses. The most famous dome, at Disney's Epcot Center, attracts millions of visitors every year.

Today, some of Fuller's lessons on how to build using tension are being used in the design of new buildings. But people have been slow to adopt many of his ideas. Fuller always tried to think 50 years into the future. He knew that his ideas—whether on new ways to build things or what people should eat or the basic geometry of the universe—were too radical to be realized during his own lifetime. Yet he succeeded in inspiring a generation of architects, designers, and others to begin thinking in new directions, examining how to build, how to live, and how to make the world a better place.

The Wichita House, a prototype of Fuller's Dymaxion House, was built in 1947. The round structure's walls and roof were supported by cables attached to a central mast, since steel can support more weight suspended from it than placed on top of it. The house was reconstructed at the Henry Ford Museum & Greenfield Village in 2001.

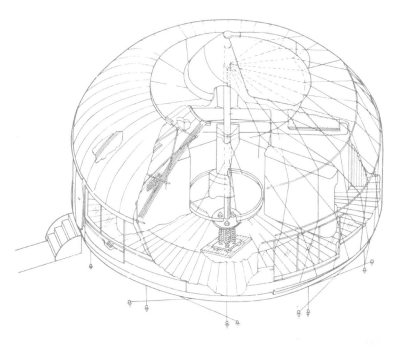

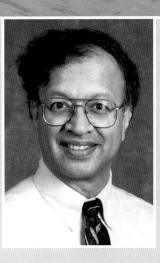

One of the world's most serious health problems is the lack of safe drinking water in developing countries. By some estimates, up to two billion people cannot get clean water. Diarrhea, cholera, hepatitis, and other diseases caused by contaminated water kill some five million people a year, including three million children. Many times that number get sick, and the growth of 60 million children is stunted by recurring diarrhea and other illnesses. Because diarrhea kills by dehydration, the lack of clean water only accelerates the process.

Although the problem is well known, it has not been easy to battle. Water becomes contaminated in many different ways, including inadequate water systems, flooding, and a lack of proper sanitation. Most solutions (such as large filtration plants or new water systems) are far too expensive or complicated for poor nations to implement. Because the problem exists primarily in poor countries, there seems to be little money to be made in fixing it, and most scientists concentrate on more profitable challenges.

In the summer of 1993, an outbreak of a new and particularly dangerous strain of cholera began in northeastern India. Dubbed "Bengal cholera," within months it had spread throughout India and into neighboring countries, killing more than 4,000 people. The tragedy inspired Ashok Gadgil, a scientist working at the Lawrence Berkeley National Laboratory in California, to look for a new way to purify drinking water. Using science no more complex than the ultraviolet light emitted by an unshielded fluorescent lamp, he built a simple, effective, and most important, inexpensive water disinfection system. Dozens of these systems are now installed around the world, and many more will be in use soon.

Born in Bombay, India, in 1950, Gadgil was interested in science from a very early age. "I finished reading all the high school books on general science by the time I was in the fourth grade," he remembers. His parents indulged his interests by buying him chemistry and mechanics sets, books, and electrical components. "One great thing my parents did was bring home *Popular Science*, *Popular Mechanics*, and *Scientific American*," Gadgil says. "So even

A Bhupalpur villager uses a hand pump to feed water into
Gadgil's purification system, housed inside the cement structure.

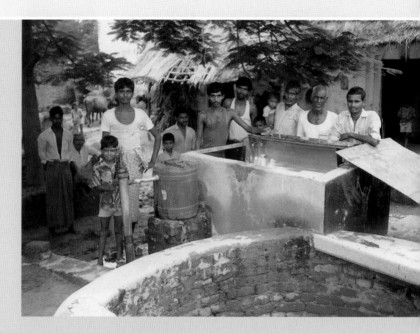

though I was in Bombay, I had access to the kind of excitement that these magazines conveyed." He and some friends also formed a small science club to perform their own investigations—they worked to build better gliders, tracked individual ants in their colonies, and even tried to collect methane gas from rotting biomass in stagnant pools left by the yearly monsoons.

Although Gadgil's parents wanted him to become a doctor, he thought it would be "extremely boring to be doing the same thing all your life." Instead, he chose to pursue physics. He received his bachelor's and master's degrees in physics in India and then, in 1973, came to the University of California at Berkeley to continue his studies.

At Berkeley, Gadgil continued to figure out how best to use his physics knowledge. But he also became aware of things outside of the classroom. "Two things really struck me while I was in graduate school," he says. "One was the high level of affluence in the United States. The second thing was getting a sense of how important it is to have science applied to address problems that are societally significant. They may not be scientifically significant, because the basic science is well understood, but nobody had bothered to take the final step to convert that into a useful technology."

"In the 1970s, when I came to Berkeley, the important thing was relevance," Gadgil notes. "Whatever you are doing, is it meaningful, is it of value?" He began to study solar energy as it applied to buildings—a discipline that had clear applications in the real world, since the United States was facing an energy crisis. After receiving his Ph.D., Gadgil worked for a while at the Lawrence Berkeley National Laboratory, then spent about eight months in Paris collaborating with scientists looking for a solar solution to heating buildings in the Peruvian mountains.

In 1983, Gadgil and his wife Anjali, who is also Indian, decided to return to their home country to try to give something back to their community. After they arrived, he says, "it was clear that the stuff I learned in the United States would not be the right thing to do in India. The problems facing the Indians, as a society or as individuals, are not even on the radar screen here." Rather, he wanted to bring to India the approach he had learned in Berkeley and Paris, to "develop the right research agenda, identify the right research problems, and roll up your sleeves and go do something about it."

For the next five years, he worked with a fledgling research institution to address some basic problems in Indian society, including how to heat water and houses, and whether the country should adopt time zones in order to conserve electricity. (The answer was no; using efficient fluorescent bulbs instead of incandescents would save far more power.) In 1988, frustrated by the shortcomings of India's bureaucracy and its higher education system, he returned to the Lawrence Berkeley Lab to work on problems of energy efficiency.

In 1997, one of Gadgil's systems was installed at this South African hospice for HIV-positive children.

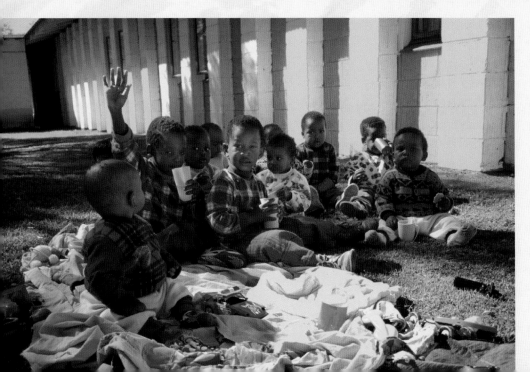

Gadgil remained involved with science back home, though, occasionally sending papers and other information to his colleagues there. One of India's problems that haunted him was that of contaminated drinking water. When Gadgil was living in India in the 1980s, he had witnessed a water-spread outbreak of hepatitis that affected at least 700 people. So in the early 1990s, he began sending information back to his colleagues in India about ultraviolet disinfection, which had some potential for cleaning up the country's water.

There are three basic ways to kill bacteria and viruses in drinking water: chlorination, boiling, and ultraviolet light. Chlorination depends on large-scale treatment plants, and thus is impractical in a country with a poor water infrastructure. Boiling water requires an impractically large amount of fuel, even more than is needed to cook food. And most of the energy used to disinfect water through boiling is wasted; all of the water needs to be boiled to kill the tiny amount of contaminants in it.

Ultraviolet (UV) light seemed like a great alternative to these methods. A certain wavelength of UV light has a profound affect on bacteria and viruses. When used for a short period of time—about 12 seconds—UV light damages their DNA, preventing them from reproducing or even making the enzymes that keep them alive. They die soon after this exposure—and, since they can't reproduce, even if live bacteria or viruses are ingested by a person, no illness will occur.

In 1993, after the Bengal cholera outbreak caused the death of more than 10,000 people in India and neighboring countries, Gadgil grew frustrated with his colleagues, who were not pursuing UV disinfection. That summer, he and a graduate student investigated the effectiveness of UV light and whether it was economically feasible. "We were completely amazed," he says. "Using the simplest engineering, we could disinfect water for half a cent per ton. That's shockingly cheap. You could disinfect one person's drinking supply for a full year for a couple of cents."

From his experiences in India, Gadgil knew that any purification system would have to require little maintenance and not take for granted basic technologies like electricity and water pressure. The system he and his student built, later named UV Waterworks, is remarkably simple. In a compact, enclosed box, a UV lamp is suspended above a shallow pan. Water runs into the pan by the force of gravity, where it is exposed to the UV light, then into a holding tank. The only power that is needed is

about 40 watts to power the light; this can come from a car battery. The system can disinfect four gallons of water a minute, killing 99.999 percent of bacteria and viruses. Run continuously, this produces enough clean water to serve more than 1,000 people.

Water Health International, the company founded to bring the technology to market, now makes several different versions of Gadgil's disinfection system, for small and large applications, for emergency use, and for locations that also need to filter out silt and other large contaminants. Prices start at about $1,500. The company also offers solar cells and small windmills that can power the UV lamp.

UV Waterworks systems have been used in India, South Africa, the Philippines, Honduras, and other countries. Since 1998, the Mexican government has installed about 100 in Guererro, a state on the Pacific in southwestern Mexico. The results have been very positive. In the summer of 2000, Gadgil reports, people from Water Health International returned with stories and data showing a dramatic decline in the incidence of diarrhea among children and adults. And preventing deaths and illness are just the most visible effects of purifying water—it also protects children from stunted physical and mental growth. "This is the kind of story that really makes my day, really makes me happy," Gadgil continues. "It makes me feel good when I get up in the morning."

Run continuously, Gadgil's UV Waterworks device can produce enough clean water to serve more than 1,000 people.

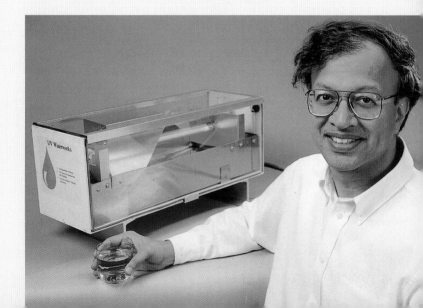

STANFORD OVSHINSKY

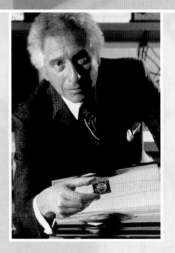

Stanford Ovshinsky built his career and several industries out of two basic ideas. The first was his concept for a completely new class of materials—disordered or "amorphous" materials. The second was a lifelong motivation: "I'd like to be able to make a better world." For more than 40 years, he has combined these two ideas in the pursuit of new kinds of electronics, batteries, and power sources that are more efficient, more powerful, and less polluting. Among the inventions that have come out of this quest are highly efficient batteries and hydrogen fuel cells to power automobiles, rewritable optical storage for computers, and solar cells that can be manufactured cheaply and in large quantities. His work, especially the batteries that powered General Motors' first production electric vehicle, the EV-1, led *Time* magazine to declare him a "Hero for the Planet."

It may be surprising that Ovshinsky, who holds almost 200 patents, is self-taught; he learned a trade during high school, and never pursued college. "I was not very much interested in school," he says. "But I was interested in learning." There were plenty of places for Ovshinsky to indulge his curiosity in Akron, Ohio, where he was born in 1922. He spent a lot of time around Akron's machine shops and foundries, and also read about all kinds of science, from anthropology and archaeology to astronomy. "At our local library, which was a small room in the poorer section of town," he recalls, "the librarians were only supposed to give out two books to every child, and only in their age bracket. They permitted me to take out as many as I wanted, of any age level."

During the depression, Ovshinsky attended high school during the day and trade school at night. After graduation, he opened his own machine shop, where he eventually began making machines that automated industrial processes. (The word *automation* hadn't been coined yet; Ovshinsky tried to get the term *automatation* to stick, although it didn't.) In the late 1940s, he brought his machines to Detroit and worked with the Big Three automakers—Chrysler, Ford, and General Motors—to improve production at their factories. In 1947 he created his first successful invention, an automatic lathe that he later sold to a large industrial company.

At Energy Conversion Devices' first laboratory, Stanford and Iris Ovshinsky discuss using solar energy to "disassociate" water, freeing hydrogen atoms.

The Ovshinskys founded Energy Conversion Devices in 1960 to further explore the amorphous materials he had been investigating and, they hoped, to create products that could better society.

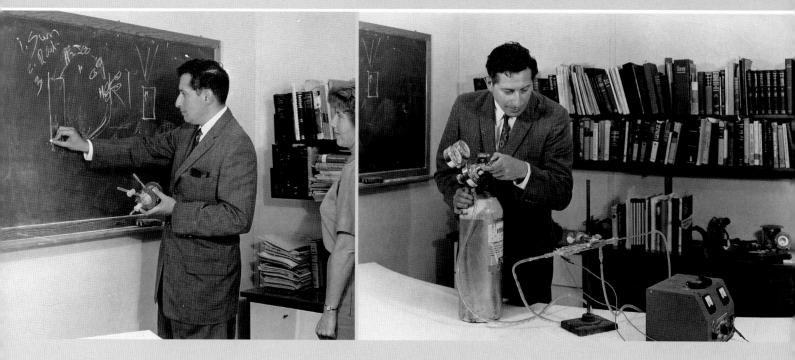

It was Ovshinsky's interest in automating machines that led him, in a roundabout way, to the science of amorphous materials. His machines could make some simple decisions as they went about their work, and Ovshinsky realized that this was a form of intelligence. But it was also clear to him that this wasn't *really* intelligence. So Ovshinsky asked, "What is the physical basis of intelligence?" He corresponded with several leading neurophysiologists about the question. "Some of them said that a nerve cell was like a crystalline material," he remembers. "One of them said that he thought that the neuron was an empty bag. And I didn't think that."

If a neuron was empty, Ovshinsky thought, then perhaps the outside of the neuron, its surface, was the important part. And while many researchers proposed that neurons worked like transistors—logic gates made out of crystalline silicon—he noticed that the neuron surface was disordered, non-crystalline. With the help of his wife, Iris, a biology and biochemistry Ph.D.,

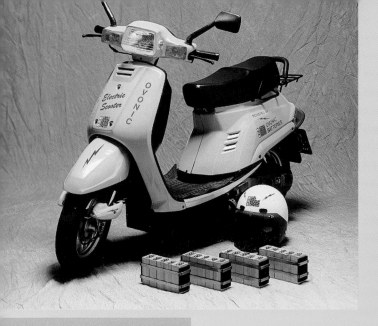

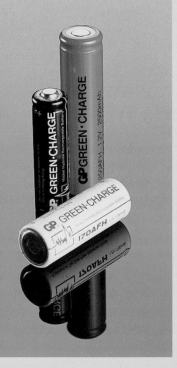

One of the major focuses of Stan Ovshinsky's career has been batteries. Licensed versions of his rechargeable nickel-metal-hydride (NiMH) batteries (above) are used in millions of laptops and other portable electronics. Four packs of NiMH batteries power this electric scooter (top), giving it a range of up to 70 miles.

Ovshinsky designed a model of a nerve cell based on this idea of a disordered surface. "It acted like a nerve cell should act," he says. "It had memory, it had the equivalent of synaptic connections."

This proved to Ovshinsky that disordered materials had interesting characteristics. Yet "I couldn't find any literature on disorder," he notes. "At that time amorphous materials were called *schmutz* materials." On January 1, 1960, he and Iris founded Energy Conversion Devices (ECD) to explore the field and, he hoped, "to have science and technology solve serious societal problems."

The most surprising and exciting property of disordered materials was that they could act as semiconductors. Until then, people thought that only crystalline solids, like the silicon that makes up computer chips, could act as semiconductors. Silicon does the job very well. But the process of manufacturing silicon chips is difficult, requiring "clean rooms" in factories that now cost upward of $1 billion, and the size of the chips is limited by the small size of a crystal. Disordered materials, as their name implies, do not have any overall structure. But their molecular structure—they are made from cesium, tellurium, or related elements—allows them to shift, in small quantities, to a more ordered state, when energy such as light or electrons hits them. This shift, called a "phase change," lets the material act like a conductive metal.

Ovshinsky's discovery that these materials could be shifted into working as a semiconductor opened up all kinds of possibilities, such as using them for computer memory. Because the phase change is a physical process—the molecules actually move into an ordered state—data can be stored even in the absence of electricity. This quality led to the invention of "flash" memory, often used in laptops and other electronic devices that need to store information when they're switched off, as well as rewritable CDs and DVDs.

In the early 1980s, Ovshinsky began applying his amorphous material science to solar panels, called photovoltaic (PV) panels. Photovoltaics had until then been made using crystalline materials like silicon. As with computer chips, the manufacturing process was expensive and demanding. In addition, these PV panels were thick and heavy, so they had to be mounted on a building or some other strong structure.

Although the PV cell Ovshinsky developed using disordered materials only produced about 50 to 60 percent of the power that conventional PV did, it had some significant advantages. The amorphous semiconductor that made them work was a thin film, rather than a thick crystalline material, so the PV cells were much lighter and more flexible. Most important, they allowed Ovshinsky to create a new PV manufacturing process. In 1983, he patented a device much like a large printing press. A long roll of thin, flexible metal is fed through the machine, which deposits the thin film of disordered materials. The most recent generation of the machine can create 1/2-mile-long rolls of PV cells up to 18 inches wide; the next version will accommodate 1 1/2-mile-long rolls.

Such large-scale production has drastically lowered the cost of PV cells, to about $1 per watt, which is comparable with power from oil, gas, or coal. In addition, the thin, lightweight material has freed designers to create new kinds of energy-producing components. The most interesting of these is the PV shingle, which not only looks like a slightly oversized version of a regular roof shingle, it works like one. "What I've done with PV is make it prosaic, bring it back down to earth," Ovshinsky says. "The shingles aren't on top of the roof, they are the roof."

To Ovshinsky, this is an important achievement. The mission of his and Iris's company is still to change the world for the better, and he believes you can't do that with niche products, as PV cells have been for decades. PV shingles are easily understandable by people who might not be interested in solar energy; they also save space, since there are already roofs all around the world ready for them.

Ovshinsky's company is also involved with another kind of energy technology: hydrogen fuel cells, which may turn out to be even more valuable than solar cells. A fuel cell uses a reaction similar to that of a battery to create electricity from hydrogen; many car makers are betting that it is the next big fuel technology. There is no pollution—the only by-product is water—and hydrogen is abundant.

Although it is an inexpensive fuel source, hydrogen is difficult to store and manage. As a gas, it has to be stored under great pressure; as a liquid, it has to be kept at −253° Celsius. Ovshinsky devised a better way to store it: in metal. Hydrogen can be pulled out of or pushed into a metal matrix, which is compact and safe and stores more hydrogen per liter than the liquid or gas forms of the element. Making hydrogen easier to use will accelerate the development of fuel-cell–powered cars.

Even though humans only recently learned how to convert sunlight into usable energy, Ovshinsky promises that hydrogen power could be even more revolutionary. "It's a complete decoupling from the earth's resources," he says. "It's pollution-free. You don't have to fight wars over oil." Still going strong at the age of 78, Ovshinsky sees his latest technological contribution as just part of the goals he and his wife set for ECD in 1960. "We're doing what we said we were going to do," he says. "What better way is there to express your ideals than to make the world better and safer and healthier?"

Ovshinsky discovered that amorphous materials could act like semiconductors; one application of this was the creation of thin, flexible solar power panels. Making the panels in large rolls lowers the cost of their power to about $1 per watt.

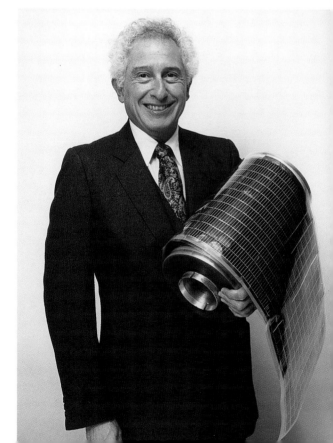

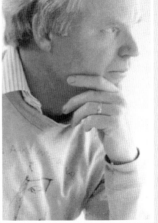

JOHN TODD

John Todd is dedicated to the idea that biology should be the model for all design. By enlisting nature's own processes, he has created new systems for farming, aquaculture, treating waste, and purifying water, among other things. These systems, which he calls Living Machines, have the potential to shift technology—and by extension the world—to a more sustainable path.

This application of biology and ecology to human systems is fitting, for Todd grew up surrounded by both nature and industry. Born in 1939, he was raised on the shores of Hamilton Bay, a center for Canadian steel and shipping. It was "a world of ships and slag and burning ovens and fires and ice," Todd says. Although his father was an executive for 3M, he was also passionate about the outdoors. "All he talked about at home was the woods and the farms and the forest and canoes and kayaks," Todd remembers. So while the local environment had been severely damaged, he was still able to develop a deep connection with nature. "We had marshes right next to our house and streams and I could follow them right up to their headwaters," he says. "It was a very mysterious world for a kid."

Todd had little interest in academics as a youth, preferring pursuits such as sailing and skiing. Two events helped change his focus. The first was his becoming depressed as the local environment was further damaged. "Some of the woods I would walk through to school were being cut down," he explains. "Orchards and market farms were being paved over to be subdivisions. Even my beloved clay pits were under siege. From all around, from the water to the hills behind, I felt threatened." Then, when Todd was 13, his father gave him a series of books written by the novelist Louis Bromfield, describing his effort to restore an agricultural region of Ohio.

Bromfield had returned from Europe after World War II to find the area depopulated and eroding. "His dream was to bring it back to life," Todd says. "He re-created an agricultural community with the holistic knowledge he had brought from [rural France]. In the midst of destruction, here was this marvelous tale of hope." Todd began working on farms and decided to study agriculture at McGill University in Montreal, Canada. What he was taught at

Todd's first attempt at using living things to clean the environment took place in Cape Cod—he set up 21 translucent tanks to cleanse sewage being dumped into an open pit.

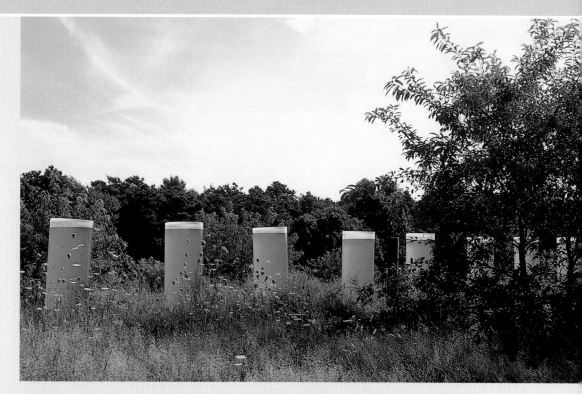

college, though, came as a shock. The agriculture program focused on chemical and mechanical farming, not sustainable or traditional practices. "We were told that most of us would be salesmen for the drug or chemical companies," he remembers.

Dispirited by the idea of institutional farming, Todd became interested in the disciplines of his favorite professors: ecology and biology. After graduating from McGill, he worked for several years as an environmental consultant, surveying damage from factories across America and Canada. Even in these affected environments, though, he found some reasons for hope. "I could see points where there was a recovery," he says. "These were my first inklings of the possibility of the regenerative forces of nature."

In graduate school, first at McGill and then at the University of Michigan, Todd studied oceanography and fisheries. After earning an award for the

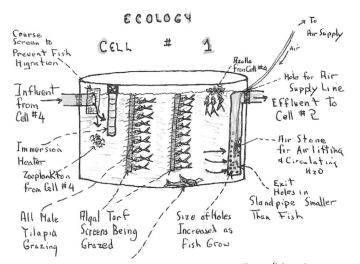

ECOLOGY CELL # 1

- Course Screen to Prevent Fish Migration
- Influent from Cell #4
- Immersion Heater
- Zooplankton from Cell #4
- All Male Tilapia Grazing
- Algal Turf Screens Being Grazed
- Size of Holes Increased as Fish Grow
- Armored Catfish as Cleaner Fish /Solids Removal
- To Air Supply
- Air
- Azolla From Cell #4
- Hole for Air Supply Line
- Effluent To Cell #2
- Air Stone for Air lifting & Circulating H2O
- Exit Holes in Standpipe Smaller Than Fish

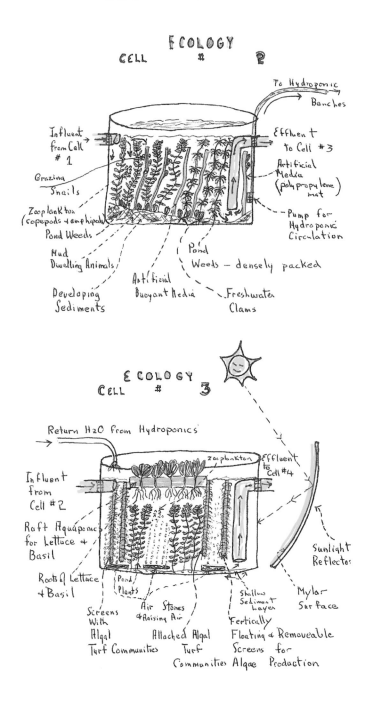

ECOLOGY CELL # 2

- Influent from Cell #1
- Grazing Snails
- Zooplankton (copepods + amphipods)
- Pond Weeds
- Mud Dwelling Animals
- Developing Sediments
- Artificial Buoyant Media
- Pond Weeds — densely packed
- Freshwater Clams
- To Hydroponic Benches
- Effluent To Cell #3
- Artificial Media (polypropylene mat)
- Pump for Hydroponic Circulation

ECOLOGY CELL # 3

- Return H2O from Hydroponics
- Influent from Cell #2
- Raft Aquaponics for Lettuce & Basil
- Roots of Lettuce + Basil
- Screens With Algal Turf Communities
- Air Stones & Raising Air
- Attached Algal Turf Communities
- Pond Plants
- Shallow Sediment Layer
- Vertically Floating & Removeable Screens for Algae Production
- Zooplankton
- Effluent to Cell #4
- Sunlight Reflector
- Mylar Surface

outstanding doctorate at Michigan in 1968, he decided to take a position at San Diego State University teaching ethology (animal behavior) so he could conduct research in the warm waters of nearby Mexico. After a couple of years of "doom watch" research—studying what's wrong with the environment—Todd felt he'd reached a dead end. With the help of his wife, Nancy, he began to look at more positive possibilities for science. "I began to have a conversation around how knowledge could be reintegrated to be reused in an earth-healing way," he says.

He, Nancy, and their colleague William McLarney began to pursue what they called "new alchemy," the science and practice of applied ecology. In a 1971 paper, Todd laid out a plan for a new science of "earth stewardship." The three of them also founded the New Alchemy Institute in Woods Hole, Massachusetts, where Todd had taken an oceanographic research job. Today, he realizes that their goals seem innocent and perhaps pompous. "Our slogan was, 'To restore the land, protect the seas, and inform the Earth's stewards,'" he recalls. "That's a lot for three people."

During the 1970s, New Alchemy's work became more concrete, as Todd and others began to establish guidelines for

John Todd's Living Machines use natural processes—from bottom-feeding fish to photosynthesis—to remove contaminants from water.

designing systems from a biological or ecological starting point. In the mid-1980s, Todd decided that one of the biggest threats to humans was water pollution. Two of his closest friends had recently died of cancer, and he noticed that a neighboring Cape Cod town was dumping its sewage and other waste in an open pit just 25 feet above the drinking water table. Looking at that pit, Todd says, he "made the connection between the environment and this epidemic that permeates our lives."

Methods for treating this kind of waste already existed, but they were chemical- and energy-intensive and expensive, and not being used at all in this case. From his own experience, Todd thought he could build a treatment system that was less expensive and based on natural processes. In the 1970s, he had built seminatural habitats to conduct research on fish from the Pacific Ocean and the Gulf of Mexico, fish that were notoriously hard to breed in captivity. In essence, he re-created their natural environment in a greenhouse. "I was asking plants and animals to play the roles of the filters and all the other things you would find in an aquarium," he explains. Todd succeeded in breeding the fish, but he wound up more interested in the system he had built. "It was clear in my mind," he continues, "that living systems, whether plant or animal, can be a substitute for energy, hardware, and manufactured chemicals. There is an analog that we can find in the natural world to carry out functions that we currently carry out with brute force."

In 1984, Todd applied these ideas to a test system to treat the waste in that open pit. He built an artificial marsh and 21 connected clear tanks, each containing various organisms, from algae and marsh plants to invertebrates and small fish. As the water made its way through these tanks the living creatures in each broke down, ate, or otherwise processed the pollutants. The process was sped up by the tanks' transparency—bright sunlight accelerated the photosynthesis that fueled many of the organisms. The cleansing process took 12 days, at the end of which 100 percent of nearly all the major pollutants had been removed.

Two companies have been founded to refine and market Todd's water treatment system. To date, it has been installed in Florida, Wisconsin, Vermont, and Nevada, among other places, to treat waste from factories, nature centers, and schools. These Living Machines work much as the first test system did. Waste water is first directed into underground tanks, where organic matter and solids are broken down by bacteria. Then, the water moves through a series of open-air tanks full of plants,

At the San Francisco Museum of Modern Art, a small Living Machine supported a species of African fish that is extinct in the wild.

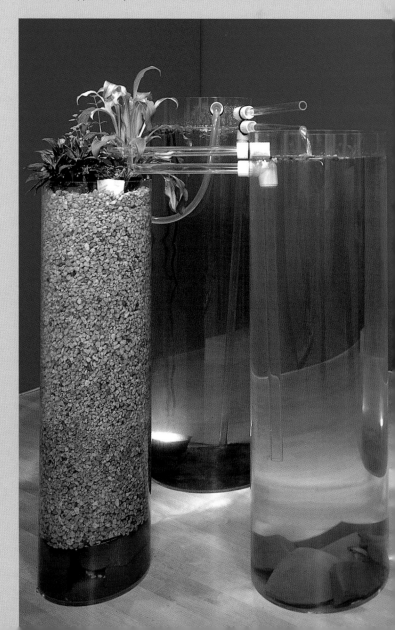

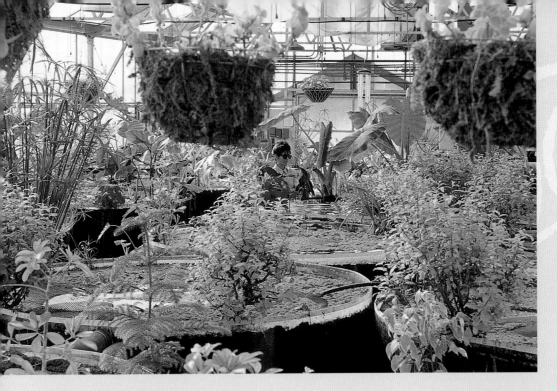

Today, a Living Machine in Providence, Rhode Island, treats millions of gallons of sewage every year.

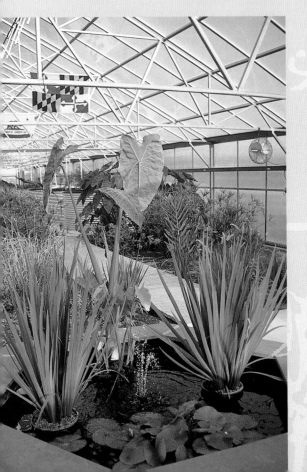

Another Living Machine was installed in Frederick, Maryland, as a demonstration of an ecologically engineered landscape.

plankton, snails, and fish, which each play a role in digesting and breaking down more of the waste. Remaining solids are collected from the water, which then moves through a natural filter such as lava rock. In the end, the water is clean enough to be reused or released into local waterways.

Todd continues to work on other designs that harness natural processes. He is currently developing a method for "compact farming" that would let people raise food in relatively small spaces. "In a sense I'm trying to reinvent a chunk of agriculture," he says. If his new method of farming is adopted, it could bring the production of food closer to urban areas and eventually open up more space for nonindustrial and nonfarming use.

Todd is also working with architect Maya Lin on the restoration of a chapel in Purchase, New York. A glass structure around the ruined church would stabilize it, and a Living Machine would be installed inside to clean the water of a nearby creek. Water "would flow up into the tower and then through the build-ing in a very formal way," he explains, "through a Living Machine, step by step, right down the middle of the building. The purified water then heads back to the stream." This marriage of nature and aesthetics encapsulates many of Todd's ecological beliefs and designs. With the Living Machine's clear tanks occupying the chapel, he adds, "the connection between other forms of life and our own lives will be rendered more visible."

"Our slogan was, 'To restore the land, protect the seas, and inform the Earth's stewards,'" he recalls. "That's a lot for three people."

COMPUTING AND TELECOMMUNICATIONS

INTRODUCTION

This group of innovative American minds works in what is perhaps the key field of endeavor when it comes to causing change in the modern world: information and communications technology. Throughout history, the greatest innovative surges seem to come after a major advance in the ability to generate, store, or distribute information. Developments in communications technology make it easier for ideas to come together in new ways and generate novelty. Innovation generated in this way then expands by a ripple effect, spreading out from the original idea to bring social change.

Witness the ripple effect of one side-product of the printing press: printed maps. In the early seventeenth century these maps, easily updated and reprinted with the latest navigation and exploratory data from ships' logs, made it safer for captains to go looking for profitable cargoes in the East. The first Dutch trading companies to use the new maps made it a legal requirement for returning crews to report all newly discovered navigational information to the company printing-house, so that the data could be included in the next edition of charts and atlases. As a result, by the second decade of the century the Dutch were bringing goods back from the East and re-exporting them all around Europe, sometimes making 600 percent profit in the process. The idea soon caught on, and demand for cash to invest in the new ventures triggered the establishment of new land registers to give formal title to land (the prime contemporary source of wealth) so as to borrow money against it, through another new entity set up for the purpose: the mortgage company. Insurance companies were then organized to reduce the

financial risk of shipwreck, and joint-stock companies were formed to reduce the risk of failure. Joint-stock companies in turn brought the emergence of the first stock market and a national bank was set up to organize extra funding through its new credit agencies. The whole enterprise was made secure with another new invention: the business contract, whose philosophy would find its way into politics with the citizen-state relationship embodied in the new Constitution of the United States.

The information/communication-technology work of this group of inventors—including the mouse, the walkie-talkie, computerized telephone switching systems, microchips, programming, computer games, and the personal computer—will help to generate perhaps the greatest ripple effect so far. By the end of the first decade of this century the communication and information industry can expect to see virtually unlimited bandwidth, handheld semi-intelligent communications devices, and supercomputers capable of a thousand trillion operations per second. What this technology will do can only be guessed at. Continuing innovation in this field will almost certainly make America the first fully virtual social and economic structure. All citizens, anywhere, will be able to enjoy the benefits of a new kind of existence, wherever they find themselves: in education, jobs, acts of self-expression, with access to anything they want to know, wherever they are, at any time of the night and day. Electronic avatars will represent them in social, political, and business decisions, making these future Americans members of the first truly informed and fully enfranchised society in history.

Perhaps the greatest moment of discontinuity that our final group of inventors is helping to facilitate, however, will come when the new technology changes the nature of innovation itself. Ever since the first flint tool, the constraints imposed by technological limitations have shaped what contemporary society could do and, above all, who could do it. Access to knowledge and the means of expression was limited to a tiny, literate minority. It is their work alone that tells us what happened in history. We know little or nothing of the vast, silent, illiterate majority. This state of affairs has lasted up to the present time and has generated what might be termed a "culture of scarcity," in which the few have always ordered and the many have always obeyed. We have lived for millennia in a culture in which talent and intelligence and innovative capabilities have come to be regarded as exceptional, because in the country of the blind the one-eyed man is king.

We have no means of knowing if those individuals whom we now regard as history's greats—Newton, Michelangelo, Franklin, Galileo, and all the others—were indeed the best. There may have been thousands of others even more talented, but, being illiterate, they were out of the loop. However, the ones we know about certainly showed what humans are capable of, given the tools and the opportunity. This is what the information and communications technology now being developed by American inventors is about to offer, to an unprecedented number of human beings, all over the planet, each of whom has a brain of the same size and complexity as Einstein's.

—JB

NOLAN **BUSHNELL**

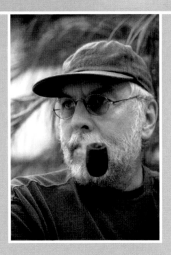

In just three decades, video games have taken a prominent and permanent place in American culture. They have more than a hundred million fans, have spawned dozens of magazines, and have even captured the attention (and disapproval) of the U.S. Senate. The demands made by games have been responsible for many improvements in computer technology, advances that have led to higher graphics and speed capabilities in today's personal computers.

The more than $6 billion Americans now spend on video games every year started with the first quarter dropped into Computer Space in 1971. That game—a small computer hooked up to a black-and-white TV, housed in a futuristic-looking plastic case—was the creation of Nolan Bushnell, a young engineer from Utah. Bushnell went on to found Atari, whose products, from Pong to Football to the Atari 2600, brought video games into every arcade and millions of homes. And while Computer Space was based on the already-classic computer spaceship battle game called Spacewar, it was Bushnell's genius to see the potential games had beyond the computer lab.

"I've always been a tinkerer," Bushnell says. As a teenager, he was one of the youngest ham radio operators in the country, and he did science experiments in his garage. At least one of those went awry: A liquid-fuel rocket attached to a roller skate crashed into the back of his garage, igniting a bright but short-lived fireball. Rockets were a side interest, though. "I loved electronics from an early age," Bushnell remembers, "But I was also always a game player." He was a tournament chess player, and a fan of the Chinese board game Go. (Atari is a Japanese word announced when a Go player has almost captured an opponent.) He also learned about business when he was young. After his father died, Bushnell took over the family's concrete business. He was just 15.

Bushnell discovered computer games in the early 1960s while studying electrical engineering at the University of Utah. The school's computer had a copy of Spacewar, the seminal game created at MIT by Steve Russell. Two starships circling a sun battled each other and the star's gravity, firing "torpedoes" and occasionally resorting to "hyperspace" to jump out of, and

In 1977, Atari released the Video Computer System, also known as the 2600. More than 25 million of the cartridge-based machines were sold, ushering in the first golden age of home video games.

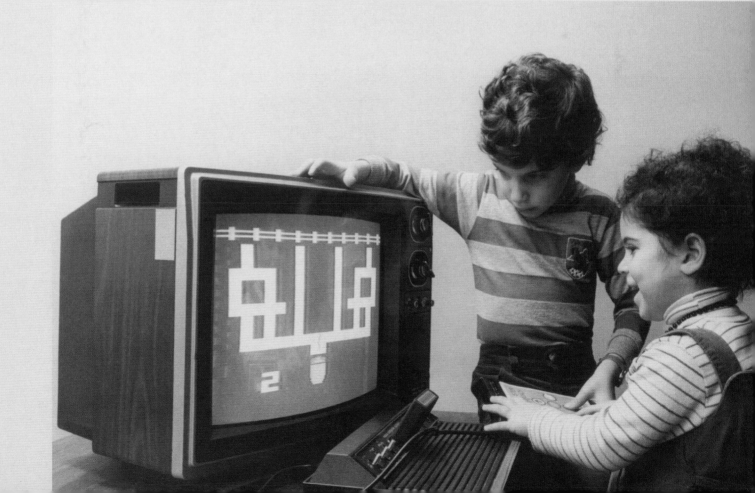

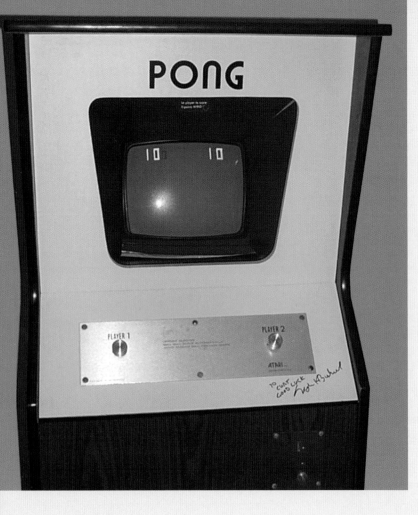

The first successful video arcade game was Atari's Pong, which debuted in 1972. The game, a simple electronic tennis match, had just one line of instructions: "Avoid Missing Ball for High Score."

THE PREHISTORY OF VIDEO GAMES

Late eighteenth century—Bagatelle, a miniature tabletop game related to billiards, becomes popular.

1871—A small version of bagatelle with a spring-loaded plunger becomes popular; it is the ancestor of the pinball machine.

1905—The first nickelodeon opens, in Pittsburgh. Customers can see a short movie by dropping a nickel in a machine's slot.

1931—The first coin-operated pinball machine is built.

1947—The pinball flipper is invented, ushering in the Golden Age of Pinball. The game is banned in New York City the following year.

1958—Willy Higinbotham, an engineer at Brookhaven National Laboratory on Long Island, New York, uses an analog computer to make a "ball" bounce back and forth across the screen of a small oscilloscope. He adds a "net" and the first computer tennis game is born. Visitors to the lab's open house line up for hours to play.

sometimes into, trouble. (Hyperspace would reappear in 1978 in Atari's Asteroids game.) Spacewar was immensely popular among computer scientists and students, and was soon being played on computers around the world. The visionary computer designer Alan Kay once declared, "The game of Spacewar blossoms spontaneously wherever there is a graphics display connected to a computer." Bushnell was hooked, and he would sneak into the computer lab late at night to play.

During his college summers, Bushnell managed the arcade at a local amusement park, where he saw how eager people were to play games. It was this experience that gave Bushnell his big idea. "It was very easy for me to see that if I could put a quarter slot on [Spacewar] and put it in the amusement park, it'd make money. It wasn't really a huge Aha!" he says. But Spacewar ran on huge, expensive computers. "You'd divide 25 cents into a $7 million computer, and you'd see, gee, this doesn't work," he continues. "But in the back of your mind, you'd say, If I can build it cheap enough it will work. And one day the costs came in such that I thought that it was possible."

By 1971, Bushnell had moved to Silicon Valley and had begun to work on his game. He took over one of his daughters' rooms and built from scratch the circuits that would run his own version of Spacewar, which he called Computer Space. The biggest technical challenge was the display. The computers that ran Spacewar used what were essentially adapted radar screens, each of which cost about $30,000. So Bushnell made circuits that would display graphics on an ordinary black-and-white television set. At his kitchen table, he sculpted a scale model of Computer Space's curvy, futuristic case out of clay. (The game looked so distinctive that it was used as a prop in the 1973 sci-fi movie *Soylent Green*.)

Computer Space was licensed to a company called Nutting Associates, which built about 1,500 of the machines. The game was a moderate success, but not a runaway hit; many people thought it was too complicated. Bushnell had a different complaint about its manufacturer. "Nutting Associates was an extremely incompetent company," he says. "I've often thought that that was a huge blessing, because it was clear that these guys were succeeding in spite of being really stupid. There's nothing like being around that to embolden yourself."

Bushnell began designing other games and he hired a staff of engineers. In 1972, Bally, a company that made pinball and slot machines, contracted him to make a video driving game. He gave the task to one of his new hires, Al Alcorn. But Alcorn didn't yet know the tricks of making a video game, so Bushnell gave him a smaller task: to make a game with a ball bouncing back and forth on the screen. (Bushnell had seen a similar game demonstrated that year as part of the Odyssey home video

1961–1962—At MIT, Steve Russell and others create Spacewar on the university's PDP-1 computer. Copies of Spacewar wind up at universities around the country, draining countless hours of expensive computer time and inspiring a generation of programmers. The first gaming controls, the ancestors of the joystick, are built by Spacewar-playing MIT students.

Mid-1960s—More games are written for the PDP-1 and other computers, including Lunar Lander, which simulated a moon landing; Hunt the Wumpus, a search-and-destroy mission; and ADVENT, the world's first adventure game.

1966–1967—Ralph Baer, a defense company engineer, builds a small computer and hooks it up to a TV set and makes two electronic dots chase each other across the screen. Within a year, he and some colleagues turn it into a system that plays Ping-Pong, football, and shooting games. When it's released as the Magnavox Odyssey in 1972, Baer's invention becomes the first home video game system.

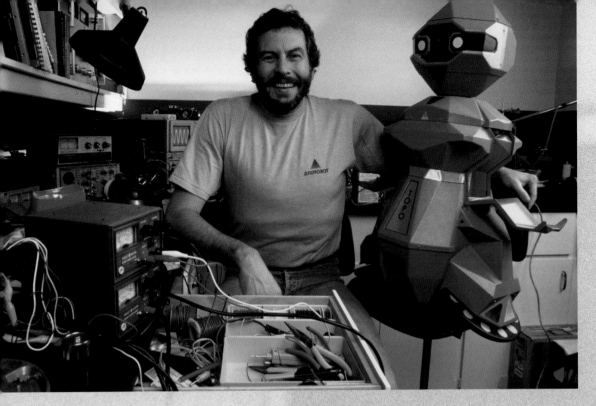

Nolan Bushnell sold Atari in 1978; since then, he has been
involved in business ranging from family restaurants to home
robots to Internet gaming.

"The brain is something that if you exercise it you can be
smarter. It turns out that games are that exercise."

game, designed by Ralph Baer and marketed by Magnavox.) "I defined this very simple game for Alcorn as a learning project," he explains. "I thought it was going to be a throwaway. It took him less than a week to get it partially running. And the thing was just incredibly fun."

Bushnell took a copy of Alcorn's game, named Pong after one of its noises, to Bally's headquarters in Chicago, hoping that they would buy it instead of the driving game. At the same time, Alcorn built a case for their other copy of Pong, complete with a 13-inch TV set and a slot for quarters. There was one sentence of instructions on the cabinet: "Avoid Missing Ball for High Score." Alcorn set Pong up at a bar in Sunnyvale, California.

In Chicago, Bally's turned Pong down. Back in California, the reaction was different. People lined up to feed quarters into Pong, and played it nonstop. The next day, the machine suddenly stopped working; Alcorn went to see what was wrong and discovered that the machine was too full of quarters—they'd spilled out of their container and shorted the game out. Pong, released by Atari rather than Bally's, became a hit and ushered in the first golden age of video games. Rich from Pong's success, the company designed dozens of successful games, first variations on Pong and later arcade hits like Atari Football, the driving games Night Driver and Sprint, and, in 1978, the best-selling Asteroids.

Bushnell also helped usher in a new era in Silicon Valley. Although the area (which extends from Palo Alto to San Jose) had long been a center for the electronics industry, most of the companies there were large and corporate. Atari was different. Bushnell always wore jeans, and he encouraged his engineers and technicians to do the same. His management style was not very rigid or hierarchical; as long as someone got his or her job done, almost anything went. These principles were proved in 1976, when Bushnell hired a young technician named Steve Jobs. The long-haired Jobs would often work barefoot, talked of going to India, and was abrasive to some of the other engineers. Bushnell gave Jobs the task of designing a game he had thought of, a new variation on Pong called Breakout. Jobs worked the night shift, and with lots of technical help from his friend Steve Wozniak, built Breakout on a very short schedule. The two would continue their collaboration that year by building and marketing the Apple computer.

In 1975, Atari introduced a version of Pong for the home, which quickly sold hundreds of thousands of copies and spawned dozens of imitators. Two years later, the company introduced the Video Computer System, also known as the Atari 2600. This was the first successful home system that used interchangeable cartridges, so players could enjoy dozens (and eventually hundreds) of different games. More than 25 million systems were sold, and the system-and-cartridge idea has been adopted by Nintendo, Sega, and Sony. "That's something I'm really proud of," Bushnell says. "I set up the economic model, the software/hardware link that's been the pattern ever since. There wasn't anything out there like it."

Bushnell sold Atari in 1978 and left the company soon after that. He has launched several businesses since then, including the Chuck E. Cheese chain of video-game pizza parlors and, in the 1980s, Axlon, which made small robots for the home. He has now returned to his video game roots, running a company called uWink that is introducing a line of arcade games that will be linked up over the Internet. Bushnell envisions game tournaments with thousands of participants linked up around the country or the world.

Almost thirty years after building that first arcade game, Bushnell remains excited about the promise of video games, as much for their effects on players as for their business opportunities. Just as Spacewar attracted him to the computer lab as a youth in Utah, today's games excite kids about technology, and even make them smarter. "I call them the training wheels of computer literacy," he says. "It's very clear that game playing grows dendrites. So people are smarter. The brain is something that if you exercise it you can be smarter. It turns out that games are that exercise."

DOUGLAS ENGELBART

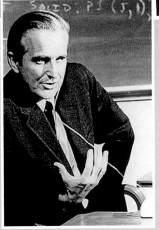

When Douglas Engelbart took the stage at the San Francisco Civic Auditorium in December 1968 to demonstrate the NLS (oN Line System), a computer he and some colleagues at the Stanford Research Institute had built, only a handful of the 2,000 people gathered for the Fall Joint Computer Conference could have imagined how prescient the demo would prove. Looking a bit like a NASA Mission Control navigator, Engelbart sat at a computer console and spoke into a headset microphone while an image of his face was projected onto a screen behind him. He explained to the crowd that he was going to show them how his system worked, not just explain it. And he began. Overlaid on the image of his talking head was a computer display, the kind of text-only display that a generation of personal computer enthusiasts would come to know, but that until then had never been seen. He typed a few words on the blank screen. And then Engelbart began to manipulate the words he had typed. A strange object appeared on the screen: a small, moving black dot.

The little dot is what we now call a cursor. Engelbart was moving it with a peculiar device under his right hand, a chunky, square box with a single button, tethered to the machine with a cord. In the lab, he and his colleagues had called it a "mouse," after its tail-like cable, and the name stuck. With this mouse, Engelbart was able to select text, move it around, and otherwise manipulate it. The mouse was not simply a pointing device, though. It was a key element of the NLS, which in turn was a key element of Engelbart's larger ideas about "Human Augmentation"—making systems and tools that would help people work smarter and better. He has been pursuing those ideas since he had an epiphany about what to do with his life in 1950, while driving to his job as an engineer at the National Advisory Committee on Aeronautics (NACA, which became NASA) Ames Research Center in Mountain View, California.

It had taken Engelbart the first 25 years of his life to get to that moment of clarity. Born in Oregon in 1925, he was the grandson of Western pioneers and the son of a radio store owner and a mother who, he remembers, was "quite sensitive, and artistic." His father passed away when Engelbart was only nine, and the family's finances were tight. After high school, he studied electrical engineering at Oregon State University for two years, then signed up with the navy. This was in 1944, the thick of World War II, though on the day he shipped out of San Francisco, Japan surrendered.

In the navy, Engelbart served as a radar technician, which gave him direct experience with how information could be conveyed directly, electronically, on a screen. While he was stationed in the Philippines, he came across a copy of *Life* magazine that included Vannevar Bush's essay, "As We May Think," which described something like the personal computer, as well as something like the World Wide Web.

After the war, Engelbart finished his degree and moved down to the San Francisco Bay area, to work at Ames. Within a few years, his work there had become less than exciting, and he began to wonder what else he could, or should, be doing. The epiphany came to him the day after he asked his future wife, Ballard, to marry him. He was driving to work, thinking, and "I had this realization that I didn't have any more goals, and that getting married and living happily ever after was the last of my goals," he told a Stanford University interviewer in 1986. "I had to figure out a good set of professional goals." He calculated how many minutes of working life he had left in him—about five and a half million—and wondered how he could maximize the use of that time, for himself but also for mankind.

So Engelbart began looking at the various avenues he could take to do something beneficial and still make a living. (He had a family to support, and memories of his modest childhood weren't far from his mind.) He thought about going into economics, or education. But then he saw, suddenly and whole, the problem that he could help solve. Engelbart realized that everything had changed. The world was moving away from old modes of work, industry, and thought. Civilization had reached a point where the problems it was facing were growing increasingly complex, and at the same time they were growing more urgent. This complexity and urgency "had transcended what humans can cope with," he explained. "It suddenly flashed that if you

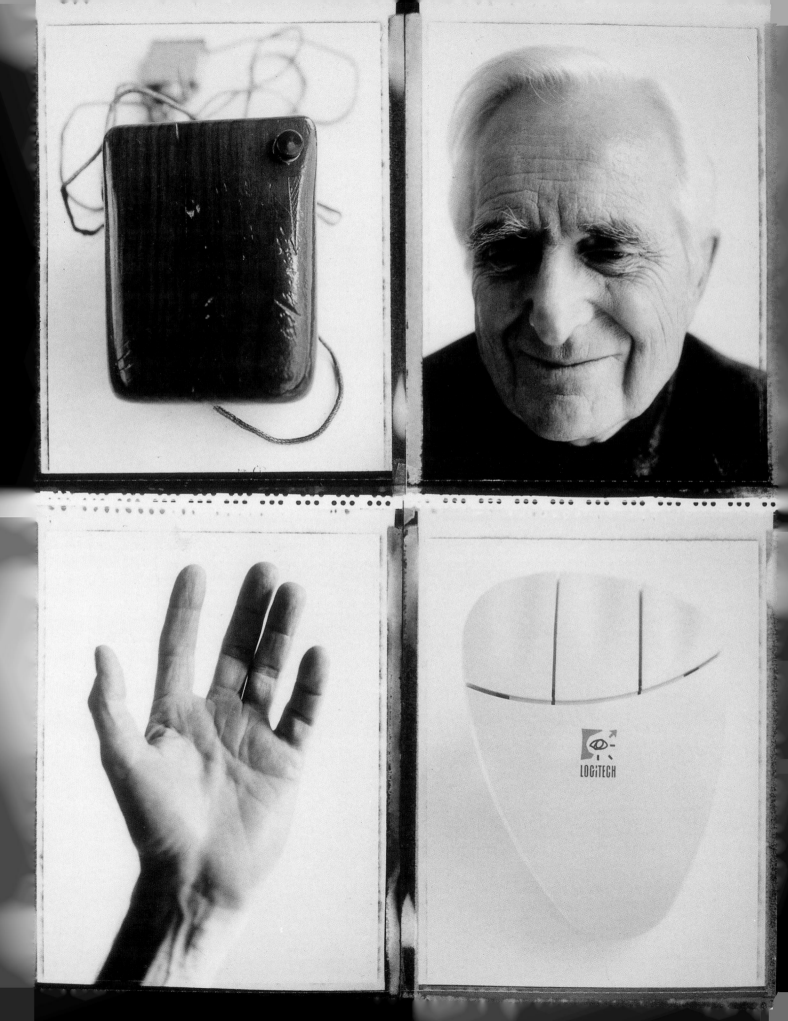

could do something to improve human capability to deal with that, then you'd really contribute something basic."

What was needed to achieve this goal was a new way to work with information and for people to work with each other. "What makes us think that the old way of looking at a book page," he asks, "or of writing, that that's the way God meant us to do it?" Engelbart, who had read about digital computers and had experience with the display screens used in radar systems, quickly envisioned what such a system would be. "I think it was just within an hour that I had the image of sitting at a big screen with all kinds of symbols, new and different symbols," he remembers. "I also really got a clear picture that one's colleagues could be sitting in other rooms with similar workstations, tied to the same computer complex, and could be sharing and working and collaborating very closely."

It took 18 years to get from that vision to the demonstration in San Francisco. Within months, Engelbart left NACA to enter the electrical engineering Ph.D. program at the University of California at Berkeley, which offered the chance to study computers, although it did not have a computer itself. With his wild ideas about computers and interaction and collaboration, however, Engelbart was not cut out for academia, and after earning his Ph.D. he joined the Stanford Research Institute (SRI), an independent think tank in Menlo Park. In 1959, he began to outline the system he had envisioned a decade earlier, and in 1963 published a paper entitled "A Conceptual Framework for the Augmentation of Man's Intellect." The paper caught the eye of the U.S. Advanced Research Projects Agency (ARPA, now DARPA), and Engelbart was able to found the Augmentation Research Center at SRI.

His research center set out to create new tools for working with ideas and words. There were two main ideas Engelbart followed in developing such a tool, which would become the NLS. First was the creation of a new "writing machine" that would let

someone revise and reorganize text and ideas on the fly. In essence, this writing machine was a word processor. But in his new way to get words down on paper, Engelbart saw a path to more advanced thinking: "If the tangle of thoughts represented by the draft becomes too complex," he wrote, "you can compile a reordered draft quickly. It would be practical for you to accommodate more complexity in the trails of thought you might build in search of the path that suits your needs." The second

The world's first computer mouse, built by Doug Engelbart in the mid-1960s. The simple wood box has a button on top and two wheels underneath, to track a user's hand movements.

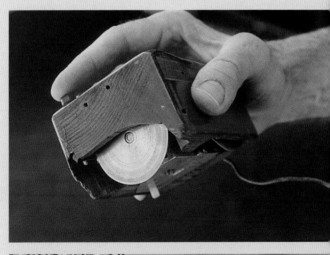

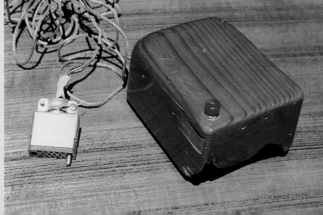

Engelbart's mouse and chord keyboard were small parts of his overall vision: to build computers that would let people work better, smarter, and in collaboration with each other.

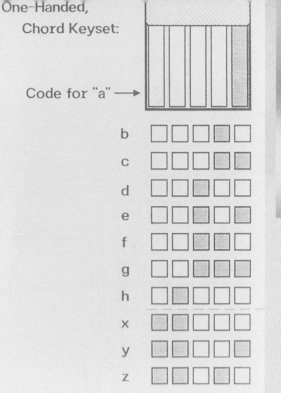

One-Handed,
Chord Keyset:

Code for "a" →

b
c
d
e
f
g
h
x
y
z

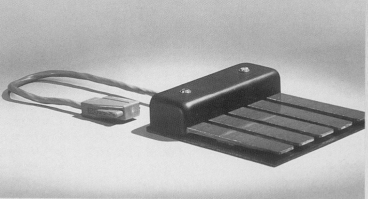

The computer system Engelbart built in the 1960s included not only a mouse but also a new kind of one-handed keyboard. A user typed by hitting a combination of its five keys, much like playing a piano chord.

AS WE MAY THINK

The essay that Douglas Engelbart happened upon in late 1945, in a Red Cross library in a native hut in the Philippines, has become a cornerstone of the Information Age, and the founding document of the World Wide Web. Published in the July 1945 issue of the *Atlantic Monthly* (and a few months later, in an abridged version, in *Life*), Vannevar Bush's "As We May Think" sketched out what the author saw as a looming problem: the inaccessibility of much of the information being produced. "We can enormously extend the record," Bush wrote, "yet even in its present bulk we can hardly consult it. This is a much larger matter than merely the extraction of data for the purposes of scientific research; it involves the entire process by which man profits by his inheritance of acquired knowledge."

Bush—a scientist, engineer, inventor, and, during World War II, the director of the U.S. Office of Scientific Research and Development—envisioned a technological solution, a new machine that would help humans navigate information in a way that mimicked the way we think. The mind works, he explained, by association. "With one item in its grasp, it snaps instantly to the next that is suggested by the association of thoughts, in accordance with some intricate web of trails carried by the cells of the brain."

The device Bush proposed was a kind of predigital personal computer that allowed an individual to store and retrieve "all his books, records, and communications." The desk-size Memex, as he named it, would have screens on which to display these records, a keyboard, and controls to move through one's store of information. This would have made for an interesting machine in

idea that guided him was that for people to work better, they had to be able to work together, to share their "trails of thought" and develop them collaboratively, in real time. The NLS allowed two or more users to work on the same document from different workstations, even from different locations. (At the 1968 San Francisco demo, a colleague in Menlo Park joined Engelbart on line, and on screen, to work on a single document.)

The early 1960s was an unlikely time to be building a computer intended for tasks such as writing and manipulating ideas. Since the digital computer's birth in the 1940s, its main work had revolved around crunching numbers. Power was more important than speed, and "ease of use" was unheard of. Computers required operators to enter programs and data slowly, by hand, on paper cards or paper tape. They would put the cards into a "reader," then wait 20 minutes or so for a result. No one imagined that computers could work instantaneously. And no one, it seemed, could see the benefits of devoting a computer's power to tasks such as writing and outlining.

Today, the spiritual descendants of Engelbart's NLS, with its mouse and graphic display and "writing machine," sit on desks around the world. And with the arrival of the Internet and local-area networks and "groupware" like Lotus Notes, it seems that much of Engelbart's vision has become reality. Yet the core

ideas of his work on "augmentation" remain unrealized. The personal computer has allowed us to work better, but we still work, for the most part, alone. "Relative to what our potential is, we can go as high as Mt. Everest, and we're only at 2,000 feet," he says.

So Doug Engelbart continues to work toward achieving those goals he articulated to himself 50 years ago. Humans still need new tools, and new methods of working, to cope with the ever-increasing complexity and urgency of the world. He now leads an organization called the Bootstrap Institute, which is dedicated to raising the awareness of the challenges facing humans, as well as the potential for new systems to meet those challenges. "Bootstrapping is sort of like compound interest," he says. With the proper approach, an organization's progress in making itself work better will build exponentially, as each advance improves on earlier improvements. Today's computers and the Internet and the Web are small advances, but the problem is still huge. "If we humans don't learn how to be collectively smarter as fast as we can," Engelbart explains, "there's going to be a better and better chance that the human race is just going to crash. That's what keeps us going."

itself, a super-microfilm reader. But what was revolutionary about the Memex was not that it stored information, but the way in which one accessed it. The essential feature of the Memex, Bush wrote, was its associative indexing, "whereby any item may be caused at will to select immediately and automatically another." Bits of information would be intertwined, becoming "a trail of [a user's] interest through the maze of materials available to him." If ideas and images and documents could be connected in this way, it might help manage the flow of that great quantity of information that threatened to smother science and business.

The "trails" and connections of the Memex are close cousins to what we now call hypertext. And just as today's Internet visionaries predict new forms of content blossoming from such connections, so too did Bush. "Wholly new forms of encyclopedias will

appear," he wrote, "ready made with a mesh of associative trails running through them. . . . The lawyer has at his touch the associated opinions and decisions of his whole experience, and of the experience of friends and authorities. The patent attorney has on call the millions of issued patents, with familiar trails to every point of his client's interest. The physician, puzzled by a patient's reactions, strikes the trail established in studying an earlier similar case, and runs rapidly through analogous case histories, with side references to the classics for the pertinent anatomy and histology." Some 50 years before its time, Bush was seeing, however faintly, the promise of the World Wide Web.

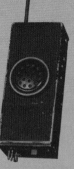
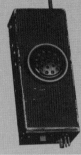

AL **GROSS**

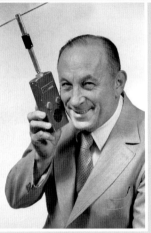

One day in the late spring of 2000, two climbers set out to scale Mount Hood, the highest peak in Oregon. The ascent did not go well—a few hours into it, a rock slide injured the two men, seriously enough that one of them couldn't move. Fortunately, they were carrying a small communication device, and they began sending out pleas for help. Seventy miles away, a seven-year-old boy was holding a similar device, and he heard a scratchy voice from the mountain. The boy and his father assured the two men that rescuers were on their way, then helped guide the Air Force Reserve's Rescue Wing to the injured climbers.

The climbers' personal communication device wasn't a satellite phone, or a cell phone, or anything particularly new. It was a walkie-talkie, little changed since its invention more than 70 years earlier.

The story of the walkie-talkie, and its inventor, Al Gross, begins with a boy almost as young as the Oregon rescuer. In 1927, when he was just nine, Gross and his family were crossing one of the Great Lakes on a steamship. The inquisitive Gross was exploring the ship and happened upon the radio operator's cabin. He was instantly enthralled. "I saw all that electrical stuff the guy had there," Gross remembered. "He put me on his lap and he put the earphones on my ears and I heard the dots and dashes and that intrigued me all over. Boy! I had to learn what he was doing and how he did it."

After some persuading, Gross's father bought him a crystal radio set, which let him listen to the airwaves. His next step was to become an amateur radio operator, so he could talk to other radio buffs miles away. By the age of 15, Gross was building and experimenting with his own radios. He also began studying the work of the radio pioneers, including Nikola Tesla, Heinrich Hertz, and Guglielmo Marconi.

When Gross walked into that ship's radio cabin, it had been barely 25 years since Marconi had sent the first wireless message across the Atlantic Ocean, an event that ushered in the modern era of telecommunications. (And it wasn't until radio distress calls had helped save some 700 people from the sinking *Titanic* in 1912 that people really started paying attention to the new

Al Gross fell in love with radios when he was just nine years old; a decade later, he built a two-way radio that could he could carry around. He called it a "walkie-talkie."

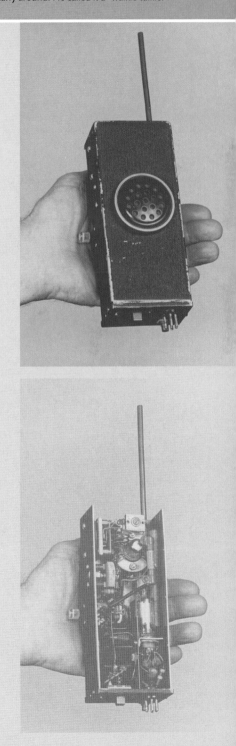

medium.) So when he began to tinker with his equipment and think of ways to make it better, there was a lot of fresh exploring to do.

By the mid-1930s, the young radio operator had in mind one particular improvement he wanted to make. "I didn't like to sit in the house and talk," he explained. "I wanted to be mobile." The solution was obvious: Build a radio transmitter and receiver (a transceiver) that was small and light enough to carry around. Gross began by searching out smaller and smaller components. He also started thinking about what radio frequency to use. At the time, broadcasters weren't using frequencies higher than 100 megahertz—about the frequency used for FM radio today. Experimenting at home, Gross was able to make miniature vacuum tubes operate at up to 300 megahertz, far higher than anything anyone else was using. (Radio signals now fill a range from about 535 kilohertz, used for AM radio, up to 2 gigahertz, used in newer cordless phones.) By 1938 he had perfected a portable radio that he could walk around with while he was talking—a walkie-talkie, his radio friends called it. The new device was just eight inches long and a little more than two inches wide.

About this time Gross began his college education, studying electrical engineering at the Case School of Applied Sciences (now Case Western University) in Cleveland. But World War II was on the horizon, and the Office of Strategic Services (or OSS, the forerunner of the CIA) was keenly interested in new kinds of communications devices. A radio operator who had heard about Gross's walkie-talkie brought it up at the OSS, and Gross traveled to Washington, D.C., to demonstrate it. Very soon he was working on the war effort, developing a top-secret communications system called Joan/Eleanor, named after his daughter and wife.

The system had two elements: Joan was a portable device much like his walkie-talkie, and Eleanor was a larger and heavier receiver that was installed in planes that could fly at high altitudes. OSS agents working behind enemy lines would carry a Joan unit, which weighed just four pounds and worked on batteries. At certain times, they would broadcast straight up into the air, where

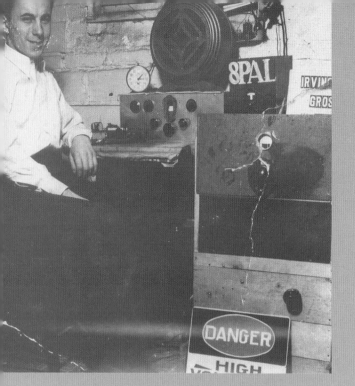

By the time he was 18 years old, Gross had built his own short-wave radio station, which he installed at his home.

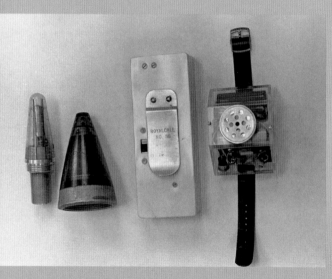

Three of Gross's inventions: from left to right, a proximity fuse for use in weapons; the world's first pager; and a two-way wristwatch radio that inspired the one worn by Dick Tracy.

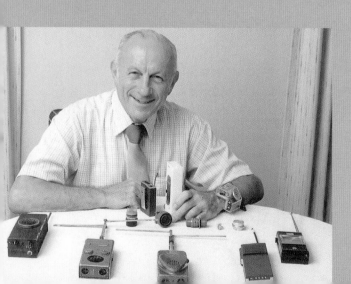

The walkie-talkie itself went though several incarnations, each getting smaller and lighter.

an unseen plane would pick up their messages and send news back down to the ground.

The Joan/Eleanor system had huge advantages over other ways for agents to communicate with headquarters. First, it was light, small, and concealable. But just as important, because it operated on the unexplored high frequencies, the enemy—in this case, Germany—couldn't listen in. And even if they did try, they'd have to be flying directly overhead, since the Joan unit was designed to transmit straight up in a very narrow band. And the portable units put out a strong signal, so the listening planes could fly as high as 30,000 feet, beyond the range of most German countermeasures. The system was put into use in Europe in late 1944, and was used successfully until the end of war. The U.S. Joint Chiefs of Staff called it one of the "most successful wireless intelligence gathering operations, saving millions of lives by shortening the war."

After the war, Gross wanted to extend his new device beyond the world of secret agents. The Federal Communications Commission (FCC) soon allocated a range of frequencies for walkie-talkie use—the Citizens Radio Frequency Band, which would eventually lead to the CB Radio craze of the 1970s. Gross began manufacturing walkie-talkies, and he sold more than 100,000 of them. The challenges and pressures of such a large operation were not what interested him, though, and he licensed the technology to other companies.

Gross was continually trying to improve on his walkie-talkies, and in 1948 he built a radio that could fit on a man's wrist. Chester Gould, who drew the daily comic strip "Dick Tracy," visited Gross's workshop and was impressed with the prototype. That October, Dick Tracy began wearing his now-famous two-way wristwatch radio.

Next, Gross created an even smaller communication device, which would become known as the pager. Essentially a miniaturized two-way radio, the little silver boxes could be set to respond to specific signals—a short message would be broadcast to every pager, but only a specific person's device would recognize it and beep. Gross had high hopes that doctors and nurses would adopt his new invention as a way to keep in touch with their hospitals or offices. But the pager met with resistance; nurses feared it might disturb patients, and one doctor, Gross recalled, complained that it would interrupt his golf game.

By 2000, Al Gross saw the world flourishing with wireless communications devices. Cell phones and pagers are constant presences in our lives, and anyone can gain access to the World Wide Web from a personal digital assistant. Although Gross was not directly responsible for cellular technology, the current wireless revolution is in many ways the culmination of his vision for instant, portable communication. In July 1945, just after World War II ended in Europe, E. K. Jett, the commissioner of the FCC, wrote a story for the *Saturday Evening Post* that described a world using a version of Gross's walkie-talkie.

The "handie-talkie," Jett explained, could be carried around by anyone, even used in cars. Its use would range from deliverymen receiving orders to families staying in touch to emergency calls for help. "One can picture a young woman motorist riding alone at night on a lonely road," Jett wrote. "A car comes roaring down an intersection, sideswipes her coupe, and crashes against an abutment. . . . She turns to the handie-talkie, which is slung camera-like over her shoulder. . . . She pulls out the antenna, spins the dial to Citizens' Radio distress frequency . . . and in a few minutes an ambulance arrives."

In 1977, Gross (center) appeared on the TV quiz show "To Tell the Truth."

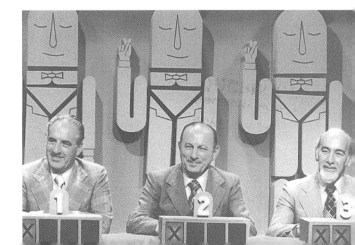

ERNA SCHNEIDER
HOOVER

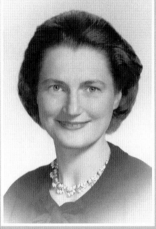

Before the 1950s, the process of making a telephone call often involved simple personal contact. In many places, when you picked up the telephone, an operator would ask, "Number please?" After you responded, the operator would make a physical connection with a wire to the switchboard and your call would go through. It was a comforting, human aspect to a relatively new technology, and it worked pretty well, at least for a while.

As the U.S. economy boomed in the decade following World War II, people and businesses began to use the telephone more and more. Technological advances increased the load on the system: Beginning in 1951, microwave relay stations increased long distance service, and in 1956 the first transatlantic telephone cables started carrying international calls. Bell Telephone's own projections made it clear that the continually increasing demand for telephone service would one day—and probably soon—overwhelm the system. The answer to this looming problem was the same as in many other industries at the time: computerized automation. Around 1954, Bell Labs, the research arm of the Bell Telephone company, began working on automating the process of connecting calls, known as switching.

More than 10 years and $500 million later, Bell Telephone unveiled the first large-scale electronic switching system, or ESS. Although the company advertised that "more than 2,000 man-years of research" had gone into ESS, one of the key figures in its development was a woman, Dr. Erna Schneider Hoover. A medievalist, logistician, working mother, and computer programmer, Hoover designed the basic architecture of the switching system, which could automatically route hundreds (and later, thousands) of calls in a few seconds. This work earned her one of the first patents ever awarded for software and a job as a research supervisor at Bell Labs, the first time a woman had held such a position.

Erna Schneider grew up in Irvington, New Jersey, where she was born in 1926, and moved to Massachusetts in 1944 to attend Wellesley College. She studied medieval history and philosophy there, earning her bachelor's degree in 1948. Since Hoover intended to both work and raise a family, she focused

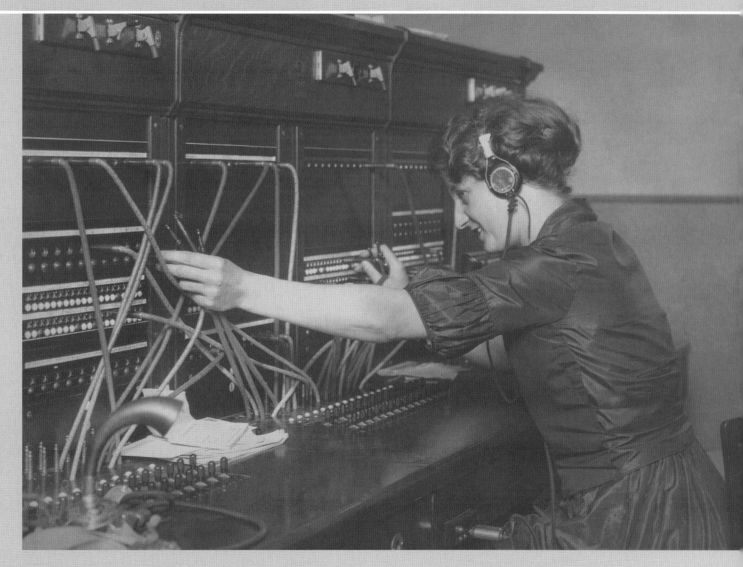

The process of "switching" (connecting) calls before automation depended on operators working at switchboards. In the 1950s, Bell Telephone introduced direct dial, and in the 1960s it added completely automated service.

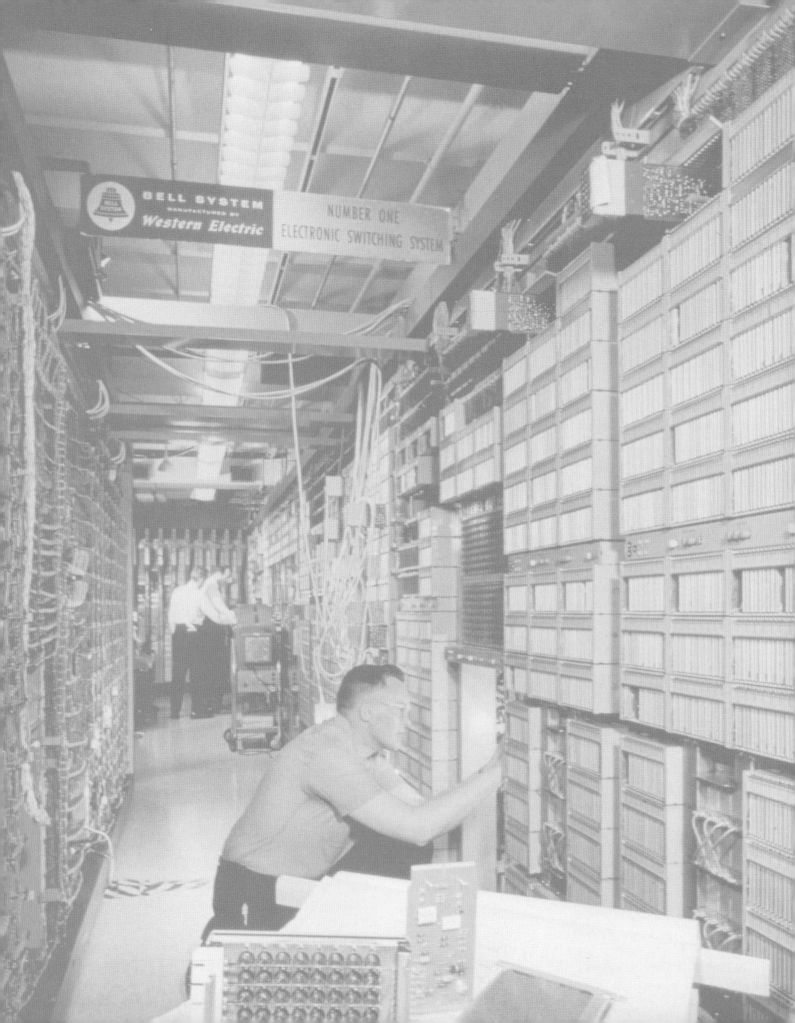

on getting a position in academia, where the hours were more flexible. In 1951, she earned her Ph.D. in logic and the philosophy of science at Yale University.

As a graduate student Hoover encountered the challenges of sexism. When she earned her doctorate at Yale, she was told that she would have been kept on to teach there "if I had been a man." However, her experience and success at college helped her deal with this prevailing attitude. "The academic grounding Wellesley gave me left me feeling that I could learn almost anything," she told the *Wellesley* in 1990. "I had a supreme sense of self-confidence from professors who were role models and students who showed they had ability to run things themselves. I found [college] liberating after high school, where girls were supposed to act dumb even if they were not."

After Yale, Hoover taught philosophy for three years at Swarthmore College in Pennsylvania. She married Charles Wilson Hoover, Jr., an engineer who had just been hired by Bell Labs, and in 1954 she, too, joined the research team at Bell. When Hoover got there, she remembered, "they were planning to develop a telephone switch that could be controlled by electronic computer." The idea of computer control was the key: Problems could be fixed and adjustments made from a central computer, rather than by altering or swapping the electromechanical components then in use. A computer could also check its own performance, testing and fixing itself.

Computer science was still in its infancy at the time, and Hoover's seemingly arcane academic specialty, symbolic logic, was suddenly in high demand. A computer is essentially made up of many logic gates; vacuum tubes were the first such gates used, although by the time Hoover got involved, Bell Labs' transistor, invented in 1947, was replacing tubes. (The integrated circuit would replace the transistor during the following decade.)

Logic gates govern how information bits, or at their most basic level, electrons, move through circuits. These gates obey strict rules of logic; the three essential gates are AND, OR, and NOT. In an AND gate, if the two arriving bits are 1s, the gate produces a 1. With an OR gate, if either (or both) of the arriving bits is a 1, it produces a 1. And with a NOT gate, a single input is reversed; a 1 produces a 0, and vice versa. There are four other gates that are variations on the basic three that combine their logic; for example, the NAND gate marries NOT and AND, producing 1s where an AND would produce 0s.

The first electronic switching system (ESS) was installed in Succasunna, New Jersey, in 1965. On the table are the ESS's major components; the square object second at left is one of its mechanical memory cards, made before silicon memory chips.

By creating sequences—circuits—of these gates, an engineer (or a logistician) can manipulate data in useful ways. A particular combination of 12 gates, for instance, makes a circuit that can add two bits; a series of eight of these circuits can add a whole byte. Today's processors, with more than 10 million gates, can quickly manipulate large quantities of data.

Since an electronic phone switching system would need to make hundreds or thousands of logical decisions every minute, Hoover was well suited to the task. (Computer programs take advantage of the same strict logic, although high-level programming languages allow programmers to use much more complex arguments.) In her description of the ESS, she noted that most of the computer's time would be spent "performing logical operations. . . . [An] arithmetic unit is not needed, but a wealth of logic instructions are."

Hoover conceived of the basic logical architecture of the Electronic Switching System while in a hospital bed, following the birth of her second child. The ESS had two main components: a large memory bank (which relied on physical, magnetic storage, since it predated memory chips) and a "central control," which contained the computer and its program.

One of the main challenges in switching calls was that they did not come in at regular intervals; at night, for example, it was simple to take care of the few connections to be made. During peak hours, though, a system could easily be overwhelmed. "Unlike a typical computation center," Hoover wrote, "in which work is scheduled in job shop fashion, the ESS cannot control the time when it must process calls, because telephone customers expect to receive prompt service at any time."

Hoover created a set of logical rules for how the system dealt with calls, and another for how the computer divided its attention among the calls coming in. The system she and her colleagues built used some timing tricks to deal with more calls than it otherwise might, by queuing extra calls and switching its attention from call to call, since the computer worked much faster than callers could. "Once having determined what sort of signal has come in," she noted, "the system can afford to take more time before making the chain of logical decisions which determines how to treat the call." Because all of those logical decisions were made by the computer's program, rather than the phone company's physical equipment, changes in phone service could be made easily and quickly.

The finished ESS system, which debuted in Succasunna, New Jersey, in 1965, was one of the first uses of large-scale computer automation to reach the public, although its function was so transparent that most callers never realized it. (Computer-controlled switching did, however, allow several notable new telephone features such as call forwarding and call waiting.) While that first installation covered only 200 phone subscribers, within a decade 6 million phones were being switched electronically. Today, virtually all phone calls are routed through computerized switching centers, although many have been upgraded to the next generation of "digital switching."

Hoover continued her research work at Bell Labs after the ESS was completed. During the 1960s, she contributed to the antiballistic missile defense system, which successfully intercepted mock ICBM warheads before the program was banned by treaty. In 1978, she became the first female head of a research division at Bell Labs, where she worked on the application of artificial intelligence to communications systems.

In 1971, Hoover was granted a patent for the software governing electronic call switching. This was not only one of the first patents ever granted for a computer program, it was also proof of one of the larger meanings behind Hoover's invention.

Although it involved a complicated computer system, the key achievement of the ESS was its software; as such it represented one of the first triumphs of software over hardware. While today software is almost always more useful, impressive, and important than the hardware it runs on, in the 1960s Hoover's work was a sharp (if not immediately noticed) contradiction of the belief that bigger computers were the answer to any information-processing problem.

GRACE MURRAY **HOPPER**

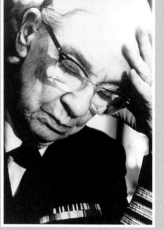

Grace Murray Hopper discovered the pleasure of finding out how things work when she was just seven years old. Intrigued by one of her family's alarm clocks, she took it apart, spilling out its springs and gears. Still curious, she opened up another clock, and another, until she had disassembled seven of them. Although it's not clear whether she was able to put any of them back together, the experience began a lifelong quest for knowledge, a quest that made her one of the great pioneers of computing. Working with some of the world's first computers, Hopper established basic methods for writing software and created the first high-level programming languages. Her ideas were applied to the development of all subsequent languages, including those used today.

Grace Murray was born in 1906 in New York City. Her father was an insurance broker with a love for books, and her mother was a housewife with a deep interest in mathematics. While many parents would be dismayed by the destruction of their alarm clocks, Hopper's encouraged her technical interests. As a young girl, she would sometimes accompany her grandfather, a civil engineer, as he surveyed the city to plan new streets. And while most young women were not then encouraged in academic pursuits, Hopper's father thought that she should get the same education as a boy. In 1924, she entered Vassar College, one of the country's top schools for women. There Hopper studied mathematics and physics and graduated in 1928 with honors; two years later she earned her master's degree in mathematics at Yale University. The same year, she married Vincent Hopper, an English professor who joined her at Vassar.

Hopper became a well-liked professor of mathematics at Vassar; at the same time she was studying for a Ph.D. in that discipline, which she received from Yale in 1934. She continued teaching for the next eight years, and she might have remained teaching at Vassar much longer but for the start of World War II. Hopper had always been deeply patriotic—her great-grandfather had been an admiral in the navy, and during World War I she had knitted caps and socks for American servicemen. In 1942, after her husband and brother had joined the air force, Hopper decided to join the navy. It was not

"Humans are allergic to change," she declared. "They love to say, 'We've always done it this way.' I try to fight that."

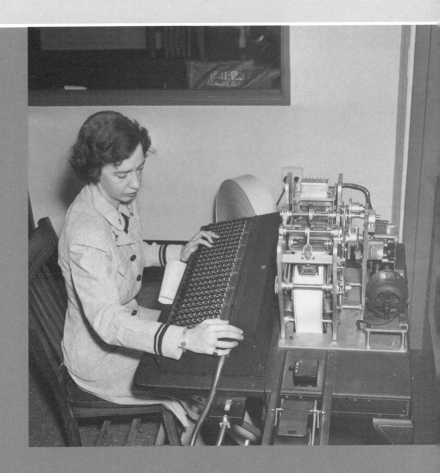

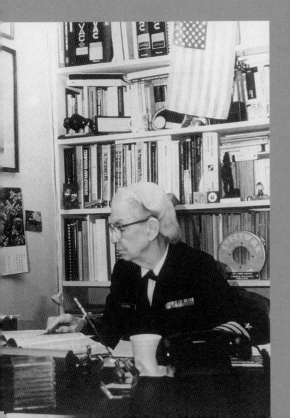

Hopper devoted much of her life to the navy. She served in
the women's reserves from 1943 to 1946, and then as an officer
from 1967 through 1986.

0800   antan started
1000   "   stopped - antan ✓   { 1.2700   9.037 847 025
        13" vc (032) MP - MC   1.9825...7000   9.037 846 995 consct
                                2.130476415 (-3) 4.615925059(-2)
        (033)   PRO 2   2.130476415
                consct   2.130676415
        Relays 6-2 in 033 failed special speed test
        In Tieday   10.000 test.
            Relays changed   Relay 3376
1100   Started Cosine Tape (Sine check)
1525   Started Mult+ Adder Test.

1545   Relay #70 Panel F
                        (moth) in relay.

       First actual case of bug being found.
   1630 antangent started.
1700   closed down.

The first computers were made before transistors and depended on relays and other mechanical devices. When the Mark II computer Grace Hopper was using during the summer of 1945 failed, she tracked down the cause: a moth caught in a relay, the first computer "bug."

easy for her to get in. In addition to being too old at 34, she was underweight, and her job as a professor was considered essential. But with special permission, Hopper joined the navy's women's reserves in 1943.

After basic training, Hopper was assigned to work on one of the world's first computers, the navy's Mark I, at Harvard University. The Mark I was a large and primitive machine. Some 51 feet long and eight feet high, the computer relied on electro-mechanical switches—relays—to process numbers. (The transistor wouldn't be invented for a few more years.) Hopper was immediately excited to work with the Mark I. "It was the fanciest gadget I'd ever seen," she later said. "I had to find out how it worked."

Hopper's job was to program the Mark I to calculate the trajectories of missiles. But the Mark I, like all early computers, was not easy to use. First, Hopper had to figure out the equa-tions that described how a missile would fly. Then she had to break those down into basic steps simple enough for the computer to understand. Next, Hopper would write these steps down as instructions for the computer, in a language it could understand, using just ones and zeroes. Finally, those instructions would be encoded onto a long piece of paper tape—a punched hole for "one," no hole for "zero." It was a time-consuming and error-prone process, but it worked most of the time, and Hopper, her colleagues, and their Mark I (and later the Mark II and Mark III) were able to produce missile trajectories much faster than human calculators could.

In the summer of 1945, Hopper was working with the Mark II when the machine stopped functioning. Searching for a me-chanical failure, she discovered a moth squashed in a switch. Hopper kept a log book of the computer's operation and taped the moth into it, noting that it was the "first actual case of a bug being found." From then on, whenever she and her colleagues were trying to fix the computer or a program, they called it debugging.

In 1946, Hopper was forced to retire from the navy. She remained at Harvard for a few years, then joined the Eckert-Mauchley Computer Corporation, which was building the first commercial computer, the UNIVAC. This machine was smaller, faster, and more flexible than the Mark I, and with it Hopper began to explore new ways to program computers. Until then, every part of a program had to be re-entered every time it was used, even if the computer had done that operation—dividing two numbers, for example—many times before. The programmer and the computer had to start from scratch each time.

Hopper thought this was a waste of time and resources. She began to collect pieces of programs that could be used again and again. "I kept them in a notebook," she recalled. "But to put them in a new program I still had to copy them [by hand]. So I decided to make a library of all these pieces of code and I'd give them each a name and then I'd tell the computer to put them together, copy them, and add them to the [computer's memory]." What Hopper had created was the first compiler—a program that translated these "libraries" into binary code for the computer. With it, a computer could "automatically" write its own programs, based on the instructions fed into Hopper's compiler.

At first, the "names" of the pieces of code were mathematical functions, since at that point most computers were used for scientific or military purposes. But Hopper realized that there were far wider applications for the machines, particularly in businesses that had to process large amounts of information. "So I decided data processors ought to be able to write their programs in English, and the computers would translate them into machine code," she explained. "I could say, 'Subtract income tax from pay' instead of trying to write that in octal code or using all kinds of symbols."

None of her colleagues believed that computers could handle programs written in English. That kind of attitude always bothered Hopper. "Humans are allergic to change," she declared. "They love to say, 'We've always done it this way.' I try to fight that." One way she fought was by hanging up a clock that ran counterclockwise; it still told time, just in a different way.

After two years of work, Hopper did make a compiler that let the UNIVAC understand English commands such as Compare, Transfer, Price, and Write. Called Flow-Matic, it was one of the very first high-level computer languages, and was soon put to use by insurance companies, the military, and other organizations.

By the late 1950s, several companies were beginning to make computers. However, Flow-Matic worked only on the UNIVAC. Hopper and others in the computer industry recognized that they needed a programming language that could be used on any computer. In 1959, Hopper became part of a committee that was planning to make just such a language, called COBOL (for COmmon Business-Oriented Language). Although she did not work on COBOL herself, her Flow-Matic served as one of its main models, and her idea about using common English commands was one of its programmers' guiding principles. Introduced in 1960, COBOL became the most common and most popular computer language, the basis for most programming as the United States and the world became more and more computerized. Today, many important large-scale programs written in COBOL are still in use; during the Y2K scare in 1999, companies had to scramble to find programmers who could work on their long-running COBOL software.

In addition to being a pioneer programmer, Hopper was a highly effective leader. One of her passions through the late 1950s and 1960s was persuading businessmen and her colleagues in the computer industry to use English-based programming languages. In 1967 she was recalled to navy service because no one else could coordinate the service's different COBOL programs; she did it by creating a standard version of the language, USA Standard COBOL. Although she was supposed to serve for only six months this time, she remained an officer until 1986; by then she had been promoted to Rear Admiral, and was the oldest active navy officer. Grace Hopper died in January 1992 at the age of 85.

One of Hopper's favorite things to teach was the importance of taking chances, of ignoring the usual way things are done. "A ship in port is safe," she liked to say to colleagues or students. "But that's not what ships are for. Be good ships. Sail out to sea, and do new things."

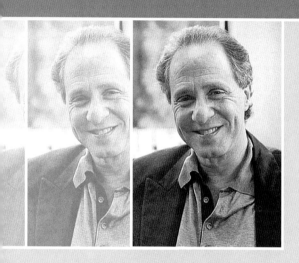

Raymond Kurzweil has been making computers smarter since he was in high school. As a teenager, he built a computer that could analyze melodies and then create new ones based on that information. In 1976, he introduced the first commercial product based on artificial intelligence, a scanner-character-recognizer speech synthesizer that could read books aloud to the blind. A decade later, he created the first large-vocabulary speech recognition system. As an inventor on the cutting edge of technology, Kurzweil has also become a student of technological change, using that knowledge to speculate on and predict the future of computing and technology.

Kurzweil grew up in Queens, New York, where he was born in 1948. Although his parents were artists—his father a musician and conductor and his mother a visual artist—academics ran in the family. "There were a lot of doctors and scientists and Ph.D.s," he notes. "Including the women. My mother's mother was one of the first female Ph.D.s in chemistry." And he had at least one inventive ancestor, his father's father, who built and marketed automation systems.

His inventive impulse was clear at the age of five, when he began building his own model boats, cars, and (failed) rocket ships. The young Kurzweil's goal was to be a scientist—an important scientist—and to him that meant being an inventor. It soon came to mean inventing things with computers. "I would go down to Canal Street in New York and buy surplus electronics," he remembers. He built a simple computing device when he was 12, and he also learned how to program. Kurzweil's uncle, an engineer at Bell Labs, helped inspire these pursuits, but Kurzweil did most of his learning and experimentation on his own.

When Kurzweil was 15, he began his first project involving pattern recognition—teaching machines how to see and understand patterns in information. The result was a computer that could write original melodies based on patterns it saw in the work of a composer. It also landed him on the game show "I've Got a Secret," where he played a machine-written composition on

In 1976, Ray Kurzweil's company introduced the Reading Machine, a combination scanner, character recognition system, and speech synthesizer that could read books aloud.

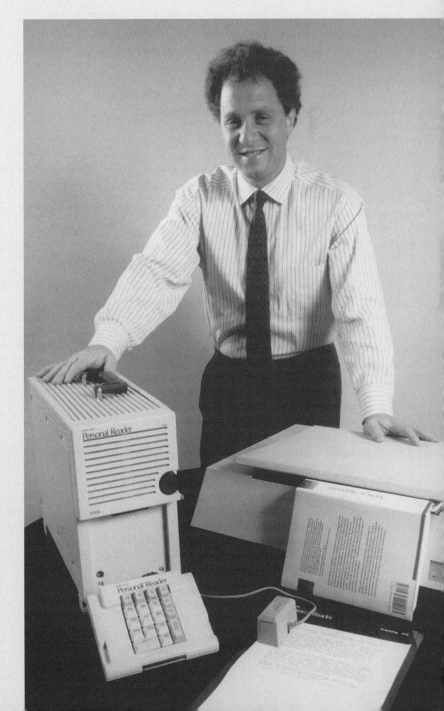

piano. (The panelists had to guess his secret, that a computer had written the piece.)

While in high school, Kurzweil began corresponding with Marvin Minsky, the pioneer of artificial intelligence at the Massachusetts Institute of Technology. This friendship helped convince him to attend MIT, where he began studying computer science. But at the time MIT had only eight or nine computer classes; Kurzweil took them all during his first two years, then added a second major in creative writing. (He continues to combine technical and literary pursuits.) The classes Kurzweil took occupied only part of his time at MIT; he was also running a company, which used a computer to match high school students with colleges. He eventually sold his company to Harcourt Brace and World for $100,000 plus royalties.

In 1974 Kurzweil founded his first major company, Kurzweil Computer Products, to tackle a long-standing challenge: creating a machine that could read printed text in any font. This was a classical problem of pattern recognition; other inventors had made reading machines, but to Kurzweil they "basically just matched pixels against a perfect template."

Kurzweil and his colleagues wanted to rely on the patterns of letters rather than a template. "We wanted to really attack the general problem of recognizing characters, to consider a character to be an image with a more abstract definition," he says. "What makes a capital A inherently a capital A?" As he explored how to achieve this, he developed some basic principles that he has followed in all subsequent pattern-recognition problems: use multiple approaches; learn from the real world; and make a system that can itself figure out patterns.

He defined several different ways of recognizing a letter; some used mathematical transformations of the image, while others analyzed invariant features—the constant properties of a character. A capital A, for example, has a triangular looped portion; line segments that run from the top to the bottom corners; and a cross bar. Then Kurzweil wrote an "expert" program that weighed the strengths and weaknesses of the different recognizers and decided from that information what the character

RAY KURZWEIL'S CYBERNETIC POET

Ray Kurzweil has applied pattern recognition to literature as well as language. By reading and analyzing a selection of an author's writing, his program "Ray Kurzweil's Cybernetic Poet" can create a "language model" of how he or she writes. Using these models, the program can write poems that replicate the rhythm, style, and structure of the original poet. It can also combine the characteristics of several poets in one work.

Here are a few examples of the program's cybernetic poetry.

A Wounded Deer Leaps Highest
(after reading poems by Wendy Dennis and Emily Dickinson)

A wounded deer leaps highest,
I've heard the daffodil
I've heard the flag to-day
I've heard the hunter tell;
'Tis but the ecstasy of death,
And then the brake is almost done,
And sunrise grows so near

sunrise grows so near
That we can touch the despair and
frenzied hope of all the ages.

The Saxophone Player
(after reading poems by Ray Kurzweil and Pat Sherman)

The saxophone player
lives alone,
blows
lives alone,
blows
a swinging door
splendid silence
prophetic poses
splendid silence
prophetic poses
of a prayer and the walls.

was. "Any of [the individual recognizers] could do the whole job," he notes, "but not as accurately as the whole system." Kurzweil's recognition system was also able to learn from the different characters it saw. "You can only get so far if you just define high-level properties and say an A has these particular features," he says. "You'll find real world images that don't have all those properties. So you need a system that can actually learn what real images are like."

Just as he was getting his system to work, Kurzweil met a blind man on a plane. As they talked, Kurzweil remembers, "he was explaining, 'Blind people aren't handicapped. I travel around the world and I participate in meetings and I talk on the phone and there's really no limitations.' Except he did have a problem accessing ordinary printed materials. If he could access ordinary print, that would really address the primary limitation he faced." The character recognition project suddenly had a much larger goal: to build a machine that would read to the blind.

Although Kurzweil's recognition system was doing a good job reading characters, two problems remained in building a system that could scan a book and speak it out loud: Neither the flat-bed scanner nor text-to-speech synthesizers had been invented yet. Within about a year, though, he and his engineers accomplished both of these tasks, using equipment that now seems very primitive. The scanner, for instance, could only see a small part of the page at a time, so it had to move back and forth and then down the text to read it all. On January 13, 1976, the Kurzweil Reading Machine was demonstrated to the press. That night, CBS news anchor Walter Cronkite did not deliver his usual sign-off, "And that's the way it is." Instead, the Reading Machine spoke it.

The musician Stevie Wonder, who is blind, heard the announcement that day and soon bought the first production model of the Reading Machine. That purchase began a long friendship between Wonder and the inventor, which, in the early 1980s, spawned Kurzweil Music Systems, a line of music syn-

Moon Child

(after reading poems by Kathleen Frances Wheeler)

Crazy moon child
Hide from your coffin
To spite your doom.

Tomcat

(a haiku, after reading poems by Randi and Kathryn Lynn)

An old yellow tomcat
lies sleeping content,
he rumbles a heart

Dark

(after reading poems by Kathryn Lynn)

I am the dark.
on
the night
The
past of love
gone stale.

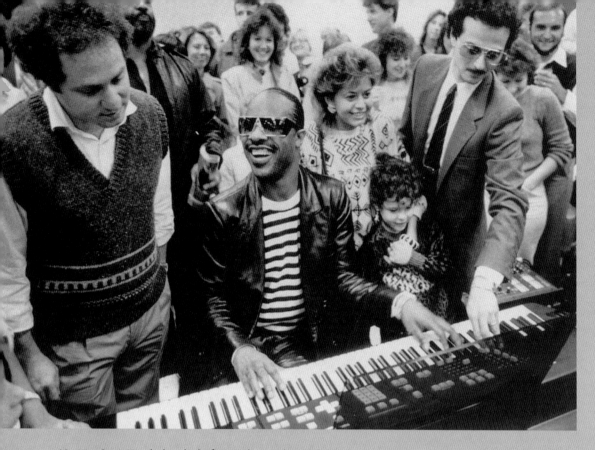

Musician Stevie Wonder bought the first Reading Machine and later worked with Kurzweil to develop a music synthesizer that accurately re-created the sounds of acoustic instruments.

thesizers that mimicked traditional instruments so well that most listeners couldn't tell the difference.

In the 1980s, Kurzweil also began working on another classic problem of pattern recognition, the opposite task of the Reading Machine's: turning speech into text. For years, a system that could manage this was thought of as a Holy Grail of artificial intelligence. "All of our intelligence is embodied in our language," Kurzweil says. "Speech embodies not only textual language but also the intelligence we put behind the inflection and the emotion we can represent and the cadence of our voice."

Kurzweil used the same principles as in character recognition. The advantage of starting ten years later was that computer speed had increased exponentially—which was essential, because speech recognition takes enormous processing power. Different ways of recognizing a sound were employed, along with an expert program to decide which sound it really was. The system Kurzweil designed was also able to develop its own models of the patterns found in speech. Rather than telling the system that there were, say, exactly 44 phonemes in the English language, he says, "we let it figure out itself how many different patterns it finds and what those patterns look like. It will actually develop different models for different dialects."

The speech-recognition system was first introduced in 1987, and its early users were people with disabilities that prevented them from typing. Doctors also began using it, since the limited vocabulary used in medical records lent itself to recognition. The technology has come into its own in the past few years, though, with about a million systems now installed. Soon, Kurzweil says, speech will become an important interface between humans and machines.

Making such predictions is another of Kurzweil's talents; many appear in his two best-selling books, *The Age of Intelligent Machines* (1990) and *The Age of Spiritual Machines* (1999). "Writing is an opportunity to invent with the resources of the future," he says. "So I can invent using the computers and communications resources of 2010 or 2020." To invent the future accurately, though, he had to have a very good idea of what technology would be available. One key was recognizing that the rate of technological change is accelerating, doubling every 10 years. So what might seem to be a 100 years in the future is really only 25 years away.

Still, this attention to how fast things change has as much to do with Kurzweil's current projects as it does to those of 2025. "I became a student of technology trends as part of the discipline of inventing," he says. "You want your project to make sense when it's finished, not when it started."

When he was only 15 years old, Ray Kurzweil appeared on the game show, "I've Got a Secret." Kurzweil's secret: the music he played on the piano had been written by a computer, which he had programmed to create new melodies from existing works by human composers.

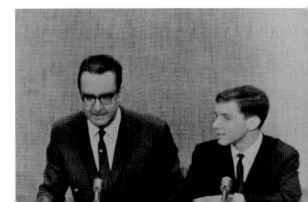

CARVER **MEAD**

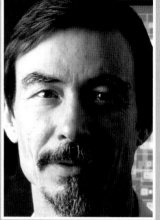

"I get interested in particular topics," explains physicist, engineer, and innovator Carver Mead, "because the way people are going at it doesn't make any sense to me. That drives me nuts, and that's what gets me motivated to figure out a better way to do it."

The "better ways" Mead has figured out have had far-reaching impacts. Some of the topics he has become interested in include the physics of semiconductors, microchip design, biological computing, and digital imaging. And in each of these realms, Mead has made tremendous advances and discoveries—developing, for instance, a method for designing chips that is now used for almost all high-performance microprocessors. One of his most recent interests, digital imaging, resulted in the recent unveiling of a digital camera far more advanced, and more like photography on film, than any previous digital camera.

Mead's childhood revolved around the technologies that would eventually become his career: electricity and electronics. Born in Bakersfield, California, in 1934, Mead grew up in Big Creek, a "camp" in the Sierra Nevada where his father ran a hydroelectric plant. His first fascination was with the power plant, where, he remembers, there was a "palpable energy." When he was about 13, though, an amateur radio operator moved into the camp and Mead was soon hooked on electronics. "There was something special about radio," he says. "That you could communicate over large distances, the whole propagation of radio waves, that was just fascinating to me."

World War II had recently ended, and the market was flooded with inexpensive surplus electronics. Mead bought as much of it as he could and spent his spare time tinkering. Between the plentiful equipment and the quick advances being made, he says, "It was just a fabulous time to be getting into electronics." In 1952 Mead began studying electrical engineering and physics at the California Institute of Technology. It was also a fabulous time to begin studying at CalTech. Physicist Richard Feynman had just joined the faculty; Mead took his mathematical physics class and also began a lifelong friendship and collaboration with him. His freshman chemistry professor was Linus

Pauling. "That [class] was my start in quantum mechanics," Mead remembers. "He just knew that stuff absolutely cold."

Mead earned all of his degrees at CalTech—a bachelor's in 1956, a master's in 1957, and a Ph.D. in 1960—and was subsequently hired as an instructor. (He is currently the school's Gordon and Betty Moore Professor of Engineering and Applied Science.) Mead's initial research project as a faculty member led to his first major invention, what is now known as the HEMT transistor. "I studied the detailed physics of the contacts between metals and semiconductors," he explains. "It doesn't sound very exciting, but it actually is." His investigation into the physics of semiconductors convinced him that he could make an entirely new kind of transistor that could work better. Mead was correct; his transistor was able to work at much higher frequencies than previous ones, and they became a key element in modern microwave communications, including satellites and cell phones.

As his research into metal-semiconductor junctions continued, Mead began to look into a phenomenon called electron tunneling. When insulating materials get thin enough, he explains, "the fact that the electron is actually a wave starts to matter. Electrons can penetrate through the very thin layers of these materials." Because circuits are based on the orderly and predictable flow of electrons, this behavior could be troublesome. One day, Mead was talking about this phenomenon with Gordon Moore, who was then at Fairchild Semiconductor. "He said, 'Carver, doesn't that mean that if you make a device sufficiently small, that it won't really work anymore?'" Mead remembers. "I said, 'Yeah, I think that's what it means.' And he said, 'Why don't you work on how small that is?'"

In the late 1960s, after he had figured out how small integrated circuit components could be made, Carver Mead realized a new system was necessary to design chips as they became more complex. His solution was Very Large Scale Integration (VLSI), a simpler and more systematic approach to chip design.

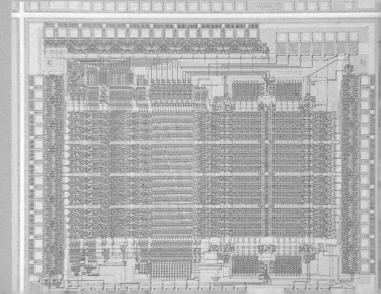

In 1965, *Electronics* magazine asked Gordon Moore, the research director of Fairchild Semiconductor, to write an article on the future of the integrated circuit industry. As Moore looked at the number of active components engineers had been able to put on chips since their invention by Jack Kilby and Robert Noyce, he noticed a linear progression. In 1959, there was one component; in 1964, there were 32; and in 1965, there were 64. He plotted these data on a piece of paper and, he recalled, "I just drew a line. It doubled every year for 10 years." This observation, that the number of components able to be put on a single chip doubled every year, became known as Moore's Law.

Moore's Law has been revised a few times. In 1975, he updated the rate of doubling to once every two years. Later, one of his colleagues at Intel, the company he helped found in 1968, applied the "law" to computer performance—speed—rather than strictly the number of components on a chip. (The two measures have always been linked.) Eventually the difference between the two predictions—doubling every year and every two years—was split, with people generally accepting a doubling rate of once every 18 months.

Moore's Law has proved remarkably accurate over the past 35 years. Continued innovations in manufacturing techniques have allowed components to be etched into silicon wafers in ever-increasing numbers. Using ultraviolet light, which has a smaller wavelength than visible light, chips are now made with features as small as .15 millionths of a meter. Current memory chips contain about a billion components; the latest generation of microprocessors has about 10 million.

Some computer scientists think that the era of Moore's Law may soon come to an end. The size limits of etching with light are being reached, and if the ultrathin connections between components get any smaller, the odd effects of quantum physics may impede the flow of electrons. However, research continues on alternative technologies, such as quantum processing, which depends on those quantum effects, and DNA computing, which may someday harness DNA helixes for data processing. If these or other new technologies pan out, the rate of change in computing might even get faster.

Carver Mead at bat during a playday in May, 1947. The schoolhouse in the background held about 20 students in grades 1–8.

Graduating class of 1948 at Chawanakee #1 school, Big Creek, California. Carver Mead is on the left.

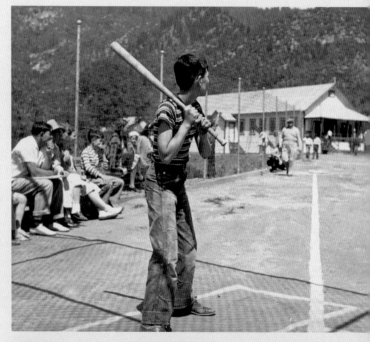

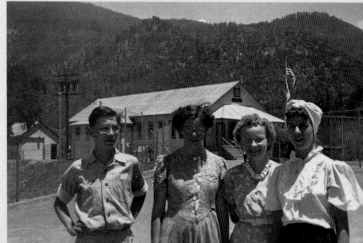

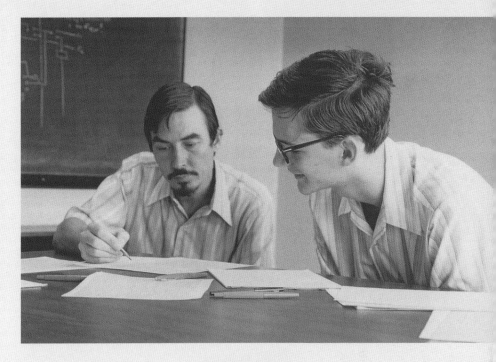

Mead speaks in awe of the professors he had at CalTech in the 1950s, and he takes pride in his teaching at that institution over the past four decades.

At the time, many physicists and computer scientists were making predictions about how small a chip's transistors could be; their estimates were in the range of 10 microns. Using his own research into electron tunneling, Mead realized that "[their numbers] just didn't make any sense. They were basically invoking the principle that you can't change anything as you make the devices smaller. And of course you have to change some things. . . . When you did that, it turns out that everything got better. The devices got smaller, the power they dissipated got a lot less so the heat generated by the chip went down, and they worked a lot faster."

Mead predicted—in a talk he gave in 1968 and papers he published a few years later—that semiconductor devices could eventually be made as small as .15 microns thick. And while his colleagues disbelieved him at first, that size is just now being reached in the most advanced semiconductor fabrication plants.

This proof of how small transistors could get—and how much faster they might become—was an enormous advance in the understanding of semiconductors. But Mead's discovery raised as many questions as it answered. With transistors shrinking to .15 millionths of an inch, designers could fit tens of millions of them on a single chip. While this promised much more powerful chips, it was also a virtual impossibility, given the state of chip design at the time. To make a chip, one had to draw the circuit, then hand-trace it with a razor blade on a special silk-screening material. "It was all done by hand and enormously labor-intensive," Mead says. "And error-prone. Terribly error-prone."

Mead explains that whenever a new technology is introduced, be it the electric motor or the transistor, people first use it as a simple replacement for the old one. "So transistors were used as replacements for vacuum tubes," he says. "It wasn't until Bob Noyce figured out how to do a true integrated circuit that we got the idea, 'This is really a different medium.' The real boundary between ordinary integrated circuits and [modern ones] was when the design problem got to be something you couldn't keep in your head anymore."

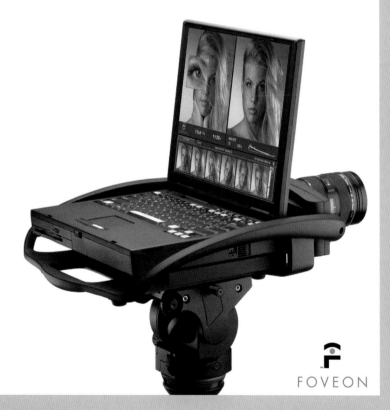

FOVEON

In 2000, Mead's company Foveon unveiled several high-end digital cameras based on his imaging technology. The color camera's pictures are as good as 35mm photographs; a black-and-white camera produces even higher quality pictures.

He began thinking about how to automate the process. The answer was to create a silicon compiler. Like a software compiler, Mead's program, devised with the help of some of his students, let a designer describe what he or she wanted on a chip in a structured, easy-to-understand language. This language was then translated by a computer into the lines that make up a silicon circuit, and was output on a high-resolution plotter. The plotted design could then be etched onto a silicon chip.

Mead's approach, now called VLSI, or very large-scale integration, was the advance that kicked integrated circuit design into high gear. Most of the microprocessors that fueled the personal computer revolution were created with VLSI, and almost all of today's advanced chips are designed using the basic method he outlined in 1971 and expanded into book form, with coauthor Lynn Conway, in 1979.

In the 1990s, Mead turned his attention—and his frustration at people doing things the wrong way—to digital imaging. Most digital cameras begin with video technology, usually a CCD (charge-coupled device) image sensor much like those used in camcorders, rather than the principles of film. "It isn't photography," Mead says. "It's an insane way to make pictures. You've thrown away two-thirds of the light, you've thrown away two-thirds of the information, and [you have to] spend all of this computing trying to get it back when the right way to do it was to not throw it away in the first place."

In September 2000, Foveon, a company Mead founded, introduced a new generation of digital cameras that use a proprietary, silicon-chip-based image sensor that allows for detail and tonal range far greater than traditional digital cameras. Mead explains that people have known that silicon was light-sensitive for decades; in the 1960s, some engineers even proposed making photo sensors with it. However, it was only when manufacturing techniques allowed for very small transistors and very dense chips—an outgrowth of Mead's own work in the late 1960s—that silicon became practical to use in photography.

Foveon's image sensor consists of a two-inch-square CMOS chip that can capture a 16-million-pixel black-and-white image. What's more, the tonal range of the chip exceeds that of professional-quality film. Foveon also makes a color version, using a filter that directs the three primary colors of light to three separate image sensors, that boasts a resolution of 4 million pixels. Mead's new cameras, made in partnership with Hasselblad, are just now reaching professional photographers.

While there are still intriguing technical challenges for Mead at Foveon, he is also working on several "next" projects, including a silicon learning system, or chips whose programming can physically change as they learn new processes or functions. This is in part a continuation of the work he began in the 1960s, looking at the basic physical properties of silicon, but it is also an extension of the research he did in the 1970s and 1980s into creating computational analogs to the human (or animal) brain. Still, after almost twenty years, this remains a huge challenge. "People have always enormously underestimated the computing power that happens in a brain," Mead says. "That's just a big mistake. There's still a huge amount we don't know about what happens in the brain. And it's very dangerous to just assume that what we're doing is just equivalent in some way."

STEVE WOZNIAK

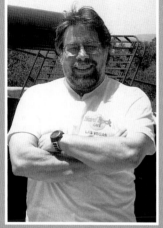

Steve Wozniak only wanted to impress his fellow enthusiasts in the Homebrew Computer Club. He and the others were building "microcomputers" with the new microprocessors just introduced by Intel and Motorola. He dubbed his first machine, built in 1976, the Apple. While it was impressive, it was his next creation, the Apple II, that was destined to bring computers into ordinary homes. Powerful, expandable, easy to use and program, and capable of displaying high-resolution color graphics, the Apple II opened people's eyes to what a computer could do, and why they should own one. By the time the last Apple II was produced in the early 1990s, there were millions of Wozniak's invention in homes, schools, and businesses.

Wozniak was born at the right time and in the right place for a future computer genius: in San Jose, California, in 1950. The area extending from San Jose north to Mountain View and Palo Alto was already a center for technology, home to Hewlett-Packard, the NACA (later NASA) Ames Research Center, and several aerospace companies. Over the next few decades, the academic draw of Stanford University and more and more technology companies brought thousands of engineers and scientists to the region.

In 1958, Wozniak's father, an electrical engineer, took a job at Lockheed and moved the family to nearby Sunnyvale, even closer to the core of what would become Silicon Valley. As he grew up, Wozniak fell in love with mathematics and electronics. He loved to read about Tom Swift, Jr., a teenage inventor/engineer who got involved in all sorts of adventures, often in outer space. He also subscribed to *Popular Electronics* and began tinkering with electronics. There were other technically minded kids in the neighborhood; together they made an intercom system to connect their houses.

When Wozniak was 11, he built his first computer, or something like a computer. With hundreds of components laid out on a three-by-four-foot piece of plywood, he made a machine that could play tic-tac-toe. Although his father would sometimes offer advice or help him get parts, for the most part Wozniak taught himself. In high school, Wozniak became even more involved with electronics. When he had advanced beyond the school's electronics class, he be-

When Wozniak was 11, he built his first computer, or something like a computer: with hundreds of components laid out on a three-by-four-foot piece of plywood, he made a machine that could play tic-tac-toe.

gan working for free at Sylvania, learning to run and program the company's minicomputer. He continued to design his own primitive computers, although by this point he had gone far beyond his friends. Nobody else "did this design stuff with me," he said later. "I had nobody to even show my designs to."

In 1968, Wozniak graduated from high school and began attending the University of Colorado in Boulder. He could only afford the school for a year, though, then returned to California, where he got a job at one of the many new electronics companies that were starting up. In his spare time, Wozniak continued to try to build his own computer. In 1971, he made one that worked so well that his mother called in the local newspaper for a demonstration. Unfortunately, when the reporter showed up, the computer shorted out with a puff of smoke.

Later that year, Wozniak returned to college, this time at the University of California at Berkeley. Although Berkeley was still a hotbed of radical politics, Wozniak devoted his time to studying electronics and computers. There were plenty of ways to get in trouble with electronics, however. He and his new friend Steve Jobs had heard about something called a "blue box," a device that emitted a tone at a particular frequency. When used correctly, the device would let users make free phone calls, and even listen in on other people's conversations. Always interested in jokes and pranks (even illegal ones), Wozniak set out to build his own blue box. One night, he tried to call the pope, and actually got through to his secretary. Fortunately, the pope was asleep.

Wozniak and Jobs had been introduced to each other by a mutual friend in Sunnyvale. In many ways, the two men were opposites; Wozniak was a dedicated geek, losing himself for hours or days in his electronics designs, while Jobs was a talkative visionary, eager to spread the word of technology, even if he

wasn't as good as his friend at creating it. Their first business partnership came about with the blue box; Wozniak was pleased just to have made it, while Jobs wanted to sell them. They eventually built and sold about 50 of them.

The key to the personal computer is the microprocessor, which is essentially a computer etched onto a small silicon chip. The first microprocessor was invented in 1971 by Ted Hoff at Intel. By the mid-1970s, prices for the chips had begun to come down and people started to find uses for them. In January 1975, a company in Albuquerque announced the world's first personal computer: the Altair. Today, an Altair would be barely recognizable as a computer. Commands and programs were input by flipping toggle switches, and a few red LEDs were its only way of communicating back. Still, it was the first computer that was meant for one person to use and cheap enough for one person to buy. Later that year, a small group of computer enthusiasts, inspired in part by the Altair, came to the first meeting of the Homebrew Computer Club in Palo Alto. At each meeting, people would talk about their own ideas and designs for computers, and often demonstrate them.

Wozniak began to build a computer he could show off at the Homebrew club. By February 1976 it was ready, able to run programs written in the BASIC programming language and display them on a small black-and-white TV set. His fellow computer designers thought it was a great computer; more important, his friend Steve Jobs thought they could sell them. Within a few months, they had an order for 100 of the computers. To raise money, Jobs sold his Volkswagen bus and Wozniak sold his calculator. (At the time, good calculators sold for hundreds of dollars.) Apple Computer was born.

Even with that first order, Apple was just another tiny company with a computer meant for hard-core geeks. (The Apple I

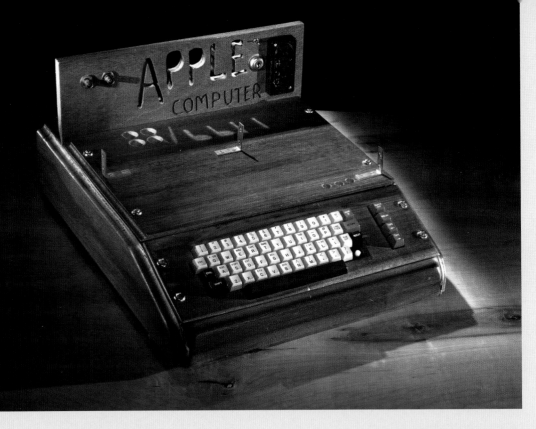

The first Apple computer, designed by Steven Wozniak in 1976, came as a kit, without a case. Some users made their own enclosures out of wood and often personalized them.

TIM BERNERS-LEE AND THE WORLD WIDE WEB

When Steve Wozniak invented the Apple II, he wanted a computer that one person could use. Previously, most computers were shared by many people, who used simple ("dumb") terminals to access a minicomputer or a mainframe, which did all the work. As more and more people used personal computers, though, they began to need ways to connect with other users. The first solution was local-area networks such as Ethernet and Appletalk, which allowed several computers in an office to communicate back and forth. In the 1990s, a much larger network came into widespread use: the Internet.

The Internet was created in the late 1960s as a way to link large university and military computer networks. For the next two decades it was used by a relatively small number of people to exchange data and messages (the first e-mail). Once information had been sent through the Internet, though, there was no easy way for others to see it.

In 1980, Tim Berners-Lee, a British computer scientist working at CERN, Europe's main physics research facility, took the first step in creating an "information space" where data could be shared. Berners-Lee wanted to be able to organize the various kinds of information he used everyday—such as CERN's phone book, his notes, and his research papers. He wrote a program that let him store different kinds of documents.

Berners-Lee also had an idea about how to access all that information. Although computers are very good at finding data stored in a logical way, they are awful at recognizing connections between documents or bits of information. Humans, on the other hand, are great at making those connections, although not partic-

didn't come with a keyboard, a display, or even a case.) But Jobs saw that Wozniak's computer had great potential, and other people in Silicon Valley did, too. Mike Markkula, a business executive Jobs met through friends at Atari, joined the company and lent it $250,000. Apple needed a better product to sell, and Wozniak was already designing it.

For the next year, Wozniak worked on the Apple II, designing it almost completely by himself. Unveiled in April 1977, it was in every way a better machine than its predecessor. It was relatively fast (it ran at 1 MHz), the BASIC programming language was built in, and through some sophisticated electronic sleight-of-hand, Wozniak had given it color graphics. Wozniak's design used the minimum number of chips, which made it both cheaper and more reliable.

The Apple II was also friendlier than other computers. Sporting the company's multicolored logo and packaged in a distinctive beige plastic case, it provoked none of the anxiety then associated with computers. With the Apple II, Wozniak explained, "the phrase 'personal computer' came to mean one that a single person used, but it also meant one that was acceptable in homes, with a non-commercial appearance."

The computer was an almost instant hit. Although it initially had only 4K of memory and its programs had to be stored on cassette tape, within a couple of years it had a full 48K of RAM and an inexpensive floppy disk drive. In 1979, it gained another crucial advantage over other personal computers: Visicalc, the first spreadsheet program. Businesses found this new tool essential. The software finally answered the question, What do I do with a computer? Visicalc was a runaway best-seller; some people give it credit for much of Apple's success.

The Apple II was Wozniak's last great computer. He stayed at Apple for several years, refining succeeding generations of the Apple II and then the Apple III. In 1981, he had just begun to work with the team that would create the Macintosh computer when he was involved in a plane crash. His injuries gave him amnesia and made it difficult for him to concentrate. When he recovered, he decided he'd rather spend his time (and money— Apple had made him a multimillionaire) with his family and on other projects.

Today, Wozniak's devotes much of his time to kids and education. In the 1980s, he helped found the Tech Museum of Innovation, a child-oriented science museum in San Jose. A few years later, he discovered the joy of teaching them himself. Starting with a small group of his son's friends, he began showing kids how to use computers, and how they work. Now he leads classes at his home and at local schools, and he has donated equipment for many of the school district's computer labs. "I was born to teach," he told a biographer. "I plan to continue to be a fifth-grade teacher of computers and just get better and better at it."

---

ularly good at holding large amounts of data. Berners-Lee wanted to make a system that allowed for a permanent "web" of connections between information.

Over the next decade, Berners-Lee refined his ideas on how to link documents, and then found a way to make them available to many people at once. There were two parts to his solution, which made up what he called the World Wide Web. He created a standardized way to make documents readable and linkable by using a simple computer language called HTML ("hypertext markup language"). And he set up a "server"—a computer that CERN users could access that would "serve up" the document they were looking for.

In 1991, Berners-Lee connected CERN's server to the Internet and told people how to access it. That summer, the server got about 100 "hits" a day; by 1993, that number had grown to 10,000. It wasn't quite the Web people know today; those early users' browsers could display only text. In early 1993, however, an American student named Marc Andreesen released a new browser, called Mosaic, which could display Web "pages" with different fonts, colors, and graphics.

In 1994, Andreesen cofounded Netscape and began distributing his new browser free of charge. Within a few years, millions (and then hundreds of millions) of people were on line. The combination of information, commerce, entertainment, and communication that the Web brought home has made computing an essential part of many people's daily lives.

SOURCES AND FURTHER READING

Much of the information in this book came from interviews with the subjects and from material in the archives of the Lemelson-MIT Program. The Lemelson-MIT Program's Website, The Invention Dimension (**web.mit.edu/invent**), contains short biographies of the inventors profiled here as well as many others.

What follows are other sources that were helpful in investigating the individual inventors profiled and in understanding some technical aspects of their work, as well as suggested reading for those interested in learning more about American inventors and inventing.

For detailed discussions of basic scientific and technical concepts and some biographical insights, **Brittanica.com** is an indispensable source. Marshall Brain's "How Stuff Works" (**www.howstuffworks.com**) is useful for thorough explanations of many things, notably Boolean logic and simple circuits.

The Innovative Lives section of the Website of the Jerome and Dorothy Lemelson Center for the Study of Invention and Innovation at the Smithsonian Institution (**www.si.edu/lemelson**) features illuminating essays on several of the inventors featured in this book, including Sally Fox, Ashok Gadgil, Wilson Greatbatch, and Stephanie Kwolek.

Kenneth Brown's book *Inventors at Work* (Tempus, 1988) was useful both for its interviews with several of the inventors in this book and for its incisive point of view on invention and innovation.

The United States Patent and Trademark Office has a searchable database of all patents issued since 1790, at **www.uspto.gov**.

Medicine and Healthcare

Adam, John. "Wilson Greatbatch." *IEEE Spectrum*, March 1995.

Cima, Michael, John Santini, Jr., and Robert Langer. "A Controlled Release Microchip." Press release. Massachusetts Institute of Technology, January 20, 1999.

Dale, W. Andrew, M.D. *Band of Brothers: Creators of Modern Vascular Surgery.* [Thomas Fogarty.] Appleton Communications, 1992.

Davies, Kevin, and Michael White. *Breakthrough: The Race to Find the Breast Cancer Gene.* [Mary-Claire King.] New York: John Wiley & Sons, 1996.

Kemper, Steve, "If you do not want to hear about what he does, do not ask." [Dean Kamen.] *Smithsonian*, November 1994.

Kleinfield, Sonny. *A Machine Called Indomitable.* New York: Crown, 1985.

Lloyd, Robin. "The Tissue Master Delivers." [Robert Langer.] *The World & I*, August 1999.

Maloney, Lawrence D., "Saga of a High-Tech Maverick." [Dean Kamen.] *Design News*, March 7, 1994.

Mattson, James, and Merrill Simon. *The Pioneers of NMR and Magnetic Resonance in Medicine: The Story of MRI.* Ramat Gan, Israel: Bar-Ilan University Press, 1996.
(Also at **www.heckel.org/pioneers/index.htm**.)

Regalado, Antonio. "Ideas Are Like Children." [Robert Langer.] *Technology Review*, January 1, 1999.

Straus, Eugene, M.D. *Rosalyn Yalow, Nobel Laureate: Her Life and Work in Medicine.* New York: Plenum Press, 1998.

Consumer Products

Bijker, Wiebe. *Of Bicycles, Bakelites, and Bulbs.* Cambridge: MIT Press, 1995.

Bruce, Roger, ed. *Seeing the Unseen : Dr. Harold E. Edgerton and the Wonders of Strobe Alley.* Cambridge: MIT Press, 1995.

Edgerton, Harold E. *Exploring the Art and Science of Stopping Time: A CD-ROM Based on the Life and Work of Harold E. Edgerton.* Cambridge: MIT Press, 2000.

Flatow, Ira. *They All Laughed.* New York: Harper Perennial, 1993.

Gallawa, J. Carlton. "Who Invented Microwaves?" in *The Complete Microwave Oven Service Handbook*, Upper Saddle River, N.J.: Prentice Hall, 2000.
(Also at **www.gallawa.com/microtech/history.html**.)

Kanigel, Robert. "One Man's Mousetraps." [Jacob Rabinow.] *New York Times Magazine*, May 17, 1987.

Murray, Don. "Percy Spencer and His Itch to Know." *Reader's Digest*, August 1958.

Rabinow, Jacob. *Inventing for Fun and Profit.* San Francisco: San Francisco Press, 1990.

Schatzin, Paul. "The Farnsworth Chronicles."
www.songs.com/philo/index.html.

Schwartz, Evan. "Who Really Invented Television?" *Technology Review*, September/October 2000.

Wolfe, Tom. "Land of Wizards," in *The Best American Essays of 1987*, edited by Gay Talese. [Jerome Lemelson.] New York: Ticknor & Fields, 1987.

Transportation

The Black Inventor Online Museum, "Garrett Morgan," at **www.blackinventor.com/pages/garrettmorgan.html**.

Federal Highway Administration/Department of Transportation, "Garrett Morgan: An American Inventor," at **www.fhwa.dot.gov/ education/gamorgan.htm**.

Grosser, Morton. *Gossamer Odyssey: The Triumph of Human-powered Flight*. New York: Dover, 1991.

Hughes, Thomas Parke. *Elmer Sperry: Inventor and Engineer*. Baltimore: Johns Hopkins Press, 1971.

Lacey, Robert. *Ford: The Men and the Machine*. Boston: Little, Brown, 1986.

Lehman, Milton. *This High Man: The Life of Robert H. Goddard*. New York: Farrar, Straus & Giroux, 1963.

Rodengen, Jeffrey. *Evinrude, Johnson and the Legend of OMC*. Ft. Lauderdale, Fla.: Write Stuff Syndicate, 1992.

Energy and the Environment

Baldwin, J. *Bucky Works: Buckminster Fuller's Ideas for Today*. New York: John Wiley & Sons, 1996.

Djerassi, Carl. *The Pill, Pygmy Chimps, and Degas' Horse*. New York: Basic Books, 1992.

Djerassi, Carl. *Cantor's Dilemma*. New York: Penguin, 1992.

Djerassi, Carl. *Steroids Made It Possible*. Washington, D.C.: American Chemical Society, 1990.

[Ashok Gadgil.] *Physics Today*, July 1996.

Fleischer, Betsy, and V.S. Arunachalam, "Order in Disorder: Stanford Ovshinsky Talks of His Materials, Methods, and Machines." *Materials Research Society Bulletin*, November 1998.

[Ashok Gadgil.] "Water, Pure and Simple." *Discover*, July 1996.

Geary, James. "Green Machines." [John Todd.] *Time* (Latin American Edition), March 23, 1999.

Hatch, Alden. *Buckminster Fuller: At Home in the Universe*. New York: Crown Publishers, 1974.

Kremer, Gary R., ed. *George Washington Carver: In His Own Words*. Columbia: University of Missouri Press, 1987.

Neil, Kathy. "Cotton's Golden Girl." [Sally Fox.] *Hemp Times*, Summer 1997.

Todd, John, and Nancy Todd. *Bioshelters, Ocean Arks, City Farming: Ecology as the Basis of Design*. San Francisco: Sierra Club Books, 1984.

Todd, Nancy Jack, John Todd, and Jeffrey Parkin. *From Eco-Cities to Living Machines: Principles of Ecological Design*. Berkeley: North Atlantic Books, 1994.

Computing and Telecommunications

Berners-Lee, Tim. *Weaving the Web*. New York: Harper San Francisco, 1999.

Bush, Vannevar. "As We May Think." *Atlantic Monthly*, July 1945. (Also at **www.theatlantic.com/unbound/flashbks/computer/ bushf.htm**.)

[Bushnell, Nolan.] There are many websites devoted to the history of video games and to Atari specifically; two of the best are Atari Gaming Headquarters (**www.atarihq.com**) and The Dot Eaters (**www.emuunlim.com/doteaters**).

[Engelbart, Douglas.] A comprehensive history of Douglas Engelbart's work on Human Augmentation, including a video of the first public demonstration of the oNLine System and the mouse, can be found at the MouseSite, **sloan.stanford.edu/MouseSite**.

[Engelbart, Douglas.] The website of Douglas Engelbart's Bootstrap Institute, **www.bootstrap.org**, explores current efforts at helping people work better, and also contains historical and biographical information about Engelbart's work.

Gemperlin, Joyce, and Tanya Scheinman. "An Interview with Nolan Bushnell," at **www.thetech.org/revolutionaries/bushnell**.

Herz, J.C. *Joystick Nation*. New York: Little, Brown, 1997.

Jett, E.K. "Phone Me by Air." [Al Gross.] *Saturday Evening Post*, July 28, 1945.

Kendall, Martha E. *Steve Wozniak*. New York: Walker and Company, 1994.

Kurzweil, Ray. *The Age of Spiritual Machines*. New York: Viking, 1999.

Leopold, George. "Beacon for the Future." [Grace Hopper.] *Datamation*, October 1, 1986.

Macdonald, Anne L. *Feminine Ingenuity: How Women Inventors Changed America*. [Erna Schneider Hoover.] New York: Ballantine, 1992.

Malone, Michael S. *Infinite Loop.* New York: Currency/Doubleday, 1999.

Mead, Carver. *Collective Electrodynamics: Quantum Foundations of Electromagnetism.* Cambridge: MIT Press, 2000.

Mink, Michael. "Inventor Al Gross." *Investor's Business Daily,* July 20, 2000.

Stanley, Autumn. *Mothers and Daughters of Invention: Notes for a Revised History of Technology.* [Grace Hopper.] New Brunswick, N.J.: Rutgers University Press, 1995.

Whitelaw, Nancy. *Grace Hopper: Programming Pioneer.* New York: W.H. Freeman and Company, 1995.

Wolfson, Jill, and John Leyba. "An Interview with Steve Wozniak," at **www.thetech.org/revolutionaries/wozniak**.

Further Reading

Basalla, George. *The Evolution of Technology.* New York: Cambridge University Press, 1988.

Brodie, James M. *Created Equal: The Lives and Ideas of Black American Innovators.* New York: William Morrow, 1993.

Brown, Kenneth A. *Inventors at Work: Interviews with Sixteen Notable American Inventors.* Redmond, Wash.: Tempus Books of Microsoft Press, 1988.

Chang, Laura, ed. *Scientists at Work: Profiles of Today's Groundbreaking Scientists from Science Times.* Introduction by Cornelia Dean and foreword by Stephen Jay Gould. New York: McGraw-Hill, 2000.

Day, Lance, and Ian McNeil, eds. *Biographical Dictionary of the History of Technology.* New York: Routledge, 1996.

Fiell, Charlotte, and Pater Fiell. *Industrial Design A–Z.* New York: Taschen, 2000.

Francis, Raymond L. *The Illustrated Almanac of Science, Technology, and Invention.* New York: Plenum Trade, 1997.

Gibbs, C.R. *Black Inventors from Africa to America.* Silver Spring, Md.: Three Dimensional Pub., 1995.

Haskins, James. *Outward Dreams: Black Inventors and Their Inventions.* New York: Walker, 1991.

Ierley, Merritt. *The Comforts of Home: The American House and the Evolution of Modern Convenience.* New York: C. Potter, 1999.

Ives, Patricia Carter. *Creativity and Inventions: The Genius of Afro-Americans and Women in the United States and Their Patents.* Arlington, Va.: Research Unlimited, 1987.

James, Portia P. *The Real McCoy; African-American Invention and Innovation 1619–1930.* Washington, D.C.: Smithsonian Institution Press, 1989.

Karnes, Frances A., and Suzanne M. Bean. *Girls and Young Women Inventing.* Minneapolis: Free Spirit Publishing, 1995.

Molella, Arthur P. "Inventing the History of Invention." *American Heritage of Invention and Technology* 4 (1988).

McKinley, Burt. *Black Inventors of America.* Portland, Ore.: National Book Company, 2000.

National Geographic Society. *Inventors and Discoverers: Changing Our World.* Washington, D.C.: National Geographic Society, 1988.

Noble, David. *America by Design: Science, Technology and the Rise of Corporate Capitalism.* New York: Knopf, 1977.

Petroski, Henry. *The Evolution of Useful Things.* New York: Vintage, 1994.

Rhodes, Richard, ed. *Visions of Technology: A Century of Vital Debate about Machines, Systems and the Human World* (The Sloan Technology Series). New York: Simon and Schuster, 1999.

Rothschild, Joan, ed. *Women, Technology and Innovation.* New York: Pergamon Press, 1982.

Science Museum of London. *Inventing the Modern World: Technology Since 1750.* New York: DK Pub., 2000.

Townes, Charles H. *How the Laser Happened: Adventures of a Scientist.* New York: Oxford University Press, 1999.

Van Dulken, Stephen. *Inventing the 20th Century—100 Inventions That Shaped the World.* London: The British Library, 2000.

Vare, Ethlie Ann, and Greg Ptacek. *Mothers of Invention: From the Bra to the Bomb, Forgotten Women and Their Unforgettable Ideas.* New York: Quill, 1989.

Vare, Ethlie Ann, and Greg Ptacek. *Women Inventors and Their Discoveries.* Minneapolis: Oliver Press, 1993.

Weber, Robert J., and David N. Perkins, eds. *Inventive Minds: Creativity in Technology.* New York, Oxford University Press, 1992.

Weber, Robert J. *Forks, Phonographs, and Hot Air Balloons: A Field Guide to Inventive Thinking.* New York: Oxford University Press, 1992.

ACKNOWLEDGMENTS

This book is a culmination of the Lemelson-MIT Program's efforts to seek out and celebrate America's scientific and technological innovators, many of them unsung heroes of modern life. We are deeply grateful for the vision and generous support of the Lemelson Foundation and its cofounders, the late Jerome Lemelson and his wife, Dorothy, and the Massachusetts Institute of Technology. Without this unique partnership to inspire the next generation of inventors and innovators, this book simply would not have been.

There were countless contributors to this project. We must first thank Lester Thurow for his leadership in "ringing the bells" about the excitement and joy of invention, and for illustrating inventiveness as a distinctly American trait in the book's foreword. We must also thank James Burke, whose introductions to our book sections place Yankee ingenuity within the broader context of world history. We are enormously indebted to David E. Brown for telling the innovators' stories through such a lively set of biographies.

Many, many hours of research helped us conquer the daunting challenge of selecting these inventors and preparing the manuscript. Here, our greatest thanks go to Carrie Capizzi and Paul Melvin for their resourcefulness, energy and persistence. For their editorial insights and repeated readings of our manuscript, we owe a thousand thanks to Mariette DiChristina, David Lucsko, and Caryn Wesner-Early. We are also thankful for the assistance of Joshua Dorchak, Wendy Murphy, Victor McElheny, Michael McNally, Kate O'Neill, Arthur Molella, Joyce Bedi, Paul Montie, Shannon Peavey, Michael Rutter, and Lori Leibovich.

Our editors at The MIT Press, Michael Sims and Larry Cohen, showed boundless enthusiasm for the project and compassion for our mission. We could not wish for better support from a publisher. We also thank Emily Gutheinz for conveying the creative nature of invention through the book's playful design and Yasuyo Iguchi for her artistic direction.

Kristin Joyce deserves special thanks for her keen eye, superb organizational talents, and unwavering dedication to seeing through the book's production. Her command of the myriad details and deadlines was vital to this project.

We would like to thank not only the innovators in this book but the innumerable scientists, engineers, and technologists who help to shape our future through their discoveries and inventions. Without their contributions, wonders might indeed cease.

Annemarie C. Amparo
Director, The Lemelson-MIT Program

PHOTO CREDITS

Numbers preceding credits are the pages on which the images appear.

Raymond Damadian
All figures courtesy of Fonar Corp.

Thomas Fogarty
12: Paul Andrew Michaels
13 (top), 17: Fogarty Research
Remaining images courtesy of Edwards Lifesciences

Wilson Greatbatch
18, 21: Courtesy of Wilson Greatbatch
19, 20: Wilson Greatbatch Ltd.
22 (top): Australian Heart Association, Melbourne, Australia; (bottom) Charles O'Rear/CORBIS

Dean Kamen
24: Dean Kamen/DEKA Research
25, 26 (bottom), 29: Dean Kamen
26 (top), 28: United States Patent and Trademark Office

Mary-Claire King
30: Harley Soltes, *Seattle Times*
31: Republished with permission of Globe Newspaper Co., Inc.
32: University of Washington

Robert Langer
34: Andrew Fingland
Remaining images: Donna Coveney/MIT

Rosalyn Yalow
38, 40: From Eugene Straus, *Rosalyn Yalow: Her Life and Work in Medicine* (Cambridge, Mass.: Perseus Books, 1998), courtesy of Dr. Eugene Straus
39: Bettmann Collection/CORBIS

Leo Baekeland
All images courtesy of the Smithsonian Institution National Museum of American History

Harold "Doc" Edgerton
52, 56: MIT Museum
Remaining images © Harold & Esther Edgerton Foundation, 2002, courtesy of Palm Press

Philo T. Farnsworth
All images courtesy of the Farnsworth Family Archives

Stephanie Kwolek
62: Photograph by Jeff Tinsley, Smithsonian Institution
63: Michael Branscom, photographer
64: Hulton/Deutsch Collection/CORBIS

66 (top): CORBIS; (middle): Richard Cooke/CORBIS; (bottom): Ken Redding/CORBIS

Jerome Lemelson
69: Smithsonian photograph by Jeff Tinsley
Remaining photographs courtesy of the Lemelson family; patent drawings courtesy of the United States Patent and Trademark Office

Jacob Rabinow
74: Courtesy of Jack Rabinow
75: John Carnett for *Popular Science Magazine*
77: United States Patent and Trademark Office
78: Jay Velez

Perry Spencer
80 (header image): PhotoDisc
Remaining images courtesy of Raytheon Co.

Ole Evinrude
86, 89: Norwegian-American Historical Association
87: United States Patent and Trademark Office
88: Courtesy of Jeffrey L. Rodengen, author, and Write Stuff Syndicate, Inc., publisher, *Evinrude, Johnson and the Legend of OMC*. With the permission of the Boats and Outboard Engines Division, Bombardier Motor Corporation of America

Henry Ford
90: From the collections of Henry Ford Museum & Greenfield Village O.4401
91: From the collections of Henry Ford Museum & Greenfield Village, 833.158 (circa 1925)
92 (left): From the Collections of Henry Ford Museum & Greenfield Village, P.O. 6522, Jervis B. Webb Co., Farmington Hills, Mich. (circa 1925), (right): From the Collections of Henry Ford Museum & Greenfield Village, P.833.38556 (1924)

Robert Goddard
All images courtesy of Clark University Archives

Paul MacCready
All images courtesy of AeroVironment/Paul MacCready

Garrett Morgan
All images courtesy of The Western Reserve Historical Society, Cleveland, Ohio

Elmer Ambrose Sperry
115 (patent drawings): United States Patent and Trademark Office
117: Computer Museum of America
Remaining images courtesy of Hagley Museum and Library

George Washington Carver
120 (header image): PhotoDisc
120 (portrait), 121, 123: Tuskegee Institute
122: Iowa State University Library/Special Collections Department